Contributors

CLAIRE E. BENDER, M.D.

THOMAS H. BERQUIST, M.D.

MANUEL L. BROWN, M.D.

MIGUEL E. CABANELA, M.D.

DONALD C. CAMPBELL, II, M.D.

JOSEPH R. CASS, M.D.

ROBERT H. COFIELD, M.D.

KAY L. COOPER, M.D.

MARK B. COVENTRY, M.D.

WILLIAM L. DUNN, M.S.

ROBERT H. FITZGERALD, JR., M.D.

GLENN S. FORBES, M.D.

BRAD B. HALL, M.D.

E. MEREDITH JAMES, M.D.

KENNETH A. JOHNSON, M.D.

CURTIS B. KAMIDA, M.D.

GERALD R. MAY, M.D.

BERNARD F. MORREY, M.D.

DOUGLAS J. PRITCHARD, M.D.

JAMES A. RAND, M.D.

LAWRENCE B. RIGGS, M.D.

JOHN STEARS, R.T., [R]

HEINZ W. WAHNER, M.D.

N.T. WINKLER, R.T., [R]

MICHAEL B. WOOD, M.D.

IMAGING OF ORTHOPEDIC TRAUMA AND SURGERY

Edited by

THOMAS H. BERQUIST, M.D.

Consultant in Diagnostic Radiology
Mayo Clinic, and
Associate Professor of Radiology
Mayo Medical School
Rochester, Minnesota

1986
W. B. SAUNDERS COMPANY
PHILADELPHIA   LONDON   TORONTO   MEXICO CITY   RIO DE JANEIRO   SYDNEY   TOKYO

W. B. Saunders Company: West Washington Square
                                Philadelphia, PA   19105

Library of Congress Cataloging in Publication Data

Main entry under title:

Imaging of orthopedic trauma and surgery.

1. Radiography in orthopedia.   2. Orthopedic surgery.
   I. Berquist, Thomas H. (Thomas Henry), 1945–   .
   II. Bender, Claire E. [DNLM: 1. Bone and Bones—
   injuries.   2. Bone and Bones—radiography.
   3. Fractures—radiography. WE 200 R129]

RD734.5.R33R33 1986   617′.15   85-1818

ISBN 0-7216-1102-8

Editor: Suzanne Boyd
Designer: Terri Siegel
Production Manager: Bill Preston
Manuscript Editor: Steve Albert
Illustration Coordinator: Walt Verbitski
Page Layout Artist: Patti Maddaloni

Imaging of Orthopedic Trauma and Surgery   ISBN   0-7216-1102-8

Last digit is the print number: 9   8   7   6   5   4   3   2   1

To my loving wife, Kay, for her kindness and understanding
and
to my sons, Aric, Matthew, and Andrew, who relinquished their
father during the preparation of this text.

Contributors

CLAIRE E. BENDER, M.D.
Assistant Professor, Department of Diagnostic Radiology, Mayo Medical School. Consultant in Diagnostic Radiology, Mayo Clinic. St. Mary's Hospital and Rochester Methodist Hospital, Rochester, MN.
Imaging Techniques: Routine Radiography, Tomography, Magnification Radiography; Femoral Shaft Fractures; Fractures of the Shafts of the Tibia and Fibula; Fractures of the Shafts of the Humerus; Fractures of the Shafts of the Radius and Ulna.

MANUEL L. BROWN, M.D.
Associate Professor, Department of Diagnostic Radiology and Laboratory Medicine, Mayo Medical School. Consultant in Diagnostic Radiology and Nuclear Medicine, Mayo Clinic. St. Mary's Hospital and Rochester Methodist Hospital, Rochester, MN.
Imaging Techniques: Scintigraphy; An Imaging Approach to Musculoskeletal Infections

MIGUEL E. CABANELA, M.D.
Associate Professor, Department of Orthopedic Surgery, Mayo Medical School. Consultant in Orthopedic Surgery, Mayo Clinic. St. Mary's Hospital and Rochester Methodist Hospital, Rochester, MN.
The Spine

DONALD C. CAMPBELL, II, M.D.
Assistant Professor, Department of Orthopedic Surgery, Mayo Medical School. Consultant in Orthopedic Surgery, Mayo Clinic. Rochester Methodist Hospital and St. Mary's Hospital, Rochester, MN.
Femoral Shaft Fractures; Fractures of the Shafts of the Tibia and Fibula; Fractures of the Shafts of the Humerus; Fractures of the Shafts of the Radius and Ulna

JOSEPH R. CASS, M.D.
Instructor, Department of Orthopedic Surgery, Mayo Medical School. Consultant in Orthopedic Surgery, Mayo Clinic. Saint Mary's Hospital and Rochester Methodist Hospital, Rochester, MN.
The Foot and Ankle

ROBERT H. COFIELD, M.D.
Associate Professor, Department of Orthopedic Surgery, Mayo Medical School. Consultant in Orthopedic Surgery, Mayo Clinic. Rochester Methodist Hospital, Saint Mary's Hospital, and Mayo Clinic, Rochester, MN.
The Shoulder

KAY L. COOPER, M.D.
Assistant Professor, Department of Diagnostic Radiology, Mayo Medical School. Consultant, Department of Diagnostic Radiology, Mayo Clinic. Rochester Methodist Hospital and Saint Mary's Hospital, Rochester, MN.
Stress Fractures

MARK B. COVENTRY, M.D.
Emeritus Professor, Department of Orthopedic Surgery, Mayo Medical School. Emeritus Consultant, Orthopedics, Mayo Clinic, Rochester, MN.
The Pelvis and Hips

WILLIAM L. DUNN, M.S.
Instructor, Nuclear Medicine Technology and Radiology, Resident Physics Program, Mayo Medical School. Technical Analyst-Physicist, Section of Diagnostic Nuclear Medicine, Mayo Clinic, Rochester, MN.
Imaging Techniques: Quantitation of Bone Mineral

ROBERT H. FITZGERALD, JR., M.D.
Associate Professor, Department of Orthopedic Surgery, Mayo Medical School. Consultant in Orthopedic Surgery, Mayo Clinic. St. Mary's Hospital and Rochester Methodist Hospital, Rochester, MN.
An Imaging Approach to Musculoskeletal Infections

GLENN FORBES, M.D.
Associate Professor, Department of Diagnostic Radiology, Mayo Medical School. Consultant in Neuroradiology, Mayo Clinic. Rochester Methodist Hospital and Saint Mary's Hospital, Rochester, MN.
Imaging Techniques: Myelography

BRAD B. HALL, M.D.
Department of Orthopedic Surgery, University of Texas Health Sciences Center. St. Luke's Lutheran Hospital, Southwest Texas Methodist Hospital, Humana Hospital, San Antonio, Santa Rosa Medical Center, and Baptist Memorial Hospital System, San Antonio, TX.
Interventional Orthopedic Radiology

E. MEREDITH JAMES, M.D.
Assistant Professor, Department of Diagnostic Radiology, Mayo Medical School. Consultant in Diagnostic Radiology, Mayo Clinic. Rochester Methodist Hospital and Saint Mary's Hospital, Rochester, MN.
Imaging Techniques: Ultrasound

KENNETH A. JOHNSON, M.D.
Associate Professor, Department of Orthopedic Surgery, Mayo Medical School. Consultant in Orthopedic Surgery, Mayo Clinic. Rochester Methodist Hospital and St. Mary's Hospital, Rochester, MN.
The Foot and Ankle

CURTIS B. KAMIDA, M.D.
Assistant Professor, Department of Diagnostic Radiology, Mayo Medical School. Consultant in Diagnostic Radiology, Mayo Clinic. Rochester Methodist Hospital and St. Mary's Hospital, Rochester, MN.
An Imaging Approach to Musculoskeletal Infections

GERALD R. MAY, M.D.
Assistant Professor, Department of Diagnostic Radiology, Mayo Medical School. Consultant in Diagnostic Radiology, Mayo Clinic. Rochester Methodist Hospital and Saint Mary's Hospital, Rochester, MN.
Imaging Techniques: Computed Tomography, Angiography

BERNARD F. MORREY, M.D.
Associate Professor, Department of Orthopedic Surgery, Mayo Medical School. Consultant in Orthopedic Surgery, Mayo Clinic. Rochester Methodist Hospital and St. Mary's Hospital, Rochester, MN.
The Foot and Ankle; The Elbow

DOUGLAS J. PRITCHARD, M.D.
Associate Professor, Department of Orthopedic Surgery, Mayo Medical School. Consultant in Orthopedic Surgery, Mayo Clinic. Rochester Methodist Hospital and St. Mary's Hospital, Rochester, MN.
Stress Fractures

JAMES A. RAND, M.D.
Assistant Professor, Department of Orthopedic Surgery, Mayo Medical School. Consultant in Orthopedic Surgery, Mayo Clinic. Rochester Methodist Hospital and St. Mary's Hospital, Rochester, MN.
Fracture Healing; The Knee

B. LAWRENCE RIGGS, M.D.
Professor of Medicine, Mayo Medical School. Rochester Methodist Hospital and St. Mary's Hospital, Rochester, MN.
Imaging Techniques: Quantitation of Bone Mineral

JOHN STEARS, R.T. (R)
Instructor, Mayo School of Health Related Sciences, Radiography Program. Quality Control Unit Supervisor, Mayo Clinic, Rochester, MN.
Imaging Techniques: Routine Radiography

HEINZ W. WAHNER, M.D.
Professor, Laboratory Medicine, Mayo Medical School. Consultant in Nuclear Medicine, Mayo Clinic. St. Mary's Hospital and Rochester Methodist Hospital, Rochester, MN.
Imaging Techniques: Quantitation of Bone Mineral

TED WINKLER, R.T. (R)
Program Director, Radiography, Mayo School of Health Related Sciences. Assistant Professor, Mayo Medical School, Rochester, MN.
Imaging Techniques: Routine Radiography, Xeroradiography

MICHAEL B. WOOD, M.D.
Associate Professor, Department of Orthopedic Surgery, Mayo Medical School. Consultant, Department of Orthopedics, Section of Hand Surgery, Mayo Clinic. Saint Mary's Hospital and Rochester Methodist Hospital, Rochester, MN.
The Hand and Wrist

Preface

Many books have been written on arthritis, neoplasms, and metabolic bone disease, yet a communication gap persists between radiologists and orthopedic surgeons in the areas of radiographic assessment of trauma and of the results of reduction, surgery, and joint reconstruction. In an effort to bridge that gap, chapters in this text were co-authored by radiologists and orthopedic surgeons. We have assembled for the reader the relevant clinical and imaging details necessary to obtain optimal information from the radiographic studies.

The text is organized as follows: Chapter 1 reviews basic concepts of imaging techniques. It provides the reader with basic principles, applications, and limitations of the various imaging techniques as they apply to orthopedic practice. Basic principles are discussed in sufficient detail to afford an understanding of the mechanics of techniques without overburdening the reader with details. This chapter is oriented toward clinicians and orthopedists rather than radiologists, who are more familiar with the imaging techniques. Conventional radiographic procedures (routine radiography, tomography, etc.) are presented as well as such newer techniques as computed tomography and magnetic resonance imaging.

An understanding of the physiology of fracture healing is essential in orthopedic practice and in evaluating radiographic studies. Chapter 2 discusses fracture definitions, systematic approaches to interpretation of musculoskeletal images, and basic concepts of fracture healing with special attention to the ways in which various forms of treatment (internal fixation, external fixation, and casting) affect the healing process. Illustrations of the common fixation plates, medullary rods, and external fixation devices are provided to assist radiologists in becoming more familiar with the tools of orthopedic practice.

The main body of the text (Chapters 3 to 13) addresses imaging in adult trauma, post-reduction follow-up, and reconstructive surgery. The respective chapters focus on anatomic regions (spine, pelvis, hips, etc.). The initial section of each chapter, which is devoted to anatomy, is also image-oriented and contains radiographs and CT scans when appropriate. Commonly-used positioning techniques are reviewed in each area. All radiographic techniques that are useful in a given anatomic area are also discussed, including arthrography, computed tomography, angiography, and magnetic resonance imaging. Technique, indications, complications, and pitfalls of arthrography, tenography, and bursography are discussed in detail for each joint. The clinical aspects of specific bone and soft tissue injuries follow these sections. Mechanism of injury, pertinent orthopedic classifications, and clinical evaluation of the patient are addressed along with the most logical imaging approaches for specific clinical situations. Illustrations and images were carefully selected to demonstrate how certain techniques are more valuable than others in identifying specific abnormalities. This provides the basis for the main thrust of the text, which is effective communication between the radiologist and orthopedist to arrive at the best strategy for evaluating musculoskeletal injury.

The final three chapters discuss infection, stress fractures, and interventional orthopedic techniques. The emphasis again concerns a logical imaging approach coupled with these clinical problems. Interventions such as facet injections, aspiration techniques, and musculoskeletal biopsy are thoroughly discussed. The imaging methods best suited to the performance of these interventional procedures vary considerably with each clinical situation, and we have tried to provide guidance for choosing the most suitable modality and the safest method for each procedure.

This text provides a comprehensive reference for radiologists, orthopedic surgeons, and other clinicians or residents in training who deal with trauma. Other texts have dealt with radiographic evaluation of the injured patient. We feel that this book provides the best coverage of the many available imaging techniques. Today it has become even more important to be familiar with each technique and how each may be applied to a variety of clinical problems.

We hope the cooperation demonstrated by radiologists and orthopedic surgeons in preparing this text will carry over into daily clinical practice. The end result of better communication and optimal use of imaging techniques will be better patient care.

Acknowledgements

The preparation of a comprehensive reference text requires the support of many individuals. The assistance of Dr. Robert H. Hattery, the chairman of Diagnostic Radiology at the Mayo Clinic, was greatly appreciated during this endeavor. His encouragement and instruction were essential.

Many colleagues provided daily assistance in obtaining representative material. I want, especially, to thank the residents in diagnostic radiology and orthopedic surgery who assisted in collecting these cases. William Munstock and Ken McEwen and their staff of technologists provided invaluable assistance in obtaining radiographs of special views frequently used in orthopedic practice. Sue Ramthun, one of our lead technologists, deserves special mention for her assistance in posing for demonstrations of the radiographic positioning techniques.

The department of photographics provided quality radiographic prints for publication. James Martin and Tom Flood were especially helpful in this regard. The expertise of Elman Hanken was valuable in filming patient positioning techniques.

The medical graphics department headed by Bob Benassi, with assistance from Tammy Bell, John Hagen, John Hutchison, and Jack Nelson provided excellent illustrations necessary to demonstrate classifications and specific injuries.

The manuscript was prepared by secretaries in diagnostic radiology and orthopedic surgery. Special thanks are due my secretaries, Debbie Roach, Nancy Kerr, and Mary Goltz for their diligence and patience in preparing the manuscript, its numerous tables, and lengthy bibliography.

Finally, I wish to thank the production staff at W. B. Saunders, specifically Steven Albert in copy editorial, Bill Preston in production, and my editor, Suzanne Boyd.

Contents

1

IMAGING TECHNIQUES 1

2

FRACTURE HEALING 51

3

THE SPINE 91

4

THE PELVIS AND HIPS 181

5

FEMORAL SHAFT FRACTURES 281

6

THE KNEE 293

7

FRACTURES OF THE SHAFTS OF THE TIBIA AND FIBULA 393

8

THE FOOT AND ANKLE 407

9

THE SHOULDER 499

10

FRACTURES OF THE SHAFT OF THE HUMERUS 567

11

THE ELBOW 579

12
FRACTURES OF THE SHAFTS OF THE RADIUS AND ULNA 631

13
THE HAND AND WRIST 641

14
AN IMAGING APPROACH TO MUSCULOSKELETAL INFECTIONS 731

15
STRESS FRACTURES 755

16
INTERVENTIONAL ORTHOPEDIC RADIOLOGY 767

INDEX.. 789

DIAGNOSTIC TECHNIQUES

There are multiple imaging techniques that are of diagnostic importance in evaluating orthopedic problems. Table 1–1 provides a list of the major techniques used in musculoskeletal evaluation.

Proper application of these techniques is essential in obtaining optimal diagnostic information. In this chapter we will provide the background information and indications for each of the modalities listed in Table 1–1. This information will be applied in subsequent chapters in discussing the radiographic evaluation of orthopedic problems.

ROUTINE RADIOGRAPHY

CLAIRE E. BENDER • THOMAS H. BERQUIST • JOHN STEARS • TED WINKLER

Routine radiography remains the mainstay for diagnostic evaluation of orthopedic problems. This section will discuss equipment, radiation protection, film identification, and other background material necessary for radiography of consistently high quality. Specific positioning techniques will be discussed in future chapters as appropriate.

Thorough radiographic evaluation of any condition requires high quality films. These cannot be obtained without properly functioning equipment, proper screen-film combinations, and technical consistency. Communication between the examining physician, the radiologist, and the technologist performing the examination is essential. The proper

TABLE 1–1. Diagnostic Techniques

Routine radiography
Tomography
Magnification
Xeroradiography
Ultrasound
Skeletal scintigraphy
Bone mineral quantitation
Computed tomography
Magnetic resonance imaging
Angiography
Myelography
Arthrography
    Routine
    Subtraction

views will be obtained only if information concerning the patient's situation is properly distributed.

EQUIPMENT

The following equipment is used in our department for routine orthopedic radiography: (1) a 3-phase, 12-pulse x-ray generator, (2) Machlett 69B x-ray tubes with a 0.6-mm focal spot, and (3) four-way floating tables. Radiography of the axial skeleton is performed at a 48-inch source-to-film distance (Bucky grid technique, 16:1 ratio), with Kodak X-omatic cassettes, regular screens, and Kodak XL film. Extremity radiographs are obtained with Dupont extremity cassettes, Cronex II screens, and Kodak XL film.

For the acutely traumatized patient we use a dedicated radiographic room adjacent to the emergency room. The equipment includes a Kermath Versitome table with a U-arm system capable of performing all routine radiographs as well as tomography in the lateral, oblique, AP, and transaxial directions (Fig. 1–1). The room is also equipped with a modern life-support system. With such a dedicated emergency unit we can obtain radiographs in all directions without moving the patient. The same film and screens are used in the trauma room.

Selection of the proper recording medium (films and screens) is essential in obtaining radiographs of consistently high quality. The choice of screen-film combinations is complicated by the number of combinations available. There are approximately 40 different screens and 80 different films on the market. Various screen-film combinations can produce radiographs with a broad spectrum of sensitivity, contrast, and resolution characteristics. Generally, the optimum combination will be a compromise between the image quality desired, available equipment, and patient-exposure factors. The ideal combination would insure high speed, high detail, high contrast, and wide latitude. However, these factors tend to oppose one another. High-speed systems tend to have lower resolution characteristics, and high-contrast systems are low in latitude. Institutions with small generators may have to sacrifice resolution for a higher-speed system because of equipment limitations.[2]

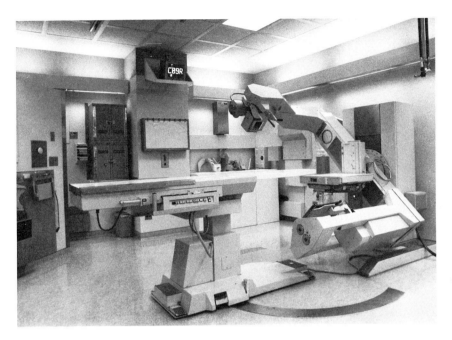

Figure 1–1. Radiographic trauma unit. Versigraph with multiple-angle tomographic capability, life-support equipment, and ample space for managing critically injured patients.

SCREEN-FILM COMBINATIONS

It is common to describe screen-film sensitivity or speed using a relative speed index (Fig. 1–2). The index is built around a par speed calcium tungstate intensifying screen and par-speed film equaling 100, assuming optimal processing conditions. For comparison, a system is assigned a number that expresses its speed relative to the standard. Therefore, systems that are twice as fast as the standard (requiring half the exposure time) are 200 speed. Systems with one half the speed (requiring twice the exposure time) are assigned a speed index of 50. Of the two components of the screen-film combination, the intensifying screen exerts the most influence on speed and resolution characteristics.

Many manufacturing processes are used in tailoring an intensifying screen for the desired character-

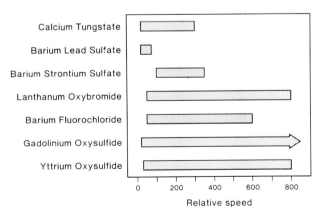

Figure 1–2. Expected system speed by phosphor material for single or pairs of intensifying screens and single or double emulsion films. Exposure conditions, film processing, and match of spectral sensitivity are assumed. The standard is the calcium tungstate screen (par speed) and par speed film equalling 100. (From Bernau, A., and Berquist, T. H.: Orthopedic Positioning in Diagnostic Radiology. Baltimore, Urban & Schwarzenberg, 1983.)

istics. However, the phosphor material used in the screen is the major variable influencing the speed of the system. The currently used phosphors vary in their ability to convert photons to usable light and can be ranged in a scale of one to nine. In general, the calcium tungstate phosphors are least efficient and the rare earth phosphors most efficient, with other materials falling in between. Figure 1–2 lists some of the commonly used phosphor materials and the anticipated relative speed of the system.

The color of light emitted by the phosphor is an important consideration. Most of the phosphors, with the exception of the rare-earth family, emit light in the blue or ultraviolet range. Rare-earth phosphors emit light in the green region of the spectrum. However, activators used in the phosphors can be altered, resulting in a shift of the color into the blue portion of the spectrum. Care must be taken in selection of film to be certain that the film is sensitive to the color emitted by the screen.

In addition to the effects of spectral sensitivity, the film selected can also alter the speed of the system and the contrast of the radiographs. Excluding single-emulsion films, most manufacturers provide film that ranges in speed by a factor of two within the spectral-sensitivity groups. This variation in the speed of the film offers control over the contrast of the images, which can be adjusted through use of different types of film. These films are designated as latitude, medium-contrast, or high-contrast. Latitude films are designed to image a broad range of radiographic densities, such as soft tissue and bone. High-contrast films are designed to enhance subtle changes in contrast, and medium-contrast films range somewhere between latitude and high-contrast films.

In selecting a screen-film combination, the intensifying screen or screens should be chosen according to the required speed and resolution. Detail or extremity systems often use one intensifying screen. Desired image contrast and control of speed are options to be considered in the selection of radiographic films.

What is considered to be an optimal system should be determined within each institution. In theory, multiple screen-film combinations would be needed to obtain optimal results for each specific radiographic examination; however, this approach increases the potential for human error and inconsistency. Many departments select one screen-film system for all examinations or purchase different types of cassettes to assist in identification of the combinations within the department. In general,

Figure 1–3. Kilovoltage versus centimeter thickness of the body part being examined. Charts available in each filming station. (From Bernau, A., and Berquist, T. H.: Orthopedic Positioning in Diagnostic Radiology. Baltimore, Urban & Schwarzenberg, 1983.)

SCALE 8	SCALE 4	SCALE 2	SCALE 1	CM	1/2 SCALE	1/4 SCALE	1/8 SCALE
				6	54	60	68
				7	55	62	71
				8	56	63	73
				9	57	65	75
				10	59	66	77
				11	60	68	80
				12	62	71	82
				13	63	73	85
				14	65	75	88
				15	66	77	91
			60	16	68	80	95
			62	17	71	82	100
			63	18	73	85	104
			65	19	75	88	109
			66	20	77	91	115
49	54	60	68	21	80	95	120
50	55	62	71	22	82	100	126
51	56	63	73	23	85	104	132
52	57	65	75	24	88	109	138
53	59	66	77	25	91	115	144
54	60	68	80	26	95	120	150
55	62	71	82	27	100	126	
56	63	73	85	28	104	132	
57	65	75	88	29	109	138	
59	66	77	91	30	115	144	
60	68	80	95	31	120	150	
62	71	82	100	32	126		
63	73	85	104	33	132		
65	75	88	109	34	138		
66	77	91	115	35	144		
68	80	95	120	36	150		
71	82	100	126	37			
73	85	104	132	38			
75	88	109	138	39			
77	91	115	144	40			
80	95	120	150	41			
82	100	126		42			
85	104	132		43			
88	109	138		44			
91	115	144		45			
100	126	150		46			
104	132			47			
109	138			48			
115	144			49			
120	150			50			
132				51			
138				52			
144				53			
150				54			

EXTREMITY CASSETTE

CM	kVp
1	47
2	51
3	54
4	57
5	60
6	63
7	66
8	69
9	72
10	75

we use a 200 speed system for the axial skeleton and proximal extremities and a 50 speed system for the distal extremities.

Proper choice of screen-film combinations will help maintain consistent radiographic quality. However, consistency in selecting proper exposure factors may be an even larger problem.

Patient size and the body part being examined specifically affect exposure factors (kVp and mA-s) required for optimal radiographs. We prefer to use a system that can be applied throughout the department and provide uniform quality. Measuring the body part to be examined and referring to standardized charts (Figs. 1–3 and 1–4) available in

EXAMINATION	TIME/SEC	mA	kVp SCALE	TFD	CASSETTE
SKULL					
SKULL, AP, Lat. 0 - 3 yrs.					
4 - 7 yrs.					
Adult					
CERVICAL SPINE					
Cervical AP 10°↑				48″	8 x 10 in
Lateral (Cross Table)				48″	24 x 30 cm
3/4 (Table Top)				48″	24 x 30 cm
Swimmer's (Grid or Bucky)				48″	24 x 30 cm
Odontoid				30″	8 x 10 in
Piller 30°↓				48″	24 x 30 cm
SHOULDER					
Shoulder AP				48″	24 x 30 cm
Neer View				48″	24 x 30 cm
Transthoracic Lateral				48″	35 x 43 cm
Axillary View (Grid)				48″	24 x 30 cm
Scapula AP & Lat				48″	24 x 30 cm
Clavical PA				48″	24 x 30 cm
Humerus AP & Lat				48″	35 x 43 cm
THORACIC					
Dorsal AP (Filter)				48″	35 x 43 cm
Lat, Dorsal (Filter)				48″	35 x 43 cm
EMACIATED THIN	AVERAGE	PORTLY	OBESE		
_____mA _____mA	_____mA	_____mA	_____mA		
Dorso-Lumbar Junction 10 ↓				48″	24 x 30 cm
Dorsal Lower Lat				48″	24 x 30 cm
Lumbar Upper Lat				48″	24 x 30 cm
LUMBAR AND ABDOMINAL					
Lumbar AP 5°↑ and Abdomen					
- 18 cm				48″	35 x 43 cm
19 - 23 cm				48″	35 x 43 cm
24 cm -				48″	35 x 43 cm
Lumbar 3/4, 42° Obl, 5°↑					
- 18 cm				48″	24 x 30 cm
19 - 23 cm				48″	24 x 30 cm
24 cm -				48″	24 x 30 cm
Lumbar Lat Meas L-2				48″	30 x 35 cm
Lumbar Loc Lat Meas L-5				48″	6 x 10 in
Lumbar Graft Lat				48″	24 x 30 cm
Lumbar Flexion & Extension				48″	30 x 35 cm

Figure 1–4. Radiographic technique chart for filming spine, abdomen, pelvis, and extremities. Charts are standardized and present in each radiographic suite. (From Bernau, A., and Berquist, T. H.: Orthopedic Positioning in Diagnostic Radiology. Baltimore, Urban & Schwarzenberg, 1983.)

Illustration continued on opposite page

each examining station results in more uniform quality. The charts remove the guesswork in deciding which exposure factors should be used.

In addition to using the proper exposure factors, certain basic principles of physics must be applied. The focal spot should be as small as practical in order to reduce geometric unsharpness or blurring. The central portion of the beam should be as perpendicular to the cassette as possible in order to minimize distortion of the object being radiographed. This also assures that adjacent structures will be recorded in their true spatial relationships

Figure 1–4. Continued

EXAMINATION	TIME/SEC	mA	kVp SCALE	TFD	CASSETTE
LUMBAR AND ABDOMINAL (cont'd)					
Pancreatic Area (AP & Both 15° Obl) 24 x 30 cm Transverse					
- 18 cm				48″	24 x 30 cm
19 - 23 cm				48″	24 x 30 cm
24 cm -				48″	24 x 30 cm
PELVIC REGION					
Pelvis & Hips AP				48″	35 x 43 cm
Hips Lat & Obl 5°↓				48″	24 x 30 cm
Sacrum AP 5°↑				48″	24 x 30 cm
Sacrum Lat				48″	24 x 30 cm
Coccyx AP 10°↓				48″	24 x 30 cm
Coccyx Lat				48″	24 x 30 cm
S-I Joints (R & LPO 20°)				48″	24 x 30 cm
FEMUR, KNEE					
Femur AP				48″	35 x 43 cm
Lat & Obl for Vessels				48″	35 x 43 cm
Knee AP, Lat				48″	24 x 30 cm
Intercondylar Notch				48″	Non-Bucky
Houston View 45°↑				48″	35 x 43 cm
CHEST					
AP Supine, All				48″	35 x 43 cm
Lateral Supine (Bucky)				48″	35 x 43 cm
Lateral Decubitus (Grid)				48″	35 x 43 cm
Lateral Sternum				48″	30 x 35 cm
RIBS					
Ribs Above Diaphragm				48″	24 x 30 cm
EMACIATED THIN AVERAGE PORTLY OBESE _____mA _____mA _____mA _____mA _____mA					
Ribs Below Diaphragm					
- 18 cm				48″	24 x 30 cm
19 - 23 cm				48″	24 x 30 cm
24 cm -				48″	24 x 30 cm
EXTREMITY					
Wrist, Hand, Forearm, Foot — Use Extremity Cassette, 48″					
Extremity — sec, mA — kV from Extremity Cassette Scale as Measured					
Wrist & Hand Finger & Toes	Small kVp	Medium kVp	Large kVp		
Ankle, Leg, Elbow, Patella, Intercondylar Notch — Use Regular Cassette					
Extremity — Regular Cassette				48″	Non-Bucky

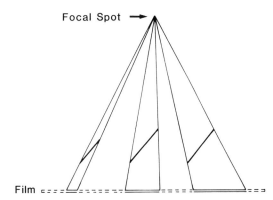

Focal Spot ➡

Film

Figure 1–5. The size and shape of an object are dependent upon its location within the x-ray beam. (From Christensen, E. E., Curry, T. S., and Dowdey, J. E.: An Introduction to the Physics of Diagnostic Radiology. Philadelphia, Lea & Febiger, 1972.)

(Fig. 1–5). The body part to be examined should be placed parallel to the film to minimize magnification, blurring, and distortion. The body part should be placed as close as possible to the cassette.[5]

Motion of either the equipment or the body part during the examination results in blurring of the image. Thus short exposure times are necessary, especially in severely injured or uncooperative patients. This will assist in reducing the lack of clarity in the image due to motion. Proper positioning as well as reduced motion can also be aided by using positioning wedges and props. This not only assists the patient in maintaining the proper position but also assures consistency in positioning. Consistency in positioning is especially desirable in orthopedic radiology, as multiple follow-up studies are often performed. Slight changes in position may make observation of fracture healing and other orthopedic problems more difficult.

RADIATION PROTECTION

Proper radiation protection must be given to the patient, radiology department staff, and any assistants who may be required to aid in patient positioning. When it is necessary to hold or position patients (as in acute trauma or when children are involved), it is often best to enlist the aid of persons not normally engaged in radiographic work. For instance, parents may be best able to calm and reassure children. Assistants should wear lead gloves and aprons during the procedure.[1, 2]

Multiple factors must be considered in discussing patient exposure. Proper positioning and exposure factors will prevent unnecessary retakes. Proper collimation not only decreases patient exposure but also increases image quality. Gonadal shielding should be undertaken when it will not obscure needed information. The Bureau of Radiological Health recommends shielding when the gonads lie within 5 cm of the primary beam in patients of reproductive age, assuming the objective of the examination will not be compromised.[4]

Filtration with a minimum of 2.5 mm of aluminum equivalent is required with fluoroscopic and radiographic units capable of generating over 70 kVp. This reduces the soft radiation that increases patient exposure but is of no diagnostic usefulness.[4] Proper choice of screen-film combination may reduce patient exposure by as much as 400 percent. Technical factors such as high kVp also reduce patient exposure. Therefore, the highest practical kVp (the kVp that produces the needed subject contrast) should be used.

Film Labeling

Radiographic films must be properly labeled with the patient's name, registration number, and the date. If multiple films are to be taken on the same date they should be properly numbered chronologically or have the times imprinted on them. In larger departments it is also helpful to include the technologist's initials on the film. The films should be labeled as to right or left, and if specific positions were used they should be indicated.[1, 4]

TOMOGRAPHY

CLAIRE E. BENDER

Tomography, or body-section radiography, provides a method of blurring out unwanted information in order to better visualize the desired structures. Laminography, planography, and stratigraphy are terms that have been applied to this technique. The technique was developed by two Dutch investigators (Ziedes des Plantes and Bartelink) in 1931.[6] During the exposure the x-ray tube and film move in two parallel planes but in opposite directions. Speeds are maintained at a constant relationship.

Most skeletal structures can be readily evaluated with routine radiographs or films obtained with fluoroscopic monitoring.[12] Tomography is a useful addition to conventional films when more detailed information is required.[7, 11] Conventional tomography provides an image of any selected plane in the body while blurring structures above and below that plane.[9, 10] Basic equipment includes (1) x-ray tube, (2) a connecting rod that moves about a fixed fulcrum, and (3) a cassette and film (Fig. 1–6). As the film moves in one direction, the tube moves in the opposite direction. The plane of interest within the patient (shaded area in Fig. 1–6) is most commonly selected by adjusting the fulcrum level. Less commonly, the apparatus includes an elevating table top to position the plane of interest at a fixed level. Only the plane of interest remains in sharp focus on the tomogram. Planes above and below (Fig. 1–6) will be blurred. Commonly used tomo-

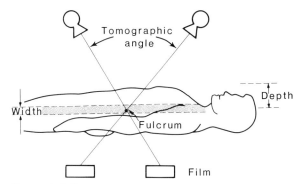

Figure 1–6. Linear tomography. The fulcrum (focal plane), tomographic angle, and motion of the tube and film are demonstrated. (From McCullough, E. C., and Coulam, C. M.: Physical and dosimetric aspects of diagnostic geometrical and computer-assisted tomography. Radiol. Clin. North Am. 14:3, 1976.)

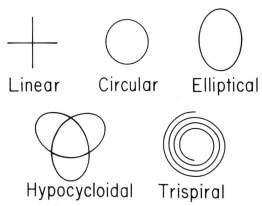

Figure 1–7. Commonly used tomographic motions. (From McCullough, E. C., and Coulam, C. M.: Physical and dosimetric aspects of diagnostic geometrical and computer-assisted tomography. Radiol. Clin. North Am. 14:3, 1976.)

graphic motions include simple (linear) and complex (circular, hypocycloidal, elliptical, and trispiral) (Fig. 1–7).

BLURRING AND SECTION THICKNESS

A better understanding of tomography requires a basic understanding of blurring and section thickness. Blurring refers to the effect of the tomographic system on objects outside the focal plane.[8] It depends upon (1) the amplitude of tube travel, (2) its orientation (Fig. 1–8), and (3) the distance of the tube from the focal plane. Section thickness refers to the plane that is in sharp focus on the film.[8] It is inversely dependent (but not proportional) to the amplitude of tube travel. Therefore, the greater the tomographic angle, the thinner the section.[8]

For evaluating skeletal structures (which have high inherent contrast), wide-angle tomography using an arc of 30 to 50 degrees is usually preferred. With the wide angle, maximum blurring of objects outside the focal plane occurs, and therefore phantom images (unwanted images) are less likely to be produced. For standard skeletal tomography we

use a CGR Stratomatic which is capable of performing linear (longitudinal, transverse, and diagonal), circular, and trispiral motions. Linear and circular tube travel may be 20°, 30°, or 45°. In trispiral studies the angle is always 45°. 3M XUD film with Lanex regular screens (200 speed system) in special carbon-fiber front cassettes are used at a 48-inch source-to-film distance. A Bucky grid with a 12:1 ratio is used. Exposure factors will vary with the body part being studied.

TUBE MOTION IN ORTHOPEDIC TOMOGRAPHY

In orthopedic practice tomography is frequently used to evaluate subtle fractures (Fig. 1–9). Fracture healing and other clinical problems are also effectively studied with tomography (Table 1–2). In most orthopedic tomography the detail is improved with trispiral or other complex motion. Occasionally, especially in patients with metal internal or external fixation devices, linear motion may be more useful (Fig. 1–10). Trispiral motion (Fig. 1–10A) can cause significant loss of bone detail adjacent to the metal. Linear motion parallel to the metal (Fig. 1–10C) and

Figure 1–8. Tomographic blur in linear tomography. The tube motion is transverse (white arrow in number 2). Both wires of the cross pattern are in the focal plane in number 1 (left). When the fulcrum is above the wire pattern, the blurring is less evident in the wire parallel to the tube motion (number 2, right). (From McCullough, E. C., and Coulam, C. M.: Physical and dosimetric aspects of diagnostic geometrical and computer-assisted tomography. Radiol. Clin. North Am. 14:3, 1976.)

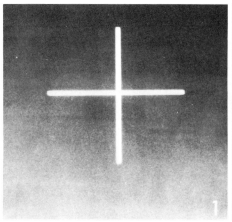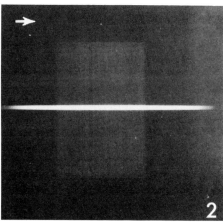

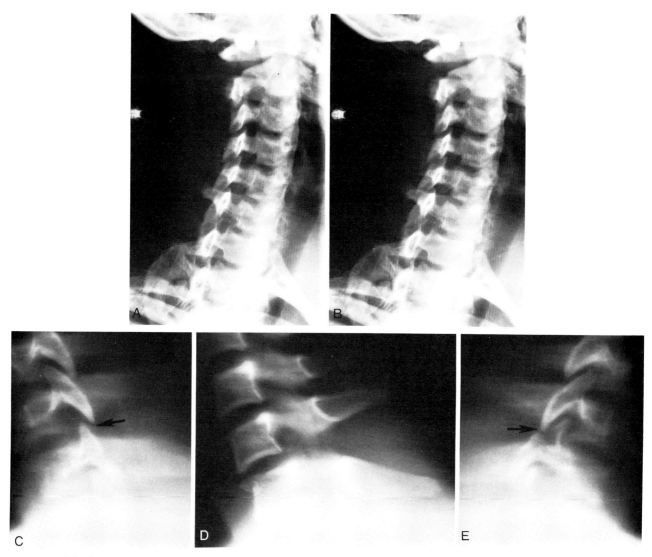

Figure 1–9. Radiographs of the cervical spine in a patient with neck pain following a motor vehicle accident. AP and lateral views were negative. The oblique views (*A* and *B*) demonstrate apparent widening of the C6–C7 facet joints with slight subluxation. Lateral tomograms (patient supine on the versigraph table) demonstrate subluxation of the left C6–C7 facet *(C)*, anterior subluxation of C6 on C7 with a fracture of the vertebral body *(D)*, and an impacted facet fracture on the right (*E*).

linear motion perpendicular to the metal (Fig. 1–10*B*) demonstrate that the metal artifact is reduced when the motion of the tube is parallel to the metal. Note that the adjacent bone and bone graft (Fig. 1–10*C*) are better defined with linear motion parallel

TABLE 1–2. Tomography: Orthopedic Indications

Trispiral or complex motion
Subtle fractures
Stress fractures
Fracture healing
Metabolic bone disease
Neoplasms
Arthritis
Linear motion
Acute trauma (Versitome)
Metal fixation devices

to the metal. In certain cases the configuration of the fixation device is such that examination choices are more difficult (Fig. 1–11). Tomography is still useful in providing increased detail in these situations.

In the immobilized patient with acute trauma we use the Kermath Versitome system (Fig. 1–1). It provides multiple-projection radiography (AP, lateral, oblique) in the supine patient; and in addition, through the use of an angulated cassette holder, it allows tomograms to be obtained in the exact plane of interest. Linear (longitudinal AP, transverse AP, transverse oblique, and transverse lateral) and transverse axial tomography are available (Fig. 1–12). This versatility is useful in the acutely injured patient, for it is often necessary to define the extent of the injury with tomography so that proper treat-

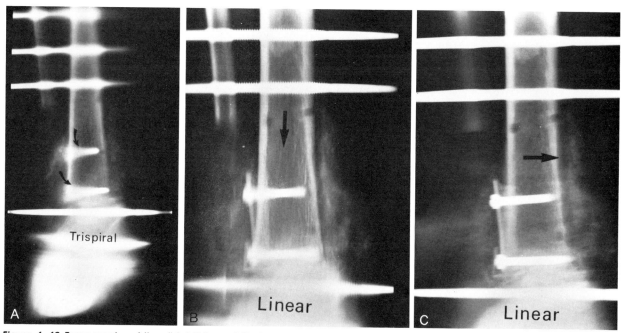

Figure 1–10. Tomography of the distal tibia and fibula with bone grafts and external fixation pins in place. Note that the trispiral motion blurs the pin more severely, resulting in some loss of bone detail adjacent to the pin *(A)*. With linear motion perpendicular to the pins, a similar problem occurs but the bone detail is improved *(B)*. When the tube motion is parallel to the pins *(C)*, the bone detail and bone graft are seen more clearly. *(Arrows* indicate direction of tube motion.)

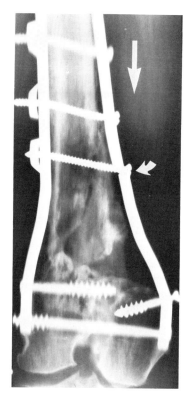

Figure 1–11. Plate and screw fixation of a supracondylar fracture of the femur. A linear tomogram parallel to the bone and the large plates causes the least reduction in bone detail. Note the fracture of the plate on the left *(curved arrow).*

ment can be instituted prior to moving the patient (see Fig. 1–9). The Versitome also provides a linear-sweep range of 8° to 50°. We commonly use the 50° angle for skeletal tomography. Narrower angles (10° amplitude) may be used in uncooperative patients, as the exposure time is reduced with narrow-angle tomography. With transverse axial tomography the tube travels 180°. Kodak OG film with Lanex regular screens (400 speed system) and a 52-inch source-film distance are used.

SUMMARY

The type of tomographic motion used may greatly influence the radiographic findings. There are advantages to simple and complex motion studies. Increased blurring of objects occurs outside the plane in focus because of the greater distance the tube-film moves during the complex motion exposure. This results in elimination of streaking (incomplete blur) in images of structures when their long axis is aligned with the tube-film motion, as seen in linear tomography.[8] Complex motion has decreased tendency to produce phantom images (unreal or unwanted images). The more complex the motion, the less the likelihood of phantom images. Linear tomography has the advantage of shorter exposure time, which may be useful in uncooperative patients. Linear motion may also be more useful when metal fixation devices are in place.

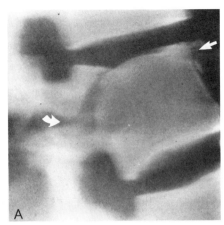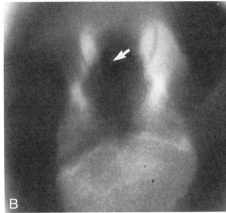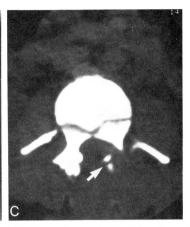

Figure 1-12. Tomograms obtained on the Versitome. A, Compression fracture of the body of L1 *(straight arrow)* with distraction of the posterior complex *(curved arrow)*. B, Transaxial tomogram demonstrating the body fracture and posterior complex fragments *(arrow)*. C, CT scan at the same level as the transaxial tomogram adds soft tissue information, but the fractures have a similar appearance.

MAGNIFICATION RADIOGRAPHY

CLAIRE E. BENDER

Magnification radiography was first introduced in 1940 but did not gain popularity until the last decade.[13] The primary indication for this technique is small vessel angiography, but it is also useful in skeletal radiography. The technique provides accurate and detailed assessment of subtle skeletal abnormalities in articular, metabolic, infectious, neoplastic, and traumatic disorders.[14-19, 22]

EQUIPMENT AND PRINCIPLES OF MAGNIFICATION

A thorough understanding of the equipment and principles of magnification is necessary in order to obtain high-quality magnification radiographs. Proper selection of the x-ray tube is the key to success. We use a Machlett DX78E tube with a 0.20 mm focal spot (as specified by the manufacturer). The actual focal spot size (grid-biased) measures 0.10 mm using a star text pattern in accordance with the specifications of the National Electrical Manufacturers Association.[13, 21] High-speed rotation of the anode is necessary to prevent x-ray tube damage under heavy exposure conditions. A three-phase generator is also preferred.

For magnification hand films we use (1) 44-inch source-film distance, (2) Kodak NMB single emulsion film, (3) Kodak single Min-r intensifying screens (used as a rear screen), and (4) exposure factors of 60 kVp, 30 mA-s, and 1.25 sec. The patient's hand is supported on a Lucite stand 24 inches above the film. This results in a 2.2 to 1 magnification factor (Fig. 1-13).

Magnification radiography is based on two geometric principles. First, the size of the image is proportional to the distance between the object and the film; and second, the smaller the focal spot of the x-ray tube, the sharper the image.[13, 20, 21] A focal spot size of 0.30 mm or less is required for magnification radiography. Increased image size occurs as the distance between the object and film increases and as the distance between the focal spot and the object decreases, other factors remaining constant.[13, 20] Geometric magnification is defined as the ratio of the source-film distance to the source-

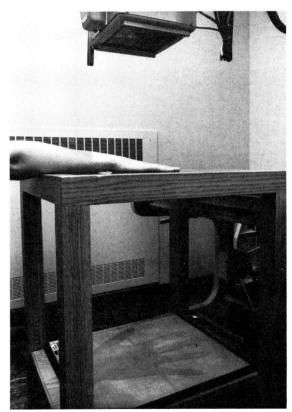

Figure 1-13. Radiographic magnification unit. X-ray tube, Lucite plate for positioning body part, and 14 × 17 cassette in lower portion of the support frame. Hand positioned for filming. Note the size of the shadow projected on the cassette.

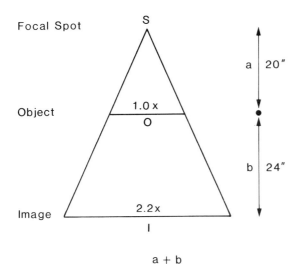

Focal Spot

S

Object   1.0 x
         O

a | 20"

b | 24"

Image   2.2 x
         I

$$\text{Magnification} = \frac{a + b}{a} = 2.2$$

Figure 1–14. Principles of magnification. Note that source (S) to image (I) distance (a + b) divided by the source (S) to object (O) distance (a) equals a magnification factor of 2.2.

object distance for a point-source focal spot (Fig. 1–14).

ADVANTAGES AND LIMITATIONS

Radiation exposure to the skin is increased in magnification radiography because of the short source-to-skin distance. However, the size of the entrance field (in skull and abdominal magnification) is significantly reduced, thereby lowering total body exposure to nearly the equivalent dose obtained with conventional techniques. Entrance exposure to the skin for the magnified hand using our technique measures 246 mR.* This exposure is higher than the routine hand films (26 mR) but is accepted, as the magnification technique is used only in selected cases.[16, 21] Also, the hand is among the least radiosensitive body parts. The overall high-quality image is the advantage of this technique (Fig. 1–15). Increased effective sharpness, reduced effective noise, increased subject contrast (the air gap reduces the scattered radiation reaching the film), and improved visual effect of the enlargement contribute to high quality radiographs. When the technique is properly performed, anatomic structures are better defined than those visualized in conventional radiographs observed with a magnifying lens. Use of a magnifying lens results in magnification of the inherent unsharpness of the screen-film combination and graininess along with magnification of the anatomic detail.[13, 19]

Limitations of magnification include the following: (1) imaging is limited to small areas, (2) proper positioning of the area of interest may be difficult, (3) high relative skin exposure and long exposure times may result in limited tube-loading capabilities.[19]

XERORADIOGRAPHY

THOMAS H. BERQUIST • TED WINKLER

Xeroradiography was first described by Carlson in 1937. Medical usage of the technique began in 1952 with John Roach.[26, 33, 38] This modality has been most frequently used in mammography and evalu-

*Webbels, W.: Exposure data, St. Mary's Hospital, 1983.

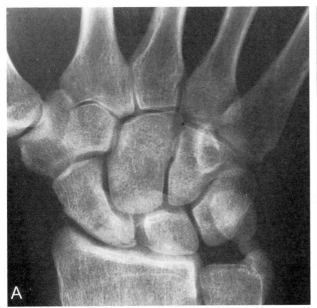

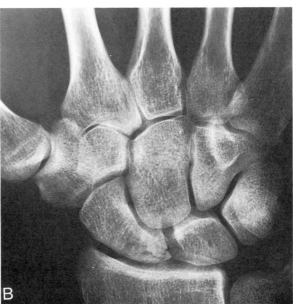

Figure 1–15. PA views of the wrist in a patient with fragmentation and avascular necrosis of the proximal scaphoid. *A,* Routine technique. *B,* Magnification technique.

ation of bone and soft tissue disorders of the extremities.[24–27, 33, 35, 38] It is also beneficial in evaluation of the upper airway and sternum and in selected dental techniques.[27, 29, 32, 37] In orthopedic radiology xeroradiography is useful in studies of bone and soft tissue trauma, arthritis, and metabolic and infectious diseases.

EQUIPMENT AND PRINCIPLES OF XERORADIOGRAPHY

In conventional radiography, the cassette contains the film, which is the final recording medium. In xeroradiography, the cassette contains a xerodiographic plate, which consists of an aluminum base with a thin (130 micron) layer of selenium (a photo conductor).[27, 37] Steps *A* to *H* in Figure 1–16 indicate the stages in xeroradiography. The xerodiographic plate (*A*) records an intermediate image electronically. To prepare the xeroradiographic plate to record the electronic image, the cassette containing the plate is inserted into a conditioner. A uniform positive charge (*B*) is applied to the selenium coating by exposing it to a corona discharge of over 1000 volts DC. The density and contrast of the xeroradiographic image may fluctuate by changing this voltage. The xeroradiographic cassette containing the charged plate is exposed to x-rays (*C*) in the same manner as conventional film techniques. The plate is discharged in proportion to the x-rays passing through the examined part and striking the plate. The electronic image is then recorded. The cassette is introduced into a xeroradiographic image processor in which a blue negatively charged powder (toner) is applied to the plate (*D*). The powder is attracted to the remaining positively charged segments of the plate. This forms a visible but nonpermanent image. A paper or plastic xeroradiographic material in sheet form is compressed against the powder-laden plate, and the image is transformed from the plate to the paper (*F*). The paper is heated, causing fixation of the powder. The image is then ready for interpretation. The entire developing process requires approximately one minute. Since the xeroradiographic plate will remain in the altered state for a period of time, it must be prepared for re-use. When the xeroradiographic cassette is inserted into the conditioner, the residual powder is automatically cleared with brushes and the plate is uniformly discharged by heating to 135° for 30 to 40 sec. The uniform charge is returned and the plate is ready for the next image. The above process describes the positive xeroradiographic mode. A negative mode may also be used.

ADVANTAGES AND LIMITATIONS

The image provided by the xeroradiograph has greater latitude than exists with conventional film techniques, and the edge enhancement that results from the electrostatic process makes xeroradiography advantageous for demonstrating abrupt changes in density. This provides better detail for viewing adjoining areas of differing density, such as bone and soft tissue adjacencies. Conventional radiography is somewhat better suited for subtle changes in density of adjoining tissues. If one compares images, the unexposed area of a xerograph appears deep blue rather than the white of conventional films. The exposed area on the xerograph is white rather than the black seen on the conventional radiograph. Areas of calcification appear as deep blue on the xerograph and white on conventional film.[37]

Advantages of the electrostatic system of xeroradiography include (1) no fog or noise, (2) control of the characteristic curve (contrast), (3) display of detail at different contrast values, (4) multiple images from a single exposure, (5) no darkroom requirements, (6) greater latitude for exposure factors, and (7) accentuated density differences due to edge

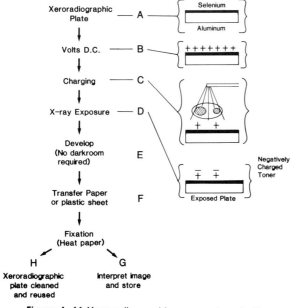

Figure 1–16. Xeroradiographic process (see text).

TABLE 1–3. Indications for Xeroradioraphy

Soft tissue evaluation
    Masses
    Foreign bodies
    Tendinitis
    Synovitis
Skeletal
    Subtle fractures
    Casted fractures
    Sternal trauma
    Metabolic bone disease
    Osteomyelitis
    Arthritis
    Xerotomography—spine
Arthrography
    Cruciate ligament evaluation

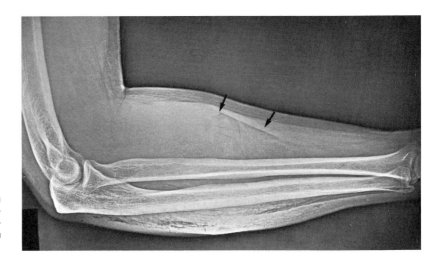

Figure 1–17. Lateral view of the forearm following a soft tissue injury. Note the subcutaneous emphysema along the extensor surface. Wood fragment *(arrows)* can be seen in the soft tissues.

enhancement. There are also disadvantages with this technique, the main disadvantage being higher radiation exposure to the patient than in conventional radiography. For example, the skin entrance exposure for radiography of the knee is 44 mR compared with 636 mR with xeroradiography.* Radiation exposure can be decreased, however, by increasing the selenium sensitivity, increasing the tube voltage, or matching the x-ray spectrum to the selenium sensitivity.[23, 30] Bryant and Julian demonstrated a dose reduction of about 50 percent by using 100 kVp and a 0.15 mm copper filter.[23] The latter prevents low-energy radiation from reaching the patient.

The paper and blue powder are also somewhat more difficult to handle than conventional films, as they are easily smudged and the powder is readily

*Webbels, W.: Exposure study. St. Mary's Hospital, 1983.

attracted to the hands and clothing of the examining physician. Also, pressure artifacts may occur if a heavy body part is placed on the xeroradiographic cassette. In-house x-ray service engineers may be less familiar with xeroradiographic equipment, requiring outside assistance from the manufacturer for maintenance of the equipment.

For many years, xeroradiography was used primarily for mammography.[37] Recent advances in screen-film combinations have resulted in lower dose systems, reducing the use of the higher dose xerographic system.[26, 31, 34] Use of xerographs in other clinical areas is not routine, but this technique is of value in selected situations (Table 1–3). Evaluation of soft tissue masses in the extremities and studies of the sternum and soft tissues of the neck are less difficult with xeroradiography. Figure 1–17 demonstrates the value of xeroradiography in detection of nonopaque foreign bodies. Selected to-

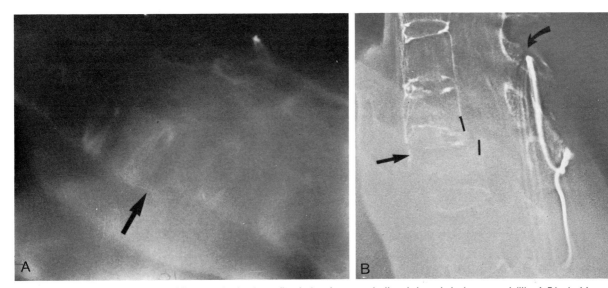

Figure 1–18. Lateral tomograms of the cervical spine after fusion for pseudarthrosis in ankylosing spondylitis. *A,* Trispiral tomogram demonstrates the fracture and subluxation *(arrow),* but the fusion site is not clearly seen. *B,* Xerotomogram in the same plane demonstrates these features more clearly. In addition, the fusion is more clearly demonstrated, and a fracture of the spinous process *(curved arrow)* at the superior aspect of the fusion is evident.

mographic sections using the xerox technique may also be useful, especially in the lower cervical and upper thoracic spine (Fig. 1–18).

The fine detail of the skeletal work in the extremities makes xeroradiography useful for detection of subtle metabolic and arthritic conditions.[24, 25, 28, 32, 36] Griffiths has described the use of this technique, combined with arthrography, in studying the cruciate ligaments.[28] Subtle changes in other ligaments and tendons may also be detected. In sports medicine dedicated to running injuries of the knee, Achilles tendon, and other structures, xeroradiography may provide a means for early detection of inflammation.

On occasion, xerographs may be useful in detecting subtle fractures. Fracture lines are accentuated owing to differences in density.[36] Also, better detail is afforded when examining casted extremities following fracture reduction.[32]

ULTRASOUND

E. MEREDITH JAMES

The term ultrasound refers to mechanical vibrations whose frequencies are above the limit of human audible perception (about 20,000 Hz or cycles per second). Medical ultrasound imaging utilizes frequencies in the range of 2 to 10 MHz.[50] A central component of any ultrasound instrument is the transducer, which contains a small piezoelectric crystal. It serves as both the transmitter of sound waves into the body and the receiver of the returning echoes. When a brief alternating current is applied to the crystal, it vibrates at a characteristic frequency. By applying this vibrating transducer to the skin surface (through an acoustic coupling medium such as mineral oil), the mechanical energy is transmitted into the body as a brief pulse of high-frequency sound waves. The advancing wave front interacts with tissues in various poorly understood ways and generates small reflected waves that return to the transducer. These cause the crystal to vibrate again, thereby generating an electrical signal that is conducted back to the machine where it is processed and displayed. With B-mode ultrasound imaging, the returning echoes are displayed as dots of light on an oscilloscope or television screen, with the position of the dot on the screen corresponding to the position in the body where the echo was generated. In this way, the ultrasound image represents a cross-sectional display of the underlying anatomy. Unlike computed tomography, in which the geometric constraints of the scanner itself limit the possible scanning planes obtainable, any conceivable plane or section can be obtained with most ultrasound instruments. Such scanning flexibility can be of great value in demonstrating the continuity or discontinuity of adjacent structures.[50, 53]

STATIC AND REAL-TIME SCANNERS

There are two basic types of B-mode ultrasound scanners. One, called a static, or articulated-arm, B-mode scanner, uses a mechanical arm with the transducer attached at one end to "construct" a static image as the transducer is moved across the skin surface. The other, called a real-time ultrasound scanner, generates rapid, sequential B-scan images that permit high-speed continuous viewing.[39, 42, 44, 50, 51, 53] This instrument can display dynamic events, such as a pulsating vessel, or can be moved across the body to provide continuous viewing of the underlying anatomy. Both types employ so-called grey-scale image processing, whereby the returning echoes (depending on their amplitude) are assigned one of up to 64 shades of grey for final display. The resulting images, therefore, demonstrate not only the major boundaries between soft tissue structures but also their internal parenchymatous texture. This permits characterization of diffuse pathologic processes as well as detection of space-occupying lesions. Certainly, the development of grey-scale processing has been a crucial factor in the recent clinical success of ultrasound imaging.

Recently, a relatively specialized type of real-time ultrasound instrument, called a small-parts scanner, has been developed, offering high-resolution images of superficial soft tissue structures.[48] This uses high-frequency sound waves (up to about 10 MHz). It is a fundamental principle of ultrasound that the higher the frequency of the sound, the better the resolution of the images. However, it is also fundamentally true that high-frequency sound waves are attenuated more rapidly in the soft tissues and therefore cannot penetrate very deeply. The result of these counterbalancing effects is that the small-parts scanner can obtain submillimeter resolution, but only for structures located within about 5 cm of the skin surface. While conventional static or real-time scanners will generally provide satisfactory results in these superficial areas, small-parts instruments are definitely superior.

APPLICATIONS TO ORTHOPEDICS

Perhaps the most severe limitation of diagnostic ultrasound imaging is due to the inability of sound waves to penetrate gas and bone. The strength of an echo generated at the boundary between any two tissues is related to differences in the acoustic impedance of the tissues (a physical property generally dependent on density). Because the acoustic impedances of bone and air are so different from those of human soft tissues, almost all sound energy is reflected off a soft tissue–bone or soft tissue–gas interface, leaving essentially no sound energy left to penetrate and thus image deeper structures. The strong echo reflected off such an interface "overwhelms" the transducer and is displayed as useless noise or artifact in the image.

Because this fundamental physical principle prevents ultrasound from passing from soft tissue into bone, the applications of this modality to orthopedics are relatively limited. In fact, they are confined solely to the soft tissues. Transcutaneous ultrasound bone imaging is impossible.

However, the remarkable sensitivity of ultrasound in distinguishing fluid from solid tissue has made it particularly useful in the characterization of the internal consistency of masses.[40] A simple fluid collection, such as an uncomplicated cyst, will be represented sonographically as an echo-free area, while solid tissue, or the cells and debris within some fluid masses (such as abscesses), will provide interfaces for sound reflection and will therefore be echogenic. Some masses, of course, will demonstrate a complex pattern with both solid and cystic elements. Thus in addition to characterizing a mass by the number of echoes generated within it, it is also important to assess the manner in which sound is transmitted through the mass. Fluid-containing structures cause little attenuation of the sound beam and thereby demonstrate a characteristic ultrasound finding: so-called "enhanced through-transmission." This finding takes the form of stronger or brighter echoes deep to the fluid structure. Solid lesions cause greater attenuation of sound and therefore lack the finding of acoustic enhancement. By evaluating both the internal echogenicity of a mass and the ease of sound propagation through it, one can in virtually all instances characterize the basic contents of the mass as fluid, solid, or mixed. While such a broad categorization is by no means histologically specific, such information, combined with appropriate clinical data, can often be very helpful in patient management.

In addition to defining the internal nature of a soft tissue mass, ultrasound can also play a useful role in defining its size and extent. For very large or deep-seated lesions, however, the major disadvantage to ultrasound imaging is the inability to demonstrate bony involvement. For this reason suspected malignant bone or soft tissue tumors are generally better evaluated with conventional radiography combined with computed tomography. For smaller and more superficially located masses ultrasound can be a useful diagnostic tool, especially when the high-frequency transducer of a small-parts scanner is employed (Fig. 1–19).

DIAGNOSTIC EVALUATION OF THE POPLITEAL FOSSA

The one anatomic region where ultrasound has come to play a key role in diagnostic soft tissue evaluation is the popliteal fossa.[41, 43, 45, 47] Masses or swelling in this area, whether pulsatile or not, can be difficult diagnostic problems for the clinician.

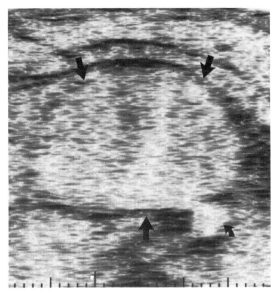

Figure 1–19. Transverse image of the upper arm using a small-parts scanner demonstrates an oval-shaped, well-circumscribed solid mass *(straight arrows).* At surgery this proved to be a benign neurofibroma of the median nerve. Small hash marks at the bottom of the image represent a 1-mm scale. Curved arrow points to the brachial artery, deep to the mass.

Ultrasound has been successful in imaging popliteal artery aneurysms, popliteal cysts, abscesses, hematomas, and malignant tumors. In addition, patients with acute calf pain can be evaluated by ultrasound to differentiate pseudothrombophlebitis (due to ruptured popliteal cyst) from true thrombophlebitis.[49, 52]

The patient is positioned prone on the examining table and both transverse and longitudinal scans are obtained on the posterior surface of the lower extremity from the lower thigh to the mid-calf. Because the popliteal artery can virtually always be visualized, an aneurysm involving this vessel is readily appreciated by noting continuity of the "mass" with the vessel above and below. A popliteal cyst usually appears sonographically as an echo-free mass exhibiting acoustic "enhancement" behind it, which is located separate from the popliteal artery (Fig. 1–20).[41, 43, 45, 47] If large, it can dissect for a considerable length into the calf. Occasionally, the cyst may contain scattered internal echoes, representing fibrin strands or other debris. Such an appearance can be indistinguishable from an abscess, but the clinical presentation usually permits differentiation.

Numerous studies have confirmed the accuracy of ultrasound in detecting popliteal cysts when compared with the results of arthrography. In patients with rheumatoid arthritis, ultrasound has also been reported to be useful in distinguishing proliferative synovial tissue from simple effusion in the suprapatellar recess of the joint space.[42, 46] The ultrasound depiction of both fluid and soft tissue within the knee joint has also been described with

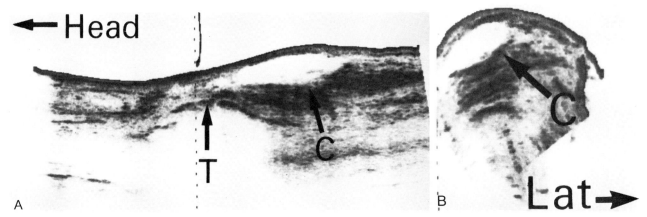

Figure 1–20. Popliteal cyst. Longitudinal *(A)* and transverse *(B)* ultrasound images of the popliteal region with the patient lying prone show an elongated echo-free cystic mass (C) posteriorly and medially. The posterior surface of the tibia (T) produces a strong acoustical interface that prevents further penetration of the sound. Small graticule marks represent 1-cm scale.

pigmented villonodular synovitis. Early work in evaluation of rotator cuff tears is also in progress.

SUMMARY

While ultrasound imaging has become a major diagnostic tool for clinical medicine in general, its applications in the field of orthopedics are limited. However, ultrasound has clearly established its usefulness in evaluation of the popliteal space, and in selected situations it can offer important information about soft tissues in other anatomic regions.

SKELETAL SCINTIGRAPHY

MANUEL L. BROWN

Bone scintigraphy developed by way of a progression that began with P-32 orthophosphate tissue distribution studies in the 1930's. Early nuclides of calcium were first used in the 1940's to study bone mineral metabolism. The earliest attempts at external detection included surface counting of the distribution of P-32 orthophosphate and manual scanning with a Geiger-Müller tube of the distribution of gallium-72, and later strontium-85. Strontium-85, strontium-87m, and fluorine-18 all played major roles in the development of clinical bone scanning in the 1960's and early 1970's. Current bone imaging is a spin-off of the early work with phosphate compounds and has its origins with Subramanian's introduction of tripolyphosphate.[79, 80]

RADIOPHARMACEUTICALS USED IN BONE SCANNING

Radiopharmaceuticals currently used in bone scanning include compounds with P=O=P bonds (methylenediphosphonate). The diphosphonates are the current agents of choice because of their better stability and soft tissue clearance rates. The phosphate and phosphonate reagents come in sterile pyrogen-free lyophilized form with stannous ion as a reducing agent. Tc-99m (technetium pertechnetate) is added to the vial. The Tc-99m is reduced from the +7 to the +4 state and forms a chelate with the diphosphonate. After compounding, the material is checked for acceptability by quality control procedures commonly using thin-layer or paper chromatography. The material is injected intravenously. Its localization in bone is dependent on blood flow and osteoblastic activity. The most widely accepted mechanism of localization is felt to be chemiadsorption to the hydroxyapatite crystals of the bone mineral matrix. Approximately 50 percent of the material is cleared by the kidneys and excreted in the urine. Good hydration and an appropriate interval between administration and scanning of approximately 3 hours allow for soft tissue clearance and improved target-to-background ratios.

Another important radiopharmaceutical in the case of orthopedic patients with suspected infection is gallium-67 citrate. In the 1950's gallium isotopes were originally studied as potential bone-scanning agents. Although they do localize in bone, the available isotopes at that time were not satisfactory for imaging. Later, gallium-67 was shown to localize in tumors and sites of infection, its major role today. The mechanism of localization of gallium in infection sites is not well understood, but it appears to be related to the binding of gallium to lactoferrin at sites of infection, leukocyte labeling, and/or direct bacterial uptake.[65] The optimal time from injection to scan is 24 to 48 hours. Since we know that gallium is deposited in bone, care must be taken in the interpretation of gallium-uptake when looking for bone or joint infections. A sequence of Tc-99m and gallium scans may be necessary to differentiate reactive bone from inflammatory lesions.

A new agent that may prove useful in bone and joint infections is indium-111–labeled autologous white blood cells. The method of cell labeling is beyond the scope of this chapter, but the primary method is based on the work of Thakur.[83, 84] White blood cells migrate to sites of infection, and localization in the area of bone implies an infectious process. Images may be taken at 4 and 24 hours after the administration of the labeled white cells.

INSTRUMENTATION

Originally the rectilinear scanner was the most common instrument used for whole-body bone surveys. The Anger-gamma camera is the instrument most frequently used at this time. The camera allows total-body surveys with a moving table or moving detector. Selected views can also be obtained with this instrument. Radioactivity from the patient passes through a lead collimator and enters a sodium iodide crystal. The photon deposits its energy in the crystal. It in turn gives off photons of light, which are converted to electrons by the photocathode of the photomultiplier tubes. These electrons are amplified by the photomultiplier tubes and processed, with the resulting data being placed on film or entered into a computer for further analysis.

Collimators are designated according to the resolution and energy levels at which they can be used (i.e., lower energy for Tc-99m agents, medium energy for indium-111 labeled white cells or gallium-67 studies, and high energy for iodine-131 agents). Collimator holes can be parallel or nonparallel; converging collimators magnify slightly. The pinhole collimator is a single hole that allows for magnification of an area of interest with some geometric distortion.

CLINICAL APPLICATIONS

Although there are many indications for the use of bone scanning in clinical practice, the most common use is in oncology for detection and follow-up of metastatic bone disease primarily from prostatic, breast, and lung cancer. The orthopedic uses of bone scanning primarily include diagnosis of trauma and infection, determination of vascularity, compartmental evaluation of degenerative arthritis of joints, and evaluation of patients with painful prosthesis. Secondary uses include evaluation of elevated alkaline phosphatase and diagnosis of patients who present with bone pain of undetermined etiology.

Tumors

Bone scanning is perhaps of greatest use in the diagnosis and delineation of metastatic diseases. In patients with prostatic carcinoma the bone scan is more sensitive for the early detection of metastasis than conventional radiographic surveys or enzyme

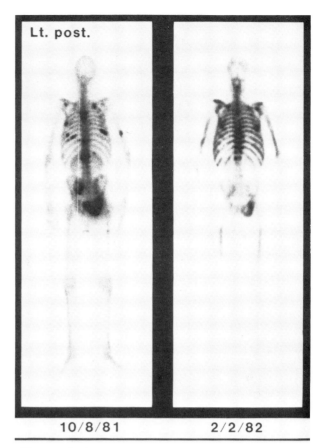

Figure 1–21. Serial isotope scans from 10/8/81 to 2/2/82 in a 77-year-old male with carcinoma of the prostate. Scan finding preceded the x-ray and clinical findings by 5 months.

determinations (Fig. 1–21). Schaffer and colleagues studied a group of patients with proven metastatic prostate carcinoma and positive bone scans.[76] In this series 43 percent had no bone pain, 39 percent had normal acid phosphatase levels, and 23 percent had normal alkaline phosphatase. The bone scan is also very sensitive in breast carcinoma; however, the utility of the preoperative scans depends on the clinical stage of the tumor. McNeil and colleagues[71] and Wilson and colleagues[89] showed that in Stage 1 and 2 disease the yield of metastasis was low. However, many feel that there is value in preoperative scans in Stage 1 and 2 as a base-line study, and of course patients with Stage 3 disease or bone pain should have preoperative bone scans.

Bone scans are also sensitive for the detection of bone metastasis in other soft tissue primary tumors and in primary bone tumors (Fig. 1–22). However, the bone scan is of very limited utility in the evaluation of multiple myeloma, a malignancy that seems to evoke little reparative response. Conventional radiographs are more sensitive in the evaluation of these patients.[90]

Bone scans can be used to locate sites for bone biopsy.[56] Some groups have localized the area in question with a gamma camera and injected methylene blue in the tissue to help guide the open biopsy.

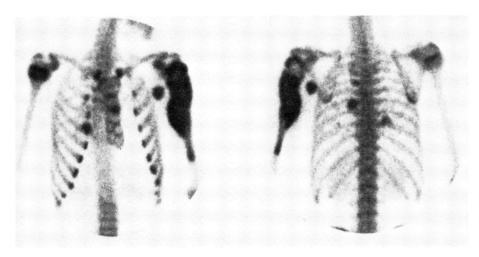

Figure 1–22. Tc-99m MDP scan in a 12-year-old male with radiographic findings of a left humeral osteogenic sarcoma. In addition to the humerus, the bone tracer can be seen in the axillary adenopathy and in the pulmonary metastasis.

Bone scintigraphy is of little use in the evaluation of benign tumors except for suspected osteoid osteoma not diagnosed with plain films. When plain films are negative or atypical, bone scanning is the procedure of choice (Fig. 1–23).[77, 82] The bone scan allows imaging of various sites, as the pain may be referred. The lesion of osteoid osteoma is quite intense and can locate the area for tomography.

Trauma

Bone scanning can provide important information in patients with known or suspected trauma. Routine radiographs will easily demonstrate the site of fracture in most patients with a clinical history of trauma. In these uncomplicated cases bone scintigraphy will not add significant additional information. However, when the initial x-rays are normal, as may occur with subtle fractures of the pelvis (Fig. 1–24), proximal femurs, or carpal bones[59] (Fig. 1–25), the bone scan may play a role in directing the course of management. Fractures will show focal areas of increased uptake early, with 80 percent visible in 24 hours and 95 percent in 72 hours,[69] though in elderly patients more time is often required for the onset of activity to occur at the fracture site. Bone scanning is also very helpful in patients suspected of having stress fractures. The scan will detect stress fractures earlier than radiography, and if cessation of the stress is instituted,

Figure 1–23. Lumbar spine films were normal in a 15-year-old male with low back pain felt mainly at night. The Tc-99m MDP scan demonstrates increased uptake at L3 on the left *(arrow).* This allowed localized tomograms to define the osteoid osteoma.

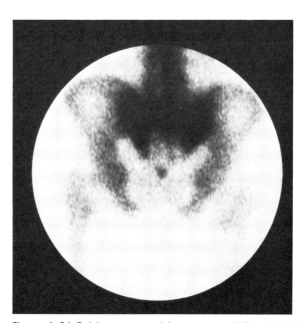

Figure 1–24. Pelvic x-rays and tomograms of the right hip were normal in a disoriented elderly female with pain following a fall. Tc-99m MDP scan shows increased uptake in the midsacrum and both sacroiliac joints due to pelvic fractures.

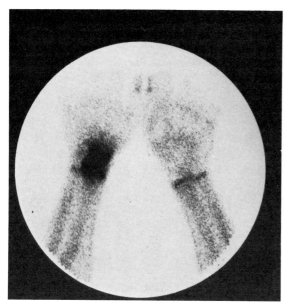

Figure 1–25. X-rays and tomograms were normal in a 16-year-old male with left wrist pain following a fall. The Tc-99m MDP bone scan shows marked focal areas of increased uptake in the distal radius and scaphoid. Repeat tomograms showed a fracture of the distal radial physis and scaphoid.

the radiographs may never become positive (Fig. 1–26).[61, 78, 88] A negative scan implies that the symptoms are not due to a stress fracture. Finally, in the battered child syndrome the bone scan may show the extent of the bone trauma, allowing for directed radiographic confirmation. The scan may also demonstrate bone contusion not seen radiographically.

Other uses for bone scanning are currently being explored. Animal models show that sequential studies can use radionuclide imaging to evaluate fracture healing,[64] although this has not yet been convincingly demonstrated in humans. There does seem to be a role for bone scintigraphy in selecting patients with non-united fractures for percutaneous electrical stimulation, however, as reported by Desai and colleagues.[58] Their study showed that when there was diffuse increased activity at the fracture site, 95 percent healed completely with percutaneous electrical stimulation. When there was a photon deficient (cold) area at the fracture site, none healed; and only 50 percent healed if there was low uptake in the fracture site. The question of bone viability following trauma, such as in the femoral neck

fracture, can also be evaluated with bone scanning[62, 63] (Fig. 1–27). Finally, focal areas of intense increased uptake in the spine may indicate pseudarthrosis in patients with ankylosing spondylitis[73] or following fusion.[70] This finding on an otherwise normal patient may indicate spondylosis.

Vascularity of Bone

The vascularity of bone can be assessed with the use of radiotracers. As mentioned above, bone scanning has a potential clinical role in evaluating femoral head vascularity following fracture. In a patient suspected of having Legg-Calvé-Perthes disease, the bone scan will demonstrate a lack of tracer earlier than the appearance of the radiographic findings[57, 60, 81] (Fig. 1–28). The results of one large series showed a sensitivity of 98 percent, a specificity of 95 percent, and an accuracy of 96 percent.[81] After revascularization the bone scan may reveal increased activity in the femoral head. Elderly patients with painful knees may show intense activity in the metaphysis of the tibia or femur due to osteonecrosis.[68] Bone scintigraphy may also play a role in the early evaluation of bone grafts, detecting vascularity in the first postoperative week.[55] Studies performed later may not be accurate, since uptake may occur in a thin area of new cortical bone, and may not demonstrate true graft viability.

Infection

Bone scanning is helpful in the evaluation of patients with suspected osteomyelitis. However, there are pitfalls in its use, especially in neonatal osteomyelitis, in patients with orthopedic appliances, and in patients with recent trauma or surgery. Gallium- and possibly indium-labeled white cells can be helpful in these instances. This topic will be covered in detail in the chapter on osteomyelitis (Chapter 14).

Further Clinical Applications

The bone scanning agents accumulate in the arthritides. Although the pattern of localization may

Figure 1–26. Tc-99m MDP scan in a 22-year-old jogger with a left lower leg pain reveals focal increased uptake in the posterior aspect of both tibias due to stress fractures.

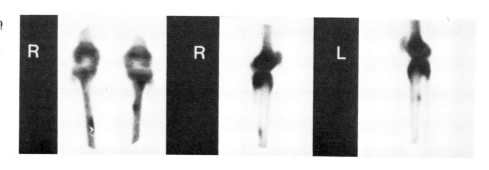

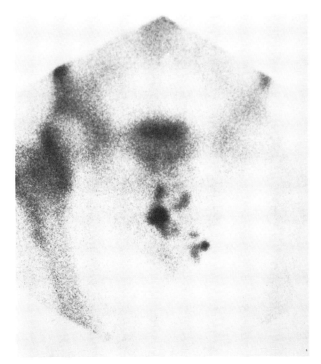

Figure 1–27. Tc-99m MDP scan in a 44-year-old female with fractured right femur from a roller skating accident shows increased uptake in the femoral neck fracture. There is also decreased activity in the femoral head indicating loss of vascularity. Several months later the typical radiographic features of avascular necrosis appeared. Findings were confirmed at surgery.

help differentiate between rheumatoid arthritis and the rheumatoid variants, the scan is less specific than radiographic findings,[87] and its ability to aid in the diagnosis and follow-up of patients with arthritis is uncertain. When it is important to assess accurately the compartmental involvement of os-

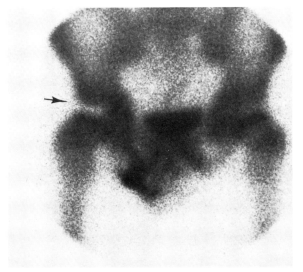

Figure 1–28. Tc-99m MDP scan in a 7-year-old male with a limp and hip pain shows a well-defined photon deficient area in the right femoral head *(arrow).* Radiographic findings were consistant with Legg-Calvé-Perthes disease.

teoarthritis of the knee, the bone scan is more sensitive than radiographs or arthrography.[83]

Following joint replacement the bone scan may show increased activity for 6 to 12 months[67] as the bone readjusts to the new stresses of the arthroplasty. Following the appropriate interval, increased uptake in the components implies loosening or infection.[60, 66, 86] The addition of a gallium scan can be helpful in making the diagnosis of infection.[72, 74, 75]

QUANTITATION OF BONE MINERAL

HEINZ W. WAHNER • *WILLIAM L. DUNN* • *B. LAWRENCE RIGGS*

Noninvasive bone mass measurements have been developed over the last several decades and are now firmly established as investigative and clinical tools in many medical centers. These methods include a wide spectrum of different techniques, such as radioscopy (biconcavity index, Smith index, Singh index, fine detail roentgenograms), radiographic morphometry (cortical thickness), radiographic photodensitometry, photon absorptiometry (single and dual photon), radionuclide uptake, quantitated computed tomography (CT), and neutron activation analysis (total or partial skeleton). The validity of these methods has been described in the literature.[92, 94, 99, 103, 104, 106–108, 112–115, 119, 120] In this review emphasis will be given to photon absorptiometry techniques which can be performed with commercially available instrumentation in any nuclear medicine or radiology department. Relevant information on the different methods is given in Table 1–4.

In contrast to most of the other radiographic and imaging techniques used to study bone disease, which are concerned with focal expression of disease, bone mineral measurements are performed to study skeletal mineralization in diseases that diffusely affect the skeleton, such as metabolic bone disease. Further applications are the study of age-related bone loss, the assessment of drug effects on bone mineralization, and the accurate assessment of fracture risk at specific bone sites, such as the spine, femoral neck, and radius. It is particularly the latter application that is of interest to the physician in orthopedic practice.

CLINICAL RELEVANCE OF BONE MINERAL MEASUREMENT

In clinical practice bone mineral measurements may be performed to assess cortical or trabecular bone mineral loss resulting from accelerated bone resorption or decreased bone formation, to predict

TABLE 1–4. Different Methods for the Assessment of Bone Mineral

Method	Type of Measurement	Remarks on Clinical Usefulness*
Radioscopy	Biconcavity index	Unreliable
	Singh index	Value debated but used in some centers
	Smith index	Unreliable
	Fine detailed radiographs	Only for osteomalacia (periosteal resorption)
Radiographic morphometry	Cortical thickness	Does not assess intracortical porosity and endosteal erosion, 5 to 10% CV
Radiographic photodensitometry	Visual inspection	20 to 40% CV
	Reference wedge	5 to 10%, 30% CV
Absorptiometry	Single photon (^{125}I)	Measures appendicular bone, 3–5% CV
	Dual photon (^{153}Gd)	Measures mainly trabecular bone of axial skeleton, 2–5% CV
Radionuclide uptake	^{47}Ca, ^{45}Ca, ^{85}Sr, ^{87}mSr, ^{131}Ba, ^{18}F, ^{203}Pb, ^{99}mTc	
Compton scattering		5% CV
Computed tomography		2–5% CV measures purely trabecular bone
Neutron activation analysis	^{48}Ca–^{49}Ca (^{241}Am-Be or ^{238}Pu-Be)	5% CV total body calcium, partial assessment of skeleton also possible

*Estimates of error are given as coefficient of variation (CV).

total body calcium, and to provide a quantitative result that can be used for the prediction of fracture risk. The relationship between abnormal bone remodeling and mineral changes, as assessed by this method, is easy to understand. Total skeletal mineralization can be estimated from these localized measurements with reasonable accuracy. The coefficient of correlation between total skeletal weight and bone mineral in different parts of the skeleton has been evaluated and is about 0.86 (r) for the distal radius as a measuring site.[96]

The relationship between fracture risk and bone mineral mass is more complex. Decreased strength of bone and increasing susceptibility to fracture are related to the quantity of bone mineral in both trabecular and cortical bone, but they are not identical. Geometric changes in compact bone with aging, predominant loss of either cortical or trabecular bone, and the occurrence of microfractures in cortical bone can alter the relationship between breaking strength and bone mineral. Despite this variability, bone mineral measurements have been used successfully to predict the breaking strength of bone as measured in the laboratory on excised bone and in epidemiologic studies.[91, 95]

REVIEW OF THE DYNAMICS OF BONE MINERAL CHANGES

The mammalian skeleton serves two sets of needs. One function is to provide a structural support for the body, and the other function is to serve as a reservoir for almost all the body calcium and phosphorus. The skeleton is never metabolically at rest. Bone is constantly renewed by the process of remodeling. Bone mineral measurements at any given time reflect long-term changes in bone turnover but give little information about the nature of these changes, i.e., either abnormal resorption or formation.

The skeleton changes with age and so does bone mineral. The amount of noncrystalline amorphous calcium phosphate, imperfect crystals and incompletely mineralized bone, tends to increase with age of the bone. With maturation, the exchange of various ions between bone and extracellular fluid decreases; and the ability of bone to take up bone-seeking elements similarly decreases. Despite these changes in age and disease, the absorption coefficient of bone for gamma rays of a given energy level remains constant for practical considerations.

Physiological bone loss as well as bone loss associated with disease ultimately affects the entire skeleton. There are, however, differences in bone loss patterns in different bones, and bone loss occurs at different rates on different bone surfaces even within the same bone. Further, it appears that these patterns vary in prominence in different individuals. These variations influence fracture patterns and have to be considered when measurements are being interpreted.

The skeleton has 80 percent cortical bone and 20 percent trabecular bone, the latter being located mainly in the axial skeleton. The distribution of cortical and trabecular bone in different parts of the skeleton is given in Table 1–5. Because of its greater surface area, trabecular bone is metabolically more active and thus more likely to change.

TABLE 1–5. Trabecular and Cortical Bone at Common Sampling Sites for Bone Mineral Measurements by Single and Dual Photon Absorptiometry

Bone Site		Cortical Bone (%)	Trabecular Bone (%)
Radius	Mid-shaft	>90	<10
	Distal	75	25
Femur	Neck	75	25
	Trochanter	50	50
Spine	Lumbar	50	50

Since magnitude and rate of bone loss are not uniformly distributed in the skeleton, the proper selection of a measuring site and its composition with respect to trabecular and cortical bone are of importance for the interpretation of bone mineral results.

Specific requirements for clinically useful measurements of bone mineral mass have been defined.[104, 108] For longitudinal measurements high precision or reproducibility is required. For the detection of osteopenia or bone loss, accuracy is very important and a good normal population study for comparison is necessary. The method should be of sufficient sensitivity to detect clinically significant bone loss. This is about 0.8 percent per year in normal women and may be up to 15 percent in the postmenopausal period in women with osteoporosis. For longitudinal studies designed to monitor treatment effects, reproducibility should be about 2 percent. This will allow detection of bone mineral changes of about 5 percent with statistical significance.[97] The method should separate measurements of regional, predominantly cortical, and predominantly trabecular sites. A combination of single and dual absorptiometry fulfills these requirements.

SINGLE PHOTON ABSORPTIOMETRY

The technique of single photon absorptiometry was developed by Cameron and Sorenson in 1963.[93] The method has evolved as the most practical method to measure bone mineral at cortical bone sites and is adapted for measurements in appendicular bone. Metacarpal bones, radius, ulna, humerus, femur, tibia, calcaneus, and also mandible have been used in different studies. For these measurements, a collimated I-125 source (200 mCi or 7.4 GBq) or americium source for humerus and femur, is scanned over the bone, and the transmitted beam intensity is measured with a scintillation detector. The thickness of bone mineral (T_b) in the path of the photon beam is given by the following equation:

$$T_b = [\ln (I_o^*/I)]/(\mu_b \rho_b - \mu_s \rho_s)$$

I_o^* is the beam intensity after passage through tissue (by convention I_o is the intensity in air). I is the beam intensity after passage through bone and tissue. The mass absorption coefficients of bone mineral and tissue are μ_b and μ_s, and the density of bone mineral and tissue are ρ_b and ρ_s, respectively. These values are constants and are assumed not to change in bone disease and to be the same in different individuals. Plotting I as a function of position across the bone under investigation gives a profile of the radius bone thickness as shown in Figure 1–29. The integration of this curve between the limits defined by I and 0.85 I_o^* yields a value proportional to the cross-sectional area of the radius

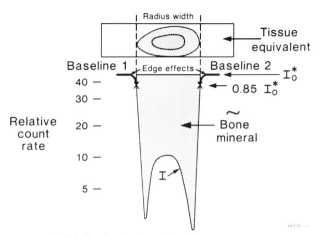

Figure 1–29. Single photon absorptiometry, with schematic illustration of scanning procedure. The plot shows the radiation beam intensity as a function of position across a bone sample. The integration of this curve between I and the detected bone edges gives a value proportional to total bone mineral. The edge is experimentally determined to be 85 percent of the base-line. Bone diameter can also be determined. (From Wahner, H. W., Dunn, W. L., and Riggs, B. L.: Noninvasive bone mineral measurements. Semin. Nucl. Med. *13*:282, 1983.)

and to the amount of bone mineral in the section of radius scanned. An absolute quantitation of mineral content is obtained by scanning a dried, defatted human radius with known mineral content in tissue-equivalent material and by using a standard curve for comparison. In this technique it is assumed that the bone is surrounded by tissue of constant thickness and absorptive property. This is approached by surrounding the bone with soft tissue-equivalent material, such as water or specific plastic material (Play-dough). This requirement restricts the technique to appendicular bones that are surrounded by predominantly muscular tissue. Greater differences in tissue fat between subjects may significantly affect the measurements. Presence of fat results in falsely low bone mineral. This should be considered when results are compared between patients but has little effect on longitudinal studies in the same patient. Several instruments are commercially available using water or plastic material as tissue-equivalent material. These instruments are primarily built for measurements of bone mineral on the forearm but can be adapted for metacarpal or phalangeal bones.

The measuring device for single photon absorptiometry used in our laboratory is shown in Figure 1–30. The NaI(T1) scintillation detector and I-125 source move in unison across the bone, which is fixed in position. The source and detector are rigidly coupled in parallel opposed motion and are motor driven in a direction transverse to the longitudinal axes of the radius. A microprocessor facilitates calculation of bone mineral and conversion of data into units of g/cm.²

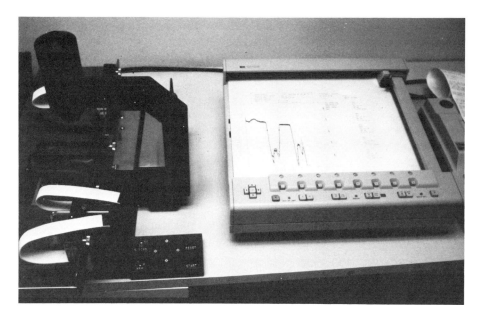

Figure 1–30. Single photon bone mineral densitometer constructed at the Mayo Clinic. The main components are the source detector assembly, a microcomputer, and a plotter. (From Wahner, H. W., Dunn, W. L., and Riggs, B. L.: Noninvasive bone mineral measurements. Semin. Nucl. Med. *13*:282, 1983.)

DUAL PHOTON ABSORPTIOMETRY

Dual photon (dichromatic) absorptiometry for clinical use has been developed in recent years and is perhaps the most important method for bone mineral measurements at the present time.[99, 103, 104, 106–108, 110, 113, 114, 120] These instruments employ two photon energies in order to correct for overlying fat and tissue. The technique allows measurements to be made in areas such as the spine and the hip. Thus this method allows a more specific evaluation of predominantly trabecular bone sites and a direct measurement of the important fracture sites.

The method is based on measurements of radiation transmission from two separate photon energies through a medium consisting primarily of two different materials, bone and soft tissue. The absorptiometer consists of a rectilinear scanner frame, a 1.5 Ci (55.5 Gbq) Gd-153 source, a NaI(Tl) detector, and a PDP-11 computer (Fig. 1–31). The gadolinium-153 energy spectrum has photoelectric peaks in the NaI(Tl) at approximately 44 and 100 keV (europium K x-rays 42, 48 keV, and gamma rays 97, 103 keV).

The following equations describe the absorption of each photon energy in a medium composed of bone and soft tissue.

$$I^{44}x, y = I_o{}^{44}\exp\left[-(\mu/\rho)_{st}{}^{44} \cdot M_{st} - (\mu/\rho_{bm}{}^{44} \cdot M_{bm}\right] \quad (1)$$

$$I^{100}x, y = I_o{}^{100}\exp\left[-(\mu/\rho)_{st}{}^{100} \cdot M_{st} - (\mu/\rho)_{bm}{}^{100} \cdot M_{bm}\right] \quad (2)$$

Figure 1–31. Dual photon bone mineral densitometer constructed at the Mayo Clinic. The frame is of a dual head scanner, used to perform total body radioisotope scans. (From Wahner, H. W., Dunn, W. L., and Riggs, B. L.: Noninvasive bone mineral measurements. Semin. Nucl. Med. *13*:282, 1983.)

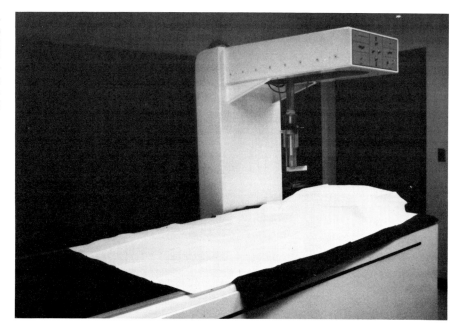

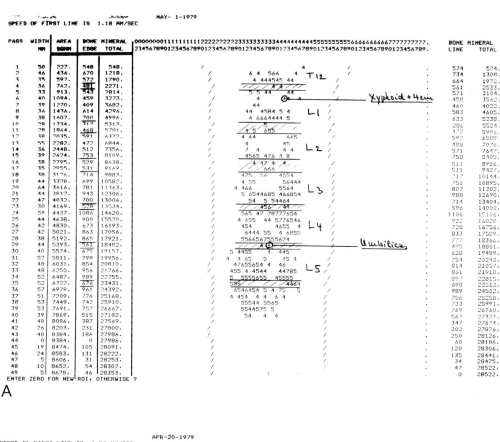

Figure 1–32. Dual photon absorptiometry bone images of human lumbar spine *(A)* and femur *(B).* Because scans are performed in a cranial direction the image of the femur is inverted.

$I^{44}x,y$ and $I^{100}x,y$ refer to the transmitted radiation beam intensity at a point x,y for 44 and 100 keV photon energies, respectively. I_0^{44} and I_0^{100} are the unattenuated photon intensities. The attenuation coefficients of soft tissue and bone mineral at energy level A are represented by $(\mu/\rho)_{st}^A$ and $(\mu/\rho)_{bm}^A$, respectively. The mass per unit area (g/cm) of tissue and of bone mineral is indicated by M_{st} and M_{bm}. The following solution for bone mineral is derived from equations 1 and 2.

$$M_{bm} = \frac{RST(\ln I^{100} x,y/I_0^{100}) - (\ln I^{44}x,y/I_0^{44})}{(\mu/\rho)_{bm}^{44} - RST \, (\mu/\rho)_{bm}^{100}} \quad (3)$$

where $RST = (\mu/\rho)_{st}^{44}/(\mu/\rho)_{st}^{100}$

In the measurement of bone mineral, a rectilinear scan of the region of interest is performed with the source detector assembly, and a point-by-point determination of bone mineral is made. The total bone mass is determined by summing the individual M_{bm} point values. The RST value is averaged over all of the extraòsseous area scanned, and the average RST is used to calculate M_{st}.

The actual absorption coefficients for soft tissue do not need to be determined. The RST is calculated from the measured radiation intensities as shown below.

$$\left. \begin{array}{l} I^{44}x,y = I_0^{44} \exp\,[-(\mu/\rho)_{st}^{44} \cdot M_{st}] \\ I^{100}x,y = I_0^{100} \exp\,[-(\mu/\rho)_{st}^{100} \cdot M_{st}] \end{array} \right\} \begin{array}{l} In\ tissue \\ only \end{array}$$

$\ln\,(I_0^{44}/I^{44}x,y) = (\mu/\rho)_{st}^{44} \cdot M_{st}$
$\ln\,(I_0^{100}/I^{100}x,y) = (\mu/\rho)_{st}^{100} \cdot M_{st}$
$(\mu/\rho)_{st}^{44}/(\mu/\rho)_{st}^{100} = \ln(I_0^{44}/I^{44}x,y)/\ln(I_0^{100}/I^{100}x,y) = RST$

In order to calculate RST accurately, the regions occupied by bone must be located. The bone surface area and edge limits are defined by an edge-detection routine based on the change in the magnitude of M_{bm} at the bone-tissue interface. Experiments with water, fat, and ashed bone in phantoms demonstrate that the RST averaging procedure corrects for the presence of varying amounts of fat.

The output is a plot of the character of intensity of bone mineral (Fig. 1–32). For the spine, the region of L1 through L4 is calculated. For the hip, bone mineral is calculated at the site of the femoral neck, trochanter, and shaft.

CLINICAL APPLICATIONS

Normal Bone Mass

In the appendicular skeleton, bone diminution with age varies with sex. In women bone loss does not occur until about age 50.[95, 102, 105, 109, 117, 118] Bone loss is accelerated from ages 51 to 65 and then decelerates somewhat after age 65. Overall bone diminution throughout life is 30 percent for the mid-radius and 39 percent for the distal radius. The slightly higher rate of bone loss at the distal radial

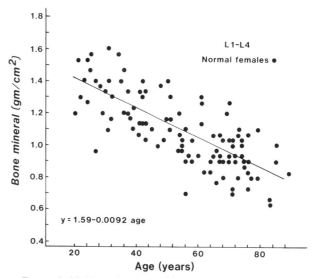

Figure 1–33. Normal values of bone mineral in 105 women determined by dual photon absorptiometry. Roos's[114] equation for regression, y = 1.59 − 0.0092 × age. (From Riggs, B. L., Wahner, H. W., Dunn, W. L., et al.: Differential changes in bone mineral density of the appendicular and axial skeleton with aging: Relationship to spinal osteoporosis. Reproduced from *The Journal of Clinical Investigation*, 1981, Vol. 67, pp. 328–335, by copyright permission of The American Society for Clinical Investigation.)

site is due to the presence of trabecular bone (see Table 1–8). In men, bone loss with age is minimal and does not show accelerated bone loss at middle age.

The bone mass and bone density of different parts of the skeleton show a considerable interindividual variation in both sexes. Attempts to normalize the data to correct for body weight, height, or span have in general not narrowed this variation. Mass and density are, however, dependent on sex and age.

In normal women, bone diminution from the vertebrae in the lumbar spine begins in young adulthood and is linear (Fig. 1–33). Overall bone diminution is 47 percent for the vertebrae in the period between young adulthood and extreme old age. In men, bone loss from the spine is also linear but minimal, overall bone loss during the lifetime being 14 percent.[111]

With three different measuring sites having varying cortical to trabecular ratios (femoral neck, trochanter region, and shaft) bone loss in the hip is also linear in both sexes but again more pronounced in women. The difference at this measuring site, however, is smaller than that for the lumbar spine. Overall bone diminution for women throughout life is 57 percent for the femoral neck and 53 percent for the intertrochanteric region, respectively. Again, bone loss is also linear with age in both sexes. For men the rate of bone mineral decrease in the hip is two-thirds of that observed in women. These differences may explain why the female/male ratio is 8:1 for vertebral fractures but only 2:1 for hip fractures.[100, 112]

There is generally good agreement on the bone

loss pattern in the appendicular skeleton as determined by different laboratories using varying methods. For bone loss in the lumbar spine, however, some authors have noted an accelerated bone loss in women at the time of menopause similar to that observed in the appendicular skeleton. Longitudinal data are presently being collected to investigate this aspect further. Our preliminary data from a longitudinal study of the lumbar spine support the finding of a slight increase in bone loss in women at the time of menopause until about age 60.

Fracture Threshold

The definition of a fracture threshold for a given skeletal site is helpful in identifying a population group at risk for bone fracture at this site. Studies designed to evaluate treatment modalities to prevent fractures are presently being conducted in such a population. It appears mandatory that bone mineral measurements be made at the exact site for which a fracture threshold is to be determined. For the lumbar spine we have chosen the 90th percentile of bone mineral content obtained in patients with nontraumatic spinal fractures (0.965 g/cm²). By age 65 half of the women and by age 85 virtually all have bone mineral values below this threshold for fracture. Similar fracture thresholds have been defined for the radius. Efforts to predict spinal or hip fractures from measurements on the radius or other appendicular bones, however, have met with limited success. This is probably due to the predominantly cortical bone that is measured at the radius site and probably also to the specific nature of metabolic bone disease, which suggest that different skeletal sites may lose bone at different rates.

Bone Mass Changes in Osteoporosis

Mean bone mineral in axial and appendicular measuring sites is lower in patients with osteoporosis than in age- and sex-normal subjects.[111] This is shown in Figure 1–34. Spinal measurements discriminated best between the two groups. The data

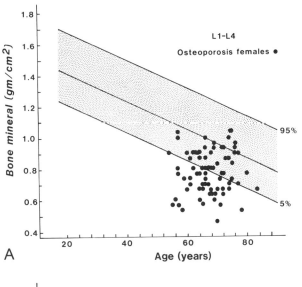

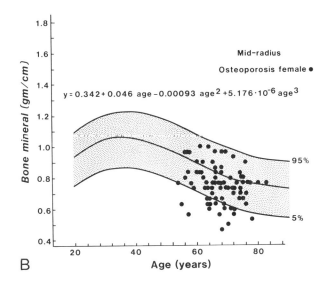

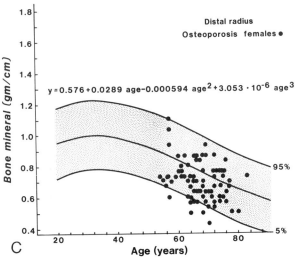

Figure 1–34. Comparison of bone mineral of spine *(A)*, midradius *(B)*, and distal radius *(C)* between 105 normal and 76 osteoporotic females. The latter group was characterized by the presence of nontraumatic compression fractures. The shaded region represents the 5th to 95th percentile range of normals. Individuals with osteoporosis are indicated by dots. The incomplete separation between these two populations is seen particularly at the radius site. Separation is best at sites of trabecular bone. (Modified from Riggs, B. L., Wahner, H. W., Dunn, W. L., et al.: Differential changes in bone mineral density of the appendicular and axial skeleton with aging: Relationship to spinal osteoporosis. Reproduced from *The Journal of Clinical Investigation*, 1981, Vol. 67, pp. 328–335, by copyright permission of The American Society for Clinical Investigation.)

suggest that in osteoporosis there is a disproportionately greater loss of trabecular bone from the axial skeleton when compared with cortical bone from appendicular sites. This may be a distinguishing characteristic of spinal osteoporosis. A measuring site in the spine should be preferred for clinical diagnosis and follow-up when osteoporosis is under consideration. Bone mineral measurements for the diagnosis of osteopenia should take into consideration the normal age-related bone loss.

Bone Mass in Metabolic Bone Disease

In patients with hyperparathyroidism bone mineral is substantially decreased in the lumbar spine, moderately decreased in the distal radius, and insignificantly decreased in the mid-radius.[116] This is consistent with clinical studies of hyperparathyroidism, which show that the occurrence of vertebral fractures is increased.[98] In patients with secondary hyperparathyroidism complicating chronic renal failure, however, bone mineral is not decreased and indeed may be elevated in the mid-radius.

The greatest disparity between values for bone mineral in the axial and trabecular skeleton is found in patients with hypercortisolism. Previously reported data obtained with other techniques support our findings that hypercortisolism causes severe and disproportionate loss of trabecular bone.

In hyperthyroidism there is little or no significant bone loss at either site. This is in contrast to the findings in the older literature. Our failure to find decreases in bone mineral in the lumbar spine may be due in part to the relatively short duration of hyperthyroidism at the time the diagnosis is made in modern medical practice.[98]

In acromegaly patients with active disease have significant increases, in bone mineral in the spine and radius. This supports previous studies by us and others with single photon absorptiometry and total-body neutron activation analysis that show an increase rather than a decrease in bone mass. Osteopenia in acromegaly probably should be explained by other complicating factors, such as hypogonadism.[98]

In patients with hypoparathyroidism following surgery, there is an increase in bone mineral in all sampling sites when compared with age- and sex-matched controls. The increase is greatest in the axial skeleton. This observation may suggest that PTH deficiency protects against age-related bone loss.[98] The data for the spine and mid-radius are summarized in Figure 1–35.

There is a differential response of appendicular and axial bone to changes in endocrine function. The reasons are unclear. We believe that regional differences in the proportional content of cortical and trabecular bone are part of the explanation and that cortical and trabecular bone react differently to hormonal stimuli.

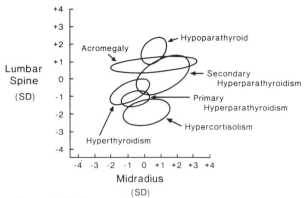

Figure 1–35. Bone mineral content of the midradius and lumbar spine for six metabolic bone diseases. The area within each ellipse represents 95 percent confidence limits for the means. Units are standard deviations from predicted mean for normal subjects. These are obtained from sex-specific regression equations that predict bone density as a function of age. (From Seeman, E., Wahner, H. W., Offord, K. P., et al.: Differential effects of endocrine dysfunction on the axial and the appendicular skeleton. Reproduced from *The Journal of Clinical Investigation,* 1982, Vol. 69, pp. 1302–1309, by copyright permission of The American Society for Clinical Investigation.)

Bone Mass in Hip Fractures

In women with hip fractures mean bone mineral in the proximal femur is less when compared with sex- and age-matched controls.[112] However, there is no discernible bone loss in the lumbar spine or radius in these patients. Similar results are obtained in men with hip fractures. The lack of bone loss in the spine in patients with hip fractures leads to speculation that spinal osteoporosis and age-related hip fractures may be two different osteoporotic syndromes.[112]

Patients with intertrochanteric fractures have lower values at the trochanter site than those with femoral neck fractures. Because the femoral neck is a predominantly cortical bone site, loss of cortical bone should be a predisposing factor for femoral neck fractures. The intertrochanteric site has more trabecular bone, and loss of trabecular bone should play a more prominent role at this site. This hypothesis is supported by the observation that intertrochanteric fractures are more likely to be associated with vertebral fractures than are femoral neck fractures, since vertebrae and the trochanteric region contain about the same amount of cortical and trabecular bone.

SUMMARY

Single and dual photon absorptiometry techniques are now available to aid the physician in diagnosis and management of generalized bone diseases. They permit an accurate and reproducible assessment of bone mineral at predominately cortical (appendicular skeleton) and trabecular (axial skeleton) bone sites. Newer findings show that cortical and trabecular bone behave differently and that the effect of endocrine dysfunction on bone appears to be specific according to both disease and site. These qualitative and quantitative differences in cortical and trabecular bone loss require that an optimal sampling site be found for a given bone problem if maximum benefit is to be derived from these tests.

COMPUTED TOMOGRAPHY

GERALD R. MAY

The introduction of computed tomography (CT) has played a major role in improving imaging of most structures in the body and has resulted in a decrease in the use of more invasive imaging modalities, such as pneumoencephalography and angiography. It has a secondary role in skeletal imaging, as in most areas it has not supplanted the routine radiograph. CT of the skeletal system, however, can add additional information to the plain film examination in a number of skeletal abnormalities.[121, 127, 128, 130, 136] Initial experience in CT scanning of the musculoskeletal system was directed mainly toward the evaluation of neoplasms. However, continued experience with this modality has demonstrated its usefulness in trauma and other orthopedic problems.

EQUIPMENT

CT scanners use highly collimated x-ray beams, highly efficient detectors, and computer-image reconstruction and display to produce images that have superior contrast resolution but slightly less spatial resolution than routine radiographs. CT thus provides better display of soft tissues than any plain film technique. In addition, the transverse axial orientation of the images is a useful supplement to the plain film examination of skeletal structures.

All CT scanners have three components: (1) the scanning gantry, (2) the computer, (3) the display console. The scanning gantry contains the x-ray source, detector system, and couch and positioning system for the patient. The patient lies on the horizontal couch and moves through a circular opening in the vertically oriented scanning gantry, passing through the x-ray source and detectors. Although many gantry systems can be tilted a few degrees from the vertical, the orientation of the system permits only transverse axial images to be obtained in most cases. Therefore, sagittal and coronal images must be obtained by computer reformatting of the transverse axial image data rather than by direct scanning. In a typical CT scanner the x-ray tube moves through 360° at small increments (as many as 1200 or more) during a single CT scan

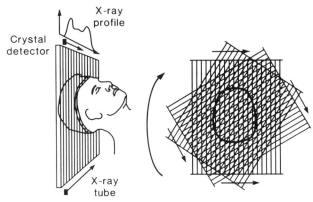

Figure 1–36. Basic data collection method used in computed tomography consists of collecting a series of contiguous pencil-beam transmission measurements (called a "profile") repeated at various angles about the subject (right). (Courtesy of E. C. McCullough, Mayo Clinic.)

slice (Fig. 1–36). The x-ray detectors (which can be fixed or rotate opposite the x-ray tube) take several hundred measurements of x-ray transmission at each increment. One slice requires from 1 to 20 sec, depending upon the scanner used. In critically injured patients or patients with respiratory difficulty, fast scanners (1 to 3 sec) are required.

The data from the x-ray detectors is processed by a computer that uses an algorithm (a series of mathematical formulas) to manipulate the data and reconstruct an image of the scanned object. Reconstruction time for a single image varies from 2 to 60 sec. The computer divides the scanned area into a matrix (e.g., 256×256 or 512×512) of small squares (picture elements or pixels). An x-ray attenuation coefficient is determined for each square by applying the reconstruction algorithm to the data obtained by the detectors. Each square is then assigned a CT number related to the attenuation coefficient (with the CT number of water being 0). The numbers are displayed on the final image as various shades of grey with the highest numbers (e.g., air) being black.

Since the x-ray beam in the scanner has a finite thickness (from 3 to 13 mm for most scanners), the x-ray attenuation coefficient calculated by the computer for each pixel actually represents the average coefficient of a volume of tissue rather than a plane. The pixel thus actually represents a volume element or voxel. This can introduce a significant artifact, called a partial volume effect, into the final image (Fig. 1–37). This occurs when two objects which have different x-ray attenuation coefficients (e.g., bone and fat) are both included in the volume scanned. Since the pixels displayed on the monitor screen are represented as the average attenuation coefficient of the contents of the voxel, the number for the voxel containing both bone and fat will be somewhere between the actual attenuation coefficients of fat and bone. This partial volume artifact can result in significant errors. For example, a fracture line in the transverse plane of the scan can

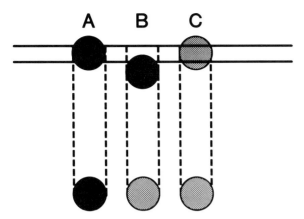

Figure 1–37. Concept of partial volume effect in which a highly attenuating structure partially occupying the scan slice width (B) appears with the same density as the lower attenuating structure fully occupying the scan slice width (C). (Courtesy of E. C. McCullough, Mayo Clinic.)

be missed because it is averaged in with the bone in the rest of the voxel.

The reconstructed image is displayed on a console that allows the operator to manipulate the window width (range of CT numbers in the grey scale) and the window level (center of the grey scale) optimally to display either bone detail or soft tissues. In addition, the operator can obtain sagittal or coronal reconstructions of the scanned object using computer reconstruction of the transverse image data.

Many CT scanners can also produce digital radiographs of any area of the body by moving the patient through the x-ray beam with sampling at intervals from the x-ray detectors. These digital images (Fig. 1–38A) are of lesser quality than routine radiographs but can be quite useful for localization purposes.

The x-ray dose delivered by a CT scan varies with a number of factors, some related to the CT unit (e.g., transverse spatial resolution, slice thickness, scan noise) and some related to the individual examination, such as the number of slices obtained and the degree of overlap of the slices. In general, the dose is greater than that for a single radiograph but less than that for conventional tomograms of the same body part. CT doses may vary from less than 1 rad to greater than 10 rads.[122, 134, 135]

TECHNIQUES

The radiologist should review the patient's history and the indication for the examination in order to tailor the procedure to the patient's problem. In most cases, contiguous slices 1 cm thick are adequate, although in evaluation of small lesions or anatomically complex areas such as the spine, thinner slices at overlapping intervals are required (especially if sagittal or coronal reconstruction is contemplated). Anatomic symmetry is very useful in evaluating CT images of the skeletal system and therefore care should be taken to position the patient symmetrically within the scanner. The contralateral side should be included whenever possible. The gastrointestinal tract can be opacified with oral or rectal contrast if a lesion in the abdomen or pelvis is suspected. Intravenous contrast by rapid infusion or bolus technique with rapid acquisition of multiple slices may be useful in detecting subtle soft tissue lesions or in detecting the relationship of pathology to major vessels. The radiologist should monitor the procedure and manipulate the display controls (window level and window width) to insure optimal display of both bones and soft tissue. Images of bones should be viewed at wide window width

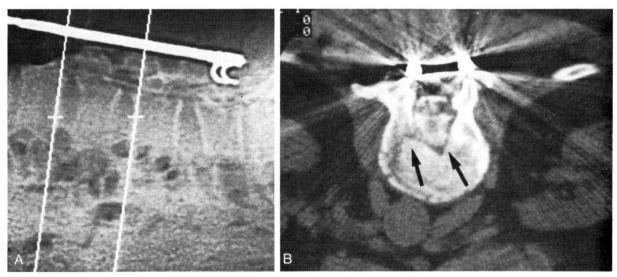

Figure 1–38. *A,* Scout view (digital radiograph) of the lumbar spine demonstrating a burst fracture of L2 and Harrington rod reduction. *B,* Transverse axial CT scan demonstrates the fracture *(arrows),* but significant artifact from the metal rods prevents evaluation of the posterior arch.

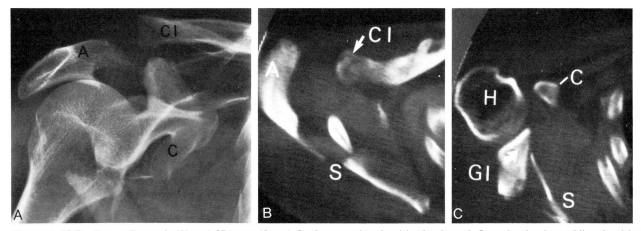

Figure 1–39. Routine radiograph *(A)* and CT scans *(B* and *C)* of a complex shoulder fracture. *A*, Complex fracture of the shoulder with disruption of the scapular spine and acromion (A). The relationship of the humeral head to the glenoid and the involvement of the articular surface are difficult to evaluate. CT scans *(B* and *C)* clearly demonstrate the relationship of the fragments and the articular surface. (H, humeral head; C, coracoid; Gl, glenoid; Cl, clavicle; S, scapula; A, acromion.)

settings and high window levels, while soft tissues are best displayed at narrower window widths and lower levels.

The quality of the CT image is affected by a number of variables beyond the control of the examiner. In general, individual muscles, vessels, and nerves are optimally imaged when surrounded by fat. Thus, the scan is less helpful in examining thin patients, infants, or the distal extremities. Patient motion produces significant degradation of image quality. This can be especially troublesome in attempting to evaluate a severely injured or uncooperative patient. Metallic objects such as joint prostheses, internal-fixation devices, and surgical clips produce artifacts that may obscure detail in the region of interest (Fig. 1–38).

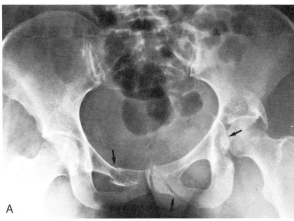

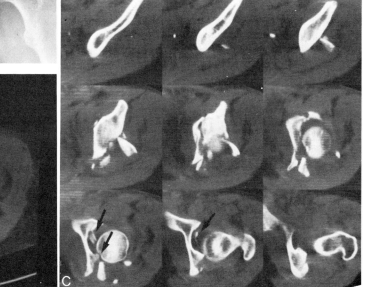

Figure 1–40. Complex pelvic fracture. *A*, Pubic rami fractures and a comminuted acetabular fracture are evident on the routine film *(arrows)*. *B*, CT scans of the acetabular fracture demonstrate fragments in the joint space *(large arrow)* and impaction of the femoral head posteriorly *(small arrow)*. Posterior subluxation and joint space widening are also clearly demonstrated. Contiguous slices through the acetabulum are demonstrated in *C*.

INDICATIONS

CT is particularly useful in examination of the bones in areas of complex anatomy such as the pelvis, hips, sacrum, spine, shoulders, and face.[130, 136] In addition, some areas that cannot be easily displayed on routine radiographs, such as the sternoclavicular joints, are optimally seen on the cross-sectional images obtained by CT.[126] Occult fractures not visible on plain film or tomography may be detected, especially in the spine.[121, 124, 125, 130, 131, 137] Some authors have found CT more useful than plain film tomography in the evaluation of the vertebral column following trauma.[121] Most have found that CT adds valuable information to routine radiographs in the majority of cases, although most cases studied by CT were selected instances rather than consecutive cases of trauma. In addition to the presence of a fracture, CT can demonstrate bone, disk, blood, or foreign bodies in the spinal canal.[131] Metrizamide or intrathecal gas may be given for better delineation of the spinal canal.[138] Plain films are still essential, as CT may miss horizontal fractures (fractures parallel to the plane of the scan slice), such as odontoid fractures, owing to the partial volume effect or improper slice selection. In addition, it is difficult to detect vertebral body compression fractures, subluxations, and increased intervertebral distance on CT scans alone.[131]

CT scans of the shoulder (Fig. 1–39), hip (Fig. 1–40), or pelvis after trauma aid in the display of the spatial relationships of the fracture fragments before and after reduction. CT may detect intraarticular fragments that prevent reduction and require operative intervention.[123, 129, 132, 133, 138]

CT can accurately detect soft tissue injuries and is especially important in evaluating the abdomen after trauma.[139] Its use in place of radionuclide scanning or ultrasonography depends upon availability, the extent of the injury, and the specific information desired. CT may also be useful in detecting some vascular injuries (such as thoracic aortic pseudoaneurysm); however, its place in relation to traditional angiographic techniques remains to be determined.

MAGNETIC RESONANCE IMAGING

THOMAS H. BERQUIST

Resonance properties of nuclei were first reported by Block and Purcell.[142, 156] Clinical interest in magnetic resonance as an imaging modality has increased rapidly in recent years. In 1971, Damadian reported differences in the relaxation times of normal and malignant tissue.[148] In 1975, Lauterbur demonstrated the capability of producing axial images using nuclear magnetic resonance techniques.[152] Technological advances have since resulted in significant improvements in magnetic resonance imaging.[140, 144–147, 150, 151, 161]

PRINCIPLES

An in-depth discussion of the physics of magnetic resonance imaging is beyond the scope of this introductory section. However, the following paragraphs will provide an overview of the factors in magnetic resonance that allow image formation.

Magnetic resonance imaging is based on the principle that nuclei with an odd number of protons or neutrons (^1H, ^{31}P, ^{13}C, ^{23}Na, ^{19}F, ^{17}O) exhibit spin.[157] Because of its abundance and favorable magnetic moment, proton imaging(^1H) is most practical at this time. When placed in a strong magnetic field (Fig. 1–41), the normally randomly oriented nuclei tend to produce a net magnetic vector parallel to the magnetic field.[147, 157] Applying a radio frequency (RF) pulse to the spinning nuclei causes displacement of the nuclei in proportion to the strength of the RF pulse. A pulse resulting in a 90° deflection (Fig. 1–41) causes the magnetic field to rotate at 90° to the static field (Z in Fig. 1–41). Following the RF pulse, the magnetization induces a signal in the receiver coil (the coils around the patient). The nuclei then regress to their original position in the magnetic field. As the nuclei return to their equilibrium position, the signal decreases and two sample-related time constants occur, the spin-lattice (longitudinal) relaxation time T1, and the spin-spin (transverse) relaxation time T2.[157] The relaxation times vary, depending upon the tissue being studied. Along with proton density, relaxation times provide the basis for image formation. In general, T1 is always longer than T2 except in liquids, where the relaxation times are nearly equal.

Currently available pulse sequences are designed to measure different factors in the tissue sample. Free-induction decay sequences (or FID, where a

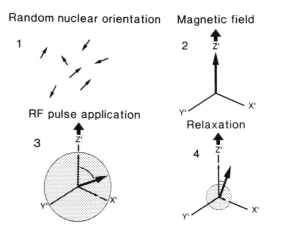

Figure 1–41. Principles of magnetic resonance imaging. (1) Nuclei are randomly oriented. (2) Static magnetic field with nuclei aligned parallel to the magnet (Z'). (3) RF pulse causes nuclei to precess to transverse position. (4) Relaxation or return to equilibrium occurs following the RF pulse.

90° pulse is applied) are proton-density–weighted images, inversion-recovery sequences (or IR, where a 180° pulse is followed by a variable interval [tau] and a 90° pulse) primarily measure T1, and spin-echo sequences (or SE, where a 90° pulse is followed by a variable interval [tau] and a 180° pulse) provide T2-weighted images. The image produced depends on the sequence chosen and the tissue being studied. For example, the lymphoma in Figure 1–42C and D appears white (high intensity) with the spin-echo sequence (T2-related) and shows low density with the inversion-recovery sequence (T1-related) because of the long relaxation times of the malignant tissue compared with those of the normal marrow.

In general, cortical bone, ligaments, and cartilage produce very little signal, which has advantages and disadvantages for MRI. The lack of a signal from cortical bone results in improved imaging of the posterior fossa and results in better visualization of pathology adjacent to bone.[161] This is a significant advantage of MRI, since the signal produced by bone in computed tomography may result in loss of adjacent detail. The main disadvantage of magnetic resonance imaging is difficulty in studying cortical bone itself and in detecting subtle periosteal

TABLE 1–6. Magnetic Resonance Imaging

Advantages:
  High contrast (soft tissue)
  No bone artifact
  Multiple pulse sequences available
  Increased tissue specificity ?
  No known biologic hazards
Disadvantages:
  Lack of cortical bone detail
  High cost
  No currently available contrast agents
  Long scan time compared with CT

changes clearly seen on conventional films or CT (see Fig. 1–42). Table 1–6 summarizes some of the advantages and disadvantages of magnetic resonance imaging. One must keep in mind that this imaging modality is still in its early investigative stages.

There is no radiation with magnetic resonance imaging and to date no known biologic hazards have been demonstrated. Saunders found no detectable cardiac effects of magnetic field strengths up to 10 tesla.[159] Animals and cell cultures exposed to magnetic fields show no evidence of malignant change or genetic mutation.[160] Care must be taken

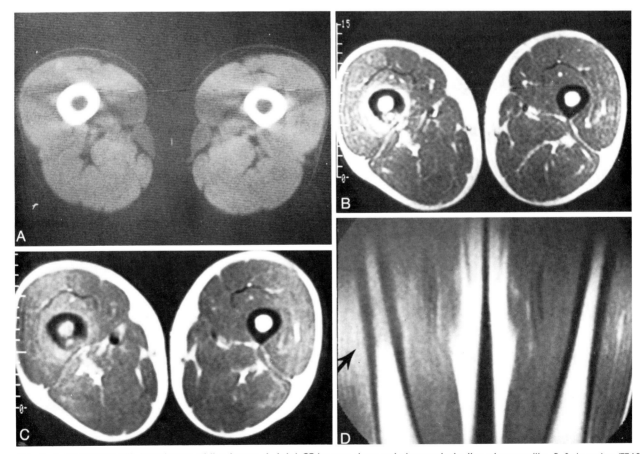

Figure 1–42. Patient with lymphoma of the femur. *A*, Axial CT image does not demonstrate the abnormality. *B*, Spin-echo (TE60, TR2000) MR images clearly demonstrate the cortical and periosteal involvement. *C*, Inversion recovery sequences (TI500, TE40, TR1500) more clearly demonstrate the medullary involvement. *D*, The extent of involvement *(arrow)* is easily evaluated on the coronal image (TE40, TR500).

in examining patients with cardiac pacemakers, however, as the devices revert to the asynchronous mode.[154, 155] In our experience, orthopedic appliances composed of stainless steel or Vitallium (prosthetic joint replacements, metal plates and screws, and vascular clips) are not magnetic and no heating of the components occurs in the magnetic field or when RF pulses are applied. Aneurysm clips used at our institution are magnetic and until further studies have been performed, patients with aneurysm clips should not be studied with magnetic resonance imaging techniques. Further investigations concerning potential hazards are continuing and in time the effects, if any, of strong magnetic fields will be better understood.

EQUIPMENT

Three types of imaging units are available at this time. These include resistive magnets, permanent magnets, and superconducting magnets. We are currently evaluating a resistive system that operates at 0.15 tesla (unit of magnetic field strength, 1 tesla = 10,000 gauss).

Installation of these imaging units is significantly more complicated than installation of other radiographic equipment. Adjacent equipment, elevators, ferromagnetic objects, and electrical wiring must be taken into consideration as they may interfere with

TABLE 1–7. Orthopedic Applications of Magnetic Resonance Imaging

Infection	Trauma
Soft tissue	Ligament tears
Osteomyelitis	Muscle tears
Neoplasms	Avascular necrosis
Soft tissue	Fracture healing
Skeletal	

the unit. Also, the unit may affect the performance of the equipment nearby.

CLINICAL APPLICATIONS

To date, the majority of clinical studies have concentrated on the central nervous system. Magnetic resonance imaging provides improved grey-white matter differentiation, allowing detection of demyelinating diseases such as multiple sclerosis. Evaluation of the posterior fossa is also superior to that provided by computed tomography.[145, 161]

Early evaluation of the body with this modality shows promise in soft tissue evaluation, marrow studies, evaluation of muscle and ligament injuries, and diagnosis of bone and soft tissue tumors.[141, 143, 144, 149, 153, 158] Table 1–7 presents these applications. The strong signal intensity of medullary bone (Figs. 1–42 and 1–43) provides excellent detail

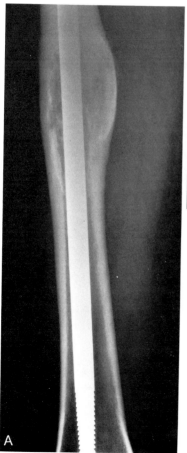
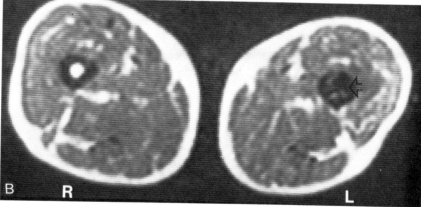

Figure 1–43. A, Radiograph demonstrating medullary rod in the femur with an old, healed fracture of the femur. *B,* Axial SE sequence image of the femur shows no significant artifact *(arrow).* Note the normal signal (white) from the medullary bone on the right.

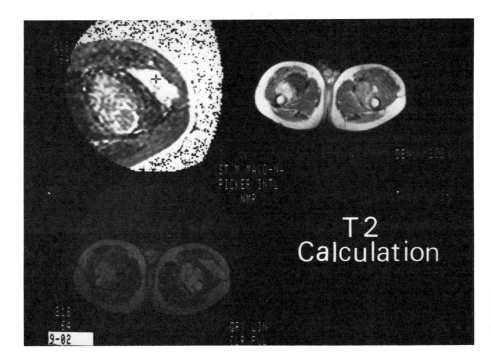

Figure 1–44. T2 calculation of an abscess in the thigh (+ left upper image). SE 20 (right upper image) and SE 60 (right lower image) sequences were used for the calculation. T2 = 202 msec.

for study of osteomyelitis, neoplasm, and avascular necrosis.[141] It is not clear at this time if changes can be detected earlier than with isotope scans. The use of relaxation times (T1 and T2) in evaluation of tissue may provide further information regarding specific pathologic conditions (Fig. 1–44). This work and study of *in vivo* spectroscopic potential are currently being investigated. Finally, while metal components in orthopedic patients result in considerable artifact formation on CT scans, the artifact created by metal on the magnetic resonance image is less significant (Fig. 1–43) and can be further reduced by using the spin-echo sequences. The degree of image-quality reduction caused by metal is also dependent upon location and size of the metal component.

At this stage, the true value of magnetic resonance imaging is still being evaluated, but early results indicate that this technique may be of great benefit in orthopedic radiology.

ANGIOGRAPHY

GERALD R. MAY

Angiography is useful in the diagnosis and treatment of vascular injuries following blunt, penetrating, or operative trauma.[169, 170] Vascular injuries include intimal injury, arterial transection or thrombosis, pseudoaneurysm, arteriovenous fistula, and venous thrombosis or transection.[176] Vascular trauma may be asymptomatic or may result in hemorrhage, pulse defects, expanding masses, bruits, or signs of distal ischemia.[172] In addition, repetitive minor trauma, usually occupationally related, may result in vascular injury as serious as

that produced by major trauma.[162] The recent introduction of digital subtraction angiography and further experience with ultrasound and computed tomography will reduce the necessity for diagnostic angiography in many of the above conditions.

In addition to diagnosis, angiography can be used to treat some of the arterial lesions by transcatheter introduction of embolic materials to produce temporary or permanent vessel occlusion.[163, 164–168, 171, 173–175, 177] These techniques are most helpful in the patient with post-traumatic pelvic hemorrhage, the majority of which is due to arterial sources. The bleeding arteries can be accurately localized and then occluded through the catheter, resulting in a high rate of successful cessation of the hemorrhage. In addition, some cases of pseudoaneurysm and arteriovenous fistula can be treated by transcatheter embolization.

EQUIPMENT

The angiogram should be performed on dedicated angiographic equipment if possible, since this results in the highest-quality films and the most flexibility in obtaining multiple views and a variety of film series. A variety of contrast media and catheter shapes are available, depending upon the type of study performed and the preference of the angiographer.

Transcatheter occlusion of blood vessels requires a variety of agents, whose use depends upon the specific clinical situation and the experience and preference of the angiographer. The occluding agents include particles of Gelfoam, Ivalon, or blood clot; mechanical devices, such as the Gianturco-Wallace-Anderson coil or detachable balloons; or tissue adhesives, such as isobutyl-2-cyanoacrylate.

Selection and preparation of the embolic material depends upon the size of the blood vessel occluded, and the duration of occlusion varies from a few days for blood clot to a few weeks for Gelfoam. Permanent occlusion can be accomplished with coils, balloons, Ivalon, and cyanoacrylate. In most cases of hemorrhage a temporary agent such as blood clot or Gelfoam is adequate. For arteriovenous fistula or pseudoaneurysm a permanent agent should be used.

A recent advance in technology that promises to make evaluation of blood vessels faster and less invasive is digital subtraction angiography. This technique links a computer to an x-ray fluoroscope and allows high-quality images of arteries to be made after peripheral or central intravenous injection of contrast medium. The information from the fluoroscopic image is digitized, and the computer then subtracts an image made before injection of contrast material from images made after injection. The only difference between the two images, the contrast in the blood vessels, is then enhanced by the computer, allowing excellent vascular images to be obtained. The contrast medium can be injected through a peripheral vein or into the superior or inferior vena cava, thus avoiding the risks of arterial puncture. The images obtained are perfectly adequate for the diagnosis of arterial occlusion in most areas of the body and in many cases will also allow detection of fine detail, such as intimal injuries. Experience in the detection of pseudoaneurysm and arteriovenous fistula is limited, but subtraction angiography should be adequate in most cases. Improvements in the quality of digital equipment have been rapid and many angiograms done after trauma will probably be replaced by digital subtraction angiography.

TECHNIQUE

The angiographic examination and all other imaging examinations should be tailored to the clinical problems of the patient. The imaging evaluation should be designed in such a way that no tests that might interfere with a subsequent angiogram are performed. For example, oral or rectal contrast media should not be administered prior to the angiogram. In addition, care should be exercised in the amount of intravenous contrast material given both before and during the angiogram, as large volumes of intravenous contrast material can have serious effects on renal function. One should be certain that the patient's other injuries can be stabilized long enough to allow angiography to be performed before surgical intervention is required. If not, the angiogram can be delayed. The angiographer should direct his attention initially to the area of greatest clinical suspicion; survey examinations of the rest of the body should be performed afterward if the patient's condition and the amount of contrast medium used permits.

In most cases a transfemoral route using the Seldinger technique with selective catheterization of the affected vessel is the preferred approach for performance of the angiographic exam. In a few cases this route is not available owing to the extent of pelvic trauma or to coexisting vascular disease. In these cases an axillary approach can be used. Complications of these techniques can occur at the puncture site (hemorrhage, arterial obstruction, pseudoaneurysm, arteriovenous fistula), or result from the guide wire or catheter (vessel perforation or intimal damage, distal embolization), or may be systemic (contrast medium reactions, cardiac and neurologic abnormalities). The incidence of complications is higher with the axillary than the transfemoral approach mainly because of an increase in the number of puncture sites and neurologic complications.[165]

Great care and attention to technical detail are required when attempting transcatheter embolization. In general, only the affected artery should be occluded and the agent used should provide a duration of occlusion that is sufficient to resolve the clinical problem (Fig. 1–45). In pelvic bleeding, which is the most common indication for embolization after trauma, only those branches of the internal iliac artery from which the hemorrhage is occurring should be occluded, although selective catheterization is not possible in all cases. In some cases, occlusion of the entire internal iliac is all that is possible. Agents that produce occlusions of short duration (blood clots and Gelfoam) should be used. If both internal iliac arteries must be occluded, the risk of such complications as impotence or ischemic necrosis of the bladder increases; but in these instances the procedure may be necessary to save the patient's life.

INDICATIONS

Angiography can accurately identify the vast majority of trauma-induced arterial lesions. Unfortunately, despite years of experience with its use, the indications for angiography after trauma are still not well defined. In extremity trauma, some physicians advocate performing angiography in every case of blunt or penetrating trauma that occurs near a major vessel, whereas others favor angiography only when physical findings such as pulse deficit or bruit are present.[172] The indications for angiography in thoracic trauma are equally varied depending on the series quoted.[164] Pelvic angiography for the diagnosis and treatment of bleeding after pelvic trauma is very useful but the exact point when it should be used in the course of treatment is poorly defined. Venography may be useful in a few cases to define venous injuries, especially in the case of expanding pelvic hematomas with negative angiograms.[174]

The performance of these examinations will probably continue to depend upon local experience and

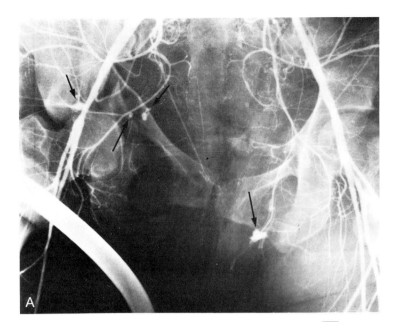

Figure 1–45. Angiographic diagnosis and treatment of pelvic hemorrhage, pre- and post-embolization. *A,* The angiogram demonstrates multiple bleeding sites bilaterally *(arrows). B* and *C,* Coned down views of the right and left side of the pelvis after Gelfoam embolization demonstrate occlusion of the involved vessels and no evidence of contrast extravasation.

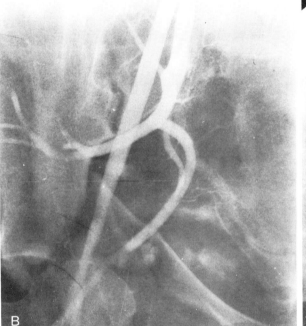
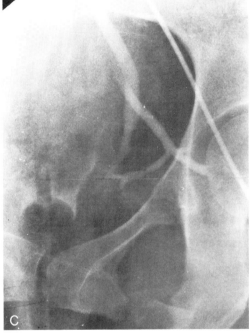

the availability of angiographic and surgical expertise. Evolving experience with angiography will continue to be modified by less invasive procedures such as ultrasound, computed tomography, and digital subtraction angiography.

MYELOGRAPHY

GLENN S. FORBES

Positive contrast myelography has been accomplished for many years and provides useful information regarding the bony spinal canal, spinal cord, and nerve roots. Until recently positive contrast examination of the spinal canal was performed with

film or fluoroscopic studies. The advent of computed tomography of the spine has added a new imaging technique. The combination of CT and intrathecal contrast medium has provided an additional technique for evaluation of the posterior spinal structures that is complementary to conventional myelography and occasionally more definitive.[181, 184]

Two contrast agents are primarily used for myelography in the United States. Iophendylate (Pantopaque) is an oil-based medium and has a long history of established use in myelography. Metrizamide (Amipaque) is a water-soluble agent that has recently gained wide acceptance. The water-soluble agent generally has more irritating side effects on the central nervous system; however, it is less viscous, thus providing better visualization of nerve roots. Also, because of its water solubility, metrizamide does not have to be removed from the spinal canal, as does its counterpart iophendylate. Both materials have advantages in different situations. Either of the contrast agents is adequate, and selection should be based on the practice and the patient's clinical situation.[183]

TECHNIQUE

Routine myelography is accomplished with the patient in the prone position on a radiographic table equipped for 90° tilt in either direction. Plain films should be thoroughly examined prior to the examination, as subtle changes on these films may dictate

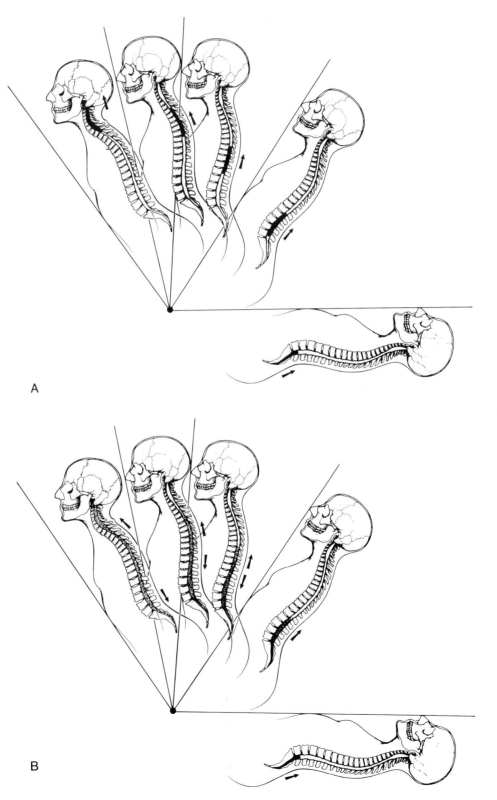

Figure 1–46. Positioning effects on opaque myelographic contrast material. *A*, Oil-based material (Pantopaque) remains in bolus form and is controlled by gravity as it passes through the spinal canal. Lumbar films are taken in the erect or near erect position; thoracic and cervical films are taken nearly horizontal. *B*, Water-soluble contrast material (metrizamide) tends to spread and dilute as it mixes with the cerebrospinal fluid. Less motion is required for control of the contrast material. (From Forbes, G.: Radiologic examination of the spine and myelography. *In*: Spittell, J.: Clinical Medicine. Philadelphia, Harper & Row, 1982.)

A

B

changes in filming sequence and the appropriate needle placement for the myelogram. Routinely an 18-gauge needle (20-gauge for metrizamide) is introduced into the L2–L3 interspace. Because of the level of the conus, puncture at a higher site is undesirable. If the needle is placed in a lower position, it may create artifacts, making it difficult to identify L4 and L5 pathology. This is, of course, a common location for lumbar disk disease. Spinal puncture should be made with fluoroscopic guidance to insure an ideal midline position for the needle. This allows better position of the needle in the subarachnoid space for injection and also for removal of contrast material, if iophendylate is used. Following a single-wall midline puncture, cerebral spinal fluid should be collected for laboratory studies. The contrast material is then injected under fluoroscopic observation to confirm its presence in the subarachnoid space. In most cases, 10 to 12 ml of contrast agent is all that is required. After filming, if iophendylate has been used, as much of the contrast as possible should be removed from the spinal canal.

Filming for myelograms using iophendylate as the contrast material consists of a series of AP, cross-table lateral, and oblique exposures through the region of potential disease. As iophendylate is heavier than cerebral spinal fluid, tilting the table under fluoroscopic control produces gravity-directed flow of the contrast material, allowing one to evaluate the site of interest (Fig. 1–46).

With metrizamide myelography, several changes in the standard technique are employed.[178, 180, 182] The patient should be well hydrated, and administration of any phenothiazine medication should be discontinued prior to the examination. Also, in patients with previous seizure activity, there is a higher risk with utilization of metrizamide. In these patients the procedure should be performed cautiously with anti-epileptic medication considered.

Unlike iophendylate, which is provided in a standard concentration and dose, metrizamide is prepared prior to the examination and the doses are tailored to the needs of the particular examination. A smaller needle is used (20 to 22 gauge), since the contrast agent is less viscous. A major advantage of metrizamide is that it need not be removed from the spinal canal following the procedure. This contrast agent is totally absorbed from the cerebral spinal fluid space and excreted through the kidneys in 24 to 48 hours. Though metrizamide is more directly irritating to the central nervous system than iophendylate, it is considered to have less potential for the feared late complication of arachnoiditis. Arachnoiditis has been attributed to iophendylate in certain cases. The lesser risk of arachnoiditis with use of metrizamide is primarily due to the total disappearance of metrizamide through its early resorption.[185]

Following myelography with metrizamide, the patient should be kept well hydrated and the head should be elevated at approximately 45° for several hours. This prevents the immediate ascent of the metrizamide into the intracranial region. Should this occur, the incidence of complications such as seizure is significantly higher. With iophendylate the patient should be kept supine, well hydrated, and still with as little head movement as possible for at least 6 to 8 hours. If headaches occur following the myelogram, they should be treated supportively.

Though myelography is rarely indicated immediately following acute spinal trauma, in such cases the procedure is conducted quite differently. The

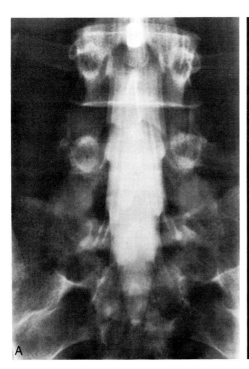 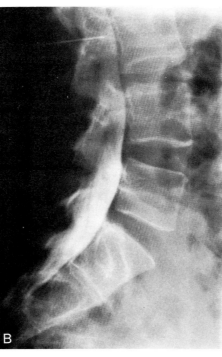

Figure 1–47. Normal metrizamide lumbar myelogram. *A,* AP view. Note the negative filling defects due to the nerve roots. *B,* Normal lateral view. Needle in place at the L3 level. (From Forbes, G.: Radiologic examination of the spine and myelography. *In:* Spittell, J.: Clinical Medicine. Philadelphia, Harper & Row, 1982.)

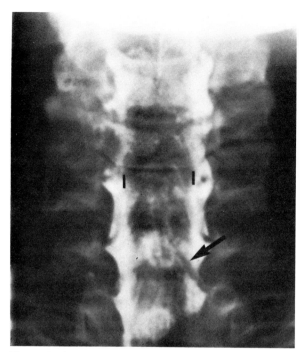

Figure 1–48. Normal AP cervical myelogram. Note the nerve roots *(arrow)* and the width of the spinal cord *(vertical lines).*

needle must be positioned away from the lesion, often resulting in a lower puncture site or a C1 puncture.[184] Only a small amount of cerebral spinal fluid should be removed in cases of potential obstruction. The fluid should be examined carefully, and if blood is present the significant risk of arachnoiditis must be recognized. In these situations, metrizamide is the contrast material of choice.[187]

Patient positioning may be a significant problem following acute injury. This may require additional equipment to stabilize the spine and assist in controlled patient motion in directing dye flow.

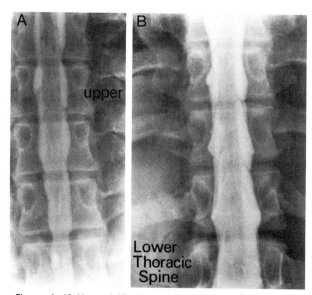

Figure 1–49. Normal AP views of the upper *(A)* and lower *(B)* thoracic spine. Note the reduced size of the cord and spinal canal.

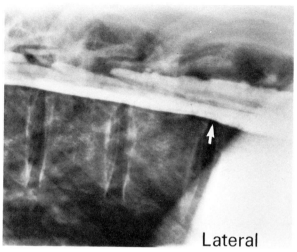

Figure 1–50. Normal lateral thoracic myelogram. Note the smooth indentations (arrow) due to the posterior longitudinal ligament.

NORMAL MYELOGRAPHIC ANATOMY

The cord and proximal nerve roots entering the neural canals are demonstrated myelographically as negative filling defects (Fig. 1–47). The spinal cord is widest at the C5–C6 level, occupying up to 75 percent of the transverse diameter of the sac on the AP view (Fig. 1–48). The spinal canal is smaller in the thoracic region and the conus is best demonstrated with the supine AP views at the T12 level (Fig. 1–49). The opacified subarachnoid space is separated from the bony walls of the canal by fat, ligaments, and the veins of the epidural space. On the lateral view smooth indentations may be seen at the interspaces owing to the posterior longitudinal ligament (Fig. 1–50). Draining veins may be seen on occasion near the conus in the thoracic region.

INDICATIONS

In practice, myelography is most commonly used for definitive diagnosis or exclusion of herniated disks. This has changed significantly in recent years owing to the increased application of computed tomography, with or without metrizamide, in eval-

TABLE 1–8. Myelography: Common Indications

Disk disease
Spondylosis and spinal stenosis
Spinal neoplasms
    Primary
    Metastatic
Congenital malformations
Arachnoid cysts
Arteriovenous malformations
Arachnoiditis
Trauma
    Epidural obstruction
    Nerve root avulsion

uation of the spinal canal.[181, 184] Other indications for conventional myelography include spondylosis or spinal stenosis, spinal tumors, congenital malformations, and arteriovenous malformations (Table 1–8). Myelography is rarely indicated following acute spinal trauma. Computed tomography and conventional tomography will usually provide the necessary information. In selected patients myelography may be useful in defining the level of epidural obstruction (Fig. 1–51) following trauma or surgery (Fig. 1–52) and in localizing cervical nerve root avulsions.[184, 186]

INTRODUCTION TO ARTHROGRAPHY

THOMAS H. BERQUIST

This section provides the necessary background information for arthrography regardless of the joint being studied. Details involving procedural techniques will be reserved for specific chapters.

Arthrography is an extremely useful, benign procedure. The technique is most frequently employed

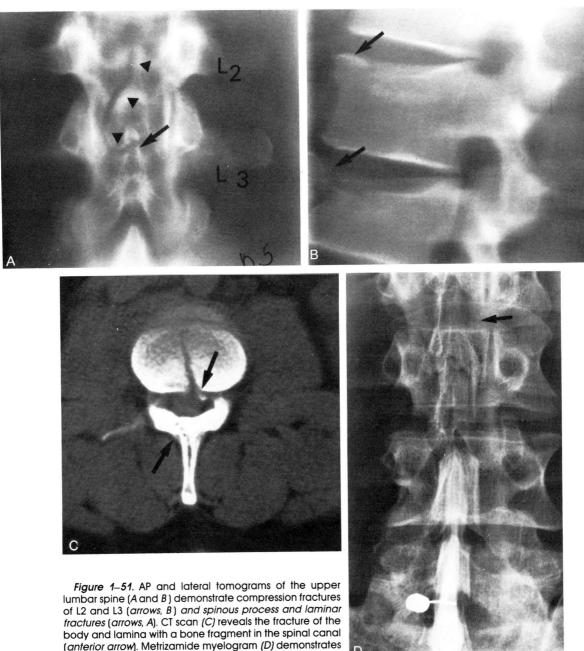

Figure 1–51. AP and lateral tomograms of the upper lumbar spine (*A* and *B*) demonstrate compression fractures of L2 and L3 (*arrows, B*) *and spinous process and laminar fractures* (*arrows, A*). CT scan (*C*) reveals the fracture of the body and lamina with a bone fragment in the spinal canal (*anterior arrow*). Metrizamide myelogram (*D*) demonstrates epidural block at the L2 disc level (*arrow*).

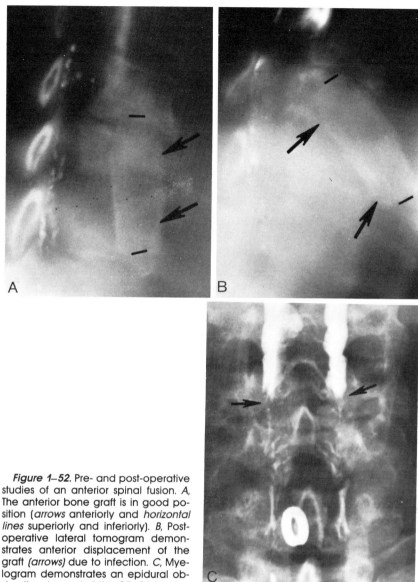

Figure 1–52. Pre- and post-operative studies of an anterior spinal fusion. *A,* The anterior bone graft is in good position (*arrows* anteriorly and *horizontal lines* superiorly and inferiorly). *B,* Post-operative lateral tomogram demonstrates anterior displacement of the graft (*arrows*) due to infection. *C,* Myelogram demonstrates an epidural obstruction (*arrows*) at the C5–C6 level.

in the knee, shoulder, and hip; however, almost any accessible articulation may be evaluated. Table 1–9 lists the joints most frequently studied at the Mayo Clinic in order of decreasing frequency.

In order to obtain the maximum information, arthrography should be performed by an experienced arthrographer with a thorough understanding of the patient's clinical situation. Review of

routine radiographs is essential. These films may provide clues that dictate subtle changes in film technique, views that may be required, and the contrast medium that may be best suited for the procedure. Simply stated, arthrography should be tailored to the individual patient and not performed as a set procedure.

EQUIPMENT

Radiographic equipment should provide excellent detail and allow adequate work space to simplify patient positioning and needle placement. We prefer an overhead fluoroscopic tube with a small focal spot (no larger than 0.6 mm) and a 48-inch source-to-target distance (Fig. 1–53). This provides better geometric positioning and resulting film quality

TABLE 1–9. Arthrography: Commonly Studied Joints

Knee	Foot
Shoulder	Tarsal
Hip	MTP
Wrist	Lumbar facet
Ankle	AC joints
Hand	Temporomandibular
Elbow	Sacroiliac
	Pubic symphysis

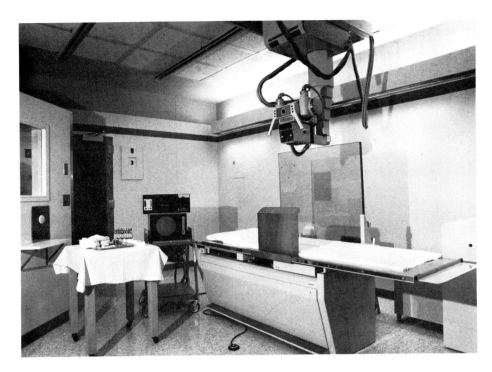

Figure 1–53. Arthrographic and interventional fluoroscopic suite with overhead fluoroscopic tube to allow greater patient access.

than a conventional fluoroscopic suite with the x-ray tube under the table. The overhead tube allows better access to the patient, making the procedure less difficult to perform. This table, which is movable, can be used for all types of arthrography and interventional orthopedic procedures.

The arthrogram set (Fig. 1–54) is devised so that all arthrograms, injections, and biopsies can be performed with the same tray. The tray includes the following items: four sterile drapes, one sterile drape with a 4-inch center hole, six absorbent 6×6 gauze sponges, one 5 ml syringe, two 10 ml syringes, one 30 ml syringe, one cup for contrast material, and extension tubing. A needle box is kept

in the room. This contains 22- and 18-gauge spinal needles, 1½-inch 18- and 22-gauge needles, and ⅝-inch 25-gauge needles. Needle selection will vary depending on the joint to be studied and the size of the patient.

Additional items include vials of nonbacteriostatic saline solution for joint aspiration and irrigation, culture vials for aerobic and anaerobic bacterial and fungal studies, specimen tubes for synovial fluid analysis, and 1 percent lidocaine (Xylocaine). Betamethasone (Celestone) and 0.25 percent bupivacaine (Marcaine) are also stocked for diagnostic and therapeutic injections. Sterile conventional and leaded surgical gloves are also available in the

Figure 1–54. Arthrogram set with syringes, needles, anesthetic vials, culture bottles, Celestone, and other items.

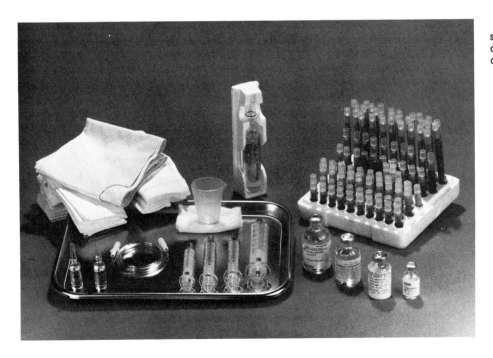

arthrographic suite. An additional necessity is an emergency tray or cart in case of contrast medium reactions or other unforeseen emergencies.

Contrast Material

Arthrography may be performed with positive-contrast material, air, or double-contrast techniques that use both a positive contrast medium and air or CO_2. Several contrast media are available. We most commonly use Hypaque-M-60 (Winthrop). Renografin-60 and Reno M-60 (Squibb) may also be used. Iodine content, approximately 47 percent with Hypaque-M-60, does not differ significantly from that in other arthrographic contrast media. However, sodium content with these contrast agents is less than with other diatrizoates, resulting in less irritation. Extracapsular injection is particularly painful if the sodium content of the contrast medium is too high.

Because of increased osmolality and rapid absorption, contrast medium becomes rapidly diluted in the joint, resulting in loss of detail on the radiographs. This may occur in 5 to 10 minutes following the injection. If an effusion is present in the joint, the detail may deteriorate even more rapidly. This can be prevented to some degree by combining 0.3 ml of 1:1000 epinephrine with the contrast material.[195] Spataro has noted enhanced film quality for up to 1 hour with this technique.[206] However, epinephrine may cause systemic side effects and should not be used in patients with cardiac disease. We generally reserve the use of epinephrine for cases that require tomography or CT in addition to the conventional views. Tomography requires significantly more time, and if epinephrine is not used the image quality may be decreased.

Improved contrast agents are being investigated but are not commonly used at this time. PhDZ 59B was studied in Sweden and demonstrated prolonged duration in the joints.[189] Metrizamide, now commonly used in myelography, is a water-soluble contrast medium which has also been investigated for arthrographic purposes. Metrizamide also remains in the joint longer and has a lower incidence of postarthrographic effusion compared to Urografin-60 and Conray-282.[200, 202]

In the shoulder, knee, and elbow, double-contrast technique provides increased articular detail. We routinely use room air rather than CO_2. Room air is less expensive and readily available, and we have not experienced any complications. Mink reported a lower incidence of postarthrographic pain with room air compared to CO_2.[203] Rarely, room air alone is used in patients with a significant history of allergy to contrast media.

COMPLICATIONS

Arthrography is a benign procedure with little risk of significant complications. Freiberger reported an incidence of infection of 1:25,000 cases.[193] Effusions may occur following arthrography, whether contrast medium or air alone is used. The effusion usually appears within 12 hours of the arthrogram and results in pain and stiffness of the involved joint.[193, 204] Murray reported transient eosinophilia in the knee following pneumoarthrography, which is often combined with a turbid fluid owing to the high eosinophil count (normally 2 percent, 75 percent following pneumoarthrography). No infection could be detected.[204, 205] Eosinophilic infiltration of the synovium has also been demonstrated[198, 205] and may explain the postarthrographic pain and swelling. Mink postulates that pH decreases in the synovial fluid following arthrography may be responsible for the discomfort experienced by some patients.[203] Regardless of the etiology of the effusion and discomfort, this is not usually a significant problem, especially when compared with the diagnostic usefulness of the procedure. This difficulty seems to be less of a problem following double-contrast studies, perhaps because of the smaller volumes of contrast medium used with this technique.[196] Also, air may remain in the joint for up to 10 days,[204] which will result in increased crepitation in the joint.

Patients should be questioned concerning allergies to iodinated contrast media prior to performing the arthrogram. Allergy to contrast agents must be considered but is extremely rare, numbering fewer than 1 per 1000 studies in Freiberger's series.[193] Urticaria is the usual reaction experienced and often no treatment is required. Antihistamines may be used in more severe cases of urticaria. Most reactions to contrast medium develop within 15 to 30 min following the injection.

SUBTRACTION TECHNIQUE

The advent of joint replacement procedures has resulted in an alteration of conventional arthrographic techniques. Subtraction techniques are almost always used in patients with joint arthroplasties.

Subtraction radiography provides a technique for photographically removing certain unnecessary information from the radiograph. This results in specific information becoming more visible. Photographic subtraction was first described by Ziedes des Plantes in 1934.[192] The technique is most frequently used in angiography to enable improved visualization of subtle changes in small vessels.[197, 199, 201] Subtraction is also valuable in arthrographic evaluation of patients with pain following joint replacement. The density of arthrographic contrast medium is about the same as the barium-impregnated methyl methacrylate used to cement the components of the joint replacements in place. Therefore, it may be difficult to detect extravasation of contrast material around the cemented components. Subtraction allows improved visualization of

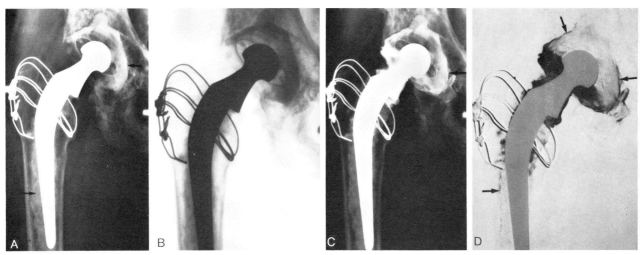

Figure 1–55. *A,* Scout film for subtraction arthrogram with barium-impregnated methyl methacrylate *(arrows). B,* Mask film is the reverse density of the scout film (black). *C,* Post-injection film demonstrates some extravasation about the acetabular component *(arrow)* and a small pseudocapsule. *D,* Subtraction arthrogram reveals loosening of both the acetabular and femoral components *(arrows).*

the bone-methacrylate interface; and thus loosening, a common cause of pain following joint replacement, can be detected more easily.[188, 194]

Subtraction technique involves obtaining (1) a scout film, (2) a mask (reversed image) of the scout film, and (3) a film following the introduction of contrast material[190, 191, 207] (Fig. 1–55).

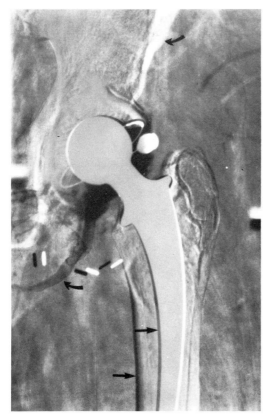

Figure 1–56. Subtraction arthrogram film with misregistration *(arrows)* that could give the false impression of loosening. Note that the ischium and femoral cortices do not cancel out.

The scout film in orthopedic studies (Fig. 1–55A) contains information regarding the components of the joint, soft tissues and bony architecture. The mask film (Fig. 1–55B) is a reverse image of the scout film; and if it is superimposed on the scout film, all information is discarded. The arthrogram film (Fig. 1–55C) must be taken as soon as possible after the scout film, with the same technical factors and the patient motionless. Any patient motion between obtaining the scout film and the positive contrast film will invalidate the subtraction. Subtraction will also be inadequate if the films are not properly overlaid to cancel the unwanted information (Fig. 1–56). If the patient is able to cooperate and the process is perfectly performed, the resulting subtraction film (Fig. 1–55D) reveals the contrast medium to better advantage, and the unwanted information is removed. In practice, because of limitations in the photographic reproduction process, problems of registration of the mask, and slight patient motion, perfect subtraction is rarely ob-

TABLE 1–10. Radiographic Techniques in Soft Tissue Evaluation

Extremities	Trunk
Low keV radiographs	CT
Soft tissue masses	MRI
Xeroradiography	Isotope scans
Soft tissue masses	Liver
Foreign bodies	Spleen
Ultrasound	Angiography
Superficial masses	Diagnosis and
Vascular structures	treatment of
Superficial tendons &	hemorrhage
ligaments	
CT	
MRI	
Angiography	
Post-traumatic	
Occlusions and fistula	
Phlebitis	

TABLE 1–11. Imaging Techniques for Articular Evaluation

Routine radiographs
Stress views
Tomography
Arthrography
    Routine
    Subtraction
    Xerograms (cruciate ligaments)
Tenography
CT
MRI
    Ligaments
    Early erosions
Ultrasound
    Popliteal cysts
Isotope scans
    Infection
    Osteonecrosis
    Early arthritis
Magnification techniques
    Infection
    Arthritis
    Metabolic diseases
    Subtle fractures
Low keV techniques
    Tendinitis
    Synovitis

TABLE 1–13. Radiographic Evaluation: Post-reduction and Internal or External Fixation Devices

Routine radiographs
Tomography
    Metal blur, direction-dependent
Magnetic resonance imaging
    Little metal artifact if nonmagnetic
CT
    Significant metal artifact
Isotope scans
    Infection
    Fracture healing
    Avascular necrosis
Myelography
    Epidural obstruction

tained. The results are nevertheless clinically useful when ordinary care is taken in the process.

The subtraction mask (Fig. 1–55*B*) is black where the scout film (Fig. 1–55*A*) is white. The density differences of the scout and mask must be exactly opposite if the subtraction is to be complete. Scout film density (+1) plus mask density (−1) cancel one another out, and therefore only the contrast material is visible. Kodak RPS X-omat subtraction film or DuPont Cronex subtraction film can be used for the mask. The mask is obtained by placing the scout film and superimposed subtraction film over a printing apparatus that exposes the film with a 15-watt bulb for approximately 5 to 10 sec. The mask film can then be developed in an ordinary processor.

Once the mask has been obtained, the subtraction print can be produced by placing the mask over the arthrogram film. The print film is then positioned over these films, and the films are exposed for 10 to 20 sec using the same printing apparatus. The longer time required is owing to the increased number of films. The print is then processed in an X-omat, resulting in the subtraction film (Fig. 1–55*D*).

Second-order subtraction may also be accomplished by producing two mask films. This process compensates for limitations of the photographic reproduction process, improving subtraction and enhancing detail further.[197, 199] Second-order subtraction is usually not required with presently available films, especially in arthrography.

SUMMARY

This chapter has provided the background information necessary to familiarize physicians with the currently available imaging techniques. Routine radiography remains the most important method for initial patient evaluation. Proper use of the numerous routine projections and other modalities (CT, angiography, MRI, etc.) is important diagnostically and in minimizing patient costs. Common applications of imaging techniques are summarized in Tables 1–10 to 1–13. Imaging approaches to specific clinical problems will be discussed in more detail in future chapters.

TABLE 1–12. Imaging Techniques in Skeletal Evaluation

Extremities	Pelvis and Hips	Spine
Routine radiographs	Routine radiographs	Routine radiographs
Tomography	AP, angled, Judet	Tomography
Isotope scans	Tomography	Odontoid
Stress fractures	Subtle fractures	Facets
Femoral neck	CT	Neural arch
Neoplasm	Posterior fractures	Xerograms
CT	Fragment orientation	CT
Bone mineral analysis	Joint fragments	Dural tears
Magnification	Soft tissue injury	Spinal fragments
Subtle fractures		Disk disease
Infection		Myelography
Metabolic disease		Obstruction
Xeroradiography		Nerve root avulsion
Subtle fractures		
Early arthritis		

REFERENCES

Routine Radiography

1. Ballinger, P. W.: Merrill's Atlas of Roentgenographic Positions and Standard Radiologic Procedures. St. Louis, C. V. Mosby, 1982.
2. Bernau, A., and Berquist, T. H.: Orthopedic Positioning in Diagnostic Radiology. Baltimore, Urban & Schwarzenberg, 1983.
3. Eastman Kodak Co.: The Fundamentals of Radiology. 12th Ed. Rochester, NY, 1980.
4. Gonadal shielding in diagnostic radiology. Publication No. (FDA) 75–8024, Rockville, Bureau of Radiological Health, 1975.
5. Orhan, H. S., Showalter, C. K., Koustenis, G. H., et al.: A sensitometric evaluation of film-screen–chemistry-processor systems in the state of New Jersey. Bureau of Radiological Health, Rockville, 1982.

Tomography

6. Berrett, A., Brunner, S., and Valvassori, G. E.: Modern Thin Section Tomography. Springfield, IL, Charles C Thomas, 1973.
7. Bokstrom, I.: Principles of vertebral tomography. Acta Radiol. Suppl., 103, 1955.
8. Christensen, E. E., Curry, T. S., and Dowdey, J. E.: An Introduction to the Physics of Diagnostic Radiology. 2nd Ed. Philadelphia, Lea & Febiger, 1978.
9. Eastman Kodak Co.: Fundamentals of Radiology. 12th Ed. Rochester, New York, 1980.
10. McCullough, E. C., and Coulam, C. M.: Physical and dosimetric aspects of diagnostic geometrical and computer assisted tomographic procedures. Radiol. Clin. North Am., 14:3, 1976.
11. Norman, A.: The value of tomography in the diagnosis of skeletal disorders. Radiol. Clin. North. Am. 8:251, 1970.
12. Resnick, D., and Niwayama, G.: Diagnosis of Bone and Joint Disorders. Philadelphia, W. B. Saunders Co., 1981.

Magnification Radiography

13. Christensen, E. E., Curry, T. S., Dowdey, J. E.: An Introduction to the Physics of Diagnostic Radiology. 2nd Ed. Philadelphia, Lea & Febiger, 1978.
14. Fletcher, D. E., and Rowley, K. A.: Radiographic enlargements in diagnostic radiology. Br. J. Radiol. 24:598, 1951.
15. Genant, H. K., Kunlo, D., Mall, J. C., et al.: Direct magnification for skeletal radiography. Radiology 123:47, 1977.
16. Gordon, S. L., Greer, R. B., and Wiedner, W. A.: Magnification roentgenographic technique in orthopedics. Clin. Orthop. 91:169, 1973.
17. Milne, E.: Magnification radiology, editorial. Applied Radiol., Jan-Feb, p. 12, 1976.
18. Nemet, A., and Cox, W. F.: The improvement of definition of x-ray image magnification. Br. J. Radiol. 29:335, 1956.
19. Resnick, D., and Niwayama, G.: Diagnosis of Bone and Joint Disorders. Philadelphia, W. B. Saunders Co., 1981.
20. Eastman Kodak Co.: The Fundamentals of Radiology. 12th Ed. Rochester, New York, 1980.
21. Wagoner, L. K., Cohen, G., Wong, W., et al.: Dose efficiency and the effects of resolution and noise detail perceptibility in radiographic magnification. Med. Phys. 8:24, 1981.
22. Weiss, A.: A technique for demonstrating fine detail in the bones of the hand. Clin. Radiol. 23:185, 1972.

Xeroradiography

23. Bryant, T. H., and Julian, W. L.: Reduction of radiation dose to patients in xeroradiography. Br. J. Radiol. 51:974, 1978.
24. Campbell, C. L., Roach, J., and Grisolia, A.: Comparative study of xeroradiography and routine roentgenography in the recording of roentgen images of bone specimens. J. Bone Joint Surg. 39A:577, 1957.
25. Campbell, C. J., Roach, J. F., and Jabbur, M.: Xeroradiography. J. Bone Joint Surg. 41A:271, 1959.
26. Chang, C. H. J., Sibala, J. L., Martin, N. L., et al.: Film mammography: New low radiation technology. Radiology 121:215, 1976.
27. Crowe, J. K.: Pulmonary application of xeroradiography and xerotomography. Thesis, Univ. of Minnesota, 1976.
28. Griffiths, H. L., and D'Orsi, C. J.: Use of xeroradiography in cruciate ligament injuries. A. J. R. 121:94, 1974.
29. Hyman, J., and Bakker, V.: Xeroradiographic detection of tooth and bone pathology. Oral Surg. 47:482, 1979.
30. John, V. B., Ewen, K., and Bringewald, B.: Dose reduction in xeroradiography: Application to chest tomography. Radiology 133:520, 1979.
31. Ostrum, B. J., Becker, W., and Isard, H. J.: Low dose mammography. Radiology 109:323, 1973.
32. Resnick, D., and Niwayama, G.: Diagnosis of Bone and Joint Disorders. Philadelphia, W. B. Saunders Co., 1981.
33. Roach, J. F., and Hilleboe, H. E.: Xeroradiography. A. J. R. 73:3, 1955.
34. Sickles, E. A., and Genant, H. K.: Controlled single blind clinical evaluation of low dose mammographic screen-film systems. Radiology 130:347, 1979.
35. Tan, C. Y., Marks, R., and Payne, P.: Comparison of xeroradiographic and ultrasound detection of corticosteroid induced dermal thinning. J. Invest. Dermatol. 76:126, 1981.
36. Wolf, J. N.: Xeroradiography of the bones, joints and soft tissues. Radiology 93:583, 1969.
37. Wolf, J. N.: Xeroradiography of the Breast. Springfield, IL, Charles C Thomas, 1972.
38. Wolf, J. N.: Xeroradiography: Image content and comparison with film roentgenograms. A. J. R. 117:690, 1973.

Ultrasound

39. Bluth, E. I., Merritt, C. R., and Sullivan, M. A.: Grey scale ultrasound evaluation of the lower extremities. JAMA 247:3127, 1982.
40. Braumstein, E. M., Silver, T. M., Martel, W., et al.: Ultrasonographic diagnosis of extremity masses. Skeletal Radiol. 6:157, 1981.
41. Carpenter, J. R., Hattery, R. R., Hunder, G. G., et al.: Ultrasound evaluation of the popliteal space. Comparison of arthrography and physical examination. Mayo Clin. Proc. 51:498, 1976.
42. Cooperberg, P. L., Tsang, J., Truelove, L., et al.: Grey scale ultrasound in the evaluation of rheumatoid arthritis of the knee. Radiology 126:759, 1978.
43. Gordon, G. V., and Edell, S.: Ultrasonic evaluation of popliteal cysts. Arch. Intern. Med. 140:1453, 1980.
44. Grompels, B. M., and Darlington, L. G.: Grey scale ultrasonography and arthrography in evaluation of popliteal cysts. Clin. Radiol. 30:539, 1979.
45. Hermann, G., Yeh, H. C., Lehr-James, C., et al.: Diagnosis of popliteal cysts: Double contrast arthrography and sonography. A. J. R. 137:369, 1981.
46. Kaufman, R. A., Tarskins, R. B., Babcock, D. S., and Crawford, A. H.: Arthrosonography in the diagnosis of pigmented villonodular synovitis. A. J. R. 139:396, 1982.
47. Lawson, I. L., and Mittler, S.: Ultrasonic evaluation of extremity soft tissue lesions with arthrographic correlation. J. Can. Assoc. Radiol. 29:58, 1978.
48. Leopold, G. R.: Ultrasonography of superficially located structures. Radiol. Clin. North Am. 18:161, 1980.
49. McDonald, D. G., and Leopold, G. R.: Ultrasound B-scanning in the differentiation of Baker's cyst and thrombophlebitis. Br. J. Radiol. 45:729, 1972.
50. Sarti, D. A., and Sample, W. F.: Diagnostic Ultrasound, Text and Cases. Boston, G. K. Hall and Co., 1980.
51. Silber, T. M., Washburn, R. L., Stanley, J. C., et al.: Grey scale ultrasound evaluation of popliteal artery aneurysms. A. J. R. 129:1003, 1977.
52. Swett, H. A., Jaffe, R. B., and McCliff, B. B.: Popliteal cysts: Presentation as thrombophlebitis. Radiology 115:613, 1975.

53. Winsberg, F., and Cooperberg, P. L.: Real Time Ultrasonography. New York, Churchill Livingstone, 1982.

Skeletal Scintigraphy

54. Ash, J. M., Gilday, D. L., and Reilly, B. J.: Pinhole imaging of hip disorders in children. J. Nucl. Med. 16:512, 1975.
55. Berggren, A., Weiland, A. J., and Ostrup, L. T.: Bone scintigraphy in evaluating the viability of composite bone grafts revascularized by microvascular anastomosis, conventional autologous bone grafts, and free nonrevascularized periosteal grafts. J. Bone Joint Surg. 64A:799, 1982.
56. Collins, J. D., Bassett, L., Main, G. D., et al.: Percutaneous biopsy following positive bone scans. Radiology 132:439, 1979.
57. Danigelis, J. A.: Pinhole imaging in Legg-Perthes disease. Semin. Nucl. Med. 16:69, 1976.
58. Desai, A., Alvi, A., Dalinka, M., et al.: Role of bone scintigraphy in the evaluation and treatment of nonunited fractures: Concise communication. J. Nucl. Med. 21:931, 1980.
59. Ganel, A., Engel, J., Oster, Z., et al.: Bone scanning and assessment of fractures of the scaphoid. J. Hand Surg. 4:540, 1979.
60. Gelman, M. I., Coleman, R. E., Stevens, P. M., et al.: Radiography, radionuclide imaging and arthrography in evaluation of total hip and knee replacement. Radiology 128:677, 1978.
61. Geslien, J. E., Thrall, J. H., Espinosa, J. L., et al.: Early detection of stress fractures using Tc-99m polyphosphate. Radiology 121:683, 1976.
62. Greiff, J.: Determination of the vitality of the femoral head with Tc-99m-SN-pyrophosphate scintigraphy. Acta Orthop. Scand. 51:109, 1980.
63. Greiff, J., Lanng, S., Høilund-Carlsen, P. F., et al.: Early detection by Tc-99m-Sn-pyrophosphate scintigraphy of femoral head necrosis following medial femoral neck fractures. Acta Orthop. Scand. 51:119, 1980.
64. Gumerman, L. W., Fogel, S. R., Goodman, M. A., et al.: Experimental fracture healing: Evaluation of radionuclide bone imaging: Concise communication. J. Nucl. Med. 19:1320, 1978.
65. Hoffer, P.: Gallium: Mechanisms. J. Nucl. Med. 21:282, 1980.
66. Hunter, J. C., Hattner, R. S., Murray, W. R., et al.: Loosening of the total knee arthroplasty: Detection by radionuclide bone scanning. A. J. R. 133:131, 1980.
67. Hutz, J. A., Galvin, A. G., and Lull, R. J.: Natural history or Tc-99m MDP bone scan in asymptomatic total hip prosthesis. J. Nucl. Med. 23(5):28, 1982.
68. Lotke, P. A., Ecker, M. L., and Alavi, A.: Painful knees in older patients: Radionuclide diagnosis of possible osteonecrosis with spontaneous resolution. J. Bone Joint Surg. 59A:617, 1977.
69. Matin, P.: The appearance of bone scans following fractures, including immediate and long-term studies. J. Nucl. Med. 20:1227, 1979.
70. McMaster, M. G., and Merrick, M. V.: A scintigraphic assessment of the scoliotic spine after fusion. J. Bone Joint Surg. 62B:65, 1980.
71. McNeil, B. J., Pace, P. D., Gray, E. B., et al.: Preoperative and follow-up bone scans in patients with primary carcinoma of the breast. Surg. Gynecol. Obstet. 147:745, 1978.
72. Reing, C. M., Richin, P. F., and Kenmore, P. I.: Differential bone scanning in the evaluation of a painful total joint replacement. J. Bone Joint Surg. 61A:933, 1979.
73. Resnick, D., Williamson, S., and Alazraki, N.: Focal spinal abnormalities on bone scans and ankylosing spondylitis: A clue to the presence of fracture of pseudarthrosis. Clin. Nucl. Med. 6:213, 1981.
74. Rosenthal, L., Lisbona, R., Hernandez, M., et al.: Tc-99m-pp and Ga-67 imaging following insertion of orthopedic devices. Radiology 133:717, 1979.
75. Rosenthal, L., Kloiber, R., Damten, B., et al.: Sequential use of radiophosphate and radiogallium imaging in the differential diagnosis of bone, joint, and soft tissue infection: Quantitative analysis. Diagn. Imaging 51:249, 1982.
76. Schaffer, D. L., and Pendergrass, H. P.: Comparison of enzyme clinical, radiographic, and radionuclide methods of detecting bone metastasis from carcinoma of the prostate. Radiology 121:431, 1976.
77. Smith, F. W., and Gilday, D. L.: Scintigraphic appearance of osteoid osteoma. Radiology 137:191, 1980.
78. Spencer, R. B., Levinson, E. D., Baldwin, R. D., et al.: Diverse bone scan abnormalities in "shin splints." J. Nucl. Med. 20:1271, 1979.
79. Subramanian, G., and McAfee, J. G.: A new complex for skeletal imaging. Radiology 99:192, 1971.
80. Subrammanian, G., McAfee, J. G., Bell, E. G., et al.: Tc-99m-labeled polyphosphate as a skeletal imaging agent. Radiology 102:701, 1972.
81. Sutherland, A. D., Savage, J. R., Patterson, D. C., et al.: The nuclide bone scan in the diagnosis and management of Perthes disease. J. Bone Joint Surg. 62B:300, 1980.
82. Swee, R. G., McLeod, R. A., and Beabout, J. W.: Osteoid osteoma. Detection, diagnosis and localization. Radiology 130:117, 1979.
83. Thakur, M. L., Coleman, R. E., Mayhall, C. G., et al.: Preparation and evaluation of 111In-labeled leukocytes as an abscess imaging agent in dogs. Radiology 119:731, 1976.
84. Thakur, M. L., Coleman, R. E., and Welch, M. J.: Indium-111-labeled leukocytes for the localization of abscesses: Preparation, analysis, tissue distribution in comparison with gallium-67 citrate in dogs. J. Lab. Clin. Med. 89:217, 1977.
85. Thomas, R. H., Resnick, D., Naomi, P. A., et al.: Compartmental evaluation of osteoarthritis of the knee. A comparative study of available diagnostic modalities. Radiology 116:585, 1975.
86. Weiss, P. E., Mall, J. C., Hoffer, P. B., et al.: Tc-99m methylene diphosphonate bone imaging in evaluation of total hip prosthesis. Radiology 133:727, 1979.
87. Weissberg, D. L., Resnick, D., Taylor, A., et al.: Rheumatoid arthritis and its variants: Analysis of scintiphotographic, radiographic and clinical examination. A. J. R. 131:665, 1978.
88. Wilcox, J. R., Moniot, A. L., and Green, J. P.: Bone scanning and the evaluation of exercise-related injuries. Radiology 123:699, 1977.
89. Wilson, G. S., Rich, M. A., and Brennan, M. J.: Evaluation of bone scan in preoperative clinical staging of breast cancer. Arch. Surg. 115:415, 1980.
90. Woolsenden, J. M., Pitt, M. J., Brian, G. M., et al.: Comparison of bone scintigraphy and radiography in multiple myeloma. Radiology 134:723, 1980.

Quantitation of Bone Mineral

91. Arnold, J. S.: Amount and quality of trabecular bone in osteoporotic vertebral fractures. Clin. Endocrinol. Metab. 2:221, 1973.
92. Bradley, J. G., Huang, H. K., and Ledley, R. S.: Evaluation of calcium concentration in bones from CT scans. Radiology 128:103, 1978.
93. Cameron, J. R., and Sorenson, J.: Measurement of bone mineral in vivo: An improved method. Science 142:230, 1963.
94. Cann, C. E., and Genant, H. K.: Precise measurement of vertebral mineral content using computed tomography. J. Comput. Assist. Tomogr. 4:493, 1980.
95. Chalmers, J., and Weaver, J. K.: Cancellous bone: Its strength and changes with aging and an evaluation of some methods for measuring its mineral content. J. Bone Joint Surg. 48A:299, 1966.
96. Christiansen, C., Rodbro, P., and Jensen, H.: Bone mineral content in the forearm measured by photon absorptiometry. Scand. J. Clin. Lab. Invest. 35:323, 1975.
97. Christiansen, C.: Bone mineral measurements with special reference to precision, accuracy, normal values, and clinical relevance. In Jequeker, J., and Johnston, C. C. (Eds.):

Noninvasive Bone Measurements: Methodological Problems. Arlington, VA, IRL Press, 1981.

98. Dauphine, R. T., Riggs, B. L., and Scholz, D. A.: Back pain and vertebral crush fractures: An unemphasized mode of presentation for primary hyperparathyroidism. Ann. Intern. Med. *83*:365, 1975.

99. Dunn, W. L., Wahner, H. W., Riggs, B. L.: Measurement of bone mineral content in human vertebrae and hip by dual photon absorptiometry. Radiology *136*:485, 1980.

100. Gallagher, J. C., Melton, J., Riggs, B. L., et al.: Epidemiology of fractures of the proximal femur in Rochester, Minnesota. Clin. Orthop. *150*:163, 1980.

101. Goldsmith, N. F.: Normative data from the osteoporosis prevalance survey, Oakland, California, 1969–1970. *In* Mazess, R. B. (ed.): Bone mineral at the distal radius: variation with age, sex, skin color, and exposure to oral contraceptives and exogenous hormones; relation to aortic calcification, osteoporosis, and hearing loss. Proceedings of the International Conference of Bone Mineral Measurements. U.S. Dept. of Health, Education, and Welfare, 1973.

102. Johnston, C. C., Smith, D. M., Yu, D. L., et al.: In vivo measurement of bone mass in the radius. Metabolism *17*:1140, 1968.

103. Madsen, M., Peppler, W., and Mazess, R. B.: Vertebral and total body bone mineral by dual photon absorptiometry. Calcif. Tissue Int. *21*:361, 1976.

104. Mazess, R. B.: Non-invasive Measurement of Bone. *In* Barzel, U.S. (ed.): Osteoporosis II. New York, Grune and Stratton, 1979.

105. Mazess, R. B., and Cameron, J. R.: Bone mineral content in normal U.S. whites. *In* Mazess, R. B. (ed.): Proceedings of International Conference on Bone Mineral Measurements. U. S. Dept. of Health, Education, and Welfare, 1973.

106. Mazess, R. B., Ort, M., Judy, P., et al.: Absorptiometric bone mineral determination using 153-Gd. *In* Cameron, J. R. (ed.): Proceedings of Bone Measurement Conference (Conf. 700515). US Atomic Energy Commission, 1970.

107. Mazess, R. B., Wilson, C. R., Hanson, J., et al.: Progress in dual photon absorptiometry of bone. *In* Schmeling, P. (ed.): Symposium of Bone Mineral Determinations (AE-489). Studsvik, Sweden, Aktiebologet Atomenergi, Vol. 2, 1974.

108. Mazess, R. B.: Measurement of skeletal status by noninvasive methods. Calcif. Tissue Int. *28*:89, 1979.

109. Meema, H. E.: Menopausal and aging changes in muscle mass and bone mineral content. J. Bone Joint Surg. *48A*:1138, 1966.

110. Reed, G. W.: The assessment of bone mineralization from the relative transmission of 241-Am and 137-Cs radiations. Phys. Med. Biol. *11*:174, 1966.

111. Riggs, B. L., Wahner, H. W., Dunn, W. L., et al.: Differential changes in bone mineral density of the appendicular and axial skeleton with aging. J. Clin. Invest. *67*:328, 1981.

112. Riggs, B. L., Wahner, H. W., Seeman, E., et al.: Changes in bone mineral density of the proximal femur and spine with aging. Differences between postmenopausal and senile osteoporosis syndromes. J. Clin. Invest. *70*:716, 1982.

113. Roos, B., Rosengren, B., and Skoldborn, H.: Determination of bone mineral content in lumbar vertebrae by a double gamma-ray technique. *In* Cameron, J. R. (ed.): Proceedings of Bone Measurement Conference (Conf 700515). US Atomic Energy Commission, 1970.

114. Roos, B.: Dual Photon Absorptiometry in Lumbar Vertebrae. Goteborg, Sweden, Akademisk Avhalning, 1974.

115. Ruegsegger, P., Elasser, U., Anlicker, M., et al.: Quantification of bone mineralization using computed tomography. Radiology 121:93:1976.

116. Seeman, E., Wahner, H. W., Offord, K. P., et al.: Differential effects of endocrine dysfunction on the axial and appendicular skeleton. J. Clin. Invest. *69*:1302, 1982.

117. Smith, D. M., Khairi, M. R. A., Norton, J., et al.: Age and activity effects on rate of bone mineral loss. J. Clin. Invest. *58*:716, 1976.

118. Wahner, H. W., Riggs, B. L., and Beabout, J. W.: Diagnosis of osteoporosis: Usefulness of photon absorptiometry at the radius. J. Nucl. Med. *18*:432, 1977.

119. Weissberger, M. A., Zamenhof, R. G., Aronow, S., et al.: computed tomography for the measurement of bone mineral in the human spine. J. Comput. Assist. Tomogr. 2:253, 1978.

120. Wilson, C. R., and Madsen, M.: Dichromatic absorptiometry of vertebrae bone mineral content. Invest. Radiol. *12*:180, 1977.

Computed Tomography

121. Brant-Zawadski, M., Miller, E. M., and Federle, M. P.: CT in the evaluation of spine trauma. A. J. R. *136*:369, 1981.

122. Brasch, R. C., Boyd, D. P., and Gooding, C. A.: Computed tomographic scanning in children: Comparison of radiation dose and resolving power of commercial CT scanners. A. J. R. *131*:95, 1978.

123. Canale, S. T., and Manugion, A. H.: Irreducible traumatic dislocations of the hip. J. Bone Joint Surg. *61A*:7, 1979.

124. Coin, C. G., Pennink, M., Ahmad, W. D., et al.: Diving-type injury to the cervical spine: Contribution of computed tomography to management. J. Comp. Assist. Tomogr. *3*:362, 1979.

125. Colley, D. P., and Dunsker, S. B.: Traumatic narrowing of the dorsolumbar spinal canal demonstrated by computed tomography. Radiology *129*:95, 1978.

126. Destouet, J. M., Gilula, L. A., Murphy, W. A., et al.: Computed tomography of the sterno-clavicular joint and sternum. Radiology *138*:123, 1981.

127. Genant, H. K.: Computed tomography. *In* Resnick, D. and Niwayama, G.: Diagnosis of Bone and Joint Disorders. Philadelphia, W. B. Saunders Co., 1981.

128. Genant, H. K., Williams, J. S., Bovill, E. G., et al.: Advances in computed tomography of the musculoskeletal system. Radiol. Clin. North Am. *19*:645, 1981.

129. Gilula, L. A., Murphy, W. A., Chandrakant, C. T., et al.: Computed tomography of the osseous pelvis. Radiology *132*:107, 1979.

130. Griffith, H. J., Hamlin, D. J., Kiss, S., et al.: Efficacy of CT scanning in a group of 174 patients with orthopedic and musculoskeletal problems. Skeletal Radiol. *7*:87, 1981.

131. Handel, S. F., and Lee, Y. Y.: Computed tomography of spinal fractures. Radiol. Clin. North Am. *19*:69, 1981.

132. Lange, T. A., and Alter, A. J.: Evaluation of complex acetabular fractures by computed tomography. J. Comp. Assist. Tomogr. *4*:849, 1980.

133. Lasada, N. A., Levinsohn, E. M., Yaun, H. A., et al.: Computerized tomography in disorders of the hip. J. Bone Joint Surg. *60A*:1099, 1978.

134. McCullough, E. C., and Payne, J. T.: Patient dosage in computed tomography. Radiology *129*:457, 1978.

135. Leo, J. S., Bergerson, R. T., Kricheff, I. I., et al.: Metrizamide myelography for cervical spinal cord injuries. Radiology *129*:707, 1978.

136. McLeod, R. A., Stephens, D. H., Beabout, J. W., et al.: Computed tomography of the skeletal system. Semin. Roentgenol. *13*:235, 1978.

137. O'Callaghan, J. P., Ulrich, C. G., Yuan, H. A., et al.: CT of facet distraction in flexion injuries of the thoracolumbar spine: The naked facet. A. J. R. *134*:563, 1980.

138. O'Connor, J. F., and Cohen, J.: Computerized tomography in orthopedic surgery. J. Bone Joint Surg. *60A*:1096, 1978.

139. Toombs, B. D., Lester, R. G., Ben-Menachem, Y., et al.: Computed tomography in blunt trauma. Radiol. Clin. North Am. *19*:17, 1981.

Magnetic Resonance Imaging

140. Alfidi, R. J., Haaga, J., Yousef, S. J., et al.: Preliminary experimental results in humans and animals with super-conducting, whole-body nuclear magnetic resonance scanner. Radiology *143*:175, 1982.

141. Berquist, T. H.: Magnetic resonance imaging: Preliminary experience in orthopedic radiology. Mag. Res. Image. 2:41, 1984.

142. Block, F.: Nuclear induction. Physical Review *70*(7 and 8), 1948.
143. Brady, T. J., Rosen, B. R., Pykett, I. L., et al.: NMR imaging of leg tumors. Radiology 149:*181*:1983.
144. Brady, T. J., Gebhart, M. C., Pykett, I. L., et al.: NMR imaging of forearms in healthy volunteers and patients with giant cell tumors of bone. Radiology *144*:549, 1982.
145. Bydder, G. M., Steiner, R. E., Young, I. R., et al.: Clinical NMR images of the brain: 140 cases. A. J. R. *139*:215, 1982.
146. Crooks, L. E., Arakawa, M., Hoenninger, J., et al.: Nuclear magnetic resonance whole-body images operating at 3.5 Kgauss. Radiology *143*:169, 1982.
147. Crooke, L. E., Ortendahl, D. A., Kaufman, L., et al.: Clinical efficacy of nuclear magnetic resonance imaging. Radiology *146*:123, 1983.
148. Damadian, R.: Tumor detection by nuclear magnetic resonance. Science *171*:1151, 1971.
149. Fletcher, B. D., Scoles, P. V., and Nelson, D. A.: Osteomyelitis in children: Detection by magnetic resonance imaging. Radiology *150*:57, 1984.
150. Goldman, M. R., Brady, T. J., Pykett, I. L., et al.: Applications of NMR to imaging of the heart. Applied Radiol. *107*:111, 1982.
151. Hricak, H., Crooks, L., Sheldon, P., et al.: Nuclear magnetic resonance imaging of the kidney. Radiology *146*:425, 1983.
152. Lauterbur, P.: Magnetic resonance zeugmatography. Pure and Applied Chem. *40*(2):40, 1975.
153. Moon, K. L., Genant, H. K., Helms, C. A., et al.: Musculoskeletal applications of magnetic resonance imaging. Radiology *147*:161, 1983.
154. New, P. F. J., Rosen, B. R., Brady, T. J., et al.: Potential hazards and artifacts of ferromagnetic and nonferromagnetic surgical and dental materials and devices in magnetic resonance imaging. Radiology *147*:139, 1983.
155. Pavlicek, W., Geisinger, M., Castle, L., et al.: The effects of magnetic resonance imaging on patients with cardiac pacemakers. Radiology *147*:149, 1983.
156. Purcell, E. M., Torrey, H. C., and Pound, R. V.: Resonance absorption by nuclear magnetic moments in a solid. Phys. Rev. *69*:37, 1946.
157. Pykett, I.: Principles of nuclear magnetic resonance imaging. Radiology *143*:157, 1982.
158. Ranade, S. S., Shah, S., Advani, S. H., et al.: Pulsed nuclear magnetic resonance studies of human bone marrow. Physiol. Chem. Phys. *9*:297, 1977.
159. Saunders, R. D.: Biological effects of NMR clinical imaging. Applied Radiol. Sept/Oct 43, 1982.
160. Schwartz, J. L., and Crooks, L. E.: NMR imaging produces no observable mutation or cytotoxicity on mammalian cells. A. J. R. *139*:583, 1982.
161. Young, I. R., Burl, M., Clarke, G. J., et al.: Magnetic resonance properties of hydrogen imaging in the posterior fossa. A. J. R. *137*:895, 1981.

Angiography

162. Conn, J., Bergan, J. J., and Bell, J. L.: Hypothenar hammar syndrome: Post-traumatic digital ischemia. Surgery 68:1122, 1970.
163. Crossland, S. G., and Slovin, A. J.: The role of arteriography in diagnosing unsuspected vascular injuries. Am. Surg. 44:98, 1981.
164. Fisher, R. G., and Hadlock, F.: Laceration of the thoracic aorta and brachiocephalic arteries by blunt trauma. Radiol. Clin. North Am. 19:91, 1981.
165. Hessel, S. J.: Complications of angiography and other catheter procedures. *In* Abrams, H. L., Angiography. Boston, Little, Brown and Co., 1983.
166. Kam, J., Jackson, H., and Ben-Menachem, Y.: Vascular injuries in blunt pelvic trauma. Radiol. Clin. North Am. 19:171, 1981.
167. Long, E. K.: Pelvic angiography. *In* Abrams, H. L., Angiography. Boston, Little, Brown, and Co., 1983.
168. Long, E. K.: Transcatheter embolization of pelvic vessels for control of intractable hemorrhage. Radiology 140:331, 1981.

169. Long, E. K.: The role of arteriography in trauma. Radiol. Clin. North Am. 14:353, 1976.
170. Love, L.: Arterial trauma. Semin. Roentgenol. 5:267, 1970.
171. Margolies, M. N., Ring, E. J., Waltman, A. C., et al.: Arteriography in the management of hemorrhage from pelvic fractures. N. Engl. J. Med. 287:317, 1972.
172. McDonald, E. J., Goodman, P. C., and Winestock, D. P.: The clinical indications for arteriography in trauma to the extremity. Radiology 116:45, 1975.
173. Ring, E. J., Athanasoulis, C., Waltman, A. C., et al.: Arteriographic management of hemorrhage following pelvic fractures. Radiology 109:65, 1973.
174. Ring, E. J., Athanasoulis, C., Waltman, A. C., et al.: Angiography in pelvic trauma. Surg. Gynecol. Obstet. 139:375, 1974.
175. Rubin, B. E., Fortune, W. P., and May, W. A.: Therapeutic embolization of post-operative hemorrhage about the hip of a patient with pseudomonas infection. J. Bone Joint Surg. 60A:988, 1978.
176. Slaney, G., and Ashton, F.: Arterial injuries and their management. Postgrad. Med. 47:257, 1971.
177. Van Urk, H., Perlberger, R. R., and Muller, H.: Selective arterial embolization for control of traumatic pelvic hemorrhage. Surgery 83:137, 1978.

Myelography

178. Ahn, H. S., and Rosenbaum, A. E.: Lumbar myelography with metrizamide supplemental techniques. Am. J. Neuroradiol. 2:91, 1981.
179. DiChiro, G., and Fisher, R. L.: Contrast radiography of the spinal cord. Arch. Neurol. 11:125, 1964.
180. Fox, A. J., Venulia, F., and Debrun, G.: Complete myelography with metrizamide. Am. J. Neuroradiol. 2:79, 1981.
181. Genant, H. K., Chefetz, N., and Helms, C. A.: Computed Tomography of the Lumbar Spine. Diagnosis and Therapeutic Implications for the Radiologist, Orthopedist, and Neurosurgeon. San Francisco, Univ. of California Press, 1982.
182. Khan, A., Marc, J. A., Chen, M., et al.: Total myelography with metrizamide through the lumbar route. Am. J. Neuroradiol. 2:85, 1981.
183. Keiffer, S. A., Binet, E. F., Esquerra, J. V., et al.: Contrast agents for myelography: Clinical and radiographic evaluation of Amipaque and Pantopaque. Radiology 129:695, 1978.
184. Leo, J. S., Bergeron, R. T., Kricheff, I. I., et al.: Metrizamide mylelography for cervical spinal cord injury. Radiology 129:707, 1978.
185. Paling, M. R., Quindlin, E. A., and DiChiro, G.: Spinal seizures after metrizamide myelography in a patient with spinal block. Am. J. Neuroradiol. 1:473, 1980.
186. Pay, N. T., George, A. E., Benjamin, M. V., et al.: Positive and negative contrast myelography in spinal trauma. Radiology 123:103, 1977.
187. Skalpe, I. O.: Adhesive arachnoiditis following lumbar radiculography with water soluble contrast agents. A clinical report with special reference to metrizamide. Radiology 121:647, 1976.

Introduction to Arthrography

188. Anderson, L. S., and Staple, T. W.: Arthrography of total hip replacement using subtraction technique. Radiology 109:157, 1973.
189. Bjork, L.: A new contrast medium in arthrography. A. J. R. 109:606, 1970.
190. Christensen, E. E., Curry, T. S., and Dowdey, J. E.: An Introduction to the Physics of Diagnostic Radiology. 2nd Ed. Philadelphia, Lea & Febiger, 1978.
191. Chynn, K.: Simplified subtraction technique. A. J. R. 95:970, 1965.
192. Ziedes des Plantes: Subtraktion: Eine roentgenographische Methode zur separaten Abbildung bestimmte Teile des Objekts. Fortschr. Rontgenstr. 52:69, 1934.
193. Freiberger, R. H., and Kaye, J.: Arthrography. New York, Appleton-Century-Crofts, 1979.
194. Gelman, M. I., Coleman, R. E., Stevens, P. M., et al.:

Radiography, radionuclide imaging and arthrography in evaluation of total hip and knee replacement. Radiology *128*:677, 1978.

195. Hall, F. M.: Epinephrine enhanced knee arthrography. Radiology *111*:215, 1974.
196. Hall, F. M.: Morbidity from shoulder arthrography. A. J. R. *136*:59, 1981.
197. Hanafee, W., and Shinno, J. M.: Second order subtraction and simultaneous bilateral carotid and internal carotid injections. Radiology *86*:334, 1966.
198. Hasselbacher, P.: Synovial fluid eosinophilia following arthrography. J. Rheumatol. *5*:173, 1978.
199. Holman, C. B., and Bullard, F. E.: The application of closed circuit television in diagnostic radiology. Mayo Clin. Proc. *38*:67, 1963.
200. Johansen, J. G.: Arthrography with Amipaque and other contrast media. Invest. Radiol. *11*:534, 1976.
201. Joyce, J. W., Dalrimple, G. V., Jungkind, F. F., et al.: Improved contrast in subtraction technique. Radiology *94*:157, 1970.
202. Katzberg, R. W.: Evaluation of various contrast agents for improved arthrography. Invest. Radiol. *11*:528, 1976.
203. Mink, J. H.: Air vs. CO_2 for knee arthrography. A. J. R. *134*:991, 1980.
204. Murray, R. C.: Transitory eosinophilia localized to the knee joint. J. Bone Joint Surg. *32B*:74, 1950.
205. Pastershank, S. P.: Effect of water soluble contrast medium on the synovial membrane. Radiology *143*:331, 1982.
206. Spataro, R. F.: Epinephrine enhanced knee arthrography. Invest. Radiol. *13*:286, 1978.
207. Winkler, N. T.: Roentgenographic subtraction technique. Radiol. Tech. *39* (6):339, 1968.

FRACTURE HEALING

JAMES A. RAND • *THOMAS H. BERQUIST*

INTRODUCTION

Trauma is a frequent occurrence in our highly mechanized society. Injuries to the axial skeleton and limbs are common problems for the orthopedic surgeon and radiologist. Fracture recognition, assessment of the etiologic mechanism, and determination of the extent of healing are essential in patient management. Accurate description of the fractures and changes noted on the post-reduction radiographs is an essential part of communication between the radiologist and the orthopedic surgeon. Recognition of the failure or orderly progress of fracture union will aid in deciding upon an appropriate course of management.

Types of Fractures

There are many common labels that describe the various types of fractures and fracture-dislocations. Terms such as clay shoveler's fracture, Monteggia fracture, and greenstick fracture may be well understood.[10, 42, 128, 145, 180] However, these labels are often misused, and proper description of the bony and ligamentous injury is preferred. The detection of fractures may be somewhat difficult, although in most situations the abnormality is readily identified. All too often, however, the interpreter of the film gives a less than complete description of the injury.

Evaluation of skeletal trauma should begin with a thorough evaluation of the soft tissues, tissue planes, and fat pads. The skin and soft tissues are intact in closed fractures. Disruption of the soft tissues results in an open or compound fracture.[180] Displacement of the fat pads of the elbow (Fig. 2–1), the pronator fat stripe of the distal radius (Fig. 2–2), and the navicular fat stripe may be the only clues to the presence of subtle fractures. Another helpful finding is the presence of a lipohemarthrosis (fat-blood level) in the joint, which indicates an intracapsular fracture (Fig. 2–3).

Fractures may be complete (both cortices interrupted) or incomplete (one cortex fractured). Incomplete fractures generally occur in children. The following is a list of the commonly encountered incomplete fractures:

1. Torus fracture. An incomplete fracture resulting in buckling of the cortex (Fig. 2–4).

2. Greenstick fracture. Interruption of one cortex with angulation resembling a broken branch (Fig. 2–5).

3. Microfracture or bowing fracture. A bending

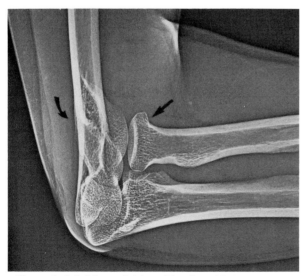

Figure 2–1. Subtle radial head fracture *(straight arrow)*. The posterior fat pad *(curved arrow)* is elevated owing to hemarthrosis. This may be the only indication of a fracture.

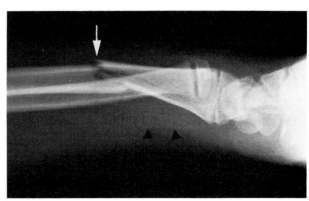

Figure 2–2. Fracture of the distal radial shaft *(arrow)*. The pronator fat stripe is displaced *(double arrows)*. In certain cases the displaced fat stripe may be the only indication of a subtle fracture.

51

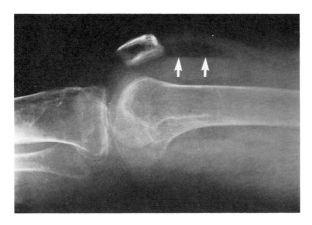

Figure 2–3. Cross-table lateral view of the knee. There is a lipohem-arthrosis in the suprapatellar region *(arrows)* indicating an intracap-sular fracture.

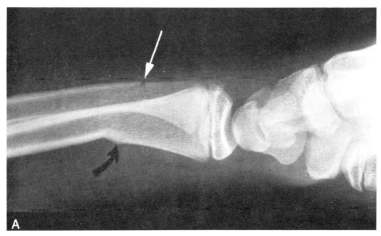

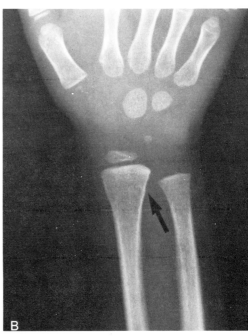

Figure 2–4. A, Lateral view of the wrist. There is a greenstick fracture of the distal ulna *(straight arrow)* and a torus fracture of the volar surface of the distal radius *(curved arrow).* Note the displaced pronator fat stripe. *B,* AP view of the wrist. Subtle torus fracture of the distal radius *(arrow).*

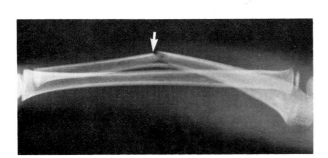

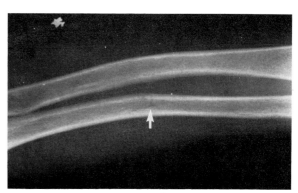

Figure 2–5   Figure 2–6

Figure 2–5. Forearm. There is a greenstick fracture *(arrow)* of the ulnar midshaft.

Figure 2–6. Forearm. Bowing fractures of both the radius and ulna are present. A small lucent fracture line *(arrow)* is evident in the midulna.

fracture that commonly involves the radius and ulna (Fig. 2–6). Often there is no obvious fracture line.[24, 25]

4. Growth plate or physeal fracture. A subtle fracture of the growth plate and associated metaphysis or epiphysis which can be easily overlooked. This group of fractures has been classified by Salter and Harris.[177] In Type I, the fracture involves the growth plate but spares the epiphysis and metaphysis (Fig. 2–7A). In Type II, the fracture involves the growth plate and exits through the metaphysis (Fig. 2–7B). In Type III, the fracture involves the growth plate and exits through the epiphysis (Fig. 2–7C). In Type IV, the fracture line extends through the epiphysis, growth plate, and metaphysis (Fig. 2–7A). Finally, in Type V, the growth plate is impacted or crushed (Fig. 2–7A).

Complete fractures involve both cortices with a

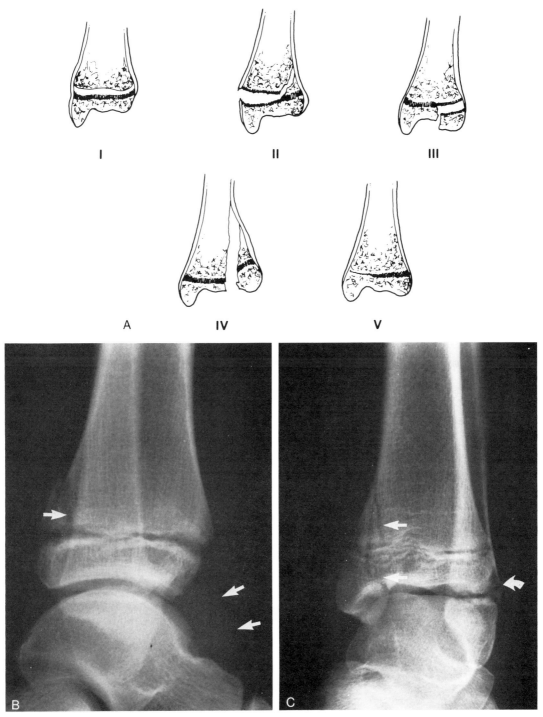

Figure 2–7. A, Illustration of Salter-Harris Types I to V. B, Lateral view of ankle. There is a Salter-Harris Type II fracture *(arrow).* Note the effusion in the joint space *(double arrow).* C, Oblique view of the ankle in different patient. Salter-Harris Type IV fracture medially *(double arrows)* and a subtle Type II fracture of the fibula *(curved arrow).*

lucent line through the medullary portion of the bone. These fractures may be transverse, oblique, spiral, or comminuted. Depression fractures, such as those seen with cancellous bone in the region of the tibial plateau, also occur (Fig. 2–8). Compression fractures occur in the vertebral body and may involve the anterior or lateral cortex (Fig. 2–9). Avulsion fractures occur at the insertion of ligaments or tendons (Fig. 2–10). Pathologic fractures involve bone with some underlying abnormality such as metabolic disease or neoplasia (Fig. 2–11). Stress fractures are incomplete fractures due to chronic overuse of normal bone and are most often seen in the metatarsals of military recruits and in the femoral necks, pubic rami, and tibias of long-distance runners (Fig. 2–12).[180] (See Chapter 15, Stress Fractures.) The insufficiency fracture is a special example of the stress fracture.[152] Abnormal bone gives way under stresses that would not be excessive under normal circumstances. An example is a stress fracture affecting the tibia or femoral neck in a patient with rheumatoid arthritis who becomes too active too soon after total joint arthroplasty.

Radiographic Description of Fractures and Fracture-dislocations

Table 2–1 offers an outline approach to the description of fractures or fracture-dislocations.[160] A general description of the fracture should be provided first. This should include the date, time of

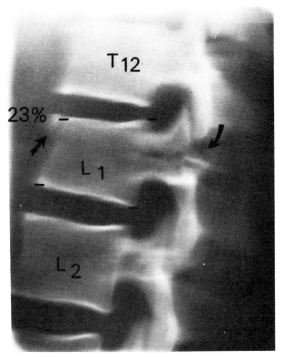

Figure 2–9. Lateral view thoracolumbar spine. A compression of the anterior aspect of the L1 vertebral body *(arrow at 23 percent)* is demonstrated. A distraction fracture of the posterior elements *(curved arrow)* is also present.

day, and projections obtained. Is the fracture transverse or oblique? Is there significant soft tissue involvement? The location should be specified (epiphysis, metaphysis, or shaft). Fractures of the shaft can be conveniently divided into mid, proximal or

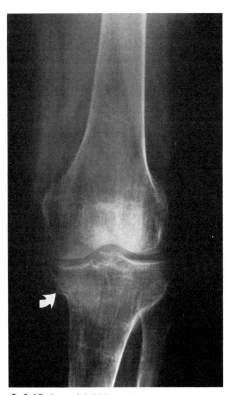

Figure 2–8. AP view of right knee. There is a depressed cortical fracture of the upper tibia *(arrow).*

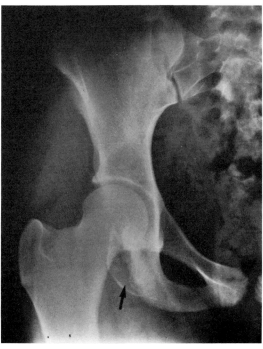

Figure 2–10. Avulsion fracture of the ischial margin *(arrow).*

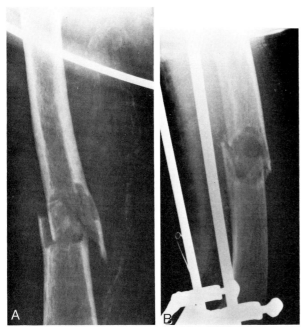

Figure 2–11. AP *(A)* and lateral *(B)* views of the femur demonstrate a pathologic fracture through a metastatic neoplasm.

distal thirds (Fig. 2–13*A*). The anatomic description of the position of the fracture fragments should be given. This includes the apposition of the fragments and whether or not there has been any change in the anatomic length of the part. Fractures may be impacted, which imparts some degree of stability (Figs. 2–14 and 2–15). Distraction or separation of the fracture fragments may be the result of traction devices or soft tissue interposition. These factors should be carefully reported.

Any angulation of the fracture fragments should

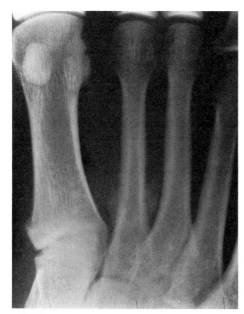

Figure 2–12. Stress fracture of the 2nd metatarsal with callus formation.

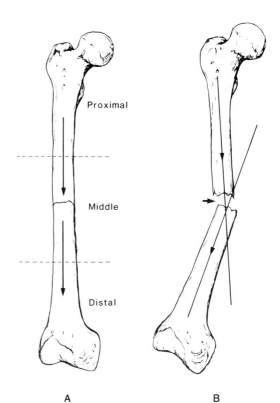

A   B

Figure 2–13. *A,* The femoral shaft and other long bones can be divided into thirds for purposes of fracture description. In discussing alignment the longitudinal axis is described *(arrow)*. *B,* A transverse fracture of the midshaft of the femur is demonstrated. Angulation may be described by the direction of the apex, in which case there is medial angulation *(arrow)* and distraction of the fracture fragments. Angulation may also be described by the direction of the distal fragment. In this illustration the distal fragment is laterally angulated.

also be discussed in the radiographic report (Figs. 2–13*B*, 2–14, and 2–16). There are two commonly used methods for describing fracture angulation.[160] We prefer to describe angulation according to the direction of the apex of the fracture fragments (Fig. 2–16). One may also report angulation according to

TABLE 2–1. Skeletal Injury. Radiographic Description of Fractures and Fracture Dislocations

 I. Fractures
  A. General description
   1. Date and time
   2. Projections obtained
   3. Type of fracture
   4. Soft tissue evaluation
  B. Location
  C. Anatomic position of fragments
   1. Length and apposition
   2. Angulation
   3. Displacement
   4. Rotation
  D. Further imaging techniques
 II. Dislocations/subluxations
  A. Degree of displacement
  B. Joint space
  C. Associated fractures
   1. Location
   2. Articular involvement

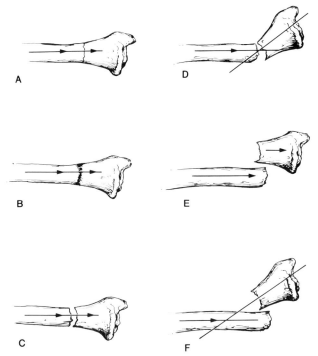

A

B

C

D

E

F

Figure 2–14. Illustration of fractures. *A,* An undisplaced fracture of the distal shaft with normal alignment and no displacement. *B,* An impacted fracture of the distal shaft with normal alignment. No angulation or rotation is present. *C,* A distracted fracture with no loss of alignment or angulation. *D,* Distal shaft fracture with angulation. *E,* Transverse fracture of the distal shaft with displacement. Alignment is maintained (*arrows* mark longitudinal axis), and there is no angulation or rotation. Shortening is evident. *F,* Distal shaft fracture with both displacement and angulation. Shortening is also evident.

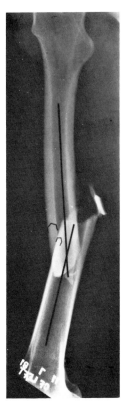

Figure 2–16. AP view of the right femur. There is a comminuted overriding fracture of the femur at the junction of the middle and distal thirds. The fracture is angulated medially, and considerable rotation of the distal fragment is evident. (Note upper shaft in AP and lower shaft in lateral position.) Cortical thickness (brackets) at the fracture site is not uniform, which is another indication of rotation.

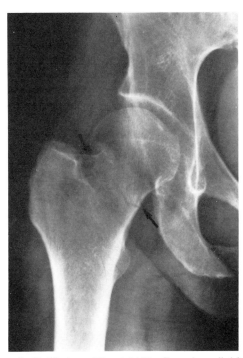

Figure 2–15. AP view of the right hip. The subcapital fracture is complete, involving both cortices *(arrows).* There is impaction of the lateral cortex *(curved arrow).*

the direction of the distal fragment. For example, fragments can be said to be angulated medially (varus) (Fig. 2–16), or alternatively, the distal fragment can be said to be angulated laterally (valgus). Displacement describes any change in the anatomic axis of the components of the fracture. Overriding or displacement of comminuted fragments should be noted. Rotation of the fragments, particularly common with spiral fractures of the metacarpals and tibia, may pose significant treatment problems. The fracture of the femur in Figure 2–16 is rotated. Note that the proximal fragment is visualized in the AP projection, and the distal fragment is seen laterally. The thickness of the cortex at the fracture site is also an important indicator of rotation.

Following complete interpretation of the radiographs, any additional views that may be helpful in further evaluation should be mentioned. In certain cases, tomography, computed tomography, and nuclear medicine studies may be indicated.

Descriptions of subluxations and dislocations should include the degree of displacement of the articular surfaces. If the subluxation involves the spine (Fig. 2–17), the upper vertebral body should be described in relation to the body below. In the peripheral skeleton the distal fragment is described

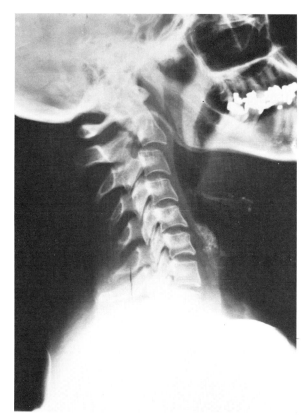

Figure 2–17. Lateral cervical spine. Pedicle fractures at the C2 level result in anterior subluxation of C2 and C3.

TABLE 2–2. Skeletal Injury. A Structured Approach to Interpretation of Post-reduction Radiographs

I. Interval change
    A. Change in apposition
    B. Change in angulation
    C. Distraction or impaction
II. Healing process
    A. Callus formation
    B. Evidence of delayed union or non-union
III. Internal fixation devices (position of rods, screws, and pins)
IV. Additional imaging techniques

demonstrate these changes as well as increased distraction (as a result of soft tissue interposition or excessive traction). Evidence of callus formation should be mentioned, though the diagnosis of fracture healing is made clinically. If an internal or external fixation device is in place, the position of the device should be compared with that of previous films. Evidence of loosening, metal fracture, or improper positioning should be noted (Fig. 2–19). Irregularity and sclerosis of the opposing fracture fragments may indicate delayed union or non-union. Serial films are most helpful in this determination. As with prereduction radiographs, additional images may be helpful in evaluating the healing process. Tomography, CT, or isotope studies may be indicated if evidence of delayed union or non-union, or infection, is present. Comments regarding direct care of the patient, such as acceptability of the position of the fragments, should be avoided.[160] Radiographs do not present the entire clinical situation.

Phases of Fracture Healing

Fracture healing may be divided into three phases: (1) inflammatory, (2) reparative, and (3) remodeling (Fig. 2–20).[47]

The inflammatory phase comprises 10 percent, the reparative phase 40 percent, and the remodeling phase 70 percent of the time to fracture union.[47] These phases are not distinct, there being a significant overlap between them. The inflammatory phase consists of hematoma formation, osteocyte death, vasodilatation, and migration of acute inflammatory cells into the wound.[47] There is a prominent hematoma present as well as necrotic fracture ends. The reparative phase consists of vascular dilatation, which involves the entire vascular bed of the affected limb, new vessel proliferation, mesenchymal cell proliferation, change from an acid to alkaline pH, and collagen production in the wound.[47] There is prominent granulation tissue present as well as early cartilage and bone formation. The remodeling phase consists of osteoblastic resorption and new bone formation.[47] During this late phase in fracture healing, there is prominent endosteal and periosteal callus formation. Revascularization of the bone occurs.

in relation to the proximal fragment. Figure 2–18 demonstrates dorsal dislocation of the middle phalanx in relation to the proximal phalanx. Evaluation of the joint space should also be discussed, as ligament interposition or osteochondral fragments may result in joint-space widening. This is especially important following reduction. The location and the degree of articular involvement of any associated fractures should also be described.

Careful reporting of post-reduction views is also important (Table 2–2). Any interval changes in position of the fracture fragments should be noted. Has there been a change in bony apposition or angulation? Fractures treated with traction may

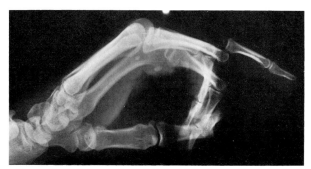

Figure 2–18. Lateral view of the middle finger. There is dorsal dislocation of the middle phalanx on the proximal phalanx. The articular surfaces are completely disrupted.

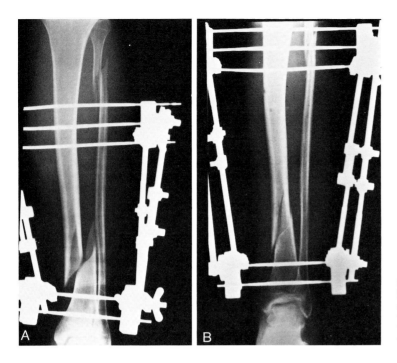

Figure 2–19. AP views of the tibia and fibula. There are spiral fractures of the distal tibia and proximal fibula with Hoffman fixation. *A,* There is considerable overriding and rotation is also evident. *B,* Adjusting the fixation device has resulted in improved position. There is good apposition and little overriding of the fracture fragments.

Figure 2–20. Phases of fracture healing. (From Cruess, R. L., and Dumont, J.: Fracture healing. Can. J. Surg. *18:*403, 1975.)

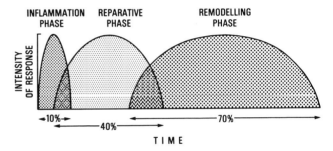

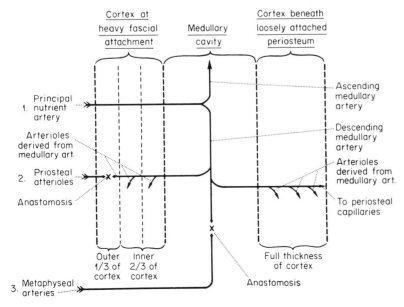

Figure 2–21. Afferent blood supply of bone and sites of anastomosis. The afferent vascular system brings blood to every portion of a long bone and includes three primary components that together form the total nutrient supply. The components include (1) the principal nutrient artery, (2) the metaphyseal arteries, and (3) the periosteal arterioles. (From F. W. Rhinelander: Circulation in bone. *In* Bourne, G. H.: The Biochemistry and Physiology of Bone, Vol. II, Chapter 1. New York, Academic Press, 1972, p. 1–77.)

Fracture repair may be conceptually divided into those events associated with the soft tissue proliferation and those related to mineralization of the callus. The initial fibroblastic proliferation is associated with an increase in proteoglycans. As chondroblasts and osteoblasts proliferate, collagen production increases and is associated with a decrease in proteoglycans. Mineralization of the matrix occurs later. Finally, bone remodeling results in a return to normal.

Vascular Supply of Bone

A knowledge of the normal blood supply of a long bone is the key to understanding fracture repair. The normal afferent blood supply to a mature, mammalian tubular bone consists of three parts: (1) the nutrient artery, (2) the metaphyseal arteries, and (3) the periosteal arteries (Fig. 2–21).[34, 102, 139, 167, 179] Upon entering the medullary cavity, the nutrient artery divides into two major branches that ascend and descend within the shaft. Arterial sub-branches form two parallel arterial supplies, one to the cortex and another to the marrow.[120, 189] The cortical branches give rise to branches oriented parallel to the shaft as well as to radially directed vessels.[124, 198] Conduit vessels connect the arteriolar system with the periosteal vessels (Fig. 2–22).[124] The smaller arterioles supply capillaries to the haversian canals.[102, 124] The haversian canals are connected to osteocytes via canaliculi.[85] Some authors have suggested that the inner two thirds to three quarters of the cortex is supplied by the nutrient system,[34, 98, 167, 172, 201] while the outer one third is supplied by the periosteal vessels.[166, 201] More recent authors state that the endosteal system supplies the majority of blood to the cortex.[124, 198] The metaphyseal arteries supply blood to the metaphysis and anastomose with the medullary arteries.[167, 201]

The efferent or venous drainage of a long bone consists of three parts: (1) the emissary veins and the vena comitans of the nutrient artery, (2) the cortical venous channels, and (3) the periosteal capillaries.[167] The emissary veins and vena comitans of the nutrient artery are derived from the central venous sinus in the medullary canal and are involved primarily in drainage of the marrow.[124, 167] The majority of the cortical bone venous drainage takes place through the periosteal capillaries.[124] In contrast, Trias and colleagues feel that the majority of the cortical venous drainage is centripetal into the sinusoidal system in the marrow.[198]

The normal circulatory pattern of diaphyseal cortex is one of centrifugal flow from the endosteum

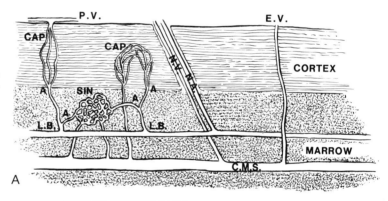

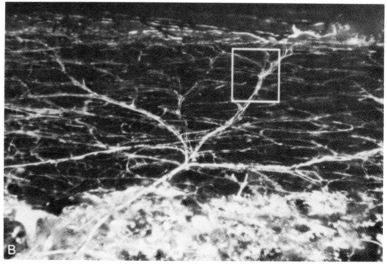

Figure 2–22. A, Circulation of the tibial diaphysis. N. A., Nutrient artery; N. V., Nutrient vein; C. M. S., Central medullary sinus; A, Arterioles; SIN, Medullary sinusoids; L. B., Lateral branches of nutrient artery; CAP, Haversian capillaries; P. V., Periosteal vein; E. V., Emissary vein. *B,* Branches of the nutrient artery in diaphyseal cortex. (From Lopez-Curto, J. A., et al.: Anatomy of the microvasculature of the tibial diaphysis of the adult dog. J. Bone Joint Surg. *62A:*1362, 1980.)

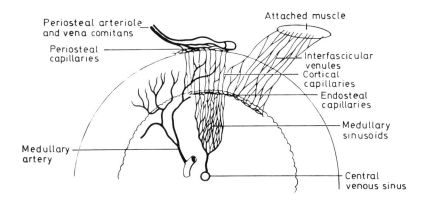

Figure 2–23. Centrifugal flow of blood from endosteum to periosteum. (From Brookes, M.: The Blood Supply of Bone. London, Butterworth, 1971, p. 119.)

to the periosteum (Fig. 2–23).[34, 167, 168] This pattern of flow may be reversed in pathologic conditions, such as after fracture.[34]

Key sites of anastomosis between the three components of the afferent vascular system exist.[139, 167, 201] An anastomosis exists between the nutrient medullary vessels and the metaphyseal vessels at the ends of the medullary cavity. An anastomosis also exists between the nutrient-medullary system and the periosteal vessels in the outer cortex. These anastomoses are of key importance when one of these vascular systems is disrupted, as in the period following fracture.

The relative importance of the three afferent components for maintenance of viability of the diaphyseal cortex has been investigated. In the adult mammal, the primary source of blood supply to the diaphyseal cortex is the nutrient system.[98, 148] Shim and colleagues have shown that the nutrient artery supplies at least 46 percent of the total blood supply of the femur.[184] The nutrient artery supplies at least 71 percent of the total blood supply of the shaft and 35 percent of the total blood supply of the metaphyseal-epiphyseal area. After nutrient-artery ligation, 63 percent of the normal flow through the upper epiphysis, 30 percent of the flow through the shaft, and 67 percent of the flow through the lower epiphysis and metaphysis are still intact.[184] The nutrient artery is responsible for 70 percent, and the epiphyseal-metaphyseal system for 30 percent, of the blood flow to a long bone.[184] The metaphyseal vessels are second in importance after the nutrient system, and the periosteal vessels are least important.[98] Although the periosteal vessels are of minor importance in supplying blood to the normal cortex, they do supply the vessels for the development of new haversian systems on the external surface of the cortex.[139]

Blood Flow in Bone

The circulation of blood through bone is necessary for osteogenesis, the maintenance of bone vitality, bone growth, and repair of fractures.[183] Blood flow in the entire skeleton of animals has been estimated to be between 4 and 10 percent of

the resting cardiac output[183] and 5.2 to 6.9 percent in the dog.[212] In the conscious dog, bone blood flow is 9.6 percent (mature) and 10.3 percent (immature) of the cardiac output.[134] In man, skeletal blood flow has been estimated as 5 percent of the resting cardiac output.[186]

Blood flow through various regions of bone varies, as does blood flow between different bones within an animal and blood flow in immature as opposed to mature animals. Weinman and colleagues noted blood flows of 7.7 ml per min per 100 gm in the tibias of immature dogs compared with 5.6 ml per min per 100 gm in mature dogs.[212] Morris and Kelly, using microspheres in mature dogs, found blood-flow values of 2.46 ml per min per 100 gm in cortical bone and 38.3 ml per min per 100 gm in cancellous bone.[134] Higher perfusion values have been noted for immature as opposed to mature dogs.[214] Kane and Grim, using potassium-42 and rubidium-86 clearance in dogs, noted considerable variation in blood-flow rates in ml per min per 100 gm between the humerus, tibia, and femur.[101] They also noted variation in blood flow in various regions of bone, with the epiphysis having a higher rate of blood flow than the shaft and the marrow having a higher rate of flow than the cortex.[101] Whiteside and colleagues noted a higher flow in the metaphysis than in the epiphysis and least flow in the diaphysis.[214] Brookes, using chromium-51–labeled red cells in the femur of rats, noted greatest to least blood flow in the following order: inferior metaphysis, marrow, superior metaphysis, inferior epiphysis, and finally cortex.[33] Since there was a variation in blood-flow rate in compact and cancellous bone, Brookes felt that vascular factors might have a major function in the local control of normal bone formation and bone repair.[33] Whiteside and colleagues, using hydrogen washout in rabbits, noted a positive correlation between blood-flow rate and the histologic level of osteoblastic activity in the skeleton.[214] Another possible function of the heterogeneity of bone blood flow might be to regulate the mineral reservoir in order to stabilize ion levels in bone.[27]

Various factors may contribute to the regulation of blood flow. Shim and Patterson have noted that the osseous circulation is affected by changes in the

TABLE 2–3. Factors Involved in Blood Flow Regulation

Systemic	Local
Cardiovascular condition	Arterial occlusion
Hypoxia	Muscle contraction
Hypercapnia	Sympathetic nerve stimulation
Hormonal	

systemic cardiovascular condition, such as local femoral arterial occlusion and systemic hypoxia and hypercapnia (Table 2–3).[187] They felt that neural, hormonal, and metabolic factors, both local and systemic, control blood flow. Shim and colleagues have also noted that sympathetic nerve stimulation and skeletal muscle contraction affect blood flow.[185]

Many different methods of studying the rate of normal blood flow have been used, and estimates of blood flow in normal bone vary widely. Direct and indirect methods of measuring blood flow in bone have been used. Excellent summaries of the various techniques and their limitations have been published by Kelly[102] and Shim.[183]

PHYSIOLOGY OF FRACTURE HEALING

The Vascular Response to Fracture

The vasculature serves a key function in fracture healing. Albrecht von Haller, in 1763, stated that "the origin of bone is the artery carrying the blood and in it the mineral elements."[83] The most important histologic elements for bony callus formation are osteoblasts and the vascular proliferation that occurs after fracture.[193] Blaisdell and Cowan felt that the manner and branching of the new blood vessels determined the orientation and position of the early bony trabeculae.[21] Osteogenesis is carried on by cells carried into the fibrocartilaginous callus by the proliferating vasculature.[206] Trueta believed that the endothelial cells of the new blood vessels divide at both ends and along large sections of the vessel walls, laying down a progeny of osteoblasts.[199] These cells remain attached by cytoplasmic processes that are retained in bone as bone matrix is laid down around the cells.[194] The new vessels invade and resorb dead bone, with new bone formation occurring adjacent to them.[158] The new vasculature appears at the fracture ends and the pericallus soft tissue.[193] As maturation of the cells occurs, the vessels are oriented parallel to the bone axis, anastomoses develop, and normal vascularization is restored.[194]

Along with vascular proliferation following fracture, blood flow also undergoes a local change. Wray and Lynch noted an increase in the vascular volume of the affected limb by the third day after fracture, with a peak at 9 days, followed by a gradual return to normal levels.[222] Laurnen and Kelly noted an increase in blood flow to bone in canine tibial fractures by the first day after fracture,

with a peak of six times normal at 2 weeks, followed by a gradual return to normal (Fig. 2–24).[118] They did not find any significant changes in oxygen, carbon dioxide, or pH levels. They concluded that an increase in blood flow in bone was the primary homeostatic mechanism responsible for supplying the increased metabolic requirements of the healing fracture. Paradis and Kelly found a significant correlation between blood flow in bone and mineral deposition in canine tibial fractures.[150] They also noted an increase in blood flow in bone with a peak 10 days after fracture. Hughes and colleagues found that the increase in blood flow following a fracture represents recruitment of capillaries.[91] Thus, following a fracture, vessels increase in size and number, and blood flow also increases.

The importance of the three afferent sources of blood supply to a long bone in contributing to fracture healing has been debated. Cavadias and Trueta performed vascular suppression of two of the three afferent sources of blood supply to healing osteotomies of the radius in rabbits.[39] When the nutrient vessels were the only source of blood supply to the fracture, no periosteal callus was noted, union occurred by endosteal callus and was delayed compared with that in controls, and there was decreased breaking strength of the callus. When the metaphyseal-epiphyseal vessels were the only source of blood supply, extensive necrosis of the cortex occurred despite patent medullary vessels on arteriograms, and union was delayed. When the periosteal vessels were the only source of blood

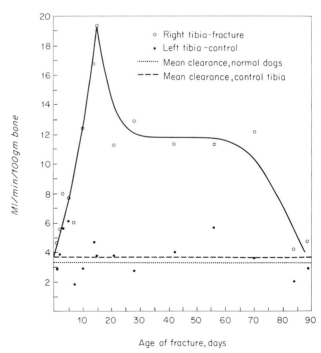

Figure 2–24. Vascular response following fracture. (From Laurnen, E. L., and Kelly, P. J.: Blood flow, oxygen consumption, carbon-dioxide production and blood-calcium and pH changes in tibial fractures in dogs. J. Bone Joint Surg. *51A:*298, 1969.)

supply, the periosteal callus appeared normally, necrosis of the inner one half of the cortex occurred, no endosteal callus was present, union occurred by periosteal callus, and a late revascularization of the inner cortex by the periosteal vessels occurred. Johnson studied the repair of canine tibial defects after suppression of blood supply to bone.[98] He found that the nutrient vessels alone would maintain viability of the inner one half of the cortex and allow active repair of the defect. The metaphyseal vessels would maintain viability of the medulla but would not support active repair of the defect. The periosteal vessels alone were not able to support any active repair or serve as a collateral source of blood supply during the 4 weeks of the experiment. Johnson concluded that the nutrient vessels were the most important, the metaphyseal vessels of intermediary importance, and the periosteal vessels of least importance in the repair of a bone defect.[98]

The relative importance of the periosteal compared with the endosteal blood supply in contributing to fracture union has been contested. Kolodny felt that the periosteal blood supply was essential for normal union of osteotomies of the radius in dogs and that the periosteal callus was more important than the endosteal callus for fracture union.[108] Destruction of the nutrient artery affected fracture healing only in cases in which the periosteal vessels had been destroyed.[108] Wray, in studying rabbit tibial fractures, felt that the periosteal vascular system as augmented by vessels from the surrounding soft tissues was the major source for vascularization of the forming callus.[221] He felt that the interosseous circulation was not important in fracture healing. Holden emphasized the importance of the vessels derived from the surrounding soft tissues.[90] In rabbits with segmental-displaced fractures of the radius, he noted that revascularization of the entire thickness of the cortex occurred by periosteal vessels prior to re-establishment of continuity of the medullary vessels. If the surrounding muscles were made ischemic, revascularization of the bone was delayed until after revascularization of the muscle had occurred.

In contrast, other authors have felt that the medullary vascular system is more important for fracture healing than the periosteal system. Ladanyi and Hidvegi, in studying osteotomies of the ulna in dogs, found that response from the medullary vascular system appeared earlier in the fracture area and was consistently richer than the periosteal response.[113] Rhinelander feels that the medullary arterial system derived from the nutrient and metaphyseal vessels remains dominant throughout fracture healing.[169] He claims that the periosteal vessels play a significant role only in the vicinity of fascial attachments and that this new external blood supply is distinct from the normal one. Rhinelander stated that the new periosteal blood supply is derived entirely from extraosseous arterial systems and is only facultative in regard to its bone function.

This extraosseous blood supply is derived from ruptured capillaries and arterioles in torn muscle that combine with torn periosteal arterioles. The extraosseous blood supply is transitory and persists only until the medullary vessels have regenerated and restored the normal centrifugal flow of blood through the cortex.

A partial explanation for the discrepancy of opinion concerning the relative importance of the periosteal and medullary systems for fracture union may be found if differences in displaced and undisplaced fractures are taken into account. The vascular changes in the healing of displaced and undisplaced diaphyseal fractures differ. In undisplaced fractures, not all vascular connections adjacent to the fracture are severed.[170] The majority of the blood supply for revascularization is derived from the medullary circulation, which furnishes the major portion of the blood supply to the uniting callus and revascularizes the necrotic cortex at the fracture.[170] The medullary vascular system remains dominant throughout all stages of healing and the periosteal vessels have only a limited role.[160] In contrast, in displaced fractures the proliferation of the disrupted endosteal vessels is initially blocked by the hematoma.[172] The periosteal circulation, augmented by vessels from the surrounding soft tissues, is the initial source of blood supply to the fracture and supplies the external callus. If stable reduction is maintained, early regeneration of the medullary vessels may occur; but if reduction is unstable, regeneration of medullary vessels is delayed by the interposition of fibrocartilage in the fracture site. As the medullary vessels regenerate, they become dominant and supply the area of earliest osseous union. Therefore, in both undisplaced and displaced fractures, the medullary circulation remains dominant and supplies the area of earliest osseous union.[172]

The function of the vascular dilatation after fracture is to supply nutrients to the healing fracture. Oxygen is a prime nutrient, yet controversy exists concerning the optimum oxygen concentrations for fracture union. Sim and Kelly, in comparing bone remodeling, oxygen consumption, and blood flow in canine tibias, found the arteriovenous oxygen difference (i.e., oxygen extraction) unchanged in high, normal, or low remodeling states.[188] However, they did note a close correlation between the rate of bone remodeling, oxygen consumption, and the rate of blood flow in bone. In high remodeling states there was an increase in oxygen consumption, which correlated with an increased rate of blood flow. They concluded that alterations in blood flow were important in meeting the nutritional demands of active tissue.

Brighton and Krebs studied oxygen tension in healing fibular fractures in the rabbit.[32] They noted the lowest oxygen tension in newly formed cartilage and fiber bone, and the highest values in fibrous tissue in the callus. Biomechanical evaluation of fracture stiffness in a three-point bending test revealed a return to control levels of stiffness prior to an increase in oxygen tension at the fracture site. Oxygen tension at the fracture site did not rise to normal diaphyseal levels until the medullary canal was reconstituted. They concluded that the low oxygen tension at the fracture site might be a stimulus to osteoblast proliferation and calcium release.

In contrast, Ham felt that osteogenic cells in the presence of an adequate blood supply and calcium would form bone but in the absence of an adequate blood supply and calcium would form cartilage.[84] Bassett, in studying chick mesenchymal cells in tissue culture, noted cellular differentiation into bone in the presence of a high-oxygen environment, whereas cartilage was formed in a low-oxygen environment.[15] Heppenstall and colleagues studied the effect of chronic hypoxia on the healing of fibular fractures in the dog.[89] They noted decreased new bone formation and decreased biomechanical strength of the fracture in the hypoxic dogs as compared with controls. They felt that the poor fracture healing in these dogs might be attributable to a loss of the normal oxygen gradient across the fracture.

Biochemical studies have shown the importance of oxidative metabolism for fracture healing. Kuhlman and Bakowski, in studying the enzyme content of fracture callus, noted that the process of bone repair relied upon oxidative carbohydrate metabolism, which indicated the importance of an adequate blood supply for fracture healing.[109] Ketenjian and Arsenis noted that a shift to oxidative glycolysis occurred with cartilage maturation in the callus.[103] They felt that this finding supported the concept of oxybiotic metabolism in the fracture during the early stages of vascular invasion.

In summary, the vascular response following fracture, which consists of new vessel proliferation and increased blood flow, serves as an important homeostatic mechanism for the supply of the increased metabolic requirements necessary for the healing fracture.

Cellular Response to Fracture

The basic requirements for bone formation are the presence of free circulatory elements, adequate surfaces on which bone formation may take place, and cells with osteogenic potency.[196] The origin of the cells involved in fracture repair and the relative contributions of the periosteum and the endosteum have been the subject of controversy. As early as 1740, Duhamel considered the periosteum as osteogenic, while Haller considered the endosteum and haversian canals as most significant for fracture union.[20] Todd and Iler felt that both the periosteal and endosteal cells were of major importance, while the cells of compact bone were of minor impor-

tance.[194] Enneking found that periosteal activity following a fracture preceded endosteal cellular activity.[65] The endosteal reaction followed the periosteal reaction by 48 hours but was of equal intensity and duration.[65] Slatis and Rokkanen stated that the intense proliferation of the periosteal osteogenic cells was responsible for the majority of the initial callus.[190]

The cells involved in the repair of a fracture include osteogenic cells derived from the cambium layer of the periosteum, from Volkmann's and haversian canals, and from the endosteum.[20, 65, 206] Undifferentiated surrounding mesenchymal cells as well as cells derived from the new vasculature may play a role (Table 2–4).[199, 206] Bassett and Ruedi have shown that bone formation may occur in a bone defect isolated from the periosteum and endosteum, indicating the osteogenic potential of cells lining Volkmann's and haversian canals.[18]

Controversy has also surrounded the relative importance of the endosteal and periosteal callus in securing fracture union. Lexer felt that the periosteal callus was most important in fracture union,[120] while Bier felt that the endosteal callus was most important.[108] The periosteum has been noted to form the earliest callus following a fracture, while the endosteum forms callus only after the intraosseous circulation has recovered.[108] Phemister thought that the periosteum was very important for fracture healing and noted that excision of the periosteum delayed callus formation and ossification and predisposed to delayed union.[158] Subperiosteal osteoblasts play a very active role in periosteal callus formation.[181] Therefore, excessive periosteal stripping at operation should be avoided to prevent damage to the blood supply of the bone.[76] Periosteal stripping may devitalize the underlying bone and damage the cambium layer of the periosteum.[194] In healing of bone defects, the presence of periosteum allows union; in the absence of periosteum, nonunion occurs.[138] It has been stated that mineralized periosteal callus is the first callus to span the fracture gap.[140] In contrast, other authors have found that the endosteal callus unites the fracture prior to the bridging of the fracture gap by the periosteal callus.[65, 169] Rhinelander stated that the medullary callus was always the first to accomplish osseous union, with the periosteal callus functioning as an ancillary external support.[169]

Thus, both periosteal and endosteal callus are important in fracture union, with their relative contributions depending upon the initial displacement

TABLE 2–4. Cells Involved in Fracture Repair

Undifferentiated mesenchymal
Cambium layer of periosteum
Volkmann's canals
Haversian canals
Endosteum
Vascular

of the fracture, the degree of initial trauma, and the stability of immobilization during treatment.

BIOMECHANICS OF FRACTURE HEALING

Biomechanics of Normal Bone

A knowledge of the effect of various stresses upon normal bone and its general mechanical properties is important for understanding the response of bone to fracture and internal fixation. As Wolff pointed out in 1892, "Every change in the form and function of a bone, or of its function alone, is followed by certain definite changes in its internal architecture and equally definite secondary alterations in the external conformation in accordance with mathematical laws."[219] The ability of bone to adapt to stress becomes progressively more apparent when the morphology of the trabecular pattern of the femoral neck and head is viewed on a phylogenetic basis.[197] A similar phenomenon may be seen during normal growth and development. A change in the posture of the human infant is reflected in changes in the trabecular pattern of the femoral head.[197]

Various theories have been advanced to explain the mechanical basis for these morphological findings. According to Scott, there are five theories concerning the mechanical structure of bone.[181] Bone may be formed along lines of tension or pressure stress. Pressure from either weight-bearing or muscle action may determine bone structure. The internal architecture of bone may follow its external conformation, with functional demands playing only a secondary role in its modification. The vascular pattern may determine bony architecture. Or, finally, the elastic recoil of bone following loading may affect bone structure. The actual mechanical structure of bone is probably affected by all of the factors mentioned in these various theories. Most importantly, bone is able to respond to applied stress. Glucksmann has shown experimentally that bone growth may be affected by applied forces.[77] *In vitro* endosteal chick cultures, when subjected to tension, form bone oriented perpendicular to the tension force; and when subjected to compression, the endosteal cultures form bone oriented parallel to the compression force.[77] If the longitudinal growth of chick rudiments is inhibited *in vitro*, ossification will always be greater on the convex side.[78] Thus bone formation responds to applied stresses. Additionally, Bassett has shown that *in vitro* mesenchymal cell differentiation is affected by the mechanical environment (Table 2–5).[15] In the presence of compression plus adequate oxygen, bone is formed. In contrast, in the presence of tension plus adequate oxygen, fibrous tissue is formed.

The material properties of bone are unique and must be considered when analyzing the mechanical

TABLE 2–5. Mechanical and Biologic Factors Affecting Osteogenic Cell Differentiation

Environment	Tissue Formed
Compression plus high O_2	Bone
Compression plus low O_2	Cartilage
Tension plus high O_2	Fibrous tissue

structure of bone. Bone is nonisotropic and viscoelastic.[37, 55] As a nonisotropic material, it has different properties in different directions. As a viscoelastic material, it is a material whose characteristic constants are affected by the rate of deformation. Any material, including bone, may be characterized by three such constants.[164] First, Young's modulus or stiffness is the slope of the stress-strain curve obtained from a uniaxial tension test. Second, Poisson's ratio is the negative of the ratio of transverse strain to longitudinal strain in the direction of uniaxial loading and is a measure of the ability of a material to conserve volume when loaded in one direction. Finally, the shear modulus is the ratio of the induced shear to the resulting shear strain and is determined from torsional testing. Values for human bone of Young's modulus (14.1×10^9 N/m²), Poisson's ratio (0.08 to 0.45), and the shear modulus (0.31×10^9 N/m²) have been reported.[164] The strength of the specimen is defined as the maximum stress sustained by the bone specimen without fracture in a given loading configuration.[164] Additionally, maximum shear stress may be obtained by torsional testing.

The nonisotropic nature of bone is reflected in variations in mechanical properties from one region to another in a given bone, differences in the same region between different individuals, and differences from one bone to another within an individual.[55, 67] Therefore, both the type of testing and the site of bone sampling influence results. Careful selection of samples, preferably mirror segments within an animal, is thus necessary for comparison testing. The physical factors that affect such variations in bone strength include the number of collagen fibrils, the axial direction of these fibrils, the number of osteones, and the mineral content of the bone.[68] Thus, bending strength increases as the ash (mineral) content of the bone increases.[48] Totally haversian bone is 30 percent weaker than lamellar bone in tensile strength.[48] Tensile strength in the longitudinal direction (i. e., oriented parallel to the haversian canals) differs from that in the transverse direction.[164] Compression strength also differs, depending upon the direction of loading, with bone being 50 percent stronger when loaded parallel to the osteones as opposed to transverse loading.[55] Age has an effect, with the tensile strength of human femoral bone decreasing approximately 4 percent per decade.[129]

Similarly, the mechanical principles involved in the initiation of a fracture vary according to the type of stress applied and its rate of application. In tension, plastic deformation is exhibited by the bone and failure occurs by a transverse fracture.[37] In pure compression, an oblique fracture occurs, with a shear initiation as the mode of failure.[37] Burstein and colleagues have noted microfractures at an angle of 45° to the direction of compressive loading along the lines of principal shear stress.[37] These cracks are more numerous if the stress-field is nonuniform.[37] Failure in both tension and compression is consistent with such a multiphasic material as bone, which exhibits yield by means of a pull-out that creates voids and crazes.[37] Torsional loading results in pure shear stress, giving rise to a spiral fracture along the plane of maximum shear stress.[37] Pugh felt that torsional loading resulted in a failure at 45° because this angle marked a tension plane.[161] Burstein noted that in torsional failure the vascular network between lamellae acted as a surface of fracture initiation.[37, 164]

In fact, bone has a high resistance to bending and torsion, largely because the bony material is located at the periphery, where the stresses are highest.[161] The rigidity-efficiency of the tissue increases with the fourth power of the distance from the center of rotation or bending.[153] Therefore, endosteal callus is less efficient than interfragmentary bone, which in turn is less efficient than periosteal callus, provided that the repair tissue is of equal quality.[153] Fractures tend to occur along planes of tension or shear because bone is weakest in tension and shear and strongest in compression.[161] If a bone is loaded purely in bending, the initiation of fracture always begins on the tensile side because its tensile strength is less than its compressive strength.[55]

Other factors besides the plane of the fracture provide information concerning the initiating forces. Flat smooth surfaces result from a quickly traveling crack or a brittle fracture process with low energy absorption.[164] Rough surfaces with pull-out of constituents indicate a slower fracture process and more energy absorption. Since bone is a viscoelastic material, it is stiffer at higher rates of loading and its fracture strength is higher.[161] Therefore, in high-loading rate injuries more energy is absorbed, resulting in a comminuted fracture.[161]

Fracture Healing

When is the fracture healed? This is the key question that confronts the surgeon when treating a patient with a fracture. Clinical criteria are useful in framing an answer but are difficult to quantitate. A knowledge of the changes in the biomechanical characteristics of a healing fracture is useful both for clinical treatment and for experimental studies in which quantitative comparisons between treatment methods can be performed.

In healing fibular fractures in rabbits, Brighton and Krebs found a progressive increase in bending strength and rigidity as healing progressed.[32] Lindsay studied healing fibular fractures in rats by subjecting the healing fractures to a simple bending test (Fig. 2–25).[123] He noted a progressive increase in strength until the twenty-first day following fracture, which correlated with increasing mineralization of the fracture and increasing callus area.[123] After the twenty-first day, there was a small decrease in strength in conjunction with a decrease in callus area. This was followed by a gradual increase in strength to control levels despite a further decrease in callus area.[123] Lindsay felt that the decrease followed by an increase in bone strength correlated with the phases of fracture remodeling.[122] In further studies, Lindsay found a direct correlation between the breaking strength of the healing fracture and the size and weight of the bone.[122] He noted that the breaking strength varied according to three phases of fracture healing: fibrosis, calcification, and structural reorganization.[122]

Figure 2–25. Healing strength of a fracture. (From Lindsay, M. K., and Howes, E. L.: The breaking strength of healing fractures. J. Bone Joint Surg. *16*:162, 1931.)

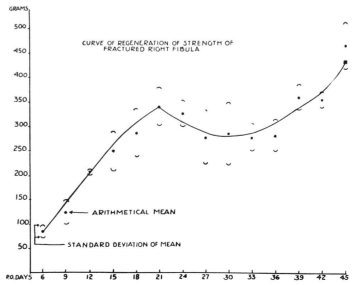

In healing osteotomies of the radius in rabbits, Falkenberg noted a peak in callus area and ash weight of the fracture between 20 and 30 days following fracture.[68] From 20 to 60 days following fracture, the callus area decreased 50 percent and the ash weight decreased 25 percent, but the absolute tensile strength of the callus increased 100 percent.[68] An increase in mineral content paralleled the increase in bone strength in the later stages of fracture healing.[68] Also, hydroxyapatite crystals were reorganized during fracture remodeling from an initially random orientation of the C-axis of the crystals to an orientation parallel to the longitudinal axis of the bone.[140] Falkenberg concluded that an initial rapid increase in the absolute tensile strength of the callus occurs with increasing callus area, but the actual quality of the callus improves more slowly in conjunction with fracture remodeling.[68] A combination of increasing mineral content, reorientation of the hydroxyapatite crystals, and secondary osteone formation contributes to the increase in strength of the healing fracture.

White and colleagues have classified fracture healing into four biomechanical stages based upon torsional testing of the healing fracture (Fig. 2–26).[713] Stage I displays failure through the original fracture site with low stiffness. Stage II displays failure through the original fracture site with high stiffness. Stage III displays failure partially through the original fracture site with high stiffness. Stage IV displays failure entirely through intact bone with high stiffness. A progressive increase in the maturity of fracture healing is present from Stages I to IV.

Different mechanical forces also have different effects upon fracture healing. Yamagishi and Yoshimura found that a neutral force resulted in healing by direct transformation of mesenchymal cells into osteoblasts, but healing was slow.[224] A compression force resulted in rapid healing by endochondral ossification unless the force was excessive, in which case healing was delayed.[224] If a distraction force was applied, fibrous tissue formed and healing was also delayed.[224] The worst loading configuration was shear combined with intermittent compression, which resulted in pseudarthrosis.[224] Friedenberg and French attempted to quantitate the effects of compression forces on fracture healing.[73] They found that an optimum range of compression existed, in which fracture union occurred in two thirds of their experimental animals.[73] Higher or lower compression resulted in a lower rate of union.[73]

Therefore, mechanical forces affect the rate of fracture union. Fracture healing progresses through several stages with a gradual increase in strength. The increase in strength correlates with callus area initially but in later stages relates to fracture remodeling.

Biologic Signal for Fracture Healing

The nature of the signal that induces fracture healing is poorly understood. Two concepts have been advanced as a potential initiating signal for fracture healing. The first is a series of electrical signals, and the second involves a bone-inductive substance. It is beyond the scope of this review to give a detailed discussion of these concepts, but they will be briefly summarized.

Electrical Signals

Two types of electrical signals or potentials are found in bone: (1) stress-generated or strain-generated potentials, and (2) bioelectric or standing potentials. Stress-generated potentials arise when bone is stressed and are not dependent upon cell viability. Areas of compression are electronegative, while areas of tension are electropositive (Fig. 2–27).[72] These electrical signals arise from the organic component of the bone and are not derived from the mineral component. In normal intact bone, Friedenberg and colleagues have shown that electrical polarity exists with the ends of the bone being electronegative in comparison to the midshaft.[72] Following fracture or osteotomy the electrical polarity will change. The entire surface of the bone becomes electronegative with a peak of electronegativity occurring over the fracture site (Fig. 2–28).[72] This change in electrical potentials will remain until the fracture heals. A second peak of electronegativity will also occur over the opposite physis.[72] The bioelectrical potentials are dependent upon cell viability. If the cells are killed or damaged there will be a significant drop in the electrical potentials in the area.

Friedenberg has shown with implantable elec-

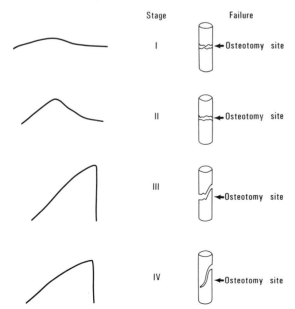

Figure 2–26. Biomechanical stages of fracture healing. (Modified after White, A. A., et al.: The four biomechanical stages of fracture repair. J. Bone Joint Surg. *59A*:188, 1977.)

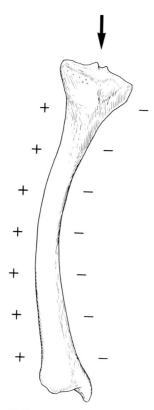

Figure 2–27. Stress-generated potential in bone.

trodes that bone will form immediately around the negative electrode or cathode.[72] However, there is an optimal amperage below which no bone will form and above which bone formation will give way to cell necrosis. Surrounding the positive electrode or anode only bone necrosis will occur. In the rabbit fibula, electrical stimulation will result in a significant increase in fracture healing, as evidenced by an increased maximum resistance to bending.[74] Using this semi-invasive technique, the amount of

new bone formed is related to the true current density and change.[31] The amount of bone formed is linearly related to charge. In fact, a variety of forms of electricity will produce osteogenesis. In addition to direct current of varying amplitude, pulse width, and frequency, noninvasive techniques using electromagnetic fields, as advocated by Bassett, have proved successful both experimentally and clinically.[16] The mechanism of action of the electrical stimulation on bone cells is poorly understood, but two potential mechanisms are (1) direct cellular changes induced by the electrical current possibly acting through cyclic AMP, or (2) indirect changes produced in the microenvironment.[75] Friedenberg and colleagues feel that a change in the oxygen concentration in the microenvironment is a probable mechanism of action.[75]

Jacobs and colleagues studied the mechanism of healing of non-unions treated by the semi-invasive technique of implanted electrodes in non-union of canine ulnae.[95] In hypertrophic non-unions, bone formation was twice as great in the electrically stimulated non-unions as compared with controls. In oligotrophic non-unions, bone formation was increased 22 percent as compared with controls. Bone did not form in fibrous tissue alone but always arose by appositional growth from existing bone. Jacobs and colleagues concluded that electrical stimulation functioned through a cell-mediated rather than physiochemical mechanism.[95]

Bassett and colleagues studied the effects of pulsating electromagnetic fields upon acute fracture repair.[19] They found that the biologic response was dependent upon a specific type of wave form. Osteogenesis was not directly stimulated. The major effect of electrical stimulation was an increased rate of mineralization of existing fibrocartilage. A similar mechanism of action has been suggested for pulsating electromagnetic fields used in treating non-unions.[17]

Bone-Inductive Signal

As mentioned earlier, bone-inducing material has been advocated as an alternative signal for fracture healing. Induction refers to the capacity of one living cell to influence the differentiation of another living cell. Three conditions must be met for bone induction to occur.[40] First, an inducing agent must be present. Second, viable osteogenic precursor cells must be available. Third, the environment must be permissive for osteogenesis. Extraskeletal implantation of decalcified bone matrix will induce surrounding pleuripotent host cells to differentiate into osteoblasts and form bone.[204] The inducer cells and the induced cells are felt to be derived from the host bed rather than from the bone graft.[204] The osteogenic cells arise from a competent mesenchymal cell population residing in the host tissues rather than from blood-borne or vascular cells.[18, 205]

A variety of substances have been sought that might act to induce bone. The concept of a bone-

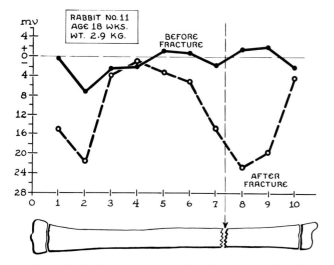

Figure 2–28. Negative potential at the fracture site. (From Friedenberg, Z. B., and Brighton, C. J.: Bioelectrical potentials in bone. J. Bone Joint Surg. *48A*:919, 1966.)

induction substance has been experimentally studied by a variety of authors. Urist has identified a substance that he terms bone morphogenic protein (BMP).[205] The bone morphogenic principle will induce the formation of new bone as old bone is resorbed. Even in the absence of living cells, the organic matrix of bone contains this protein, which can induce formation of new bone adjacent to living bone. BMP has a molecular weight of approximately 10,000 and can diffuse across a Millipore filter. It appears to play a role in osteoinduction, which depends upon a substrate-cell interaction that induces competent mesenchymal cells to differentiate into osteoblasts. More generally, a variety of factors have been noted to influence bone induction. Induction is accelerated by the demineralization, freezing, and heat denaturation of bone; and it is inhibited by irradiation, proteolytic enzyme degradation, or the presence of minerals.[205] Heterotopic ossification is an example of bone induction in muscle.

The most frequent use of the bone-induction principle in orthopedics involves bone grafting. Three factors act in bone grafting: cellular proliferation, prevention of fibrous ingrowth, and induction.[88] Both the host and graft contribute cells that form new bone about the transplant.[88] Some of the potential sources of osteogenic cells include surface osteoblasts in the graft and recipient bone, marrow cells, soft tissues in the recipient bed, and free circulatory elements in the blood.[35] The contribution of each osteogenic cell population in the cancellous bone graft has been studied by Gray and Elves.[81] Endosteal lining cells and marrow stroma contribute 60 percent to osteogenesis and periosteal cells 30 percent.[81] The least osteogenic tissues are marrow cells and osteocytes.[81] The rate of osteogenesis is 2.2 times higher in cancellous than in cortical bone grafts.[81]

The type of bone graft used has an effect upon the results. Autogenous bone graft is the most osteogenic, followed by freeze-dried homogenous bone.[87] The least osteogenic graft material is deproteinized homogenous bone.[87] Autogenous cancellous or corticocancellous grafts contribute to bone formation, are free from immunologic response, and allow bone induction in the recipient bed.[35]

FRACTURE FIXATION

Compression-Plate Fixation of Fractures

Plate fixation of fractures is designed to immobilize the fracture while allowing mobility of the soft tissues of the injured limb. The first use of a bone plate has been attributed to Hansmann in 1886.[86] A variety of bone plates subsequently became available in the early part of the twentieth century, such as the Lane and Sherman plates. Many modifications of bone plates have been devised in an attempt to improve the quality of fixation (Fig. 2–29).

The significance of compression in promoting bone union was first advocated by Key in 1932 in arthrodesis of the knee.[104] Key felt that the factors acting in compression arthrodesis were apposition of the bone surfaces, fixation of the fragments, and compression itself. In 1946, Eggers made the first attempt to use compression to aid healing of fractures immobilized by plates.[61] He devised a plate termed the "contact splint" that allowed sliding contact of the fracture fragments and physiologic compression of the fragments from muscular action.[62] According to Eggers, excessive compression would cause necrosis of bone, while lack of compression would fail to stimulate osteogenesis; physiologic compression from muscular action, however, would be optimal for stimulating bone union.[63, 64] Key and Reynolds found slightly more rapid union with an Eggers plate than with a

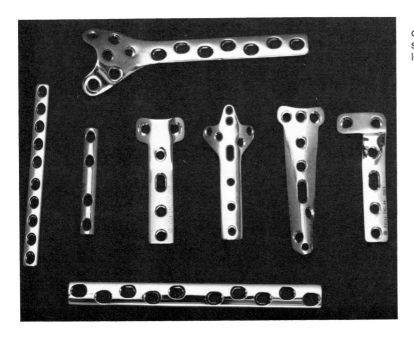

Figure 2–29. Types of bone plates. Upper: condylar buttress; middle (left to right): 3.5 mm DCP, semitubular, T-plate, cloverleaf, spoon, L-plate; lower: 4.5 mm DCP.

standard bone plate.[105] Close approximation and continuous immobilization of the fracture ends were felt to be advantages of the Eggers plate. In fact, primary bone union without an intermediary cartilaginous stage was noted in some fractures treated with the Eggers plate.[105] The major difficulty with the Eggers contact splint, however, was inability to control the quantity of compression and degree of immobilization of the fracture site.

Danis, in 1947, stated that the key principles of internal fixation were rigid immobilization, axial pressure, and coaptation of the bone fragments.[52] In 1949, Danis described the first true compression plate and reported satisfactory results in its use in treating forearm fractures.[53] Venable felt that impacted coaptation of the fracture fragments was essential for early healing and that excessive callus was evidence of insufficient stability or insufficient blood supply to the fracture.[208] Venable also devised a compression plate to achieve rigid stabilization of the fracture. Bagby devised a plate that was self-compressing upon application owing to impaction of the screws against the screw holes in the plate.[11] He found that union occurred earlier in experimental fractures treated with a compression plate than in those treated with a standard bone plate. Bagby felt that the effect of compression on fracture healing might be either a direct effect of the compression or more likely an indirect effect. Compression would result in close approximation of the fracture fragments, which would decrease the fracture gap and might stimulate osteogenesis, and would also provide rigid immobilization.[11, 12, 13]

Muller, in 1962, reported on primary bone healing using the AO compression plate.[135] There was no resorption of the fracture site, no radiologically evident callus, and primary bone healing occurred in 79 percent of 188 tibial fractures. He felt that compression improved stability but was unable to prove that compression actually stimulates bone union. Allgower and Perren reported on the dynamic compression plate (DCP) in 1969, which was similar in principle to the plate previously designed by Bagby.[6, 155, 157] The major advantages of the DCP when compared with the standard AO compression plate include improved engineering, which allows greater versatility in the angle of screw placement and compression between any two screw holes in the plate; compression with limited surgical exposure; and absence of unpredictable change in compression, a problem in the removal of the standard compression device.[154] The advocates of the DCP and standard AO compression plates stress the advantages of maintaining rigid fixation of the fractures with these implants.

Mechanism of Action of Compression-Fixation

The mechanism of action and the optimum quantity of compression for fracture healing have been investigated. In experimental fractures, it has been suggested that there is an optimal range of compres-sion in which union is stimulated. Higher pressures cause bone necrosis and lower pressures fail to stimulate bone union.[63, 73, 114] Friedenberg and French found an increased rate of union from compression-fixation, which was attributed to enhanced mobility of the fracture fragments, enhanced immobility of the fracture combined with close contact of fragments, and a possible stimulation of osteogenesis at the fracture site from the pressure.[73] In contrast, Laurin was unable to demonstrate more rapid union in experimental fractures subjected to compression.[116] Lettin found a similar rate of union in fractures fixed with a bone plate, whether or not compression was applied.[118a] Ford and Key were unable to demonstrate more rapid union with compression across experimental canine fractures of the ilium and did not observe bone necrosis from high pressure.[70] Anderson, in comparing compression- and noncompression-plate fixation of canine femoral osteotomies, found more rapid union and less periosteal callus in those fractures treated with compression.[8] Prominent endosteal callus was responsible for the area of earliest osseous union with both types of plate fixation. However, there was no significant difference in tensile strength between those fractures treated with compression and those without.[8] Allgower and Perren, in studying compression-plate fixation of experimental fractures, noted that despite the high loads applied to the bone by the compression plate and at the screw-bone interface, no bone necrosis occurred.[5]

The biomechanical properties of bone help explain the variable effects of compression. The pressure beneath a compression plate decreases approximately 20 percent initially owing to the viscoelastic behavior of bone and then gradually decreases by 50 percent over the next 8 weeks in conjunction with haversian remodeling.[155] Coletti found that bone loaded with compression of greater than 318 psi responded with formation of bone beneath the pressure site.[41] The area of bone formation correlated with areas of tensile stress, and there was no evidence of bone necrosis. Given this relation between pressure and bone formation, a unique mechanical explanation for the mechanism of action of compression has been suggested by Pinter.[159] X-ray diffraction studies of bovine bone *in vitro* revealed an association between an increase in the total quantity of crystalline material in bone and a decrease in the quantity of amorphous material present when the bone was subjected to compressive loading.[159] Pinter felt that the beneficial action of compression might be a purely physical process of oriented crystal growth superimposed upon cellular activity.

Morphologic Findings of Primary Bone Healing with Compression-Plate Fixation

The morphologic findings and characteristics of fracture union after compression-plate fixation have been termed *soudre autogène,* or primary fracture healing.[178] Some authors consider primary fracture healing the ideal mode of healing. Under rigid internal fixation, primary angiogenic ossification may occur, in which the ingrowing capillary network is protected from motion and thus disruption. This allows osteoblastic proliferation and direct bone union of the fracture gap.[178] Histologically, secondary osteones directly cross the fracture site without the presence of intervening cartilage. New osteone formation is estimated to occur within 5 to 6 weeks in the dog and within 3 months in man.[127, 178] The osteoblastic "cutter head" forming the secondary osteone progresses at a rate of 50 to 80 microns in 24 hours.[178] The advantage of primary fracture healing is that the restoration of the original bone structure of the cortex begins earlier than in fracture healing without rigid fixation. Therefore, the main features of primary bone healing include primary bone union in interfragmental gaps, minimal resorption of the bone ends without widening of the fracture gap, longitudinally directed secondary osteones crossing the fracture, and minimal external callus.[178] Minimal external callus is seen on radiographs associated with a gradual obliteration of the fracture line.

Primary bone healing has been observed by several authors using other modes of fixation than the compression plate, including external fixation with pins and a compression spring.[73, 224] Blockey, as well as Burwell, reported primary fracture healing using a noncompression Burns plate which provided rigid internal fixation.[22, 38] Primary bone healing similar to that observed with the standard AO compression plate has been reported using the DCP plate.[6, 155]

Bone healing beneath a compression plate occurs in two distinct forms. Immediately beneath the plate, primary bone healing occurs where the cortical fragments are in direct contact. This involves the direct bridging of the fracture by secondary osteones with minimal periosteal callus but significant bridging medullary callus. This is contact healing.[156, 169] Union of the cortex opposite the plate involves a different mechanism. A slight gap exists between the fracture fragments, and union here is termed gap healing.[156, 162, 169] In gap healing, direct bone formation occurs oriented perpendicular to the long axis of the bone and must later be remodeled into longitudinal osteones. The vascular supply for gap healing receives an important contribution from the periosteal circulation, whereas in contact healing the endosteal circulation is most important.[162] In both cases primary bone healing occurs only in the presence of an adequate blood supply and rigid stabilization of the fracture.[169] Enhancement of stabilization that protects the regenerating blood vessels is the major contribution of compression-fixation.[167]

Effect of a Plate on Bone Blood Flow

The effect of internal fixation on the blood supply of a long bone has been the subject of extensive investigation. Rhinelander feels that of the methods of secure internal fixation, plating disturbs the blood supply least.[169] He has noted reconstitution of medullary vessels across an osteotomy within 1 week of internal fixation with a plate.[169] However, because it blocks the venous drainage from the bone, the plate does reduce vascularization of the entire thickness of the cortex immediately beneath the plate.[167, 169, 172] Screws do not significantly disturb the circulation.[169] Olerud found avascular regions extending over one-half the thickness of the cortex beneath a compression plate.[142] He noted revascularization occurring from periosteal, endosteal, and haversian vessels. Endosteal vessels are responsible for 80 percent of the revascularization of a fracture fixed with a compression plate.[125, 126]

Biomechanics of Plate Fixation

Biomechanical analysis of the fixation achieved with various plates has been performed. Lindahl found that the AO plate ranked among the top three plates tested for resistance to bending and torsion.[121] He felt that the anchorage of a plate should satisfy the following requirements: the rigidity and shape of the plate should be such that the strength of immobilization is roughly equal to bone; enough screws must be used and the shear area should be large; and the material should be as little irritant as possible.[121] According to Lindahl, the AO plate best fulfilled these requirements. The cross-sectional area of the plate is important. The broader the plate, the greater the rigidity of fixation without regard to the other aspects of fixation.[141] More rapid healing of experimental fractures has been observed with use of a broad as opposed to narrow compression plate.[141]

The mechanical effect of a compression plate is to create compression of the cortex beneath the plate and a bending moment in which tensile forces lead to distraction of the cortex opposite the plate.[216, 217] Therefore, only 17.4 to 21.6 percent of the total cross-sectional area of the bone is in actual contact.[216, 217] Rybicki and colleagues, using a finite-element analysis, predicted a 9 percent contact of the fracture surfaces for an oblique fracture treated with a compression plate.[176] Stabilization with a compression plate is based upon local pressure and transmission of force between the implant and bone.[156] In addition to friction between the implant and bone, friction between the fracture surfaces is also important. If a plate is placed on the tension side of the bone as a "tension band" and is applied with a "prebend," compression will tend to be applied to the cortex opposite the plate as well as to the cortex beneath the plate, resulting in greater bony contact and stability.[156] If prebending and compression are used, a gap may occur on the cortex beneath the plate, but the potential gap on the cortex opposite the plate is closed.[141] Prebending of the plate generates interfragmental friction in the opposite cortex, which results in increased torsional load stability. An increased rate of histologic union has been observed using prebending of the plate combined with compression as opposed to use of compression alone.[141] Compression of any two surfaces produces friction that preloads the surfaces, keeping them in motionless coaptation. The friction generated by compression protects against the shearing forces generated by torsional stresses.[153] In a transverse fracture, Rybicki noted that in the ideal compression-loading configuration 80 percent of the applied load was supported by the bone.[175] He found that the cortex beneath the plate was protected from 75 percent of the applied stress, while the cortex opposite the plate was subjected to 1.5 times the applied stress value.

Adverse Effects of a Compression Plate

Adverse effects on the underlying bone have been observed in fractures treated with rigid compression plates. A major clinical concern is a diminution of bone strength according to Wolff's law due to stress protection of the bone by the plate. Spongious transformation of the cortex may occur beneath a compression plate because the rate of bone resorption exceeds the rate of bone formation.[114, 143, 155] In experimental canine femoral fractures treated with rigid compression plates, Uhthoff and colleagues noted that there was osteopenia of the cortex beneath the plate, a reduction in shaft caliber, and persistent woven bone at the fracture site (Fig. 2–30).[203] Eighteen months after compression-plate fixation of forearm fractures, Mathews found satisfactory mineralization of the bone but also atrophy of cortical bone.[127] In contrast, Stromberg felt that a decrease in bone mineral occurred beneath the plate with an increase in bone mineral proximal to the plate.[191, 192] A 50 percent decrease in thickness of the cortex from intracortical resorption and a 15 percent decrease in calcium content beneath the plate were observed in intact rabbit femora 17 weeks following application of an ASIF compression plate.[146] A decrease in cortical thickness by 11.2 percent due to endosteal resorption and a 15.9

percent decrease in ash weight (mineral content) has been reported in unfractured canine femora following application of a compression plate for 7 months.[146]

These changes in underlying bone have biomechanical consequences. Tonino and colleagues found a 17 percent decrease in bone mineral and a 30 percent decrease in mechanical strength in bending tests in intact canine femora treated with a steel AO compression plate as opposed to a plastic plate.[195] A reduction in torque moment of 53 percent and angular deformation of 26.3 percent was observed after application of a rigid DCP plate to intact rabbit tibias with or without compression.[148] Stromberg found a reduction in maximum torque capacity of 18 percent and maximum angle of torsion of 22 percent in plated bones compared with those in controls.[191, 192] Akeson and colleagues found that a bone treated with a compression plate showed no change in its mechanical properties, such as the ultimate bending strength or modulus of elasticity; but significant alterations were visible in the structural properties of the bone, such as the maximum bending load and energy absorption.[2] They did not find any change in the porosity of the bone but did find a thinning of the cortical wall.

In comparing plates with different degrees of stiffness and therefore rigidity of fixation, less adverse structural changes were noted with a less stiff plate.[1, 2] A 70 percent reduction of bone stress occurs near a steel plate and a 60 percent reduction of stress near a less stiff titanium plate.[156] Double plating results in a marked reduction in bone strength.[107] Woo and Akeson reported that a special composite plate with a low modulus of elasticity (i.e., stiffness) resulted in healed fractures that did not display any significant differences from controls upon biomechanical testing.[220] However, Hutzschenreuter found that a thick (i.e., stiff) plate allowed bone union without resorption of the fragment ends and minimal callus, whereas a thin (i.e., less stiff) plate resulted in marked bone resorption and marked callus formation.[92]

The effect of rigid plates on intact bone has also been investigated. Woo and colleagues noted a decrease in the structural properties of the bone due to thinning of the cortex, whereas mechanical properties remained unchanged from controls.[224] Slatis and colleagues performed a study of the effect of the DCP plate on intact rabbit tibias. They found an increase in bone porosity within 3 weeks, and by 36 weeks resorption cavities occupied 40.6 percent of the cortex.[189] A thinning of the cortical wall occurred along with an increase in the diameter of the bone. These changes in the bone were more marked in the cortex beneath the plate than in the opposite cortex. Similar morphologic changes occurred in the presence of a standard rigid plate or a compression plate. Slatis and colleagues concluded that the morphologic bone changes were a product of the rigid plate and were not influenced by compression.[189] Application of a plate to intact

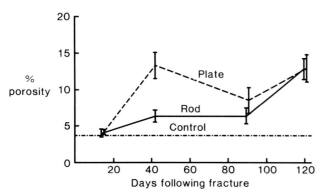

Figure 2–30. Bone porosity following internal fixation of canine tibial fractures. (From Rand, J. A., et al.: A comparison of the effects of open intramedullary nailing and compression-plate fixation on fracture-site blood flow and fracture union. J. Bone Joint Surg. *63A:*427, 1981.

bone also results in an acceleration of bone turnover rates.[46] The addition of compression or distraction does not significantly change this effect of the plate. Bone porosity increases above control values regardless of the mode of plate application.[46] The hydroxyproline content increases with a decrease in the calcium-hydroxyproline ratio, indicating active remodeling of bone tissue.[147] Two explanations for the increase in porosity observed beneath a plate have been suggested. The porosity may reflect mechanical unloading or the remodeling process.[153]

Since adverse structural changes occur in bone subjected to rigid internal fixation, the danger of bone refracture exists. Therefore, the timing of removal of the internal fixation device must be considered. Bone refracture may occur following plate fixation by two mechanisms.[71] First, bone may fail at its weakest section. Second, local stress risers may be present near the fracture site. Stress risers include screw holes, which induce local stresses two to three times greater than those present in adjacent bone areas, and compact dense callus with a different modulus of elasticity (Fig. 2–31).[71] Hutzschenreuter and colleagues reported early refracture of the bone at the end of the plate in an animal fixed with a rigid plate.[92] They attributed the fracture to increased stress at the junction of the rigidly plated bone segment with the normal elastic bone. Stromberg cautioned concerning refracture after plate removal because the load distribution on the bone underlying the plate will suddenly alter.[191] Since the bone will be unprepared to deal with the normal load, the possibility of refracture exists.

Convent felt that any implant material should be removed in younger persons and that removal should be carefully timed.[43] An overly late removal might lead to refracture because of spongious transformation of the bone. However, he felt that a period of 1 to 2 years should elapse prior to plate removal, and a period of protected usage for 6 to 8 weeks should follow removal of the plate. Convent stated that the majority of refractures were due to screw holes acting as stress risers in the bone.[43] Huys and colleagues stated that plates should be routinely removed only in athletes or children, or in cases in which they are symptomatic.[93] If an implant is removed, the limb should be protected for a period of time to prevent refracture. In the lower extremity, the AO group recommends routine removal of the implant after 1 to 2 years because of stress protection of the bone by the implant.[137]

In summary, the advantages of compression-plate fixation include rigid immobilization of the fracture and a decrease in the fracture gap. The regenerating blood supply is protected, allowing primary bone healing across the fracture at an early time following injury. The disadvantages are local interference with the venous drainage of the bone, stress protection of the bone by the rigid implant, and the need for exposure of the bone with resultant disturbance of its blood supply and risk of infection.

Intramedullary Nail Fixation of Fractures

The technique of intramedullary nail fixation of fractures was used as early as 1897 by Nicolayson, in 1906 by Delbet, and in 1913 by Lambotte.[209] The use of massive nails in the medullary cavity was introduced by Hey Groves in 1916.[209] A variety of materials were used for the early intramedullary nails, including ivory, bone, and metal, but caused tissue reaction to the implant. Rush and Rush used a round Steinmann pin for intramedullary fixation in 1939.[174] However, intramedullary nail fixation was not popularized until the reports of Küntscher in the early 1940's. Since that time, many different designs of intramedullary nails have been devised and this method of fracture treatment is widely used (Fig. 2–32). The reports of Lauritzen and Watson-Jones give excellent historical reviews.[117, 209]

Effect of an Intramedullary Nail on Bone Blood Flow

The effect of an intramedullary nail on the blood supply of a healing fracture has been a source of concern and investigation. Trueta and Cavadais compared intramedullary nail-fixed and unfixed osteotomies of the radius in rabbits, in which the metaphyseal blood supply in each had been suppressed.[200] The nutrient artery was never reconstructed in the nailed fractures, and necrosis of the marrow and inner one third to two thirds of the cortex occurred. Large portions of necrotic cortex persisted for up to 8 months following nailing.

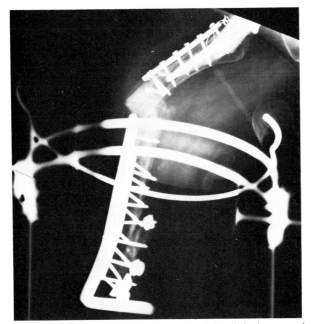

Figure 2–31. Stress riser between two rigid plated segments of femur. (From Rand, J. A., et al.: Biomechanical factors in fracture healing. Minn. Med. 65:558, 1982.

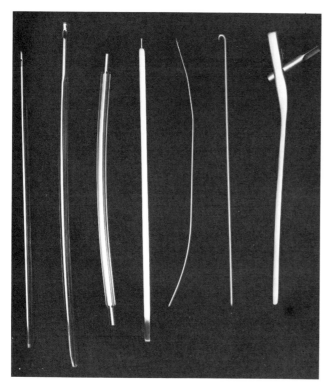

Figure 2–32. Types of intramedullary nails. Left to right: Küntscher, ASIF, Sampson, Hansen-Street, Enders, Rush, Zickel.

However, the number of small vessels at the fracture site appeared similar in both the nailed and unfixed fractures. The new vessels on the nailed side were derived from the periosteal circulation. Large quantities of periosteal callus but no endosteal callus formed on the nailed side. In contrast, large quantities of endosteal callus formed on the unfixed side. In spite of differences in vascularity and callus formation, delayed union did not occur in any of the nailed fractures.

Gothman studied intramedullary nailing of the tibia in rabbits.[80] In unfractured tibias subjected to intramedullary nailing, active medullary vessels were noted to persist after introduction of the nail. One week following fracture and intramedullary nailing, the cortex showed evidence of a vascular reaction derived largely from the periosteal circulation and to a small extent from the persisting medullary arteries. The arterial reaction displayed a peak response between 2 and 4 weeks following nailing, with the majority of vessels being derived from the surrounding soft tissues. Minimal vascular reaction was noted from the medullary vessels. In tibial fractures in monkeys treated with intramedullary nail fixation, the vascular response was similar to the case of the rabbit, with vessels derived from the surrounding soft tissues being of major importance.[79, 80] Although segments of the medullary vessels remained patent via anastomoses with metaphyseal vessels, they frequently did not reach

the fracture site. Callus formation largely followed the new vessels derived from the soft tissues.

Rhinelander studied the effect of loose- and tight-fitting intramedullary nails on fracture-site revascularization.[167–170, 172] In the presence of a loose-fitting intramedullary nail, the inner two thirds to three fourths of the cortex in contact with the nail became avascular. The outer one third of the cortex remained vascularized by vessels derived from the periosteal circulation. Medullary vessels were regenerated in spaces surrounding the nail to revascularize the cortex. If medullary reaming was performed and a tight-fitting nail inserted, the cortex became devascularized except for areas of fascial attachments and a small external layer of the cortex. Revascularization occurred through a regenerative endosteal membrane formed around the nail, through the external callus at its junction with the cortex via the periosteal circulation, and through the substance of the cortex via regenerating nutrient vessels. Six weeks following intramedullary reaming and tight nailing, the significant component of the regenerative blood supply was derived from the medullary circulation. Since a tight nail results in almost total medullary blockade, regeneration of the nutrient vascular supply occurs through intracortical arteries.

Rhinelander also noted that intramedullary nailing delays fracture healing because nailing results in almost total devascularization of the fracture ends, damaging the medullary vessels, and also strips away the fascial attachments that carry the periosteal arterioles. In addition, an intramedullary nail inhibits the endosteal callus formation that is responsible for the area of earliest osseous union.[169] Delayed union was observed frequently with a Küntscher nail, whereas union occurred earlier with a four-fluted Schneider nail. The nutrient artery was able to regenerate between the flutes, providing a more favorable situation for revascularization than the cloverleaf nail. Danckwardt-Lilliestrom and colleagues found that osteotomy plus intramedullary reaming resulted in total avascularity of the fracture ends.[50] Initially, the normal centrifugal flow of blood through the cortex was replaced by a centripetal flow derived from the periosteal circulation. If stable fixation was maintained, revascularization occurred by way of longitudinally directed vessels penetrating through the cortex (the so-called "cutter head" formation), by connections with pre-existing intracortical vessels, by vessels surrounding the nail, and by vessels penetrating through the fracture gap. Immediate bone formation occurred in the fracture gap followed by remodeling of the fracture area by longitudinal secondary osteones.

The effects of intramedullary reaming have been studied.[49, 50, 169] Intramedullary reaming, in the absence of fracture or nailing, almost completely destroys the medullary blood vessels of the diaphysis. Three days following reaming of the medullary cavity, from 10 to 60 percent of the cross-sectional area of the cortex is avascular.[50] High intramedullary pressures of up to 300 mg of Hg are generated during reaming, resulting in fat embolization into the cortex that obstructs the intracortical vessels. Some marrow is forced subperiosteally, resulting in increased periosteal new bone formation.[49] However, if low intramedullary pressures are maintained during reaming by applying a negative pressure to the medullary cavity, intracortical fat embolism may be minimized, allowing more rapid bone revascularization.[51]

Morphologic Findings in Union through Intramedullary Nail Fixation

Morphologic studies of fracture union have revealed several differences between nailed and unfixed fractures. In nailed fractures, Fitts and colleagues found extensive periosteal callus at a distance from the fracture site.[69] Maximum callus at the fracture site was greater in the unfixed than in the nailed fractures. However, callus appeared earlier and union occurred more rapidly in the nailed fractures. They concluded that the immobilization provided by the nail was the factor determining more rapid union in the nailed group. Sharma and Kumar noted greater periosteal callus formation in unfixed than in nailed fractures.[182] Nailed fractures united by periosteal callus because the nail blocked endosteal callus formation. Union generally occurred by endochondral ossification, but one fracture, in which rigid fixation was maintained, displayed union by direct bone formation. In fractures treated with an intramedullary nail, Rhinelander found that greater periosteal callus formed when rotation was not controlled compared with fractures with rotational stability.[171] Anderson and colleagues noted excessive periosteal new bone formation with sequestration of the cortical fracture ends and delayed union in the presence of a loose intramedullary nail. Union occurred by endochondral ossification.[9] In the presence of a tight intramedullary nail, there was less periosteal new bone formation, minimal cortical bone resorption, and rapid fracture union. Union occurred by direct bone formation. Anderson concluded that the insertion of an intramedullary nail is basically unsound physiologically because it destroys the medullary blood supply and prevents endosteal callus formation.[8] Varma and Mehta found that union was delayed in nailed fractures when compared with unfixed fractures.[207] However, union occurred more rapidly in nailed fractures with secure fixation than in fractures without adequate fixation. In the presence of stable fixation, union occurred by direct bone formation. In the presence of unstable fixation, union occurred by endochondral ossification. They stressed the importance of stable intramedullary fixation.

In clinical studies, Küntscher recognized that endosteal callus was inhibited by the intramedullary nail and that union occurred by more extensively formed periosteal callus.[110] Küntscher felt that periosteal callus was most important for fracture repair.[112] He felt that even complete destruction of the endosteum during intramedullary nailing did not prevent fracture union. In experimental studies in dogs, he noted that endosteal callus completely encircled the intramedullary nail.[112] The technique of closed intramedullary nailing was developed to avoid damaging the periosteum, which might interfere with periosteal callus formation. In an extensive review of clinical material, Lauritzen was unable to find evidence of more rapid or delayed callus formation due to intramedullary nailing.[117] Rhinelander stated that an intramedullary nail always results in a delay in fracture healing because it limits the formation of the medullary bridging callus that is responsible for the earliest osseous union.[169] Union is effected by periosteal bridging callus that requires an abundance of extraosseous blood supply. Since stripping of the periosteum and fascial attachments from the fracture ends may occur at the time of injury or surgery, revascularization of the fracture site may be delayed.

Danckwardt-Lilliestrom studied the effect of intramedullary reaming on the healing of a cortical defect.[49] When the medullary cavity was intact, the defect was rapidly bridged and filled by woven bone. However, if the medullary cavity had been destroyed by intramedullary reaming, the defect was bridged by periosteal callus, which occurred at a later time than if the medullary cavity were intact.

Biomechanics of Intramedullary Nail Fixation

Biomechanical evaluation of intramedullary nails and the mechanical aspects of nail fixation have been performed. Küntscher felt that the basic principle of stable intramedullary fixation was flexible impingement of the nail in the bone.[110] Reaming of the canal might be necessary to achieve stable fixation. Küntscher stated that a nail must be strong enough to resist the stresses caused by muscle contraction, joint movement, and weight bearing. It must have sufficient elasticity to be compressed during insertion and to re-expand once in place, both to prevent rotation of the fracture and to fill the medullary cavity if bone resorption occurs around the nail.[111] Küntscher felt that a V-profile or cloverleaf pattern best fit these criteria. The intramedullary nail has been suggested as a favorable method of fixation because the nail absorbs shearing and bending stress but allows compressive stress across the fracture line.[112] Lauritzen felt that a good nail should have flexibility to allow oblique insertion in curved bones, strength to provide fracture stability, and resistance against corrosion.[117] The thickness of the nail should not be so large that the nail becomes inflexible, which would increase the risk of impaction.

One of the difficulties with intramedullary nails

has been bending and breaking of the implant. Intramedullary reaming was introduced to allow the use of larger, stronger nails, as well as to improve contact between the nail and the bone. An 11-mm Küntscher nail has twice the resistance to bending as a 9-mm nail.[215] The strength of a nail depends not only on its design but also on its orientation in the bone and the mode of testing.[4] A diamond-shaped or Schneider nail is more rigid in torsion than a Küntscher nail, though a Küntscher nail is stronger in bending. Placing the slot of the Küntscher nail on the tension side of the bone results in greater strength than placing the slot on the compression side. The "working length" of the nail (that portion of the nail crossing the fracture between the two areas of contact in the proximal and distal fracture fragments) affects the rigidity of fixation.[4] The stiffness in bending and torsional rigidity are inversely proportional to the working length. Doubling the working length will halve the rigidity in torsion.

The most recently developed intramedullary nail is a fluted nail that is extremely rigid and provides rotational control. Allen and colleagues stated that the fluted nail was designed to overcome the following difficulties of conventional nails: too much flexibility for optimum healing; poor torsional load transmission; poor fixation of the nail in the intramedullary canal; and an appreciable incidence of non-union, malunion, and implant failure if the canal is not reamed to the larger sizes.[3] This nail has greater bending rigidity and bending strength than conventional nails and provides significant torsional rigidity, which no other nail provides. However, the bending stiffness of this nail remains 25 percent less than that of the femur. The stiffness of the nail allows three-point fixation with a secure fit even if the canal is reamed to a larger diameter than the nail. The rigidity of fixation with the fluted nail is approached only by dual-compression plating.

Comparative biomechanical evaluation of the quality of fracture union in either unfixed fractures or fractures fixed with an intramedullary nail was performed by Falkenberg.[68] A linear increase in the tensile strength of both the nailed and unfixed fractures occurred beginning on the tenth day following fracture. In the initial phases of healing, the nailed fractures were stronger than the unfixed fractures. This was attributed to the improved stability of the nailed fractures. After the fortieth day following fracture, the absolute tensile strength of the unnailed fracture was greater than the nailed fracture; and by the sixtieth day, the difference was highly significant ($p < 0.001$). Callus formation was 25 percent less in the nailed than in the unfixed fractures 30 days following fracture, and a marked retardation of endosteal callus was noted in the nailed fractures. When adjustments for cross-sectional area were made, the strength of the nailed fractures remained less than that of the unfixed fractures.

Complications of Intramedullary Nailing

Many complications of intramedullary nailing have been reported. Reported complications include infection, impaction of the nail, impaction of the guide wire, vascular injury, neural injury, distraction of the fracture, splintering of bone, migration of the nail, penetration of the joint by the nail, bending of the nail, failure to engage the distal fragment, radiation burns, delayed union, nonunion, bursitis around the protruding portion of the nail, and fat embolism. Böhler felt that most complications were related to use of too thick, thin, short, or long a nail.[23] Dencker reported the complications encountered in open intramedullary nailing in 432 fractures of the femur.[56] Technical errors were encountered in 14 percent of the cases, with too short a nail as the most frequent error. Complications included inadequate fixation in 5.7 percent, nail impaction in 5.5 percent, splintering of the femur in 1.4 percent, penetration of the joint by the nail in 0.7 percent, and failure to engage the distal fragment in 0.5 percent of the cases. The incidence of infection following intramedullary nailing has been estimated at 5 percent.[209] Refracture following intramedullary nailing may occur. Convent stated that the risk of refracture over a 10 year period was 1 percent in nail-fixed fractures compared with 5 percent with plate-fixed fractures.[43] Böhler felt that an intramedullary nail inhibited callus formation and therefore that nail removal should be delayed for at least 1 year to minimize the risk of refracture.[23] Huys and colleagues noted that osteoporosis due to stress protection of the bone occurs with intramedullary nail fixation as well as with plate fixation.[96]

In summary, intramedullary nail fixation has proved useful in the clinical treatment of fractures. However, intramedullary nailing and reaming damage the nutrient vessels and medullary circulation as well as inhibit endosteal callus formation. Rotational stability is a problem with nails other than the new fluted nail. In the presence of secure fixation with an intramedullary nail, union with primary bone healing may occur.

Comparisons of Intramedullary Nail and Plate Fixation of Fractures

Few comparisons between intramedullary nail and plate fixation of experimental fractures have been reported. Barron and colleagues studied blood flow and fracture healing in osteotomies of the ulna in dogs treated with either a standard plate or an intramedullary Steinmann pin.[14] At 14 days following fracture, they found that fracture-site blood flow was greater on the plate side, whereas whole-bone blood flow was greater on the nail side. At 14 days, new bone formation was greater on the plate than the nail side. However, at 90 days following fracture, there was no difference in blood flow, new bone formation, or fracture union between the two sides. Barron and colleagues concluded that an intramedullary nail decreases blood flow to a fracture site and that plate fixation results in increased quantities of endosteal and periosteal new bone. Therefore, they felt that a plate was a more physiologically sound method of fixation than an intramedullary nail.[14]

Mihula compared the intramedullary nail to plate fixation in osteotomies of the canine radius.[131] Revascularization of plate-fixed fractures occurred by medullary vessels, while nail-fixed fractures were revascularized both by medullary vessels and by vessels derived from the periosteal system and soft tissues. The most rapid union occurred in the fractures treated with a plate. He concluded that plate fixation was the more physiologically sound mode of internal fixation. Rhinelander, on the other hand, noted that both plates and intramedullary nails have an adverse effect on fracture-site revascularization.[172] He stated that the cortex beneath a tightly applied plate becomes avascular and the endosteum in contact with a tight-fitting intramedullary nail becomes avascular.

Reynolds and Key compared healing of canine femoral osteotomies treated with standard plates, slotted Eggers plates, and intramedullary nails.[165] They noted an inhibition of endosteal callus formation by the intramedullary nail. If the nail fixation was secure, only a small quantity of periosteal callus formed; but if the nail was loose, large quantities of periosteal callus formed. Union occurred most rapidly in the fractures treated with the Eggers plate. However, they concluded that if approximation and continued immobilization of the bone ends was achieved, union would occur in approximately the same time regardless of the type of internal fixation employed.[57]

Gustilo and colleagues compared intramedullary nail and plate fixation in femoral osteotomies in the dog.[82] On the nail side, avascularity of almost the entire diaphyseal cortex occurred, with cortical necrosis persisting for 6 to 12 weeks following fracture. The nailed fracture displayed marked periosteal proliferation and an inhibition of endosteal callus formation. Union occurred within 3 months on the plate side compared with 6 months on the nail side.

Braden and Brinker studied healing of canine femoral osteotomies fixed with an intramedullary pin alone, an intramedullary pin plus a one-half Kirschner wire (to control rotation), and a compression plate.[27] Fractures treated with a plate displayed less callus, earlier revascularization, and earlier union than fractures treated with the other methods of fixation. The overall success rate was 91 percent with the plate (one plate loosened owing to screw failure), 100 percent with the intramedullary pins plus a one-half Kirschner wire, and 64 percent with the intramedullary pin alone. They concluded that plate fixation was the best mode of treatment. A comparative study of fractures of the radius in rabbits treated with either an intramedullary nail or a subperiosteal plate or left unfixed did not reveal any significant differences in return of mechanical strength as evidenced by a four-point bending test.[177] Fracture stiffness returned more rapidly than strength.

Anderson compared various methods of fracture treatment in canine femoral osteotomies.[7] The femora treated without fixation displayed a large quantity of callus. Delayed union and non-union occurred frequently. In the presence of a loose-fitting intramedullary nail that did not control rotation, necrosis of the fracture ends occurred, a large quantity of periosteal callus formed, and endosteal callus was severely inhibited. Healing occurred by endochondral ossification, with delayed union and non-union occurring frequently. In the presence of a tight-fitting intramedullary nail, little periosteal or endosteal callus formed. Union occurred by direct primary bone formation at the fracture site. Fractures treated with a standard non-compression plate displayed moderate periosteal callus and a large quantity of endosteal callus. Union occurred by cartilaginous endosteal callus. The fractures treated with compression plates united with minimal periosteal callus, a large quantity of endosteal callus, and direct primary bone formation. Therefore, union occurred by direct bone formation in the tight-fitting intramedullary nail group and the compression-plate group. In both groups, rigid immobilization of the fracture was present.

Comparative biomechanical evaluation of the quality of fixation provided by intramedullary nails and plates was performed by Laurence and colleagues.[115] Küntscher intramedullary nails provided greater bending stiffness than any onlay plate but were unable to provide rotational stiffness. Addition of a keel to the nail did not significantly improve torsional resistance. Biomechanical evaluation of the quality of bone union after either intramedullary nail or plate fixation was performed by Braden and colleagues.[28] Upon torsional testing 10 weeks following fracture, the fractures fixed with an intramedullary pin plus a one-half Kirschner wire to control rotation had regained 80.2 percent of the control value for ultimate strength. The group fixed with only an intramedullary pin regained 61.9 percent, and the plate group regained 36 percent of the control value for ultimate strength. A significant difference ($p < 0.01$) was noted between the intramedullary pin combined with a one-half Kirschner wire group and the plate group. Braden and colleagues attributed the lower strength of the plate group to stress protection of the bone by the plate.

Rand and colleagues compared open intramedul-

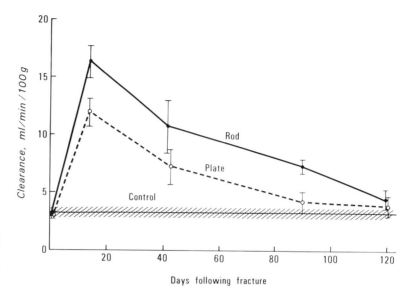

Figure 2–33. Increased blood flow on the rod-fixed side of a canine tibial fracture as opposed to the plate-fixed side. (From Rand, J. A., et al.: A comparison of the effects of open intramedullary nailing and compression-plate fixation on fracture-site blood flow and fracture union. J. Bone Joint Surg. *63A*:427, 1981.)

lary nailing after reaming and compression-plate fixation with regard to fracture-site blood flow, rate of fracture union, and biomechanical quality of fracture union.[163] The rod-fixed side displayed significantly higher whole-bone and fracture-site blood flow (Fig. 2–33). Significantly more endosteal new bone was present on the plate side than on the rod side, while more periosteal new bone was seen on the rod side rather than the plate side (Fig. 2–34). There was a general tendency for the rod side to display a less mature biomechanical stage of union than the plate side at all three time interval studies

(Fig. 2–35). The conclusion from this study was that fractures fixed with an intramedullary rod displayed higher values for a longer time for bone blood flow than do those fractures fixed by a rigid plate. The high prolonged blood flow on the rod side may reflect a compensatory mechanism to increase blood flow to bone because the medullary circulation is blocked by the intramedullary rod.[163] The delay in biomechanical maturation of a rod-fixed fracture may reflect an inhibition of endosteal callus formation rather than an effect upon bone blood flow.[163]

The appropriate management of the fracture with

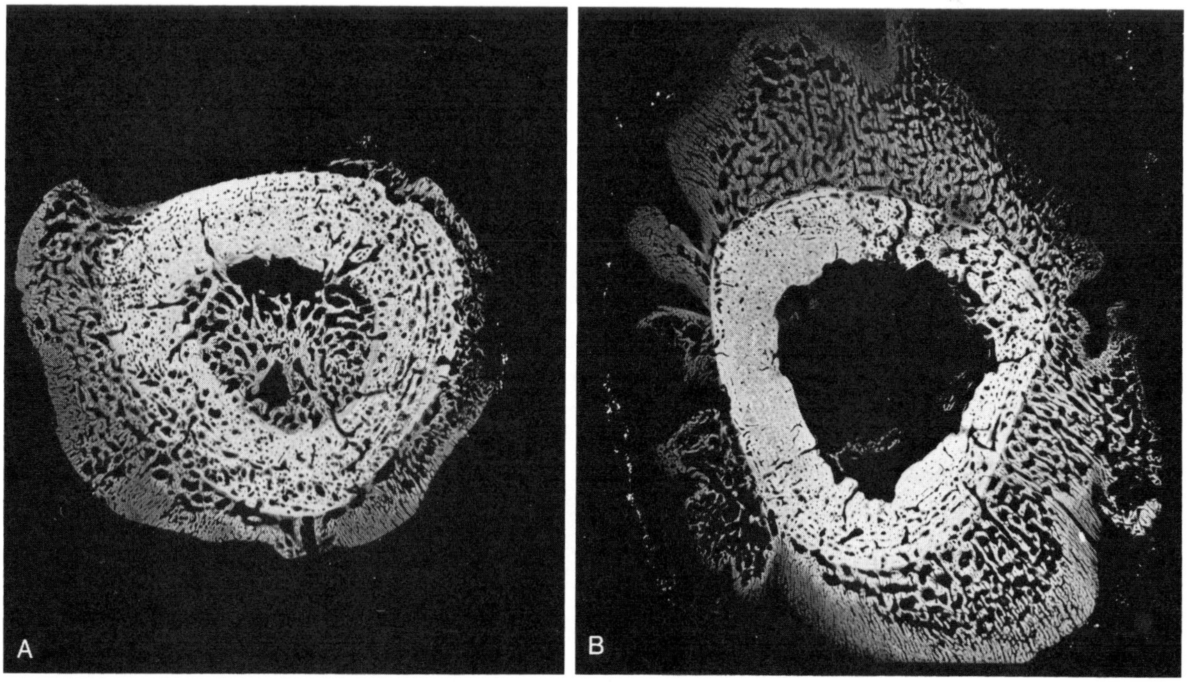

Figure 2–34. *A,* Moderate periosteal and extensive endosteal callus seen in a transverse section of a 90-day plate-fixed canine tibial fracture. *B,* Extensive periosteal and minimal endosteal callus seen in a transverse section of a 90-day rod-fixed canine tibial fracture. (From Rand, J. A., et al.: A comparison of the effects of open intramedullary nailing and compression-plate fixation on fracture-site blood flow and fracture union. J. Bone Joint Surg. *63A*:1981.)

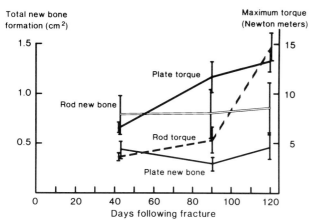

Figure 2–35. Increased strength of a plate-fixed compared to a rod-fixed canine tibial fracture at 42 and 90 days despite greater new bone formation on the rod side. (From Rand, J. A., et al.: A comparison of the effects of open intramedullary nailing and compression-plate fixation on fracture-site blood flow and fracture union. J. Bone Joint Surg. *63A*:1981.)

failed internal fixation depends upon identifying the reasons for failure, whether mechanical or biologic. Secondary surgical intervention must obtain adequate mechanical stability while minimizing adverse biologic consequences. Karlstrom and Olerud have studied the biologic effects of secondary internal fixation.[100] They studied the effects of primary plate fixation followed by intramedullary nailing after reaming in osteotomies of the rabbit tibia. They then compared these results with primary intramedullary nailing after reaming followed by secondary plate fixation. The vascular damage of each procedure was not additive. The reparative process of revascularization following the first operation limited the area of cortical avascularity after the second operation. They concluded that in clinical practice secondary internal fixation by an intramedullary nail was preferable to a plate because it protected against refracture of the bone owing to cancellous transformation of the bone.

The clinical correlation of these studies is evident. The requirements for fracture healing include accurate reduction and close contact of the fracture fragments, an adequate blood supply, the presence of osteogenic cells, and stability of the fracture site. If internal fixation of a fracture is performed, accurate reduction, close contact, and stability may be obtained. However, the internal fixation will significantly alter bone blood flow with possible adverse consequences on fracture healing. One should avoid excessive internal fixation with damage to periosteal and endosteal vascular supplies, as nonunion may result (Fig. 2–36).

External Fixation

External fixation is in frequent use for stabilizing fractures (Fig. 2–37). Indications for external fixation include open fractures, severely unstable comminuted fractures, infected non-unions, arthrodesis, and leg lengthening. External fixation is advantageous in that it requires minimal operative trauma for application, is remote from the fracture, requires a minimum of foreign material, and is adjustable after application. External fixation also allows wound care, preserves joint motion, and provides mobilization of the patient. However, complications of pin loosening, pin infection, and neurovascular injury may occur. The majority of reports concerning external fixation of fractures are clinical with little scientific basis.

Yamagishi and Yoshimura studied rabbit tibial fractures treated with external fixation using varying mechanical conditions.[224] For optimal healing, moderate intermittent compression was the preferred mechanical environment. Laurin and colleagues studied a similar model, using pins and plaster supplemented by an intramedullary pin.[116] They found three phases in fracture healing: (1) hematoma with instability; (2) periosteal callus formation with increasing strength; and (3) endosteal callus that provided little additional stability. They concluded that compression did not hasten callus formation.[116] A comparison between cast immobilization and unilateral single-sidebar external fixation in rabbit tibial osteotomies revealed increased blood flow at 7 weeks on the cast-immobilized side.[45] The relative rigidity of the fixation was felt to decrease the tendency to form callus and thus to lessen the need for blood supply.[45]

A comparison of unilateral external fixation and compression-plate fixation in canine tibial osteoto-

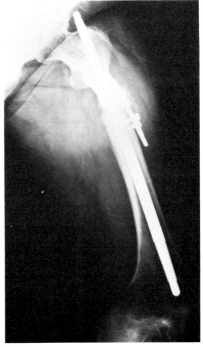

Figure 2–36. Delayed union of femur fracture following combined fixation with a plate and intramedullary nail.

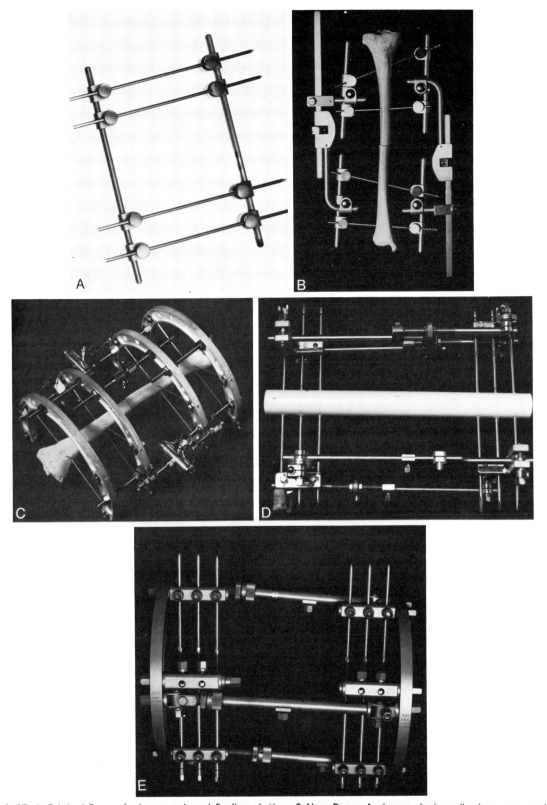

Figure 2–37. *A,* Original Roger Anderson external fixation device. *B,* New Roger Anderson device allowing compression of the fracture surfaces. *C,* Volkov-Oganision device. *D,* Hoffman quadralateral frame. *E,* Fischer apparatus.

mies revealed less rigid fixation with the external fixation device.[119] The less rigid external fixation correlated with a persistently elevated blood flow and less mature biomechanical strength.[119] In an-

other study, the effect of varying rigidity of external fixation devices was analyzed using a canine tibial-fracture model.[223] The less rigid external fixation resulted in an increased periosteal callus and increased bone porosity but no difference in bone blood flow or mechanical strength.[223] Finally, cyclic loading has been compared with constant compression using external fixation in rabbit tibial osteotomies.[149, 218] The cyclic compression–treated bones exhibited improved mechanical strength and a 27 percent saving in healing time compared with the constant-compression group.[149, 218]

Mechanical monitoring of fracture healing has also been performed in fractures treated with external fixation devices. In sheep tibial osteotomies, there was an initial slow decrease followed by a rapid decrease in ability to displace the fracture upon stress.[97] The changes in mechanical properties were attributed to progressive mineralization of the fracture callus.[97] Jorgenson has used a similar technique to study healing human tibial fractures treated with external fixation.[99] Five different shapes of healing curves were found and could be related to the type of fracture, extent of weight bearing by the patient, and quality of treatment. He felt that this technique was applicable to determine the appropriate time for weight bearing and removal of the external device.[99] Burny identified eight types of deformation curves in healing human tibial fractures.[36] He recognized three segments in the healing of a fracture treated with external fixation. There was an initial increase in mobility during the first 3 weeks related to resorption of the bone ends. Next, there was a decrease in mobility related to interfragmentary union. Finally, a plateau level was reached, in which the mechanical properties of the callus were approximately 50 percent that of normal bone.[36]

In summary, although external fixation is in frequent use, additional information is required in order to determine the optimal external-fixation configuration, mode of application, and duration of use. Mechanical monitoring of the fracture site may prove to be a useful technique for assessing the appropriate timing for weight bearing and removal of the external device. Monitoring can also be used for demonstrating problems in fracture union at a time that will allow early intervention by the treating physician.

FRACTURE UNION AND NON-UNION

Definition of Union and Non-union

One of the most difficult decisions facing the clinician is the determination of fracture union. Union may be defined in many ways. Clinically, union may occur when there is no local tenderness and the fractured bone ends can no longer be moved by the examining physician. Union may also be defined as the time when the individual is able to bear full weight with or without aids. The problem with both of these definitions of clinical union is that a firm fibrocartilaginous union can prevent motion between the fractured bone ends and allow weight bearing even when true bony union has not occurred. While a fracture does not obtain adequate strength without bone bridging and fracture remodeling, clinical weight bearing can occur when the fracture has regained only approximately 50 percent of the strength of normal bone. Thus clinical union frequently precedes radiographic union and may be present as early as 6 to 8 weeks after injury.[210] Therefore, though clinical union is useful in deciding treatment options such as the time of weight bearing, it is inadequate as an end point for following the patient's fracture.

Union may also be defined radiographically. Is bridging callus across a fracture an adequate end point for deciding union? How much callus should be present? Does the presence of a fracture line affect the decision regarding union? Even with radiographic information many questions can be raised regarding the end point for union. Unfortunately, fixed criteria that are applicable to all situations are difficult to define. Complete obliteration of the fracture line with evidence of fracture remodeling is a strict criterion for union. For practical purposes, a fracture with bridging callus surrounding 50 percent of the fracture site with no pain or motion on clinical testing may be considered united. However, such fracture strength, although adequate for function without external splintage, may be inadequate for vigorous sports activities without a risk of refracture. Fracture remodeling with obliteration of the fracture line is essential for optimal mechanical strength. Thus, stating a standard time for fracture union for even a specific bone with a single fracture type is difficult.[210] Only the minimal period can be defined and fixed. The rate of union is never constant. It is affected by a variety of biologic variables.

Non-union may be easier to define. One must consider the definition of delayed union, nonunion, and pseudarthrosis. A delayed union occurs when a fracture has not united at the average time for the location and type of fracture.[29] It is important to specify the type of fracture in deciding upon the definition of a delayed union (Fig. 2–38). A nondisplaced transverse fracture without comminution may be expected to heal more rapidly than a severely displaced comminuted fracture in the same location. A non-union exists when the repair process has completely stopped and union will not occur without surgical intervention.[29] The term "pseudarthrosis" is often used synonymously with the term "non-union." A more limited and perhaps more accurate usage would limit use of the term "pseudarthrosis" to a true synovial-lined cavity, the synovial pseudarthrosis. The distinction between fibrous tissue interposition and a true synovial pseudarthrosis is important. Electrical stimulation as a treatment method has a high failure rate in the presence of a synovial pseudarthrosis.[30, 66] The AO group has divided non-unions into two types, hy-

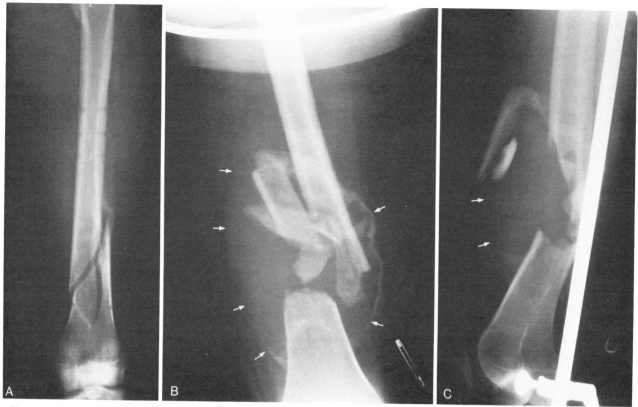

Figure 2–38. A, Early union of nondisplaced spiral femur fracture. AP *(B)* and lateral *(C)* x-ray of comminuted femur fracture with callus forming.

pertrophic and avascular.[137] The distinction is based upon radiographic appearance and the need for bone grafting to obtain union.

Etiologic Factors in the Pathogenesis of Non-union

The etiologic factors contributing to failure of fracture union may be considered as either systemic or local (Table 2–6). Systemic factors of importance include nutritional level, age, endocrine status, and medications. While nutrition is not really a significant problem in the United States, severe vitamin deficiencies, especially those of A, C, and D, can alter fracture healing.[88] Fractures tend to heal more

TABLE 2–6. Factors Affecting Fracture Healing

Systemic	Local
Nutrition	Displacement
Age	Open or closed
Endocrine status	Infection
Medications	Comminution
	Quality of fixation
	Surgical intervention
	Angulation
	Blood supply
	Soft tissue interposition
	Distraction
	Time

slowly in the elderly than in the young. Endocrine abnormalities such as hypothyroidism can lead to a delay in fracture union.[106] Systemic treatment with diphosphonate for Paget's disease may lead to delayed mineralization and thus to a delay of union of normal bone that has sustained a fracture. Systemic metabolic bone disease may result in poor fracture healing due to inadequate mechanical strength but usually does not lead to a delayed rate of union.

Local factors are of much greater importance than systemic factors in the pathogenesis of non-union. Local factors of importance are displacement of bone ends, open fractures, infection, comminution with loss of bone substance, inadequate fixation, inappropriate surgical intervention, persistent angulation, inadequate blood supply, segmental fracture, soft tissue interposition, and distraction.[29, 88, 210]

Distraction of the fracture ends allows fibrous tissue ingrowth and interposition of soft tissues, which mechanically interfere with bridging callus.[84] Distraction may also lead to tension at the fracture site that impedes bone formation.[18] By preventing bone contact, distraction leads to inadequate immobilization. The converse of distraction, compression, leads to close bony contact and improved immobilization.[52, 53]

The importance of an adequate blood supply for fracture healing has been well emphasized.[183] In the segmental or displaced fracture, the endosteal blood supply to the fracture site has been disrupted.[172] This leads to a delayed rate of revascularization and subsequent union. Motion at the fracture site from inadequate immobilization may disrupt the initial endosteal vessels attempting to bridge the fracture site.[88] Ill-performed open reduction and internal fixation may further disrupt the blood supply and provide insufficient stability to allow healing.

The advantages of open reduction in obtaining close contact and anatomic alignment must be weighed against the increased soft tissue damage incurred and risk of infection. If internal fixation is chosen, an excellent reduction and stable internal fixation must be achieved. Displacement and comminution of the fracture as well as the soft tissue damage associated with an open fracture probably contribute to non-union by interfering with the local blood supply to the fracture.[88] Jackson and MacNab correlated the time to union with the extent of displacement in tibial fractures.[94] They found that fractures with minimal displacement healed in 4 months, whereas those with marked displacement frequently were not united before 6 months. Eighty-six percent of the closed tibial fractures united within 6 months as compared with 66 percent of the open fractures.[94] The type of fracture correlates with the time to union, requiring 13 weeks in transverse, 17 weeks in oblique, and 20 weeks in spiral and comminuted fractures of the tibia.[94] Infection of the fracture site leads to a delayed rate of union. Infection may damage the local blood supply as well as interfere with callus formation.[88]

Diagnosis and Classification of Non-union

The diagnosis of non-union can frequently be made by routine radiographs obtained in two planes. The roentgenographic findings in non-union are sclerosis of the bone ends, sealing off of the medullary cavity, and sclerotic marginal proliferation of bone that does not bridge the fracture site (Fig. 2–39).[29] A lucency or gap may be present between the bone ends. Serial roentgenograms over a period of several months that fail to show progression of union are most helpful in the diagnosis.[29] Additional stress roentgenograms and tomograms are also helpful (Fig. 2–40).[29] Bone scintigraphy has been advocated as a useful technique for diagnosis of non-union (Fig. 2–41).[58, 66] Three specific bone-scan patterns have been identified: (1) an intense activity at the fracture site, (2) a cold cleft between two intense areas of uptake, and (3) an indeterminate pattern in which a cold cleft cannot be identified with certainty.[58, 66] The pattern displaying a cold cleft between the bone ends is indicative of a synovial pseudarthrosis with a false positive rate of 10.8 percent.[58, 66] In the series of Esterhai and colleagues, an intense uniform uptake was present in 69.5 percent, the cold cleft type in 23.4 percent, and an indeterminate pattern in 7.1 percent

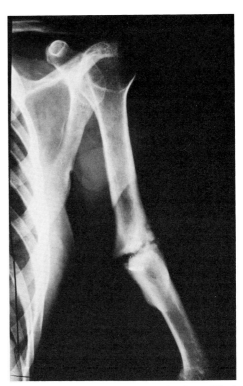

Figure 2–39. Non-union of a transverse fracture of the humerus with sclerosis of the bone ends, plugging of the medullary cavity, and a residual fracture line.

of 157 scans.[66] A synovial pseudarthrosis was most frequently present in non-unions of the humerus (57.1 percent).[66]

Non-unions may be divided into several types.

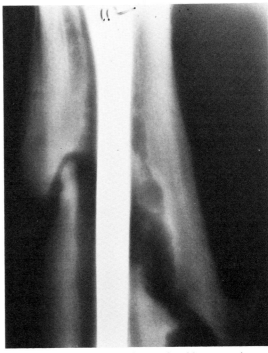

Figure 2–40. Tomogram of hypertrophic non-union of the femur with a poorly fitting Zickel nail.

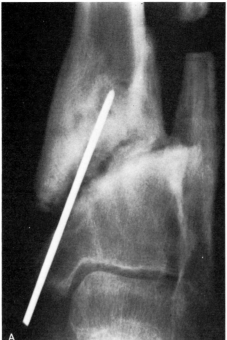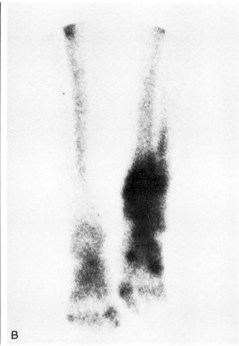

Figure 2–41. Radiograph of ankle *(A)*, and bone scan of hypertrophic non-union of distal tibia *(B)*.

Non-union may be considered with respect to the presence or absence of complicating infection, i.e., noninfected, previously infected, or infected.[137] Non-unions may also be classified according to location, whether they are diaphyseal and metaphyseal.[137] The diaphyseal pseudarthrosis may be subclassified into hypervascular and avascular types.[137, 211] The hypervascular non-union is vascular and capable of biologic reaction (Fig. 2–42).[211] The hypervascular non-union may be further subdivided into elephant foot, horse hoof, and oligotrophic types based upon the radiographic appearance.[211] The elephant foot type has hypertrophy of the bone ends and exuberant callus formation. It represents 85 to 90 percent of non-unions following nonoperative treatment.[137] The horse hoof type has only mild callus formation and sclerosis is frequently present. This type is commonly associated with unstable internal fixation. The oligotrophic non-union has minimal callus formation. This type occurs following major displacement of a fracture, distraction of the fragments, or internal fixation.

The avascular non-union has poor vascularity and is incapable of biologic reaction (Fig. 2–43). It may be subdivided into torsion wedge, comminuted, defect, and atrophic types.[211] The torsion wedge non-union has an avascular intermediate fragment that is healed to one main fragment but not to the other. The comminuted non-union is characterized by one or more necrotic intermediate fragments with absence of callus. A defect non-union is present when fibrosis seals the fracture ends, which remain osteoporotic and atrophic.[211]

Treatment Modalities

A detailed discussion of the treatment of nonunited fractures is beyond the scope of the present chapter. However, the available treatment modalities and their indications related to the type of nonunion will be briefly reviewed. The principles of treatment of non-union are firm fixation, apposition

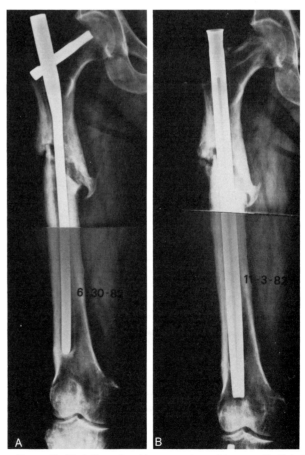

Figure 2–42. A, Hypertrophic non-union of femur with Zickel nail. *B,* Radiograph after repeat internal fixation with a large ASIF intramedullary nail.

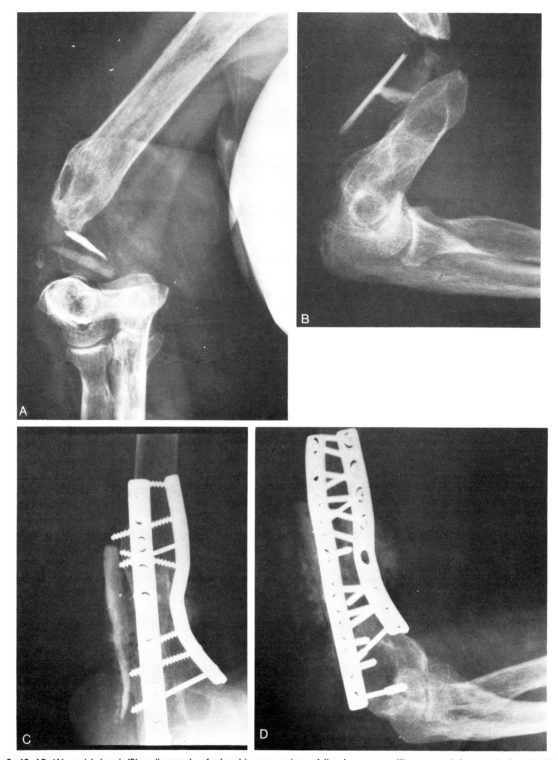

Figure 2–43. AP *(A)* and lateral *(B)* radiograph of atrophic non-union of the humerus with a synovial pseudarthrosis. AP *(C)* and lateral *(D)* x-rays following resection, dual compression-plate fixation, and bone grafting.

of the fragments, and osteogenesis.[27] The commonly used methods of treatment of the non-united fracture include bone grafting, rigid fixation (either internal or external), and electrical stimulation. A combination of these modalities may be used (Fig. 2–44). The hypervascular non-union is capable of biologic reaction and does not require bone graft-

ing.[136, 137] The well-aligned hypervascular pseudarthrosis may be adequately treated with rigid internal fixation alone (Fig. 2–42). There is no need for removal of the intervening fibrous tissue and no need for external cast immobilization. In contrast, the avascular non-union requires rigid fixation plus extensive decortication and an autogenous cancel-

7. Anderson, L. D.: Compression plate fixation and the effect of different types of internal fixation on fracture healing. J. Bone Joint Surg. *47A*:191, 1965.

8. Anderson, L. D.: Compression plate fixation and the effect of different types of internal fixation on fracture healing. Instruct. Course Lect. *18*:224, 1969.

9. Anderson, L. D., Gilmer, W. S., and Tooms, R. E.: Experimental fractures treated with loose and tight fitting medullary nails. Surg. Forum *13*:455, 1962.

10. Bado, J. L.: The Monteggia Lesion. Springfield, IL, Charles C Thomas, 1962.

11. Bagby, G. W.: The effect of compression on the rate of fracture healing using a special plate. Thesis, University of Minnesota, 1956.

12. Bagby, G. W., and Janes, J. M.: An impacting bone plate. Proc. Staff Meetings, Mayo Clin. *32*:55, 1957.

13. Bagby, G. W., and Hanes, J. M.: The effect of compression on the rate of fracture healing using a special plate. Am. J. Surg. *95*:761, 1958.

14. Barron, S. E., Robb, R. A., Taylor, W. F., et al.: The effect of fixation with intramedullary rods and plates on fracture-site blood flow and bone remodeling in dogs. J. Bone Joint Surg. *59A*:376, 1977.

15. Bassett, C. A. L.: Current concepts of bone formation. J. Bone Joint Surg. *44A*:1217, 1962.

16. Bassett, C. A. L.: Augmentation of bone repair by inductively coupled electromagnetic fields. Science *184*:575, 1974.

17. Bassett, C. A. L., Mitchell, S. N., and Gaston, S. R.: Pulsing electromagnetic field treatment in ununited fractures and failed arthrodesis. JAMA *247*:623, 1982.

18. Bassett, C. A. L., and Ruedi, T. P.: Transformation of fibrous tissues to bone *in vivo*. Nature *209*:988, 1966.

19. Bassett, C. A. L., Valdes, M. G., and Hernandez, E.: Modification of fracture repair with selected pulsing electromagnetic fields. J. Bone Joint Surg. *64A*:888, 1982.

20. Bast, T. H., Sullivan, W. E., and Geist, F. D.: The repair of bone. Anat. Rec. *31*:255, 1925.

21. Blaisdell, F. E., and Cowan, J. F.: Healing of simple fractures. Arch. Surg. *12*:619, 1926.

22. Blockey, N. J.: The value of rigid fixation in the treatment of fractures of the adult tibial shaft. J. Bone Joint Surg. *38B*:518, 1956.

23. Böhler, J.: Results in medullary nailing of ninety-five fresh fractures of the femur. J. Bone Joint Surg., *33A*:670, 1951.

24. Borden, S., IV: Traumatic bowing of the forearm in children. J. Bone Joint Surg. *56A*:611, 1974.

25. Borden, S., IV: Roentgen recognition of acute plastic bowing of the forearm in children. A. J. R. *125*:524, 1975.

26. Boyd, H. B., Anderson, L. D., and Johnston, D. S.: Changing concepts in the treatment of non-unions. Clin. Orthop. *43*:37, 1965.

27. Braden, T. D., and Brinker, W. O.: Radiologic and gross anatomic evaluation of bone healing in the dog. J. Am. Vet. Med. Assoc. *169*:1318, 1976.

28. Braden, T. D., Brinker, W. O., Little, R. W., et al.: Comparative biomechanical evaluation of bone healing in the dog. J. Am. Vet. Med. Assoc. *163*:65, 1973.

29. Brasher, H. R.: Diagnosis and prevention of non-union. J. Bone Joint Surg. *47A*:174, 1965.

30. Brighton, C. T., Black, J., Friedenburg, Z. B., et al.: A multicenter study of the treatment of non-unions with constant direct current. J. Bone Joint Surg. *63A*:2, 1981.

31. Brighton, C. T., Friedenberg, Z. B., Black, J., et al.: Electrically induced osteogenesis: Relationship between charge, current density, and the amount of bone formed. Clin. Orthop. *161*:122, 1981.

32. Brighton, C. T., and Krebs, A. G.: Oxygen tension of healing fractures in the rabbit. J. Bone Joint Surg. *54A*:323, 1972.

33. Brookes, M.: Blood flow rates in compact and cancellous bone and bone marrow. J. Anat. *101*:533, 1967.

34. Brookes, M., Elkin, A. C., Harrison, R. G., et al.: A new concept of capillary circulation in bone cortex: Some clinical applications. Lancet *1*:1078, 1961.

35. Brown, K. L. B., and Cruess, R. L.: Bone and cartilage transplantation in orthopedic surgery. J. Bone Joint Surg. *64A*:270, 1982.

36. Burny, F. L.: Strain gauge measurement of fracture healing. *In* Brocker, A. F., and Edwards, C. C.: External Fixation: The Current State of the Art. Baltimore, Williams and Wilkins, 1979.

37. Burstein, A. H., Reilly, D. T., and Frankel, V. H.: Failure characteristics of bone and bone tissue. *In* Kenedi, R. M.: Perspectives in Biomedical Engineering. Baltimore, University Park Press, 1973.

38. Burwell, H. N.: Plate fixation of tibial shaft fractures. J. Bone Joint Surg. *53B*:258, 1971.

39. Cavadias, A. X., and Trueta, J.: An experimental study of the vascular contribution to the callus of fracture. Surg. Gynecol. Obstet *120*:731, 1965.

40. Chalmers, J., Gray, D. H., and Rush, J.: Observations on the induction of bone in soft tissues. J. Bone Joint Surg. *57B*:36, 1975.

41. Coletti, J. M., Jr.: Effects of sustained compression loading of cortical bone *in vivo*. Surg. Forum *20*:471, 1969.

42. Coltart, W. D.: "Aviator's Astragalus." J. Bone Joint Surg. *34B*:545, 1952.

43. Convent, L.: On secondary fracture after removal of internal fixation material. Acta Orthop. Belg. *43*:89, 1977.

44. Copp, D. H., and Shim, S. S.: Extraction ratio and bone clearance of Sr85 as a measure of effective bone blood flow. Circ. Res. *16*:461, 1965.

45. Court-Brown, C. M.: An analysis of the Sukhtian-Hughes external fixation device and its effect on bone blood flow and healing. Unpublished data.

46. Coutts, R. D., Harris, W. H., and Weinberg, E. H.: Compression plating: Experimental study of the effect on bone formation rates. Acta Orthop. Scand. *44*:256, 1973.

47. Cruess, R. L., and Dumont, J.: Fracture healing. Can. J. Surg. *18*:403, 1975.

48. Currey, J. D.: The mechanical properties of bone. Clin. Orthop. *73*:21, 1970.

49. Danckwardt-Lilliestrom, G.: Reaming of the medullary cavity and its effect on diaphyseal bone. Acta Orthop. Scand. Suppl. *128*:1, 1969.

50. Danckwardt-Lilliestrom, G., Lorenzi, G. L., and Olerud, S.: Intramedullary nailing after reaming. Acta Orthop. Scand. Suppl. *134*:1, 1970.

51. Danckwardt-Lilliestrom, G., Lorenzi, G. L., and Olerud, S.: Intracortical circulation after intramedullary reaming with reduction of pressure in the medullary cavity: A microangiographic study on the rabbit tibia. J. Bone Joint Surg. *52A*:1390, 1970.

52. Danis, R.: The operative treatment of bone fractures. J. Chir. *7*:318, 1947.

53. Danis, R.: Théorie et pratique de l'ostéosynthèse. Paris, Masson & Cie, 1949.

54. D'Aubigne, R. M.: Infection in the treatment of un-united fractures. Clin. Orthop. *143*:77, 1965.

55. Dempster, W. T., and Liddecoat, R. T.: Compact bone as a non-isotropic material. Am. J. Anat. *91*:331, 1952.

56. Dencker, H.: Shaft fractures of the femur. Acta Chir. Scand. *130*:173, 1965.

57. Dencker, H.: Technical problems of medullary nailing. Acta Chir. Scand. *130*:185, 1965.

58. Desai, A., Alavi, A., Dalinka, M., et al.: Role of bone scintigraphy in the evaluation and treatment of non-united fractures. J. Nucl. Med. *21*:931, 1980.

59. Devas, M.: Stress Fractures. Edinburgh, Churchill Livingstone, 1975.

60. Duhamel, H. L.: Cited by Keith, A. in Br. J. Surg. *5*:685, 1917.

61. Eggers, G. W. N.: The contact splint. Trans. South. Surg. Assoc. *58*:418, 1946.

62. Eggers, G. W. N.: Internal contact splint. J. Bone Joint Surg. *30A*:40, 1948.

63. Eggers, G. W. N., Ainsworth, W. H., Shindler, T. O., et al.: Clinical significance of the contact-compression factor in bone surgery. Arch. Surg. *62*:467, 1951.

64. Eggers, G. W. N., Shindler, T. O., and Pomerat, C. M.:

The influence of the contact-compression factor on osteogenesis in surgical fractures. J. Bone Joint Surg. *31A*:693, 1949.

65. Enneking, W. F.: The repair of complete fractures of rat tibiae. Anat. Rec. *101*:515, 1948.
66. Esterhai, J. L., Brighton, C. T., Heppenstall, R. B., et al.: Detection of synovial pseudarthrosis by Tc⁹⁹ scintigraphy. Clin. Orthop. *161*:15, 1981.
67. Evans, F. G., and LeBow, M.: Strength of human compact bone under repetitive loading. J. Appl. Physiol. *10*:127, 1957.
68. Falkenberg, J.: An experimental study of the rate of fracture healing. Acta Orthop. Scand. Suppl. *50*:1, 1961.
69. Fitts, W. T., Roberts, B., Spoont, S. I., et al.: The effect of intramedullary nailing on the healing of fractures. Surg. Gynecol. Obstet. *89*:609, 1949.
70. Ford, L. T., and Key, J. A.: Experimental study of the effect of pressure on healing bone. Arch. Surg. *69*:627, 1954.
71. Frankel, V. H., and Burstein, A. H.: The biomechanics of refracture of bone. Clin. Orthop. *60*:221, 1968.
72. Friedenberg, Z. B., and Brighton, C. T.: Bioelectrical potentials in bone. J. Bone Joint Surg. *48A*:915, 1966.
73. Friedenberg, Z. B., and French, G.: The effects of known compression forces on fracture healing. Surg. Gynecol. Obstet. *94*:743, 1952.
74. Friedenberg, Z. B., Roberts, P. G., Didizian, N. H., et al.: Stimulation of fracture healing by direct current in the rabbit fibula. J. Bone Joint Surg. *53A*:1400, 1971.
75. Friedenberg, Z. B., Zemsky, L. M., Pollis, R. P., et al.: The response of non-traumatized bone to direct current. J. Bone Joint Surg. *56A*:1023, 1974.
76. Gallie, W. E., and Robertson, D. E.: The repair of bone. Br. J. Surg. *7*:211, 1919.
77. Glucksmann, A.: Studies on bone mechanics *in vitro*. Anat. Rec. *72*:97, 1938.
78. Glucksmann, A.: The role of mechanical stresses in bone formation *in vitro*. J. Anat. *76*:231, 1941.
79. Gotham, L.: Arterial changes in experimental fractures of the monkey's tibia treated with intramedullary nailing. Acta Chir. Scand. *121*:56, 1961.
80. Gotham, L.: Vascular reactions in experimental fractures. Acta Chir. Scand. Suppl. *284*:1, 1961.
81. Gray, J. C., and Elves, M. W.: Donor cell's contribution to osteogenesis in experimental cancellous bone grafts. Clin. Orthop *163*:261, 1982.
82. Gustilo, R. B., Nelson, G. E., Hamel, A., et al.: The effect of intramedullary nailing on the blood supply of the diaphysis of long bones in mature dogs. J. Bone Joint Surg. *46A*:1362, 1964.
83. Haller, A.: Cited by Keith, A. in Br. J. Surg. *5*:685, 1917.
84. Ham, A. W.: A histological study of the early phases of bone repair. J. Bone Joint Surg. *12*:827, 1930.
85. Ham, A. W.: Histology. 8th ed. Philadelphia, J. B. Lippincott Co., 1979.
86. Hansmann, H.: Cited by Bagby, G. W. (13).
87. Heiple, K. G., Chase, S. W., and Herndon, C. H.: A comparative study of the healing process following different types of bone transplantation. J. Bone Joint Surg. *45A*:1593, 1963.
88. Heiple, K. C., and Herndon, C. H.: The pathologic physiology of non-union. Clin. Orthop. *43*:11, 1965.
89. Heppenstall, R. B., Goodwin, C. W., and Brighton, C. T.: Fracture healing in the presence of chronic hypoxia. J. Bone Joint Surg. *58A*:1153, 1976.
90. Holden, C. E. A.: The role of blood supply to soft tissue in the healing of diaphyseal fractures. J. Bone Joint Surg. *54A*:993, 1972.
91. Hughes, S. P. F., Lemon, G. J., Davis, D. R., et al.: Extraction of minerals after experimental fractures of the tibia in dogs. J. Bone Joint Surg. *61A*:857, 1979.
92. Hutzschenreuter, P., Perren, S. M., and Steinemann, S.: Some effects of rigidity of internal fixation on the healing pattern of osteotomies. Injury *1*:77, 1969.
93. Huys, F., Martens, M., and Mulier, J. C.: Should surgical implants be removed? Acta Orthop. Belg. *43*:Fascicle 1, 1977.
94. Jackson, R. W., and MacNab, I.: Fractures of the shaft of the tibia. Am. J. Surgery. *97*:543, 1959.
95. Jacobs, R. R., Lueth, U., Dueland, R. T., et al.: Electrical stimulation of experimental non-unions. Clin. Orthop. *161*:146, 1981.
96. Jensen, J. S., Johansen, J., and March, A.: Middle third femoral fractures treated with medullary nailing or AO compression plates. Injury *8*:174, 1977.
97. Jofe, M. H., Hayes, W. C., Beaupre, G. S., et al.: Biomechanical monitoring of healing with external skeletal fixation. Transactions (28th annual meeting), Orthop. Res. Soc., 1982.
98. Johnson, R. W.: A physiological study of the blood supply of the diaphysis. J. Bone Joint Surg. *9*:153, 1927.
99. Jorgenson, T. E.: A simple mechanical method of assessing fracture healing. *In* Brooker, A. F., and Edwards, C. C.: External fixation: The Current State of the Art. Baltimore, Williams and Wilkins, 1979.
100. Karlstrom, G., and Olerud, S.: Secondary internal fixation: Experimental studies on revascularization and healing in osteotomized rabbit tibias. Acta Orthop. Scand. Suppl. *175*:3, 1979.
101. Kane, W. J., and Grim, E.: Blood flow to canine hind-limb bone, muscle and skin. J. Bone Joint Surg. *51A*:309, 1969.
101a. Keith, A.: Bone growth and bone repair. Br. J. Surg. *5*:685, 1917.
102. Kelly, P. J.: Anatomy, physiology and pathology of the blood supply of bones. J. Bone Joint Surg. *50A*:766, 1968.
103. Ketenjian, A. Y., and Arsenis, C.: Morphological and biomechanical studies during differentiation and calcification of fracture callus cartilage. Clin. Orthop. *107*:266, 1975.
104. Key, J. A.: Positive pressure in arthrodesis for tuberculosis of the knee joint, South. Med. *25*:909, 1932.
105. Key, J. A., and Reynolds, F. C.: Contact splints vs. standard bone plates in the fixation of experimental fractures. Ann. Surg. *137*:911, 1953.
106. Khomullo, G. V.: Regeneration of bone tissue in animals depending on the basal metabolic rate. Biull. Eksp. Biol. Med. *53*:97, 1962.
107. Kinzl, L.: Cited by Perren, S. M., Matter, P., Ruedi, R., et al.: Biomechanics of fracture healing after internal fixation. Surg. Ann. *7*:361, 1975.
108. Kolodny, A.: The periosteal blood supply and healing of fractures. J. Bone Joint Surg. *5*:698, 1923.
109. Kuhlman, R. E., and Bakowski, M. J.: The biomechanical activity of fracture callus in relation to bone production. Clin. Orthop. *107*:258, 1975.
110. Kuntscher, G. B. G.: The Kuntscher method of intramedullary fixation. J. Bone Joint Surg. *40A*:17, 1958.
111. Kuntscher, G. B. G.: Intramedullary surgical technique and its place in orthopaedic surgery: My present concept. J. Bone Joint Surg. *47A*:809, 1965.
112. Kuntscher, G. B. G.: The intramedullary nailing of fractures. Clin. Orthop. *60*:5, 1968.
113. Ladanyi, J., and Hidvegi, F.: Blood supply of experimental callus formation. Acta Morphol. *4*:35, 1954.
114. Laros, G. S.: Fracture healing: Compression vs fixation. Arch. Surg. *108*:698, 1974.
115. Laurence, M., Freeman, M. A. R., and Swanson, S. A. V.: Engineering considerations in the internal fixation of fractures of the tibial shaft. J. Bone Joint Surg. *51B*:754, 1969.
116. Laurin, C. A., Sison, V., and Roque, N.: Mechanical investigation of experimental fractures. Can. J. Surg. *6*:218, 1963.
117. Lauritzen, F.: Medullary nailing. Acta Chir. Scand. Suppl. *147*:1, 1949.
118. Laurnen, E. L., and Kelly, P. J.: Blood flow, oxygen consumption, carbon-dioxide production and blood-calcium and pH changes in tibial fractures in dogs. J. Bone Joint Surg. *51A*:298, 1969.
118a. Lettin, A. W. F.: The effects of axial compression on the healing of experimental fractures of the rabbit tibia. Proc. Roy. Soc. Med. *58*:30, 1954.
119. Lewallen, D. G., Chao, E. Y. S., Kasman, R. A., et al.: Comparison of compression plates and external fixation on early bone healing. J. Bone Joint Surg. *66A*:1084, 1984.

120. Lexer: Cited by Kolodny, A.: The Periosteal blood supply and healing of fractures. J. Bone Joint Surg. 5:698, 1923.
121. Lindahl, O.: The rigidity of fracture immobilization with plates. Acta Orthop. Scand. 38:101, 1967.
122. Lindsay, M. K.: Observations on fracture healing in rats. J. Bone Joint Surg. 16:162, 1934.
123. Lindsay, M. K., and Howes, E. L.: The breaking strength of healing fractures. J. Bone Joint Surg. 13:491, 1931.
124. Lopez-Curto, J. A., Bassingthwaighte, J. B., and Kelly, P. J.: Anatomy of the microvasculature of the tibial diaphysis of the adult dog. J. Bone Joint Surg. 62A:1362, 1980.
125. Lottes, J. O.: Medullary nailing of the tibia with the triflange nail. Clin. Orthop. 105:253, 1974.
126. MacEwen, W.: Cited by Keith, A. in Br. J. Surg., 5:685, 1917.
127. Mathews, R. S., and Cooper, E. M.: Cortical bone atrophy secondary to compression plate fixation: A clinical and pathophysiologic study. Surg. Forum 27:523, 1976.
128. McKellar-Hall, R. D.: Clay shovelers fracture. J. Bone Joint Surg. 22:63, 1940.
129. Melick, R. A., and Miller, D. R.: Variations of tensile strength of human cortical bone with age. Clin. Sci. 30:243, 1966.
130. Meyer, S., Weland, A. J., and Willenegger, H.: The treatment of infected non-unions of fractures of long bones. J. Bone Joint Surg. 57A:836, 1975.
131. Mihula, A.: The sources of healing of a fracture of tubular bone in different types of osteosyntheses from the standpoint of vessel supply. Rozhl. Chir. 52:35, 1973.
132. Milner, J. C., and Rhinelander, F. W.: Compression fixation and primary bone healing. Surg. Forum 19:453, 1968.
133. Morris, J. M., and Blickenstaff, L. D.: Fatigue Fractures. Springfield, IL, Charles C Thomas, 1967.
134. Morris, M. A., and Kelly, P. J.: Use of tracer microspheres to measure bone blood flow in conscious dogs. Calcif. Tiss. Int. 32:69, 1980.
135. Muller, M. E.: Internal fixation for fresh fractures and for non-union. Proc. R. Soc. Med. 56:455, 1963.
136. Muller, M. E.: Treatment of non-unions by compression. Clin. Orthop. 43:83, 1965.
137. Muller, M. E., Allgower, M., and Willenegger, H.: Manual of Internal Fixation. New York, Springer-Verlag, 1970.
138. Narang, R., and Laskin, D. M.: Experimental osteogenesis at fracture sites and gaps. J. Oral. Surg. 34:225, 1976.
139. Nelson, G. E., Kelly, P. J., Peterson, L. F. A., et al.: Blood supply of the human tibia. J. Bone Joint Surg. 42A:625, 1960.
140. Nilsonne, V.: Biophysical investigations of the mineral phase in healing fractures. Acta Orthop. Scand. Suppl 37:1, 1959.
141. Nunamaker, D. M., and Perren, S. M.: A radiological and histological analysis of fracture healing using prebending of compression plates. Clin. Orthop. 138:167, 1979.
142. Olerud, S., and Danckwardt-Lilliestrom, G.: Fracture healing in compression osteosynthesis in the dog. J. Bone Joint Surg. 50B:844, 1968.
143. Olerud, S., and Danckwardt-Lilliestrom, G.: Fracture healing in compression osteosyntheses. Acta Orthop. Scand. Suppl. 137:1, 1971.
144. Ollier, L.: Cited by Keith, A., in Br. J. Surg. 5:685, 1917.
145. Ozonoff, M. B.: Pediatric Orthopedic Radiology. Philadelphia, W. B. Saunders Co., 1979.
146. Paavolainen, P., Karaharju, E., Slatis, P., et al.: Effect of rigid plate fixation on structure and mineral content of cortical bone. Clin. Orthop 136:287, 1978.
147. Paavolainen, P., Slatis, P., Ahonen, J., et al.: Changes in calcium and hydroxyproline content of cortical bone after compression and neutral plate fixation. Acta Orthop. Scand. 49:492, 1978.
148. Paavolainen, P., Slatis, P., Karaharju, E., et al.: Studies on mechanical strength of bone. Acta Orthop. Scand. 49:506, 1978.
149. Panjabi, M. M., White, A. A., and Wolf, J. W.: A biomechanical comparison of the effects of constant and cyclic compression on fracture healing in rabbit long bones. Acta Orthop. Scand. 50:653, 1979.
150. Paradis, G. R., and Kelly, P. J.: Blood flow and mineral deposition in canine tibial fractures. J. Bone Joint Surg. 57A:220, 1975.
151. Paterson, D. C., Lewis, G. N., and Cass, C. A.: Treatment of delayed union and non-union with an implanted direct current stimulator. Clin. Orthop. 148:117, 1980.
152. Pentecost, R. L., Murray, R. A., and Brindley, H. H.: Fatigue, insufficiency and pathological fractures. JAMA 187:1001, 1964.
153. Perren, S. M.: Physical and biological aspects of fracture healing with special reference to internal fixation. Clin. Orthop. 138:175, 1979.
154. Perren, S. M., Allgower, M., Cordey, J., et al.: Developments of compression plate techniques for internal fixation of fractures. Prog. Surg. 12:152, 1973.
155. Perren, S. M., Huggler, A., Russenberger, M., et al.: The reaction of cortical bone to compression. Acta Orthop. Scand. Suppl. 125:19, 1969.
156. Perren, S. M., Matter, P., Ruedi, R., et al.: Biomechanics of fracture healing after internal fixation. Surg. Annu. 7:361, 1975.
157. Perren, S. M., Russenberger, M., Steinmann, S., et al.: A dynamic compression plate. Acta Orthop. Scand. Suppl. 125:31, 1969.
158. Phemister, D. B.: Bone growth and repair. Ann. Surg. 102:261, 1935.
159. Pinter, J., Rischak, G., and Lenart, G.: The effect of compression on bone mineral. Clin. Orthop. 83:286, 1972.
160. Pitt, M. J., and Speer, D. P.: Radiologic reporting of orthopedic trauma. Med. Radiogr. Photogr., 58:14, 1982.
161. Pugh, J.: An introduction to the biomechanics and biomaterials of bone, joints, and implants. Bull. Hosp. Joint Dis. 37:124, 1976.
162. Rahn, B. A., Gallinaro, P., Baltensperger, A., et al.: Primary bone healing. J. Bone Joint Surg. 53A:783, 1971.
163. Rand, J. A., An, K. N., Chao, E. Y. S., et al.: A comparison of the effects of open intramedullary nailing and comparison-plate fixation on fracture-site blood flow and fracture union. J. Bone Joint Surg. 63A:427, 1981.
164. Reilly, D. T., and Burstein, A. H.: The mechanical properties of cortical bone. J. Bone Joint Surg. 56A:1001, 1974.
165. Reynolds, F. C., and Key, J. A.: Fracture healing after fixation with standard plates, contact splints and medullary nails. J. Bone Joint Surg. 36A:577, 1954.
166. Rhinelander, F. W.: The normal microcirculation of diaphyseal cortex and its response to fracture. J. Bone Joint Surg. 50A:784, 1968.
167. Rhinelander, F. W.: Circulation in bone. In Bourne, G. H.: The biochemistry and physiology of bone, Vol. II, Chapter 1. New York, Academic Press, 1971, pp. 1–77.
168. Rhinelander, F. W.: Effects of medullary nailing on the normal blood supply of diaphyseal cortex. Instruct. Course Lect. 22:161, 1973.
169. Rhinelander, F. W.: Tibial blood supply in relation to fracture healing. Clin. Orthop. 105:34, 1974.
170. Rhinelander, F. W., and Baraby, R. A.: Microangiography in bone healing. I. Undisplaced closed fractures. J. Bone Joint Surg. 44A:1273, 1962.
171. Rhinelander, F. W., Gracilla, R. V., Phillips, R. S., et al.: Microangiography in bone healing. III. Osteotomies with internal fixation. J. Bone Joint Surg. 49A:1006, 1967.
172. Rhinelander, F. W., Phillips, R. S., Steel, W. M., et al.: Microangiography in bone healing. II. Displaced closed fractures. J. Bone Joint Surg. 50A:643, 1968.
173. Rosen, H.: Compression treatment of long bone pseudarthrosis. Clin. Orthop. 138:154, 1979.
174. Rush, L. V., and Rush, H. L.: A technique for longitudinal pin fixation of certain fractures of the ulna and of the femur. J. Bone Joint Surg. 21:619, 1939.
175. Rybicki, E. F., Mills, E. J., Hassler, C. R., et al.: Mathematical and experimental studies on the mechanics of plated transverse fractures. J. Biomech. 7:377, 1974.

176. Rybicki, E. F., and Simonen, F. A.: Mechanics of oblique fracture fixation using a finite-element model. J. Biomech. *10*:141, 1977.

177. Salter, R. B., and Harris, R.: Injuries involving the epiphyseal plate. J. Bone Joint Surg. *45A*:587, 1963.

178. Schenk, R., and Willenegger, H.: Morphological findings in primary bone healing. Symp. Biol. Hung. *7*:75, 1967.

179. Schneider, M., Hansen, S. T., and Winquist, R. A.: Closed intramedullary nailing of fractures of the femoral shaft. Instruct. Course Lect. *27*:88, 1978.

180. Schultz, R. J.: The language of fractures. Baltimore, Williams and Wilkins, 1972.

181. Scott, J. H.: The mechanical basis of bone formation. J. Bone Joint Surg. *39B*:134, 1957.

182. Sharma, O. P., and Kumar, R.: An experimental study of fracture healing after intramedullary nailing. Ind. J. Surg. *37*:260, 1975.

183. Shim, S. S.: Physiology of blood circulation of bone. J. Bone Joint Surg. *50A*:812, 1968.

184. Shim, S. S., Copp, D. H., and Patterson, F. P.: Measurement of the rate and distribution of the nutrient and other arterial blood supply in long bones of the rabbit. J. Bone Joint Surg. *50B*:178, 1968.

185. Shim, S. S., Hawk, H. E., and Yu, W. Y.: The relationship between blood flow and marrow cavity pressure of bone. Surg. Gynecol. Obstet. *135*:353, 1972.

186. Shim, S. S., McPherson, G. D., and Schwigel, J. F.: The rates of blood flow of bones and skeleton in man with emphasis on a radioisotopic method of measurement. Ann. R. Coll. Phys. Surg. Can. *3*:74, 1970.

187. Shim, S. S., and Patterson, F. P.: A direct method of qualitative study of bone blood circulation. Surg. Gynecol. Obstet. *125*:261, 1967.

188. Sim, F. H., and Kelly, P. J.: Relationship of bone remodeling, oxygen consumption, and blood flow in bone. J. Bone Joint Surg. *52A*:1377, 1970.

189. Slatis, P., Karaharju, E., Holstrom, T., et al.: Structural changes in intact tubular bone after application of rigid plates with and without compression. J. Bone Joint Surg. *60A*:516, 1978.

190. Slatis, P., and Rokkanen, P.: The normal repair of experimental fractures. Acta Orthop. Scand. *36*:221, 1965.

191. Stromberg, N. E. L.: Diaphyseal bone in rigid internal plate fixation: Experimental study of the weakening of canine long bone. Acta Chir. Scand. Suppl. *456*:1, 1976.

192. Stromberg, N. E. L., and Dalen, N.: Influence of a rigid plate for internal fixation on the maximum torque capacity of long bones. Acta Chir. Scand. *142*:115, 1976.

193. Teneff, S.: Experimental studies on vascularization of bony calluses. J. Intern. Coll. Surg. *13*:186, 1950.

194. Todd, T. W., and Iler, D. H.: The phenomena of early stages in bone repair. Ann. Surg. *86*:715, 1927.

195. Tonino, A. J., Davidson, C. L., Klopper, P. J., et al.: Protection from stress on bone and its effects. J. Bone Joint Surg. *58B*:107, 1976.

196. Tonna, E. A., and Cronkite, E. P.: Cellular response to fracture studied with tritiated thymidine. J. Bone Joint Surg. *43A*:352, 1961.

197. Townsley, W.: The influence of mechanical factors on the development and structure of bone. Am. J. Phys. Anthropol. *6*:25, 1948.

198. Trias, A., and Fery, A.: Cortical circulation of long bones. J. Bone Joint Surg. *61A*:1052, 1979.

199. Trueta, J.: The role of the vessels in osteogenesis. J. Bone Joint Surg. *45B*:402, 1963.

200. Trueta, J., and Cavadias, A. X.: Vascular changes caused by the Kuntscher type of nailing: An experimental study in the rabbit. J. Bone Joint Surg. *37B*:492, 1955.

201. Trueta, J., and Cavadias, A. X.: A study of the blood supply of the long bones. Surg. Gynecol. Obstet. *118*:485, 1964.

202. Udupa, K. N., and Prasad, G. C.: Chemical and histochemical studies on the organic constituents in fracture repair in rats. J. Bone Joint Surg. *45B*:770, 1963.

203. Uhthoff, H. K., and Dubuc, F. L.: Bone structure changes in the dog under rigid internal fixation. Clin. Orthop. *81*:165, 1971.

204. Urist, M. R.: Bone formation by auto-induction. Science *150*:893, 1965.

205. Urist, M. R., Hay, P. H., Dubue, F., et al.: Osteogenic competence. Clin. Orthop. *64*:194, 1969.

206. Urist, M. R., and McLean, F. C.: Calcification and ossification. I. Calcification in the callus in healing fractures in normal rats. J. Bone Joint Surg. *23*:1, 1941.

207. Varma, B. P., and Mehta, S. H.: Fracture healing with intramedullary nail fixation of the long bones: An experimental study. Acta Orthop. Scand. *38*:419, 1967.

208. Venable, C. S.: An Impacting bone plate to attain closed coaptation. Ann Surg. *133*:808, 1951.

209. Watson-Jones, R., Bonnin, J. G., King, T., et al.: Medullary nailing of fractures after 50 years. J. Bone Joint Surg. *32B*:694, 1950.

210. Watson-Jones, R., and Coltart, W. D.: Slow union of fractures with a study of 804 fractures of the shafts of the tibia and femur. Clin. Orthop. *168*:2, 1982.

211. Weber, B. C., and Chech, O.: Pseudarthrosis. Bern, Hans Huber, 1976.

212. Weinman, D. T., Kelly, P. J., Owen, C. A., et al.: Skeletal clearance of Ca^{47} and Sr^{85} and skeletal blood flow in dogs. Proc. Staff Meet. Mayo Clin. *38*:559, 1963.

213. White, A. A., Panjabi, M. M., and Southwick, W. O.: The four biomechanical stages of fracture repair. J. Bone Joint Surg. *59A*:188, 1977.

214. Whiteside, L. A., Simmons, D. J., and Lesker, P. A.: Comparison of regional bone blood flow in areas with differing osteoblastic activity in the rabbit tibia. Clin. Orthop. *124*:267, 1977.

215. Wickstrom, J., and Corban, M. S.: Intramedullary fixation for fractures of the femoral shaft. J. Trauma *7*:551, 1967.

216. Wirth, C. R., Campbell, C. J., Askew, M. J., et al.: Biomechanics of compression plating. Surg. Forum *24*:470, 1973.

217. Wirth, C. R., Campbell, C. J., Askew, M. J., et al.: The biomechanical effects of compression plates applied to fractures. J. Trauma *14*:563, 1974.

218. Wolff, J. W., White, A. A., Panjabi, M. M., et al.: Comparison of cyclic loading versus constant compression in the treatment of long bone fractures in rabbits. J. Bone Joint Surg. *63A*:805, 1981.

219. Wolff, J.: Das Gesetz der Transformation der knochen. Berlin, Hirschwold, 1892.

220. Woo, S., Akeson, W. H., Levenetz, B., et al.: Potential application of graphite fiber and methyl methacrylate resin composites as internal fixation plates. J. Bomed. Mater. Res. *8*:321, 1974.

221. Wray, J. B.: Vascular regeneration in the healing fracture. Angiology *14*:134, 1963.

222. Wray, J. B., and Lynch, C. J.: The vascular response to fracture of the tibia in the rat. J. Bone Joint Surg. *41A*:1143, 1959.

223. Wu, J. J., Shyr, H. S., Chao, E. Y. S., et al.: Comparison of osteotomy healing under external fixation devices with varying stiffness. J. Bone Joint Surg. *66A*:1258, 1984.

224. Yamagishi, M., and Yoshimura, Y.: The biomechanics of fracture healing. J. Bone Joint Surg. *37A*:1035, 1955.

3

THE SPINE

THOMAS H. BERQUIST • *MIGUEL E. CABANELA*

ANATOMY

Review of the anatomic features of the spine is critical for proper interpretation and utilization of imaging techniques. However, a complete review of the spine's complex anatomy is beyond the scope of this text.

Osteology

The vertebral column is composed of 7 cervical, 12 thoracic, 5 lumbar, 5 sacral, and 4 coccygeal segments (Fig. 3–1). The lateral masses of C1 (atlas) articulate with the occipital condyles at the base of the skull. The sacrum articulates with the innominate bones of the pelvis. The vertebral column supports the weight of the trunk and provides a bony protective covering for the spinal cord.[3, 4, 9, 10] Two major structures, the anterior body and posterior neural arch, make up the typical vertebra. The anterior body develops from one ossification center and the neural arch from two symmetric ossification centers (Fig. 3–2).[4] The neural arch normally fuses dorsally at 1 year of age. Fusion of the two posterior components with the anterior body usually occurs by 3 years of age. During puberty secondary ossification centers appear on the spinous process, on the transverse processes, and at the margins of the superior and inferior articular facets. Ring epiphyses develop on the superior and inferior margins of the vertebral body. These centers usually fuse by age 25.[3–5] Failure of ossification centers to fuse can be difficult to differentiate from fractures (Fig. 3–3).

The typical vertebral body (Fig. 3–4) consists of the anterior body with the vertebral arch, which is composed of two pedicles and two paired laminae. The laminae join posteriorly to form the spinous process. In addition, there are transverse processes bilaterally. Four extensions from the lamina-pedicle junction form the apophyseal or facet joints. The facets articulate with the vertebrae above and below. These apophyseal joints play an important role in determining the range and direction of motion of the vertebral column.[3] Most of the weight-bearing function is provided by the vertebral bodies and interposed elastic vertebral disks. However, the apophyseal joints are also involved in weight-bearing, especially when one changes from the sitting to the standing position.

There are several anatomic features that distinguish the regions of the spine. The bodies of the cervical and lumbar vertebrae are wider in transverse than in AP diameter (Fig. 3–5). The thoracic vertebral body is more uniform in AP and lateral diameter. In the upper thoracic region the vertebral bodies are somewhat heart-shaped. The spinal canal

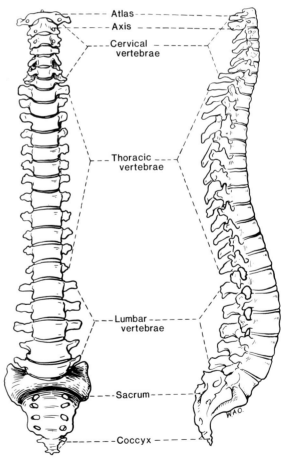

Figure 3–1. Illustration of the AP and lateral views of the spinal column. The normal cervical and lumbar lordotic curves are demonstrated. (From Hollinshead, W. H.: Anatomy for Surgeons, Vol. 3: The Back and the Limbs. 3rd Ed. New York, Harper & Row Publishers, 1982.)

Within the figure labels: Atlas, Axis, Cervical vertebrae, Thoracic vertebrae, Lumbar vertebrae, Sacrum, Coccyx

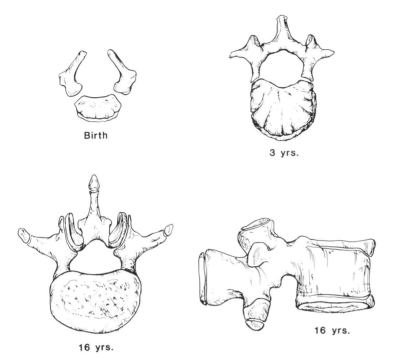

Birth

3 yrs.

16 yrs.

16 yrs.

Figure 3–2. Ossification centers of the vertebra.

in the cervical and lumbar region is triangular compared with the smaller circular configuration in the thoracic region.[4, 5, 8] The transverse processes in the cervical region contain anterior and posterior tubercles as well as a distinguishing feature, the foramen transversarium. The vertebral artery traverses this foramen from C7 to C1. The transverse processes in the thoracic region are directed dorsally, and T1 through T10 contain facets for rib articulation (Fig. 3–5*B*). Transverse processes in the lumbar region project almost straight laterally and increase in size from L1 to L3. The L4 transverse

process is shorter and directed more cephalad. The transverse process of L5 is broader, more sturdy, and also directed dorsally (Fig. 3–6).

Spinous processes are short and often bifid in the cervical spine. The spinous process of C7 is the longest and most prominent, whereas the spinous process of C2 is short and bulbous (see Figs. 3–5 and 3–9). Spinous processes in the thoracic region are directed sharply caudad; they are long and narrow as compared with the broad-based short spinous processes in the lumbar region.

The articular facets differ significantly in the cer-

Figure 3–3. Tomogram of the lumbar spine. There is an unfused ossification center *(arrow).* This should not be confused with a fracture.

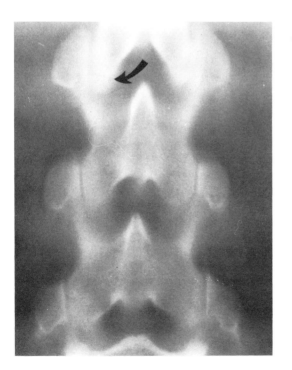

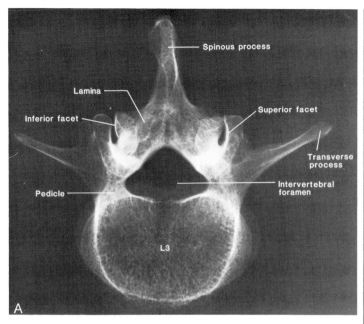
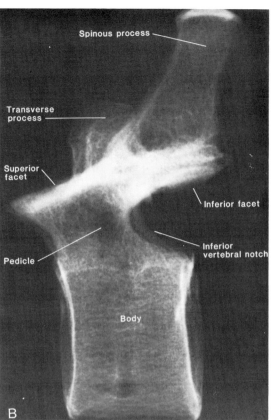

Figure 3–4. Radiographs of dried skeletal specimens. *A,* Axial view of L3. *B,* Lateral view of L1.

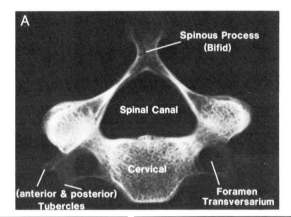

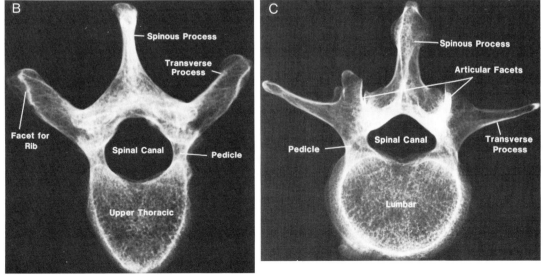

Figure 3–5. Axial radiographs demonstrating features of the cervical *(A),* thoracic *(B),* and lumbar *(C)* vertebrae.

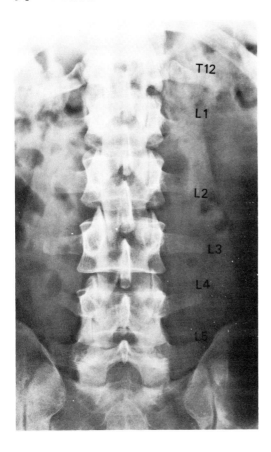

Figure 3–6. AP radiograph of the lumbar spine demonstrating the typical appearance of the transverse process.

vical, thoracic, and lumbar region. In the cervical spine the articular facets angle approximately 20° in a caudad direction with the facet directed posteriorly. A similar but steeper angle is present in the thoracic region, and the facets are angled slightly dorsolaterally. The facet joints in the lumbar region change abruptly, with the superior facets directed dorsally and medially and the inferior facets directed ventrally and laterally (see Fig. 3–4A). This results in restricted rotation in the lumbar region.[3-5, 9]

Cervical Vertebrae

The distinguishing feature of the cervical vertebrae is the foramen transversarium. In addition, there are several significant anatomic differences between C1, C2, C7, and the remaining cervical vertebrae (C3 to C6). The atlas (Fig. 3–7) has no vertebral body and lacks a true spinous process.[1, 3, 4, 5] C1 (atlas) is a ringlike structure with a large vertebral foramen bounded by the anterior and posterior arches. There are two large lateral masses that contain a superior articular facet. This facet articulates superiorly and medially with the occipital condyle. The inferior facet is directed medially and articulates with the superior facet of C2. Medial to the lateral masses are tubercles for the attachment of the strong transverse ligament. The transverse processes of C1 are also much larger when compared with the remaining cervical vertebrae (Fig. 3–7A).

C2 has several distinguishing features. These include a prominent but short spinous process that is helpful in differentiating the level of the upper cervical spine when the entire spine is not included on a radiographic film (Fig. 3–8). The odontoid or dens projects superiorly from the body of C2 and articulates with the anterior ring of C1. The spinal canal at C2 is significantly smaller and rounder than C1. The articular facets of C2 are also atypical when compared with the remaining cervical spine. The superior facets are directed in a superior lateral direction with an angle of approximately 20° in a lateral and caudad direction (Fig. 3–8).[1, 3]

The C3 through C6 vertebrae are typical cervical vertebrae (Fig. 3–9) with triangular vertebral foramina, and typically the facet joints are directed inferiorly approximately 20°. C7 can be distinguished by its prominent spinous process (Fig. 3–9). In 2 percent of cases there is a tubercle on the transverse process of C7 for a cervical rib.[4, 5]

Thoracic Vertebrae

The upper and lower thoracic vertebrae have some features similar to the cervical or lumbar vertebrae. Thus, the middle four thoracic vertebral bodies are most typical. In the upper thoracic spine the vertebral bodies are more triangular or heart-shaped, with the apex of the triangle directed ventrally (see Fig. 3–5). The vertebral bodies in the thoracic spine are typically larger in AP than in transverse diameter. The height of the thoracic

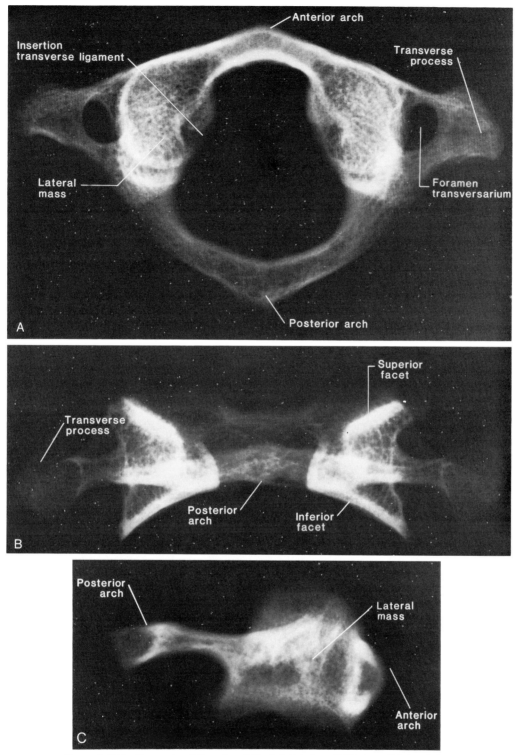

Figure 3–7. Radiographs of the atlas (C1). *A,* Axial view; *B,* AP view; *C,* lateral view.

vertebral body is 1.5 to 2 mm less ventrally than dorsally (Fig. 3–10). This normal feature should not be confused with a compression fracture.[1, 3, 4, 5] A distinguishing feature of the thoracic spine is costal facets for the articulations of the ribs. These are located on the inferior or ventral surface of the transverse process from T1 to T10 and at the junc-tion of the body and pedicle from T1 to T12. The last two ribs do not typically articulate with the transverse processes. The pedicles in the thoracic spine are short and thin, and the vertebral foramina are smaller and more circular than those in either the cervical or lumbar region. The transverse proc-esses typically decrease in length as one progresses

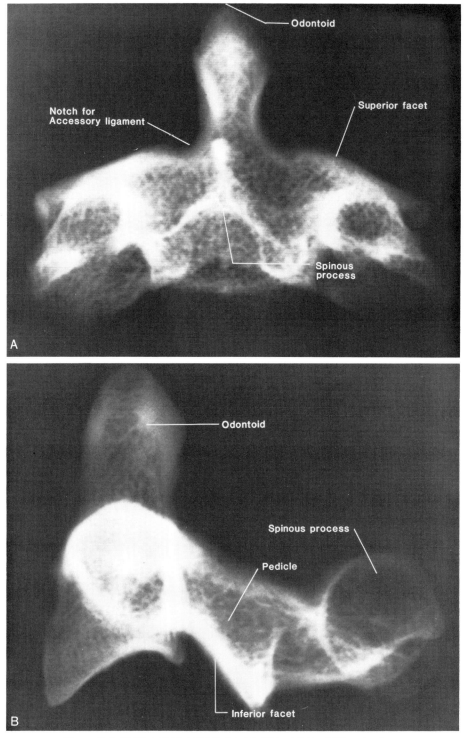

Figure 3–8. Radiographs of C2 in the AP *(A)* and lateral *(B)* projections.

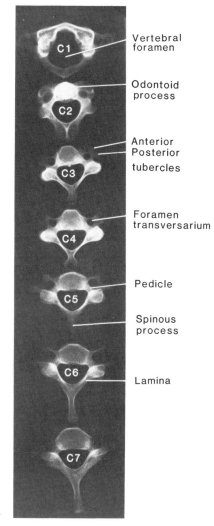

Vertebral
foramen

Odontoid
process

Anterior
Posterior
tubercles

Foramen
transversarium

Pedicle

Spinous
process

Lamina

Figure 3–9. Axial radiographs of the cervical vertebrae.

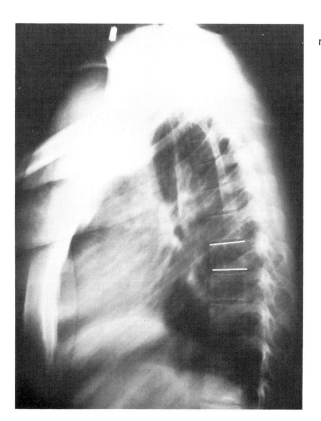

Figure 3–10. Lateral view of the thoracic spine demonstrating the reduced height of the anterior vertebral body.

from T1 to T12. Orientation of the facets in the thoracic region is almost vertical. They are directed posteriorly and slightly laterally throughout the thoracic spine except at the T12 level. Here the inferior facets face laterally to articulate with the superior facets of L1.

Lumbar Vertebrae

The lumbar vertebral bodies are larger and kidney-shaped, with the transverse diameter greater than the AP diameter (see Figs. 3–4 and 3–5). The body of L5 is taller anteriorly than posteriorly (Fig. 3–11). As in the case of the cervical spine, the spinal canal or the vertebral foramen is triangular in the lumbar region. The laminae in the lumbar region are strong and often asymmetric. The pedicles are short and thick. The apophyseal joints arise from the lamina-pedicle junction. The superior facets are directed posteriorly and medially and the inferior facets posteriorly and laterally. The lumbar vertebrae have no costal facets and no foramen transversarium. The transverse processes of the first three lumbar vertebrae are straight and project almost directly laterally, increasing in length from L1 through L3. At L4 and L5 the transverse processes are shorter, with the transverse process of L4 being directed somewhat dorsally and superiorly com-

pared with the short, stout transverse process of L5 (Fig. 3–6).[3, 4, 5, 9]

Sacrum

In adults the sacrum is composed of 5 nonmovable segments (Fig. 3–12). The disks are ossified and fused. The first sacral segment and C1 are the only vertebrae with true lateral masses.[3, 4] The sacrum articulates with the ilia, forming paired synovial sacroiliac joints. Superiorly, two facets articulate with the inferior facets of L5. Of the five sacral segments, the first is the largest. The size of the segments diminishes as one progresses inferiorly. The costal elements and transverse processes are fused. On the AP or frontal view the ventral sacral foramina (four pairs) can be clearly visualized.[1, 5]

Ligamentous Anatomy

The fibrocartilaginous intervertebral disks are the main connecting segments between the vertebral bodies from C2 through the sacrum. There may be rudimentary disks at the sacral levels; however, these are usually completely fused.

The nucleus pulposus and annulus fibrosus are derived from the notochord embryologically. The disks, composed of the nucleus pulposus and an-

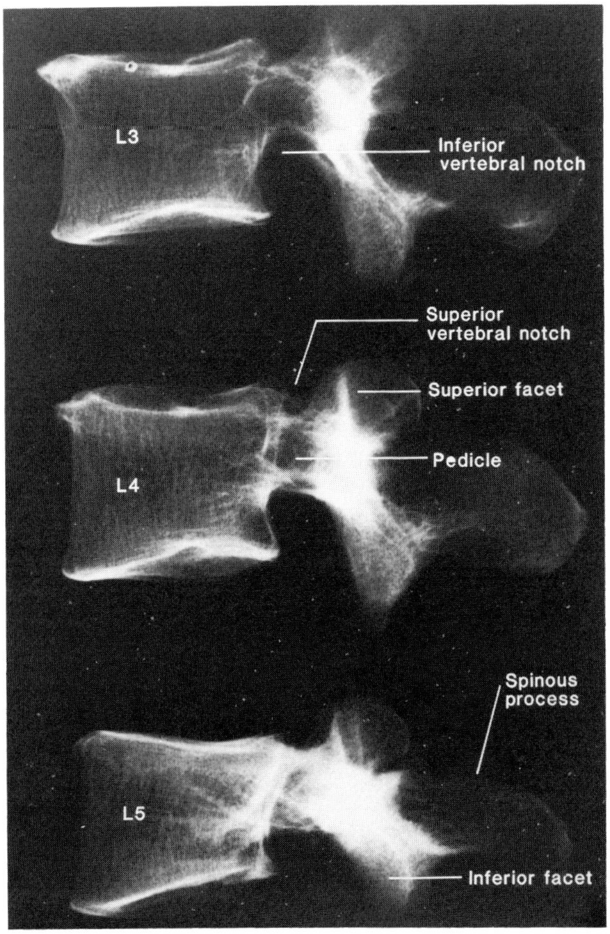

Figure 3–11. Lateral radiographs of L3–L5.

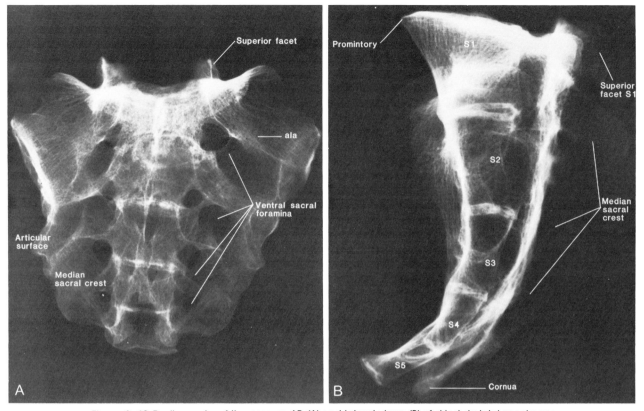

Figure 3–12. Radiographs of the sacrum. AP *(A)* and lateral views *(B)* of dried skeletal specimens.

nulus, contribute approximately one fourth to one third of the height of the vertebral column.[4] The configuration of the disk varies somewhat, depending upon the region of the vertebral column in which it is located. In the cervical region the disks are taller ventrally than dorsally. A similar situation is present in the lumbar region (see Figs. 3–19, 3–31, and 3–32). In the thoracic region the disks are approximately equal in height anteriorly and posteriorly (Fig. 3–10). The thickness of the disk in the lumbar region increases slightly as one progresses from L1 to L4 with the disk at the L4 level being the largest (see Fig. 3–31B). The L5–S1 disk is triangular and much thicker ventrally. The fibers of the annulus fibrosus develop in concentric rings running obliquely, with the superficial fibers blending into the anterior and posterior longitudinal ligaments.[1, 3, 4, 5, 9]

The anterior longitudinal ligament is stronger and wider than the posterior longitudinal ligament (Fig. 3–13). It is narrowest at its origin at the base of the skull and gradually widens to the level of its insertion on the pelvic surface of the sacrum.

The posterior longitudinal ligament lies within the vertebral foramen along the posterior surface of the vertebral body (Fig. 3–13). This ligament is contiguous with the tectorial membrane superiorly and extends caudally into the sacral canal. The posterior longitudinal ligament blends with the fibers of the annulus fibrosus but is separated from the vertebral body by a venous plexus.[5] The narrow

width and central location of the posterior longitudinal ligaments may explain the increased incidence of posterolateral disk protrusions as opposed to central disk protrusions.

The ligamentum flavum is an elastic, thick, paired ligament that extends between the lamina of the adjacent vertebra. The ligaments blend with the articular capsules of the apophyseal joints (Fig. 3–13). Posterior to the ligamentum flavum is the thinner intraspinous ligament, which joins the spinous processes and blends superficially with the supraspinous ligament. (Fig. 3–13). The supraspinous ligament in the cervical region is stronger and is called the ligamentum nuchae (Fig. 3–14). The latter structure extends from the external occipital protuberance to the spinous process of C7. Extending between the transverse processes are the intertransverse ligaments, which are best developed in the thoracic and lumbar region and essentially nonexistent in the cervical region. Also, in the cervical region the interspinous ligament may be sparse and disappear with age, resulting in a questionable significance if this ligament were torn secondary to trauma.[3, 4, 5, 7]

The apophyseal or facet joints are synovial joints with a fibrous capsule. Internally there are meniscuslike tabs composed primarily of synovium and fatty tissue that project from the capsule into the joints. The articular capsules are more lax in the cervical spine, allowing more motion than in the remainder of the spine.

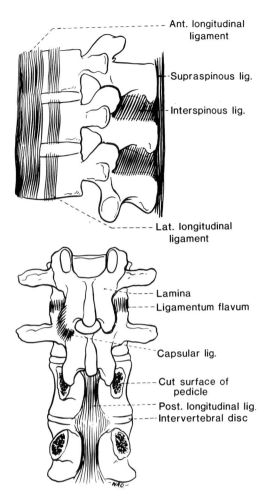

Figure 3–13. Illustration of the ligament anatomy. (From Hollinshead, W. H.: Anatomy for Surgeons, Vol. 3: The Back and the Limbs. 3rd Ed. New York, Harper & Row Publishers, 1982.)

The ligamentous anatomy in the atlantoaxial region is more complex, requiring more emphasis (Fig. 3–15). The posterior longitudinal ligament is continuous with the tectorial membrane that extends cephalad to the inner aspect of the foramen magnum. The transverse ligament lies ventral to the tectorial membrane. It is a strong fibrous band that connects the tubercles of the lateral masses of

C1 posteriorly and maintains the relationship of the odontoid to the anterior ring of C1. There are synovial joints between the odontoid and anterior ring at C1 and between the odontoid and transverse ligament. In addition, there are three ligaments extending vertically from the tip of the odontoid (Fig. 3–15). The apical ligament extends superiorly and attaches to the occipital bone. The two alar or

Figure 3–14. Ligaments of the cervical spine. (From Janes, J. M., and Hooshmand, H.: Severe extension-flexion injuries of the cervical spine. Mayo Clin. Proc. 40:353, 1965.)

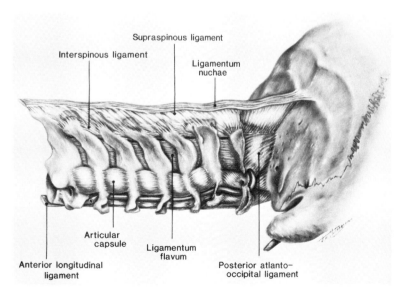

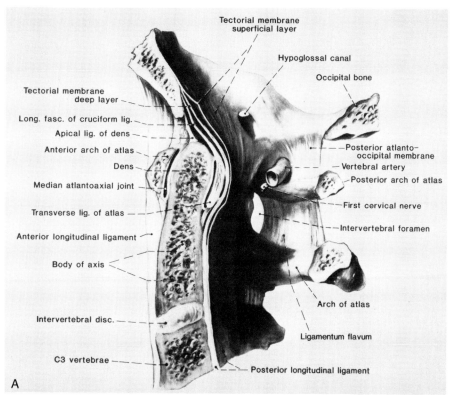

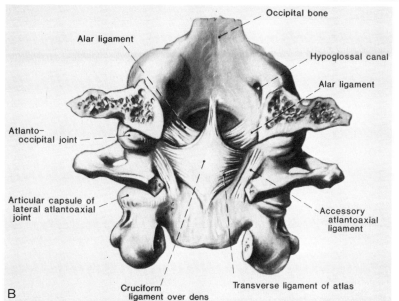

Figure 3–15. Ligament anatomy of the upper cervical spine. *A*, Sagittal illustration with anatomy labeled. *B* and *C*, Posterior coronal illustrations. (From Hollinshead, W. H.: Anatomy for Surgeons, Vol. 3: The Back and the Limbs. 3rd Ed. New York, Harper & Row Publishers, 1982.)

Illustration continued on following page

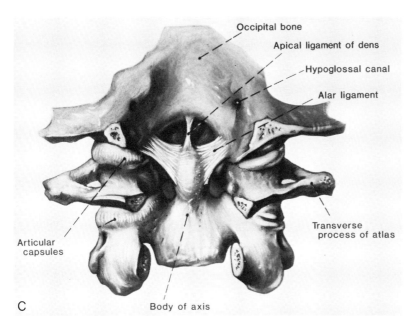

Occipital bone

Apical ligament of dens

Hypoglossal canal

Alar ligament

Transverse process of atlas

Articular capsules

C

Body of axis

Figure 3–15 Continued

check ligaments extend from the apex of the odontoid in a dorsilateral direction. The accessory ligament is a significant structure attaching at the base of the odontoid on either side. It is through this ligament that the odontoid receives part of its blood supply.[3–5, 7, 9]

Neurovascular Anatomy

The blood supply of the spinal cord is derived from the anterior and posterior spinal arteries.[2, 6] In the cervical region these branches are supplied by the vertebral arteries. In the thoracic and lumbar

Figure 3–16. Illustration of the vascular supply of the spinal cord. (From Jablicki, C. K., Aguilo, J. J., Piepgras, D. G., et al.: Paraparesis after renal transplantation. Ann. Neurol. *2*:154, 1977.)

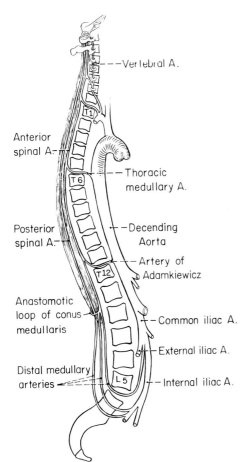

Vertebral A.

T1

Anterior spinal A.

T6

Thoracic medullary A.

Posterior spinal A.

Decending Aorta

Artery of Adamkiewicz

T12

Anastomotic loop of conus medullaris

Common iliac A.

External iliac A.

Distal medullary arteries

L5

Internal iliac A.

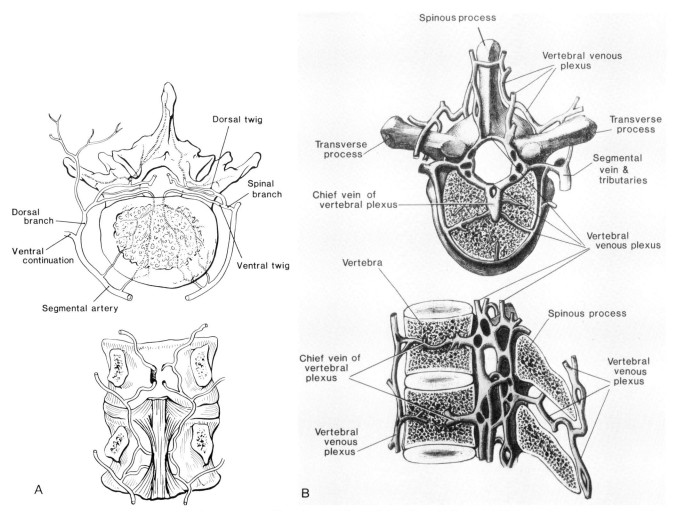

Figure 3–17. Illustration of arterial *(A)* and venous *(B)* anatomy of the vertebra. (From Hollinshead, W. H.: Anatomy for Surgeons, Vol. 3: The Back and the Limbs. 3rd Ed. New York, Harper & Row Publishers, 1982.)

region the arterial supply is derived from the paired intercostal and lumbar vessels. The artery of Adamkiewicz is generally the largest anterior spinal artery. This vessel arises from a lower intercostal or upper lumbar artery (Fig. 3–16).[4, 6] The blood supply in the sacral region is supplied by paired sacral vessels (Fig. 3–16). Multiple perforating arteries arise from these major vessels and supply the anterior portion of the vertebral body. Lateral to the vertebral body there is a dorsal segmental branch that supplies the posterior musculature (Fig. 3–17).

A portion of the venous drainage of the vertebral body occurs through the middle posterior surface in the same region as the chief entrance of the arterial supply (Fig. 3–17). The venous plexus is a valveless plexus lying between the spinal cord and bony neural arch. The previously described plexus lying between the posterior longitudinal ligament and posterior aspect of the vertebral body drains the central tributaries from the vertebral body. There is also an internal plexus anteriorly and posteriorly that is connected to a series of circular venous channels. The internal plexus is continuous with the external plexus via the intervertebral foramina.

The spinal cord with its meningeal envelope lies within the vertebral foramen and extends in the adult from the foramen magnum to the upper border of L2.[2, 3] The vertebral foramen is bordered by the body anteriorly, the pedicles laterally, and the lamina posteriorly. The size of the vertebral foramen is largest in the lumbar and cervical regions, which coincides with the nerve distribution to the upper and lower extremities. The spinal cord occupies approximately 50 percent of the vertebral foramen. The remainder of the space is occupied by the epidural venous plexus, which is intermixed with fat, connective tissue, and the protective meningeal portions of the spinal cord. The dura is a dense fibrous tube contiguous with the foramen magnum and extends to the level of the third sacral segment. The dural sleeves surround each set of spinal nerve roots as they exit the dural sac. The pia mater is the thin innermost layer of the men-

TABLE 3–1. Radiographic Techniques In Cervical Spine Trauma

Routine radiography
    Lateral
    Swimmer's
    Obliques
    AP Views
        Routine
        Angled views
    Odontoid
    Pillar views
    Fluoroscopic flexion and extension views
Tomography
    AP, lateral, oblique, transaxial
Computed tomography
Myelography

inges that is applied to the spinal cord and nerve roots as they cross the subarachnoid space. More peripheral to the pia mater is the arachnoid, which encloses the subarachnoid space. The arachnoid, pia, and dura are united by the dentate ligaments that pass from the spinal cord to the dura. In the adult the spinal cord proper terminates at the conus medullaris. The filum terminale continues caudally until it blends with the posterior ligament and sacral canal. Both structures are enveloped in the dural sac to the S2 level.

There are 31 pairs of spinal nerves: 8 cervical, 12 thoracic, 5 lumbar, 5 sacral, and 1 coccygeal. Cervical nerve roots exit above the level of the adjacent vertebral body (C8 exits between C7 and T1). In the remainder of the spine the nerve roots exit below the adjacent bodies (T1 exits at the intervertebral foramen between T1 and T2).

RADIOGRAPHIC EVALUATION OF THE SPINE FOLLOWING TRAUMA

Acutely injured patients with suspected spinal trauma must be properly immobilized until the radiographic examination is complete and treatment instituted. Radiographic evaluation can be accomplished only when close communication between the radiologist and clinicians (orthopedic surgeons and neurosurgeons) is maintained. A well-organized approach will ensure optimal use of routine films, tomography, CT, and other techniques in determining the extent of injury and stability of the lesion (Table 3–1).

A simple radiographic table with an overhead tube capable of being positioned at different angles is sufficient for evaluation of the spine. The necessary views for evaluation of the cervical, thoracic, and lumbar spine can be easily obtained. We utilize a C-arm Versigraph, which allows AP, lateral, and oblique views without moving the patient. In addition, tomograms can be obtained in the AP, lateral, oblique, and transaxial projections. Conventional radiographic equipment would require the patient to be placed in the oblique or lateral position in order to obtain tomograms in these projections.

Routine Radiography of the Cervical Spine

Radiographic evaluation of the cervical spine should be thoroughly and completely monitored by the radiologist until the degree of injury has been

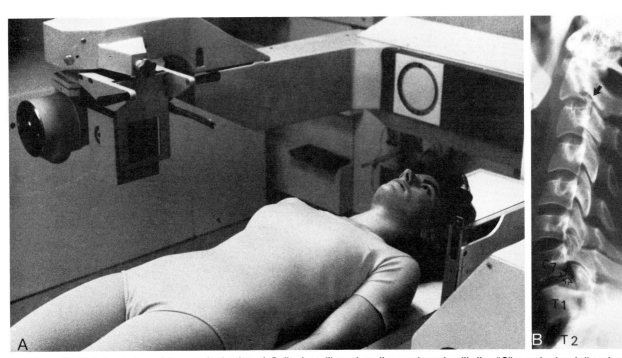

Figure 3–18. Lateral view of the cervical spine. *A,* Patient positioned on the versigraph with the "C" arm horizontally oriented for the lateral view. *B,* Lateral view of the cervical spine demonstrating the difference in size of C7 and T1. Note also the normal subluxation of C2 and C3 on this teenage patient *(upper arrow).*

established. Such an evaluation demands that the examination be tailored to the patient's clinical symptoms. The initial evaluation should include lateral, oblique, AP, and odontoid views. Pillar views may also be indicated. However, the head must be turned for pillar views. Therefore, the other views should be studied first to determine if it is safe or necessary to move the head for pillar views.[18, 21, 25]

Lateral View

The initial lateral view is obtained with the patient supine using a cross-table lateral technique (Fig. 3–18). This view is the most important radiographic view, as most significant pathology can be detected on it.[23, 25] In our review of 420 cervical spine fractures, the lateral view was positive in approximately 90 percent.

There are many features that should be carefully examined on the lateral view. It is essential that all seven cervical vertebrae be well-demonstrated. Ideally T1 should also be visible on the lateral view. The lateral view allows assessment of the following structures: the anterior and posterior arches of C1, the odontoid, vertebral bodies, disk spaces, facet joints, and spinous processes. The lateral radio-

TABLE 3–2. Cervical Spine Trauma: Lateral Radiographic Evaluation

Upper cervical spine (occipital condyles to C2)
    Clivo-odontoid relationship
    C1 lamina—foramen magnum
    C1 odontoid measurement
        2–2.5 mm in adults
        4–4.5 mm in children
    Retropharyngeal space
        Posterior pharyngeal wall to anterior inferior body of C2—7 mm.
Lower cervical spine (C3–C7)
    Prevertebral fat stripe
    Retrotracheal space (posterior tracheal wall to anterior inferior body of C6)
        Normal in adults ≤ 22 mm
        Normal in children ≤ 14 mm
    Anterior spinal line
    Posterior spinal line
    Spinolaminar line
    Disk spaces
    Facet joints
    Spinous processes and interspinous distance

graph shows that the body of T1 is larger than C7, which can give the false impression of subluxation (Fig. 3–18). This fact must be kept in mind in evaluating patients with flexion injuries.

The features demonstrated on the lateral view

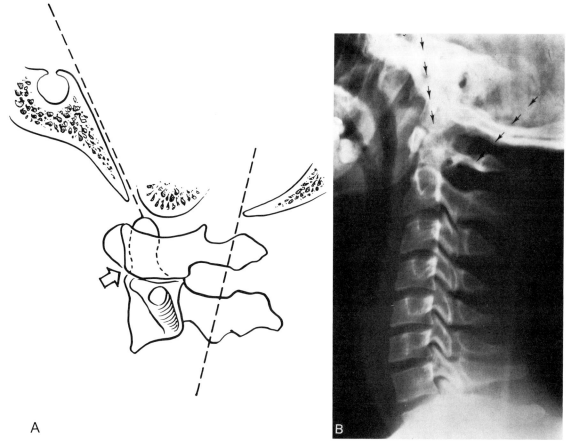

A

B

Figure 3–19. A, Illustration of normal anatomic relationship in the upper cervical spine. B, Normal lateral cervical spine showing the lines of the lamina and clivus (arrows) and normal retrotracheal soft tissues.

must be studied systematically as shown in Table 3–2. In the upper cervical region there are several relationships and measurements that must be checked routinely. These are better demonstrated on the lateral view of the head owing to better centering of the radiographic beam. A line drawn along the clivus to the tip of the odontoid should point to the tip of the odontoid at the junction of the anterior and middle thirds (Fig. 3–19). A line drawn tangentially to the lamina of C1 should intersect the posterior foramen magnum.[18] The space between the odontoid and anterior ring of C1 measured at its most inferior margin should not exceed 2 mm in adults.[18, 23, 25] This measurement may be as much as 4.5 mm in children.[17, 23]

Careful attention should also be paid to the soft tissues in the prevertebral space. In the adult the measurement of the soft tissue from the anterior inferior margin of C2 to the retropharyngeal wall should not exceed 7 mm.[9, 23] The distance from the posterior wall of the trachea to the anterior inferior margin of C6 should not exceed 14 mm in children or 22 mm in adults.[23] Care must be taken in measuring this distance in young people and children, because change in inspiration can simulate swelling. Nasogastric and endotracheal tubes invalidate measurements of the retropharyngeal space (Fig. 3–20).[23] The posterior portions of the maxillary antra and mandible may also provide a clue to the mechanism of injury. These structures can be partially studied on most lateral views of the cervical spine. Mandibular fractures are often associated with hyperextension injuries.[26]

Perhaps a more useful and readily accessible tool than these varied measurements is the prevertebral fat stripe. This can be identified in most adults as it courses along the anterior margin of the anterior longitudinal ligament. At the C6 level it deviates anteriorly over the scalene muscles (Fig. 3–21).[23, 41] Hemorrhage from hyperextension injuries will displace the fat stripe anteriorly.[21, 41] This may be the only indication of injury. The fat stripe is less frequently seen in children.

The normal lordotic curve of the cervical spine

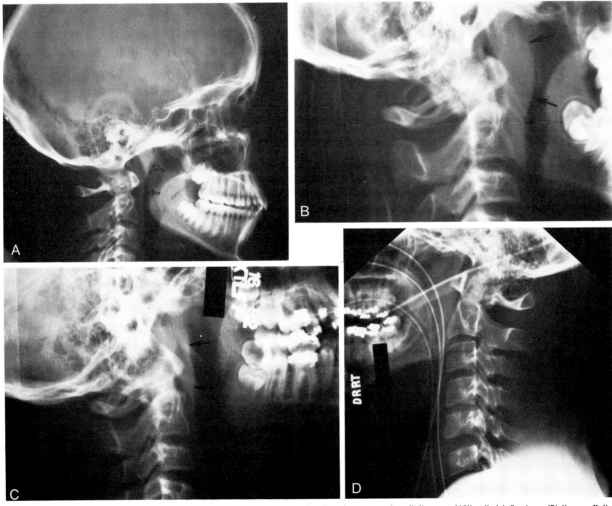

Figure 3–20. Lateral view *(A)* of the skull demonstrating normal retropharyngeal soft tissues. With slight flexion *(B)* the soft tissue appears prominent. In extension *(C)* the tissue is normal. If nasogastric or endotracheal tubes *(D)* are in place, accurate measurement is not possible.

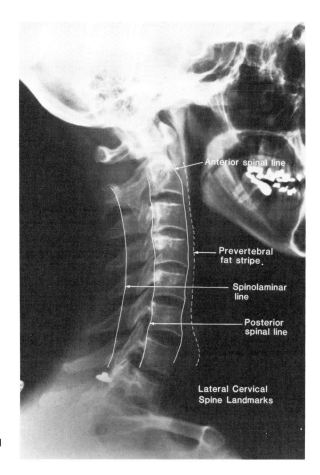

Figure 3–21. Lateral view of the cervical spine demonstrating normal cervical lines and prevertebral fat stripe.

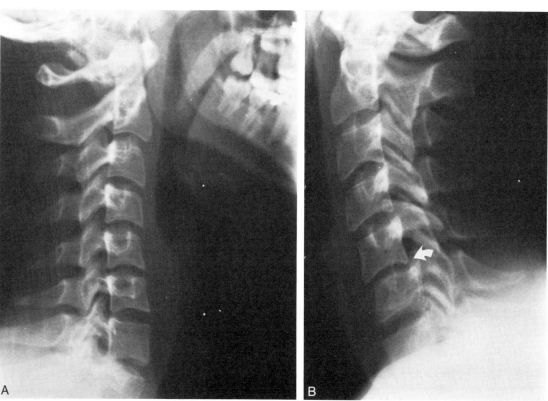

Figure 3–22. A, Loss of the normal cervical lordotic curve in the supine position. Note that the neck is slightly flexed. No lesions were present. B, Subtle subluxation on C5 and C6. There is interruption of the posterior spinal line *(arrow)* and narrowing of the disk space. The pillar of C5 is fractured and rotated off axis.

can be followed along the anterior margins of the vertebral bodies (anterior spinal line), the posterior margins of the bodies (posterior spinal line), and the laminal spinolaminar line (Fig. 3–21).[24] Disruption in these lines can indicate instability or ligament injury with resulting subluxation (Fig. 3–22). One must be careful, however, not to confuse normal positional changes with pathology. In the supine position, patients have a tendency to lose the normal cervical lordotic curve, which can be misinterpreted as evidence of a ligament injury (Fig. 3–22*A*). Muscle spasm may result in straightening of the normal cervical lordotic curve. In addition, there is normally slight ligament laxity at C2–C3 and C3–C4 in children and teenagers (see Fig. 3–18*B*). This can result in slight anterior subluxation of C2 on C3 or C3 on C4 until at least age 18.

Evaluation of the disk spaces, facet joints, and spinous processes is an important factor in determining treatment and prognosis of spinal injury.[23, 24] This factor can be fairly accurately assessed on the lateral view (Figs. 3–22*B* and 3–23). Lateral radiographs reveal instability, which can be defined as abnormal motion between vertebrae whether or not clinical symptoms are present.[23, 42] Findings indicating instability include narrowing of the disk space, compression of the vertebral body exceeding 25 percent, subluxation of greater than 3 mm, and increase in the rotational angle of adjacent vertebrae beyond 11°.[26, 37, 42] An additional feature is widening of the interspinous distance, which normally decreases as one progresses caudally from C1 to C7 (Fig. 3–23).

Sometimes it is difficult to obtain a radiograph that includes the entire cervical spine. Penetration of the shoulders may be difficult owing to muscle spasm in the neck or shoulder injuries. However, the arms can be pulled distally in some patients, which may allow better visualization of the lower cervical spine (Fig. 3–24). This requires more attendants in the room and exposes the "puller" to radiation. Kaufman has stated that this technique should not be used unless there is a low suspicion of injury.[27] Distraction of the arms can cause hyperextension of the cervical spine, thereby exacerbating an existing injury.

We routinely obtain swimmer's views on all patients if C7 and T1 are not visible on the lateral view (Fig. 3–25). This view is taken with the patient supine and the arm closest to the film elevated above the head (Fig. 3–25*A*). Occasionally even this technique is inadequate. In such cases lateral tomography can be performed with the Versigraph without moving the patient.

AP View

The AP view is obtained by angling the tube 5° to 20° to the head. The beam is centered just below the thyroid cartilage.[12, 13] The cassette (8 × 10 cm) is placed under the cervical spine, either in a Bucky tray or in the lower C-arm of the Versigraph. This view allows visualization of the vertebral bodies, uncinate processes, articular pillars, and spinous processes from C7 to C3 (Fig. 3–26). The upper cervical spine is rarely visualized on this view. In

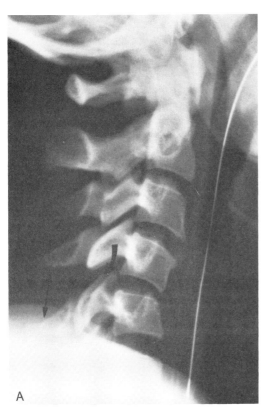
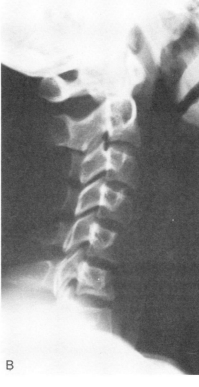

A

B

Figure 3–23. *A*, Disruptive hyperflexion injury with widening of the interspinous distance, facet joints and narrowing of the disk space at C4–C5. *B*, Subtle subluxation of C5 and C6 (widened interspinous distance and facet joints, and slight disk space narrowing) due to a posterior ligament tear.

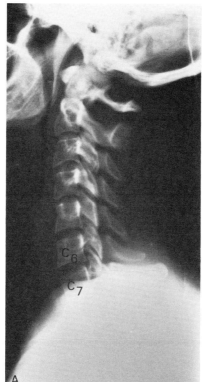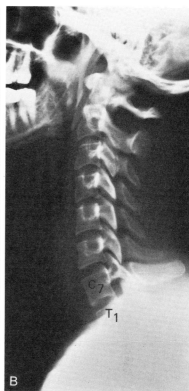

Figure 3–24. *A,* Lateral view of the cervical spine. *B,* Lateral view after pulling down on the arms.

the normal cervical spine, the articular pillars should form a smooth undulating margin bilaterally, and the spinous processes should be centered and equally spaced (Fig. 3–26B). Deviation of the spinous process from the midline (Fig. 3–26C) may indicate a unilateral locked facet secondary to a flexion-rotation injury. These injuries can be subtle and are frequently missed.[34] Widening of the interspinous distance may indicate subluxation or dislocation (Fig. 3–26D). Naidich and colleagues have stated that an interspinous distance 1.5 times that of the interspinous distance above and below indicates dislocation.[31] A double spinous process may be seen on the AP view in spinous process fractures (Fig. 3–26E and F).[16] Careful attention to detail on the AP view of the lower cervical spine may be most helpful. Changes detected may be the only clue to more serious, unstable injuries that may be partially obscured on the lateral view.

Odontoid View

The odontoid view is obtained with the patient's mouth open as wide as possible. The beam is centered over the open mouth and aligned perpendicularly to the cassette (Fig. 3–27A).[12, 13, 33]

The neck should not be extended or the posterior occiput may obscure the odontoid.[18] This view (Fig. 3–27B) allows one to study the odontoid, lateral masses, and transverse processes of C1. If the patient and tube are properly aligned, the spinous process of C2 will be midline. Spaces between the

teeth and the inferior margin of the posterior arch of C1 may overlap the odontoid and should not be confused with fractures.[18]

Oblique Views

The oblique views, following acute trauma, are obtained by angling the C-arm 45° from the horizontal (Fig. 3–28A). In the upright position the patient is rotated (Fig. 3–28B), so that the side away from the film is demonstrated.[12, 13] Detail is improved on the Versigraph. Also, magnification caused by the distance between the patient and film may assist in detecting subtle fractures. The oblique views provide excellent detail of the uncinate processes, pedicles, lamina, and alignment of facet joints (Fig. 3–28C). These views are particularly important in detecting facet subluxations and dislocations.[13, 18, 23, 24]

Pillar Views

A significant number of cervical spine fractures (50 percent in Gehweiler's series) involve the posterior arch.[23] Pillar views are useful in evaluation of the articular pillars and lamina. This view is obtained by angling the tube 25° to 30° toward the feet and can be performed with the patient's neck extended or rotated 45° (Fig. 3–29A). The central beam is centered on C7 and enters near the thyroid cartilage. The AP, lateral, and oblique views must be reviewed first to be certain there is no unstable

Text continued on page 114

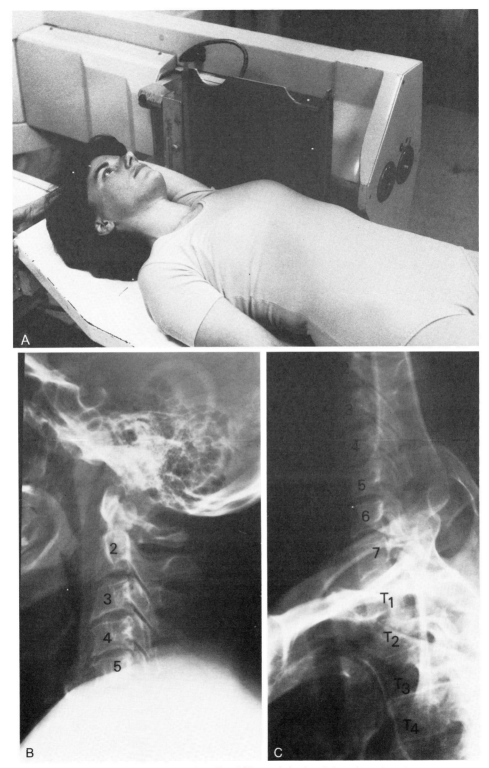

Figure 3–25. A, Patient positioned for the swimmer's view. The "C" arm is horizontal and centered on the lower cervical spine. The arm closest to the film is elevated. B, lateral view demonstrating only five cervical vertebrae. C, The swimmer's view demonstrates the entire cervical spine and upper thoracic spine.

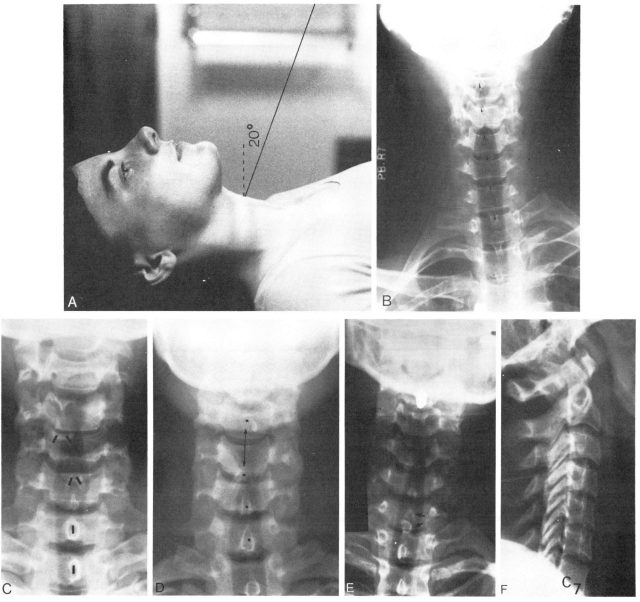

Figure 3–26. A, Patient positioned for the AP view. Beam is angled 20° toward the head. *B,* Normal AP view of the spine. The spinous processes are equidistant. *C,* Normal positioning of the spinous processes from T1 to C6. The C5 spinous process is rotated to the right due to a unilateral locked facet. *D,* Increased interspinous distance between C4 and C5 due to anterior subluxation. *E,* Double spinous process due to fracture of C7. *F,* Fracture is not well seen on the lateral view.

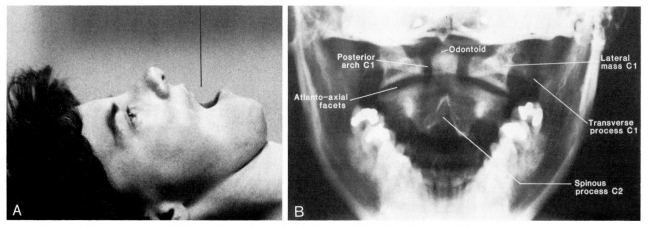

Figure 3–27. Open mouth AP view of the odontoid. *A,* Patient positioned for the odontoid view. *B,* Normal radiograph.

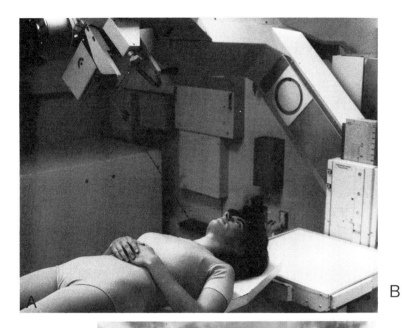

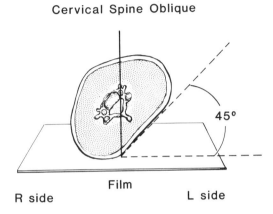

Cervical Spine Oblique

45°

Film

R side   L side

B

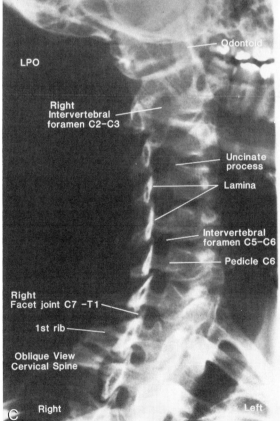

LPO

Odontoid

Right
Intervertebral
foramen C2–C3

Uncinate
process

Lamina

Intervertebral
foramen C5–C6

Pedicle C6

Right
Facet joint C7 –T1

1st rib

Oblique View
Cervical Spine

Right   Left

C

Figure 3–28. A, Patient positioned for oblique view
with the "C" arm angled 45°. The posterior elements
closest to the film will be noted on the film. *B,* Routine
oblique view demonstrates the posterior elements farthest from the film. *C,* Oblique view of the cervical spine
taken on the versigraph.

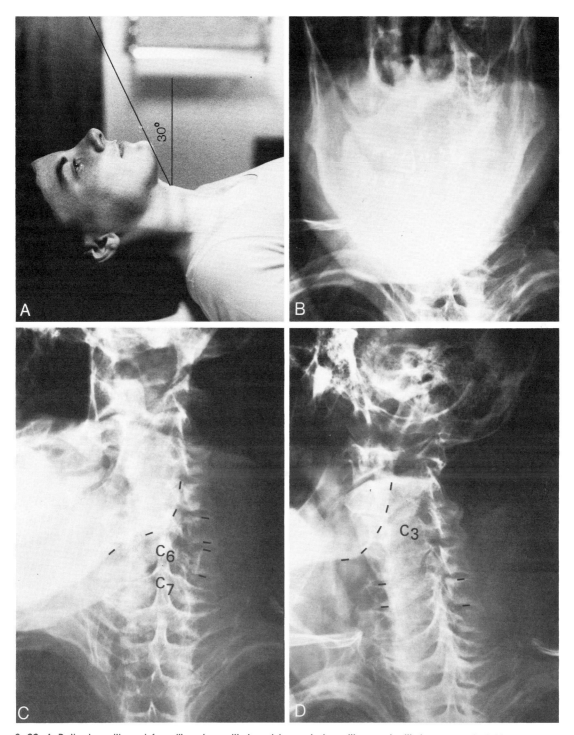

Figure 3–29. *A,* Patient positioned for pillar view with head in neutral position and with beam angled 30° toward the feet. *B,* Radiograph with the head in anatomic position. The mandible obscures the cervical spine. *C,* Radiograph with the head rotated 45° to the right. The lower articular pillars on the left are demonstrated, but the pillars on the right are obscured (the broken line marks the mandible). *D,* Elevating the chin alleviates this problem to some degree. Normally views should be taken with the head rotated both right and left.

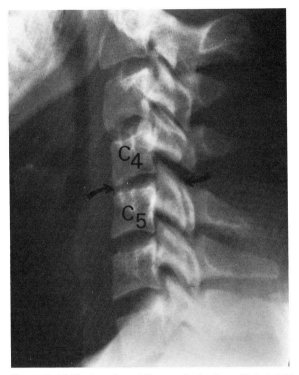

Figure 3–30. Flexion view of the cervical spine with instability. There is widening of the facet joint and disk space narrowing at C4–C5.

or significant injury. Rotation of the head or extension of the neck should be avoided if a significant injury is evident on initial views (Fig. 3–28). Pillar fractures, if present, are almost always stable but can result in significant pain and radiculopathy.[11, 30, 37, 39] The articular pillars should be symmetric in height. A difference in height of 2 mm in the same vertebral unit may indicate a fracture.[39] Changes in height and wedging can be seen frequently in elderly patients with chronic degenerative changes, and it is best not to diagnose a fracture unless an actual fracture line can be seen (Fig. 3–29C and D). The measurements given here may be helpful as a secondary sign.

It is obvious from Figure 3–29 that obtaining high-quality pillar views can be difficult. Wales and colleagues found tomography more useful.[40] They reported pillar views missed 65 percent of posterior-element fractures demonstrated by tomography.

Flexion and Extension Views

Flexion and extension views of the cervical spine are performed to evaluate stability. The examination is most often indicated to exclude ligament instability following trauma or to determine if fractures are healed and stable. This examination should be performed fluoroscopically, so that a true lateral posi-

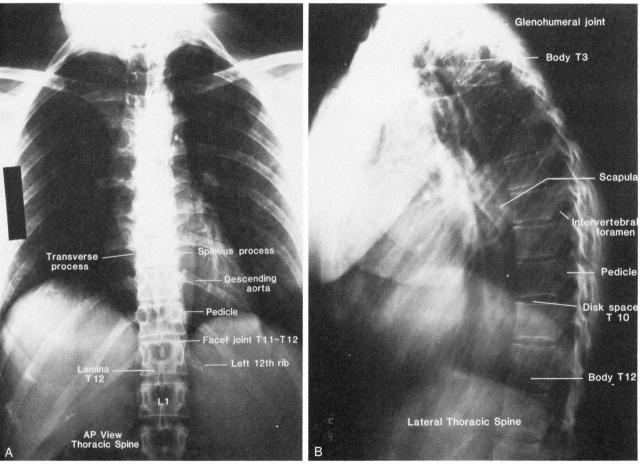

Figure 3–31. AP *(A)* and lateral *(B)* views of the thoracic spine.

tion can be properly attained and the degree of motion monitored.

The patient should sit or stand. Physiologic extension and flexion in the lateral position are monitored fluoroscopically. The extension maneuver is performed initially, and alignment of the vertebrae and anterior ligament structures are studied. The patient is then asked to flex the cervical spine slowly so that alignment, subluxation, facet joint widening, and spinous process motion can be carefully observed. The criteria discussed in routine evaluation of the lateral cervical spine (see Table 3–2) can be applied (Fig. 3–30). However, subtle changes may be important, and care must be taken not to overlook posterior ligament damage. Vertebral body subluxation in flexion should not exceed 1 mm.[19, 23, 34]

Flexion and extension views are often inaccurate immediately following injury. Muscle spasm can result in a false negative examination. Therefore, this examination should not be performed until the spasm has subsided. This may require use of a cervical collar for several days.

Routine Radiography of the Thoracic and Lumbar Spine

In the acutely injured patient AP and lateral views of the thoracic and lumbar spine are routinely obtained. Occasionally, oblique views and tomography are required. The AP thoracic view is ob-

tained with the tube centered over the midthoracic spine. The greater thickness of structures in the lower spine often produces underexposure; overexposure is more common in the upper thoracic spine. Fuchs places the anode at the superior portion of the spine, utilizing the "heal effect" to obtain a more uniform radiograph.[22]

In examining the AP view of the thoracic spine (Fig. 3–31A), one should pay careful attention to the alignment and configuration of the vertebral bodies. Traumatic compression may be asymmetrical. Occasionally, lateral wedging can occur, which may be subtle and best seen on the AP view. Also, changes in the interpedicular distance should be observed, as this may indicate fracture of the posterior elements. The spinous processes can also be seen in the midline posteriorly. The transverse processes in the thoracic spine are best seen on the AP view and normally decrease in length as one progresses caudally. Careful evaluation of the intracostal distances may be helpful, especially in the upper thoracic spine. This may provide the only clue to subluxation in a patient in whom lateral views may be difficult to obtain. Finally, on the AP view the height of each disk space in the thoracic region is usually the same.

The lateral view of the thoracic spine can be obtained using cross-table technique if rotating the patient is not possible. On the lateral view (Fig. 3–31B), one can evaluate the alignment of the vertebral bodies, pedicles, lamina, and spinous processes. The height of the posterior edge of the

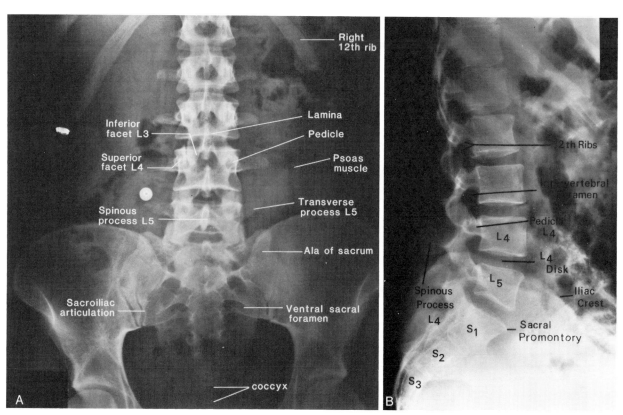

Figure 3–32. AP *(A)* and lateral *(B)* views of the lumbar spine.

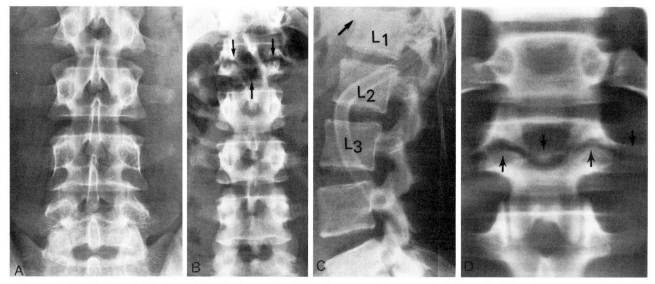

Figure 3–33. A, Normal AP view of the lumbar spine. Note the normal increase in interpediculate distance and "butterfly" configuration of the lamina and articular processes. The spinous process is the "body of the butterfly." *B,* AP view of the lumbar spine demonstrating a transverse fracture through the neural arch at L1 *(arrows). C,* Lateral view demonstrates mild compression of L1 with cortical collapse anteriorly. *D,* Tomogram clearly demonstrates the transverse fracture extending through the pedicles and transverse processes bilaterally *(arrows).*

vertebral body is 1 to 1.5 mm greater than that of the anterior edge.[18] This should not be misinterpreted as acute traumatic compression.

The AP view of the lumbar spine is obtained with the tube centered over the umbilicus (Fig. 3–32*A*). To avoid distortion from the lordotic curve, the knees can be flexed 45° or more.[13, 18] Often, this may not be possible in a severely injured patient. In the lumbar spine, the interpedicular distance normally widens slightly as one progresses from L1 to L5. Careful attention must also be given to the spinous processes and "butterfly" configuration of the lamina and apophyseal facets. Interruption of these structures may be the only clue to a posterior fracture-dislocation (Fig. 3–33). The transverse proc-

esses are clearly seen and usually increase in length from L1 to L3. The transverse processes of L4 are directed slightly cephalad, and those of L5 are much shorter and also directed slightly cephalad (Fig. 3–34; see also Figs. 3–6 and 3–32). The lateral view of the lumbar spine can be obtained with a cross-table technique, turning the patient (if possible) to the lateral position or utilizing the C-arm Versi-graph. The cross-table technique is preferred following trauma.

On the lateral view of the lumbar spine the bodies, pedicles, facet joints, and spinous processes can be clearly demonstrated. It should be noted that the body of L1 is often slightly wedged anteriorly. On occasion this may be difficult to differ-

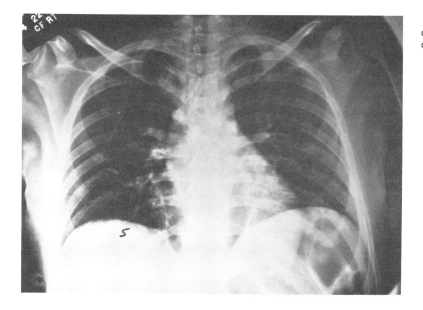

Figure 3–34. AP view of the spine demonstrates asymmetry in the intercostal distance on the right due to anterior subluxation of T5 on T6.

entiate from an acute injury (Fig. 3–32). As in the remainder of the spine, alignment of the vertebral bodies is also well-demonstrated on the lateral view. A coned-lateral view of L5–S1 is also helpful, as better detail can be obtained. There is less scatter and geometric resolution is improved with this technique.

Oblique views are commonly obtained in the lumbar region and are extremely helpful in evaluating the facet joints, lamina, and pars interarticularis. Oblique views are obtained by angling the tube on the Versigraph or rotating the patient 45° into both the left posterior and right posterior oblique positions. The left oblique view demonstrates the left side of the posterior arch and the right oblique the right side (Fig. 3–35).

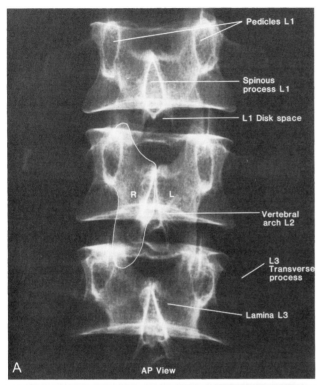

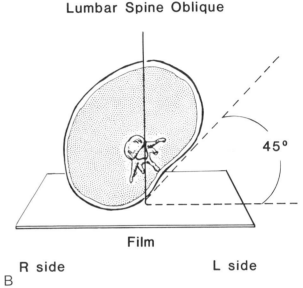

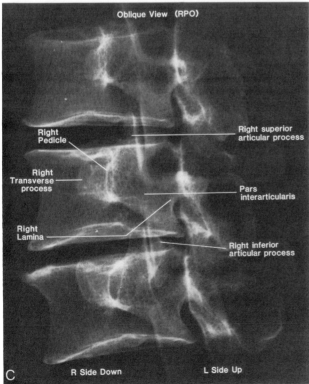

Figure 3–35. *A*, AP view of skeletal specimens L1 to L3. The right side of the posterior arch is marked *(white line)* at L2. *B*, Illustration of position for oblique view. *C*, Oblique view with right side closest to the film. The right side of the posterior arch forms the head, neck, and front leg of the "Scotty dog."

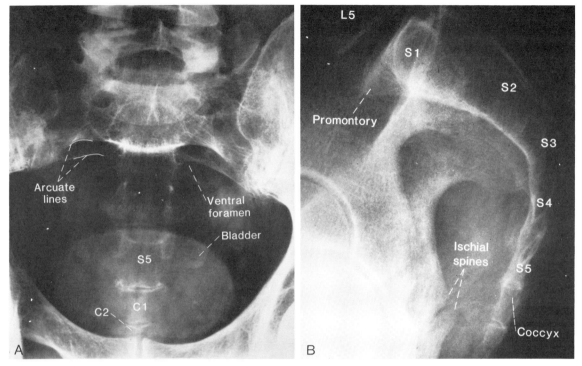

Figure 3–36. AP *(A)* and lateral *(B)* views of the sacrum.

This view demonstrates the "Scotty dog."[18] The nose is the transverse process, the eye is the pedicle, the ear is the superior facet, and the neck is the pars interarticularis. The lamina is the body, and the inferior facet is the front leg. The opposite superior facet (side farthest from the film) is the tail, and the opposite inferior facet is the hind leg.[18]

AP and lateral views of the sacrum can be obtained by centering the tube over the sacrum with the central beam perpendicular to the cassette (Fig. 3–36). On the AP view, the arcuate lines and ventral sacral foramina should be carefully studied. Interruption of the arcuate lines may be the only sign of fracture (see Chapter 4, The Pelvis and Hips). The lateral view is useful in demonstrating displacement of sacral fractures and in detecting fractures or dislocations of the coccyx.

Conventional and Computed Tomography

Tomographic techniques and CT are often helpful in determining the full extent of injury.[14, 15, 20, 28, 32, 36, 38, 43, 44] Tomograms are usually obtained in the AP and lateral projections. This usually necessitates moving the patient, which may not be possible; and, as mentioned earlier, patients with spinal injuries should not be moved until treatment is instituted. Therefore, tomograms and CT may be impossible to perform unless the patient has a stable lesion and can be carefully moved. In this case the orthopedic surgeon or neurosurgeon should assist. As the Versigraph allows tomograms to be per-

formed in the AP, lateral, oblique, and transaxial directions without moving the patient, it presents obvious advantages.

In our experience tomography is helpful in evaluating suspected odontoid (Fig. 3–37) and lateral mass (C1) fractures as well as subtle fractures of the articular facets (Fig. 3–38). These injuries may go undetected unless tomograms are obtained. Woodring and Goldstein described 16 cases of facet fracture.[44] Only two were identified on routine views. Vertebral arch fractures may also be difficult to detect without tomographic assistance. Tomography is also often required to visualize the lower cervical spine, to study a possible fracture, or to exclude fracture in a situation in which the anatomy may be confusing.

Computed tomography has greatly assisted the radiologist in detecting pathology in the vertebral foramen. This finding, namely bone fragments in the spinal canal, is the one certain indication for operative intervention.[14, 38] Tomography may be helpful as well, but CT is more definitive (Fig. 3–39). CT is also helpful in evaluating the upper cervical spine (ring of C1 atlantoaxial, rotary fixation) (Fig. 3–40) and in detecting sagittal fractures of the vertebral bodies. Epidural hematomas and dural tears have also been detected with CT.[14, 15, 32, 38]

CT is extremely helpful but does not replace tomography at our institution. The patient must be stabilized to some degree prior to moving to the CT gantry. In certain conditions this is not possible, and the Versigraph provides the essential information in most cases. This allows clinical judgment on

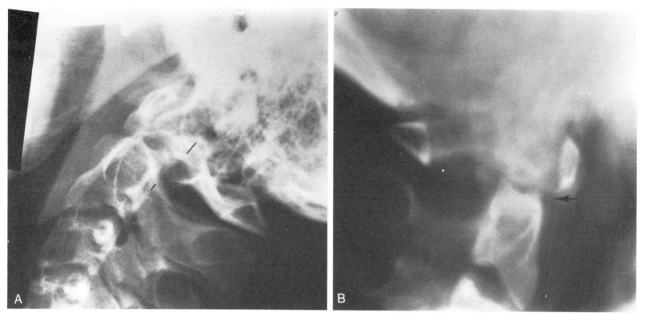

Figure 3–37. A, Lateral view of the upper cervical spine. The odontoid appears normal, and alignment *(lines)* with the body of C2 is normal. *B,* Lateral tomogram demonstrates an undisplaced Type II odontoid fracture *(arrow).* There is soft tissue swelling anteriorly.

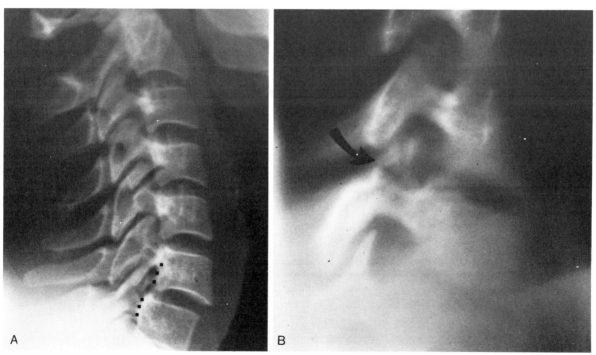

Figure 3–38. A, lateral view of the cervical spine demonstrates slight anterior subluxation of C6 on C7. *B,* Lateral tomogram reveals a comminuted fracture of the right superior facet of C7.

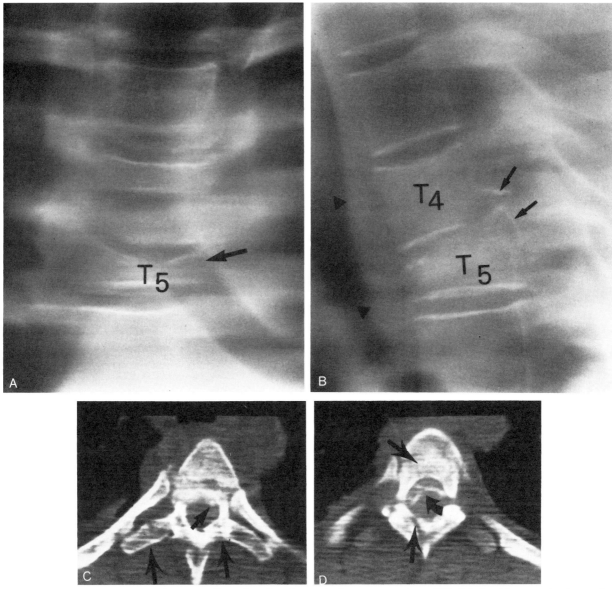

Figure 3–39. A, AP tomogram of the upper thoracic spine demonstrating compression of T5. *B,* Lateral tomogram demonstrates fragments posteriorly with anterior subluxation of T4 on T5 and hematoma anteriorly *(arrows). C* and *D,* CT scans more clearly demonstrate the degree of compromise in the spinal canal and fractures of the transverse processes *(arrows).*

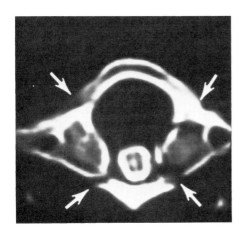

Figure 3–40. CT scan demonstrating a Jefferson fracture.

whether CT is required or whether the patient should be placed in halo traction, with the CT performed later.

As noted in Chapter 1, myelography is rarely indicated in the period immediately following injury. Occasionally, localization of an epidural block will be necessary. In this situation a metrizamide myelogram may be necessary.

CERVICAL SPINE TRAUMA

A team approach is essential in proper management of patients with acute cervical spine fracture or fracture-dislocation. This dictates that radiologists and clinicians must thoroughly discuss the patient's clinical condition. Delay in diagnosis of the severity of the lesion may result in instability and neurologic complications. Subtle posterior ligament injuries are particularly difficult and if initially missed, these may result in significant deformity and neurological sequelae.[50]

Mechanism of Injury

A thorough understanding of the mechanism of injury is essential in proper management of cervical spine trauma. Unfortunately, the classifications available in the literature are numerous and often confusing.[45–49, 52, 54, 55, 58, 59, 63, 67] In-depth discussions of this topic have been presented by Gehweiler,[54] Brackman and Penning,[48] and Holdsworth.[58] The details described in these studies are extremely valuable in understanding fractures and fracture-dislocations of the cervical spine. However, at times the classifications proposed are cumbersome. The mechanism of injury is rarely pure (e.g., flexion or extension alone without compression or rotation). One must guard against oversimplification, but categories of injury can become so complex that they become impractical. Classifications should be easily understood and yet remain accurate. The ultimate goal should be a standard classification that is accurate for determining the proper treatment and prognosis of the injury.

In our series of 420 cervical spine fractures and fracture-dislocations, most injuries could be classified into four groups (Table 3–3). Hyperextension occurred in 38 percent of patients. Hyperflexion injuries were somewhat more common (46 percent). Most were flexion-compression or disruptive hyperflexion injuries. This group included 12 percent of the total series who had unilateral facet locking or perching. Vertical compression injuries occurred in 4 percent of 420 patients. Radiographic classification could not be accomplished in 10 to 12 percent of cases. These patients presented with radiographic findings that did not allow exact determination of the mechanism of injury. Injuries included nondisplaced odontoid fractures, in which the radiographic features were insufficient to determine the mechanism of injury even when combined with

TABLE 3–3. Radiographic Classification of Cervical Spine Injuries[48, 54, 57]

Type of Injury	Incidence (%)* in 420 Patients
Hyperflexion injuries	46
A. Disruptive hyperflexion injuries	
Hyperflexion sprain (transient dislocation)	
Hyperflexion dislocation	
Locked facets (12% unilateral† locked facets)	
Spinous process fracture	
B. Compressive hyperflexion	
Vertebral wedge fracture	
Teardrop fracture	
Fracture-dislocation	
C. Shearing injuries	
Anteriorly displaced odontoid fracture	
Hyperextension injuries	38
A. Disruptive hyperextension	
Hangman's fracture	
Hyperextension sprain	
Anterior inferior vertebral body fracture	
B. Compressive hyperextension	
Posterior arch fractures	
Hyperextension fracture-dislocation	
C. Shearing injuries	
Posteriorly displaced odontoid	
Axial compression injuries	4
Jefferson's fracture	
Burst fractures of the vertebral body	
Hyper-rotation injuries	
Rotary fixation C1 on C2	
Anterior and posterior ligament ruptures	
Lateral flexion injuries	
Uncinate process fracture	
Transverse process fracture	
Lateral wedge fracture of vertebral bodies	
Brachial plexus avulsion	
Indeterminate	10-12

*10 to 12% indeterminate from radiograph alone (undisplaced odontoid, isolated spinous process, etc.)

†12% of hyperflexion injuries were due to flexion-rotation, resulting in unilateral locked facets.

clinical data. Spinous process fractures may result from flexion, extension, or direct trauma. If there are no associated fractures, classification is difficult in this case as well.

Hyperflexion Injuries

There are many descriptive terms in the literature that attempt to define the motion of the cervical spine and the direction of the force that results in injury. Certain of these terms are extremely helpful and others are confusing. Flexion injuries have been classified as (1) disruptive, (2) compressive, and (3) shearing in nature (Table 3–3).[45, 48, 54] Disruptive hyperflexion indicates that the blow was directed upward toward the occipital region, resulting in forward flexion of the head. The major force is applied to the posterior ligaments and spinous processes, resulting in distraction of the spinous processes (Fig. 3–41). If the force is sufficient and the motion of the head continues, the posterior ligaments are interrupted, resulting in an unstable

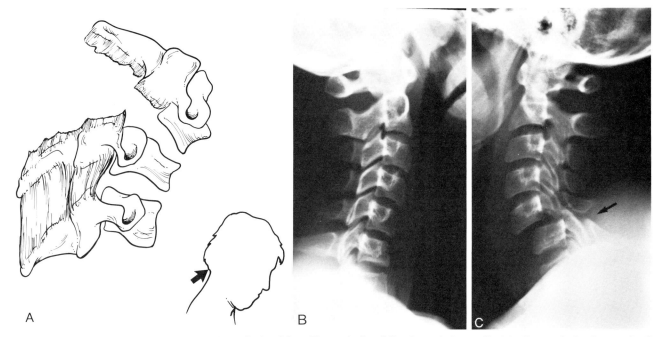

A

B

C

Figure 3–41. A, Illustration of disruptive hyperflexion injury. The majority of the force is transmitted to the posterior ligaments. *B,* Posterior ligament injury with subtle kyphotic angulation to C5–C6. *C,* Bilateral locked facets due to disruptive hyperflexion. The subluxation (C5 on C6) is typically at least one half the AP diameter of the vertebral body.

injury. The cervical spine may then return to its near normal position, depending upon the extent of force applied. In this case, the lateral radiograph may demonstrate kyphosis, with widening of the interspinous distance and facet joints. If the disrup-

tive force continues, however, unilateral or bilateral locking of the facets occurs, depending on the degree of associated rotation (Fig. 3–41). We prefer to consider unilateral locking as a flexion-rotation injury (Fig. 3–42). As mentioned earlier, this type

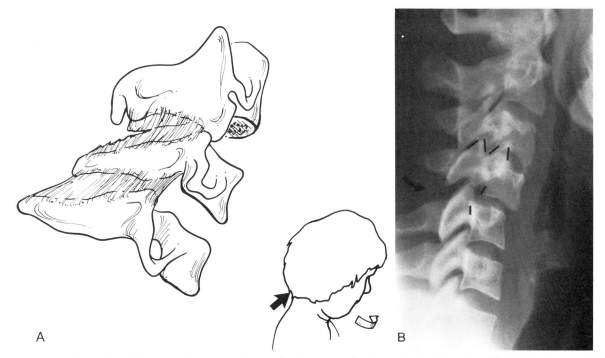

A

B

Figure 3–42. A, Illustration of flexion-rotation injury. *B,* Lateral radiograph of unilateral locked facet at C4–C5. The facets of C4 are rotated with a "bow tie" configuration. There is widening of the interspinous distance *(curved arrow)* and subluxation due to ligament disruption.

Illustration continued on opposite page

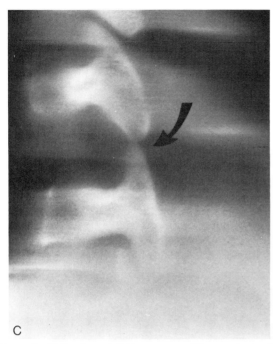

Figure 3–42 Continued. C, Tomogram of the cervical spine following a flexion-rotation injury. The facets are perched *(arrow)* but not locked.

of injury occurred in 12 percent of 420 patients in our series. Flexion-rotation injuries may be subtle, with only minimal anterior subluxation.[61] On the lateral view the facet joints at the level of the injury rotate, giving a "bow tie" appearance (Fig. 3–42B).[56] Oblique views will usually demonstrate the injury more clearly. Tomography is frequently needed for complete evaluation of these injuries (Fig. 3–42C).

Compressive hyperflexion injuries occur when a force is applied to the top of the head, resulting in forward arching of the head (Fig. 3–43). The main force is distributed along the vertebral bodies. As

Figure 3–43. Illustration of flexion-compression injury. More force is transmitted to the anterior vertebral body.

described earlier, the force is mainly compressive and thus the posterior ligaments may remain intact. Wedge fractures of the bodies, teardrop fractures, and fracture-dislocations may result. Harris states that the flexion teardrop injury is the most unstable lesion of all.[57] In this situation the vertebrae above the injury move anteriorly, and the vertebrae below posteriorly, in a circular direction (Fig. 3–44).

Compressive shearing forces result from a force directed to the back of the head with the head moving forward. The end result may be an anteriorly displaced fracture of the odontoid. Atlantoaxial and atlanto-occipital dislocations are rare but may also occur in this type of injury.

Gehweiler[55] classified hyperflexion injuries as follows: Type I, anterior fracture-dislocation of the odontoid; Type II, hyperflexion sprain; Type III, locked facets; Type IV, teardrop fracture-dislocation. These injuries are all basically due to hyperflexion. The important feature is the potential instability and frequency of neurologic complications, especially in the low cervical injuries. It has been reiterated many times in the literature that flexion alone will not result in disruption of the posterior ligaments.[58, 59, 67] The mechanism of injury is rarely pure. In our experience (420 cases) most hyperflexion injuries were of the flexion-compression variety. Regardless of the exact mechanism, one must be aware of the potential significance of hyperflexion injuries. They are frequently unstable and require aggressive treatment. This usually indicates halo immobilization frequently followed by posterior fusion. In our series the incidence of significant neurologic complications following flexion-compression injuries was 72 percent. Other series have also reported a high incidence of neurologic complications with flexion injuries.[59] Delayed instability is also a feared complication of subtle posterior ligament injuries.[46, 50, 62, 64]

Radiographic findings on the lateral view are

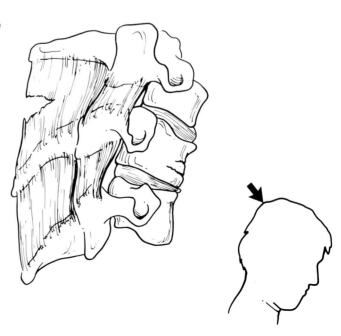

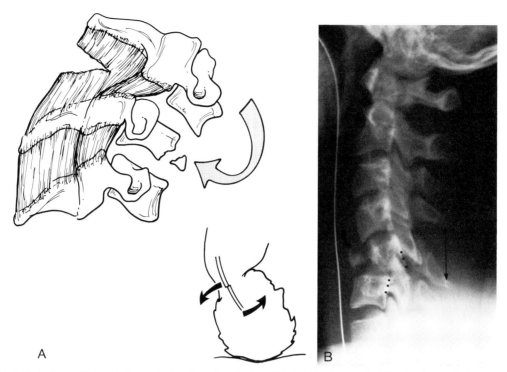

A   B

Figure 3–44. A, Illustration of forces in hyperflexion "teardrop" injury. B, Lateral radiograph following hyperflexion-compression injury with teardrop fracture of C5. Note the subluxation of C5 on C6 and the marked widening of the interspinous distance owing to tearing of the posterior ligaments. This degree of widening would not be seen with a hyperextension injury.

useful in evaluating instability (Table 3–4). These findings include anterior subluxation of greater than 3.5 mm, angular deformity of greater than 11°, widening of the interspinous distance, compression of the vertebral body greater than 25 percent, and disk space narrowing. Harris has classified bilateral locked facets and hyperflexion-teardrop injuries as unstable.[57] Both injuries fulfill the above criteria, and the latter injury is fraught with frequent neurologic complications.

Hyperextension Injuries

Hyperextension injuries were once thought to be uncommon; however, in our experience and according to other authors as well, hyperextension injury is nearly as common as hyperflexion.[45, 53–55, 67] In our series 38 percent of the patients sustained hyperextension injuries (see Table 3–3).

If a force is applied to the mandible in an upward direction, disruption of the anterior longitudinal

TABLE 3–4. Cervical Spine Trauma: Indications of Instability on the Lateral Radiograph

Significant anterior disruption
Vertebral subluxation > 3.5 mm
Angular deformity > 11°
Increased interspinous distance
Narrowed disk space
Facet joint widening
Vertebral body compression > 25%

ligament and disk may result (Fig. 3–45). The lateral radiograph may be normal or reveal soft tissue swelling with displacement of the prevertebral fat stripe.[54, 65] Widening of the anterior disk space may also be evident (Fig. 3–45).[51] A small chip fracture, usually from the anterior inferior aspect of the vertebral body, may be noted (Fig. 3–46). Unfortunately, the radiographic changes may be very subtle, with further confusion added by the presence of significant neurologic deficits. Neurologic damage often is the result of anteroposterior compression of the cord, leading to a decrease in the AP diameter of the spinal canal and vascular compromise to the cord (central cord syndrome). This could occur in spondylotic or normal spines (see Fig. 3–44).[47, 54, 67] Marar suggested that infolding of the ligamentum flavum may also play a part in the cord impingement.[60] The incidence of cord compromise with hyperextension injury from C3 to C7 was 22 percent in our series. In the upper cervical spine the most common hyperextension injury is the "hangman's" fracture, in which neurologic findings are uncommon. No permanent neurologic deficits were evident in upper (C1–C2) cervical injuries, though 10 percent did develop transient neurologic symptoms.

Hyperextension may also result from blows directed to the vertex of the skull, when most of the force is absorbed by the posterior arch. Fractures of the spinous processes, lamina, pedicles, and articular pillars may result (Fig. 3–47). Anterior subluxation may occur, which on the lateral radiograph

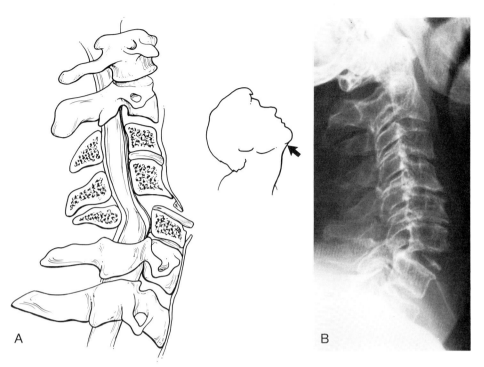

Figure 3–45. A, Illustration of disruptive hyperextension injury. The cord may be compressed with this injury. *B*, Lateral radiograph demonstrating anterior widening of the interspace with a chip fracture due to disruptive hyperflexion.

could be mistaken for a flexion injury. Oblique and pillar views will demonstrate the posterior arch fractures and aid in differentiating the mechanism of injury.[54, 67] In these cases, conventional tomography or computed tomography is often needed to evaluate the neural arch (Fig. 3–47). Facial injuries are also common in patients with hyperextension injuries.[53, 67] Finally, anterior shearing forces result in posterior fracture-dislocations in the upper cervical spine.

Most hyperextension injuries are stable. Unstable injuries include some of the hangman's fractures, hyperextension fracture-dislocations, and hyperextension sprain. The last is stable in flexion but unstable during extension.[57]

Vertical-Compression Injuries

Pure vertical compression may result in a typical Jefferson fracture (see Fig. 3–40) or a burst fracture in the lower cervical spine. The spine must be in near neutral positions at the time the vertical force is applied. These injuries are uncommon. In our series only 4 percent of injuries were due to vertical compression. Usually there is asymmetrical vertical compression with lateral flexion (Fig. 3–48). This may result in a compression fracture of one of the lateral masses of C1 or a pillar fracture. Fractures of the uncinate process or a transverse process fracture may also occur.[1]

Summary

A thorough understanding of the mechanism of injury and stability of the injury is imperative in proper management of cervical spine trauma. This discussion has reviewed a more simplified approach to the mechanism of injury (Table 3–3).

In our series of 420 cervical spine fractures and fracture-dislocations, the injuries could be classified into five basic groups. Again, remembering that the

Figure 3–46. Lateral radiograph demonstrating a subtle anterior inferior fracture of the body of C2 *(straight arrow)*. There is a congenital defect in the posterior ring of C1 *(curved arrow)*.

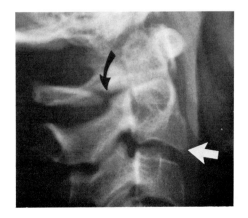

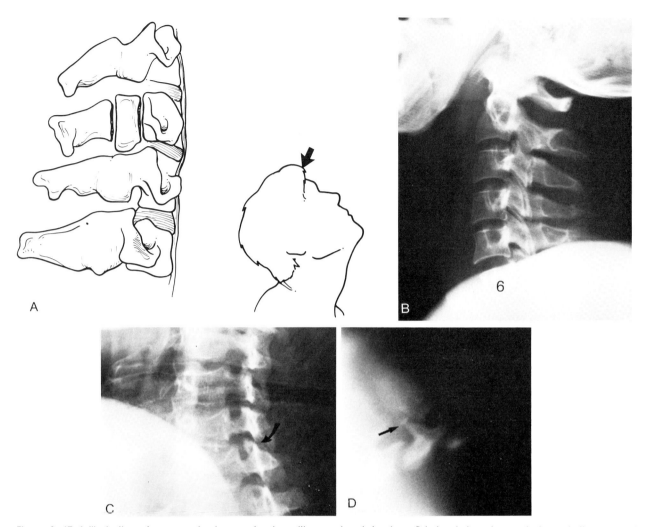

Figure 3–47. A, Illustration of compressive hyperextension with neural arch fracture. *B,* Lateral view demonstrates only the upper six cervical vertebrae with widening of the C5 interspace. *C,* Oblique view demonstrates a fracture of the superior facet of C5. *D,* Tomogram demonstrates a pedicle fracture *(arrow),* which assists in the diagnosis of an extension injury.

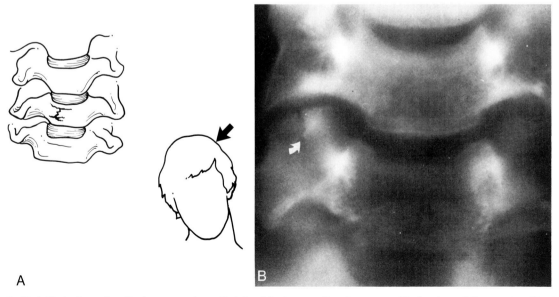

Figure 3–48. A, Illustration of vertical compression with lateral flexion resulting in asymmetric fracture. *B,* Tomogram demonstrating lateral compression injury with compression of C6 *(arrow).*

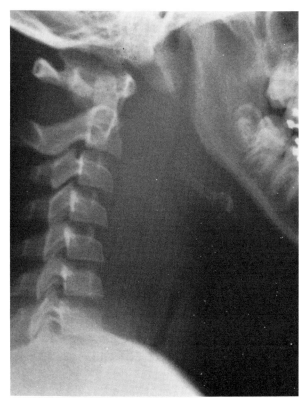

Figure 3–49. Lateral view of the cervical spine demonstrating a huge prevertebral hematoma and anterior subluxation of the occipital condyles on C1.

mechanisms of injury are rarely pure, especially in the case of axial compression, hyperextension or hyperflexion injuries occurred in 88 percent of patients. Flexion-rotation injuries (unilateral locked facets and anterior subluxations) were detected in 12 percent of patients. Only 4 percent could be classified as having vertical compressive injuries. Certain patients with undisplaced odontoid or isolated spinous process fractures could not be definitively categorized. No neurologic symptoms were present in the undisplaced odontoid group. Solitary spinous process fractures may be the result of flexion, extension, or direct trauma. These fractures are stable and of little clinical significance.

The above approach, when accompanied with assessment of radiographs for indications of instability (Table 3–4), is simple and reliable in determining the mechanism of injury and proper method of open or closed stability of the fracture.

CERVICAL SPINE FRACTURES AND FRACTURE-DISLOCATIONS

Cervical spine injuries in adults most frequently involve the lower cervical spine (81 percent in our series of 420 patients). Nineteen percent of injuries involved the upper cervical spine (from the occipital condyles to C2). Multiple injuries are common. The average number of injuries per patient is 2.2.

The anatomic relationships of the upper cervical spine are unique, and the mechanisms of injury differ somewhat from those affecting the lower cervical spine. Therefore, in discussing cervical spine injuries the upper and lower segments will be presented separately.

Upper Cervical Spine

Atlanto-occipital Region

Injuries involving the occipital condyles and atlanto-occipital articulation are rare. We noted no fractures of the occipital condyles in our series of 420 patients. The mechanism of injury that results in condyle fractures is a blow to the calvarium from above, similar to the mechanism that results in a Jefferson fracture.[73] These injuries may disrupt the hypoglossal canal, injuring the jugular vein and the 9th, 10th, and 11th cranial nerves. As with other upper cervical spine injuries, tomography (AP and lateral projections) is extremely valuable in demonstrating these injuries.

Atlanto-occipital dislocations are also rare. This injury usually occurs in high-velocity motor vehicle accidents. The lesion is usually the result of shearing forces directed either to the face or to the occipital region. Others have suggested flexion or hyperextension and distraction as the mechanism of injury.[69, 131] Death is due to brainstem injury. Two cases of atlanto-occipital dislocation were noted in our series. Both patients were in their teens. Atlanto-occipital dislocation is more common in children owing to their smaller condyles and the more horizontal articular relationship of the condyles with the lateral masses of the atlas.[133] Though the injury is almost always fatal, 15 survivors have been reported in the literature.[131]

Radiographically, the diagnosis is evident on the

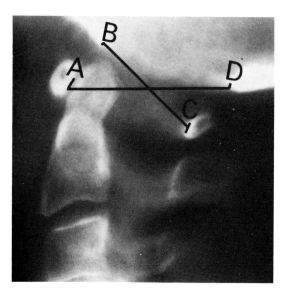

Figure 3–50. Radiograph of the upper cervical spine demonstrating the normal occipitoatlantal relationship.

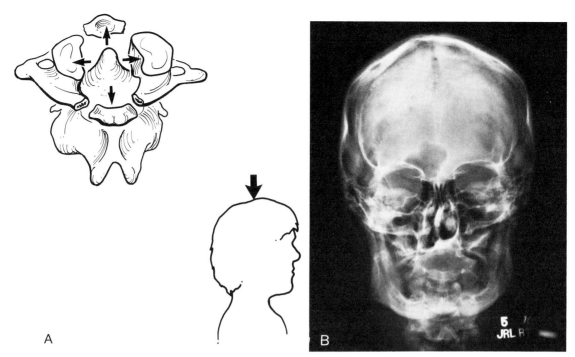

Figure 3–51. *A*, Illustration demonstrating the effect of vertical force on the ring of C1. *B*, AP radiograph demonstrates wide lateral displacement suggesting disruption of the transverse ligament.

lateral view of the skull or cervical spine (Fig. 3–49). The occipital condyles lose their normal articular relationship with the atlas, and a large hematoma is present in the retropharyngeal space. Powers devised a ratio that may be helpful in diagnosing anterior dislocations on routine lateral views.[108] The distance from the basion to the spinolaminar line of C1 (BC) divided by the distance from the posterior margin of the anterior arch of C1 to the posterior margin of the foramen magnum (DA) should be less than 1 (Fig. 3–50). If this ratio is greater than 1, a dislocation is present. Since the measurement is a ratio, the technique does not require standardization of target-film distance. Odontoid fractures have been described in association with atlanto-occipital dislocations and should be carefully checked on radiographic examination.[84]

Atlas (C1)

In our experience fractures of the atlas account for approximately 4 percent of all spinal injuries. Others report a similar incidence.[84, 93, 94, 101] Fractures most commonly involve the lateral masses and the posterior arch (Fig. 3–51). Shick and Nicholson reported that posterior arch fractures account for 67 percent of fractures of the atlas.[119] Posterior arch fractures are the result of hyperextension injuries in which the arch is compressed between the occiput and spinous process of the axis.[93, 94] Associated injuries are common (Table 3–5). Hangman's fractures were noted in 15 percent of these patients. Spinous process fractures of C7 were evident in 25 percent of patients with posterior arch fractures of

C1. Other skeletal fractures were noted in 18 percent of patients, frequently in the upper thoracic spine. As this is a hyperextension injury, one should not be surprised by the frequently associated facial injuries. Care must be taken not to mistake a normal congenital cleft (2 to 4 percent of the normal population) for a fracture (Fig. 3–52).[9] Transverse process fractures due to lateral flexion forces have been described.[73, 93]

Pure Jefferson fractures result from a force directed vertically to the skull.[99] The force is transmitted to the occipital condyles, which leads to lateral displacement of the lateral masses of the atlas (Fig. 3–51). The lateral displacement is a result of the anatomic configuration of these articulations, and fractures occur in the anterior and posterior arches (see Fig. 3–40). The anterior and, more specifically, the posterior arch are the weak points in the ring of the atlas. In our experience asymmetrical compression of the lateral mass with an associated ring fracture is more common than double breaks in the anterior and posterior arch. This is due to some degree of lateral or rotary motion along with the vertical force (Fig. 3–52). Pure vertical

TABLE 3–5. Hangman's Fractures (6% of 420 cases)

Associated Features	Incidence (%)
Spinal injuries	
C1	15
T1–T4	10
Neurologic symptoms	
Complete	0
Transient	10

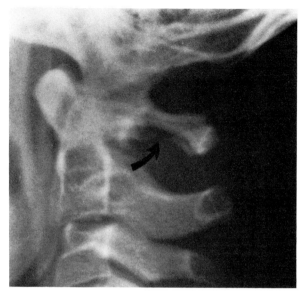

Figure 3–52. Normal congenital cleft in the posterior ring of C1. Note the sharp sclerotic images.

compression with the neck in neutral position is required for the symmetric four-part break in the ring. In either situation the cord is protected owing to the outward displacement of the fracture fragments. Less commonly, horizontal fractures of the anterior arch occur. This injury also results from hyperextension and avulsion at the insertion of the longus colli.[94, 109]

Neurologic complications with atlas fractures are rare.[84, 93, 94, 96, 99] However, significant retropharyngeal hemorrhage resulting in difficulty in breathing has been reported.[96] Delayed basilar invagination may also occur if proper treatment is not instituted.[81]

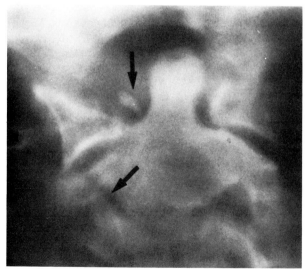

Figure 3–53. AP tomogram demonstrates a lateral compression injury with comminution of the right lateral mass of C1 *(upper arrow)* and a vertical fracture on the right facet of C2 *(lower arrow).*

Radiographically, most injuries of C1 can be detected on the AP odontoid view or on the lateral view of the cervical spine or skull. Several significant features noted on the AP odontoid view or AP tomograms should be stressed (Figs. 3–51B and 3–52). Outward displacement of the lateral masses of the atlas of greater than 6.9 mm indicates a tear or avulsion of the transverse ligament.[123] However, normal features such as the insertion of the transverse ligament and bipartite superior facets should not be confused with fractures.[100] Subtle changes may require conventional or computed tomography for complete evaluation (Fig. 3–53). Computed tomography is especially useful in evaluating the ring of the atlas (see Fig. 3–40).[101]

Atlantoaxial Dislocations

Traumatic dislocations of the atlas on the axis are rare. The transverse ligament will normally maintain the relationship of the odontoid with C1 unless the dens is fractured or the ligament is avulsed from its insertion (Figs. 3–53 and 3–54). Subluxations of the atlas on the axis are most often related to inflammatory conditions such as rheumatoid arthritis, Beçhet's syndrome, retropharyngeal infection, and congenital abnormalities.[81, 96, 100, 103, 109, 118, 123] Traumatic dislocations may be anterior, posterior, or rotary in nature. This lesion is uncommon, accounting for only 1 percent (4 of 420) of cervical spine injuries in our series. The transverse ligament was intact in all cases. In each instance the trauma resulted in an avulsion fracture at the insertion of the ligament from the lateral mass of the atlas. Measurement of the C1–odontoid distance exceeded 3 mm in the neutral position in all cases (Fig. 3–55). Associated fractures of the lateral mass of the atlas and the upper facet of the axis were present in 25 percent of the cases (Fig. 3–53). This confirmed the asymmetrical vertical compression as the mechanism of injury. If the lateral radiograph is normal, carefully performed flexion and extension fluoroscopic studies may be necessary to demonstrate the lesion (Fig. 3–54). Also, measurement of the AP diameter of the spinal canal is helpful. If the distance from the posterior aspect of the odontoid to the spinolaminal line of the atlas is less than 18 mm, neurologic symptoms are more likely to occur.[94]

Posterior and rotary dislocations are even more uncommon than anterior dislocations. These injuries were not detected in our series, and reports in the literature are infrequent.[74, 98] Rotary dislocation requires 45° of rotation of C1 on the axis for locking to occur.[94] This condition differs from the rotary fixation described by Fielding and Hawkins.[88] Sixty-five degrees of rotation is required for fixation to occur if the transverse ligament and odontoid are anatomically normal.[88] If the ligament is interrupted, less rotation is required. Cord injury and vertebral artery injury have been reported with

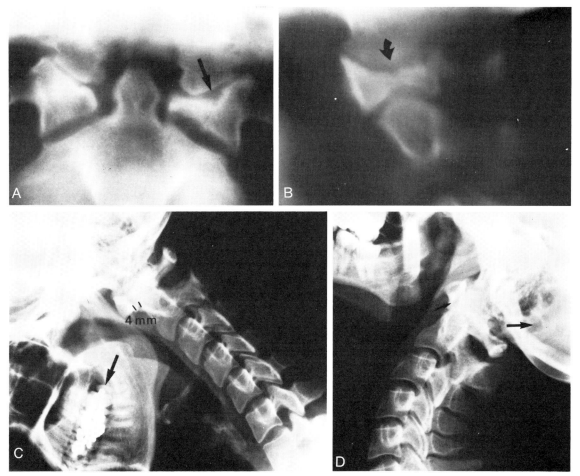

Figure 3–54. Upper cervical spine injury following a motor vehicle accident. Routine views were normal. AP *(A)* and lateral *(B)* tomograms demonstrate a compression fracture of the lateral mass of C1. Flexion *(C)* and extension *(D)* views show instability with 4-mm anterior subluxation during flexion. Transverse ligament injury was not suspected on routine views.

rotary fixation. In describing 17 cases of rotary fixation, Fielding and Hawkins defined the following four types of injuries[88] (Fig. 3–56).

Type I. Rotary fixation without anterior subluxation of the atlas on the axis (transverse ligament intact).

Type II. Rotary fixation with 3 to 5 mm of atlantoaxial subluxation.

Type III. Rotary fixation with greater than 5 mm of atlantoaxial subluxation.

Type IV. Rotary fixation with posterior atlantoaxial subluxation (deficient dens required).

Type I is the most common lesion reported.[88] Clinically, these lesions have been noted following trauma and dental procedures and in association with retropharyngeal infections. The patient usually

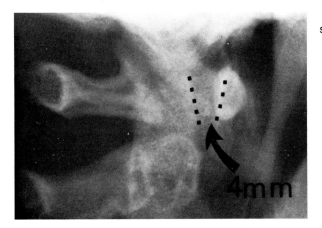

Figure 3–55. Lateral view of the upper cervical spine. Atlantoaxial subluxation *(arrow,* 4 mm).

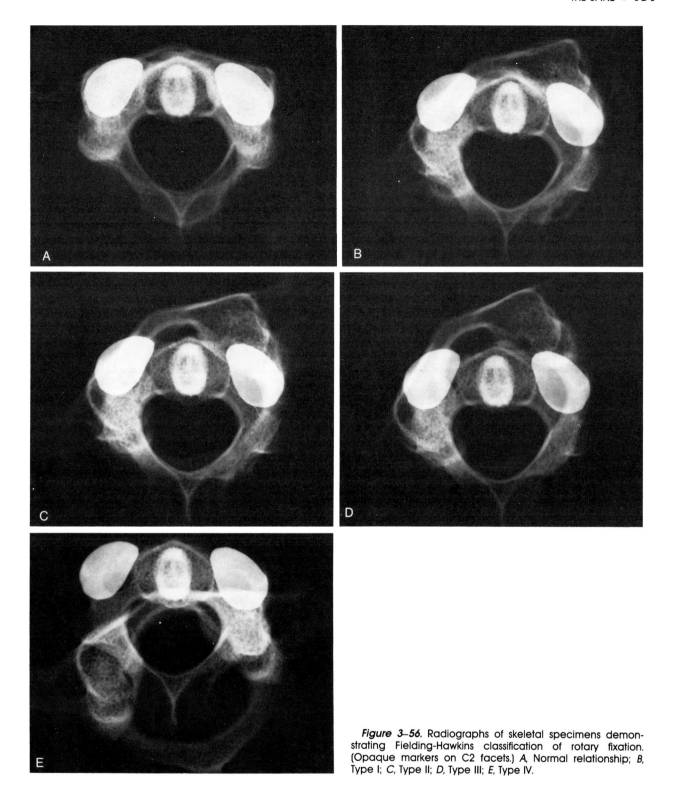

Figure 3–56. Radiographs of skeletal specimens demonstrating Fielding-Hawkins classification of rotary fixation. (Opaque markers on C2 facets.) *A,* Normal relationship; *B,* Type I; *C,* Type II; *D,* Type III; *E,* Type IV.

presents with the head rotated to the side. Neurologic deficits are rare. The exact etiology is unclear, but fixation may be related to capsular entrapment in the atlantoaxial facets.[88]

Radiographically, the AP and lateral odontoid views may be sufficient for diagnosis (Fig. 3–57). However, 15°-rotation AP odontoid views are more definitive. Normally the motion of C1 and C2 is independent on rotation-AP views. If rotary fixation is present, C1 and C2 maintain a constant relationship when rotated. Computed tomography is most accurate for evaluation and allows differentiation from torticollis or simple rotation more readily than routine radiographs (Fig. 3–58).

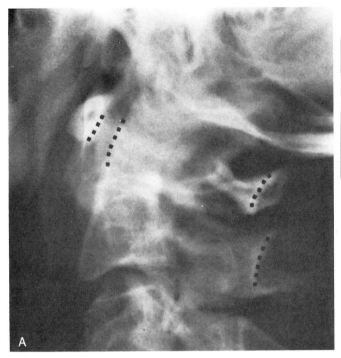

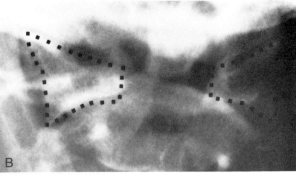

Figure 3–57. Lateral *(A)* and AP *(B)* views demonstrating Type II rotary fixation.

Axis

Fractures of the axis are common, accounting for 15 percent of cervical spine injuries. Others report the incidence of fracture of the axis to be as high as 27 percent.[94] Fractures of the odontoid and pedicles account for 80 percent of the injuries to the axis. The vertebral body is involved in about 15 percent of cases, usually through an anterior inferior chip fracture. The facets, lamina, and spinous processes are less frequently involved.

Odontoid fractures may result from anterior shearing (hyperextension), posterior shearing (hyperflexion), or lateral flexion injuries. Patients with odontoid fractures usually present with neck pain and rarely have neurologic symptoms.[112] Even if

there is displacement of the fractures, there is usually sufficient space to prevent cord injury. Although mortality in such cases has been reported to be as high as 30 percent, associated head injuries make exact mortality figures difficult to interpret.[111] Associated fractures of the atlas are not uncommon (8 percent in our series). Forty-one percent of our patients sustained associated head, facial, and extraspinal injuries.

In a significant number of cases odontoid fractures are undisplaced and subtle, requiring tomography for definitive diagnosis and classification (see Fig. 3–63). The mechanism of injury in these cases is often difficult to determine. If the fracture is slightly displaced, the mechanism of injury is more easily established. When the fracture is displaced,

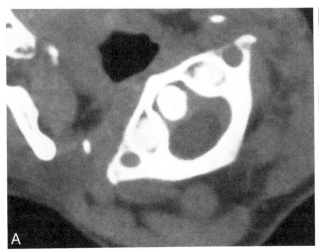

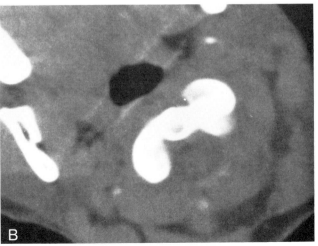

Figure 3–58. CT scans of C1 *(A)* and C1–C2 articulation *(B)* demonstrating rotation due to torticollis but no fixation.

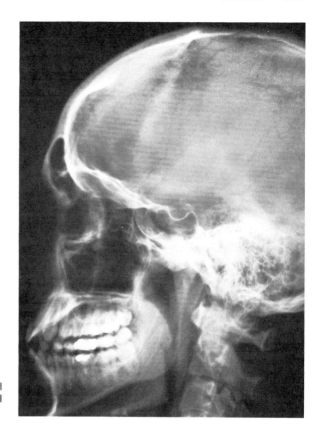

Figure 3–59. Lateral view of the skull. There is slight prevertebral swelling and a subtle buckling of the anterior cortex of C2 (Type III odontoid fracture).

the lateral view of the skull or cervical spine and the open-mouth odontoid view are usually adequate for diagnosis.

Radiographically, one should check carefully for retropharyngeal soft tissue swelling, which may be the only clue to an odontoid fracture (Fig. 3–59). Tomography is frequently required for diagnosis and classification of the fractures. Anderson's classification is commonly utilized and is helpful in determining proper management and prognosis of the fracture (Fig. 3–60).[70, 97, 132] The classification divides odontoid fractures into three types: Type I, oblique fracture of the tip of the odontoid; Type II, fracture of the base of the odontoid; Type III, fracture enters the body of the axis.

Type I fractures may be due to avulsion of the alar ligament. These are the least common odontoid fractures (Table 3–6) and usually require tomography for diagnosis (Figs. 3–61 and 3–62).

Type II fractures usually occur above the insertion of the accessory ligament, which provides at least a portion of the blood supply to the odontoid (Fig. 3–63). This may explain the high incidence of non-union with this fracture. Type II fractures are the

most common type of odontoid fracture, accounting for 59 percent of odontoid fractures. Non-union with these injuries may be as high as 72 percent if displacement is present (Fig. 3–64).[111] Posterior displacement appears to indicate a poorer prognosis.[112]

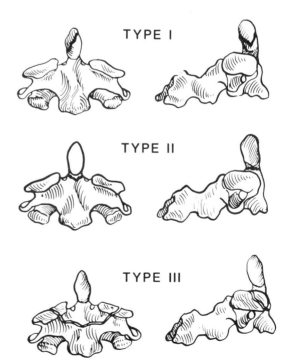

Figure 3–60. Classification of odontoid fractures. Type I, upper odontoid; Type II, base of odontoid; Type III, involves the body of C2.

TABLE 3–6. Odontoid Fractures (6% of 420 cases)

Type	Incidence (%)	
Type I	8	
Type II	59	
Non-union		54
Type III	33	

Text continued on page 136

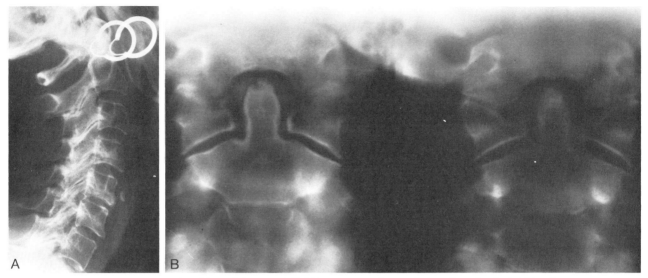

Figure 3–61. A, Lateral radiograph is normal. *B,* AP tomograms demonstrate a Type I odontoid fracture.

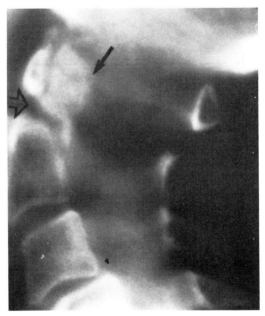

Figure 3–62. Lateral tomogram demonstrating Type I *(black arrow)* and Type II fractures *(open arrow).*

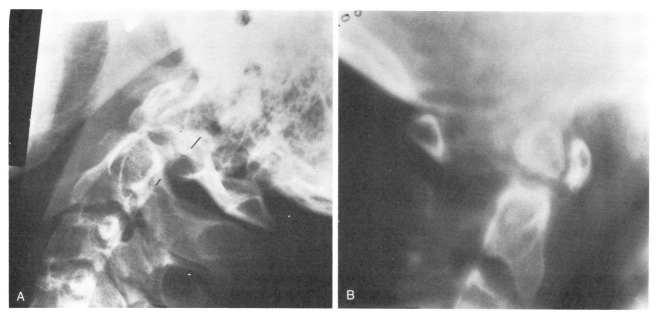

Figure 3–63. Normal lateral radiograph *(A)* and tomogram *(B)*. The tomogram clearly demonstrates the Type II fracture.

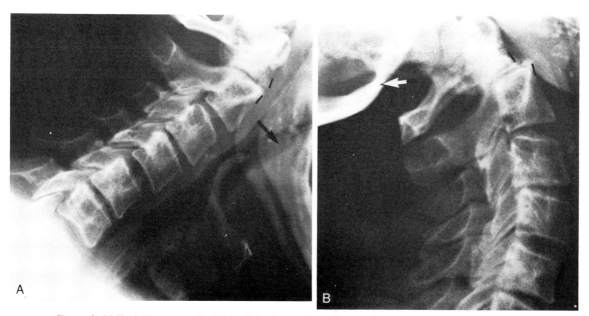

Figure 3–64. Unstable, non-united Type II fracture with motion on flexion *(A)* and extension *(B)* views.

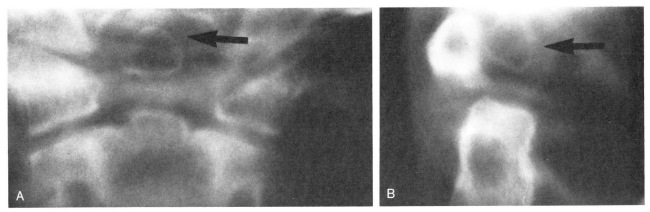

Figure 3–65. AP *(A)* and lateral *(B)* tomograms demonstrate the well-marginated os odontoideum.

Type III fractures account for about 33 percent of odontoid fractures (see Fig. 3–59). These fractures are frequently impacted anteriorly, and again tomography is usually more definitive than routine views. Type III fractures almost always unite with proper treatment.[70, 111, 122, 132]

Care must be taken not to mistake a normal variant or overlying structure for a fracture. Normally, the cortex of the odontoid is contiguous vertically with the body of the axis. The odontoid may deviate posteriorly, resulting in a convex anterior margin. This is normal. Anterior bowing of the odontoid is not normal, and in this case one should suspect a Type III fracture. On the open-

mouth odontoid view, overlying structures may be confused with fracture lines. These include the posterior arch of the atlas, the occiput, the base of the tongue, and clefts in the teeth.[80] The os odontoideum (Fig. 3–65) is well-marginated and should not be mistaken for an acute fracture. This odontoid change may be a congenital variant, but many believe this represents an old non-united Type II fracture.[94]

In our experience, fractures of the pedicles of the axis (hangman's fractures) occur as frequently as odontoid fractures. The injury results from hyperextension, and usually anterior subluxation of C2 on C3 is evident on the lateral radiograph (Fig.

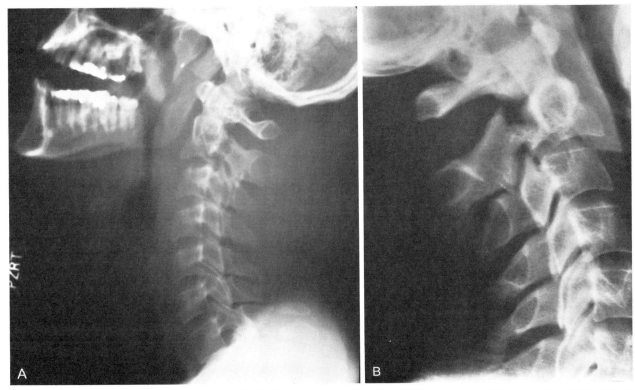

Figure 3–66. Fractures of the vertebral arch of C2 ("hangman's fractures"). *A,* Subtle fracture of the pedicles of C2 with little subluxation but marked prevertebral swelling. *B,* Displaced fracture with disruption of the disk and anterior ligaments.

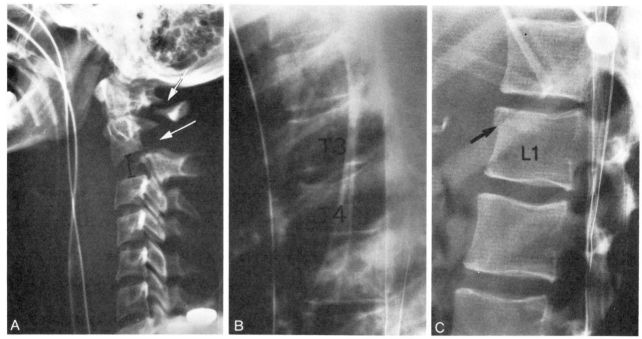

Figure 3–67. Multiple spinal injuries following a motor vehicle accident. Lateral view *(A)* of the cervical spine with distraction of the C2 disk space and fractures of the C2 pedicle and posterior arch of C1. Lateral views of the thoracic *(B)* and lumbar *(C)* spine show associated compression of T3–T4 and L1.

3–66). The lesion, as originally described, occurred as a result of judicial hanging.[129] This mechanism of hyperextension and sustained distraction resulted in death. Flexion-compression and flexion-distraction have also been implicated in hangman's fracture.[83, 90] Most of these injuries today are the result of motor vehicle accidents with transient hyperextension, and therefore neurologic damage is not common. In our series 10 percent of patients experienced transient neurologic deficits, but no permanent damage occurred. Other authors have reported a higher incidence of neurologic complications (30 to 35 percent).[85, 89, 105]

Associated cervical and distal spinal fractures are also not uncommon (Fig. 3–67). Fifteen percent of our patients sustained associated C1 arch fractures (see Table 3–5). In one case the posterior arch fracture was more obvious than the pedicle fracture of the axis. Knowledge of the C1 hyperextension injury should make one search more diligently for pedicle fractures of the axis. Fractures of the upper thoracic spine were noted in 10 percent of patients with hangman's fractures (Fig. 3–67). Fractures in this region are more likely to be associated with neurologic injury and should not be overlooked.

Fractures of the body of the axis occurred in 15 percent of patients. These fractures were all the result of hyperextension injuries and usually involved the anterior inferior margin of the vertebral body (Fig. 3–68). Soft tissue swelling was common and often marked. No neurologic symptoms were present.

Fractures of the lamina, spinous process, and facets of the axis are uncommon. Facet fractures of

the axis are often associated with compression-rotation or lateral compression injuries, which result in associated lateral mass fractures of the atlas.[68] Odontoid fractures have also been reported with articular fractures of the axis.[105]

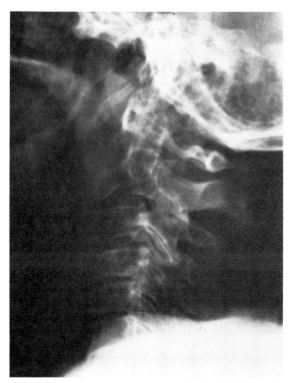

Figure 3–68. Hyperextension injury of the cervical spine with an anterior inferior body fracture of C2 and a less obvious C2 pedicle fracture.

TABLE 3–7. Cervical Spine: Location of Injury in 420 Patients*

Location	Incidence (%)
Vertebral arch	42
Vertebral body	31
Disk	27
Posterior ligaments	22
Anterior ligaments	4

*Multiple injuries result in total > 100%

TABLE 3–8. Vertebral Arch Fractures*

Location	Incidence (%)
Lamina	28
Pedicle	25
Spinous Process	22
Pillar	16
Facet	9
Transverse Process	2

*Multiple injuries result in total > 100%

Lower Cervical Spine (C3–C7)

In adults, injuries to the lower cervical spine occur four times more frequently than upper cervical spine fractures. In our experience 81 percent of 420 injuries were located at the C3–C7 level. Fractures of the posterior vertebral arch were most common, occurring in 42 percent of the injuries (Table 3–7). Fractures of the vertebral bodies were the second most common, occurring in 31 percent of patients. The average number of injuries was 2.2 per patient.

Vertebral Arch Fractures

Vertebral arch fractures have been well-discussed by other authors.[94, 116] Our experience differs slightly from the distribution of fractures described by Gehweiler.[94] Fractures observed in our series are set out in Table 3–8.

Fractures of the lamina were the most common in our series. The mechanism of injury was almost always hyperextension (Fig. 3–69). Spinous process fractures were commonly associated with these fractures. The majority of the laminar fractures occur in the C5–C7 region. Pillar views and tomography are often necessary to detect laminar fractures (Fig. 3–70). CT may also be helpful; however, several cases of undisplaced fractures not evident on CT were easily demonstrated with conventional tomography. This is true of any undisplaced fracture in which the fracture is aligned parallel to the slice. The increased utilization of tomography in our practice may be at least partially responsible for the higher incidence of laminar fractures in our series. Fractures of the lamina frequently extend into the base of the spinous process, resulting in a displaced spinous process. This should not be confused with the more benign clay shoveler's fracture. Laminar fractures with spinous process involvement have been reported frequently with hyperextension injuries of the Type V classification (comminuted vertebral arch fracture with hyperextension fracture-dislocation.[94, 96]

Pedicle fractures were present in 25 percent of vertebral arch injuries (Table 3–8). Most pedicle fractures were noted with hangman's fractures. However, pedicle fractures were also noted at the lower cervical spine with hyperextension injuries.

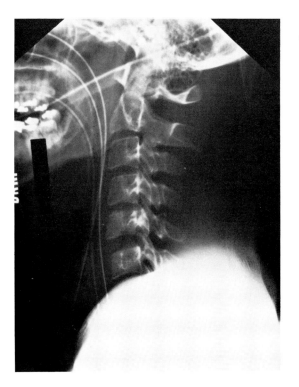

Figure 3–69. Hyperextension injury with widening of the C5 disk space and a chip fracture anteriorly. The lamina of C5 is fractured.

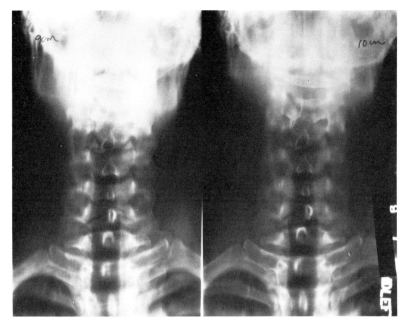

Figure 3–70. AP tomogram demonstrating an undisplaced fracture of the lamina at C6.

Thus pedicle fractures are rarely noted unless a hyperextension injury is present. These injuries may be visible on the lateral or oblique views (Fig. 3–71). Conventional or computed tomography is frequently necessary for diagnosis.

Spinous process fractures account for 22 percent

of vertebral arch injuries. Most spinous process fractures occur at the C5–T1 level. This fracture may result from direct trauma, hyperextension, or hyperflexion; and it is only through careful evaluation of the remaining vertebral units that the mechanism of injury may be established. Solitary spinous proc-

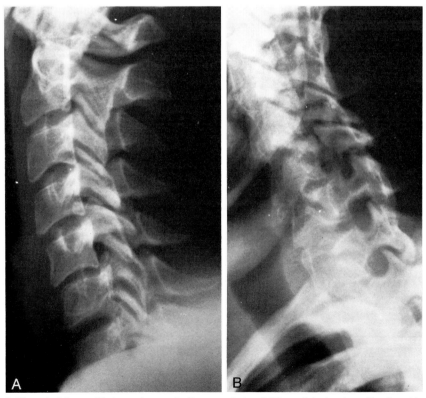

Figure 3–71. Lateral *(A)* and oblique *(B)* views demonstrating a unilateral C5 pedicle fracture. The facet is rotated anteriorly.

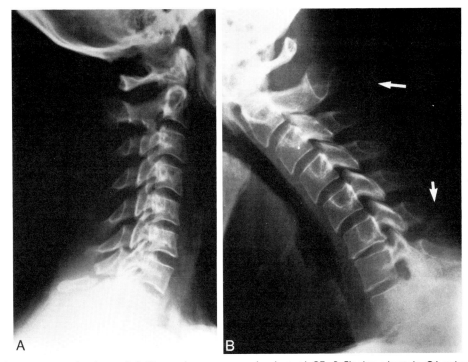

Figure 3–72. Spinous process fractures. *A*, Solitary spinous process fracture at C7. *B*, Flexion views in C6 spinous fracture *(lower arrow)*. There is no instability.

ess fractures may be difficult to classify (Fig. 3–72).[76, 82, 94, 97] On the AP view a double spinous process may be the only clue to an unsuspected spinous process fracture (see Fig. 3–26E and F).[76] In other cases the lateral view is usually most useful.

Fractures of the articular pillars have been reported to be the most common arch fracture.[94] These injuries usually occur at the C6 level. In our series pillar fractures occurred in 16 percent of vertebral arch fractures (Table 3–8). The mechanism of injury is usually hyperextension (hyperextension fracture-dislocation of Type IV or Type V) or lateral flexion. Occasionally, the AP view will demonstrate the lesion. These fractures are best demonstrated with pillar views or tomography (Fig. 3–73). There is usually no cord injury with a pillar fracture, but radiculopathy may result, especially if proper treatment is not instituted.

Several types of pillar fractures have been described. The most common is the easily overlooked simple compression fracture (Fig. 3–73).[121, 126] Smith[121] has described several signs that may be of

TABLE 3–9. Radiographic Signs of Pillar Fracture*

Feature	View
Foraminal narrowing	Oblique
Triangular articular mass	Oblique
Unilateral facet displacement	Oblique
Double lateral mass	Lateral
Subluxation	Lateral

*After Smith, G. R., Beckly, D. E., and Abel, M. S.: Articular mass fracture: A neglected cause of post-traumatic neck pain? Clin. Radiol. 27:335, 1976.

value in detecting pillar fractures; these are presented in Table 3–9. Foraminal narrowing was the most common sign detected. This radiographic feature was present in 31 percent of patients.[121] Asymmetry of the pillars of greater than 2 mm in vertical height has also been described with pillar fractures.[126] Asymmetry and degenerative changes in the pillars are common in older patients, which adds to the confusion. These patients are usually totally asymptomatic.

Facet fractures comprised 9 percent of vertebral arch fractures. These were most common with hyperflexion and flexion-rotation injuries. Oblique and lateral views may demonstrate this lesion, but tomography is usually required (Fig. 3–74). Radicular symptoms are common with solitary facet fractures.[130] Facet fractures are usually detected with multiple injuries, including injuries of the posterior ligaments and disk.

Finally, transverse process fractures are uncommon, occurring in only 2 percent of our patients (Fig. 3–75). The injury results from lateral flexion or direct trauma, such as from the chest strap of a seatbelt.[71] Associated upper rib fractures are common with seatbelt injuries. Hyperextension injuries in the lower cervical spine, odontoid fractures, and hangman's fractures have also been reported in relation to seatbelt injuries.[125]

Vertebral Body Fractures

Thirty-one percent of cervical spine injuries involved the vertebral body. Seventy-five percent of

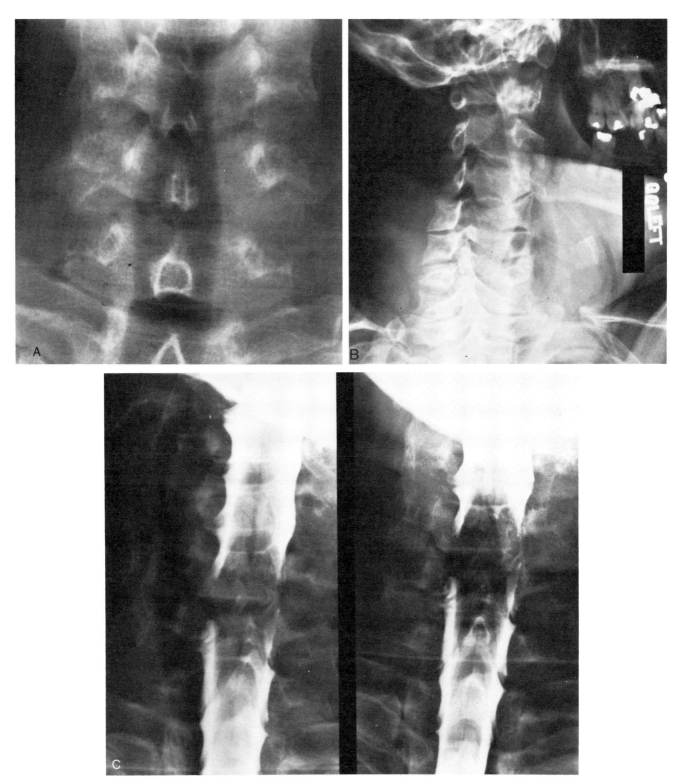

Figure 3–73. *A*, AP view in a patient with a pillar fracture of C6 on the right. The only clue to the abnormality is a subtle change in the configuration of articular pillars. *B*, Pillar view demonstrating a compression fracture of right C6 articular pillar. *C*, Myelogram in the same patient demonstrates an extradural defect at C6 on the right due to a traumatic disk protrusion.

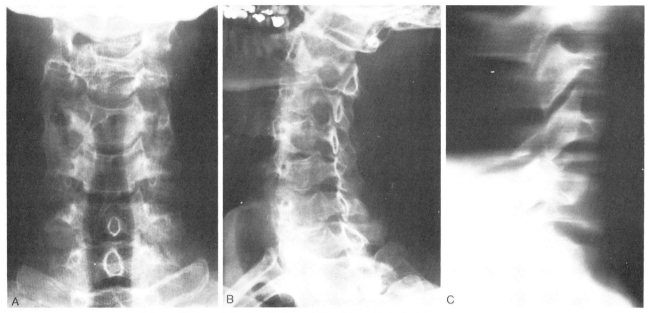

Figure 3–74. AP *(A)* and oblique *(B)* views following flexion-rotation injury. Note that the malalignment of the spinous process on the AP view *(A)* and the oblique view *(B)* suggests perching at C4–C5. The tomogram *(C)* demonstrates the inferior facet fracture at C4.

the fractures were in the C5–C7 region (Table 3–10). Fractures were demonstrated on the AP and lateral views, with oblique views adding additional information. Tomography and CT are less frequently required for detection of vertebral body fractures.

Vertebral body fractures have several radio-

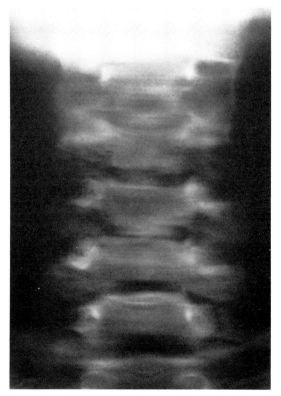

Figure 3–75. AP tomogram demonstrating a fracture of the left transverse process of C7.

graphic presentations: (1) chip fractures, usually of the anterior superior or anterior inferior margin; (2) triangular fractures; (3) burst fractures; (4) wedge fractures, usually anterior but also lateral; (5) uncinate process fractures; and (6) sagittal fractures.

Chip fractures are commonly due to hyperflexion injuries (anterior superior margin) and hyperextension injuries (anterior inferior margin). Following hyperextension injury, the fracture fragment is avulsed with the anterior longitudinal ligament and in most instances enters the disk space (Fig. 3–76).[82, 94, 117] Hyperflexion injuries are often associated with posterior ligament disruption and are therefore unstable. Hyperextension injuries are usually stable unless the fracture of the body is associated with a posterior arch fracture, in which case the lesion is unstable.[97]

Larger triangular or teardrop fractures of the vertebral body are more significant. Lee reviewed 109 patients with triangular fractures.[104] Seventy-two percent involved the anterior inferior body and 16 percent the anterior superior margin of the body. The anterior inferior fracture is the typical teardrop fracture defined by Schneider and Kahn (Fig. 3–77).[117] The majority of triangular fractures involved the lower cervical spine (67 percent). Neurologic involvement, usually quadriplegia, was present in 87 percent of patients.[104]

Simple compression fractures are most often anterior and result from flexion-compression injuries (Fig. 3–78). The posterior ligaments may be intact, depending upon the degree of associated posterior element distraction. The posterior ligaments must be evaluated at some point in the stage of treatment to be certain that the lesion is stable. This requires fluoroscopically controlled flexion and extension views.

TABLE 3–10. Fractures of the Cervical Vertebral Body in 420 Patients

Location	Incidence (%)	
C2	8	
C3	7	
C4	10	
C5	30	
C6	22	75 C5–C7
C7	23	

Lateral wedge fractures and uncinate fractures are the result of asymmetric vertical compression or lateral flexion injuries. These fractures are rare.[94]

Burst fractures in the cervical spine result from vertical compression forces with the spine in neutral position. The ligaments are intact and the lesions are usually stable. However, fragments in the spinal canal result in neurologic deficits.[94, 117] CT is extremely helpful in evaluating these injuries and in localizing the number and size of intraspinal fragments and epidural hematomas (Fig. 3–79).

Sagittal fractures of the vertebral bodies may be associated with triangular fractures.[104] The diagnosis may be difficult on the AP and lateral views. Tomography and, more importantly, CT are usually required. There is almost always an associated posterior arch fracture.[120] These fractures are uncommon,[106, 120] but neurologic damage is usually severe,

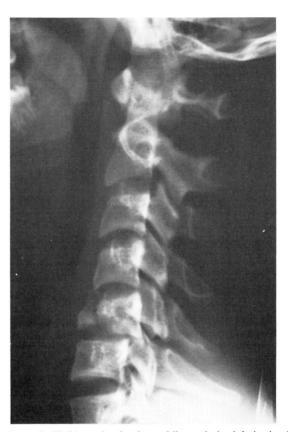

Figure 3–77. Triangular fracture of the anterior inferior body of C5. The major fragment is displaced posteriorly into the spinal canal.

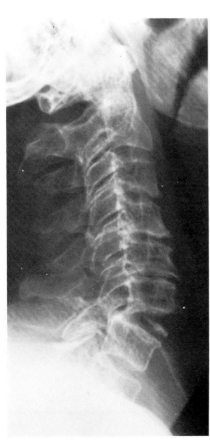

Figure 3–76. Hyperextension injury with widening of the anterior interspace and a "flake" fracture from the inferior body of C6.

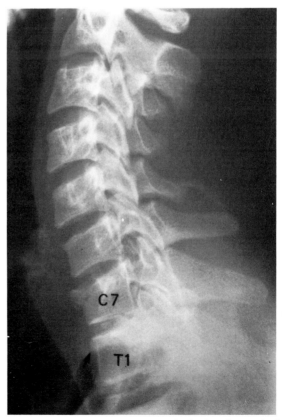

Figure 3–78. Lateral view of the cervical spine demonstrating compression fractures of C7 and T1 *(arrow)*.

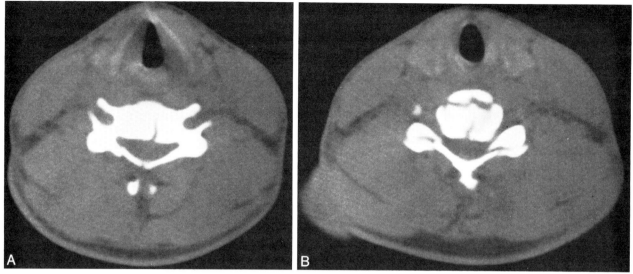

Figure 3–79. CT scans *(A* and *B)* demonstrating a complex fracture of the body and neural arch of C5.

resulting in quadriplegia.[91] Sagittal fractures are also unstable and may require surgical stabilization.[106] CT is particularly valuable in differentiating burst fractures with fragments in the spinal canal from sagittal fractures.[79]

Subluxations and Fracture-Dislocation

Most significant ligament injuries involve the posterior complex. In our series 73 percent of these injuries occurred at the C5–C7 level. Anterior ligament injuries are most common in the C2–C4 and the C6–C7 intervals. Often the changes noted radiographically (body fractures, disk space narrowing or widening, widening of the interspinous distance, and subluxation) will aid in determining if ligament injury has occurred. Posterior ligament injuries are unstable if complete disruption has occurred, and one must guard against overlooking the often subtle changes associated with this injury (Fig. 3–80).

Posterior ligament injuries may occur without associated fracture (hyperflexion sprain) and may result in widened interspinous distance, disk space narrowing, and subluxation (see Fig. 3–88). These findings may be evident on the upright lateral view but obscured on the supine lateral. For this reason if the supine views are negative, it has been suggested that an upright lateral be obtained in patients with suspected flexion injuries.[94] The ligament disruptions result from a flexion-rotation or disruptive hyperflexion injury.[74, 86, 94, 102, 115, 127] These injuries are uncommon but easily overlooked. Delay in diagnosis may result in cervical deformity and neurologic deficits.[86, 102, 115, 127] Cheshire noted persistent instability in 21 percent of patients with subluxation when the instability was treated conservatively.[77] Signs of instability (angulation of greater than 11° and subluxation greater than 3 mm) must be kept

in mind. Flexion and extension views may be required for diagnosis (Fig. 3–81). This technique should not be performed acutely, as spasm often results in a false negative study.

The same forces that result in isolated ligament disruption, if continued, may lead to unilateral or bilateral facet dislocation or locking. In our experience actual locking is less common than perching of the facets. This phenomenon is due to partial reduction of the hyperflexion process combined with osteochondral impaction of the inferior facet into the superior facet of the vertebra below. This is especially common with bilateral facet dislocation.

Unilateral locking or perching of the facets is common. This injury was noted in 12 percent of our patients (420 cases). Scher reported unilateral facet locking in 16 percent of 525 spinal injuries.[113] The injury occurs most frequently at the C4–C6 levels. Associated fractures have been reported in 35 percent of patients.[113] There is often only minimal subluxation, and if only the lateral view is obtained this lesion may be easily missed. The oblique view is most helpful in detecting facet dislocations (Fig. 3–82). Radiographically the AP view will demonstrate lateral displacement of the spinous process at the level of the lesion, with the spinous process rotated to the side of the involved facets. On the lateral view there will appear to be a true lateral appearance below the lesion and an oblique view above. This results in the "bow tie" sign[95] (see Fig. 3–42). As mentioned earlier, the oblique view is most helpful, but tomography is usually necessary to evaluate the degree of locking or perching and to exclude an associated facet fracture (Fig. 3–80). Radiculopathy is common with this lesion. The injury results from disruption of the capsule and interspinous ligaments, with minor involvement of the disk and posterior longitudinal ligament.[72, 110]

Bilateral facet locking has been reported to be

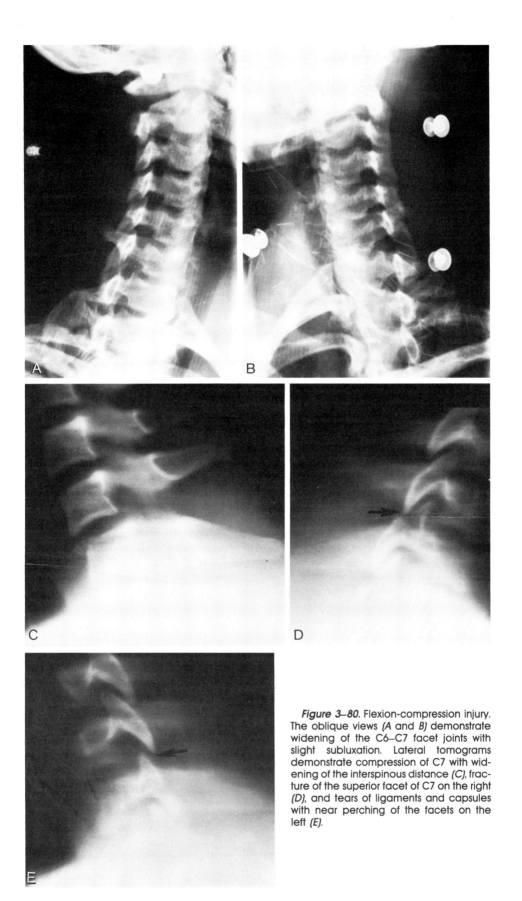

Figure 3–80. Flexion-compression injury. The oblique views *(A* and *B)* demonstrate widening of the C6–C7 facet joints with slight subluxation. Lateral tomograms demonstrate compression of C7 with widening of the interspinous distance *(C)*, fracture of the superior facet of C7 on the right *(D)*, and tears of ligaments and capsules with near perching of the facets on the left *(E)*.

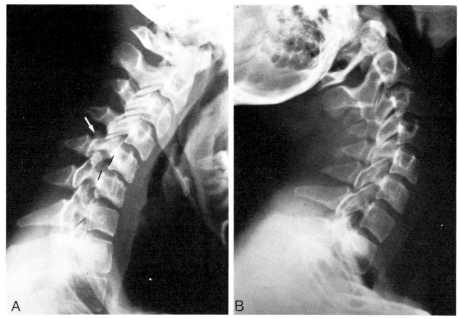

Figure 3–81. Ligament injury with chronic mild instability. Flexion *(A)* and extension *(B)* views show slight widening of the C4–C5 interspinous distance with 3 mm of anterior subluxation. Note the partially ossified ligaments in [A] *(arrow)*.

twice as common as unilateral locking of the facets.[94] In our experience, however, the two lesions occurred with equal frequency. This may be due to the patient population or to increased awareness of the subtle changes present with unilateral facet locking.[72, 94, 95, 110] With bilateral facet locking or perching there is no significant rotary component. The degree of subluxation, as noted on the lateral radiograph, is usually more than 50 percent of the

AP diameter of the vertebral body below (Fig. 3–83). There is also marked widening of the interspinous distance, widening of the apophyseal joints, and narrowing of the disk space. On the AP view there is widening of the interspinous distance at the level of the injury. Oblique views offer the most diagnostic information, revealing either locking or perching of both facets. Bilateral locked facets are associated with a high incidence of cord damage

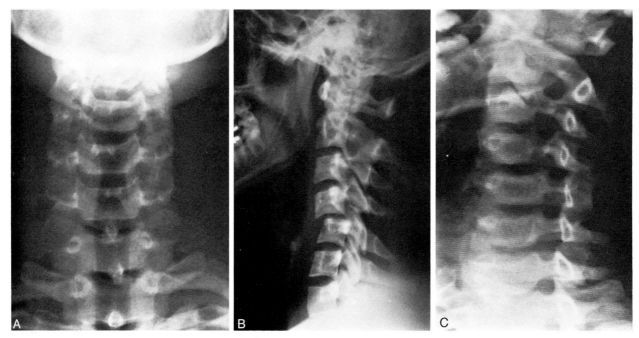

Figure 3–82. Unilateral posterior locked facet. *A,* AP view demonstrating rotation of the spinous process at C4–C5. *B,* Lateral view shows anterior subluxation with rotation at the C4–C5 level. *C,* The locking is clearly demonstrated at C4–C5 on the oblique view.

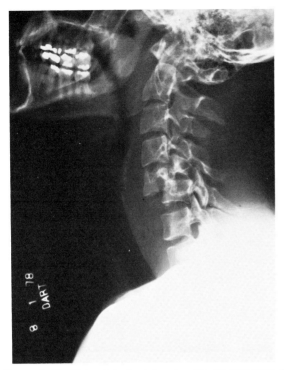

Figure 3–83. Bilateral locked facets with greater than 50 percent subluxation of C5 on C6.

(72 percent quadriplegic), and the injury is unstable.[97]

The flexion teardrop (hyperflexion fracture-dislocation) is uncommon but is one of the most unstable cervical spine injuries.[94, 97] The injury results from a flexion-compression force with an anterior triangular fracture and posterior displacement of the major body fragment into the spinal canal.

Anterior ligament injuries are often associated with anterior inferior chip fractures of the vertebral body. The mechanism of injury is disruptive hyperextension. These injuries are most common at the C2–C4 and C6–C7 levels. Changes may be subtle, with hematoma or displacement of the prevertebral fat stripe being the only indications of injury. As noted previously, on the lateral view hyperextension injuries may be difficult to differentiate from hyperflexion injuries. Oblique views may indicate that the mechanism of injury is hyperextension with neural arch fractures, or hyperflexion with facet locking or perching and facet joint widening and interspinous distance changes.

Cervical Spine Trauma—Associated Injuries

Cervical spine injuries are frequently associated with fractures of the thoracic and lumbar spine (15 percent) (Table 3–11). Head injuries (18 percent), facial injuries (4 percent), and other extraskeletal injuries are also common and may be helpful in determining the mechanism of cervical injury.

TABLE 3–11. Cervical Spine Trauma in 420 Patients: Associated Injuries

Location	Incidence (%)
Head	18
Thoracolumbar spine	15
Thoracic spine	12
Lumbar spine	3
Extremities	13
Chest	5
Facial bones	4
Abdomen	3
Pelvis	2

The possibility of overlooking a second distal spine injury may result in significant risk to the patient and improper management. Examination of the entire spine has been advocated and should be carried out in patients with significant cervical spine injury.[75, 114] Calenoff reported that in 30 patients with multiple level injuries, 80 percent sustained two separate lesions while in 20 percent there were injuries at three or more levels[75] (see Fig. 3–67).

In examining the distribution of cervical spine lesions related to injuries in the thoracic and lumbar spine, certain patterns evolved. Of the 420 patients with cervical spine fractures, 12 percent (50 patients) sustained associated thoracic fractures and 3 percent (13 patients) associated lumbar fractures. Table 3–12 describes the patterns noted in these patients. Patients with upper cervical lesions (C2 and above) tended to have associated fractures in the upper thoracic and upper lumbar region. The upper thoracic lesions are easily overlooked owing to the soft tissues of the shoulders. Significant neurologic deficit is often present with these fractures. There was also a high incidence of upper and lower cervical spine injuries. Patients with lower cervical spine injuries sustained a more uniform distribution of thoracic and lumbar fractures but tended to have midthoracic and upper lumbar fractures.

In patients with spinal trauma, especially if they are comatose or uncooperative, radiographs of the entire spine are essential. Tomography may be necessary to evaluate the lower cervical and upper thoracic region as well as other questionable areas that are not clearly demonstrated with routine

TABLE 3–12. Distribution of Cervical Spine Lesions Related to Injuries in the Thoracolumbar Spine

Extracervical Location	Incidence (%)
With C1–C2 Lesions	
T1–T4	None
T5–T8	67
T9–T12	33
L1–L3	100
L4–L5	0
With C3–C7 Lesions	
T1–T4	27
T5–T8	46
T9–T12	77
L1–L3	57
L4–L5	43

views. Unsuspected neurologically significant lesions can be overlooked if the entire spine is not evaluated in the acutely injured patient.

CERVICAL SPINE INJURIES—ESSENTIALS OF MANAGEMENT

Injuries to the Atlas and the Axis

Because of the unique anatomy of the first two cervical vertebrae, their injuries have characteristics that set them apart from injuries to the rest of the cervical spine. If fatality does not occur, proper diagnosis and treatment usually produces good results with relatively few sequelae. We will discuss briefly the management of the most important and frequent lesions in this area.

Occipitocervical Dislocations

A few cases of survival have been reported after this usually fatal injury. The treatment of choice is surgical stabilization by occipito–C2 arthrodesis followed by halothoracic immobilization for a minimum of 12 weeks.[107, 124]

Injuries to the Atlas

These consist of fractures of the posterior or anterior arch and transverse ligament tears.

Injuries to the Posterior and Anterior Arches. Fractures through the posterior arch of the atlas are the most common lesions of these vertebrae. If fractures through the anterior arch can be ruled out by tomography or preferably by CT scan, simple immobilization with a collar will suffice. If, however, fractures have occurred through both posterior and anterior arches of the atlas (Jefferson injury), halothoracic immobilization for 8 to 12 weeks will be necessary to ensure proper healing. As previously discussed, this injury is the result of an axially directed force that squeezes the lateral masses of the atlas between the occipital condyles and the lateral masses of the axis; the resulting effect is an explosion failure of the atlas with separation of its lateral masses. An uncommonly associated injury that needs to be ruled out is a tear through the transverse ligament of the axis. Spence has noted that a pathognomonic sign of this tear is a separation of the lateral masses of the atlas from the odontoid greater than 6.9 mm in the open-mouth odontoid view.[123] If this lesion is present, a two-stage treatment is mandatory: first, a halothoracic device for 8 to 12 weeks to allow the fracture to heal; second, a posterior atlantoaxial fusion to treat the ligament injury.

Transverse Ligament Tears. The potential for cord compression in this injury is high. The diagnosis is usually made by flexion-extension lateral x-rays obtained under fluoroscopy.[8] If the distance between the odontoid and the anterior arch of C1 is greater than 5 mm, insufficiency of the transverse ligament is present and operative stabilization by C1–C2 posterior arthrodesis is the treatment of choice.

Injuries to the Odontoid

These are probably the most commonly missed injuries of the cervical spine in the emergency evaluation of neck injuries.

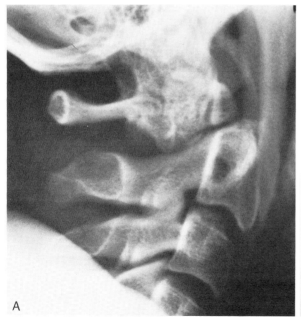 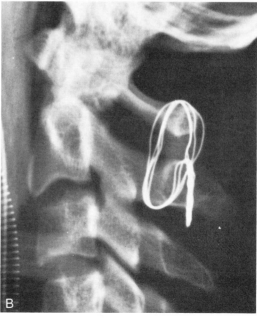

Figure 3–84. A, Lateral x-ray of cervical spine of a 20-year-old male involved in a motorcycle accident. No neurologic deficit. Note 100 percent posterior displacement of the odontoid. *B,* Same patient after early posterior atlantoaxial fusion.

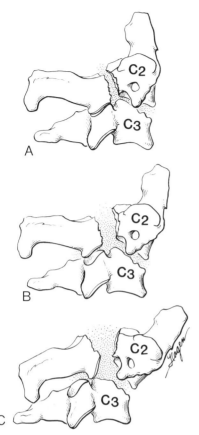

Figure 3–85. "Hangman's fractures," following classification of Effendi, et al.[83] A, Type I: pedicle fractures with no displacement. B, Type II: pedicle fractures with displacement of the anterior fragment. C, Type III: fracture-dislocation.

Type I fractures are uncommon and usually are the result of an avulsion force that does not place the stability of the atlantoaxial area in jeopardy; therefore, simple collar immobilization suffices.

Type II fractures, or fractures through the base of the odontoid, can be difficult to diagnose. Usually the open-mouth view and the lateral cervical spine x-rays will suffice to procure the diagnosis. But if the fracture is undisplaced, tomography may be necessary. These fractures, particularly if displaced, have a high incidence of non-union.[122, 124] The high mechanical stresses in this area, the small surface area of the fracture, and the partial interruption of the blood supply to the odontoid may all play a role in the failure to heal. If the fracture is undisplaced, or if anterior displacement of less than 4 mm can be reduced by gentle manipulation, halo-thoracic immobilization for 12 weeks produces satisfactory healing in the majority of the cases, especially if the patient is under 40 years of age. If, however, anterior displacement cannot be reduced, or if posterior displacement of the odontoid has occurred (Fig. 3–84), early atlantoaxial fusion should be the treatment of choice. Posteriorly displaced odontoid fractures are relatively rare, but when they are seen in elderly patients, they carry a particularly bad prognosis, primarily related to the often associated respiratory complications. If surgery is contraindicated because of the general condition of the patient, application of a halo-vest and early mobilization of the patient offers the best possible means to avoid the commonly seen respiratory complications.

Type III odontoid fractures occur through the body of the axis. As a rule, these are stable injuries through cancellous bone, and they heal promptly with halothoracic immobilization.

Injuries to the Axis[83, 89]

The most common injury is the so-called "hangman's fracture," or fracture through the pedicles of the axis. Today, this injury is most commonly seen in multiple-system trauma victims and is usually the result of an extension force. These injuries have been classified by Effendi and colleagues (Fig. 3–85).[83] Basically, injuries can be classified according to whether there is displacement of C2 on C3. If no forward displacement of the body of the axis on the

Figure 3–86. A, Lateral roentgenogram of cervical spine of a 27-year-old male involved in an automobile accident. No neurologic deficit. Note significant forward subluxation of C2 on C3, indicating damage to the anterior ligamentous and disk structures. B, Same patient 3 months after injury. Treatment has been immobilization with a halo cast for 8 weeks. Note healing of the pedicle fractures as well as anterior interbody ossification.

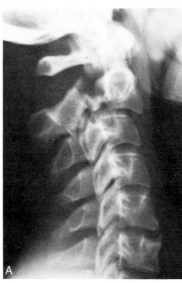 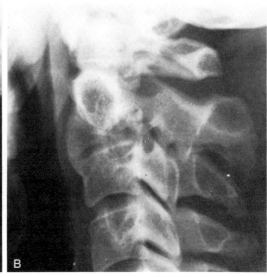

150 • THE SPINE

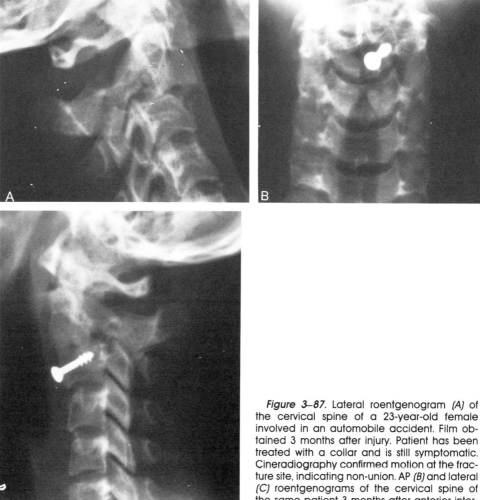

Figure 3–87. Lateral roentgenogram *(A)* of the cervical spine of a 23-year-old female involved in an automobile accident. Film obtained 3 months after injury. Patient has been treated with a collar and is still symptomatic. Cineradiography confirmed motion at the fracture site, indicating non-union. AP *(B)* and lateral *(C)* roentgenograms of the cervical spine of the same patient 3 months after anterior interbody fusion C2-C3. The patient is asymptomatic.

third cervical vertebra is noted—that is, if there is no damage to the C2–C3 disk and anterior longitudinal ligament (Type I)—then the damage is confined to the posterior elements of the axis and simple immobilization with a collar will suffice. However, if significant displacement of the body of C2 on C3 is present (Type II), or if in addition C2–C3 facet dislocation has occurred (Type III) (Fig. 3–86), then the injury is unstable and in this instance halothoracic immobilization is indicated until healing occurs. Type III injuries are very rare and require reduction of the dislocated facets. Nonunion of this injury is uncommon (Fig. 3–87), and if it occurs, it is best treated with anterior C2–C3 arthrodesis.[124] Posterior C1–C3 arthrodesis, the obvious alternative, unnecessarily restricts the rotation available at the C1–C2 level and is not advisable.

Injuries to the Lower Cervical Spine

The management of injuries to the lower cervical spine is based on the clinical assessment of the

integrity of the neurologic structures and on the radiologic assessment of stability.[128] The goals of treatment are to decompress the neurologic structures and to stabilize the spine. Decompression is usually achieved by realignment, but it may at times require removal of bony fragments from the canal (most commonly from the anterior aspect of the canal). In general, stable lesions without neurologic deficit require only the minimal support provided by a collar. Unstable or potentially unstable lesions require more aggressive treatment. When the injury involves primarily ligamentous structures, early surgical stabilization is preferred, since conservative treatment often produces late instability. However, if the injury is predominantly bony, more conservative treatment with halothoracic immobilization followed by a late stability assessment is justified.

Sprains

Posterior ligamentous injuries can have very serious consequences. They are the result of a flexion mechanism, commonly occur between the ages of

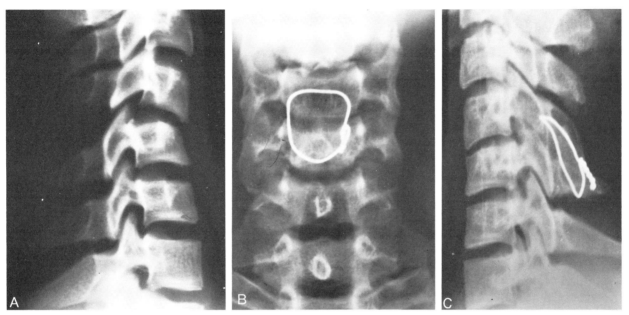

Figure 3–88. Lateral roentgenogram *(A)* of the cervical spine of a 17-year-old boy who sustained a flexion injury in a diving accident. Note the increased distance between the spinous processes of C4 and C5, the kyphotic angulation at this level, and the subluxation of the facet joints. No neurologic deficit. Anterior *(B)* and lateral *(C)* roentgenograms of the cervical spine of the same patient 1 year after posterior interspinous wiring and fusion. The patient is asymptomatic.

14 and 22, and usually involve a single interspace between C4 and T1. They have been named "hidden" injuries because they often are not recognized.[127] The pathologic lesion consists of tears of the ligamentum nuchae, the interspinous ligament, and often the ligamenta flava. The characteristic radiologic features of these injuries include (1) an

increase in the distance between the spinous processes of the two involved vertebrae, (2) a small compression fracture of the superior and anterior corner of the inferior vertebra, (3) an often subtle intervertebral subluxation, and (4) a loss of the normal cervical lordosis (Fig. 3–88). If the ligament damage is small, simple collar immobilization usu-

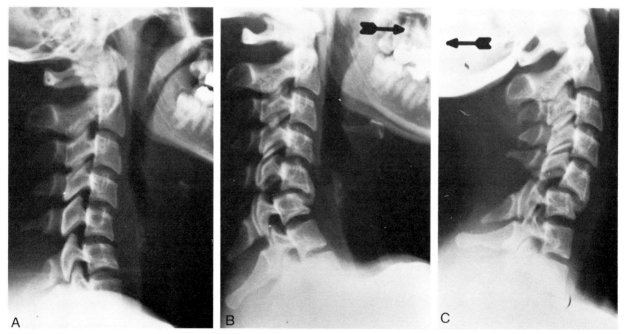

Figure 3–89. Lateral roentgenogram *(A)* obtained immediately after this 25-year-old female was involved in an automobile accident. The obvious ligamentous injury at the C5–C6 interspace was missed. The patient was not treated. Flexion *(B)* and extension *(C)* lateral roentgenograms of the same patient obtained 6 months after injury. The patient has now developed neurological symptoms (Lhermitte's sign) and has significant neck pain. Note the perching of the facet joints that has occurred as well as the precarious stability achieved by calcification and ossification of the anterior longitudinal ligament.

ally suffices. However, if the subluxation shows a tendency to increase in a controlled flexion lateral x-ray of the cervical spine, wiring of the spinous process and posterior arthrodesis is the treatment of choice (Fig. 3–88B and C). Failure to recognize these injuries early may have disastrous consequences, as cases of late dislocation have occurred with subsequent neurologic compromise (Fig. 3–89).

Dislocations and Fracture-Dislocations

In the cervical spine pure flexion or flexion associated with rotation can produce either a unilateral or a bilateral dislocation of the facets. The radio-graphic features of these two injuries have been described. Beatson[72] has clearly shown in his cadaver experiments that if forward displacement encompasses less than 50 percent of the anteroposterior diameter of the vertebral body, the lesion is a unilateral facet dislocation, whereas if the displacement is 50 percent or more of the anteroposterior diameter of the body, the lesion is always a bilateral dislocation (Fig. 3–90).

Management in this case should be no different from that of dislocations of any other joint in the body. Whether or not neurologic deficit is present, reduction of the dislocation should be undertaken if the diagnosis is made early.[107, 124] This is accomplished usually by directed traction through cranial

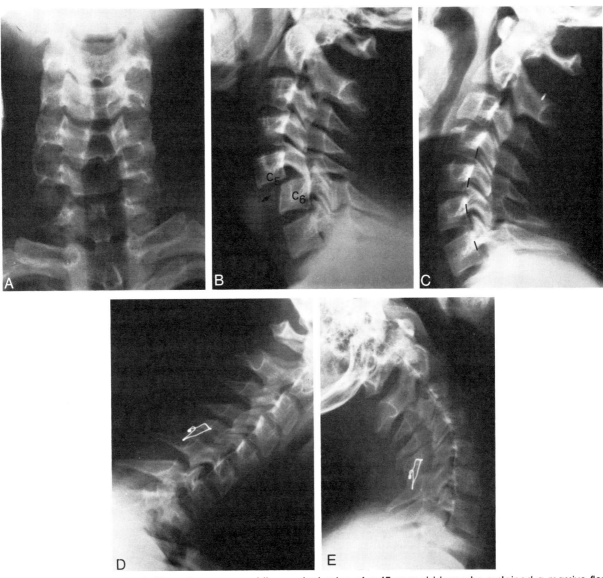

Figure 3–90. AP *(A)* and lateral *(B)* roentgenograms of the cervical spine of a 17-year-old boy who sustained a massive flexion injury during a wrestling match. Profound paraparesis is present. This is clearly a bilateral facet dislocation. Lateral roentgenogram *(C)* of the same patient obtained 2 hours after admission and immediately after reduction has been achieved by halo traction. The alignment of the cervical spine has been restored. Flexion *(D)* and extension *(E)* lateral roentgenograms of the cervical spine of the same patient obtained 3 months after posterior interspinous wiring and fusion. One year after injury the patient has regained normal neurologic function and leads a very active life in sports. Early realignment of the spine has been essential in achieving this recovery.

tongs or a halo (Fig. 3–90C). Since these injuries encompass primarily ligamentous disruptions, it is now believed that healing with stability seldom is achieved, and this explains the current tendency to stabilize these injuries surgically with early interspinous wiring and fusion of the dislocated vertebral segment (Fig. 3–90D and E).

If closed reduction cannot be achieved, as frequently occurs in the case of unilateral facet dislocations, open reduction followed by stabilization is recommended. The technique of closed manipulation[107] of the dislocated facet has been popular elsewhere but is not frequently practiced in the United States.

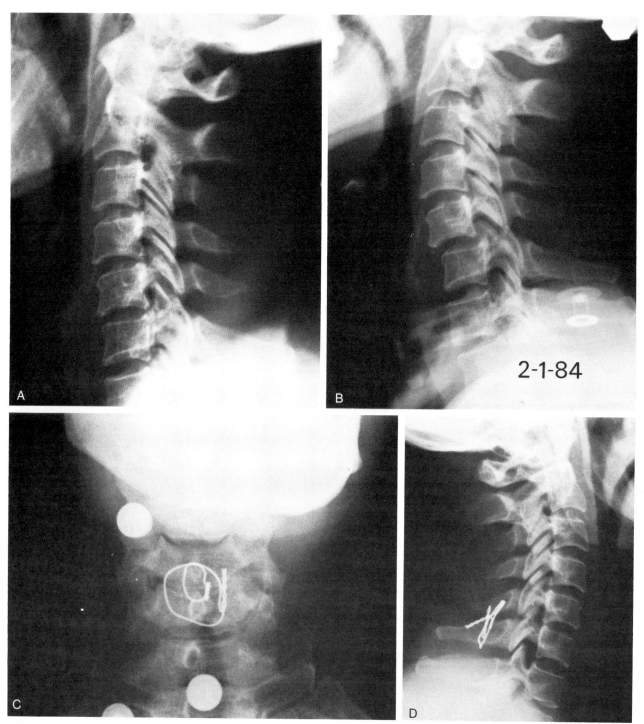

Figure 3–91. Lateral roentgenogram *(A)* of the cervical spine of a 52-year-old female involved in a single car accident. The patient presents with an acute left C6 radiculopathy. Note fracture of the superior facet of C6. Lateral roentgenogram *(B)* obtained two days after admission of the same patient. The patient has been treated with halo vest immobilization. Note the forward subluxation of C5 on C6. The patient continues to have severe symptoms and her root deficit has not improved. AP *(C)* and lateral *(D)* roentgenograms of the same patient shortly after removal of the facet fragment and posterior interspinous wiring and fusion. Two months postoperatively, the patient was free of symptoms and no longer experienced neurological deficit.

When subluxation or dislocation is associated with fractures of the tip of the inferior facet (Fig. 3–91A), a rather common occurrence resulting in isolated root deficits, reduction is difficult to achieve and even more difficult to maintain (Fig. 3–91B). The root deficit often lingers with conservative management, but early decompression of the involved root by removal of the loose facet fragment followed by surgical stabilization has produced very satisfactory results in our hands (Fig. 3–91C and D).

When dislocations or fracture-dislocations have occurred in patients with pre-existing cervical spon-

dylosis and reduction has been achieved, late instability after conservative management with halothoracic immobilization for a period of 8 to 12 weeks has produced very satisfactory results. Thus when these lesions occur in patients afflicted with cervical spondylosis, conservative rather than surgical management is justified.

Extension Injuries

These are relatively common injuries, resulting frequently from falls or automobile accidents. Often these patients are of middle or advanced age and

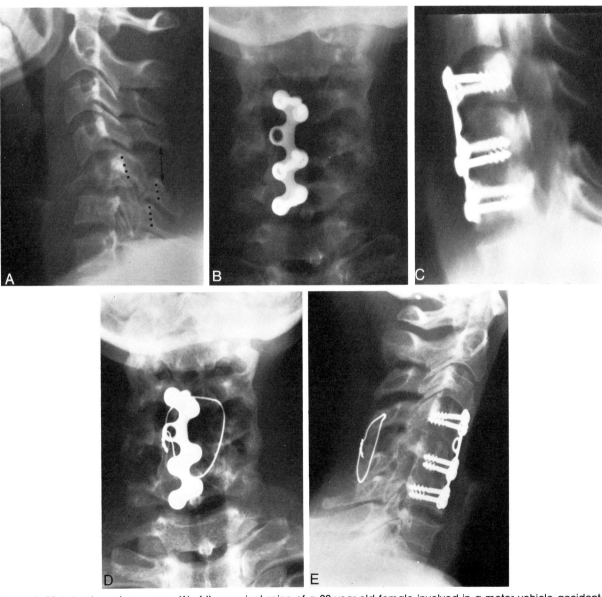

Figure 3–92. Lateral roentgenogram *(A)* of the cervical spine of a 22-year-old female involved in a motor vehicle accident. The patient presents with a profound anterior cord syndrome. Note the coronal fracture of the vertebral body and the posterior displacement of the body of C5 into the canal as well as the posterior element fracture and interspinous widening. AP *(B)* and lateral *(C)* roentgenograms of the same patient treated immediately after admission with anterior decompression of the spinal canal by removal of the comminuted vertebral body and replacement with a bone graft with internal fixation. AP *(D)* and lateral *(E)* roentgenogram of the same patient 6 months after injury. Because of significant posterior disruption, a delayed posterior wiring and bone grafting was carried out on this patient. Neurologic recovery was very satisfactory. The patient is now walking 3 years after injury, although with some residual deficit in the lower extremity.

are afflicted with cervical spondylosis, and often no evidence of skeletal damage can be encountered. Typically, these patients will present with a central cord syndrome. It is well known that the antero-posterior diameter of the spinal canal decreases significantly in extension, and it is postulated that an anteroposterior compression of the cord either by osteophytes or by the hypertrophic ligamenta flava causes a temporary interruption of the blood supply to the central part of the cord, resulting in edema or infarction of this area. The treatment of these injuries should be conservative with support by a collar for a period of 6 weeks. If there is no improvement, or if deterioration occurs, a myelogram should be considered.

Vertebral Body Fractures

Most vertebral body fractures can be treated conservatively and will heal with support by a cervical orthosis. This applies to chip fractures, minor wedge fractures, uncinate process fractures, and triangular fractures.

However, the comminuted vertebral body fracture resulting from a flexion-compression mechanism, and also known as the flexion teardrop fracture-dislocation, is a rather unstable injury (Fig. 3–92A). The vertebral body is usually split into two portions—the anterior one is displaced forward like a teardrop, and the posterior portion protrudes into the spinal canal and impacts the cord. In addition, there is usually a fracture through the posterior arch and widening of the interspinous distance. As a rule, the neurologic deficit is profound, but often it involves only the anterior part of the cord. In this injury, traction through cranial tongs or a halo can often realign the spinal canal and decrease the pressure on the anterior spinal cord. However, maintaining this reduction requires prolonged traction in the recumbent position for a period of 12 to 16 weeks. Thus the current trend is to effect surgical removal of the comminuted vertebral body through an anterior approach and replacement with a bone graft with or without internal fixation (Fig. 3–92B and C).[92, 124]

This approach gives the best chance to maximize neurologic recovery and guarantee stability. If posterior element disruption is minimal, anterior stabilization followed by early mobilization in a cervical orthosis may suffice. However, if posterior ligament disruption is significant, anterior grafting and stabilization should be followed by halothoracic immobilization for 6 to 12 weeks, or by a second-stage posterior wiring and bone grafting as well (Fig. 3–92D and E).

Summary

The current philosophy of management of cervical injury is based upon a careful assessment of the neurologic deficit and a careful study of x-rays. Early decompression of the neural elements, achieved most often by realignment of the spinal canal and occasionally by removal of bone fragments, followed by early stabilization provides the best chance for recovery of the neural elements, assures stability, facilitates rehabilitation, and minimizes late sequelae.

THORACIC AND LUMBAR SPINE TRAUMA

Anatomic differences in the cervical, thoracic, and lumbar spine must be considered in any discussion of trauma to these regions. Thus the cervical spine is more prone to injury than the thoracic and lumbar spine by virtue of its increased range of motion and fewer supporting structures.

In the thoracic spine a slight kyphotic curve is normally present. This is in contrast to the lordotic curves evident in the cervical and lumbar regions. Also, the spinal canal in the thoracic region is circular and smaller in diameter than the cervical or lumbar portions of the spine. As one progresses inferiorly, the vertebral bodies increase in size and the disks increase in height, resulting in an increasing resistance to vertical compression forces.

The lumbar segment is similar to the cervical segment in that both contain a greater potential for motion than the thoracic segment. However, the large paraspinal muscles in the lumbar region provide more stability than the cervical musculature.[151] Owing to differences in range of motion, transition in the facet joints, and other anatomic factors, the thoracolumbar junction is the area most susceptible to injury. Thus the majority of injuries occur at this level. Nicoll reported that 66 percent of the thoracolumbar fractures occurred between T12 and L2.[165]

Mechanism of Injury

Discussion of thoracolumbar trauma can best be accomplished by utilizing a mechanism of injury approach.[147, 156, 157] The majority of fractures and fracture-dislocations are due to hyperflexion, flexion-rotation, vertical compression, hyperextension, and shearing forces (Table 3–13).[137, 144, 151, 156, 165]

The mechanism of injury in the thoracolumbar

TABLE 3–13. Thoracolumbar Spine Trauma: Mechanism of Injury

Hyperflexion
    Flexion-compression
    Lateral flexion
    Flexion-rotation
    Flexion-distraction
    Seatbelt injuries
Vertical compression
Hyperextension
Shearing

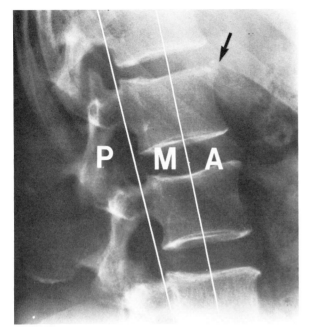

Figure 3–93. Lateral view of the thoracolumbar junction demonstrating the three column approach. A, anterior; M, middle; P, posterior. Note the normal variant *(arrow)* in L1. This should not be confused with a fracture.

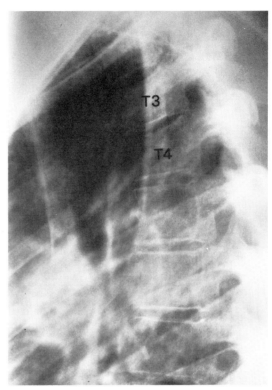

Figure 3–94. Anterior compression fractures of T3 and T4. Compression fractures are frequently multiple.

spine is similar to that in the cervical spine, but because of significant anatomic differences the results and presentation may vary. Holdsworth established his classification of spinal injury based on two columns, the anterior and posterior.[156] More recently, Denis described a three-column approach to evaluating spinal injury (Fig. 3–93).[146] The anterior column includes the anterior longitudinal ligament, anterior annulus and disk, and the ventral half of the vertebral body. The middle column consists of the posterior half of the vertebral body, disk, annulus, and posterior longitudinal ligament. The posterior column includes the neural arch and posterior ligament complex (Fig. 3–93).[146] It has been demonstrated that rupture of the posterior longitudinal ligament and annulus is necessary for instability to occur.[147]

Hyperflexion Injuries

Hyperflexion injuries are by far the most common injury in the thoracic and lumbar spine. Most often the injury is due to flexion-compression forces that result in a simple anterior wedge fracture of the vertebral body. The posterior complex is almost always intact; therefore, this is a stable injury.

The axis of the force in hyperflexion injuries is centered in the nucleus pulposus or in the midportion of the intervertebral disk. Thus the appearance of the injury may vary, depending upon the spinal level involved. In the upper thoracic region the disks are narrower and the fracture is more typically a true anterior wedge fracture (Fig. 3–94). In the thoracic region, especially the upper thoracic spine,

the anterior height of the vertebral bodies is normally 1.5 mm less than the posterior height. In the lower thoracic and lumbar region the disks are larger and more effective as shock absorbers. Thus herniation into the cartilaginous end-plates is more likely to occur in the lower thoracic and lumbar regions (Fig. 3–95). If the flexion force continues, the anterior body is more likely to be compressed.[151]

The degree of compression and changes in the disk space are important in wedge fractures of the vertebral bodies. If compression is greater than 50 percent and if the disk space is narrowed, the prognosis is less favorable.[143] These findings along with multiple contiguous wedge fractures may lead to delayed instability. Multiple contiguous wedge fractures in the upper thoracic region may lead to cord deficits (Fig. 3–96).[137]

Radiographic evaluation of anterior wedge fractures is almost always complete with AP and lateral projections of the involved areas (Table 3–14). On the AP view one should check for evidence of paraspinal soft tissue swelling, which is often pres-

TABLE 3–14. Radiographic Features in Anterior Wedge Fractures

Soft tissue swelling
Anterior superior cortical impaction
Loss of height anteriorly
Trabecular condensation
End-plate fracture
Disk space narrowing

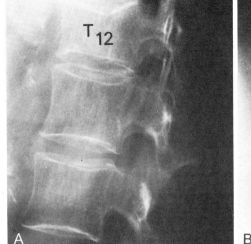
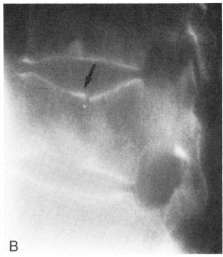

Figure 3–95. Elderly female with osteoporosis and pain following a fall. *A,* There is loss of height at T12. ? Acute versus senile osteoporosis. *B,* Lateral tomogram clearly demonstrates an acute fracture *(arrow)* with end plate involvement.

ent with anterior compression fractures (Fig. 3–97). The interpedicular distance and posterior elements are normal with a simple wedge fracture. The same force that results in a wedge fracture may disrupt the posterior ligaments or bony structures if the magnitude of the force is sufficient. Occasionally, the loss of height and trabecular compression can be detected on the AP view (Fig. 3–97), but diagnosis is better accomplished on the lateral view (Fig. 3–94). Compression or buckling of the anterior superior cortex of the vertebral body is the most common feature. Disk-space narrowing and vertebral end-plate fracture may be present. However, these features are more commonly noted with burst fractures. Occasionally, tomography (Fig. 3–95) is

required to detect a subtle compression fracture or to visualize a suspicious area. Lateral tomograms are especially important in the upper thoracic region, where penetration of the shoulders is often difficult (Fig. 3–96). This can easily be accomplished with the Versigraph without moving the patient. AP tomograms should also be obtained to exclude vertebral arch injury, which may result in instability and quite different management of the patient. With simple anterior wedge fractures computed tomography is rarely necessary.

The list of differential diagnostic possibilities that may be confused with anterior wedge fractures is extensive (Table 3–15). Diagnostic problems are common in elderly patients with osteopenia (Fig.

Figure 3–96. Patient with upper thoracic pain and neurologic deficit in the lower extremities. Routine AP view *(A)* was thought to be normal. The upper thoracic region could not be evaluated on routine lateral views. Tomogram *(B)* demonstrates 75° compression of T3, mild compression of T4, and marked kyphotic deformity.

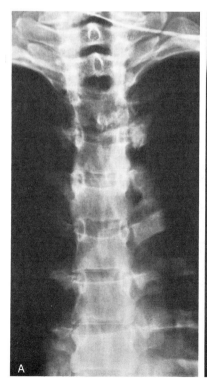
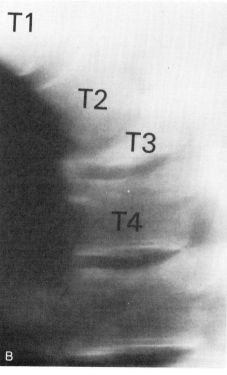

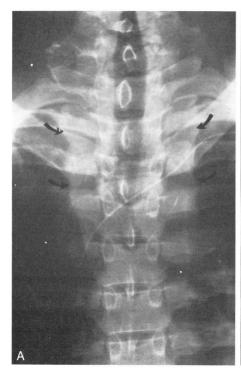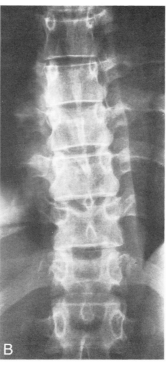

Figure 3–97. Thoracic compression fractures. *A,* Marked soft tissue swelling *(arrows)* due to multiple upper thoracic compression fractures. This is a particularly useful sign as the lateral view is often underinterpreted in this region. *B,* More subtle paraspinal swelling due to mild compression of T12.

3–95), in pathologic conditions that are difficult to differentiate from simple traumatic lesions, and occasionally in infectious conditions or cases of nuclear herniation.

Lateral flexion injuries may result in lateral vertebral wedge fractures. This injury is stable,[137] though it has been reported to result in a somewhat poorer prognosis than a simple anterior wedge fracture.[165] Radiographically there is almost always some degree of paraspinal soft tissue swelling, especially in the thoracic region. The asymmetric compression is best appreciated on the AP view (Fig. 3–98).

The same forces responsible for anterior wedge fractures, if continued, result in distraction of the posterior complex. Ligament disruption or vertebral arch fractures may occur, resulting in an unstable fracture-dislocation.[168, 169] Though it is common in the cervical spine, locking of the facets is rare in the thoracic and lumbar spine.[156] The facets and large paraspinal muscles in the lumbar region, and

the costal elements and chest in the thoracic region, provide more stability.[8]

The majority of flexion-distraction injuries occur at the thoracolumbar junction. Usually the compres-

TABLE 3–15. Anterior Wedge Fractures: Differential Diagnosis[151]

Congenital
    Hemivertebra
Pathologic
    Infectious
    Neoplasm
        Primary
        Metastatic
        Metabolic
Scheuermann's disease
Kümmell's disease
Schmorl's nodes

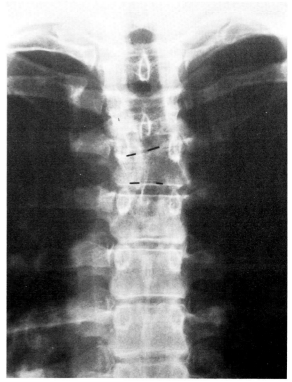

Figure 3–98. Lateral wedge fracture of T4 *(broken lines).* The degree of wedging is best demonstrated on the AP view or AP tomography.

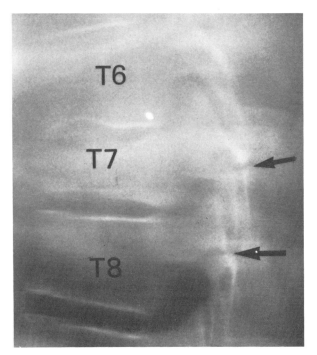

Figure 3–99. Flexion-distraction injury with compression of T7 and posterior arch fractures at T7 and T8 *(arrows)*. The posterior element fractures were not seen on CT or routine views. CT slices were in the plane of the fracture and overlooked owing to partial volume effect.

sion force is centered in the midportion of the body and nucleus pulposus with distraction posteriorly. The incidence of neurologic complications may be as high as 70 percent.[151] Flexion-distraction injuries with disruption of the posterior ligament complex or fractures of the arch are unstable (Fig. 3–99).[172, 174] The degree of compression may be minimal; and therefore not only the compression but, more importantly, the posterior injury may be overlooked. Tomography in the AP and lateral projections can be accomplished with ease in the acutely injured patient without changing the position of the patient. Computed tomography is also of value but may require more patient manipulation than can be tolerated during the early assessment period. If the patient can be moved to the CT gantry, valuable information regarding the status of the spinal canal can be obtained (Fig. 3–100). Other authors have also noted CT to be of value in examining the facet joint,[167] but in our experience tomography is preferred for undisplaced horizontal fractures and facet evaluation. Myelography is occasionally required to determine the level of obstruction due to the fractures.

Seatbelt injuries result from a mechanism similar to flexion-distraction trauma except for the fact that the fulcrum is located anteriorly at the abdominal wall and the injuries more commonly involve the

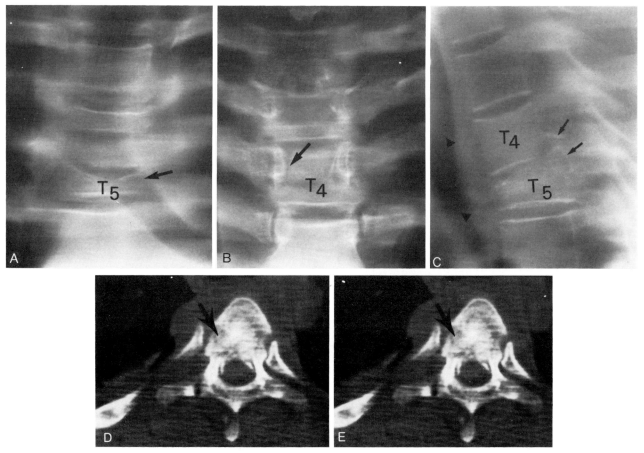

Figure 3–100. Upper thoracic spine fracture. The AP *(A and B)* and lateral *(C)* tomograms demonstrate the fractures at T4–T5. There is also soft tissue swelling. CT scans *(D and E)* clearly demonstrate the bony fragments in the spinal canal.

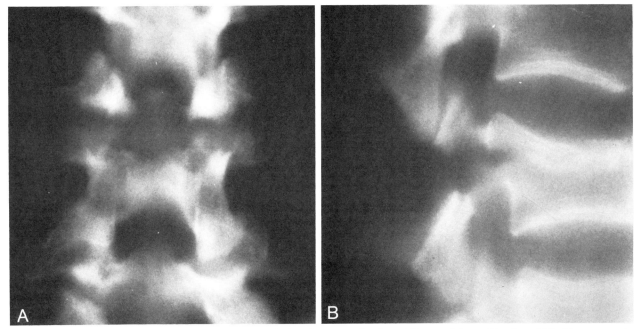

Figure 3–101. AP *(A)* and lateral *(B)* tomograms demonstrate a transverse fracture of the pedicle and lamina of L2 with compression of the vertebral body.

midlumbar region (L1–L3).[140, 151, 171] This injury was initially described by Chance in 1948.[142] Rogers[171] has described three different patterns of fulcrum injury:

1. Disruption of the posterior ligaments, facets,

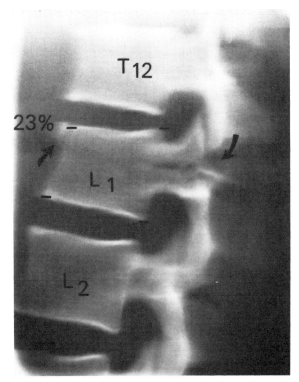

Figure 3–102. Tomogram of the upper lumbar spine with a seatbelt fracture. Note the minimal compression of L1 with obvious posterior distraction *(curved arrow).*

and disks occurs with the spinous process, transverse processes, and pedicles intact.

2. A transverse fracture of the posterior arch occurs and may involve the posterior superior body.

3. Transverse fractures are present in the posterior arch and body. The lamina, transverse processes, and pedicles are usually involved (Fig. 3–101).

The location (L1–L3), lack of significant vertebral compression, and increased incidence of abdominal injury are the major differences between the seatbelt injury and the flexion-distraction injury previously discussed. Several large series have discussed the complications associated with seatbelt or anterior fulcrum injuries.[142, 145, 150, 160, 171] Abdominal wall hematomas as well as intra-abdominal pathology may result. Lacerations in the bowel, especially the ileum, duodenum, and antimesenteric border of the jejunum, are common. Lacerations of the liver, spleen, and pancreas may also occur.[151, 171] The incidence of neurologic involvement is lower (less than 20 percent) than in the case of flexion-distraction injuries, in which the fulcrum is at the midvertebral body level.[151] The degree of vertebral compression may be minimal and occasionally no anterior injury is detectable (Fig. 3–102). Evaluation of the arch on the AP views should be performed with great care (Fig. 3–103). In our experience 25 percent of seatbelt injuries were not detected on the lateral view. This is the result of absence of significant compression. Also, the posterior elements are often not entirely included on the supine lateral projection. The AP view may provide the only clue to this significant unstable injury. Radiographic evaluation frequently requires tomography

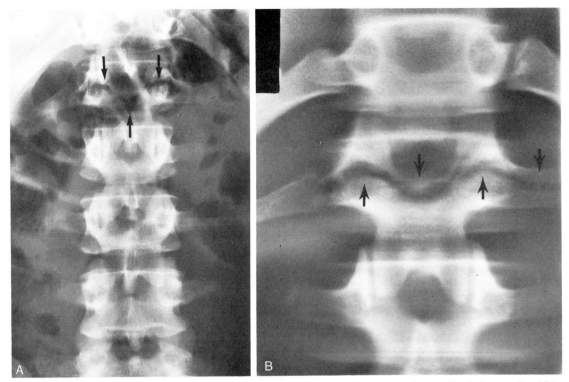

Figure 3–103. L1 posterior arch fracture *(arrows)* seen only on the AP *(A)* view. The fracture *(arrows)* is obvious on the AP tomogram *(B)*.

or CT to determine the extent of the injury (Fig. 3–103).

Flexion-Rotation Injuries

Fortunately, flexion-rotation injuries of the thoracolumbar spine are uncommon.[63] When it occurs, the lesion is among the most unstable of spinal injuries.[137, 156] The injury usually occurs at the thoracolumbar junction owing to the transition in the facet joints.[137] The incidence of neurologic deficit approaches 70 percent.[137] This injury is easily overlooked, as it is uncommon, and, more importantly, reduction of the dislocation tends to occur in the supine position.[156]

Radiographic features of the injury are similar to a unilateral locked facet in the cervical spine. On the AP view the spinous process may be rotated to the side of the involvement, and a fracture through the upper end-plate may be present. The disk space may appear asymmetric or tilted to one side. On the lateral view the disk space is often narrowed and the interspinous distance increased. A "slice fracture"[156] of the upper vertebral body is usually more obvious on the lateral view. Fractures of the articular processes and lamina frequently require tomography for detection (Fig. 3–104). Computed tomography is most useful in evaluating the degree of involvement of the spinal canal (Fig. 3–105).

Vertical Compression Injury

Vertical compression injuries result in burst fractures of the vertebral bodies with outward displacements of fracture fragments, herniation of the disk into the end-plates, and posterior extension of the disk and fracture fragments into the spinal canal. This is a stable injury, as the ligaments remain intact.[137, 149, 151, 156] Most injuries occur at the T12–L2 level. Though stable, the incidence of neurologic involvement is high owing to displacement of bone fragments into the spinal canal.[149]

Burst fractures can usually be seen on the AP and lateral views (Fig. 3–106). Such fractures involve multiple body fragments and compression of the body and disk space. The interpedicular distance is increased on the AP view, and if tomograms are obtained arch fractures are also common. Though the degree of spinal canal involvement can often be appreciated on the lateral view or lateral tomogram, CT is the technique of choice for the best evaluation of the spinal canal (Fig. 3–107).[101, 136, 173, 176, 179] Bony fragments, dural tears, and epidural hematomas may be detected with this modality.[138, 159, 166, 177]

Hyperextension Injury

Hyperextension injuries in the thoracolumbar spine are rare. Roaf demonstrated posterior arch fractures but could not disrupt the strong anterior

Text continued on page 164

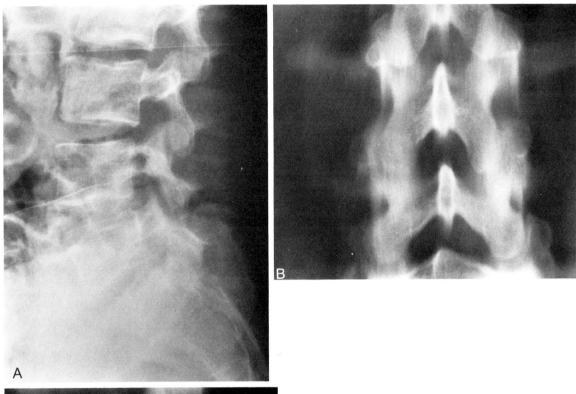

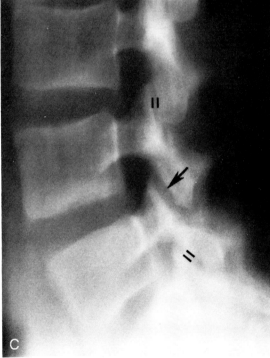

Figure 3–104. Flexion-rotation injury in the lower lumbar spine. The lateral view *(A)* shows apparent widening of the L4–L5 facet joints. The AP tomogram *(B)* was normal. Lateral tomogram *(C)* clearly demonstrates the widened facet joint *(arrow)* on the left.

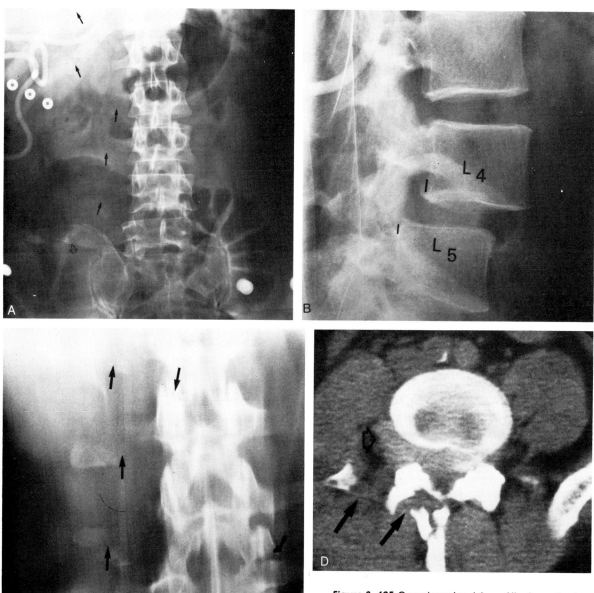

Figure 3–105. Complex rotary injury of the lower lumbar spine. *A,* AP view demonstrates multiple transverse process and rib fractures *(arrows)* with displacement of L4 on L5 to the left. *B,* Lateral view shows anterior subluxation of L4 on L5 with slight disk space narrowing. *C,* AP tomogram demonstrates the transverse process fractures and right iliac crest fracture *(vertical arrows).* There are also facet fractures at L5 on the left *(curved arrow)* and L2 on the right *(upper arrow). D,* CT scan more clearly demonstrates the canal and hemorrhage around the intervertebral foramina *(open arrow).*

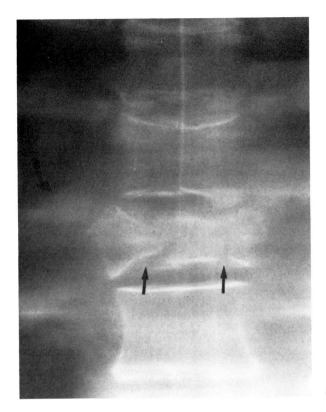

Figure 3–106. AP tomogram of a burst fracture in the lower thoracic spine *(arrows)*. There is marked soft tissue swelling *(curved arrow)*.

longitudinal ligament with pure hyperextension.[170] He felt rotary motion was required for ligament disruption. The forces applied result in posterior compression and anterior distraction, the opposite of hyperflexion injuries. The incidence of neurologic complications with this injury is also high.[139, 155, 162] De Oliveira described ten patients with dorsal blows to the back that resulted in hyperextension of the segment above the level of the injury.[144] The majority of the injuries occurred in the midlumbar region. Lateral radiographs revealed posterior subluxation of the vertebral body above the level at which the trauma occurred. The incidence of neurologic injury in these patients was not significant, and healing occurred without residual pain.

Radiographic findings with hyperextension injuries are similar to those noted in the cervical spine. The features are best detected on the lateral view. The disk space may be widened anteriorly, and the posterior structures may be fractured owing to compression forces. If subluxation is noted, CT is useful in evaluation of the spinal canal.

Shearing Injury

Shearing forces result in anterior dislocation of the vertebra at the level of the injury onto the vertebra below.[137, 151, 156, 158] In our experience this injury is more common in the thoracic region. The posterior complex is usually disrupted, resulting in

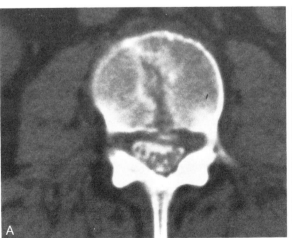
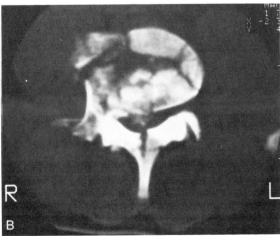

Figure 3–107. A, Subtle burst fracture. CT with metrizamide demonstrates the fracture with a fragment displacing the dural sac posteriorly. B, Complex burst fracture of L3 with marked fragmentation and compromise of the spinal canal.

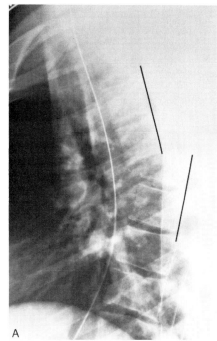 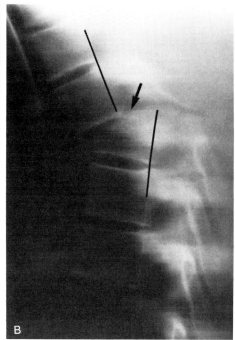

Figure 3–108. Thoracic dislocation seen on the lateral view *(A)* and lateral tomogram *(B)*.

a very unstable lesion.[137, 152, 156] Neurologic injury is common. Lateral views and tomography are most helpful in evaluation of this injury (Fig. 3–108). Often the patient's condition is such that movement to the CT gantry is not wise or essential in the acute situation.

Minor Fractures

Fractures of the posterior arch without an associated fracture-dislocation are uncommon.[134, 152, 153, 162, 168, 174] Fractures of the articular processes may result from twisting injuries and have been described in skiers.[168] Smith described posterior arch fractures involving the lamina and pars following jumping injuries; all patients presented with neurologic deficits.[174] Murray has determined that pars interarticularis fractures may actually be stress fractures.[164] Fractures of the transverse processes are most common in the lumbar region and are usually due to direct trauma or muscle contraction (Fig. 3–109).[136] These fractures are usually not significant by themselves, but associated retroperitoneal hematoma and renal injury may result. Fractures of the spinous processes may be due to flexion, extension, or direct trauma. The most common location is the lower cervical and upper thoracic region. This injury is rare in the lumbar spine.

The most difficult problem in isolated arch fractures is differentiating these findings from congenital clefts and spondylolysis.[134] Clinical history, previous films, and tomography are essential for proper evaluation of these injuries (Fig. 3–110). Congenital clefts and old non-united fractures have well-defined sclerotic margins. Acute fractures have irregular nonsclerotic margins.

Thoracic and Lumbar Injuries—Essentials of Management

About one third of these spinal injuries will result in neurologic deficit. At least in the United States

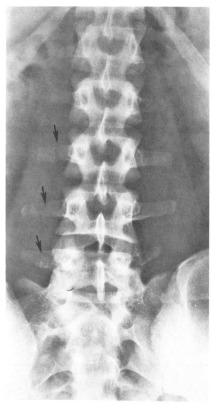

Figure 3–109. Multiple transverse process fractures *(arrows).* These are best seen on the AP view.

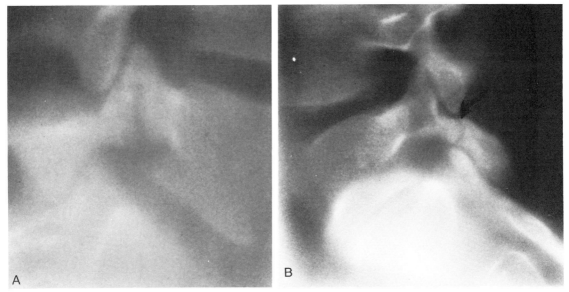

Figure 3–110. *A,* Tomogram demonstrating an acute pedicle fracture entering the L5 facet. *B,* Tomogram demonstrates sclerosis of the pars at L5 due to a stress fracture *(curved arrow).*

the incidence of incomplete injuries is on the increase—perhaps owing to improvement in the emergency medical system.[146] Proper early evaluation and treatment can have a vast impact on the future of the patient—not only from the point of view of ultimate function but also from that of lifetime cost of follow-up treatment.

Initially, the critical questions are again those of the extent of neurologic deficit and spinal instability. The answer to the first question is based on careful clinical evaluation. Complete neurologic deficit at the level of T10 or above will be the result of cord injury and is therefore irreversible. However, deficit below the skeletal level of T10 would necessarily involve the conus medullaris and/or the roots of the cauda equina. Cauda equina lesions behave like peripheral nerves, and therefore they have a better prognosis for neurologic recovery. This justifies a more aggressive approach to management of injuries at the thoracolumbar junction and below.

Evaluation of spinal instability is based on a careful study of radiographs. In general, lesions that involve the anterior and posterior elements of the spine, whether or not they are associated with neurologic deficits, should be considered unstable, particularly if significant displacement or significant angulation is present at the injury site. On the other hand, injuries that involve only the anterior or the posterior elements alone are generally considered stable. In addition, late instability can occur as a result of late kyphotic angulation, which is more common after multiple compression fractures or after bursting injuries treated with inadequate external support for an insufficient period of time. Late progressive angulation can result in progressive neurologic deterioration related to tethering of the cord around the kyphotic deformity.

Management of injuries to the thoracic and lumbar spine remains controversial. The goals of treatment are decompression of the neural elements and stabilization of the spine. Decompression can usually be achieved by realignment of the spinal canal. Postural realignment followed by prolonged recumbency has been favored by European spinal cord injury centers.[135] In the United States, on the other hand, early surgical intervention[148, 175] and spinal instrumentation have been preferred. Although no hard data are yet available comparing the results of nonoperative and operative treatment methods, evidence is accumulating that shows superior results with properly executed operative techniques that achieve decompression and stabilization simultaneously.

Decompression is often achieved by simple realignment using Harrington rod instrumentation, but with specific injuries such realignment may require removal of bony fragments from the spinal canal. Preoperative assessment of the spinal canal compromise can be done by tomography or myelography, and the advent of CT scanning has provided a superb tool to achieve this goal; CT scanning can also be used to evaluate the quality of the decompression postoperatively. Decompression can be carried out through a posterolateral approach or, more commonly, through an anterior approach. In either instance, it needs to be combined with stabilization and bone grafting.

It is now well-established that decompressive laminectomies for spinal trauma are seldom indicated.[147] Neurologic deterioration has been reported after laminectomy. Also, an increased incidence of kyphosis following laminectomy has been reported, along with chronic spinal instability. Laminectomy for trauma offers no advantages and many risks.

There are many questions at the moment that require answers. For example, the correlation be-

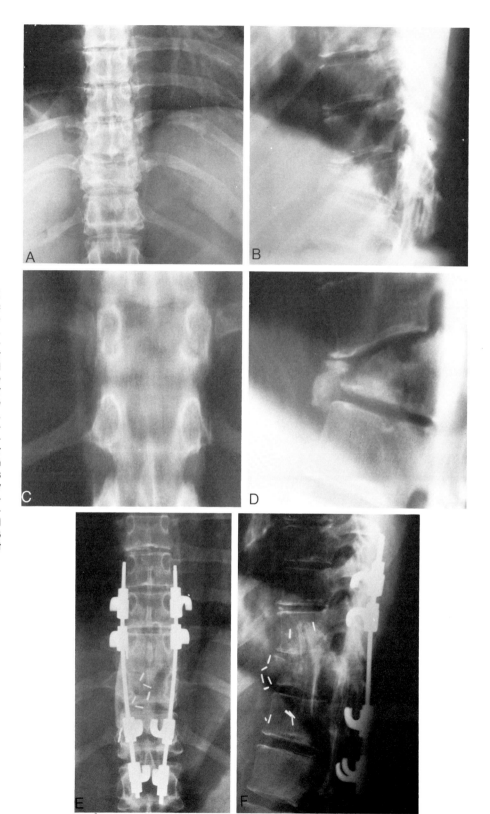

Figure 3–111. AP *(A)* and lateral *(B)* roentgenograms of the thoracic spine of a 33-year-old female involved in a motor vehicle accident. Injury is now 5 months old. The patient is having significant pain but no neurologic deficit. AP *(C)* and lateral *(D)* tomograms of the same patient. Note bilateral pedicular fracture as well as coronal fracture through the vertebral body of T11. Because of significant pain the patient required surgical management. As a first stage, an anterior correction of the kyphosis with anterior interbody fusion was undertaken. This was followed by a second stage of posterior decompression, Harrington rod instrumentation, and fusion. AP *(E)* and lateral *(F)* roentgenograms obtained 3 months after surgery. The patient has minimal symptoms.

tween neural canal compromise as seen on CT scan and its effects on neurologic recovery is not clear. There is emerging evidence, however, that indicates that canal decompression correlates with neurologic recovery. Other questions that need answers concern the type of instrumentation to be utilized, the length of the instrumentation, the length of the bony fusion necessary in healing, and the need for urgent as opposed to delayed surgical intervention. These questions are a focus of current research efforts that may offer answers in the near future.

Management of Specific Injuries

Flexion Injuries

Compression Fractures. Simple compression fractures require little treatment. Usually they are stable injuries, since the posterior elements are intact and there is no neurologic deficit. In the elderly osteoporotic patient the use of a corset or another similar orthosis is advisable.

Severe compression fractures involving more than 50 percent of the vertical dimension of the vertebral body or multiple contiguous compression fractures should be managed in a hyperextension cast or orthosis for a prolonged period of time. If significant kyphosis is present, Harrington distraction instrumentation and a spinal fusion might be the treatment of choice. Neglected injuries of this type can often be very painful and may require combined anterior and posterior procedures for treatment (Fig. 3–111).

Flexion-Distraction Injuries. These injuries occur more commonly in the thoracolumbar junction or in the upper lumbar spine. If the injury has occurred through the bony elements (Chance fracture), management with a hyperextension body cast usually suffices. However, if a fracture-dislocation has occurred that primarily involves the disk and posterior ligamentous complex (Fig. 3–112A and B), open reduction and internal fixation of the level involved combined with bone grafting are necessary (Fig. 3–112C and D).

Flexion-Rotation Injuries. These very unstable lesions occur almost exclusively at the thoracolumbar junction—a transitional area between the fixed thoracic spine and the more mobile lumbar segments (Fig. 3–113A to D). The typical, very unstable slice fracture-dislocation often associated with neurologic deficit requires spinal instrumentation and spinal fusion (Fig. 3–113E and F). Surgery here may not assist neurologic recovery but serves to stabilize the spine and allow early rehabilitation.

The quality of the reduction should be assessed both by conventional radiographs and CT scanning (Fig. 3–113G and H).[159, 179] Recent evidence indicates that the reduction of the spinal canal improves significantly with early surgical intervention.[178]

Bursting Fractures

The result of a vertical compression mechanism, bursting fractures can be stable if no damage to the posterior elements occurs. However, quite often an associated element of rotation produces fractures through the laminae, rendering these injuries unstable (Fig. 3–114). Neurologic compromise occurs frequently, and even in those injuries that do not initially produce neurologic deficits, late neurologic changes have been reported with a frequency of about 20 percent. CT scanning is the technique of choice both to evaluate the initial degree of spinal

Text continued on page 172

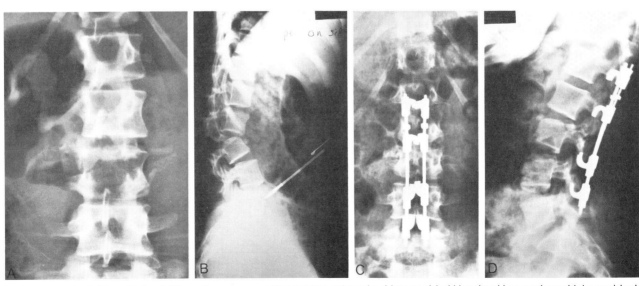

Figure 3–112. AP *(A)* and lateral *(B)* roentgenograms of the lumbar spine of a 14-year-old girl involved in a motor vehicle accident. Note the complete ligamentous disruption both anteriorly and posteriorly with significant separation of the spinous processes and disruption of both columns of the spine. No neurologic deficit. AP *(C)* and lateral *(D)* roentgenograms obtained 1 month after open reduction and internal fixation of the previous lesion, utilizing compression Harrington instrumentation. The patient has remained asymptomatic.

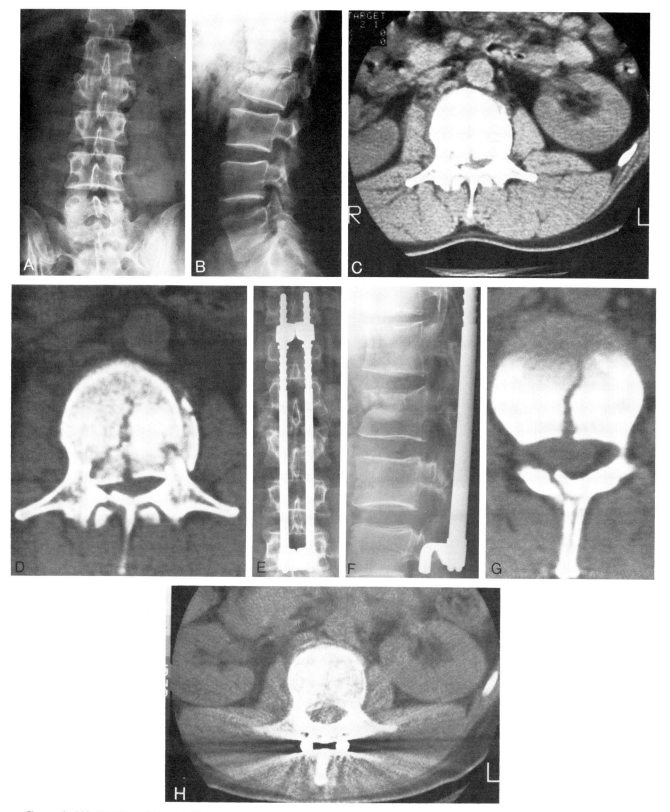

Figure 3–113. AP *(A)* and lateral *(B)* roentgenograms of the lumbar spine of a 38-year-old male with a typical slice fracture-dislocation of L1 on L2. Preoperative CT scans *(C and D)* at the level of the injury on the same patient. Note the significant compromise of the spinal canal. AP *(E)* and lateral *(F)* roentgenograms of the same patient after realignment of the spinal canal and reduction of the fracture-dislocation with Harrington distraction instrumentation. Minimal neurologic deficit present pre-operatively has been eliminated. Postoperative CT scan *(G and H)* confirms the quality of the decompression of the canal.

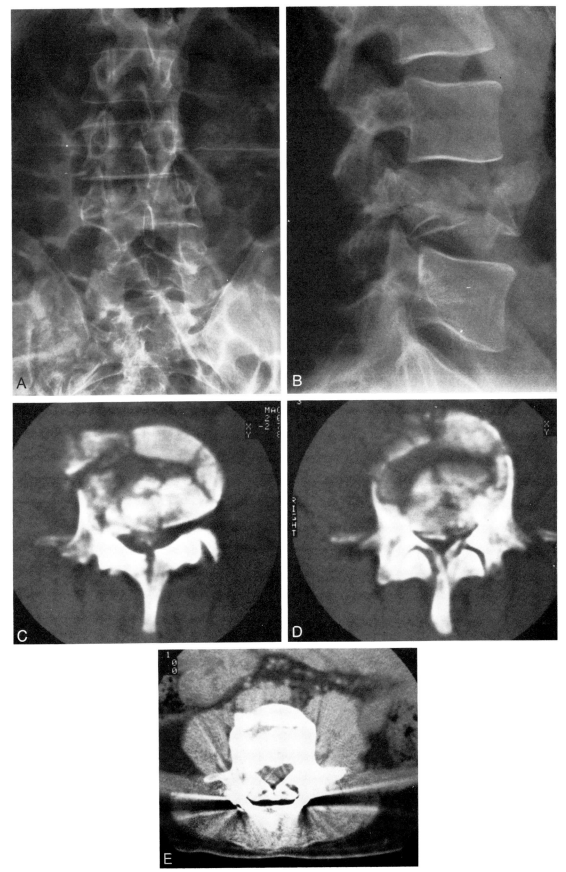

Figure 3–114. See legend on opposite page

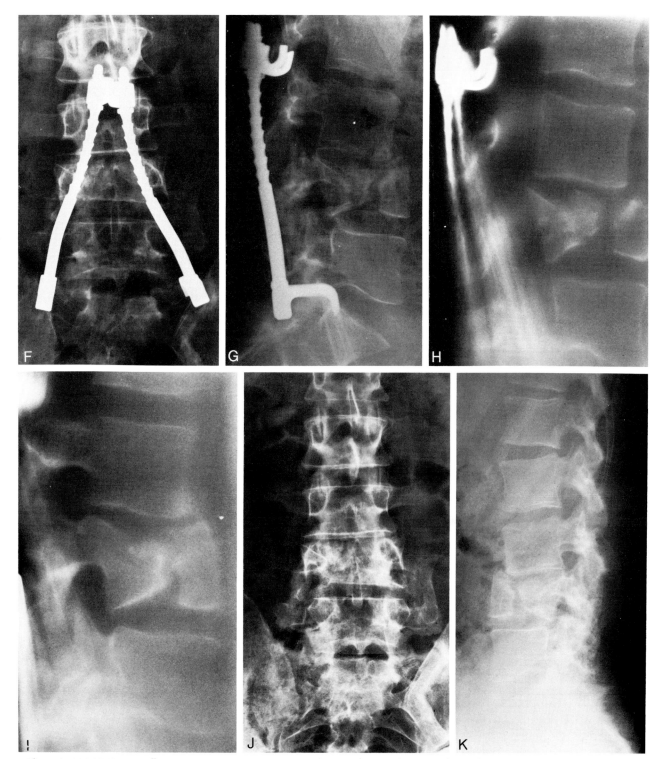

Figure 3–114. AP *(A)* and lateral *(B)* roentgenograms of the lumbar spine of a 40-year-old male who sustained this bursting fracture of L4 in a parachuting accident. The patient has significant cauda equina compression. CT scans *(C* and *D)* of the same patient, confirming both the canal compromise and the fracture through the posterior elements that render this injury unstable. Postoperative CT scan *(E)* obtained 1 year after posterior instrumentation on the same patient. Note the quality of the decompression achieved by treatment of the spinal canal. Roentgenograms of the lumbar spine *(F* and *G)* of the same patient 1 year after distraction Harrington instrumentation achieved realignment of the spine and decompression of the spinal canal. Patient has had a satisfactory clinical recovery. Lateral tomograms *(H* and *I)* of the same patient obtained one year after injury *H,* cut obtained through the right of the vertebral body; *I,* cut obtained through the left of the vertebral body. When comparing these with the CT scan *(E),* one can see that union has not occurred on the right of the vertebral body but is firm on the left. Anteroposterior *(J)* and lateral *(K)* roentgenograms of the same patient obtained 1½ years after injury after removal of the Harrington instrumentation. Note the posterolateral bone grafting that accompanied the decompression.

canal compromise (Fig. 3–114*C* and *D*) and to assess the degree of canal decompression achieved by treatment (Fig. 3–114*E*). Metal artifact can be significant (Fig. 3–114*E*), and in these situations magnetic resonance imaging may be more useful than CT. In our experience artifacts from nonferromagnetic materials occur less often with MRI than with CT.

The treatment of these injuries remains controversial. If no neurologic deficit is present, and if the degree of canal compromise is moderate, conservative treatment with external immobilization (a body cast) is justified.[147] Careful follow-up, however, is essential. For those injuries that have significant canal compromise or are associated with neurologic deficit, surgical decompression is the treatment of choice. Some authors prefer anterior decompression followed by anterior interbody fusion.[180] Others prefer posterior instrumentation utilizing Harrington distraction rods (Fig. 3–114*F* and *G*) followed by postoperative assessment of the decompression achieved and, if necessary, a late anterior decompression and fusion.[147] Regardless, postoperative support with a body cast or a thoracolumbosacral orthosis is necessary until evidence of bony healing is present radiologically.

Shear Injuries

These injuries occur primarily in the thoracic spine and usually result in complete disruption of both anterior and posterior elements. Also, severe neurologic deficit is usually present (Fig. 3–115). In addition, associated injury to the intrathoracic structures (for example, aorta, vena cava, esophagus) is common, and the treatment of the associated injuries can delay treatment of the spine and spinal cord injury.

Because of the stabilizing effect of the rib cage, some of these injuries can be treated conservatively; healing will occur even with rather marked translational deformities (Fig. 3–115*B*). The tendency, however, is to stabilize these injuries with rigid internal fixation by means of Harrington rod instrumentation and sublaminar wires (Fig. 3–116).

The object of treatment in thoracic and lumbar injuries, as in the case of cervical injuries, is to restore the dimensions of the spinal canal in order to achieve neural decompression and to stabilize the spine. It appears evident today that this can be achieved more expeditiously utilizing surgical means. This technique allows the added advantages of a shortened hospital stay and a more prompt and easier rehabilitation.

SPONDYLOLYSIS AND SPONDYLOLISTHESIS

Spondylolysis is a defect in the pars interarticularis. The defect is usually bilateral (74 percent) and occurs in 5 to 7.2 percent of the general popula-

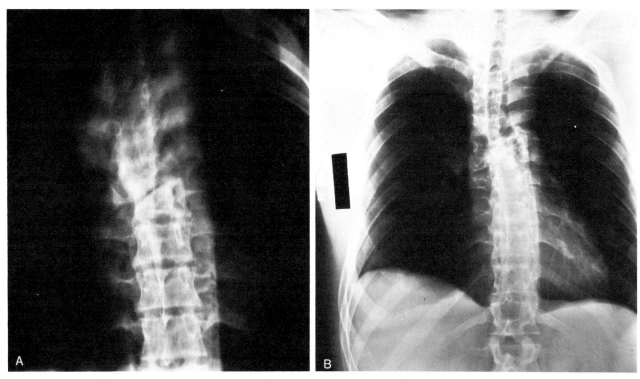

Figure 3–115. A, AP roentgenogram of the thoracic spine of a 22-year-old male involved in a car-train collision. Complete neurologic deficit is present at the level of T9. In addition, there was an associated tear of the thoracic aorta. *B*, Roentgenogram of the thoracic spine of the same patient 3 months after admission. The patient had been treated with recumbency for 6 weeks followed by simple immobilization with a brace. Note complete healing of the injury with significant deformity, which causes no discomfort.

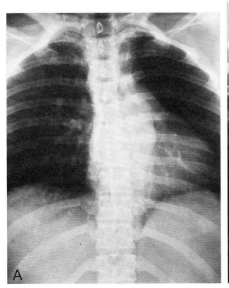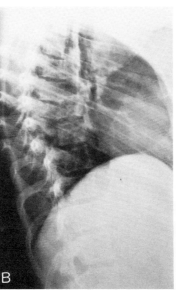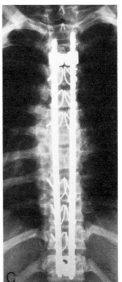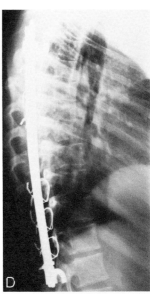

Figure 3–116. (A) and lateral (B) roentgenograms of the thoracic spine of a 27-year-old female involved in an automobile accident. Complete paraplegia at the level of T6 is present. Note complete dislocation of T6 on T7. AP (C) and lateral (D) roentgenograms of the same patient after spinal realignment and stabilization have been achieved with Harrington instrumentation and sublaminar wiring. Note the almost anatomic reduction of the dislocation.

tion.[192, 202] In patients with low back pain the incidence is increased to approximately 10 percent.[192] The incidence of spondylolysis increases with age and is more common in whites than in blacks. There is also a strong familial tendency.[202]

Individuals in certain professions, such as football linemen and weight lifters, also demonstrate an increased incidence of spondylolysis.[182, 192] The defect is most commonly noted at the L5 (67 percent) and L4 (10 percent) levels. Congenital spinous process defects are encountered 5 to 10 times more commonly in patients with spondylolysis.[182]

Spondylolisthesis is anterior slippage or subluxation of the vertebral body. This is most commonly related to spondylolysis but may also be present without a true interruption of the pars interarticularis.

Many theories have been formulated in an attempt to define the etiology of spondylolysis (Table 3–16). The suggestion that this may be congenital has been widely disputed and most clearly discussed by Newman and Stone.[194] Evidence against the congenital theory includes the following: (1) the defect has never been found in a fetus or stillborn,

(2) the incidence increases with age and is rarely noted in infants prior to walking, and (3) the defect occasionally heals.[182, 194] Others have suggested various acquired etiologies (Table 3–15).[193, 196, 198, 199] Most authors agree, however, that the defect is due to a combination of (1) an hereditary defect in the cartilage model of the arch and (2) the strain placed on the lower back due to the upright posture and lumbar lordosis.[182, 200, 202]

Spondylolisthesis may result from causes other than spondylolysis, such as degenerative facet disease, changes in the facet angles, or degenerative disk disease.[185, 195, 200] Table 3–17, based on the work of Wiltse, Newman, and MacNab,[201] summarizes the possible etiologies of spondylolisthesis. Spondylolisthesis of the nonspondylolytic variety usually occurs in patients over 50 years of age and is five times more common in females than in males. The location of the lesion also differs, being more common at the L4–5 level (80 percent). Multiple levels are involved in 5 percent of patients, with the degree of slippage rarely exceeding 30 percent.[182, 199] The incidence of neurologic involvement in degenerative spondylolisthesis is also higher than in

TABLE 3–16. Spondylolysis: Etiologic Theories

Separate ossification centers
Postnatal fractures
Exaggerated lordosis
Weak supporting structures
Dysplasia
Birth fracture
Stress fractures
Articular facet impingement
Pathologic fractures

TABLE 3–17. Spondylolisthesis: Etiology

Upper sacral dysplasia
Degenerative changes
Pathologic fractures
Pars defects
    Acute fractures
    Stress fractures
    Elongated pars
    Posterior arch fracture

spondylolytic spondylolisthesis. Rosenberg noted neurologic complications in 30 percent of patients in this category.[197]

Patients with spondylolysis and spondylolisthesis may be asymptomatic. This is especially common in children, in whom up to 50 percent of cases are noted incidentally.[188] Symptomatic patients usually present with a low back pain that may radiate into the legs or buttock. On physical exam an exaggerated lumbar lordotic curve and occasionally a dimple may be evident, if the changes are advanced.[182]

Radiographic evaluation is usually complete with the AP, lateral, coned-down lateral, and oblique views. Angling the tube 30° to the head on the AP view may also assist in demonstrating the pars defect.[182] Findings on the AP view include sclerosis of the opposite pedicle if the lesion is unilateral,[187] and foreshortening of the spine in cases of advanced spondylolisthesis (Figs. 3–117 and 3–118).[182] The lateral view is usually best for detection of the pars defects, adjacent sclerosis, and the often associated degenerative disk disease (Fig. 3–119). The degree

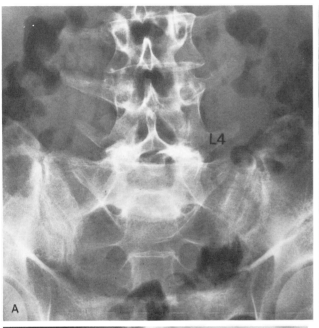

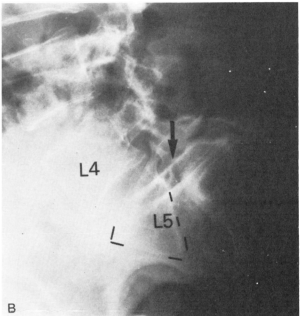

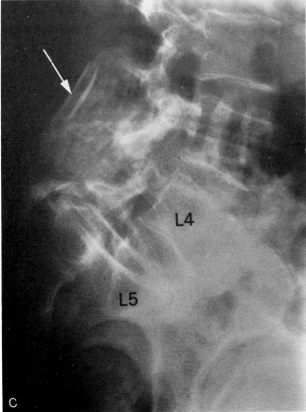

Figure 3–117. Spondylolysis with complete dislocation of L5 on S1. There is foreshortening of the lumbar spine on the AP view *(A)*. Only 4 lumbar vertebrae are seen. The degree of displacement is best seen on the lateral view *(B)*. The patient was treated with bone graft fusion from L3 to the sacrum *(C)*.

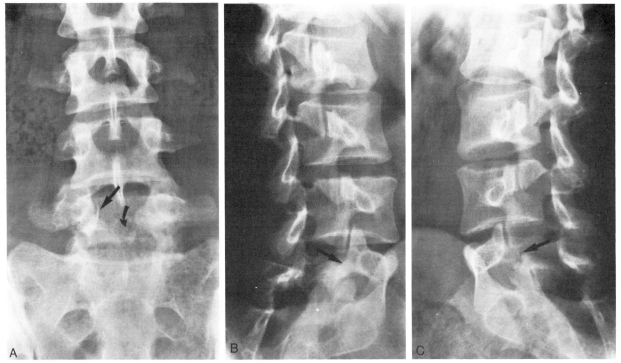

Figure 3–118. Pars defect at L5 on the right. The AP view *(A)* demonstrates spina bifida at L5 with sclerosis of the right pedicle. The left oblique view *(B)* shows sclerosis and elongation of the pars. The right oblique view *(C)* demonstrates that the L5–S1 facet "steps back" owing to a pars defect at L5.

of subluxation is usually graded according to the system established by Meyerding.[191] The vertical body is divided into four equal segments from anterior to posterior, and the degree of slippage is graded I through IV according to these measurements (Fig. 3–120). In nonspondylolytic spondylolisthesis the defect is most commonly at the L4–L5

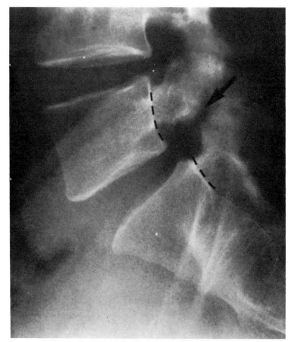

Figure 3–119. Coned lateral view of the lumbar spine demonstrating a pars defect at L5 *(arrow)* with slight subluxation of L5 on S1.

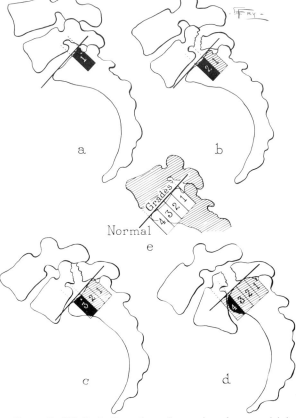

Figure 3–120. Illustration of grading system for spondylolysthesis: a, Grade 1; b, Grade 2; c, Grade 3; d, Grade 4; e, normal. (From Meyerding, H. W.: Spondylolisthesis. Surg. Gyn. Obstet. *54*:371, 1932. By permission of Surgery, Gynecology & Obstetrics.)

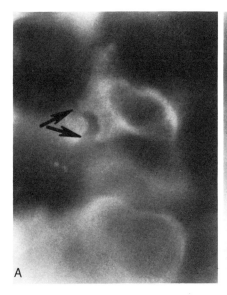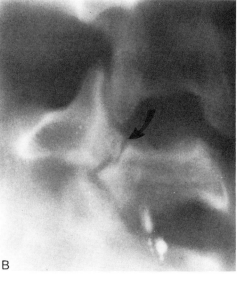

Figure 3–121. Oblique tomograms *(A* and *B)* demonstrating bilateral pars defects at L5.

level, and the degree of associated degenerative change is obvious on the lateral view (Fig. 3–120). The lumbosacral angle is also decreased in these patients compared with patients with spondylolytic spondylolisthesis. In normal patients this angle measures approximately 34°. In patients with non-spondylolytic spondylolisthesis the angle is about 20°, and if spondylolysis is present the angle is increased to about 60°.[182] Oblique views are often confirmatory and increase one's confidence in detecting pars defects (Fig. 3–118). The facet joints are also seen to better advantage.

Tomography is frequently of value in studying spondylolysis and other defects in the posterior arch (Fig. 3–121). Computed tomography may be helpful in selected cases but can also present a confusing picture. Because of their alignment, the facet joints may be confused with a pars defect (Fig. 3–122). A vacuum sign has been described in the facet joints in patients with degenerative spondylolisthesis.[184] Conventional myelography or CT studies with metrizamide may be useful in patients with evidence of neurologic involvement.[182, 192]

Posterior displacement of the vertebral body may also occur (retrolisthesis).[182, 190] This entity is commonly seen with degenerative disk disease.[183] The incidence in the general population is 4.7 percent, which is about the same as that of spondylolysis.[190] There is a tendency for retrolisthesis to occur in the upper lumbar region, especially L2, as well as in the cervical spine. Most of the features are evident on the lateral view and have been well summarized by Melamed (Fig. 3–123).[190] Degenerative disk changes, abnormal lordosis, narrowing of the intervertebral foramina, prominent spinous processes, and facet joint abnormalities are usually present.[190]

Treatment of Spondylolysis and Spondylolisthesis

Most patients with spondylolysis have little or no symptoms and require no or only conservative treatment.

If symptoms are significant and especially if they are associated with neurologic signs of root irritation

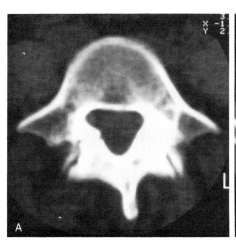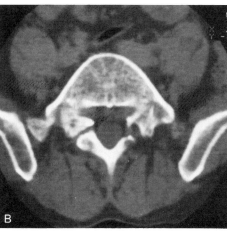

Figure 3–122. CT scans demonstrating degenerative facet disease *(A)* and bilateral pars defects *(B).*

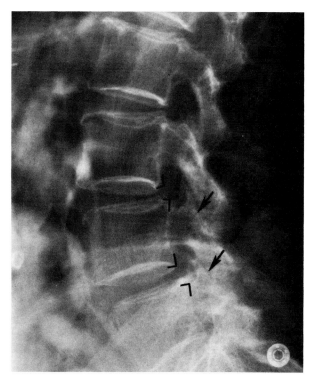

Figure 3–123. Lateral view of the lumbar spine. There are degenerative changes in the facet joints *(arrows)* with subluxation of L4 on L5 and L3 on L4. No pars defects.

or cauda equina claudication, surgical treatment is justified. Spondylolysis of L5 or grades I and II spondylolisthesis can be managed successfully with posterolateral L5–S1 fusion when low back pain is the only presenting complaint, or with removal of the posterior loose element of L5 and posterolateral fusion when leg pain is also a problem; in the latter instance, decompression of the involved root (usually the L5 or S1 root) may require a rather extensive bony removal on the involved side.

Grades III and IV spondylolisthesis require more extensive surgical procedures. Posterior decompression combined with L4–S1 lateral mass fusion is the procedure of choice. Attempts to effect reduction of the spondylolisthesis have by and large been unsuccessful, but in severe spondylolisthesis anterior and posterior procedures may be necessary.

Evaluation of the mechanical success of the fusion procedure requires flexion and extension lateral radiographs of the lower lumbar spine. Right and left side-bending views have also been utilized but are difficult to interpret.

Degenerative spondylolisthesis occurs more commonly, as noted, at the L4–L5 interspace. If associated with symptoms of spinal stenosis, posterior decompression and lateral mass fusion of the L4–L5 space is indicated. If posterior decompression alone is carried out, further spondylolisthesis commonly will be observed. Even when a lateral mass fusion follows the decompression, further forward displacement occurs in the early postoperative period before the fusion becomes solid.

REFERENCES

Anatomy

1. Christensen, P. C.: The radiologic study of the normal spine. Radiol. Clin. North Am. *15*:133, 1977.
2. Chusid, J. G.: Correlative Neuroanatomy and Functional Neurology. Los Altos, CA, Lange Publishers, 1970.
3. Gehweiler, J. A., Osborne, R. L., and Becker, R. F.: The Radiology of Vertebral Trauma. Philadelphia, W. B. Saunders Co., 1980.
4. Gray, H., and Goss, C. M.: Anatomy of the Human Body. Philadelphia, Lea and Febiger, 1966.
5. Hollinshead, W. H.: Anatomy for Surgeons. Vol 3: The Back and the Limbs, 3rd Ed. Philadelphia, Harper and Row Publishers, 1982.
6. Jablecki, C. K., Aguilo, J. J., Piepgras, D. G., et al.: Paraparesis after renal transplantation. Ann. Neurol. *2*:154, 1977.
7. Janes, J. M., and Hooshmand, H.: Severe extension-flexion injuries of the cervical spine. Mayo Clin. Proc. *40*:353, 1965.
8. Lee, B. C. P., Kazam, E., and Newman, A. D.: Computed tomography of the spine and spinal cord. Radiology *128*:95, 1978.
9. Vakili, H.: The Spinal Cord. New York, Intercontinental Medical Book Corp., 1967.
10. Wicke, L.: Atlas of Radiologic Anatomy. 3rd Ed. Baltimore, Urban and Schwarzenberg, 1982.

Radiographic Evaluation of the Spine Following Trauma

11. Abel, M. S., and Teague, J. H.: Unilateral lateral mass compression fractures of the axis. Skeletal Radiol. *4*:92, 1979.
12. Ballinger, P. W.: Merrill's Atlas of Radiographic Positions and Radiologic Procedures. 5th Ed. St. Louis, C. V. Mosby Co., 1982.
13. Bernau, A., and Berquist, T. H.: Orthopedic Positioning in Diagnostic Radiology. Baltimore, Urban and Schwartzenberg, 1983.
14. Brandt-Zawadzki, M., Jeffrey, R. B., Minagi, H., et al.: High resolution CT of thoracolumbar fractures. A. J. R. *138*:699, 1982.
15. Brandt-Zawadzki M., Miller, E. M., and Federle, M. P.: CT in evaluation of spine trauma. A. J. R. *136*:369, 1981.
16. Calcelma, J. J.: Clay shoveler's fracture. A helpful diagnostic sign. A. J. R. *115*:540, 1972.
17. Cheshire, D. J. E.: The stability of the cervical spine following conservative treatment of fractures and fracture-dislocations. Paraplegia *7*:193, 1969.
18. Christensen, P. C.: Radiographic study of the normal spine. Radiol. Clin. North Am. *15*:133, 1977.
19. Fielding, J. W.: Cine radiography of the normal cervical spine. J. Bone Joint Surg. *39A*:1280, 1957.
20. Fielding, J. W., Stillwell, W. T., and Spyropoulus, E. C.: Use of CT for diagnosis of atlanto-axial rotary fixation. J. Bone Joint Surg. *60B*:1102, 1978.
21. Forsyth, H. F.: Extension injuries of the cervical spine. J. Bone Joint Surg. *46A*:1792, 1964.
22. Fuchs, A. W.: Thoracic vertebrae. Radiol. Clin. Photo. *17*:2, 1941.
23. Gehweiler, J. A., Osborne, R. L., and Becker, R. F.: The Radiology of Vertebral Trauma. Philadelphia, W. B. Saunders Co., 1980.
24. Gerlock, A. J., Kirchner, S. G., Heller, R. M., et al.: The Cervical Spine in Trauma. Philadelphia, W. B. Saunders Co., 1978.
25. Harris, J. H.: Acute injuries of the spine. Semin. Roentgenol. *13*:53, 1978.
26. Hokl, M.: Normal motion in the upper portion of the cervical spine. J. Bone Joint Surg. *46A*:1777, 1964.
27. Kaufman, H. H., Harris, J. H., Spencer, J. A., et al.: Danger of traction radiography for cervical trauma. Letter to the editor. JAMA *247*:2369, 1982.
28. Keene, J. S., Goletz, T. H., Lilleas, F., et al.: Diagnosis of vertebral fracture: A comparison of conventional radiography, conventional tomography, and computed-axial tomography. J. Bone Joint Surg. *64A*:586, 1982.

29. Morar, B. C.: Fracture of the axis arch: Hangman's fracture. Clin. Orthop. *106*:155, 1975.
30. Miller, M. D., Gehweiler, J. A., Martinez, S., et al.: Significant new observations in cervical spine trauma. A. J. R. *130*:659, 1978.
31. Naidich, J. B., Naidich, T. P., Garfein, C., et al.: The widened intraspinous distance. A useful sign of anterior cervical dislocation in the supine frontal projection. Radiology *123*:113, 1977.
32. Raub, L. W., and Drayer, B. P.: Spinal computed tomography: Limitations and applications. A. J. R. *133*:267, 1979.
33. Roush, R. D., and Salciccioli, G. G.: Fracture of the anterior tubercle of the atlas. J. Bone Joint Surg. *64A*:626, 1982.
34. Scher, A. T.: Unilateral locked facet in cervical spine injuries. A. J. R. *129*:45, 1977.
35. Scher, A. T.: Anterior cervical subluxation: An unstable position. A. J. R. *133*:275, 1979.
36. Sköld, G.: Sagittal fractures of the cervical spine. Injury *9*:294, 1978.
37. Smith, G. R., Beckly, D. E., and Abel, M. S.: Articular mass fracture: A neglected cause of post-traumatic neck pain? Clin. Radiol. *27*:335, 1976.
38. Tadmor, R., Davis, K. R., Roberson, G. H., et al.: Computed tomography in evaluation of traumatic spinal injuries. Radiology *127*:825, 1978.
39. Vines, F. S.: The significance of "occult" fractures of the cervical spine. A. J. R. *107*:493, 1969.
40. Wales, L. R., Knopp, R., and Streetwieser, D. R.: Acute cervical spine trauma: Efficacy of supine oblique and pillar (vertebral arch) views. Presentation, ARRS meeting. Atlanta, April 1983.
41. Whalen, J. P., and Woodruff, C. L.: The cervical prevertebral fat stripe. A. J. R. *109*:445, 1970.
42. White, A. A.: Biomechanical analysis of clinical stabilization of the cervical spine. Clin. Orthop. *109*:85, 1975.
43. White, R. R., Newberg, A., and Seligson, D.: CT assessment of the traumatized dorsolumbar spine before and after Harrington instrumentation. Clin. Orthop. *146*:150, 1980.
44. Woodring, J. H., and Goldstein, S. J.: Fractures of the articular process of the spine. A. J. R. *139*:341, 1982.

Cervical Spine Trauma

45. Babcock, J. L.: Cervical spine injuries: Diagnosis and classifications. Arch. Surg. *116*:646, 1976.
46. Bedbrook, G. M.: Spinal injury with tetraplegia and paraplegia. J. Bone Joint Surg. *61B*:267, 1979.
47. Bedbrook, G. M.: Stability of spinal fractures and fracture dislocations. Paraplegia *9*:23, 1971.
48. Brackman, R., and Penning, L.: Injuries of the Cervical Spine. Amsterdam, Excerpta Medica, 1970.
49. Bradford, D. S., and Thompson, R. C.: Fractures and dislocations of the spine. Minn. Med., *59*:711, 1976.
50. Cheshire, D. J. E.: The stability of the cervical spine following the conservative treatment of fractures and fracture-dislocations. Paraplegia *7*:193, 1969.
51. Cintron, E., Gilula, L. A., Murphy, W. A., et al.: The widened disk space: A sign of cervical hyperextension injury. Radiology *141*:639, 1981.
52. Dolan, K. D.: Cervical spine injuries below the axis. Radiol. Clin. North Am. *15*:247, 1977.
53. Forsyth, H. F.: Extension injury of the cervical spine. J. Bone Joint Surg. *46A*:1792, 1964.
54. Gehweiler, J. A., Osborne, R. L., and Becker, R. F.: The Radiology of Vertebral Trauma. Philadelphia, W. B. Saunders Co., 1980.
55. Gehweiler, J. A., Clark, W. M., and Schaff, R. E.: Cervical spinal trauma: The common combined conditions. Radiology *30*:77, 1979.
56. Gerlock, A. J., Kirchner, S. G., Heller, R. M., et al.: The Cervical Spine in Trauma. Philadelphia, W. B. Saunders Co., 1978.
57. Harris, J. H.: Acute injuries of the spine. Semin. Roentgenol. *13*:53, 1978.
58. Holdsworth, F.: Fractures, dislocations and fracture-dislocations of the spine. J. Bone Joint Surg. *52A*:1534, 1970.
59. Jacobs, B.: Cervical fractures and dislocations (C3–C7). Clin. Orthop. *109*:18, 1975.

60. Marar, B. C.: Hyperextension injuries of the cervical spine. J. Bone Joint Surg. *56A*:1655, 1974.
61. Scher, A. T.: Unilateral locked facet on cervical spine injuries. A. J. R. *129*:45, 1977.
62. Scher, A. T.: Anterior cervical subluxation: An unstable position. A. J. R. *133*:275, 1979.
63. Selecki, B. R., and Williams, H. B. L.: Injury to the cervical spine and cord in man. Aust Med Assoc., 1970.
64. Webb, J. K., Broughton, R. B. K., McSweeney, T., et al.: Flexion injury of the cervical spine. J. Bone Joint Surg. *58B*:322, 1976.
65. Whalen, J. D., and Woodruff, C. L.: The cervical prevertebral fat stripe. A. J. R. *109*:445, 1970.
66. White, A. A.: Biomechanical analysis of clinical stabilization of the cervical spine. Clin. Orthop. *109*:85, 1975.
67. Whitley, J. E., and Forsyth, H. F.: The classification of cervical spine injuries. A. J. R. *83*:633, 1960.

Cervical Spine Fractures and Fracture-Dislocations

68. Abel, M. S.: Unilateral mass compression fracture of the axis. Skeletal Radiol. *4*:92, 1979.
69. Alker, J. J., Young, O. S., and Leslie, E. V.: High cervical spine and cranio-cervical junction injuries in fatal traffic accidents: A radiologic study. Orthop. Clin. North Am. *9*:1003, 1978.
70. Anderson, L. D., and D'Alonzo, R. T.: Fractures of the odontoid process of the axis. J. Bone Joint Surg. *56A*:1663, 1978.
71. Arndt, R. D.: Cervical transverse process fractures: Further observations of the seat belt syndrome. J. Trauma *15*:600, 1975.
72. Beatson, R. T.: Fractures and dislocations of the cervical spine. J. Bone Joint Surg. *45B*:21, 1963.
73. Bolender, N., Cromwell, L. D., and Wendling, L.: Fracture of the occipital condyle. A. J. R. *131*:729, 1978.
74. Brackman, R., and Penning, L.: Injury of the Cervical Spine. London, Excerpta Medica, 1970.
75. Calenoff, L., Chessare, J. W., Rogers, L. F., et al.: Multiple level spinal injuries: Importance of early recognition. A. J. R. *130*:665, 1978.
76. Canalmo, J. J.: Clay shoveler's fracture. A. J. R. *115*:540, 1972.
77. Cheshire, D. J. E.: The stability of the cervical spine following the conservative treatment of fractures and fracture-dislocations. Paraplegia *7*:193, 1969.
78. Clyburn, R. A., Lionberger, D. R., and Tullos, H. S.: Bilateral fracture of the transverse process of the atlas. J. Bone Joint Surg. *64A*:948, 1982.
79. Coin, C. G., Pennink, M., Ahmad, W. D., et al.: Diving type injury to the cervical spine. Contribution of CT to management. J. Comput. Assist. Tomogr. *3*:362, 1979.
80. Daffner, R. H.: Pseudo-fracture of the dens: Mach bands. A. J. R. *128*:607, 1977.
81. Day, G. L., Jacoby, C. G., and Dolan, K. D.: Basilar invagination resulting from untreated Jefferson fracture. A. J. R. *133*:529, 1979.
82. Dolan, K. D.: Cervical spine injuries below the axis. Radiol. Clin. North Am. *15*:247, 1977.
83. Effendi, B., Roy, D., and Cornish, B., et al.: Fractures of the ring of the axis. J. Bone Joint Surg. *63B*:319, 1981.
84. Eismont, F. J., and Bohlman, H. H.: Posterior atlanto-occipital dislocation with fracture of the atlas and odontoid process. J. Bone Joint Surg. *60A*:397, 1978.
85. Elliot, J. M., Rogers, L. F., Wissinger, J. P., et al.: The hangman's fracture. Radiology *104*:303, 1972.
86. Evans, D. K.: Anterior cervical subluxation. J. Bone Joint Surg. *58B*:318, 1976.
87. Fielding, J. W., Cochran, G. V., Lawsing, J. F., III, et al.: Tears of the transverse ligaments of the atlas. J. Bone Joint Surg. *56A*:1683, 1974.
88. Fielding, J. W., and Hawkins, R. J.: Atlanto-axial rotary fixation. J. Bone Joint Surg. *59A*:37, 1977.
89. Francis, W. R., and Fielding, J. W.: Traumatic spondylolysis of axis. Orthop. Clin. North Am. *9*:1011, 1978.
90. Francis, W. R., Fielding, J. W., Hawkins, R. J., et al.: Traumatic spondylolisthesis of the axis. J. Bone Joint Surg. *63B*:313, 1981.

91. Friedman, R. S.: Vertical fractures of the cervical vertebral bodies. Radiology 62:536, 1954.
92. Gassman, J., and Selingson, D.: The anterior cervical plate. Spine 8:700, 1983.
93. Gehweiler, J. H., Duff, D. E., Martinez, S., et al.: Fractures of the atlanto-vertebra. Skeletal Radiol. 1:97, 1976.
94. Gehweiler, J. H., Osborne, R. L., and Becker, R. F.: The Radiology of Vertebral Trauma. Philadelphia, W. B. Saunders Co., 1980.
95. Gerlock, A. J., Kirchner, S. G., Heller, R. M., et al.: The Cervical Spine in Trauma. Philadelphia, W. B. Saunders Co., 1978.
96. Hanj, S. Y., Witten, D. M., and Musselman, J. P.: Jefferson fracture of the atlas. J. Neurosurg. 44:368, 1976.
97. Harris, J. H.: Acute injury of the spine. Semin. Roentgenol. 13:11, 1978.
98. Jackson, R. H.: Single uncomplicated rotary dislocations of the atlas. Surg. Gynecol. Obstet. 45:126, 1927.
99. Jefferson, G.: Fracture of the atlas vertebra. J. Bone Joint Surg. 7B:407, 1920.
100. Kattan, K. R.: Two features of the atlas vertebra simulating fracture by tomography. A. J. R. 132:963, 1979.
101. Kershner, M. S., Goodman, C. A., and Perlmutler, G. S.: CT in diagnosis of an atlas fracture. A. J. R. 128:688, 1977.
102. Kessler, L. A.: Delayed traumatic dislocation of the cervical spine. JAMA 224:124, 1973.
103. Koss, J. C., and Dalinka, M. A.: Atlanto-axial subluxation in Beçhet's syndrome. A. J. R. 134:392, 1980.
104. Lee, C., Kim, K. S., and Rogers, L. F.: Triangular cervical vertebral body fractures. Diagnostic significance. A. J. R. 138:1123, 1982.
105. Marar, B. C.: Fracture of the axis arch. Clin. Orthop. 106:155, 1975.
106. McCoy, S. H., and Johnson, K. A.: Sagittal fractures of the cervical spine. J. Trauma 16:310, 1976.
107. McSweeney, T.: Fractures, fracture-dislocations, and dislocations of the cervical spine. In Jeffreys, T. E., et al.: Disorders of the Cervical Spine. London, Butterworths, 1980, pp. 48–80.
108. Powers, B., Miller, M. D., Kramer, R. S., et al.: Traumatic anterior atlanto-occipital dislocation. J. Neurosurg. 4:12, 1979.
109. Roush, R. D., and Salciccioli, G. G.: Fracture of the anterior tubercle of the atlas. J. Bone Joint Surg. 64A:626, 1982.
110. Roaf, R.: A study of the mechanics of spinal injuries. J. Bone Joint Surg. 42B:810, 1960.
111. Roberts, A., and Wickstrom, J.: Prognosis of odontoid fractures. Acta Orthop. Scand. 44:21, 1973.
112. Schatzker, J., Rorabeck, C. H., and Waddell, J. P.: Fracture of the dens (odontoid process). J. Bone Joint Surg. 53B:392, 1971.
113. Scher, A. T.: Unilateral locked facet in cervical spine injuries. A. J. R., 129:45, 1977.
114. Scher, A. T.: Double fractures of the spine: An indication for routine radiographic examination of the entire spine after injury. S. Afr. Med. J. 53:411, 1978.
115. Scher, A. T.: Anterior cervical subluxation: An unstable position. A. J. R. 133:275, 1979.
116. Scher, A. T.: Cervical lamina fractures. Radiological identification. S. Afr. Med. J. 58:76, 1981.
117. Schneider, R. C., and Kahn, E. A.: Chronic neurologic sequelae of acute trauma to the spine and spinal cord: The sign of acute flexion or tear drop fracture dislocation of the cervical spine. J. Bone Joint Surg. 38A:985, 1956.
118. Sherk, H. H.: Lesions of the atlas and axis. Clin. Orthop. 109:33, 1975.
119. Sherk, H. H., and Nicholson, J. T.: Fracture of the atlas. J. Bone Joint Surg. 52A:1017, 1970.
120. Sköld, G.: Sagittal fractures of the cervical spine. Injury 9:294, 1978.
121. Smith, G. R., Beckly D. E., and Abel, M. S.: Articular mass fracture: A neglected cause of post-traumatic neck pain? Clin. Radiol. 27:335, 1976.
122. Southwick, W. O.: Management of fractures of the dens. J. Bone Joint Surg. 62A:482, 1980.
123. Spence, K. F., Decker, S., and Sell, K. W.: Bursting atlantal

fracture associated with rupture of the transverse ligament. J. Bone Joint Surg. 52A:543, 1970.
124. Stauffer, E. S.: Cervical spine trauma. In Orthopaedic Knowledge Update I. Home Study Syllabus. Chicago, American Academy of Orthopaedic Surgeons, 1984, pp. 199–208.
125. Taylor, T. K., Nade, S., and Bannister, J. H.: Seat belt fractures of the cervical spine. J. Bone Joint Surg. 58B:328, 1976.
126. Vines, F. S.: The significance of "occult" fractures of the cervical spine. A. J. R. 107:493, 1969.
127. Webb, J. K., Broughton, B. K., McSweeney, T., et al.: Hidden flexion injury of the cervical spine. J. Bone Joint Surg. 58B:322, 1976.
128. White, A. A., Southwick, W. O., and Panjabi, M. M.: Clinical stability in the lower cervical spine. A review of past and present concepts. Spine 1:15, 1976.
129. Wood-Jones, F.: The ideal lesion produced by judicial hanging. Lancet 1:53, 1913.
130. Woodring, J. H., and Goldstein, S. J.: Fractures of the articular process of the spine. A. J. R. 139:341, 1982.
131. Woodring, J. H., Selke, A. C., and Duff, D. E.: Traumatic atlanto-occipital dislocation with survival. A. J. R. 137:21, 1981.
132. Yates, A.: Odontoid fracture. Semin. Roentgenol. 173:233, 1977.
133. Zilch, H.: Traumatische atlantooccipital Verrenkung. Chirurg. 48:417, 1977.

Thoracic and Lumbar Spine Trauma

134. Bailey, W.: Anomalies of fracture of the vertebral articular process. JAMA 108:266, 1973.
135. Bedbrook, G. M.: Fracture dislocations of the spine with and without paralysis. The case for conservatism and against operative techniques. In Leach, R. E., et al. (eds.): Controversies in Orthopedic Surgery, pp. 423–445. Philadelphia, W. B. Saunders Co., 1982.
136. Bowerman, J. W., and McDonnell, E. J.: Radiology of athletic injuries: Football. Radiology 117:33, 1985.
137. Bradford, D. S., and Thompson, R. C.: Fractures and dislocations of the spine. Indications for surgical intervention. Minn. Med., p. 711, Oct. 1976.
138. Brandt-Zawadzki, M., Jeffrey, R. B., Minagi, H., et al.: High resolution CT of thoracolumbar fractures. A. J. R. 138:699, 1982.
139. Burke, D. C.: Hyperextension injuries of the spine. J. Bone Joint Surg. 53B:3, 1971.
140. Burke, D. C.: Spinal cord injuries and seat belts. Med. J. Aust. 2:801, 1973.
141. Calenoff, L., Chessare, J. W., Rogers, L. F., et al.: Multiple level spinal injuries. Importance of early recognition. A. J. R. 130:665, 1978.
142. Chance, G. Q.: Note on a type of flexion fracture of the spine. Brit. J. Radiol. 21:452, 1948.
143. Day, B., and Kokan, P.: Compression fractures of the thoracic and lumbar spine from compressor injuries. Clin. Orthop. 124:173, 1977.
144. De Oliveira, J. C.: A new type of fracture-dislocation of the thoraco-lumbar spine. J. Bone Joint Surg. 60:481, 1978.
145. Dehner, J. R.: Seat belt injuries of spine and abdomen. A. J. R. 111:833, 1971.
146. Denis, F.: The three column spine and its significance in classification of acute thoracolumbar spinal injuries. Spine 8:817, 1983.
147. Denis, F.: Thoracolumbar spine trauma. In Orthopedic Knowledge Update I: Home Study Syllabus. Chicago, American Academy of Orthopaedic Surgeons, 1984, pp. 227–236.
148. Flesh, J. R., Leider, L. L., Erickson, D. L., et al.: Harrington instrumentation and spine fusion for unstable fractures and fracture dislocations of the thoracic and lumbar spine. J. Bone Joint Surg. 59A:143, 1977.
149. Frederickson, B. E., Yaun, H. A., and Miller, H.: Burst fracture of the 5th lumbar vertebra. J. Bone Joint Surg. 64A:1088, 1982.

150. Garrett, J. W., and Braunstein, D. W.: Seat belt syndrome. J. Trauma 2:220, 1962.
151. Gehweiler, J. A., Osborne, R. L., and Becker, R. F.: The Radiology of Vertebral Trauma. Philadelphia, W. B. Saunders Co., 1980.
152. Gertzbein, S. D., and Offierski, C.: Complete fracture-dislocation of the thoracic spine without spinal cord injury. J. Bone Joint Surg. 61A:449, 1979.
153. Ghormley, R. K., and Hoffman, H. O. E.: Fracture of the vertebral process. Proc. Staff Meetings, Mayo Clinic 17:17, 1962.
154. Golimbu, C., Firooznia, H., Rafii, M., et al.: Computed tomography of thoracic and lumbar spine fractures that have been treated with Harrington instrumentation. Radiology 151:731, 1984.
155. Griffin, J. B., and Sutherland, G. H.: Traumatic posterior fracture-dislocation of the lumbosacral joint. J. Trauma 20:426, 1980.
156. Holdsworth, F.: Fracture and fracture-dislocations of the spine. J. Bone Joint Surg. 52A:1534, 1970.
157. Hubbard, D. D.: Fractures of the dorsal and lumbar spine. Orthop. Clin. North Am. 7:605, 1976.
158. Jacobs, R. R.: Bilateral fractures of pedicles through the 4th and 5th lumbar vertebrae with anterior displacement of the vertebral bodies. J. Bone Joint Surg. 59A:409, 1977.
159. Keene, J. S., Goletz, T. H., Lilleas, F., et al.: Diagnosis of vertebral fractures: A comparison of conventional radiography, conventional tomography, and computerized axial tomography. J. Bone Joint Surg. 64A:586, 1982.
160. MacLeod, J. H., and Nocholson, D. M.: Seat belt trauma to the abdomen. Can. J. Surg. 12:202, 1969.
161. McAfee, P. C., Yaun, H. A., Frederickson, B. E., et al.: The value of computed tomography on thoracolumbar fractures. J. Bone Joint Surg. 65A:461, 1983.
162. Mitchell, L. C.: Isolated fracture of the articular process of the lumbar vertebra. J. Bone Joint Surg. 15:608, 1933.
163. Morris, B. A.: Unilateral dislocation of a lumbosacral facet. J. Bone Joint surg. 63A:1645, 1981.
164. Murray, R. O., and Colwell, M. R.: Stress fractures of the pars interarticularis. Proc. Roy. Soc. Med. 61:555, 1968.
165. Nicoll, E. A.: Fractures of the dorso-lumbar spine. J. Bone Joint Surg. 31B:376, 1949.
166. Nykamp, P. W., Levy, J. M., Christenson, F., et al.: Computed tomography for bursting fractures of the lumbar spine. J. Bone Joint Surg. 60:1108, 1978.
167. O'Callahan, P. J., Ulrich, C. G., Hansen, A. Y., et al.: CT of facet distraction in flexion injuries of the thoraco-lumbar spine: The "naked" facet. A. J. R. 134:563, 1980.
168. Omar, M. M., and Levinsohn, M. E.: An unusual fracture of the vertebral articular process in a skier. J. Trauma 19:212, 1979.
169. Rennie, W., and Mitchell, N.: Flexion distraction fractures of the thoracolumbar spine. J. Bone Joint Surg. 55A:386, 1973.
170. Roaf, R.: A study of the mechanism of spinal injuries. J. Bone Joint Surg. 42B:810, 1960.
171. Rogers, L. F.: The roentgenographic appearance of transverse or Chance fractures of the spine: The seat belt fracture. A. J. R. 111:844, 1971.
172. Rogers, L. F., Thayer, C., Weinberg, P. E., et al.: Acute injuries of the upper thoracic spine with associated paraplegia. A. J. R. 134:67, 1980.
173. Roub, L. W., and Drayer, B. P.: Spinal computed tomography: Limitations and applications. A. J. R. 133:267, 1979.
174. Smith, E. R., Northrup, C. H., and Loop, J. W.: Jumper's fractures: Pattern of thoracolumbar injuries associated with vertical plunges. Radiology 122:657, 1977.
175. Stauffer, E. S.: Open reduction and internal fixation of unstable thoracolumbar fractures and dislocations. In Leach, R. E., et al. (eds.): Controversies in Orthopaedic Surgery, Philadelphia, W. B. Saunders Co., 1982, pp. 446–454.

176. Tadmor, R., Davis, K. R., Roberson, G. H., et al.: Computed tomography in evaluation of traumatic spinal injuries. Radiology 127:825, 1978.
177. Thoen, D. D., and Huggins, I. G.: Diagnostic subtleties in CT evaluation of the LS spine: Insights in digital imaging, 1:14, 1982.
178. Villem, J., Lindahl, S., Irstam, L., et al.: Unstable thoracolumbar fractures: A study by CT and conventional roentgenology of the reduction effect of Harrington instrumentation. Spine 9:214, 1984.
179. White, R. R., Newberg, A., and Seligson, D.: Computerized tomographic assessment of the traumatized dorsolumbar spine before and after Harrington instrumentation. Clin. Orthop. 146:150, 1980.
180. Whitesides, T. E., and Shah, S. G. A.: On the management of unstable fractures of the thoracolumbar spine. Rationale for anterior decompression and fusion and posterior stabilization. Spine 1:99, 1976.
181. Zoltan, J. D., Gilula, L. A., and Murphy, W. A.: Unilateral facet dislocation between the fifth lumbar and first sacral vertebrae. J. Bone Joint Surg. 61A:767, 1979.

Spondylolysis and Spondylolisthesis

182. Gehweiler, J. A., Osborne, R. L., and Becker, R. F.: The Radiology of Vertebral Trauma. Philadelphia, W. B. Saunders Co., 1980.
183. Gillespie, H. W.: Vertebral retroposition (reversed spondylolisthesis). Brit. J. Radiol. 24:193, 1951.
184. Grogan, J. A., Hemminghytt, S., Williams, A. L., et al.: Spondylolysis studied with computed tomography. Radiology 145:737, 1982.
185. Junghanns, H.: Spondylolisthesis. Beitr. Klin. Chir. 148:554, 1930.
186. Lefbowitz, W. M., and Quencer, R. M.: Vacuum facet phenomenon: A CT sign of degenerative spondylolisthesis. Radiology 144:562, 1982.
187. Maldaque, B. E., and Malghen, J. J.: Unilateral arch hypertrophy with spinous tilt: A sign of arch deficiency. Radiology 121:576, 1976.
188. McKee, B. W., Alexander, W. J., and Dunbar, J. S.: Spondylolysis and spondylolisthesis in children: A review. J. Can. Assoc. Radiol. 22:100, 1971.
189. MacNab, I.: Spondylolisthesis with an intact neural arch—so-called pseudo-spondylolisthesis. J. Bone Joint Surg. 32B:325, 1950.
190. Melamed, A., and Ansfield, D. J.: Posterior displacement of lumbar vertebra. A. J. R. 58:307, 1947.
191. Meyerding, H. W.: Spondylolisthesis as an etiologic factor for backache. JAMA 111:1971, 1938.
192. Moreton, R. D.: Spondylolisthesis. JAMA 195:671, 1966.
193. Nathan, H.: Spondylolysis. Its anatomic mechanism of development. J. Bone Joint Surg. 41A:303, 1959.
194. Newman, P. H., and Stone, K. H.: The etiology of spondylolisthesis. J. Bone Joint Surg. 45B:39, 1963.
195. Newman, P. H.: Spondylolisthesis. Its cause and effect. Ann. R. Coll. Surg. Engl. 16:305, 1955.
196. Roberts, R. A.: Chronic Low Back Ache Due to Lumbar Structural Derangements. London, H. K. Lewis, 1947.
197. Rosenberg, N. J.: Degenerative spondylolisthesis. J. Bone Joint Surg. 57A:467, 1975.
198. Rower, G. G., and Roche, M. B.: The etiology of separate neural arch. J. Bone Joint Surg. 35A:602, 1953.
199. Sullivan, C. R., and Bickel, W. H.: The problem of traumatic spondylolysis. A report of 3 cases. Am. J. Surg. 100:698, 1960.
200. Taillard, W. F.: Etiology of spondylolisthesis. Clin. Orthop. 117:30, 1976.
201. Wiltse, L. L., Newman, D. H., MacNab, I.: Classification of spondylolysis and spondylolisthesis. Clin. Orthop. 117:23, 1976.
202. Wiltse, L. L.: The etiology of spondylolisthesis. J. Bone Joint Surg. 44A:539, 1962.

4

THE PELVIS AND HIPS

THOMAS H. BERQUIST • MARK B. COVENTRY

ANATOMY

The pelvis is a weight-bearing structure for the trunk and lower extremities and also serves to protect the lower abdominal viscera. The pelvic ring consists of two innominate bones that articulate posteriorly with the sacrum. Anteriorly the pubic portions of the innominate bone articulate at the pubic symphysis. The pelvis is divided by the iliopectineal line into an upper false and a lower true pelvis. The false pelvis is actually a part of the abdomen. The true pelvis contains the organs of reproduction, the lower urinary and digestive tracts, and the vessels and nerves to the lower extremities.[6, 8, 9, 22]

The weight-bearing function of the pelvis is particularly important in orthopedic practice. In the erect position, the weight-bearing forces are directed from the femurs to the acetabula and then to the spinal column via the iliac wings, the sacroiliac joints, and the sacrum, respectively.[9, 22] This forms the major or femorosacral arch. Secondary support is derived from the tie arch formed by the horizontal pubic rami (Fig. 4–1A). In the sitting position, the weight is distributed from the spine to the sacroiliac joints and then through the ilia to the ischial tuberosities, forming the ischiosacral arch. Again, a secondary tie arch is formed by the ischial rami and the inferior pubic rami (Fig. 4–1B). Following trauma the tie arches usually fracture prior to the major arches.[9]

Skeletal Anatomy

The innominate bone is composed of the ilium, ischium, and pubis (Fig. 4–2), which during childhood are separated by the triradiate cartilage. During the second decade these three bones fuse, forming the acetabulum.[9, 22]

The ilium is composed of a wing and body. The wing is large, with three palpable structures that are helpful in clinical evaluation and radiographic positioning. These structures are the anterior superior iliac spine, the iliac crest (which extends from the anterior superior iliac spine to the posterior superior iliac spine), and the posterior superior iliac spine (Fig. 4–3). The iliac wing is covered by muscles medially and laterally. Medially the wing serves as the origin of the iliacus, the quadratus lumborum, the erector spinae, and the transversus abdominis.[6, 9, 22] The gluteal muscles originate from the lateral aspect of the ilium, the sartorius from the anterior superior iliac spine, the rectus femoris from the anterior inferior iliac spine, and the tensor fascia lata from the anterior iliac crest.[6, 9, 22] The posterior superior aspect of the ilium contains a large rough area for attachment of the posterior sacroiliac ligaments (Fig. 4–3). This area is termed the iliac tuberosity. Anterior to the tuberosity is the cartilage-covered surface that articulates with the sacrum, forming the sacroiliac joint. Immediately inferior to the articular surface of the ilium is the greater sciatic notch.

The body of the pubic bone articulates with its mate via the pubic symphysis. The superior pubic ramus extends superolaterally to the acetabulum and forms the upper margin of the obturator foramen. The inferior pubic ramus courses posteriorly and laterally and is contiguous with the ischium. The inferior pubic ramus forms the lower margin of the obturator foramen (Fig. 4–3). The bodies of the pubic bones have small projections anteriorly and superiorly (pubic tubercles), which along with the symphysis are palpable in most patients and are valuable as anatomic landmarks for radiographic positioning. Multiple muscle groups originate from the inferior pubic ramus near the pubic symphysis. These include the muscles of the pelvic floor (deep transversus perinei, levator ani, and sphincter urethrae), the adductor longus, adductor brevis, gracilis, adductor magnus, and obturators internus and externus. The pectineus and rectus abdominis are attached to the superior pubic ramus.[6, 8, 9]

The ischium (Figs. 4–2 and 4–3) consists of a large body that forms the posterior inferior portion of the acetabulum, a tuberosity (directed inferiorly), and a ramus which is contiguous with the inferior pubic ramus. The ischial spine projects posteromedially and forms the lower margin of the greater sciatic notch. The coccygeus and levator ani attach to the ischial spine. The large ischial tuberosity serves as

181

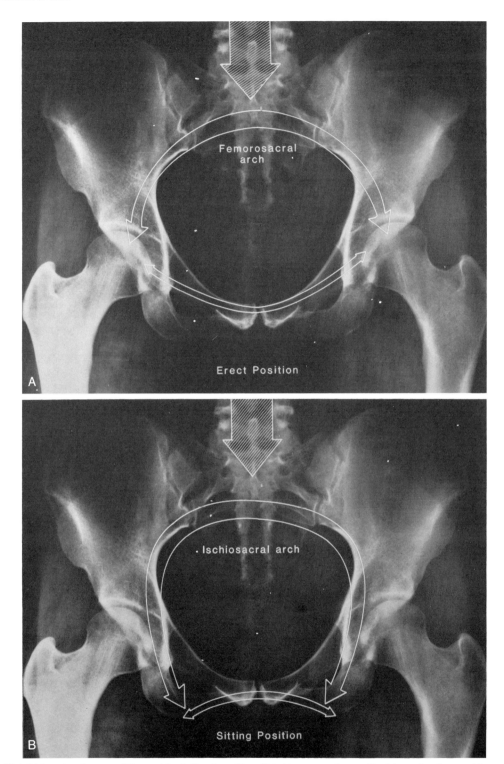

Figure 4–1. Weight-bearing forces of the pelvis. *A,* Erect position: The forces are transmitted from the femoral heads to the spine via the ilia. The secondary arch is formed by the pubic rami. *B,* Sitting position: The forces are directed from the spine to the ischial tuberosities via the sacroiliac joints. A secondary arch is formed by the ischial and inferior pubic rami. (After Kane, W. J.: Fractures of the pelvis. *In:* Rockwood, C. A., and Green, D. P.: Fractures. Philadelphia, J. B. Lippincott Co., 1975.)

the origin of the semimembranosus, semitendinosus, biceps femoris, quadratus femoris, and a portion of the adductor magnus.[5, 6]

The sacrum consists of five fused vertebral segments, which decrease in size inferiorly. The sac-

rum articulates with the coccyx inferiorly and with the ilia laterally. Superiorly the sacrum articulates with the body of L5 via the lumbosacral disk. Posteriorly it articulates with the apophyseal joints of L5. The surface of the sacrum is concave ventrally and convex dorsally. Four pairs of sacral foramina allow passage of the dorsal and ventral rami of the spinal nerves. The large lateral mass of the sacrum is formed by the fused lateral articular processes of the first three sacral segments.

The coccyx consists of four to five rudimentary segments that articulate with the last sacral segment. Four muscles attach to the coccyx. These include a portion of the gluteus maximus, the coccygeus, levator ani, and the sphinctor ani.[11] (See Chapter 3 for more detail on the anatomy of the sacral and coccygeal vertebrae.)

Ligaments and Articulations

The articulations of the pelvis and hips are summarized in Table 4–1. The sacroiliac joint is supported by the strong posterior sacroiliac ligaments (short and long fibers). The anterior sacroiliac ligaments provide much less support and serve as little more than a capsule for the sacroiliac joint. The

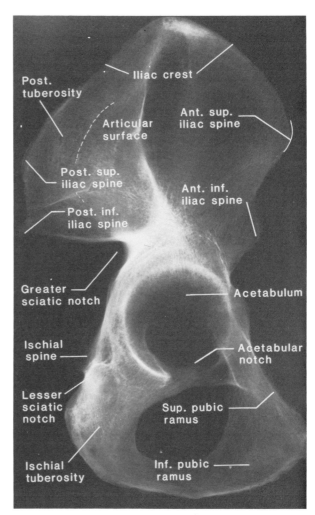

Figure 4–3. Lateral specimen radiograph of the innominate bone with anatomic labels.

sacrotuberous and sacrospinous ligaments connect the lower lateral aspects of the sacrum to the ischial tuberosity and ischial spine, respectively. These ligaments prevent posterior displacement of the sacrum.[2, 4] The articular anatomy and surrounding ligaments combine to produce minimal motion at the sacroiliac joints.[2, 4, 9] The iliolumbar and sacrolumbar ligaments restrict the rotary and ventral motion of the lower lumbar spine (Fig. 4–4).

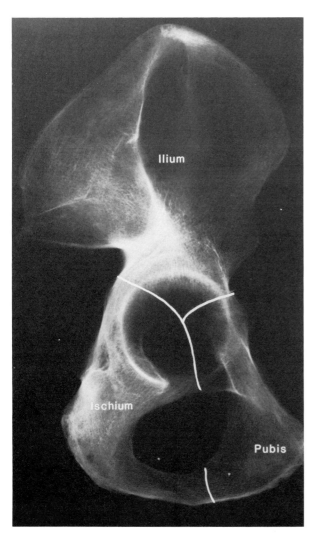

Figure 4–2. Specimen radiograph of the innominate bone demonstrating the three components (ilium, ischium, pubis).

TABLE 4–1. Articulations of Pelvis and Hips

Articulation	Type	Motion
Lumbosacral		
Facet joints	Diarthrodial	Gliding
Disk space	Amphiarthrosis	Minimal
Sacroiliac	Diarthrodial	Gliding minimal
Sacrococcygeal	Amphiarthrosis	Minimal
Pubic Symphysis	Amphiarthrosis	Minimal
Hip	Spheroidea (ball and socket)	Around central axis

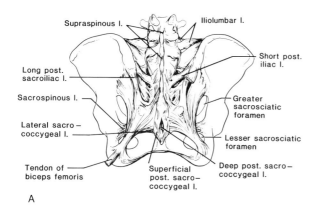

A

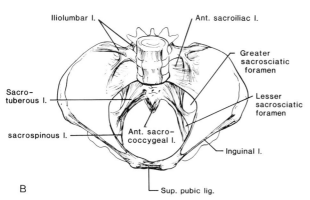

B

Figure 4–4. Posterior ligaments *(A)* and anterior ligaments *(B)* of the pelvis.

The articulation of the pubic bones is separated by a fibrocartilaginous disk that is contiguous with the superior and inferior pubic ligaments. The superior and inferior ligaments blend with the stronger anterior pubic ligament. These ligaments allow only slight motion at the pubic symphysis. Though minimal, such motion at the pubic symphysis and sacroiliac joints allows single undisplaced fractures to occur near these structures. Displaced fractures are usually multiple, as one would expect with the ring configuration of the pelvis.

The femoral head articulates with the acetabulum, forming a spheroidea (ball and socket) joint. The acetabulum is formed by the ischium (45 percent), the ilium (35 percent), and the pubic bone (20 percent) and is directed in an anterior, laterocaudad direction.[20] The bony acetabular rim is incomplete inferiorly (the acetabular notch) and is bridged in this region by the transverse ligament. The transverse ligament is contiguous with the cartilaginous acetabular labrum, which forms a supporting lip around the remainder of the acetabular margin. The synovial-lined capsule is supported by several ligaments as well as by the surrounding muscle groups. The iliofemoral ligament (Fig. 4–5) is shaped like an inverted "Y" and lies anterior to the pubofemoral ligament and just inferior to the rectus femoris.[5–7]

A weak area may be present at the crossing point of these two ligaments. This weak area allows communication between the iliopsoas bursa and the hip joint, and arthrography demonstrates such communication in up to 20 percent of patients.[7] The iliofemoral and ischiofemoral ligaments (Fig. 4–5) are thicker posteriorly and cross inferiorly, creating the zona orbicularis. The fibers of the capsule and capsular ligaments attach 5 to 6 cm beyond the acetabular labrum posteriorly as compared with the perilabral attachment anteriorly. More detailed articular anatomy will be discussed in the section on Hip Arthrography in the Adult later in this chapter.

The periarticular anatomy of the hip is important to the clinician and radiologist (Fig. 4–6). Knowledge of the various muscle groups and their fat planes and recognition of the relationship between the neurovascular anatomy and the hip joint are of great clinical significance. For example, four fat planes have been identified radiographically, and displacement of these fat planes may indicate intra-articular or periarticular disease[7, 12, 15, 16] (Fig. 4–7).

The fat plane of the obturator internus lies medial to this muscle in the bony pelvis. The iliopsoas fat plane is medial and parallel to the iliopsoas muscle as it inserts into the lesser trochanter. The two other fat planes lie lateral to the hip. The more medial of the two was originally thought to be adjacent to the capsule and therefore of great value in detecting joint pathology. However, Guerra[7] demonstrated that the largest portion of this fat plane (the portion demonstrated on the AP radiograph) is between the rectus femoris and the tensor fasciae latae and is, in fact, anterior to the capsule of the hip. It is this portion of the fat plane that is visible on the AP radiograph of the hip. The small juxtacapsular portion of this fat plane, on the other hand, is not visible radiographically. The more lateral of the two fat planes lies between the gluteus medius and gluteus minimus. According to Guerra,[7] the two fat planes nearest the hip (Fig. 4–7) are seen in 75 percent of patients. Our experience indicates that the iliopsoas and pericapsular fat planes are visible in 95 percent of patients, the obturator internus in 79 percent, and the gluteal in 53 percent. Thus significant joint pathology must be present before distortion of the fat planes will be detectable radiographically.

Muscle insertions related to the hip (Fig. 4–6) include the following: (1) The iliopsoas inserts in the lesser trochanter; (2) the gluteus maximus inserts into the tensor fasciae latae over the greater trochanter and into the linea aspera of the upper femur; (3) the gluteus medius, gluteus minimus, and the piriformis insert into the greater trochanter; and (4) the quadratus femoris inserts just below the posterior aspect of the greater trochanter.[5, 6]

Finally, the sciatic nerve courses posterior to the femoral head (Fig. 4–6), and the femoral artery and veins lie just medial and anterior to the femoral head.

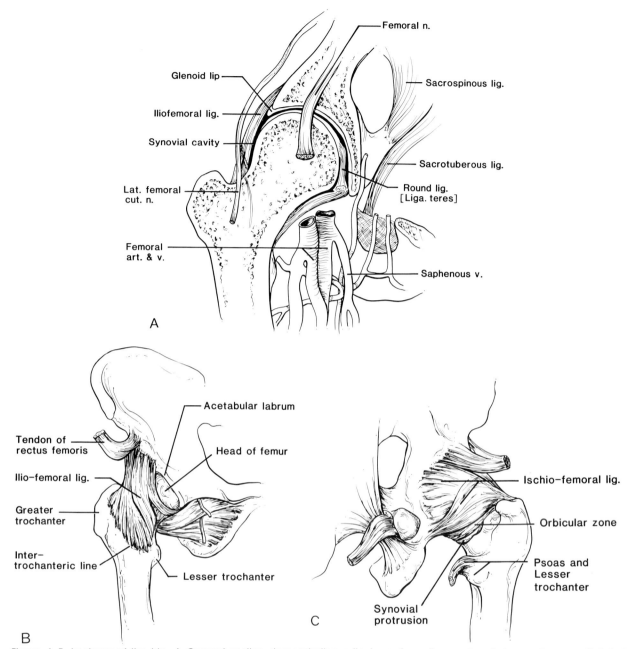

Figure 4–5. Anatomy of the hip. *A,* Coronal section demonstrating articular surface, ligaments, arteries, and nerves. *B,* Anterior ligaments. *C,* Posterior ligaments.

Vascular Anatomy

The rich vascular supply of the pelvis is partly responsible for the fact that the most frequent and most significant complication of pelvic trauma is hemorrhage.[10, 17, 18, 21] The relationship of certain vessels to the bones and joints of the pelvis and hips are particularly important for the angiographer and surgeon.

Typically the abdominal aorta bifurcates at the L4 level, forming the common iliac arteries (Fig. 4–8). The common iliac arteries divide again to form the internal iliac (hypogastric) and external iliac. This division occurs just anterior to the sacroiliac joints.

The external iliac passes inferiorly to the inguinal ligament, forming the common femoral artery. The common femoral then divides once again, forming the superficial and deep femoral (profunda) arteries. The deep femoral provides the major source of blood supply to the hip through the medial and lateral femoral circumflex branches. The femoral head receives a lesser portion of its vascular supply from the branches of the obturator internus. These smaller branch vessels follow the ligamentum teres femoris to the femoral head.

The internal iliac artery supplies the major portion of the pelvis. Knowledge of the anatomic distribution of its branches is important for proper angio-

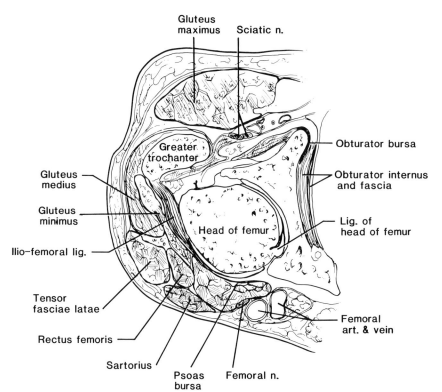

Figure 4–6. Axial illustration of periarticular anatomy of the hip.

graphic diagnosis and treatment of pelvic hemorrhage.[9, 10, 19, 21] The first major branch of the internal iliac is the iliolumbar artery, which follows the wing of the ilium superiorly. The superior gluteal artery runs posteriorly just inferior to the sacroiliac joint. Because of its location and course, it is susceptible to injury with sacroiliac fracture-dislocations.[13] The lateral sacral arteries and their branches are at risk with sacral or sacroiliac trauma.[21] The anterior pelvic branches of the internal iliac are more frequently injured in cases of displaced fractures of the obturator ring. These vessels include the obturator, internal and external pudendals, and the rectal and vesical branches.

The vessels of the pelvis have a rich anastomotic network with vessels from the contralateral hemi-

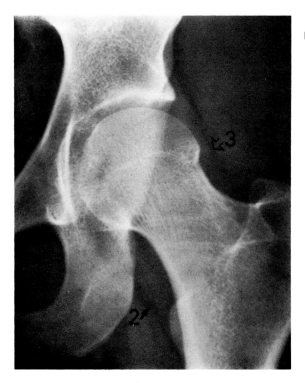

Figure 4–7. Fat planes of the hip. 1, obturator internus; 2, iliopsoas; 3, pericapsular; 4, gluteal.

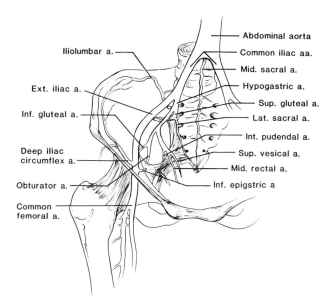

Figure 4–8. Diagram demonstrating the blood supply to the pelvis and hips.

pelvis. Venous hemorrhage may also result in significant blood loss following pelvic trauma.[14]

Neuroanatomy

The nerve supply of the pelvis and hips is derived from the lumbosacral plexus (Fig. 4–9). The lumbosacral plexus in turn is formed by the ventral rami of L1–S2. Portions of the ventral rami of T12 and S3 also contribute to this plexus. Certain neuroanatomic relationships become clinically significant in dealing with trauma to the pelvis and hips. The sacral branches exit through the ventral sacral foramina and may be injured with sacral trauma, as sacral fractures frequently involve these foramina.

The largest branch of the sacral plexus, the sciatic nerve (L4–S3), exits the bony pelvis and passes just posterior to the femoral head (Figs. 4–6 and 4–9). This nerve is thus susceptible to injury in patients with posterior dislocations of the hip. Injury to the branches supplying the genitourinary tract (S2–S4) may result in bladder and bowel incontinence and impotence in males. These aspects will be discussed further in the section dealing with complications of pelvic fractures.

Genitourinary and Gastrointestinal Anatomy

The bladder lies immediately dorsal to the pubic symphysis in both males and females. The perito-

Figure 4–9. Diagram of pelvic neuroanatomy.

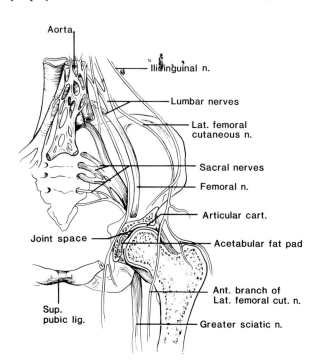

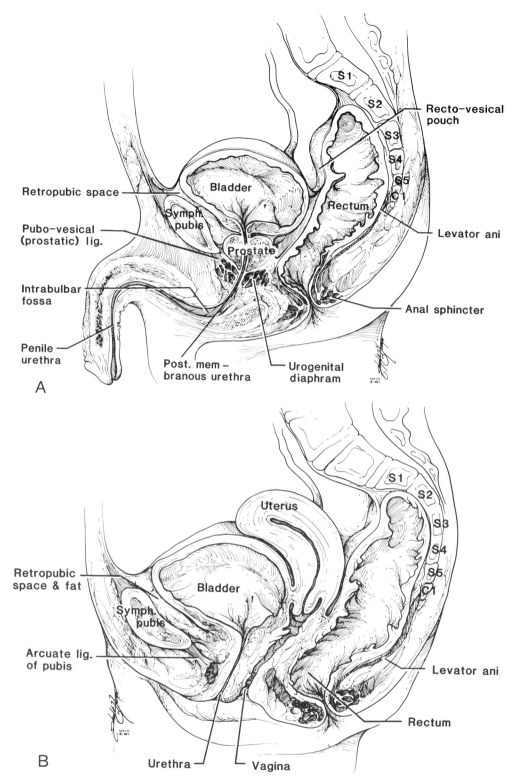

Figure 4–10. Diagrams of the genitourinary tract: *(A)* Sagittal section of the male genitourinary tract. *(B)* Sagittal section of the female genitourinary tract.

neum is reflected over the dome of the bladder and then takes a caudad course, forming the vesicorectal pouch (Fig. 4–10).

In the male (Fig. 4–10A), the urethra passes through the prostate (prostatic urethra). The pros-

tatic urethra is continuous with the membranous urethra just above the urogenital diaphragm. This area has been classically described as the part of the urethra most susceptible to injury.[15] The membranous urethra is the shortest portion of the posterior urethra and lies within the urogenital diaphragm. The anterior portions of the urethra (bulbus and cavernous) lie below the urogenital diaphragm. Both the bladder and the prostate are fixed anteriorly by the pubovesicle and puboprostatic ligaments. The ligamentous attachments of the prostate allow less motion inferiorly (i.e., near the urogenital diaphragm) than superiorly.[3] The urogenital diaphragm is stronger in males than in females and is suspected between the ischial rami to form the anterior floor of the pelvis.

In the female (Fig. 4–10B), the urethra is 3 to 5 cm in length and fixed to the vagina posteriorly and to the urogenital diaphragm inferiorly. The female urethra is not as immobile as the male urethra and is therefore less frequently injured following pelvic trauma.

The rectum and a short segment of the distal sigmoid colon are located in the true pelvis. The rectum occupies the presacral space approximately 1 cm ventral to the sacrum. The sigmoid colon is situated near the psoas muscle. Because of its well developed mesentery, the sigmoid colon is mobile and is rarely injured following pelvic fracture. The rectum has no mesentery and is more rigidly fixed. However, in our experience injury to the rectosigmoid is rare.

ROUTINE RADIOGRAPHY OF THE PELVIS AND HIPS

Newer imaging modalities, especially computed tomography, have greatly influenced the radiographic approach to diagnostic problems of the pelvis and hips. However, routine radiography remains the major technique for initial evaluation. Radiographic assessment of these patients should enable the physician to identify the area of injury and also provide sufficient anatomic information for the institution of proper therapy, at least in the period immediately following the injury. In most cases fulfillment of these goals requires that more than one radiographic projection be obtained. This section will discuss the commonly employed routine radiographic procedures used in evaluation of acute trauma.

Pelvis

AP View

Prior to positioning the patient for any view of the pelvis or hips certain palpable landmarks must be considered. These anatomic landmarks include the (1) anterior superior iliac spine, (2) iliac crest, (3) pubic symphysis, and (4) greater trochanter (Fig. 4–11).[25]

The AP view of the pelvis and hips should be the initial examination in patients with suspected trauma. It provides sufficient information for detection of most pelvic fractures. The findings on the AP view can then be applied to decisions regarding further views. The AP view is obtained with the patient in the supine position on the radiographic table (Fig. 4–12A). The feet should be internally rotated 15°, so that the medial borders of the great

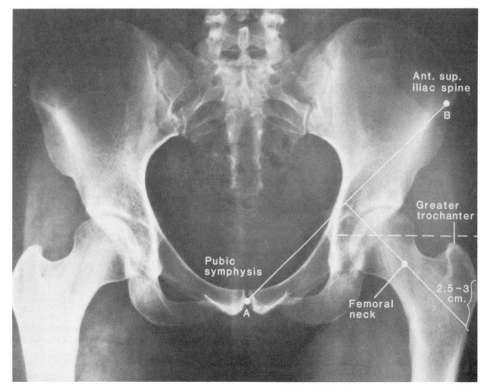

Figure 4–11. AP radiograph of the pelvis. Note the palpable anterior superior iliac spine *(B)*, pubic symphysis *(A)*, and greater trochanter. These landmarks are useful in localizing the femoral head and neck.

Ant. sup. iliac spine

B

Greater trochanter

Pubic symphysis

Femoral neck

2:5 – 3 cm.

A

toes are approximated. In certain cases, such as a hip fracture, this may not be possible for the patient. This positioning is important and should be used when possible, for it overcomes the natural anteversion of the femoral necks and allows visualization of the neck and greater trochanter (Fig. 4–12*B*). Improper positioning of the feet (Fig. 4–12*C*) results in the greater trochanter obscuring the femoral neck and clear demonstration of the lesser trochanter alone. Proper positioning may be facilitated by the use of sand bags.

A 14 × 17 inch cassette (crosswise) is positioned in the Bucky tray with the top of the cassette 1½ inches above the iliac crest (palpable). The central beam is centered on the cassette and aligned perpendicular to the cassette (Fig. 4–12*A*). Gonadal shielding should be used only if it will not obscure possible pathology. Thus it is rarely used in patients with suspected pelvic fractures. Gonadal shields may obscure the sacrum in females and the anterior arch in males.

The AP view of the pelvis and hips provides a

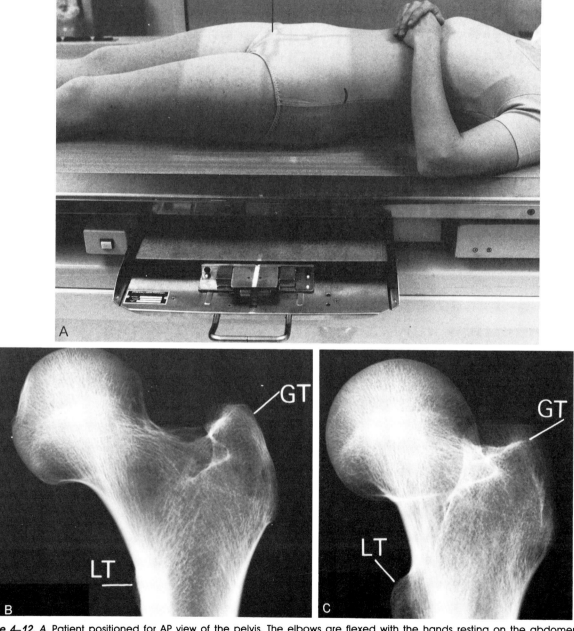

Figure 4–12. A, Patient positioned for AP view of the pelvis. The elbows are flexed with the hands resting on the abdomen. The upper margin of the 14 × 17 cassette is 1 to 1½ inches above the iliac crest *(curved line)* with the beam *(vertical line)* perpendicular to the center of the cassette. *B,* Specimen radiograph with proper amount of internal rotation (15°). Note the position of the greater and lesser trochanters. *C,* Specimen radiograph in external rotation changes the greater and lesser trochanteric appearance and obscures the femoral neck.

illustration continued on opposite page

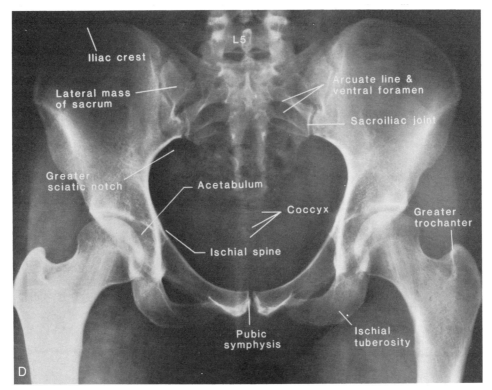

Figure 4–12 Continued. D, Normal AP view of the pelvis with anatomic labels.

significant amount of bone and soft tissue information, and the radiograph should be systematically reviewed. When this view is properly obtained, the entire pelvis, sacrum, and proximal fourth of the femurs are included on the film (Fig. 4–12D). The integrity of the pubic symphysis and obturator rings (formed by the pubic and ischial rami) should be studied, and any displaced anterior fracture should alert the physician to the possibility of a second fracture (usually posterior and near the sacroiliac joint or sacrum). The joint spaces of both

hips can also be assessed. The sacroiliac joints should be compared for symmetry, and the arcuate lines of the sacrum should be carefully compared to exclude subtle fractures of the sacrum. The lower lumbar spine is usually also visible on this view, and any transverse process fracture should alert one to the need for more careful study of the anatomy immediately above and below the fracture.

Soft tissue structures may be extremely helpful in detecting subtle fractures.[35] Slight displacement of the obturator fat plane may be the only clue to

Figure 4–13. AP view of the pelvis. There is an obvious displaced fracture of the left ilium *(open arrows).* The fat planes are all visible (1, gluteal; 2, pericapsular; 3 iliopsoas; 4, obturator internus) on the right. The obturator internus is displaced medially, providing a clue for detection of the central acetabular fracture *(curved arrow).*

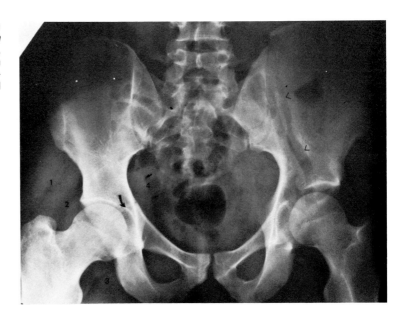

an adjacent fracture (Fig. 4–13). Views of the other fat planes about the hip (iliopsoas, lateral pericapsular, and gluteal fat stripes) may be helpful, but usually a large amount of fluid must be present in the hip joint before these structures are altered on the AP radiograph. The bladder is often visible in the midpelvis near the symphysis,[30] and elevation or deviation of the soft tissue shadow of the bladder may be present with pelvic hematoma or posterior urethral rupture. In complex pelvic fractures large hematomas may obscure the bladder and perivesical fat entirely.

AP Angled Views

Clarification of findings on the AP view of the pelvis may be accomplished with inlet and tangential projections.[25, 40, 45] The inlet projection is obtained with the patient in the supine position (as in the AP projection). The tube is angled 40° toward the feet (Fig. 4–14A). The midpoint of the 14 × 17 cassette should be centered with the central beam. This view assists in evaluation of the internal architecture of the pelvic ring (Fig. 4–14B and C). Displaced fracture fragments are more easily assessed with this view.

The tangential view is taken with the patient supine and the tube angled 25° (males) or 40° (females) toward the head (Fig. 4–15A). The cassette is positioned with its center at the midpoint of the x-ray beam.[40, 43, 45] This view allows better evaluation of the anterior pelvis, ventral foramina, and margins of the sacrum. Superior or inferior displacement of fracture fragments is evident on this view.[45] An additional advantage of the AP angled views is that they are obtained without moving the patient. This is especially important in evaluating the severely injured patient.

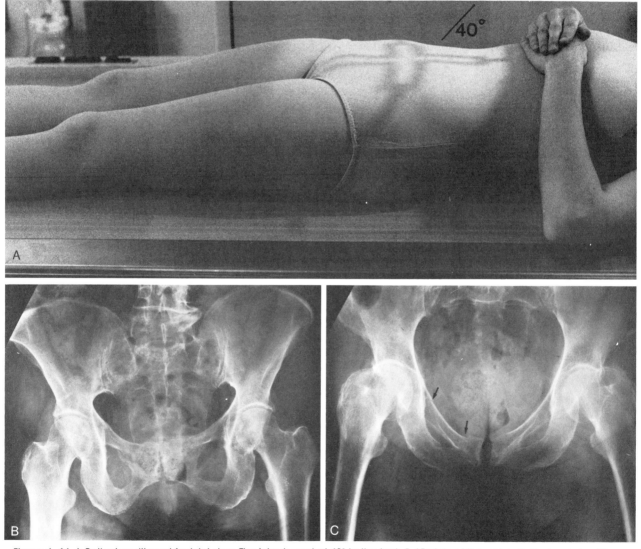

Figure 4–14. A, Patient positioned for inlet view. The tube is angled 40° to the feet. B, AP view of the pelvis. Patient sustained trauma to the pelvis with pain anteriorly. C, Inlet view. There are two minimally displaced fractures of the pubic ramus on the right (arrows). These were not evident on the AP view.

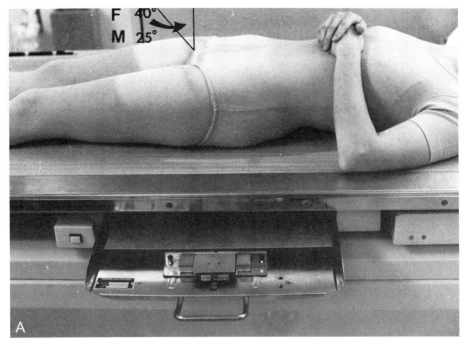

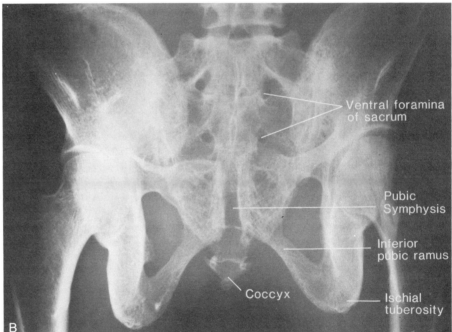

Figure 4–15. A, Patient positioned for tangential view. The tube is angled to the head (25° for males, 40° for females) and centered just below the pubic symphysis. *B,* Note that the radiograph improved visualization of the anterior pelvis.

Lateral View

The inlet and tangential views essentially fulfill the necessary requirement of obtaining two views at 90° angles. However, occasionally a lateral view of the pelvis is necessary for evaluation of the acetabulum or femoral head.[26] This view can be obtained in several ways. The patient can be positioned on his side, though this may not be possible following trauma. In this situation the lateral view can be obtained using the cross-table technique (Fig. 4–16*A*). When possible, a support cushion should be placed under the hip to assure that the posterior structures are included on the film (Fig. 4–16*B*). The central beam is centered just above the greater

trochanter (palpable) and aligned perpendicular to the cassette. The image obtained is demonstrated in Figure 4–15*C*.

An important alternative technique is performed by angling the tube and cassette (Fig. 4–16*D*).[25, 26, 33] This is a modification of the technique described by Johnson.[33] The tube is angled 25° to the table with the patient supine. The beam is centered just above the greater trochanter, with the cassette angled so that it is perpendicular to the beam. This results in an excellent view of the hips and acetabular domes (Fig. 4–16*E*). The patient's condition and the prior results of the AP view dictate which of the above views will be most useful.

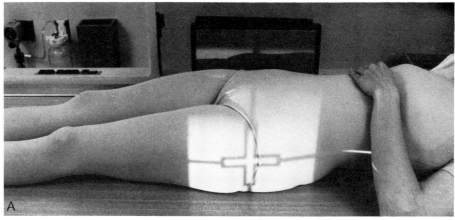

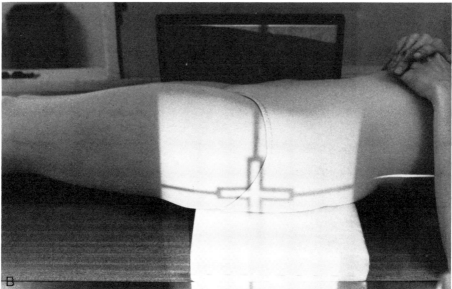

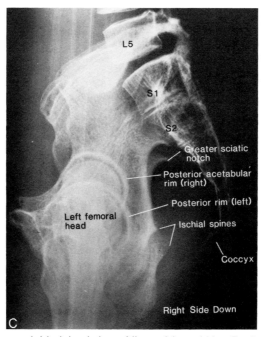

Figure 4-16. A, Patient positioned for cross-table lateral view of the pelvis and hips. The beam is perpendicular to the center of the upright cassette and centered just above the palpable greater trochanter. *B,* Patient positioned for cross-table lateral view with cushion in place to optimize posterior structural detail. Centering is the same as in *A. C,* Lateral view of the pelvis with right side closest to the film. Note the magnification of the left femoral head.

Illustration continued on opposite page

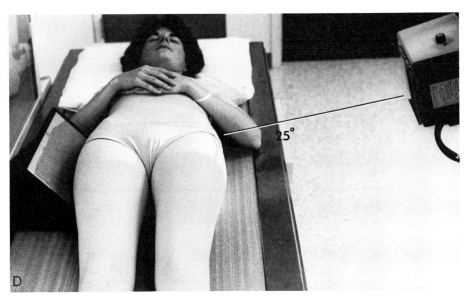

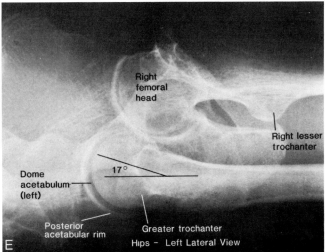

Figure 4–16 *Continued. D,* The patient is supine with the tube angled 25° above the horizontal table. Centering is just above the greater trochanter with the cassette angled perpendicular to the beam. *E,* Both hips are visualized with this technique.

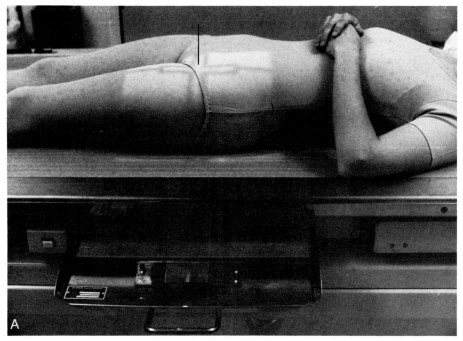

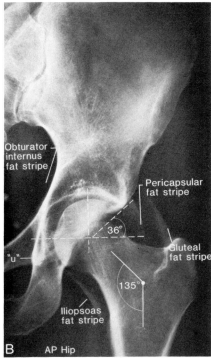

Figure 4–17. *A*, Patient positioned for AP view of the hip. The beam is perpendicular to the 10- × 12-inch cassette and centered 2 inches medial to the anterior superior iliac spine (palpable) and just above the greater trochanter (palpable). *B*, AP view of the hip with radiographic data illustrated. See Table 4–2.

Hip

AP View

The patient is supine on the radiographic table. The sagittal plane of the central beam should be centered 2 inches medial to a line longitudinal to the anterior superior iliac spine (palpable). Trans-

verse centering should be at the level of the greater trochanter (palpable).[25] A 10 × 12 inch cassette is placed in the Bucky tray with the center perpendicular to the central beam (Fig. 4–17A). This view provides better visualization of the hip and surrounding structures than the AP view of the pelvis. Table 4–2 lists the skeletal, soft tissue, and radiographic angles that should be evaluated on the AP view of the hip (Fig. 4–17).[24, 42] A single AP view of the hip is inadequate for complete evaluation. This is especially true if a complete evaluation of the acetabulum and anterior and posterior columns is required.[38, 46] Oblique views of the hip are particularly helpful in this regard. These projections were popularized by Judet.[34]

Judet Views

Judet views are obtained with the involved hip rotated posteriorly 45° toward the film (Fig. 4–18A). This view clearly demonstrates the iliac wing (iliac view). The anterior rim of the acetabulum is projected laterally to the posterior rim. The posterior column is also seen to better advantage. The anterior oblique view is obtained with the involved hip rotated 45° away from the film[34] (Fig. 4–18C). The anterior oblique view clearly demonstrates the posterior rim of the actabulum and the anterior column. The obturator foramen is clearly seen. Therefore, this view is often referred to as the obturator oblique (Fig. 4–18D).

Both views begin with the patient in the supine position. To obtain consistency in positioning, 45° wedges should be placed under the patient's hip and back (Figs. 4–18A and C). The central beam is perpendicular to the cassette and centered on the hip. The oblique views are particularly useful in detecting subtle fractures of the acetabulum (especially the central acetabulum) and pelvic columns (Fig. 4–19).[34, 46]

Lateral View

Evaluation of the upper femur often requires a lateral view to provide a second view at an angle of 90° to the AP view. The commonly used technique for obtaining a lateral view of the hip is demonstrated in Figure 4–20.[28, 39] The patient is

TABLE 4–2. Radiographic Evaluation of the Hip—AP View

Skeletal anatomy
  Iliopubic line
  Ilioischial line
  Radiographic "U"
  Acetabulum
    Posterior rim
    Anterior rim
    Dome
Angles
  CE angle of Wibert (normal 20°–40°, average 36°)
  Neck shaft angle (135° normal, >135° = coxa valga, <135° = coxa vara)
Fat planes
  Obturator internus
  Iliopsoas
  Pericapsular
  Gluteal

supine with the uninvolved hip flexed 90° and the ankle supported to assist in positioning. The foot on the injured side is internally rotated 15° if possible (patients with acute fractures of the femoral neck may be unable to maintain this position). The cassette (10 × 12 inch) is positioned perpendicular both to the table and to the central beam (Fig. 4–20A). The cassette should be aligned perpendicular to a line from the pubic symphysis to the anterior superior iliac spine (palpable). The central beam is centered just below the greater trochanter (palpable). The radiograph demonstrates the hip joint, femoral neck, and trochanters (Fig. 4–20B). An alternative method is to position a curved cassette medial to the involved hip, with the tube lateral to the patient and angled toward the feet.[25, 37]

In severely injured patients these techniques may be impossible. In this situation the Johnson method[33] is often very helpful. The cassette (10 × 12) is placed next to the hip to be examined, forming a 65° angle with the radiographic table. Angling the tube 25° to the table and perpendicular to the cassette results in a lateral view of both hips (similar to Fig. 4–16D). If the tube is also angled toward the head 25°, only the hip next to the film is obtained. An alternative to these methods is to position the patient at an oblique angle of 20° to 25° oblique to the table, with the cassette perpendicular to the table and the tube perpendicular to the film (Fig. 4–16). The resulting radiograph is similar to that produced by the other techniques. The hip closest to the film will be less magnified, and the radiographic detail will be sharper.

Oblique View

The patient is positioned with the affected side of the hip toward the 10 × 12 inch cassette. The opposite hip is supported by a cushion wedge (Fig. 4–21A). The knee should be flexed and the thigh raised about 45°. The beam is centered between the symphysis and anterior superior iliac spine (Figs. 4–11 and 4–21A).[25, 36] This view allows improved visualization of the femoral neck, acetabulum, and lesser trochanter. It is also often helpful in detecting subtle femoral neck fractures (Fig. 4–21B and C).

Other Radiographic Techniques

There are many other techniques available for study of the pelvis and hips.[25, 27, 29, 31, 32, 36, 41, 44] In addition to routine radiography, tomography, radionuclide scans, and computed tomography are often of value in complete evaluation of trauma to the pelvis and hips. The applications of these techniques will be discussed later in this chapter as they apply to the evaluation of specific problems.

Text continued on page 202

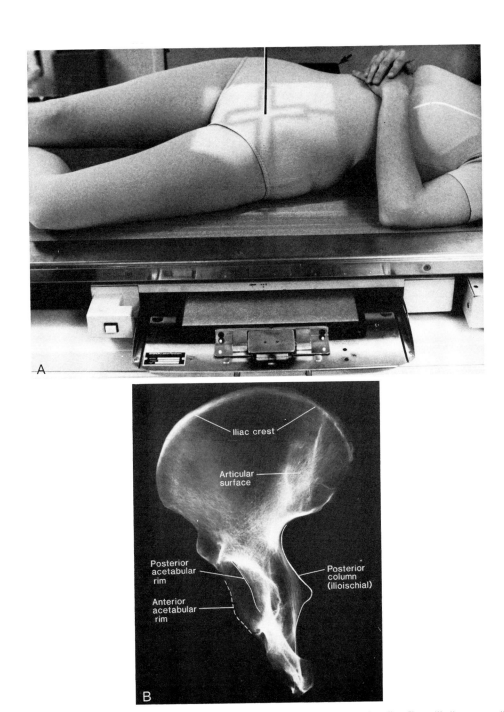

Figure 4–18. *A,* Patient positioned for posterior oblique view. The involved hip is closest to the film with the opposite hip elevated 45°. To gain this elevation, a 45° wedge is placed under the hip *(arrow)*. *B,* Specimen radiograph of the innominate bone demonstrating the anatomy depicted with the posterior oblique view (labeled).

Illustration continued on opposite page

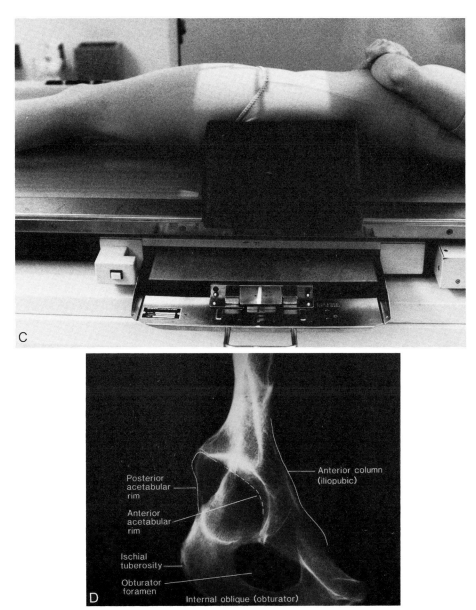

Figure 4-18 Continued. C, Patient positioned for anterior oblique views. The involved hip is rotated 45° away from the film. *D*, Specimen radiograph of anterior oblique view. Note that the anterior column is clearly demonstrated. The posterior acetabular rim is projected laterally free of overlying structures. The obturator foramen is clearly seen.

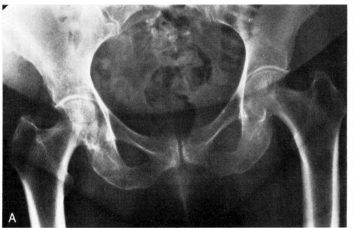

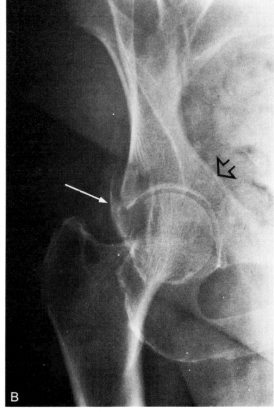

Figure 4–19. A, AP view of the pelvis in a patient with right hip pain following trauma. No definite fracture is visible. B, Anterior oblique view clearly demonstrating the posterior acetabular rim fracture *(arrow)*. The central acetabular region and anterior column are intact *(open arrow)*.

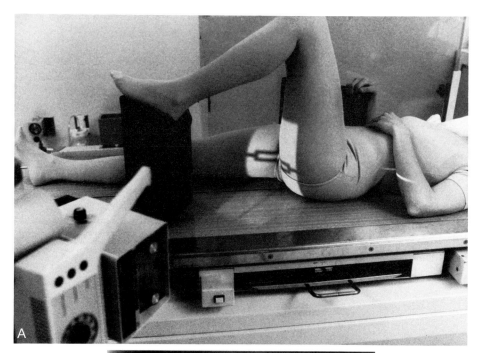

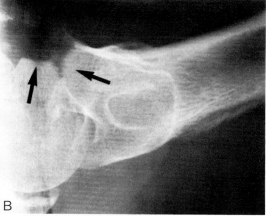

Figure 4–20. A, Patient positioned for lateral view of the right hip. The left knee is flexed 90° and supported by a prop or cushion. The central beam is centered just below the greater trochanter (palpable) with the cassette and beam perpendicular to a line from the anterior superior iliac spine to the symphysis (see Fig. 4–11). *B,* Lateral view of the hip. Subcapital fracture with rotation of the head *(left arrow)* and position of the neck *(right arrow)*. This view is particularly useful for position and evaluation of the posterior cortex.

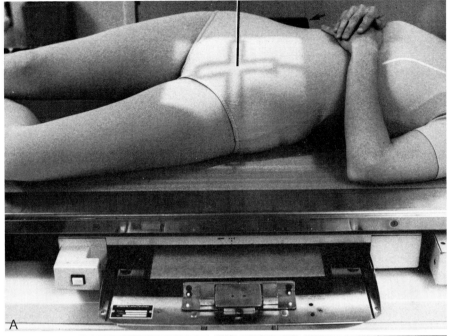

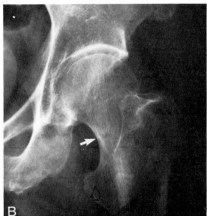

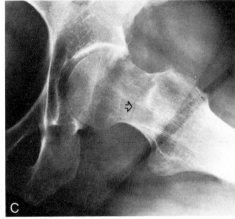

Figure 4–21. A, Patient positioned for oblique view of the hip. The patient's opposite hip is elevated and supported by a cushion wedge *(arrow).* The knee is flexed and the thigh slightly raised toward the head. The beam is perpendicular to the cassette and centered between the symphysis and anterior superior iliac spine. *B,* AP view. The hip is externally rotated with the lesser trochanter *(open arrow)* totally seen. There may be a subtle fracture *(white arrow). C,* Oblique view demonstrates an undisplaced fracture of the femoral neck *(open arrow).*

PELVIC FRACTURES

Pelvic fractures represent a small percentage (2 to 3 percent) of all skeletal fractures.[94] The severity of the fracture depends upon the mechanism of injury. Minor pelvic fractures (fractures of individual bones or single breaks in the pelvic ring) are fairly common in older individuals following simple falls. Severe pelvic injury is usually the result of high-velocity motor vehicle accidents, industrial accidents, or falls of a significant distance. Table 4–3

summarizes the etiology and associated mortality rates of severe pelvic injury in patients treated in our department. Complex pelvic fractures tend to occur in younger individuals (50 percent under 30 and 77 percent under 50 years of age), with males outnumbering females 3:1 (Table 4–4).[99] In our series of over 100 patients with complex pelvic fractures (Key and Conwell Class III), the overall mortality rate was 22 percent. Massive hemorrhage was the most common and potentially life-threatening complication.

TABLE 4–3. Complex Pelvic Fractures

Etiology	% Patients	Mortality Rate
Motor vehicle accident	43	26%
Farm accident	18	0%
Pedestrian accident	17	41%
Motorcycle accident	8	38%
Falls	6	17%
Other	8	0%

TABLE 4–4. Complex Pelvic Fractures: Age Distribution

Age (yrs.)	% Male	% Female
15–20	13	13
21–30	16	8
31–40	8	2
41–50	15	2
51–60	5	1
61–70	7	0
>70	4	4

Proper management of pelvic fractures requires complete radiographic assessment of the pelvic ring. This requires multiple radiographic views and, in certain cases, computed tomography and angiography. Detection of posterior fractures is particularly important, as complications (hemorrhage, instability, etc.) increase significantly with double breaks in the pelvic ring.[83, 91, 94, 99, 112]

Classification of Pelvic Fractures

A thorough understanding of the classification of pelvic fractures is essential for effective communication between the orthopedist or examining physician and the radiologist. Multiple classifications of pelvic fractures have been developed, each of which is designed to help the physician determine the proper management and prognosis of the pelvic fracture (Table 4–5).

Tile[112] proposed a classification based on Pennal's study of 354 pelvic fractures (Table 4–5). This classification is based on the forces that result in the pelvic fracture. Such forces include anteroposterior compression, lateral compression, and vertical shearing injuries. Lateral compressive and vertical shearing injuries are more likely to result in pelvic instability and usually present with more significant complications.[112] Connally and Hedberg proposed that pelvic fractures be considered major if the weight-bearing surface of the acetabulum is involved or if both obturator rings are fractured.[56] Watson-Jones[114] divided pelvic fractures into three categories, with Type II being the most significant (Table 4–5). We prefer to use the classification proposed by Key and Conwell[72] and modified by Kane.[94] This classification, shown in Table 4–6, will be applied to facilitate the following discussion of pelvic fractures. The incidence of each fracture class is included in Table 4–6. These numbers are based on a review of 750 pelvic fractures over a 14-year period at the Mayo Clinic.[98]

TABLE 4–5. Pelvic Fracture Classifications

Tile-Pennal[90, 111, 112]
  Anteroposterior compression
    Open book
    Straddle fractures
  Lateral compression
    Ipsilateral double fractures
    Bucket-handle fractures
    Straddle fractures with posterior disruption
  Vertical shearing fractures

Connally-Hedberg[56]
  Major
    Bilateral ramus fractures
    Acetabular dome fractures
  Minor

Watson-Jones[114]
  Type I.   Avulsion fractures
  Type II. Fracture and dislocation of the pelvic ring
  Type III. Sacrococcygeal fractures

TABLE 4–6. Key and Conwell Classification (Kane Modification) 750 Patients Mayo Clinic

Class	% Patients	Description
I	25	Fractures of individual bones without interruption of the pelvic ring. Includes: Single ramus fracture Avulsion fracture Duverney fracture Transverse sacral fracture Coccyx fracture
II	36	Single break in the pelvic ring. Includes: Fracture of two ipsilateral rami Fracture near or subluxation of pelvic symphysis or sacroiliac joint
III	15	Double breaks in the pelvic ring. Includes: Straddle fracture Sprung pelvis Malgaigne Bucket-handle fracture Complex fracture
IV	24	Acetabular fractures. Includes: Undisplaced Displaced

Class I Fractures

Class I fractures include breaks in individual bones without interruption of the pelvic ring (Fig. 4–22). This type of fracture occurred in 25 percent of patients in our series (Table 4–6). Several types of fracture fall within this category, including avulsion fractures. These fractures (Fig. 4–23) commonly occur in young athletes. Avulsion fractures result from sudden muscle contraction, with the break occurring at the origin or insertion of the muscle.[48, 50, 71, 94] Common locations for avulsion fractures include the following areas (Fig. 4–23): (1) anterior superior iliac spine by the sartorius (Fig. 4–24), (2) anterior inferior iliac spine by the rectus femoris (Fig. 4–25), (3) ischial tuberosity by the hamstrings, (4) greater trochanter by the gluteal muscles, and (5) lesser trochanter by the iliopsoas muscle. These fractures usually heal satisfactorily unless displacement exceeds 2 cm.

Fractures of the individual bones of the obturator ring (ischium and pubic rami) (Fig. 4–22) are usually caused by minor falls in elderly patients, but they may also occur with the stress of overactivity in the osteopenic patient. Rankin reported that these fractures of the individual bones were the most common type of fracture in his series of 449 patients.[92] Such fractures may be overlooked, as the patient usually presents with hip pain, and the history leads one to search for a subcapital fracture of the femur or an intertrochanteric fracture. Fractures of the ischial ramus are particularly troublesome, as they are often associated with subtle central aceta-

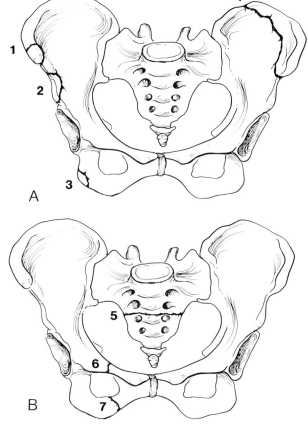

A

B

Figure 4–22. Illustration of Class I fractures, individual breaks without interruption of the pelvic ring: *A,* Avulsion fractures of the anterior superior iliac spine *(1),* anterior inferior iliac spine *(2),* ischial tuberosity *(3),* and ilium *(4)* (Duverney fracture). *B,* Transverse fractures of the sacrum *(5),* superior pubic ramus *(6),* and inferior pubic ramus *(7).* If both rami are fractured the ring is interrupted, a Class II fracture.

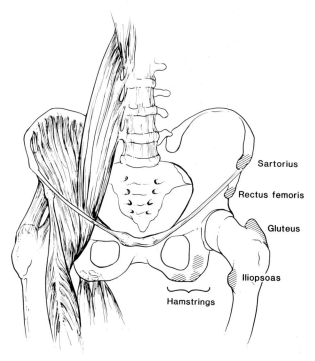

Sartorius

Rectus femoris

Gluteus

Iliopsoas

Hamstrings

Figure 4–23. Diagram of muscle insertions and origins relevant to avulsion fractures of the pelvis and hips.

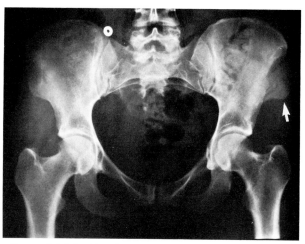

Figure 4–24. Avulsion fracture of the left anterior superior iliac spine with a large ilial fragment *(arrow).*

bular fractures.[95] In these situations careful examination of the acetabulum with Judet (oblique) views, isotope scans, or tomography should be performed (Figs. 4–26 and 4–27). This type of subtle fracture may be difficult to detect with computed tomography.

Fractures of the iliac wing without involvement of the acetabulum or sacroiliac joint (Fig. 4–22A) were described by Duverney in 1751.[61] This fracture occurs following a direct blow to the ilium or with lateral compressive forces.[59, 94, 112] As in the case of avulsion fractures and fractures of the rami, Duverney fractures are usually evident on the AP radiograph of the pelvis. In subtle cases further views, tomography, or radioisotope studies may be required.

Isolated transverse fractures of the sacrum and coccyx are due to direct trauma. These fractures have not been commonly reported in the literature.

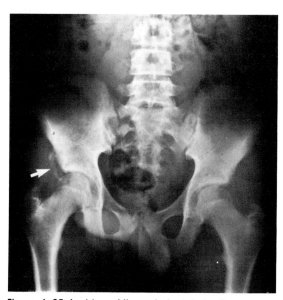

Figure 4–25. Avulsion of the anterior inferior iliac spine.

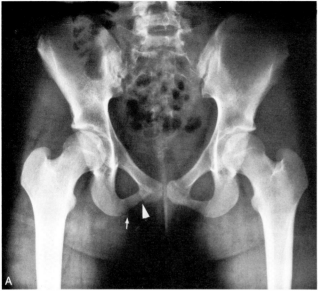

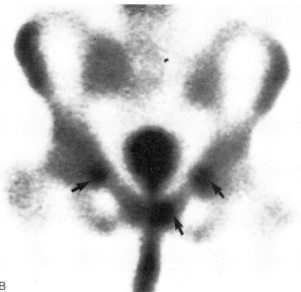

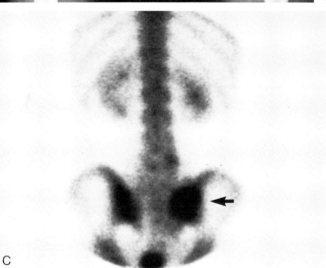

Figure 4–26. Patient with anterior pelvic pain following a motor vehicle accident. *A,* AP view of the pelvis shows a subtle fracture of the inferior pubic ramus *(large white arrow)* with avulsion of the ischial epiphysis *(small arrow). B,* Anterior radioisotope scan (technetium) demonstrates undisplaced superior rami fractures bilaterally. *C,* Posterior scan demonstrates diastasis of the sacroiliac joint. This is really a Class III fracture. Complications are much more common with such fractures.

Figure 4–27. The anterior oblique view of the hip is also very useful in evaluating the obturator ring for double fractures *(arrows).*

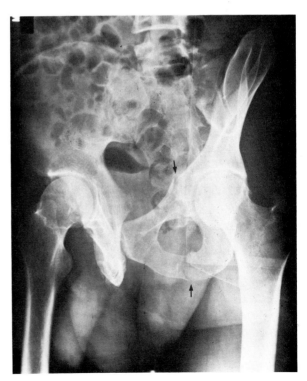

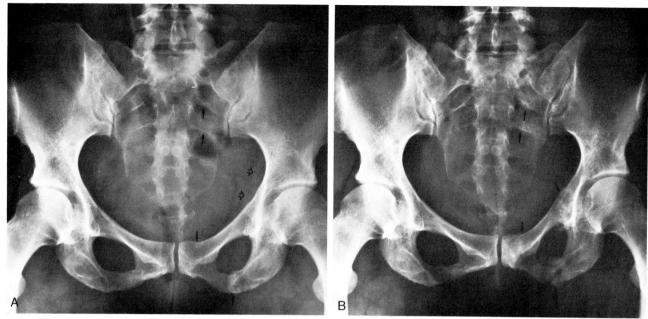

Figure 4–28. Patient with pelvic pain and blood loss following pelvic trauma. *A*, There are subtle fractures of the obturator ring on the left *(lower black arrows)* with displacement of the obturator fat stripe due to hematoma *(open arrow)*. Subtle torus fractures of the arcuate lines *(upper arrows)* were missed on this examination. *B*, Follow-up exam 3 months later. The sacral fractures *(black arrows)* are more obvious owing to callus formation.

Furey[63] reported an incidence of 8 percent and Connally and Hedberg[56] reported an incidence of 7 percent in their reviews of pelvic fractures. Identification of transverse sacral fractures on the AP view of the pelvis is often difficult owing to overlying bowel content or bladder distention. Careful attention must be given to the lateral cortical margins and the arcuate lines so that subtle fractures are not overlooked (Fig. 4–28).[69] Jackson reported that up to 70 percent of sacral fractures were overlooked on initial examination.[69] In our experience

50 percent of sacral fractures were missed in more severe pelvic injury (Class III fractures).[98] Lateral views may be helpful, especially if slight displacement is present. Computed tomography has also been successful in detecting fractures of the sacrum (Fig. 4–29).[102]

Fractures and fracture-dislocations of the coccyx occur with falls to the sitting position and are more common in females. The fracture site is extremely tender. Pain may be exaggerated on rising from the sitting position as a result of gluteal muscle contraction.[94] Lateral radiographs are most useful for identification of coccygeal fractures and dislocations.

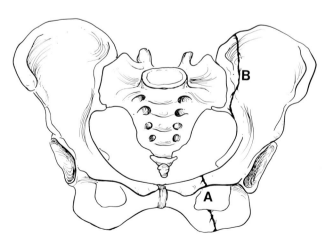

Figure 4–29. CT scan of the right sacroiliac area. Note the buckle fracture of the sacrum near the sacroiliac joint *(white arrow)*.

Figure 4–30. Class II pelvic fracture with a single break in the pelvic ring usually occurs near the symphysis *(A)* or the sacroiliac joint *(B)*.

Class II Fractures

Class II fractures, characterized by a single break in the pelvic ring, are the most common type of pelvic fracture in our series (36 percent of 750 pelvic fractures).[99] Single breaks in the pelvic ring usually occur near the pubic symphysis (Figs. 4–27 and 4–30) or, more rarely, near the sacroiliac joint.[112] The minimal motion in these articulations allows a single break to occur. Thus, according to Taylor, normal motion at the pubic symphysis is 1 mm in males and 1.5 mm in females.[108] In Rankin's series fractures of the left obturator ring were more common than the right.[92] Class II fractures may be due to direct blows, crush injury, or indirect trauma through the femur.[94]

Radiographically, identification of anterior Class II fractures is usually accomplished on the AP view of the pelvis. Unfortunately, a great many Class III fractures (anterior and posterior fractures) remain undiagnosed because of the examiner's focus on this obvious anterior injury. If the posterior fracture goes undiagnosed, a stable and relatively uncomplicated Class II fracture will be treated when the patient may actually have a much more serious Class III fracture. Class III fractures are unstable and more likely to lead to serious complications.[79, 83, 91, 94, 98]

In our review of pelvic fractures we noted that 33 percent of posterior fractures were overlooked on the initial interpretation of the radiographs (usually only an AP view of the pelvis).[98] Careful review of these cases and all Class III fractures resulted in an approach that assists in locating potential posterior fractures. Fractures of the anterior rami were graded according to the degree of displacement. A Grade 1 fracture is an anterior ramus fracture with no displacement (Fig. 4–31A). None of these patients had posterior fractures, even in retrospect. A Grade 2 fracture is a ramus fracture with displacement of one half or less than one half of the width of the ramus (Fig. 4–31B). In these patients only 20 percent had fractures posteriorly, and all these fractures involved the ipsilateral sacroiliac joint or ilium near the sacroiliac joint. A Grade 3 fracture is an anterior ramus fracture with displacement greater than one half the width of the ramus (Fig. 4–31C). In patients with Grade 3 fractures there was always a second fracture, and about 80 percent were on the ipsilateral side. If both obturator rings are fractured, the fracture is by definition already an instance of the Class III type. However, symmetrical sacroiliac joint diastasis or adjacent fractures were found in 40 percent of the patients with Grade 3 fractures. Diastasis of the pubic symphysis with no vertical displacement usually results in bilateral posterior fractures or sacroiliac separations (Fig. 4–32). If the diastasis includes a vertical displacement, the posterior injury is usually on the elevated side.

The above categories may not be entirely ade-

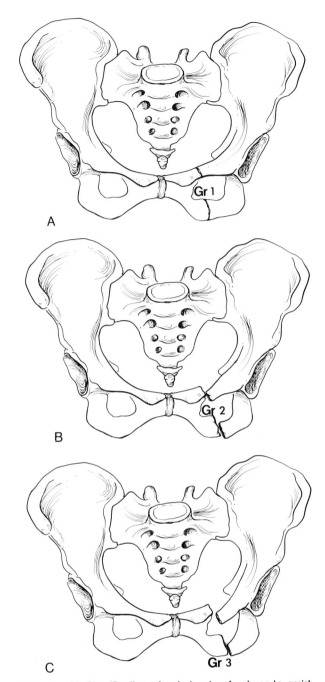

Figure 4–31. Classification of anterior ring fractures to assist in detection of a posterior fracture. *A,* Grade 1 fracture, no displacement; *B,* Grade 2 fracture, displaced one-half the width of the superior ramus; *C,* Grade 3 fracture, displaced the full width of the upper ramus or more.

quate, but they help point the way to detection of posterior injuries. Therefore, if an anterior fracture is identified and falls within Grades 2 or 3, one must search diligently for a posterior fracture. For this task computed tomography is the procedure of choice at our institution. This modality can successfully identify unsuspected fractures as well as provide valuable information regarding soft tissue injury.

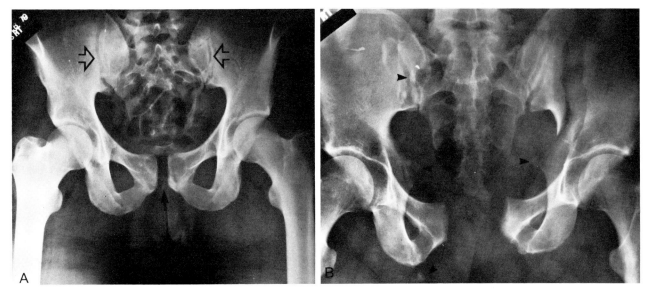

Figure 4–32. Diastasis of the pubic symphysis with bilateral posterior injuries. *A,* Slight diastasis of the pubic symphysis with no articular step-off *(black arrow).* There is diastasis of both sacroiliac joints *(open arrows). B,* Wide separation of the pubic symphysis resulted in avulsion of the ischial spines *(arrows),* ischial tuberosity on the right *(arrow),* separation of the right sacroiliac joint *(arrow),* and a displaced iliac fracture on the left near the sacroiliac joint.

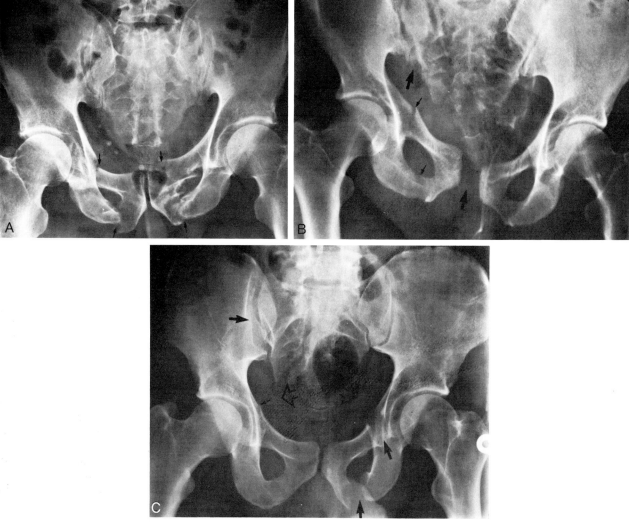

Figure 4–33. See legend on opposite page

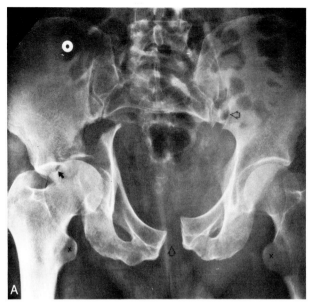 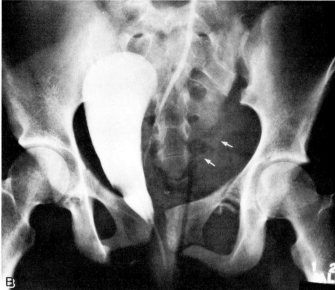

Figure 4–34. Complex pelvic fractures. *A,* There is separation of the pubic symphysis and left sacroiliac joint *(open arrows).* In addition, there is a displaced acetabular fracture on the right with an osteochondral fracture on the right femoral head *(black arrow).* Both hips are externally rotated *(x)* on the lesser trochanter. *B,* Bilateral obturator ring fractures with separation of the left sacroiliac joint. There is comminution of the lower sacrum *(white arrows),* and the bladder is deviated to the right by the large pelvic hematoma.

Class III Fractures

Class III fractures result in two or more breaks in the pelvic ring. Fifteen percent of 750 patients were included in this category.[98] These injuries are usually unstable compared with the stable Class I and Class II fractures. Significant morbidity and mortality also result from Class III fractures. In our series the mortality rate in patients with Class III fractures was 22 percent.[98]

Class III fractures tend to occur in younger individuals (52 percent less than 30 years of age) and are more common in males than females by a 3:1 ratio. The etiology is most often a high-velocity motor vehicle accident, farm accident, or pedestrian accident.

Multiple fracture patterns may result in a Class III fracture. Straddle fractures, i.e., bilateral fractures of both pubic rami (Fig. 4–33), occurred in 33 percent of patients with unstable fractures in Dunn and Morris's series.[59] This fracture occurs with direct trauma to the region of the pubic symphysis or with lateral compression.[94]

Malgaigne fractures, first described in 1859, are double vertical breaks in the pelvic ring (Fig. 4–33B). By definition this type of fracture requires an ante-

rior disruption of the pelvic ring with a second fracture posterior to the acetabulum. The posterior fracture may involve the ilium adjacent to the sacroiliac joint, or diastasis of the sacroiliac joint may be present. Anteriorly, there may be fractures of the rami or diastasis of the pubic symphysis. Malgaigne fractures have been reported to be the most common of Class III fractures.[109] In our series 38 percent of Class III fractures were Malgaigne fractures.[98] This fracture may be caused by lateral compression, anteroposterior compression, or indirect trauma from the lower extremity. A variant of the Malgaigne fracture, the bucket-handle fracture, is the result of an oblique force. The end result in this case is an anterior fracture with the posterior fracture or dislocation on the contralateral side of the pelvis (Fig. 4–33C).

Severe multiple fractures are very unstable, and significant complications almost always result (Fig. 4–34).[94, 98] In our group of over 100 Class III fractures, three subgroups of fractures could be distinguished. The largest subgroup was characterized by severe multiple fractures and consisted of 46 percent of the patients. The two other subgroups were characterized by straddle fractures, occurring in 16 percent of the patients, and Malgaigne frac-

Figure 4–33. Class III fractures. *A,* Straddle fracture with fractures of both pubic rami bilaterally. *B,* Malgaigne fracture with disruption of the pubic symphysis *(lower large arrow),* elevation of the right hemipelvis, and fracture-dislocation of the right sacroiliac joint *(upper large arrow).* There are also minimally displaced fractures *(small arrows)* of the right pubic ramus. The bladder and Foley catheter are deviated to the left by a large pelvic hematoma. *C,* Bucket-handle fracture with fracture of the left obturator ring *(lower large black arrows)* and separation of the contralateral sacroiliac joint *(upper large arrow).* Bilateral pelvic hematomas *(open arrows)* with a central acetabular fracture on the right *(small arrow).*

tures, occurring in 38 percent of patients. Also of importance were the high incidence of associated sacral fractures (Fig. 4–34*B*), evident in 23 percent of patients with Class III fractures, and the unfortunate fact that 50 percent of these fractures were missed on initial radiographic evaluation. Solitary sacral fractures are much less common.

Routine radiographic evaluation is often all that is required to identify complex displaced fractures. Initial management decisions can be made with AP and oblique or angled views. Computed tomography is useful for complete evaluation of Class III fractures or to differentiate Class II from Class III.

Class IV Fractures

Class IV fractures are fractures of the acetabulum. Acetabular fractures have been described with increasing frequency in recent years.[60, 62, 70, 75, 89, 97, 98, 107, 113] In our experience, acetabular fractures make

TABLE 4–7. Acetabular Fracture Classification Based on Position of Femoral Head

Stewart and Milford[107] (1954)

Grade I:	Linear or stellate fracture of the acetabular floor with no displacement of the femoral head
Grade II:	Comminuted fracture with mild to moderate central displacement of the femoral head and acetabular fragments
Grade III:	Marked displacement of the fracture fragments and protrusion of the femoral head into the pelvis; with or without comminution of the superior acetabulum
Grade IV:	Central dislocation with associated fracture of the head or neck of femur

Rowe and Lowell[97] (1961)

Group I:	Linear undisplaced acetabular fracture with single or multiple lines
Group II:	Posterior fracture with small or large posterior fragment
Group III:	Central acetabular fracture with displacement of femoral head
Group IV:	Superior or burst fracture with disruption of the acetabulum

Eichenholtz and Stark[62] (1964)

Type IA:	Little or no central displacement of the femoral head
Type IB:	Little or no central displacement of the femoral head and anterior pelvic fracture
Type IIA:	Central head displacement with no anterior pelvic fracture
Type IIB:	Central head displacement and anterior pelvic fracture
Type III:	Head dislocated centrally without anterior fracture

TABLE 4–8. Acetabular Fracture Classification Based on Anterior and Posterior Column

Judet, Judet, Letournel[70] (1964)
  Elementary
    Posterior acetabular rim
    Ilioischial (posterior) column
    Iliopubic (anterior) column
    Transverse fractures
  Complex
    Fracture with femoral head dislocation
    Both columns disrupted

Tile[111] (1980)
  Simple
    Anterior column
    Posterior column
    Transverse
  Complex
    "T" fractures
    Dome fractures
    Acetabulum and iliac wing
    Acetabulum and adjacent sacroiliac joint

up about 24 percent of all pelvic fractures. Key and Conwell divided these fractures into undisplaced and displaced. However, a more complex and accurate approach is required for the proper evaluation and management of acetabular fractures. We will therefore deviate from the Key and Conwell classification at this point.

Multiple approaches to the classification of acetabular fractures have been proposed. Certain authors have classified acetabular fractures according to the position of the femoral head (Table 4–7).[60, 62, 97, 107] Judet and colleagues[70] classified fractures according to the involvement of the anterior and posterior columns (Table 4–8). Tile,[111] describing the experience of Pennal, Davidson, and Plewes, found that the prognosis of acetabular fractures depends upon the degree of involvement of the weight-bearing surface, the degree of displacement, and the presence or absence of anterior pelvic ring fractures. This classification (Table 4–8) distinguishes simple fractures from more complex frac-

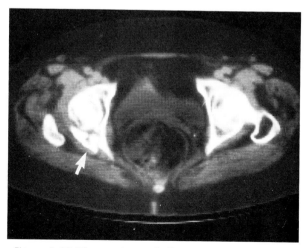

Figure 4–35. CT scan demonstrating a comminuted posterior acetabular fracture *(arrow).*

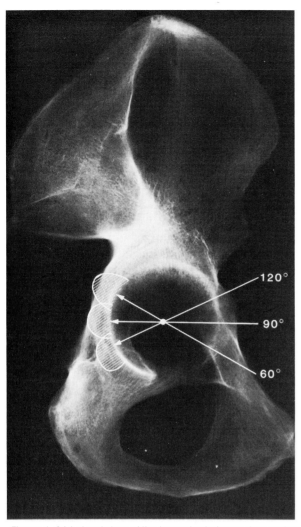

Figure 4-36. Lateral view of the innominate bone demonstrating how the position of the femur (120° to 60° flexion) results in posterior acetabular fractures.

tures, with the latter characterized by involvement of the dome, "T" fractures, iliac wing fractures, and disruption of the adjacent sacroiliac joint. The Judet approach will be used in the following discussion of acetabular fractures.

Elementary or single acetabular fractures (Table 4–8) were the most common in Judet's series (111 of 173 patients).[70] However, Tile[111] reported complex fractures to be more common, a finding confirmed in our series of cases. Acetabular fractures result from force transmitted to the femoral head via the greater trochanter or lower extremity.[70] Radiographic evaluation of acetabular fractures requires high-quality AP and Judet views at a minimum. Computed tomography is especially helpful in evaluating complex fractures. This technique allows more accurate assessment of the size, relationship, and degree of displacement of the fracture fragments. This is particularly important in choosing the proper approach if open reduction is contemplated.

Elementary Acetabular Fractures. Posterior acetabular fractures may involve a single fragment or multiple fragments and on occasion may result in impaction of the acetabular articular surface.[70] These fractures are easily seen on the anterior oblique view, as the posterior acetabulum is more clearly visualized. With large or multiple fragments CT is the technique of choice for more complete evaluation (Fig. 4–35).[64, 80] The fracture usually results from lower extremity trauma (usually at the knee) with the hip flexed approximately 90° (Fig. 4–36). The size of the fragment is also related to the degree of femoral abduction. The greater the abduction, the larger the fragment (Fig. 4–37).[70]

Fractures of the posterior (ilioischial) column usually begin above the acetabulum, extend through the posterior aspect of the acetabulum, and include

Figure 4-37. CT scan of the pelvis through the femoral heads. The degree of adduction or abduction of the femur also affects the size of posterior acetabular fragments.

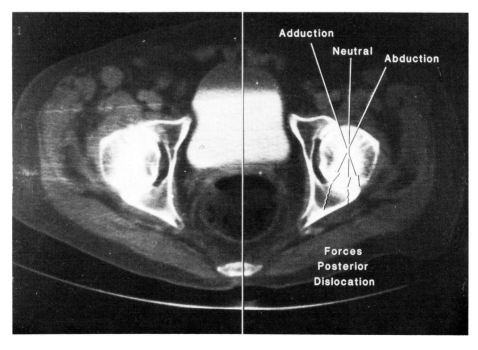

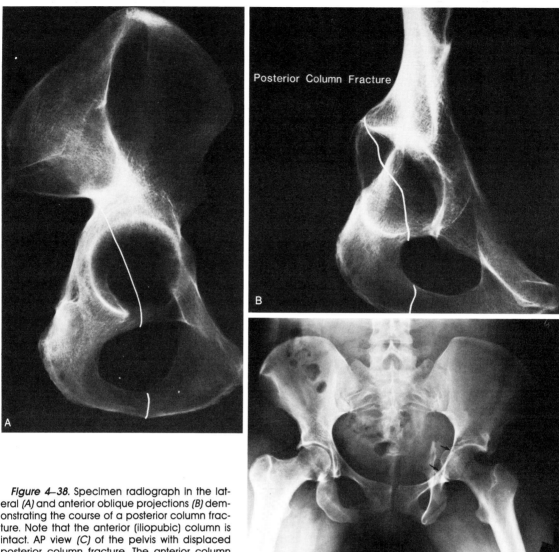

Figure 4–38. Specimen radiograph in the lateral *(A)* and anterior oblique projections *(B)* demonstrating the course of a posterior column fracture. Note that the anterior (iliopubic) column is intact.[70, 77, 111] AP view *(C)* of the pelvis with displaced posterior column fracture. The anterior column *(arrows)* is intact.

the ischial ramus (Fig. 4–38). The iliopubic line and radiographic "U" remain intact on the AP radiograph, allowing one to attribute the fracture to the posterior column. The dome of the acetabulum remains intact.[70, 77, 111] This fracture results from a blow to the knee with the hip flexed 90° and abducted about 20°.[70] Posterior dislocation or subluxation of the hip is frequently associated with this fracture, and sciatic nerve injury may result.[70, 77, 111]

Transverse fractures involve both the anterior and posterior column and frequently the ischial spine (Fig. 4–39). The mechanism of injury is a blow to the lateral aspect of the greater trochanter or the posterior aspect of the pelvis, with the hip flexed and abducted.[70] Radiographically these fractures are easily missed on the AP view, especially when no displacement is present. Judet (oblique) views (Fig. 4–40) are required and occasionally conventional tomography or radioisotope scans as well. Computed tomography may miss this type of fracture if

the fracture line is parallel to the slice. This may be the one situation in which CT is not the technique of choice in evaluation of the pelvis.

Fractures of the anterior column (iliopubic column) are less common than posterior column fractures.[111] The prognosis with these injuries is reportedly better compared with posterior column fractures.[111] These fractures usually begin just above the anterior inferior iliac spine and extend inferiorly to involve the inferior pubic ramus near the junction with the ischium (Fig. 4–41). The iliopubic line is disrupted on the AP radiograph, and once again the oblique views will clearly demonstrate the disruption of the anterior column and intact posterior column. The injury is thought to be the result of a blow to the greater trochanter with the hip externally rotated, an uncommon situation indeed.[70, 111]

Complex Acetabular Fractures. Complex acetabular fractures result in multiple fracture lines and increased morbidity. Fractures with significant cen-

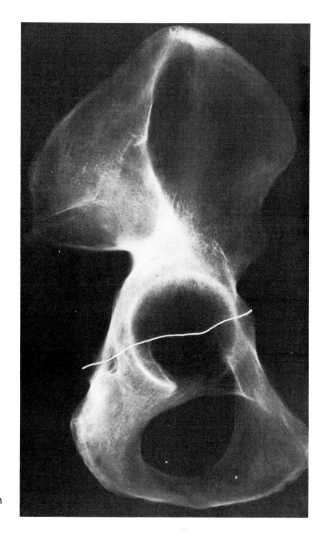

Figure 4–39. Transverse acetabular fractures typically involve both columns and the ischial spine *(white line)*.

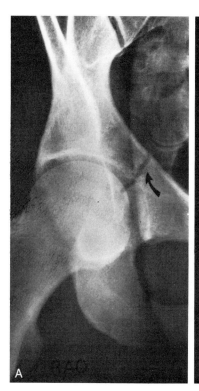 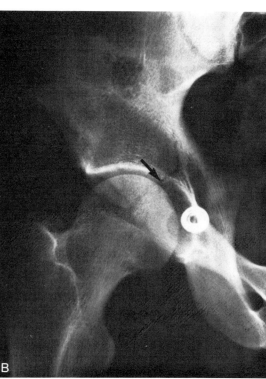

Figure 4–40. Transverse undisplaced acetabular fracture demonstrated with anterior *(A)* and posterior *(B)* oblique views.

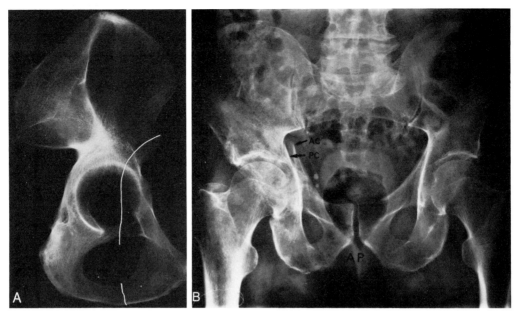

Figure 4–41. A, Specimen radiograph demonstrating the typical course *(white line)* of the anterior column fracture. B, AP radiograph demonstrating an anterior column (AC) fracture. Note that the posterior column (PC) or ileoischial line is intact.

tral displacement of the femoral head and acetabular fragments lead to complications similar to those of Class III pelvic fractures (Fig. 4–42). The complications will be discussed in detail later in this chapter.

Comminution of the acetabulum may result in a "T" pattern, with splitting of the anterior and posterior columns as well as a transverse fracture. Recognition of the division of the columns is important, as surgical correction of one column alone will not result in anatomic reduction of the acetabulum.[111] Vertical cleft fractures that separate the anterior and posterior columns are particularly well

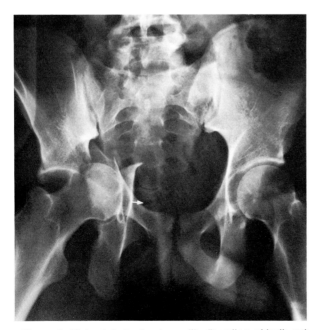

Figure 4–42. Acetabular fracture with disruption of both columns and central displacement of the femoral head. Note the dislocation of the first and second coccygeal segments *(white arrow).*

demonstrated with computed tomography. The plane of the fracture is almost perpendicular to the scan slice (Fig. 4–43).

Fragmentation or displacement of the weight-bearing surface of the acetabulum is of particular importance (Fig. 4–43). Any malrotation or comminution of the dome of the acetabulum must be corrected. This may be the most important indication for surgical intervention.[70, 77, 111] Complex fractures with involvement of the iliac wing or adjacent sacroiliac joint also result in a poorer prognosis. The sacroiliac joint involvement may be subtle and difficult to detect even with comparison of the joints. Computed tomography is particularly valuable in these situations (Fig. 4–44). Evaluation of the sacrum, sacroiliac joint, acetabular dome, and the joint space is better accomplished with CT than with routine films or conventional tomography.[64, 80, 98] The evaluation of the position of the acetabular fragments (Fig. 4–44) and intra-articular fragments is particularly effective with CT.[64]

Treatment of Pelvic Fractures

Detailed radiographic examination, as outlined in this chapter, is essential for the orthopedic treatment of pelvic fractures. Proper radiographic definition of the injury is a prerequisite to effective treatment. The four classes of pelvic fractures lend themselves to a number of generalizations regarding treatment. These will be discussed in this section.

Class I Fractures

In the acute phase of the Class I fracture there is really no treatment indicated. These fractures will

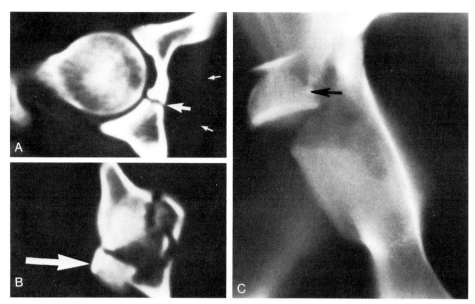

Figure 4–43. A, CT scan of vertical cleft fracture *(large arrow)* with associated hematoma *(small arrow).* B, A higher section demonstrates comminution of the dome of the acetabulum with a rotated fragment *(large arrow).* C, AP tomogram demonstrates the large fragment seen in B but is much less useful in planning treatment and in the exact positioning of the fragments.

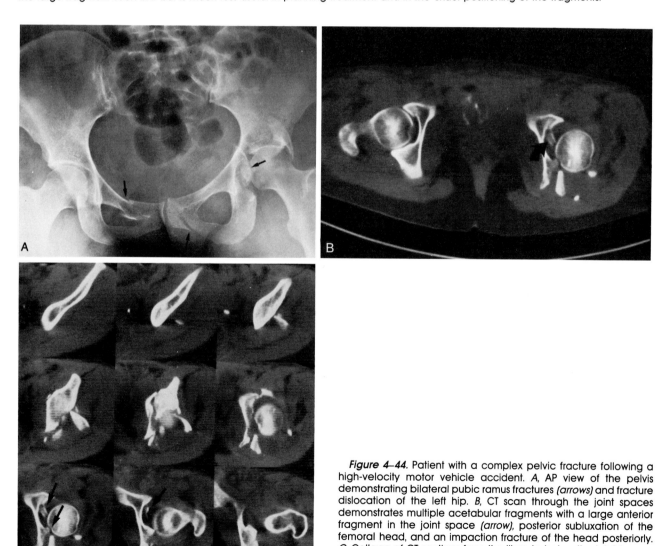

Figure 4–44. Patient with a complex pelvic fracture following a high-velocity motor vehicle accident. A, AP view of the pelvis demonstrating bilateral pubic ramus fractures *(arrows)* and fracture dislocation of the left hip. B, CT scan through the joint spaces demonstrates multiple acetabular fragments with a large anterior fragment in the joint space *(arrow),* posterior subluxation of the femoral head, and an impaction fracture of the head posteriorly. C, Collage of CT sections from the ilium to below the joint (moves top left to right).

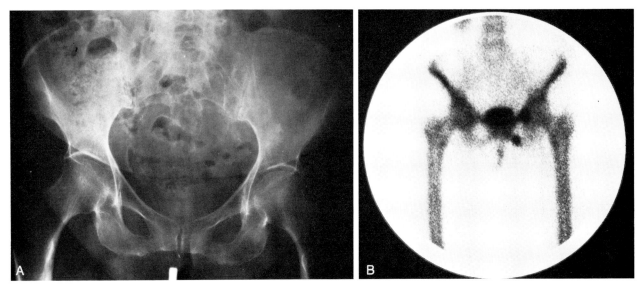

Figure 4–45. Radiograph of a 76-year-old woman with 6 weeks of pain in left groin and hip region. No history of injury. Osteoporosis. *A*, Questionable stress fracture in the superior and inferior pubic rami on the left. *B*, Confirmation with technetium scanning. Healing was uneventful.

heal and usually do not involve residual deficits. Occasionally crutches or a cane may be necessary as an aid while pain is present. An exception to this would be the fracture-dislocation of the coccyx, which needs immediate reduction. This can be performed through rectal manipulation of the fragment, usually best done with the patient under anesthesia.

Often not diagnosed is the stress fracture of the pelvis. This is most commonly seen in elderly patients with osteopenia (Fig. 4–45). A long spell of walking or a fall or even a slight twist may result in a fracture of the pubic ramus, usually the inferior element, or a fracture of both pubic rami. No radiographic findings are present. The symptoms are sometimes diffuse, and the diagnosis may only be confirmed with TC-99m scanning. This should be positive within 2 to 3 days of the injury and certainly by 1 week. The management of the patient and the prognosis depend on the diagnosis. While these patients will usually recover fully, union may be delayed for up to 2 years if tension forces act on the fracture instead of the usual compressive forces.

Residual deficits in Class I fractures are usually minimal. However, fracture of the coccyx may result in continued discomfort and may even in extreme cases require coccygectomy. Fractures through the sacrum are notorious also for residual nerve injuries. The initial fracture may even be undiagnosed until the patient presents with sacral nerve deficits.

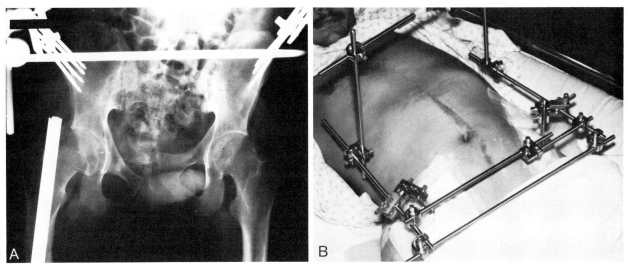

Figure 4–46. *A*, Radiograph of a 19-year-old male after motor vehicle accident. Unstable vertical fracture left side of pelvis and fracture in shaft of right femur. Preliminary traction followed by application of Hoffman-Vidal apparatus. Pins in place in iliac crest and apparatus applied. *B*, The patient in bed with the external fixation device in place.

Class II Fractures

Treatment is usually minimal for a single break in the pelvic ring, a fracture that is basically stable. The most common Class II fracture involves both the superior and inferior pubic ramus. Treatment in this case is symptomatic, with rest, often crutches, and sometimes a pelvic support if the sacroiliac joint appears involved.

Residual deficits of Class II fractures typically relate to the sacroiliac joint. Although the joint will usually stabilize, it may remain unstable and produce symptoms. Radiographic visualization of the joint is difficult. Films taken with the patient standing and with alternate weight bearing will often demonstrate instability if both the pubic symphysis and sacroiliac joint are involved. Oblique views may show sclerosis. Isotope scans will demonstrate in-

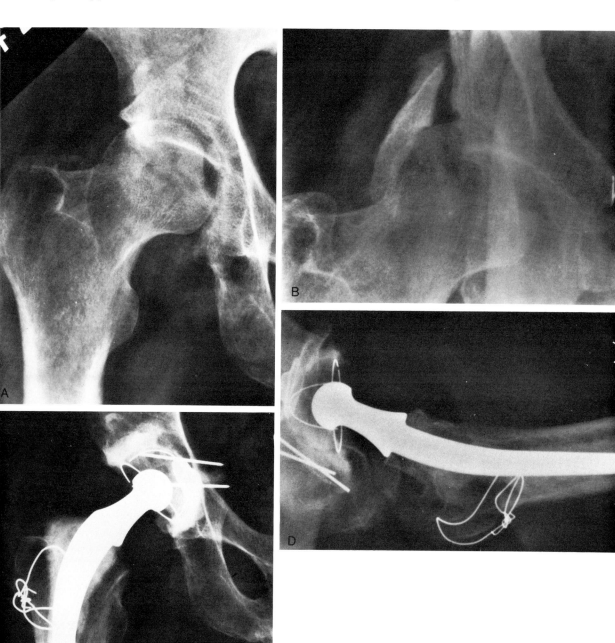

Figure 4–47. Radiographs of a 45-year-old male following motor vehicle accident. Original x-rays were interpreted in local emergency room as being negative. Patient returned 2 days later and x-rays were still called negative. Patient was put on crutches, and 9 weeks later the diagnosis was made. *A,* Anterior posterior view of the right hip. *B,* Oblique view showing the posterior fragment. *C,* AP view following open reduction and internal fixation of the fractured fragment. The dome of the acetabulum posteriorly showed damage of the cartilage, as did the head of the femur. A primary total hip arthroplasty was done. *D,* Lateral x-ray 1 year after surgery.

creased uptake in the sacroiliac joint. CT scans are most useful in the demonstration of sacroiliac joint incongruity. Local injection of anesthetic agents into the joint will often localize the source of pain to the joint. Ultimately, if other methods fail, fusion of the joint may be necessary.

Class III Fractures

These are unstable fractures and require a vigorous approach by the orthopedist. The first consideration is always the accompanying visceral and vascular complications that may be present, and these take priority over the skeletal treatment. If, however, the bladder or urethra requires surgical repair, the orthopedist can concurrently stabilize the pubis and occasionally remove or stabilize comminuted fractures in the region of the lower urinary tract.

The use of external fixation is a fairly recent innovation that has made the handling of unstable pelvic fractures less difficult (Fig. 4–46). As soon as the patient's general condition allows, fixation is applied. This will stabilize the fragments and lessen hemorrhage and other visceral trauma. In a recent review of 45 patients with fractures of the pelvis, the Baylor group reduced the time from injury to application of the Hoffman apparatus to 2.2 days in their last 25 patients.[116] Use of external fixation provides comfort to the patient and allows more rapid mobilization. It must be emphasized, however, that external fixation will do very little in the way of reduction, and closed reduction must precede or accompany its application. Lower extremity traction alone or as an adjunct is indicated in vertical shear (Malgaigne) fractures. If possible, the fixation device is left in place for 8 weeks. Walking may be allowed, depending on the type of fracture. If the injury is primarily unilateral, the opposite extremity can bear weight with the aid of crutches after 3 weeks. Bilateral unstable shear fractures, on the other hand, are best treated in recumbency for 8 weeks following stabilization with external fixation.[74, 106]

Other methods of partially stabilizing and reducing these unstable fractures have in the past included manipulation and spica casting, traction, and the pelvic compression sling. While the sling can reduce the diastasis of the pelvis, pressure against the bony prominences creates skin problems. If used, the sling must be padded with thick layers of foam, and the patient must be carefully monitored.

Residual deficits of Class III fractures are common. Continued pain due to instability, especially in the sacroiliac joint and low back, is often present. Leg length discrepancy may also occur.

Class IV Fractures

These fractures primarily involve the acetabulum, though frequently other pelvic fractures accompany such fractures. Similarly, Class III fractures may have acetabular involvement, making them merge with the Class IV type.

The same principles apply here as in other fractures involving a joint; namely, the normal anatomic configuration must be restored. Fractures that result in intrapelvic protrusion of the femoral head have been treated in the past with lateral and distal traction combined with pins in the femur and greater trochanter area. This treatment may reduce some of these fractures; and if the dome of the acetabulum is intact, this may be all that is necessary. Traction may also be used as a preliminary to open reduction under anesthesia. Stability must then be assessed. If the hip is unstable in flexion, open reduction and fixation of the posterior fragment is indicated (Fig. 4–47). The next stage resulting from forces in the anteroposterior direction is the posterior column fracture. These are the most common of the severe acetabular fractures. They must be opened, reduced, secured by plate and screws, and bent to conform. If this is done during the first 10 days to 3 weeks, a satisfactory result should occur; but the ultimate course depends in part on how badly the femoral head is damaged (Figs. 4–48 and 4–49).

Transverse fractures are more complex, making internal fixation more difficult. But, again, it is essential to restore the acetabulum to its normal configuration if possible. Anterior column fractures

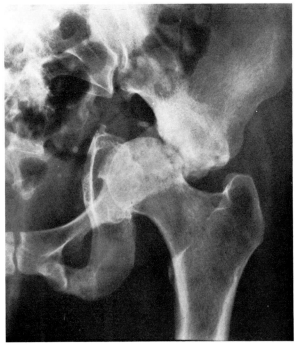

Figure 4–48. Radiograph of a 28-year-old woman following motor vehicle accident. Patient was treated in traction for 6 weeks, and union failed to occur. This is the appearance 1 year later with frank non-union of the posterior pillar and traumatic arthritis of the head and acetabulum. Early open reduction and internal fixation of the posterior pillar would probably have obviated the need for subsequent total hip arthroplasty.

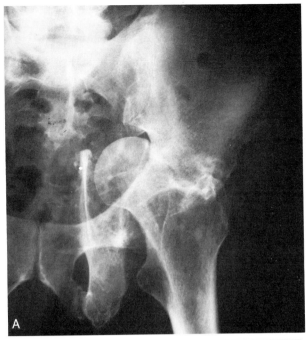

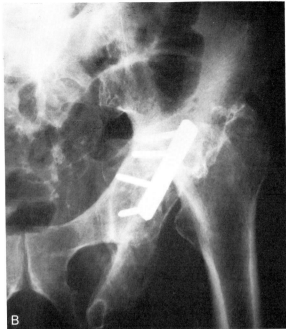

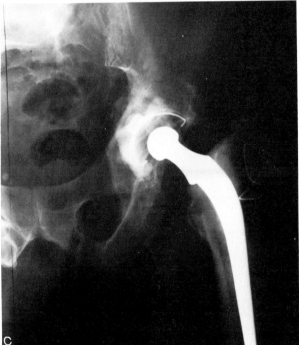

Figure 4–49. Radiographs of a 68-year-old male. Untreated fracture of the left pelvis with non-union of the posterior pillar. *A,* Seven months post-injury. *B,* Open reduction, internal fixation of acetabular fracture, removal of head and neck of femur, and pin traction in distal femur. *C,* Six weeks after internal fixation, hip explored and fracture found to be united, plate removed, and total hip arthroplasty performed. Radiograph shows appearance 8 weeks following total hip arthroplasty.

are fortunately rare. They require an anterior surgical approach and internal fixation.

Treatment of the complex central fracture-dislocation and the comminuted dome fracture does not always result in anatomic reduction. Thus, lateral-distal traction seems about all one can do initially, and the hip is then reconstructed at a later date through total hip replacement (Fig. 4–50).

The pioneer work of Judet and Letournel has shown that restoration of the acetabulum should be carried out if at all possible by open reduction and internal fixation.[76] Careful evaluation of the anatomic aspects of the fracture must be carried out prior to any surgery. Routine radiographs and Judet views should always be obtained (Fig. 4–51). These

can be complemented with CT scans. If the patient's general status does not permit surgery, it can be delayed. Letournel, for example, has recently described the surgical repair of acetabular fractures more than 3 weeks after injury.[76]

Incongruence between the femoral head and the acetabular crescent is a strict indication for open reduction and internal fixation. One must use a fracture table that allows adequate positioning and traction of the limb. The transverse fractures pose the more difficult aspects of the operation. Complete reconstruction of the hip could be achieved with good clinical and radiographic results in 50 percent of these cases. Twenty percent showed some lateral arthritic changes radiographically. It

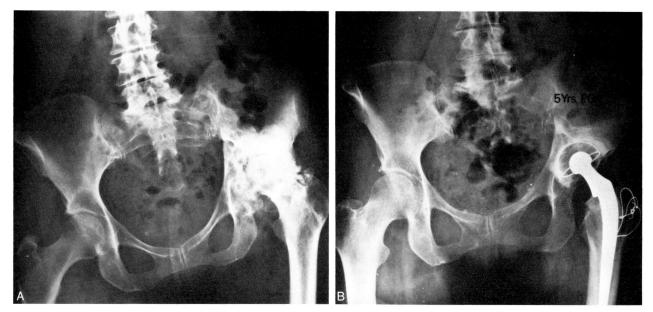

Figure 4-50. Radiographs of a 54-year-old woman. In motor vehicle accident 21 years earlier, patient suffered fracture of femoral neck and acetabulum, and femoral neck fracture was "pinned." Now pain, deformity, and very limited motion. A, Appearance of the left hip and pelvis. B, Total hip arthroplasty performed; appearance 5 years later.

seems preferable when possible to reduce and internally fix these fractures rather than to proceed with a primary total hip arthroplasty.

The residual deficits of Class IV pelvic fractures include fractures that remain unreduced as well as fractures that result in traumatic arthritis. As mentioned, unreduced fractures can often be reduced at a later date, and this is especially true of non-united posterior column fractures. These of necessity will require total hip arthroplasty in conjunction with reduction, usually as a second stage. As we have emphasized elsewhere, total hip arthroplasty in the presence of an unstable acetabulum is

doomed to failure.[58] Stable, secure foundation for placement of the acetabular prosthesis is imperative. This will often require not only open reduction but bone grafting as well, and once union is obtained the reconstruction can be done.

Occasionally the fracture is impossible to reduce, so that total hip arthroplasty cannot be performed. In such cases fusion will be necessary (Fig. 4-52).

Complications of Pelvic Fractures

The complications associated with pelvic fractures are directly related to the degree of trauma. There-

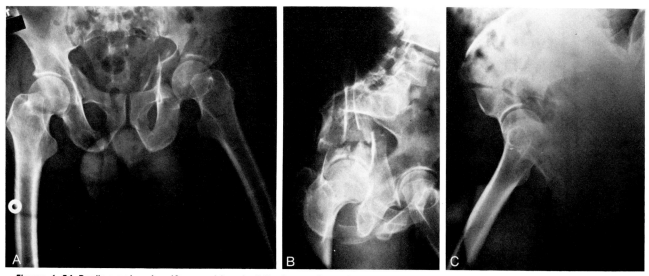

Figure 4-51. Radiographs of a 49-year-old male following motorcycle accident. A, Appearance of pelvic fractures on AP view. Note that the dome of the acetabulum appears intact. B, Obturator oblique view. Fracture into dome of acetabulum now evident. C, Iliac oblique view. Dome of acetabulum appears basically intact.

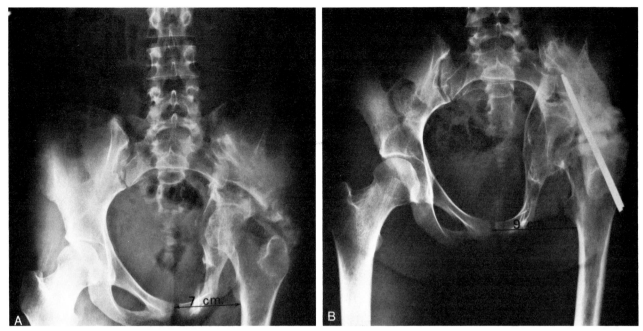

Figure 4–52. Radiographs of a 19-year-old woman following motor vehicle accident. Severe compound fracture of pelvis untreated. Four months following injury, patient experienced severe pain and walked on crutches, 45° flexion-contracture, minimal motion. A, AP view of pelvis. B, View 8 months following arthrodesis. Hip solid, extremity in neutral position, pain relieved, femur lateralized by 2 cm, 1½ cm added length, full activity without walking aid.

fore, the classification presented here assists in determining prognosis. Complications associated with Class I and Class II pelvic fractures are usually minor. Hematoma formation adjacent to the fracture site is usually the only abnormality noted. This is a very helpful finding that may lead one to identify an undisplaced fracture. With Class I and Class II fractures more significant injuries may occur to other areas, but the pelvic injury in these situations is usually not a significant clinical problem. The most severe complications result from Class III fractures (double breaks in the pelvic ring) and displaced Class IV (acetabular) fractures. Table 4–9 summarizes the incidence of immediate complications in these fracture categories at the Mayo Clinic.[98]

Pelvic Hemorrhage

The most common and significant complication is pelvic hemorrhage. All patients with Class III fractures demonstrated a significant drop in their hemoglobin. Seventy-one percent of patients with Class III or displaced Class IV fractures required over 10 units of blood.[98] The overall mortality rate was 22 percent, but in patients requiring more than 5 units of blood the mortality rate increased to 45 percent. Renal failure is commonly related to the shock resulting from massive hemorrhage, and this adds significant morbidity and mortality.[79, 83, 98] A less common but significant complication is infected hematoma, which occurred in 3 percent of our patients with complex pelvic fractures. Infection is

more common with open pelvic fractures, but it has also been reported with closed fractures.[85] The mortality rate is as high as 50 percent in these patients.[96]

The radiographic evaluation should be performed with as little movement of the patient as possible. Patient motion may increase the hemorrhage.[95] Fortunately, with complex pelvic injuries the classification and significance of the injury can almost always be determined with the AP view of the pelvis. Occasionally angled views (with the tube angled caudad or cephalad) are helpful and can be obtained without moving the patient.

Treatment choices depend upon the status of the patient. The use of antishock garments may be of great benefit.[84] However, immediate surgical or angiographic intervention may be necessary.

Angiography will usually identify multiple bleeding sites (Fig. 4–53). The sites can also be somewhat localized by assessing the fracture sites and the degree of displacement. Once the bleeding sites

TABLE 4–9. Complex Pelvic Fractures: Immediate Complications[98, 99]

Complication	Incidence* (%)
Hemorrhage	71 (Required > 10 units blood transfusion)
Associated fractures	65 (Average 2.2/pt)
Neurologic	21
Genitourinary	19
Head	11
Chest	11
Abdomen	11

*Incidence is greater than 100% owing to overlap of complications.

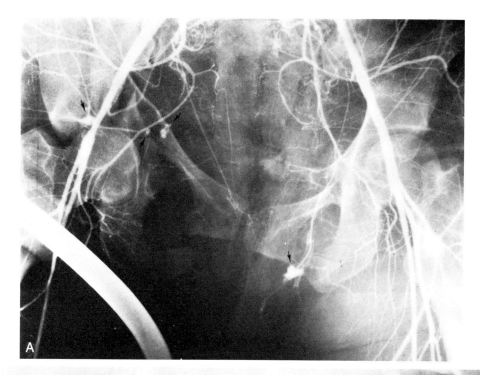

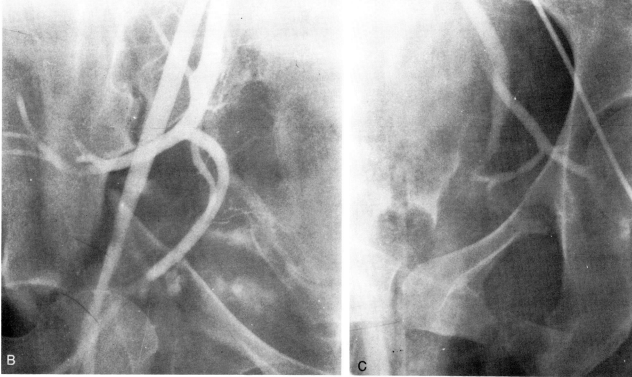

Figure 4–53. Complex pelvic fracture with active pelvic arterial bleeding. Contrast extravasates from the bleeding vessels (A, arrows). Repeat angiograms on the right (B) and left (C) following Gelfoam embolization. The bleeding is now controlled.

have been identified, embolization with autogenous clotting material or Gelfoam will usually control the bleeding.[81, 82, 93, 110] In larger vessels occlusion with inflated balloon catheters may be required.[86, 104] In patients with sacral fractures posterior bleeding sites may present a granular appearance rather than the more easily identifiable extravasation that is usually seen. This must be kept in mind for optimum control of all bleeding sites.[103]

Adjacent or Distant Fractures

The frequency with which additional adjacent or distant fractures occur with pelvic fractures is not

TABLE 4–10. Complex Pelvic Fractures: Associated Skeletal Injury[98, 99]

Location		Fractures
Skull		8
Facial bones		8
Upper extremity		32
Clavicle	4	
Scapula	2	
Humerus	9	
Forearm	15	
Wrist	2	
Chest		24
Ribs	22	
Sternum	2	
Spine		14
Lower extremity		60
Femur	24	
Tibia-fibula	30	
Foot	6	

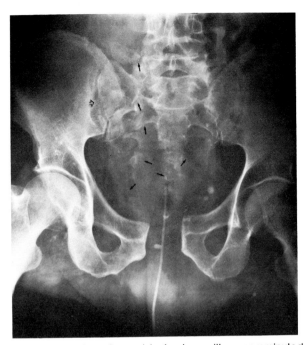

Figure 4–54. Complex pelvic fracture with a comminuted sacral fracture *(black arrows)*. There is also separation of the right sacroiliac joint *(open arrow)* and a fracture of the right transverse process of L5.

surprising. Sixty-five percent of patients with complex pelvic fractures sustained other fractures. The average number of fractures was 2.2 per patient (Table 4–10). As would be expected, lower extremity fractures were especially common.

Neurologic Complications

Neurologic complications are also common (Table 4–11), occurring in 21 percent of patients with complex pelvic injury. Injury to the lumbosacral plexus is especially common if the sacrum is fractured (Fig. 4–54).[49, 87] Sacral fractures were involved in 23 percent of our Class III pelvic fractures. The diagnosis is usually not made initially; rather, the injury is detected during the convalescent period. Leg weakness, incontinence, and impotence may result. Sciatic nerve injuries occurred in 4 percent of our patients.[99]

Injuries to the Genitourinary System

Injuries to the genitourinary system have been reported to occur in 10 to 20 percent of patients with pelvic fractures.[78, 83, 89, 99] Hartmann reported an incidence of 15.5 percent with unilateral pubic rami fractures, but the incidence increased to 41 percent with double anterior fractures.[68] There is no doubt that the incidence of lower urinary tract injury (urethra and bladder) is much higher with displaced fractures of both obturator rings or diastasis of the pubic symphysis. However, evaluation of the genitourinary system is warranted in almost any patient with a pelvic fracture.[95]

Damage to the urethra is the most common injury.[55, 78, 83, 89] The anatomy of the male genitourinary system results in the male urethra being more prone to injury than the female (Fig. 4–10). The prostatic urethra is fixed in the prostate and extends from the bladder neck to the urogenital diaphragm. The membranous urethra lies within the urogenital diaphragm. These two portions of the urethra make up the posterior urethra. The short segment between the prostate and the urogenital diaphragm has been described as the area most susceptible to injury.[55, 100] The anterior urethra (bulbous and cavernous portions) is located below the urogenital diaphragm and is less likely to be injured. The female urethra is short and the urogenital diaphragm less well developed, allowing greater mobility and less susceptibility to injury.

Clinical evaluation of the urethra with rectal examination and assessment of the classic triad of blood at the urethral meatus, inability to void, and bladder distention are useful in proper management of the patient. The radiographic evaluation is essential for complete evaluation of the entire urinary tract. If angiography is necessary (diagnosis and treatment of massive hemorrhage), it should be performed prior to retrograde studies of the urethra and bladder. Contrast medium in the bladder or extravasate in the pelvis will obscure bleeding sites on the angiogram.[101] In patients in whom urethral injury is suspected because of clinical history or

TABLE 4–11. Complex Pelvic Fractures: Neurologic Complications (21% of Patients)[98, 99]

Complication	Incidence (%)
Quadriceps (fem. nerve)	6
Gluteal (sup. & inf. gluteal nerve)	6
Sciatic nerve	4
Dorsiflexors of foot (peroneal nerve)	2
Cord injury	2
Hamstring (sciatic branches)	1

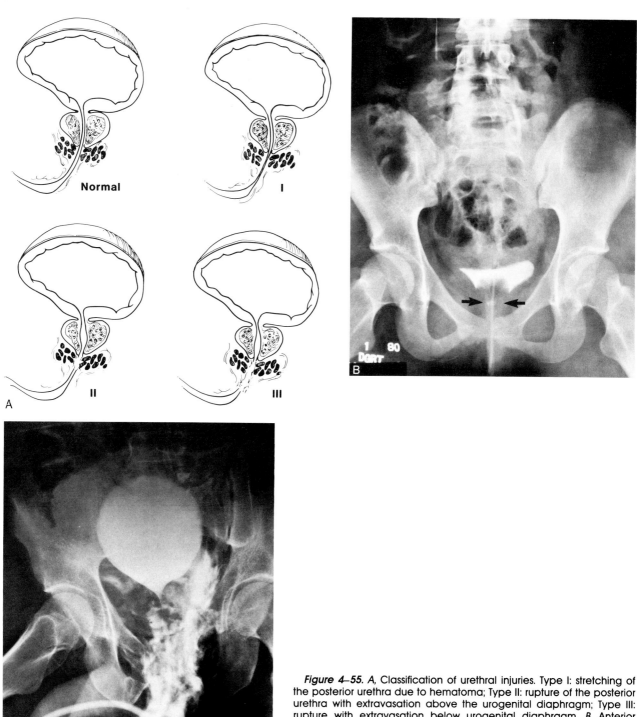

Figure 4–55. A, Classification of urethral injuries. Type I: stretching of the posterior urethra due to hematoma; Type II: rupture of the posterior urethra with extravasation above the urogenital diaphragm; Type III: rupture with extravasation below urogenital diaphragm. *B*, Anterior pelvic fracture with elevation of the bladder, stretching the posterior urethra (Type I). Foley catheter in the bladder. *C*, Type III rupture of the posterior urethra with extravasation of contrast above and below the urogenital diaphragm. There is marked elevation of the bladder due to hematoma.

from radiographic features of the fracture, a retrograde urethrogram must be performed prior to urethral catheterization. This procedure is easily accomplished by placing a Foley catheter in the distal urethra and gently injecting contrast material into the urethra. The procedure should be performed with fluoroscopic guidance if possible. If no defect in the urethra is evident, a Foley catheter can be placed in the bladder and a cystogram performed to exclude the possibility of bladder rupture. It is too difficult to fill the bladder during the urethrogram, and distention with 200 to 300 ml of contrast is required to assess the bladder.[65, 95] Radiographs of the urethra and bladder should be obtained in the AP and oblique positions. Following completion of filming with the bladder distended, the contrast medium should be allowed to drain. This prevents overlooking small tears. At this stage in the examination the excretory urogram can be performed to evaluate the upper urinary tract.

Sandler and colleagues have proposed a classification for urethral injuries based on the patterns of extravasation during retrograde urethrography (Fig. 4–55).[100] Type I injuries involve stretching of the posterior urethra due to hematoma with no actual tear. Type II injuries result from rupture of the posterior urethra just above the urogenital diaphragm (previously considered the most common injury). In Type III injuries the urethra and urogenital diaphragm are ruptured, resulting in extravasation of contrast medium below the urogenital diaphragm. Sandler's results indicated that the Type III injury was in fact the most common and occurred four times as frequently as the Type II injury.[100] This has also been our experience. The incidence of urethral rupture in our cases was 9 percent, with only 1 case of disruption of the female urethra. Additional complications involving these injuries included impotence in 78 percent of males and stricture formation requiring dilatation in 89 percent of male patients. Fistula formation occurred as a late complication of urethral rupture in 1 patient (Fig. 4–56).[98, 99]

Bladder injuries have been reported to be the most common injury of the genitourinary system following pelvic fracture. Injuries include contusions, extraperitoneal rupture, intraperitoneal rupture, and both intra- and extraperitoneal tears.[51] A rupture must be present for bladder injury to be

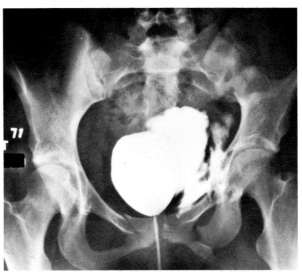

Figure 4–57. Pelvic fracture with extraperitoneal bladder rupture. There is extravasation of contrast material from the left side of the bladder. Contrast remains in the pelvis.

visible on the radiograph. Contusions are more difficult to detect. Rupture of the bladder occurred in only 4 percent of patients. The rupture was extraperitoneal in all cases (Fig. 4–57). The incidence of extraperitoneal rupture is usually 70 to 80 percent.[54] Extraperitoneal rupture is the result of penetration of the bladder by fracture fragments or shearing of the pubovesical ligaments. Intraperitoneal rupture usually results from blunt trauma to the abdomen with a distended bladder (Fig. 4–58). Significant renal trauma (laceration) was noted in 3

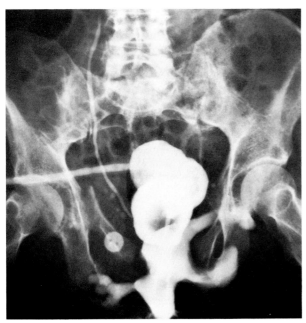

Figure 4–56. Old pelvic fracture. Fistulas have developed around the area of the ruptured urethra. Suprapubic tube in place.

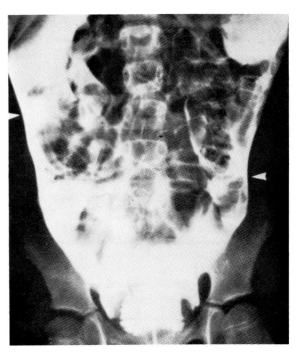

Figure 4–58. Intraperitoneal rupture with contrast outlining loops of bowel (white arrows).

TABLE 4–12. Complex Pelvic Fractures: Genitourinary Complications (19% of Patients)[98, 99]

Kidney	3%
Laceration	
Contusion	
Arteriovenous malformations	
Bladder rupture	4%
Extraperitoneal	
Intraperitoneal	
Urethral rupture	9%
Impotence (78% of urethral ruptures)	
Urethral stricture (89% of urethral ruptures)	
Vaginal laceration	2%
Neurogenic bladder	1%

percent of patients. Table 4–12 summarizes the genitourinary complications that occurred in patients with complex pelvic fractures.

Other injuries related to the genitourinary tract have been reported by Cooke.[57] For example, septic arthritis involving the hip may occur following rupture of the bladder or urethra if the urinary tract is not sterile. This is usually seen with straddle fractures and associated acetabular fractures.[57]

Injuries to the Head, Chest, and Abdomen

Injuries to the head, chest, and abdomen were associated with pelvic fractures in 33 percent of patients, 11 percent in each category (Table 4–9). Significant chest injuries included pneumothorax and rupture of the diaphragm. Ruptured diaphragms have been reported to occur more frequently with Malgaigne fractures.[78]

Abdominal injuries included ruptured liver, spleen, small bowel, and colon, all occurring with an incidence of 2 percent. Intrapelvic rupture of the rectum and anus occurred in 3 patients. This is significant in that infection of the pelvic hematoma and an abscess may result. Actual entrapment of the bowel by pelvic fracture fragments has also been reported.[52] The small bowel is most frequently involved. Injury to the pelvic viscera and open pelvic fractures deserve further discussion owing to the severity of this complication. Perry defines an open fracture as a fracture that communicates with the vagina, rectum, or perineum, or with a cutaneous laceration.[91] Postoperative sites with surgical drains in place should be included in this category. Patients with open pelvic fractures have severe pelvic and extrapelvic injuries, and the mortality rate may be as high as 42 percent.[91] The mechanism of injury also differs somewhat in that the majority of open fractures are the result of motorcycle or pedestrian accidents rather than motor vehicle accidents. Open pelvic fractures have more significant hemorrhage owing to the lack of tamponade normally seen with closed injuries. The incidence of sepsis and renal failure is also significantly increased.[55]

Delayed Complications

Delayed complications are also a significant problem in patients with pelvic fractures (Table 4–13). Such complications occurred in 47 percent of patients with complex pelvic fractures. Adult respiratory distress syndrome (ARDS), pulmonary emboli, and myocardial infarcts were not uncommon (Table 4–13). However, no deaths occurred in our group of patients as a result of these complications.[98, 99]

Long-term orthopedic complications can also occur. For example, leg length discrepancy was evident in 10 percent of our patients with Class III pelvic fractures. These were all patients with double vertical or shearing fracture-dislocations of the Malgaigne type. Other orthopedic problems include instability of the sacroiliac joint and pubic symphysis, avascular necrosis of the femoral head, malunion, and non-union.

DISLOCATIONS AND FRACTURE-DISLOCATIONS OF THE HIP

Dislocations of the hip account for only about 5 percent of all skeletal dislocations.[134] Motor vehicle accidents, motorcycle accidents, and falls from significant heights are responsible for the majority of hip dislocations.[132] These injuries are most frequent in young adults (average age, 31 years in Reigstad's study[132]), with males outnumbering females 3:1. Because of the degree of trauma necessary to cause this injury, severe multiple injuries are found in up to 75 percent of patients.[135] In Rosenthal's series 50 percent of patients were unable to return to their former type of employment.[135] Thus, there is significant economic impact associated with dislocation of the hip.

Dislocations may occur centrally (Fig. 4–48), posteriorly (Fig. 4–59), or anteriorly (Fig. 4–60). Central dislocations have already been discussed in the section of this chapter dealing with pelvic and acetabular fractures. Of the other two types, posterior dislocations are much more common than anterior dislocations.[121, 134, 140] Fractures of the femoral head and acetabulum may be associated with either type of dislocation.[126]

TABLE 4–13. Complex Pelvic Fractures: Delayed Complications (47% of 120 Patients)[98, 99]

Complication		% Patients
ARDS		8
Pulmonary embolus		10
Myocardial infarct		1
Stress ulcers		4
Incontinence		3
Infection		9
Pelvic hematoma	3	
Other	6	
Orthopedic		12
Leg length discrepancy	10	
Avascular necrosis, femoral head	2	

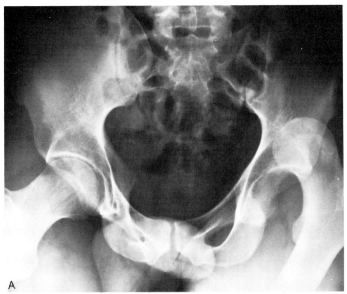 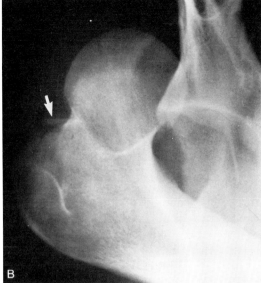

Figure 4–59. Posterior dislocation of the left hip. The AP view *(A)* demonstrates the empty acetabular fossa with the femoral head projected superiorly. The anterior oblique view *(B)* clearly demonstrates the posterior dislocation. There is a small fracture fragment *(arrow)* near the greater trochanter.

Classification of Dislocations and Fracture-Dislocations of the Hip

Posterior Dislocations

Posterior dislocations occur seven to ten times more frequently than anterior dislocations.[121, 134, 140] This injury results when a compressive force is applied to the knee or foot with the hip in the flexed position (for example, striking the knee against the dashboard of a car in a motor vehicle accident).[121] Fractures of the posterior acetabulum are frequently associated with posterior dislocations

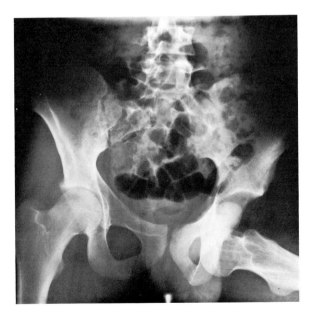

Figure 4–60. Anterior dislocation of the left hip seen on the AP view of the pelvis. The femoral head typically lies over the ischium or obturator foramen.

of the hip. The size of the fragment is dependent upon the position of the femur at the time of injury (Fig. 4–37). If the hip is flexed in a neutral position, a posterior rim fracture may result. With the hip abducted, a larger posterior fragment or comminution is more likely to occur. Adduction may result in a tiny chip fracture or pure dislocation of the hip.

TABLE 4–14. Classifications of Posterior Dislocations of the Hip

Stewart and Milford[139] (1954)

Grade I	Posterior dislocation without an associated fracture
Grade II	Posterior dislocation with a small posterior acetabular rim fracture (Fig. 4–61)
Grade III	Posterior dislocation with a large posterior acetabular fragment (Fig. 4–62)
Grade IV	Posterior dislocation with an associated fracture of the femoral head, neck, or shaft (Fig. 4–63*B* and *C*)

Thompson and Epstein[127, 141] (1974)

Type 1	Posterior dislocation with no fracture or a minor acetabular fracture (Fig. 4–61)
Type 2	Posterior dislocation with a single large acetabular fragment (Fig. 4–62)
Type 3	Posterior dislocation with a comminuted or major acetabular fragment
Type 4	Posterior dislocation with a rim and floor fracture of the acetabulum
Type 5	Posterior dislocation with a fracture of the femoral head with or without other associated fractures (Fig. 4–63)

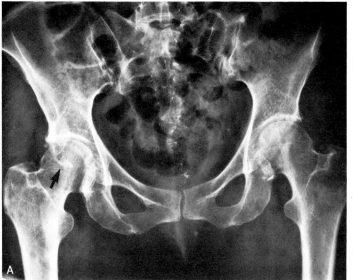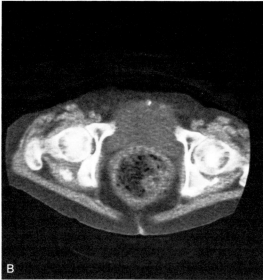

Figure 4–61. Posterior dislocation of the right hip in an elderly patient. Patient experienced continued pain several days following reduction. This was felt to be uncomplicated at the time of reduction. *A,* AP radiograph of pelvis with no evidence of joint widening. There is a density *(arrow)* projected over the femoral head. *B,* CT scan reveals small acetabular fragments bilaterally, larger on the right. Thus this would be classified as Stewart-Milford Grade 2 or Thompson-Epstein Type I.

Clinically, patients with posterior dislocations usually present with four findings: (1) the hip flexed and externally rotated; (2) elevation of the trochanter; (3) a palpable prominence in the gluteal region; (4) bruising of the buttock.[130]

Classifications of posterior dislocations have been devised by Stewart and Milford[139] and Thompson and Epstein (Table 4–14).[127, 141] These classifications are quite similar in many respects. They are both based upon the associated fractures of the acetabulum and femur, and both correlate closely with clinical results and prognosis (Figs. 4–61 and 4–62). Dislocations with more complex acetabular fractures

or femoral head fractures carry a more guarded prognosis compared with simple dislocations or dislocations with minimal acetabular involvement.

Femoral head fractures with posterior dislocations of the hip were once considered rare.[120] Recent advances in imaging techniques and increased awareness of this association, however, have resulted in improved detection of femoral head injuries.[127, 129, 133, 138] The incidence of femoral head fractures with posterior dislocations of the hip is 7 to 10 percent (Fig. 4–63).[129, 133, 138] Fracture of the femoral head occurs more frequently if the hip is flexed less than 90° (especially at about 60°). This forces

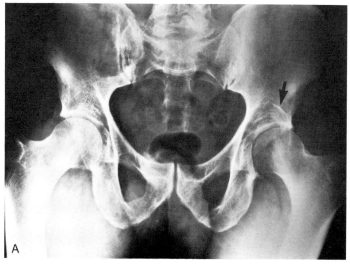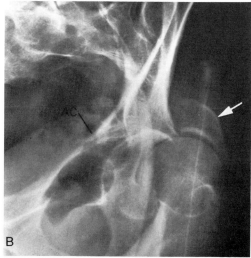

Figure 4–62. Radiographs of patient with hip pain following a motor vehicle accident. *A,* AP view of the pelvis shows widening of the joint spaces on the left with a white cortical line in the region of the acetabulum *(arrow). B,* Judet (anterior oblique) view demonstrates the posterior dislocation with a large posterior acetabular fragment *(arrow).* The femoral head appears intact. This **represents a Stewart-Milford Grade III or Thompson-Epstein Type 2 dislocation.** AC = anterior column.

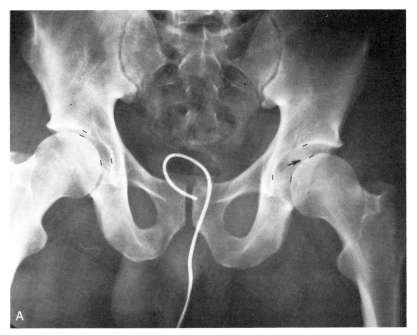

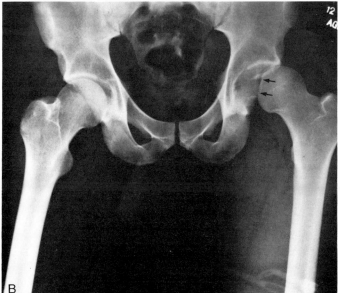
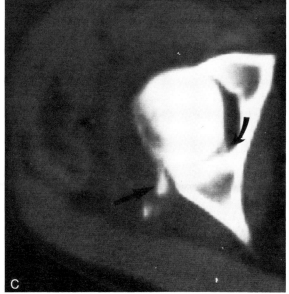

Figure 4–63. Posterior dislocations with intra-articular fragment. *A,* Post-reduction AP film following dislocation of the left hip. The joint space is widened, indicating an intra-articular fragment. Subtle density *(arrow)* appears, but the origin is not clear. *B,* Dislocation with small fragments in the joint space that appear to arise from the flattened area on the femoral head *(arrows).* Stewart-Milford Grade IV or Thompson-Epstein Type 5. *C,* CT scan following reduction of what was thought to be an uncomplicated dislocation. Note the small head fragment in the joint space *(curved arrow)* and small posterior acetabular fragments *(arrow).* In this situation what appeared to be a Grade I or Type 1 dislocation was actually a Stewart-Milford Grade IV or Thompson-Epstein Type 5.

the femoral head against the stronger posterior superior margin of the acetabulum and may result in an osteochondral shearing or impacted fracture.[133]

Identification of intra-articular fragments from the femoral head or the acetabulum is essential in determining the method of treatment. The size, location, and degree of involvement of the weight-bearing surface of the femoral head and acetabulum must be clarified (Fig. 4–63). Pipkin[131] based his classification of femoral head fractures on the rela-

TABLE 4–15. Posterior Dislocations with Associated Femoral Head Fractures: Pipkin Classification[131] (1957)

Type I	Fracture of the femoral head inferior to the fovea
Type II	Fracture of the femoral head cephalad to the fovea
Type III	Either Type I or Type II with an associated femoral neck fracture
Type IV	Type I, II, or III with an associated acetabular fracture

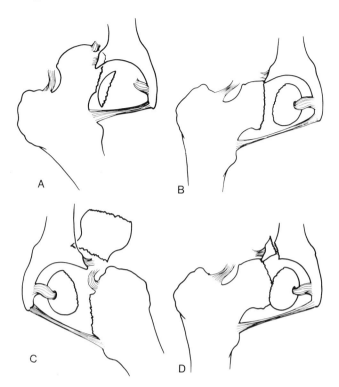

Figure 4–64. Pipkin classification of femoral head fractures. *A,* Type I: Posterior dislocation of femoral head fracture inferior to the fovea. *B,* Type II: Posterior dislocation with femoral head fracture above the fovea. *C,* Type I or II with associated femoral neck fracture. *D,* Types I, II or III with an associated acetabular fracture. (From Roeder, L. F. Jr., and DeLee, J. C.: Femoral head fractures associated with posterior hip dislocations. Clin. Orthop. *147*: 121, 1980.)

tionship of the fracture to the fovea and the presence or absence of associated acetabular or femoral neck fractures (Table 4–15) (Fig. 4–64). Femoral neck fractures associated with posterior dislocations are particularly troublesome and may interfere with reduction.[131]

Anterior Dislocations

Anterior dislocations (Fig. 4–60) account for 13 to 18 percent of hip dislocations.[123, 128, 134, 140] This injury results from forced abduction and external rotation of the hip. The neck or greater trochanter impinges on the acetabulum and forces the femoral head to dislocate in an anterior inferior direction.[121] The type of dislocation is often described by the position of the femoral head on the AP radiograph of the pelvis and hips. With the hip in extension the head may overlie the pubis or ilium. In flexion the head is seen over the obturator foramen. This is the most common presentation.[123, 124]

Fractures of the femoral head occur frequently with anterior dislocations of the hip (Fig. 4–65). Dussault[124] reported femoral head fractures in 8 of 11 anterior dislocations, and DeLee[123] noted associated femoral head fractures in 17 of 22. Shearing fractures of the femoral head may result as the femoral head passes the inferior acetabulum. Impaction fractures of the posterior superior and lateral aspect of the head have an appearance similar to a Hill-Sachs defect (Fig. 4–66). This defect may be seen on the AP view if the hip is properly positioned (15° of internal rotation).[124] The lesion occurs when the head impinges on the anterior inferior acetabulum during the dislocation.[124] The degree of impaction is significant. DeLee reported

an increased incidence of osteoarthritis if the depression exceeded 4 mm.[123] Tomography may be helpful in evaluating the degree of impaction of these fractures (Fig. 4–66C). Fractures of the anterior inferior margin of the acetabulum have also been described (3 of 11 cases in Dussault's series.)[124]

Radiographic Evaluation of Dislocations and Fracture-Dislocations of the Hip

In the severely injured patient the AP view of the pelvis and hips may be all that is possible. The patient's condition and the urgency of attending to

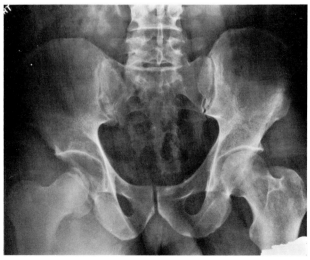

Figure 4–65. AP view of the pelvis following anterior fracture and dislocation of the right hip. There are multiple femoral head fragments.

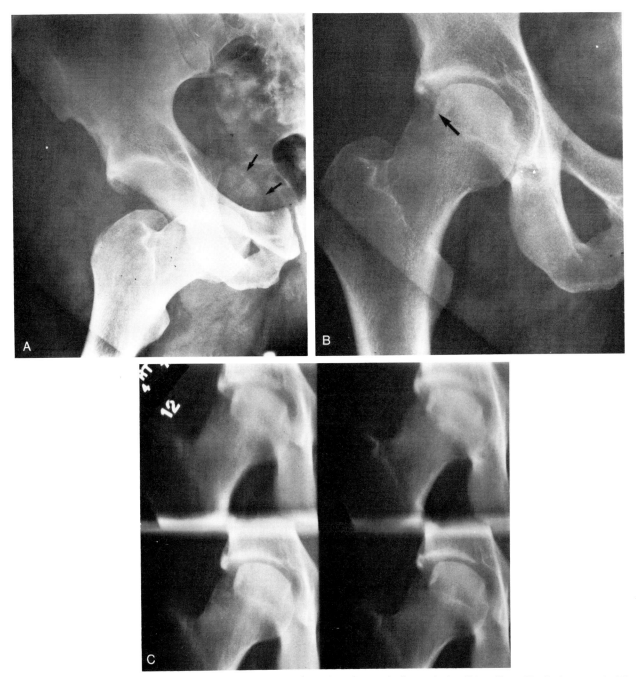

Figure 4–66. Anterior dislocation of the right hip. *A*, Iliac oblique view demonstrating anterior dislocation with displacement of the obturator fat stripe *(arrows)*. *B*, AP view of the right hip after reduction. There is an osteochondral impaction on the superior lateral aspect of the femoral head *(arrow)*. *C*, AP tomograms demonstrate the defect in the head more clearly.

severe hemorrhage or head injuries may also result in inadequate examination of the hips. Despite these difficulties, a thorough examination of this single view can yield significant information and assist in determining which additional studies may be most helpful.

Most complete dislocations are obvious on the AP view. The femoral head lies superior and lateral to the acetabulum following posterior dislocation (Fig. 4–59). The femoral head is usually projected over the obturator foramen when anterior disloca-

tion has occurred (Fig. 4–60). Careful attention to detail is necessary in more subtle injuries and in evaluation of associated injury. Shenton's line may be interrupted on the involved side and may be one of the only clues for detection of subluxation or a subtle dislocation. The joint spaces should be compared. An increase in the joint space of more than 2 mm compared with the normal side should indicate the possibility of intra-articular fracture fragments or soft tissue interposition (Fig. 4–63). This is particularly important following reduction

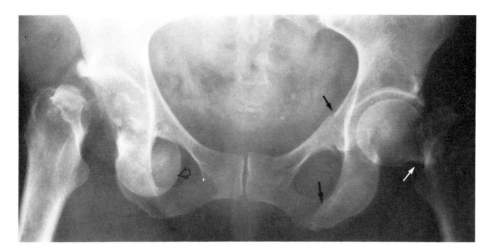

Figure 4–67. AP view of the pelvis following high-velocity motor vehicle accident demonstrates bilateral femoral neck fractures with anterior dislocation of the right femoral head *(open arrow)*. Pubic ramus fractures on the left *(arrows)*.

of a dislocation.[138] With the hip removed from the acetabulum, bone fragments may be evident in the region of the joint space. These should be carefully evaluated for position changes following reduction. The femoral head should maintain its normal smooth configuration with uniform density. Impacted or displaced osteochondral fractures will alter the surface configuration (Figs. 4–63*B* and 4–66). Density differences may indicate an overlying fracture fragment (Fig. 4–61). Fractures of the femoral neck may also be associated with anterior dislocations (Fig. 4–67).

Ideally, oblique views of the hip (Judet views) should always be obtained (Table 4–16). Also, because of the mechanism of injury, it is essential that the femur and knee on the involved side be examined to exclude associated fractures. Unfortunately, fractures of the ipsilateral knee and femur, though uncommon, often mask the hip dislocation. As a result, the pelvis is not radiographed or is less than thoroughly evaluated.[122, 125]

Femoral head fractures are often seen on the AP view when associated with anterior dislocations. They appear as depressed defects on the superior lateral margin.[124] However, identification of fragments in the joint space and evaluation of both the acetabular margins and the weight-bearing surface of the femoral head are best accomplished with tomography or computed tomography. The latter is much more informative. In certain cases, moving the patient to the CT scanner is not desirable, and in these cases we have used conventional tomography on the Versigraph. Axial tomograms can also be obtained with the Versigraph. Though the detail does not match that obtained with CT, the information gained can be of great value. Complete evaluation is essential to proper treatment. Smith and Loop have shown that over 70 percent of their initial classifications were incorrect when based on initial radiographic studies.[138] Tomography and computed tomography greatly reduce these errors. Detection of unsuspected intra-articular fragments

TABLE 4–16. Fracture-Dislocations of the Hip: Pre- and Post-Reduction Radiographic Evaluation

A. Initial evaluation
    1. AP pelvis and oblique views
    2. Femur and lower extremity views
       as indicated

B. Following closed reduction

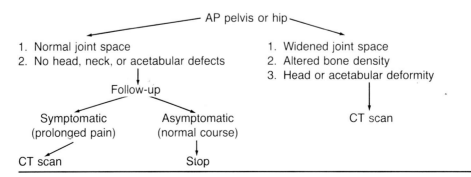

is especially important, as open reduction is often indicated.[126, 133] Table 4–16 summarizes the radiographic approach to fracture-dislocations of the hip.

Treatment of Dislocations and Fracture-Dislocations of the Hip

If the hip dislocates and no fracture is detected through careful radiographic study, including analysis of oblique views, then the matter is relatively simple. Reduction should be accomplished as soon as possible. The incidence of avascular necrosis is high if the hip remains dislocated for more than 12 hours. Reduction usually requires an anesthetic. The reduction should be checked for stability, with the hip in 90° of flexion and posterior forces placed on the femur. If it is stable, the patient can be put in traction. After the acute pain subsides, mobili-

zation can begin with partial weight bearing. There seems to be little evidence to justify a long period on crutches. Crutches should be used only until the pain subsides. Then gradual resumption of normal activities should begin. Subsequent degenerative arthritis is rare if there has been no fracture of either the head or the acetabulum.

If the dislocated femoral head is accompanied by a fracture, the fracture may involve the head itself, the acetabulum, or the femoral neck. The femoral head is usually involved in a shear type of fracture (Fig. 4–68). Open reduction is indicated if more than one third of the head is involved or if a fragment is interposed between the head and acetabulum. If the fracture fragment is relatively small and lies inferiorly in the "axilla" of the hip, traction and early ambulation is all that need be done. These small fragments need not be removed if they do not lie between the femoral head and acetabulum.

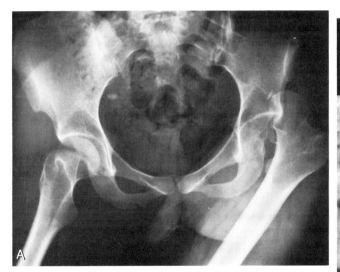
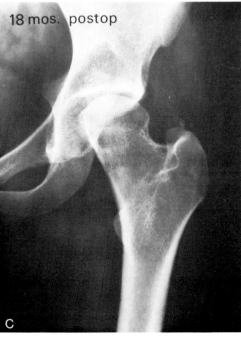
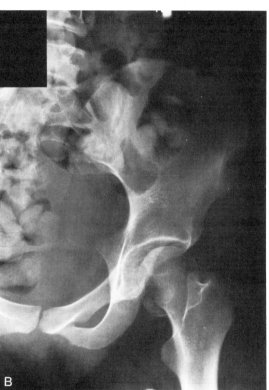

Figure 4–68. Radiographs of a 23-year-old female with multiple lacerations and head injury following motor vehicle accident. *A,* AP view of the pelvis with shearing fracture of the femoral head and posterior dislocation of the hip. *B,* Following reduction the femoral fragments are inferior. The head is slightly lateral in the acetabulum. *C,* Radiograph 18 months following open reduction and removal of three osteochondral fragments. There is deformity of the head and early avascular necrosis.

Larger fragments can be returned to their bed in the femoral head and held with a screw. If this is not possible, they must be removed.

If the fracture accompanying the dislocation involves the acetabulum and not the head, small posterior fragments can be neglected, provided that the hip is stable. If there is instability, which implies a larger posterior fragment, then open reduction and internal fixation of the fragment is necessary (see Fig. 4–62). The head can be inspected at this time for obvious injury to the cartilage, but primary arthroplasty is seldom necessary with these types of fractures. If the acetabular fragment is large or central, it should be treated with open reduction and internal fixation, as described for Class IV pelvic fractures. As in fractures of the femoral head, acetabular fractures accompanied by dislocation may lead to degenerative arthritis at a later date. Sciatic nerve palsy may accompany the fracture-dislocation. The nerve should be inspected if open reduction is performed.

If the fracture-dislocation is accompanied by a fracture of the femoral neck, treatment is a much more complicated problem (Fig. 4–67). All acetabular fragments must be reduced and internally secured; in addition, the femoral neck fracture must be reduced and secured by primary internal fixation. If reduction and stable fixation is not possible, then a primary endoprosthesis (either one-piece or bipolar) should be inserted at the time of the open reduction.

Complications of Dislocations and Fracture-Dislocations of the Hip

Regardless of the type of dislocation, it is important to obtain early reduction (i.e., within 24 hours).[121, 134] Delay in reduction leads to an increase in the complication rate, particularly with regard to avascular necrosis (Table 4–17). The incidence of avascular necrosis is reported to be 5 to 26 percent.[121, 134] Results are uniformly poor if reduction is delayed beyond 48 hours.[119] Though the incidence of avascular necrosis is highest in more severe injuries, avascular necrosis occurs in children even with Grade I dislocations (Stewart and Milford classification).[133] The incidence is reported to be lower

TABLE 4–17. Complications of Fracture-Dislocations of the Hip

Common complications
    Osteoarthritis
    Avascular necrosis of the femoral head
    Sciatic nerve injury
    Associated fractures
Uncommon complications
    Infection
    Myositis ossificans
    Redislocation
    Thrombophlebitis
    Pulmonary embolus

(8 percent) in patients with anterior dislocations.[119] Incidence also varies with the method of treatment. Clawson reported avascular necrosis in 15.5 percent of patients following closed reduction and in 40 percent of patients following open reduction.[121] One must keep in mind that patients requiring open reduction usually have more significant injuries. The average time of appearance for avascular necrosis is 17 months following injury; however, it may develop even later.[121, 133]

The sciatic nerve (especially the peroneal portion) is susceptible to injury with posterior dislocations owing to its relationship to the posterior acetabulum and femoral head. The incidence of injury with posterior dislocations is reported to be 10 to 17 percent.[121, 123, 134] Significant sciatic nerve injury usually indicates prompt surgical reduction of the dislocation.[118, 126] Epstein indicated that the internal rotation of the hip normally associated with posterior dislocation caused stretching of the sciatic nerve and was an important factor in producing the injury.[128]

Fractures associated with dislocations of the hip are common owing to the severity of trauma necessary to cause the primary lesion. Associated fractures of the adjacent femur are of particular importance, as they may result in the dislocation being overlooked.[122, 125] Femoral shaft fractures mask the clinical signs of dislocation. Rosenthal reported ipsilateral fractures of the femur (4 percent) and patella (4 percent).[135] The hip injury was unrecognized initially in all patients with femoral shaft fractures. Roeder reported major associated injuries in over 75 percent of the patients in his study.[133] These injuries included (1) lower extremity fractures, (2) craniofacial trauma, (3) upper extremity trauma, (4) chest injury.

Rosenthal also reported an 11 percent incidence of abdominal injury (ruptured spleen and liver laceration) requiring laparotomy.[135]

Arthritis may be the most common complication and may develop as late as 15 years after the injury.[120, 121, 128, 133] Epstein reported post-traumatic arthritis in 23 percent of patients.[128] The incidence of arthritis increased to 35 percent in patients with closed reductions compared with 17 percent in the case of open reductions. The incidence of arthritic complications also strongly depends on the patient's weight and activity. The complication is more common in patients with acetabular fractures or fractures involving the weight-bearing surface of the femoral head.[133, 142]

Less common complications include infection, myositis ossificans, and redislocation.[133, 135] Thrombophlebitis and pulmonary embolus have also been noted during the initial hospitalization phase.[121, 135]

FEMORAL NECK FRACTURES

Femoral neck fractures occur predominantly in the elderly and are more common in females than

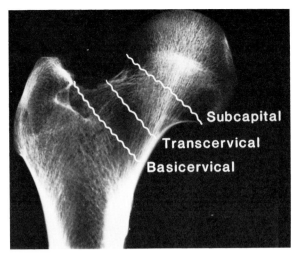

Figure 4-69. Femoral specimen demonstrating the location of common femoral neck fractures.

TABLE 4-18. Classifications of Femoral Neck Fractures

Pauwell[164] (1935)

Type I	Femoral neck fracture with an angle of 30° or less
Type II	Femoral neck fracture with an angle of between 30° and 70°
Type III	Femoral neck fracture with an angle greater than 70°

Garden[155, 156] (1974)

Stage I	Incomplete fracture of the femoral neck with no displacement of the medial trabeculae
Stage II	Complete fracture of the femoral neck with no displacement of the medial trabeculae
Stage III	Complete fracture of the femoral neck with varus angulation and displacement of the medial trabeculae
Stage IV	Complete fracture with the femoral head in normal position; the trabeculae are interrupted but maintain normal alignment

in males. The femoral neck is frequently demineralized in this patient population. Thus, neck fractures have been considered pathologic.[173] Bone mineral analysis clearly demonstrates decreased mineralization in females over 65 years of age.[153] Spontaneous fatigue fractures have also been described.[160]

The fracture usually occurs following minimal trauma. The following theories have been proposed to explain how this fracture occurs: (1) it may follow direct trauma from a fall; (2) a microfracture may become complete with minor trauma (microfractures are present in osteoporotic bone and result from chronic stress); (3) the fracture may derive from rotational forces during a fall.[157, 173]

Classification of Femoral Neck Fractures

Fractures of the femoral neck may be subcapital (most common), transcervical, or basilar (Fig. 4–69). Fractures may be complete or incomplete. Stress fractures are common in young athletes and in patients with metabolic bone disease.[150, 173] These will be discussed in Chapter 15.

Various classifications have been established for femoral neck fractures (Table 4–18). Pauwell's classification[164, 169] was based on the angle of the fracture (Fig. 4–70). Type 1 fractures formed an angle of 30° or less, Type 2 fractures formed an angle of between 30° and 70°, and Type 3 fractures formed an angle of greater than 70°.[169] Fractures that are more horizontal (Type 1) tend to impact, which imparts some degree of stability and enhances healing. If the fracture is more vertical (Type 3), the weight-bearing forces will tend to cause varus shearing, and instability will result.[155, 169] Garden stated that the angle described by Pauwell is based on the radiographic angle of the fracture.[156] The angle is more applicable following reduction.

Garden's classification is more commonly used (Table 4–18). This classification is based upon whether stable reduction can be achieved or whether instability will occur following reduction.[155] Four stages of fracture were described, with nonunion and instability confined to Stage III and IV fractures. Stage I fractures are incomplete, with valgus positioning of the femoral neck (see Fig. 4–73). Stage II fractures are complete, but the medial trabecular pattern is not displaced (see Fig. 4–74). Stage III fractures are complete with varus angulation, and the medial trabeculae are also displaced (see Fig. 4–76). Stage IV fractures are completely displaced, and the femoral head fragment returns to its normal position in the acetabulum. The medial trabeculae are disrupted and displaced but maintain their normal angulation.

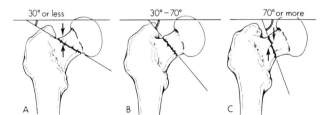

Figure 4-70. Diagram of femoral neck fractures based on Pauwell's classification. A, Class I: Fracture line is 30° or less from vertical. B, Class II: Fracture line is between 30° and 70°. C, Class III: Fracture line is greater than 70°. (From Schultz, R. J.: The Language of Fractures. © 1972, The Williams & Wilkins Co., Baltimore.)

Radiographic Evaluation of Femoral Neck Fractures

The trabecular pattern should be carefully evaluated on the AP view. The margins of the femoral

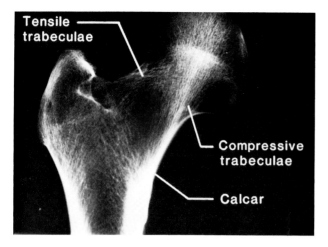

Figure 4–71. Specimen radiograph of the upper femur demonstrating the trabeculae in the femoral neck.

neck and junction with the head are also important (Fig. 4–71). If degenerative lipping is present, a line may project over the neck, mimicking a fracture. On the oblique view (Fig. 4–72) care must be taken not to mistake the cortical margin of the greater trochanter for a fracture.

Incomplete fractures (Garden Stage I, Fig. 4–73), stress fractures, and subtle undisplaced fractures (Garden Stage II, Fig. 4–74) require multiple views, tomography, and occasionally isotope studies (Fig. 4–75) for diagnosis and accurate classification. Isotope scans are positive in 80 percent of patients within 24 hours and positive in 95 percent after 72 hours. Isotope studies provide a means for earlier detection of stress fractures than routine radiographs (see Skeletal Scintigraphy section in Chapter 1). Computed tomography is of little value in undisplaced horizontal fractures. This type of fracture may be missed with CT, and in any case the above modalities are adequate. The more complex fractures (Garden Stage III and IV) can be classified on the AP view, but at least one additional view

(preferably the lateral view) is required for complete evaluation (Fig. 4–76).

Treatment of Femoral Neck Fractures

The treatment of femoral neck fractures depends on many factors, the most important being whether the fracture is stable or unstable. An initially stable fracture would include stress or fatigue fractures and Garden Stage I and most Garden Stage II fractures. Unstable fractures would include Garden Stage III and IV. This division into stable or unstable fractures classifies the fracture at the time of its occurrence or at least at the time of its treatment; it does not classify the fracture after treatment. Unless an unstable fracture is stabilized in the course of treatment, it will remain unstable and thus require a form of treatment different from that applied to the stable fracture. The stable fracture will either remain stable after injury or will tend to become unstable because of stresses placed upon it.

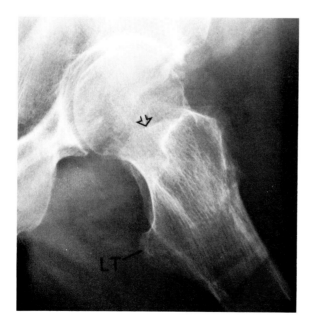

Figure 4–72. Oblique view of the hip. The greater trochanter (open arrow) overlies the femoral neck and should not be mistaken for a fracture. LT: lesser trochanter.

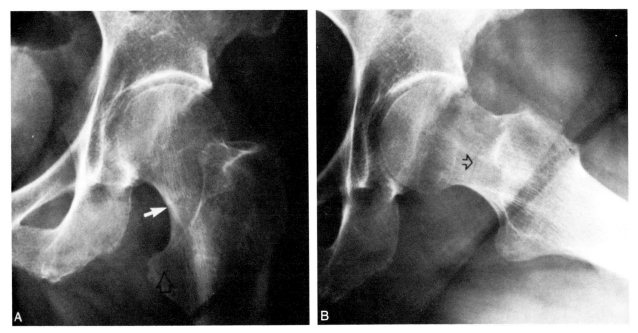

Figure 4–73. Radiographs of an elderly female with left hip pain. *A,* AP view demonstrates subtle lucent line through the medial trabeculae *(white arrow)* and slight external rotation *(open arrow)* on lesser trochanter. *B,* The oblique view clearly demonstrates the undisplaced fracture (Garden Stage I).

Over the years controversy has centered on whether an impacted fracture, or even a stress fracture, should be internally fixed or whether it can be treated without surgery. The definition of exactly what constitutes an impacted fracture has further confused the issue. A strict definition would make the impacted fracture one that is undisplaced but complete, which allows the patient to walk and to raise the limb unaided while lying in the supine position (Figs. 4–77 and 4–78). Hanson and Solgaard used a slightly more liberal definition.[158] Their definition of impacted fractures included both subcapital and transverse cervical fractures that showed some displacement but which were still basically impacted. They further defined the fracture as one in which the patient could raise the straight leg 2 days after the injury. They found that 80 percent of these healed without any intervention. They al-

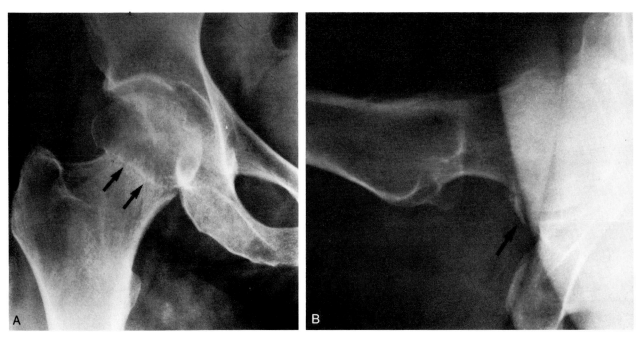

Figure 4–74. Radiographs of an elderly female with Garden Stage II fracture. *A,* AP view demonstrates a complete fracture *(arrows)* with no change in the medial trabeculae. *B,* The lateral view demonstrates comminution of the posterior cortex *(arrow).*

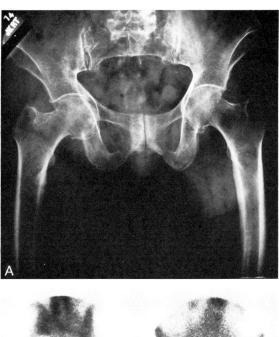

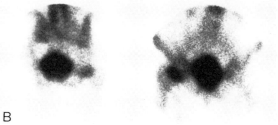

Figure 4–75. Femoral neck fracture in an elderly female with hip pain following a fall. *A,* AP view of the pelvis and hip is negative. Tomogram and oblique views were also normal. *B,* 99-MTC scan demonstrates a femoral neck fracture on the right.

lowed walking with aids from the onset. Eight of their 42 patients did show some secondary displacement, and most of these required operation. Meyers[161] on the other hand, feels, as do most orthopedists, that all fractures should be secured with pins to insure against such impacting. These two views represent the present thinking among orthopedists. However, if the impacted fracture

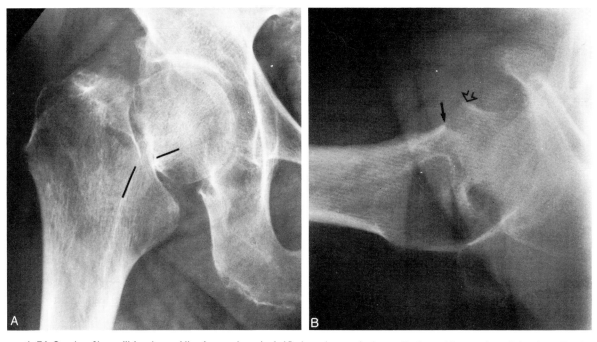

Figure 4–76. Garden Stage III fracture of the femoral neck. *A,* AP view demonstrates a displaced femoral neck fracture. The femoral head is rotated and the trabecular pattern *(black lines)* malaligned. *B,* The lateral view demonstrates the position of the distal *(black arrow)* and proximal *(open arrow)* cortical margin.

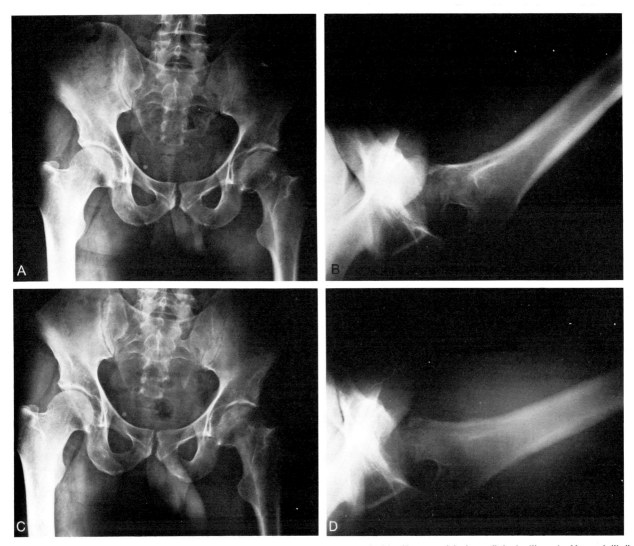

Figure 4–77. Radiographs of a 44-year-old farmer who fell off haybaler onto hip. He was able to walk but with pain. X-rays initially read negative but subsequently showed impacted subcapital fracture of the left femoral neck. *A* and *B,* AP x-ray. *C,* AP view 4 months later. Patient was treated nonsurgically, and fracture healed. *D,* Lateral x-ray appearance.

disimpacts and loses position, it can be treated with an endoprosthesis or even with reduction and internal fixation. Thus, perhaps internal fixation of this fracture is not truly necessary. In our series of 23 impacted fractures, defined according to the more strict criteria, only one became disimpacted. These patients were not given a general anesthetic or subjected to an open operation with its minimal but definite risks. Nor is there any advantage in treating an impacted fracture with prolonged bed rest, as advocated by some. If the fracture is truly impacted, the patient should be able to move about with partial weight-bearing any time after the injury, taking care only to avoid rotational forces or a subsequent fall (which is not likely in this group of patients).

Controversy also surrounds treatment of unstable femoral neck fractures, as in the case of Garden Stage III and IV fractures. Debate centers on whether these fractures should be reduced and

internally fixed or whether the femoral head should be replaced with an endoprosthesis. Many series have been reported comparing the two methods. All agree that a well-reduced, united femoral head is better for the patient than a prosthesis. However, a stable, anatomic reduction with secure internal fixation is not easily obtained, especially in Garden Stage IV types or in the patient with osteoporosis. In the old person who is less active (with age 70 as a criterion), primary femoral head replacement continues to be the more commonly used method for unstable fractures. Söreide and colleagues found that patients who had endoprosthestic replacement fared better at 1 year than those treated with internal fixation.[172]

Sikorski and Barrington compared the Thompson prosthesis with closed reduction and internal fixation achieved by two crossed Garden screws.[170] They too found that the end results were better with the use of endoprostheses, with less overall

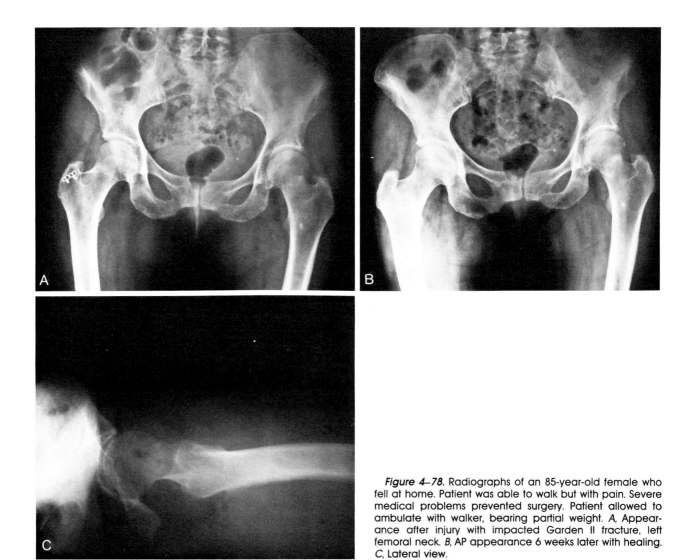

Figure 4–78. Radiographs of an 85-year-old female who fell at home. Patient was able to walk but with pain. Severe medical problems prevented surgery. Patient allowed to ambulate with walker, bearing partial weight. *A,* Appearance after injury with impacted Garden II fracture, left femoral neck. *B,* AP appearance 6 weeks later with healing. *C,* Lateral view.

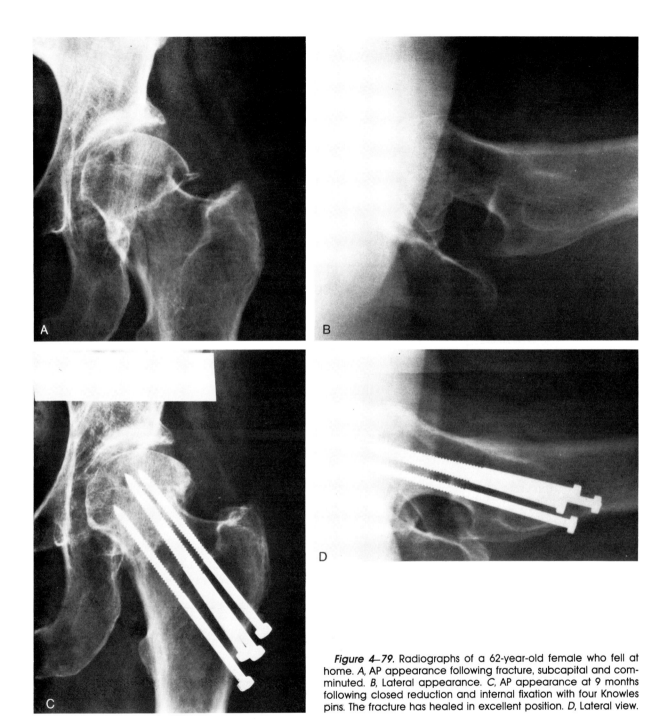

Figure 4–79. Radiographs of a 62-year-old female who fell at home. *A,* AP appearance following fracture, subcapital and comminuted. *B,* Lateral appearance. *C,* AP appearance at 9 months following closed reduction and internal fixation with four Knowles pins. The fracture has healed in excellent position. *D,* Lateral view.

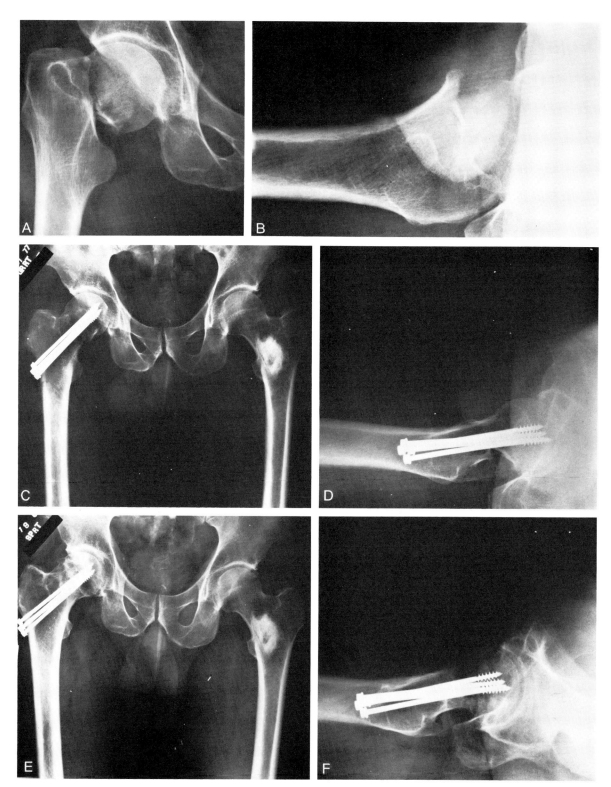

Figure 4–80. Radiographs of a 49-year-old male who fell 15 feet while working on a scaffold. Patient suffered a transcervical fracture of the right femoral neck with complete displacement. Closed reduction and internal fixation with four Knowles pins. *A* and *B,* AP and lateral views before reduction. *C* and *D,* AP and lateral appearance following closed reduction and internal fixation. *E* and *F,* AP and lateral views 6 years following fracture. Minimal early degenerative changes and avascular necrosis. The osteoblastic lesion in the left intertrochanteric area has remained unchanged, producing no symptoms. It probably represents an ossified chondroma.

complications. Their patients, however, were all over 70. Our present feeling is that unstable fractures in this older, less active age group are better treated with the endoprosthetic replacement, both in the immediate and long-term time frame. But in the younger patient, or at least in the more physically active patient, pin fixation is preferable if it can secure stable anatomic reduction.

In addition, there are certain patients who might profit from primary total hip arthroplasty rather than endoprosthetic replacement. Coats and Armour have outlined their limited indications for total hip replacement in the patient with a femoral neck fracture.[151] One candidate is the rare patient who has degenerative arthritis prior to the fracture of the femoral neck. In this case total hip arthro-

plasty is indicated if stable reduction and internal fixation cannot be obtained. Coats and Armour believe that the more active, younger patient may be a candidate for total hip arthroplasty rather than endoprosthesis if operative intervention is necessary because stable reduction cannot be obtained.

If internal fixation is used, multiple parallel pins (at least four in number, which are threaded into the proximal fragment, and with a smooth shaft distally) is preferred today rather than heavy screws, Smith-Petersen nails, and so forth (Figs. 4–79 and 4–80). Rubin and colleagues found pins to be fully effective in their laboratory studies. Their next preference was a sliding screw-plate. The sliding screw-plate will securely hold the fracture, does not cause undue trauma during insertion, supplies

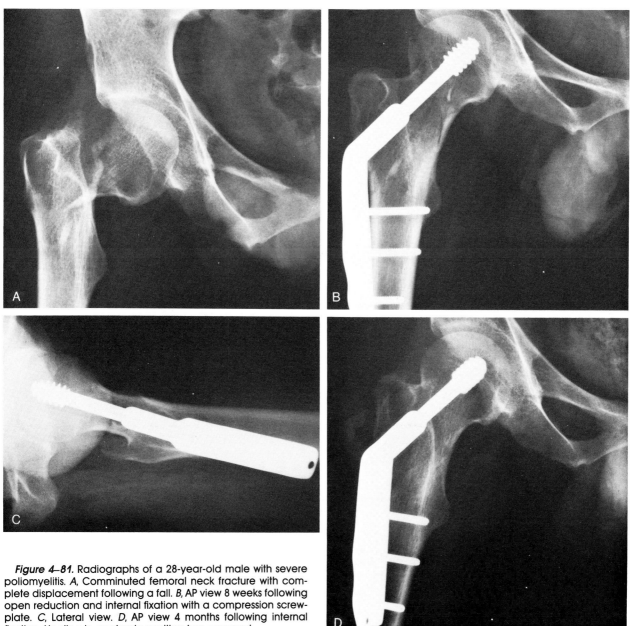

Figure 4–81. Radiographs of a 28-year-old male with severe poliomyelitis. *A,* Comminuted femoral neck fracture with complete displacement following a fall. *B,* AP view 8 weeks following open reduction and internal fixation with a compression screw-plate. *C,* Lateral view. *D,* AP view 4 months following internal fixation. Healing in anatomic position has occurred.

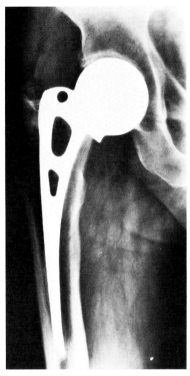

Figure 4–82. Radiograph of a 43-year-old male with alcoholic avascular necrosis. Original Moore prosthesis 11 years after insertion. Note sclerosis (stress concentration) at tip of prosthesis. Patient is symptomless and there is no sign of motion of the prosthesis in the femur.

compression, and allows for slight absorption at the fracture site without holding the fracture apart (Fig. 4–81).

Types of endoprostheses are also controversial at this time. Should a prosthesis be cemented or not?

The Thompson prosthesis is usually cemented. The classic Moore type should not be cemented because of its fine fenestrations. Recent Moore prostheses are available without fenestrations, however, and various stem sizes are available to fit the intramedullary canal better if a press-fit rather than cementing is desired (Figs. 4–82 and 4–83). Again, should a prosthesis be bipolar, the so-called articulated endoprosthesis (Fig. 4–84), to decrease wear and load stresses on the acetabular cartilage? These matters have not been completely resolved. Finally, porous-coated prostheses are appealing in that they allow bony ingrowth. What will their place be in the management of femoral neck fractures?

Complications of Femoral Neck Fractures

Complications of femoral neck fractures depend in part on whether they are intracapsular or extracapsular, whether they are comminuted, whether they are stable or unstable, and of course, very importantly, whether the circulation to the femoral head has been impaired.

Avascular necrosis is the most significant problem following subcapital fractures. The incidence approaches 24 percent.[148] Barnes reported a higher incidence in females (24 percent) than in males (15 percent).[147] This complication most commonly occurs following Garden Stage III and IV fractures.[143]

Blood is supplied to the femoral head through the retinacular artery, which ends as the lateral epiphyseal artery (Fig. 4–85). Further vascular supply is derived from the medial epiphyseal artery, a branch of the inferior retinacular artery. Arterial damage is increased with rotation and displacement

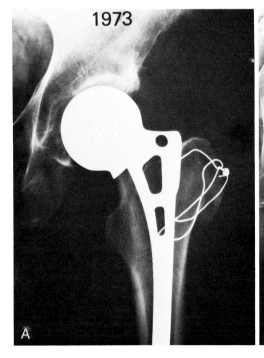

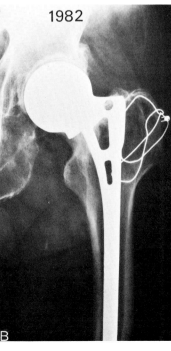

Figure 4–83. Radiographs of a 62-year-old male. Straight-stem Moore prosthesis for avascular necrosis. *A,* AP appearance 8 weeks after insertion of endoprosthesis. *B,* AP view 9 years after surgery. There has been some adaptive sclerosis at the medial femoral neck and calcar and some thinning of the acetabular cartilage but no evidence of loosening and no pain.

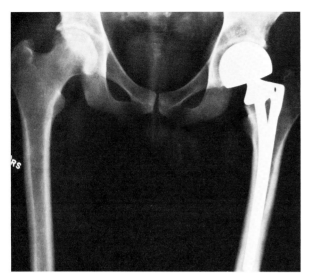

Figure 4–84. A Bateman-type bipolar endoprosthesis in a 48-year-old male.

of the fracture fragments.[147] Poor contact, unstable reduction, and disruption of the retinacular vessels are the most significant factors leading to avascular necrosis. Arnoldi noted sufficient vascular supply to the femoral head from the foveal artery in only 4 percent of patients.[144]

The average onset is 9 to 12 months following the fracture.[148] Changes may occur in 3 to 5 months or as late as 3 years following the injury. Meyers has taken the important step of performing technetium scans on all femoral neck fractures and has reported 34 undisplaced or impacted fractures with technetium scans performed within 48 hours of admission.[161] He concluded that if the scan shows an absence of circulation in the femoral head (as it did in 3 of his patients), then a primary muscle pedicle graft should be used in addition to an *in situ* pinning of the fracture. With this limited experience he has so far been able to prevent late

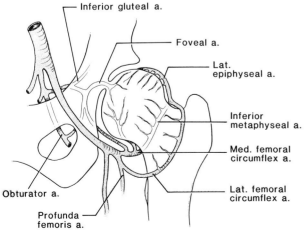

Figure 4–85. Diagram of blood supply to the femoral head.

TABLE 4–19. Stages of Avascular Necrosis (After Ficat[154])	
I	Normal radiograph; positive isotope scan
II	Abnormal radiograph with altered densities in the femoral head; positive isotope scan
III	Early collapse; sequestra formation
IV	Severe collapse and degenerative arthritis

segmental collapse. Certainly scanning is helpful in diagnosing avascular necrosis.

Ficat[154] has defined the stages of avascular necrosis (Table 4–19). Initially the radiograph is negative and the technetium scan positive. The earliest radiographic finding is increased density of the femoral head (Stage II).[147] This may occur as early as 3 months or as late as 36 months, with the average time of appearance 10 months. With early ambulation and more aggressive therapy the density difference may be less obvious. Previously the density of the head was thought to result from disuse osteoporosis, which caused the neck to appear less dense than the femoral head.[147, 149] However, the frequent use of a prosthesis in patients with femoral neck fractures has provided a greater pathologic correlation with the radiographic changes. De Haas[152] and Phemister[165] stated that the increased density of the femoral head is due to appositional new bone formation on the necrotic trabeculae. If necrotic bone does not lose calcium, the addition of new bone would increase the density. Bobechko studied pathologic changes in rabbit femurs and correlated them with the radiographic appearance.[149] His findings confirmed the statements of De Haas and Phemister. The increased density of the femoral head is due to reossification and not to increasing necrosis.

Structural collapse of the femoral head (Stage III) results in irregularity of the head. This occurs as early as 5 months and as late as 24 months following the injury. This is the most common sign of avascular necrosis.[148] Early radiographic changes consist of a subchondral lucency (the crescent sign, Fig. 4–86).[163] This is often best seen on the oblique view of the hip.

Early diagnosis and prereduction prediction of avascular necrosis would be helpful in determining which patients may require total hip arthroplasty. Isotope studies have met with some success, and magnetic resonance imaging shows early promise in the detection of avascular necrosis (Fig. 4–86).[161, 162]

Treatment of Stage I and II fractures has traditionally relied upon a watch and wait approach. Not all cases progress, but most do; and Ficat[154] and Hungerford[159] have encouraged core decompression in this group. Bonfiglio continues to treat these patients with drilling and bone grafting.[171] Owing to shear fractures of the bone underlying the carti-

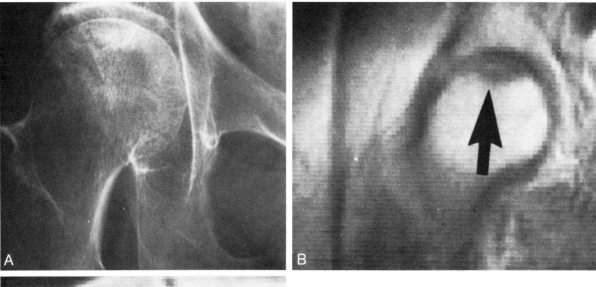

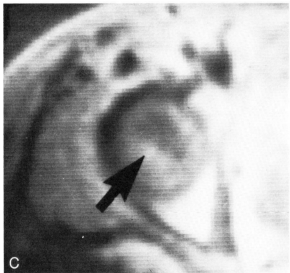

Figure 4–86. AP radiograph *(A)* demonstrating subchondral lucency and sclerosis due to avascular necrosis. The coronal *(B)* and axial *(C)* MRI images demonstrate classic avascular necrosis.

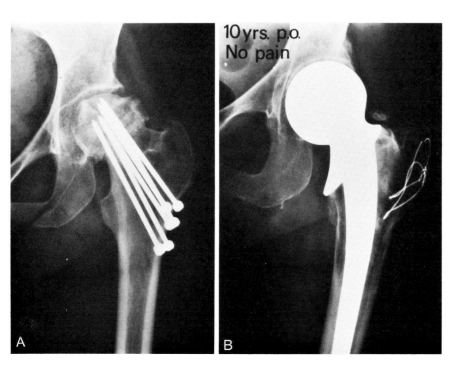

10 yrs. p.o.
No pain

Figure 4–87. Avascular necrosis in a 49-year-old female. Patient fell from a horse 2 years previously and had closed reduction and internal fixation with multiple pins. *A,* Appearance 2 years following fracture and pinning. Avascular necrosis. At this time the head was replaced with a cemented Thompson prosthesis. *B,* Appearance 10 years following Thompson prosthesis with no evidence of loosening or acetabular migration, and no pain.

lage, replacement becomes necessary in the case of Stage III fractures. These will not heal, and pain persists because of the synovitis caused by this intra-articular fracture. Finally, the treatment of Stage IV fractures (Table 4–19) is either endoprosthesis or total hip arthroplasty (Fig. 4–87).

Other complications include malunion, nonunion, and later degenerative arthritis. Nonunion can be defined as failure to demonstrate bony growth across the fracture site 4 months after injury. Non-union may result from inadequate fixation or interruption of blood supply. In this case synovial fluid interferes with callus formation, possibly by preventing normal clot formation at the fracture site. The incidence of non-union is lower if proper fixation is obtained and the fractures are impacted. In displaced fractures non-union may occur in 25 to 33 percent of patients.[143, 148] Factors increasing the degree of instability include the obliquity of the fracture line (Pauwell's Type III) and the degree of comminution of the posterior cortex.[168] The lateral view is most useful in assessing the degree of posterior cortical involvement (Fig. 4–74B).

Careful radiographic assessment of the fracture line will demonstrate widening and irregularity in early non-union. This progresses to sclerosis of the fracture margins during the later stages. Comparison views from the time of initial injury are extremely helpful in evaluation of potential nonunion. Tomography, isotope scans, and magnetic resonance imaging may also be useful.

In the past, subtrochanteric valgus osteotomy was performed to create compressive rather than shear forces at the fracture site. Non-union has also been treated with bone grafting. Currently, replacement with an endoprosthesis or total hip arthroplasty is considered most effective.

TROCHANTERIC FRACTURES

Trochanteric fractures generally follow the trochanteric line. These fractures may extend into the subtrochanteric region. Avulsion fractures of the greater and lesser trochanter may occur separately or in association with intertrochanteric and subtrochanteric fractures. For purposes of discussion three categories can be distinguished: (1) intertrochanteric fractures, (2) subtrochanteric fractures, and (3) avulsion fractures.

Classification of Trochanteric Fractures

Intertrochanteric Fractures

Unlike subcapital fractures, intertrochanteric fractures are extracapsular. The vascular supply is rarely at risk. Thus, non-union and avascular necrosis are uncommon complications.[175] Intertrochanteric fractures also occur most commonly in elderly patients with an almost equal incidence among males and females.[177, 188]

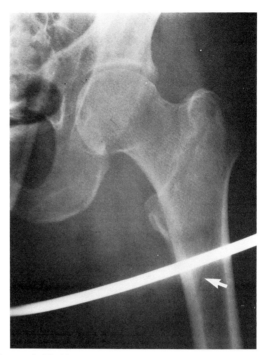

Figure 4–88. AP view of the left hip with traction device in place. There is an undisplaced intertrochanteric fracture with subtrochanteric involvement *(arrow).*

The fracture line usually extends between the greater and lesser trochanters (Fig. 4–88). In certain cases an intertrochanteric fracture may be difficult to differentiate from a basicervical fracture. Comminution of the fracture with detachment of the greater and lesser trochanters (four-part fracture) is common (Fig. 4–89). Though a single fracture in the region of the calcar is usually stable, comminution of the calcar or displacement with the lesser

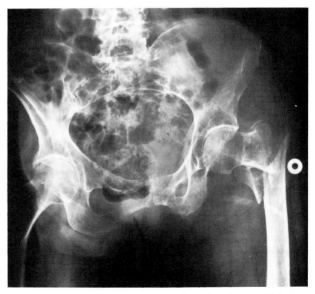

Figure 4–89. AP view of the pelvis. There is a four-part intertrochanteric fracture. Varus angulation is present. The vertical orientation of the major fracture line increases instability.

trochanter is unstable. Fractures with a nearly vertical orientation also tend to be unstable.

The fracture usually results from a fall, with direct trauma and the muscle forces about the hip both playing a part in the mechanism of injury. The external rotators tend to remain with the proximal fragment and the internal rotators with the distal fragment.[176]

Table 4–20 summarizes the commonly used classifications of intertrochanteric fractures. Fractures may be simply classified as displaced or undisplaced.[181, 195, 201] Clawson considered an intertrochanteric fracture stable if there was a single medial cortical fracture or if the medial cortex was in contact with the calcar.[176] Comminution of the medial cortex and more vertically oriented fractures were considered unstable. Dimon and Hughston stressed these two factors along with the presence of a large posterior fragment as indicators of instability.[177] Ender's classification was based on the mechanism of injury.[178] However, the most commonly used classification is the Evans' system, as modified by Jensen and Michaelsen in 1975.[184, 185] This classification is based on the prognosis for anatomic reduction and the likelihood of post-reduction instability (Fig. 4–90).[185] The primary considerations are the degree of comminution of the calcar region and the greater trochanter. Involvement of these structures increases the chances of instability following

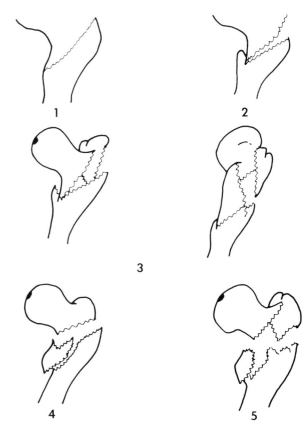

Figure 4–90. Classification of trochanteric fractures by Evans modified by Jensen and Michaelson. Type I: Undisplaced two-fragment fracture. Type 2: Displaced two-fragment fracture. Type 3: Three-part fracture with dislocated greater trochanter. Type 4: Three-fragment fracture with loss of medial support due to loss of the lesser trochanter or calcar fragment. Type 5: Four-part fracture with loss of medial and posterolateral support. Types 1 and 2 are stable. Types 3 to 5 are unstable. (From Jensen, J. S.: Classification of trochanteric fractures. Acta Orthop. Scand. *51*:803, 1980.)

TABLE 4–20. Intertrochanteric Fracture Classifications

Ender[178] (1978)

Type 1   Eversion fracture

Type 2   Impaction fracture

Type 3   Diatrochanteric fracture

Tronzo (1975, 1980)[184, 185]

Type 1   Fracture involving one of the trochanters

Type 2   Simple trochanteric fracture with or without minimal displacement; posterior neck intact

Type 3   Comminution of the posterior wall with a calcar spike; large lesser trochanteric fragment

Type 4   Same as Type 3 with associated displacement of the greater trochanter

Type 5   Comminution of the posterior cortex with a telescoping fragment

Evans[179] (1949)

Type 1   Undisplaced 2-part fracture

Type 2   Displaced 2-part fracture

Type 3   Three-part fracture with greater trochanter displaced

Type 4   Three-part fracture with displaced calcar and lesser trochanter

Type 5   Four-part fracture with medial and posterior lateral cortex fractures (combines Types 3 and 4)

reduction. Using this classification, Type 1 and 2 fractures are stable fractures that can be reduced in 94 percent of cases.[184] The remaining types are unstable. When the greater trochanter was detached (Type 3), only 33 percent could be reduced. If the calcar was involved (Type 4), only 21 percent could be reduced. Also following reduction, stable Type 1 and 2 fractures dislocated in only 9 percent of cases compared with 58 to 90 percent for Types 3, 4, and 5.[184]

Radiographic evaluation requires high-quality AP and lateral views. This allows evaluation of the calcar and posterior and medial cortex. Subtle undisplaced fractures may require further evaluation with tomography and radioisotope scans.

Significant mortality and morbidity may occur with intertrochanteric fractures unless early reduction and immobilization are obtained. Boyd and Griffin reported mortality rates of 18 percent in 300 patients with trochanteric fractures.[175] Most patients are elderly, and prolonged bed rest may result in such complications as pulmonary emboli, phlebitis,

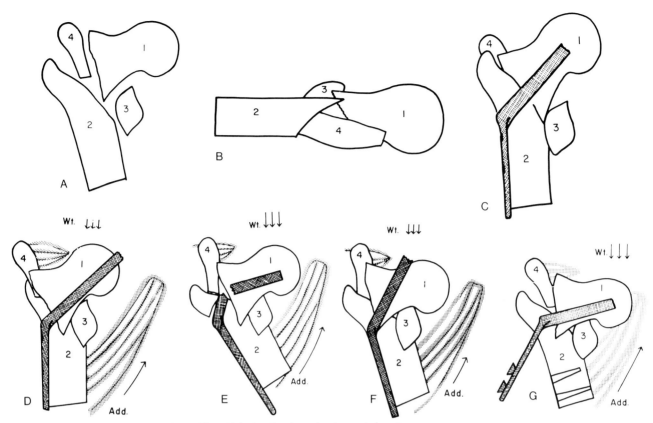

Figure 4–91. Forces leading to instability of intertrochanteric fractures. *A* and *B*, AP and lateral views of four-part intertrochanteric fracture (1, head; 2, shaft; 3, medial fragment or lesser trochanter; 4, posterior fragment or greater trochanter). *C*, Complications resulting from weight-bearing and muscle forces. *D*, Nail penetrating femoral head. *E*, Nail fracture. *F*, Nail penetrates the femoral neck. *G*, Screw fracture with varus collapse. (From Dimon, J. H., and Hughston, J. C.: Unstable intertrochanteric fractures of the hip. J. Bone Joint Surg. *49A:*440, 1967.)

and infection. Even when healing occurs, many patients are unable to return to normal full activity.[192]

Non-union and avascular necrosis are uncommon complications of intertrochanteric fractures. These complications are more frequent with femoral neck fractures. Post-reduction instability, however, occurs commonly with complex fractures (Evans' Types 3 to 5).[184] Figure 4–91 demonstrates the forces responsible for failure to maintain reduction following internal fixation. Location of the fracture (calcar and posterior cortex involvement) and muscle forces play a significant role in this post-reduction instability.[177]

Subtrochanteric Fractures

Subtrochanteric fractures involve the cortical bone below the lesser trochanter. Associated involvement of the shaft and intertrochanteric region is common. Boyd and Griffin reviewed 300 patients with trochanteric fractures, excluding avulsion fractures.[175] Thirty-three percent of the fractures involved the subtrochanteric region. Fractures tend to occur in younger patients following significant trauma (motor vehicle accidents), in elderly patients with intertrochanteric involvement. and in patients with un-

derlying pathology. Pathologic fractures tend to be transverse. Rogers suggests that any transverse subtrochanteric fracture be studied carefully for underlying pathology.[196] Evaluation may require tomography or isotope scans.

Fielding divided subtrochanteric fractures into three zones (Fig. 4–92).[180] Zone 1 included the lesser trochanter, Zone 2 the 1 to 2 inches distal to the lesser trochanter, and Zone 3 the 2 to 3 inches below the lesser trochanter (Table 4–21). The significant factor is the involvement of the diaphysis (cortical bone). Cortical bone heals more slowly. Also biomechanical studies have demonstrated that the subtrochanteric region is a high stress area, which makes treatment difficult.[186, 197]

The Boyd and Griffin classification was based upon the prognosis and ease of obtaining and maintaining reduction (Table 4–21).[175] In the case of Type I fractures, which are characterized by linear breaks in the intertrochanteric region (Figs. 4–88 and 4–93), reduction was least difficult. Type III and IV fractures were subtrochanteric, and in these cases loss of reduction was common. Medial migration of the distal fragment as a result of adductor muscle forces was a significant factor in reduction failures.

Seinsheimer[200] divided subtrochanteric fractures

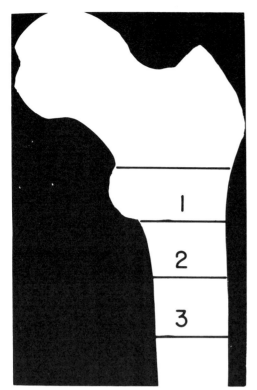

Figure 4–92. Fielding's classification. (From Fielding, J. W., et al.: Classification of subtrochanteric fractures. Surg. Obstet. Gyn. *122*:555, 1966. By permission of Surgery, Gynecology & Obstetrics.)

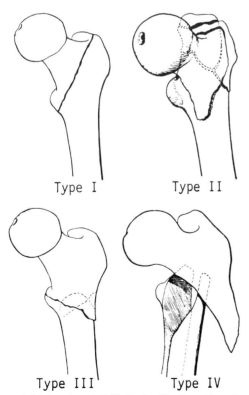

Figure 4–93. Boyd and Griffin's classification. (From Boyd, H. B., and Griffin, L. L.: Classification and treatment of trochanteric fractures. Arch. Surg. *58*:853, 1949. Copyright 1949, American Medical Association.)

TABLE 4–21. Subtrochanteric Fracture Classifications

Fielding[180] (1973)

Zone 1	Fracture includes the lesser trochanteric region
Zone 2	Fracture 1 to 2 inches distal to the lesser trochanter
Zone 3	Fracture 2 to 3 inches distal to the lesser trochanter

Boyd and Griffin[175] (1949)

Type I	Linear intertrochanteric fracture
Type II	Comminuted fracture with the main fracture along the intertrochanteric line
Type III	Subtrochanteric fracture with at least one fracture line passing through or just below the lesser trochanter
Type IV	Comminuted trochanteric fracture extending into the shaft; fracture lines in at least two planes

Seinsheimer[200] (1978)

Group I	Undisplaced fracture (less than 2 mm displacement)

Group II	Two-part fracture
	  A. Transverse fracture
	  B. Spiral fracture
	  C. Spiral fracture with lesser trochanter involvement

Group III	Three-part fractures
	  A. Spiral fracture with lesser trochanter involvement
	  B. Spiral fracture with butterfly fragment

Group IV	Four-part fractures
Group V	Subtrochanteric fractures with extension into the intertrochanteric region and involvement of the greater trochanter

into eight categories (Table 4–21). If bone-to-bone contact can be established medially, the fracture is considered stable. Most treatment failures involved Group III fractures. These are three-part fractures with involvement of the lesser trochanter or an associated butterfly fragment. The longer the spiral (greater than 8 cm), the poorer the prognosis.[200]

Radiographic evaluation requires AP and lateral views. Both projections (see section on Routine Radiography of the Pelvis and Hips) can be obtained without moving the patient. Thus, risk of further displacement of the fracture fragments is not of concern. If transverse fractures are present, tomography may be required to exclude pathologic fractures.

Complications associated with subtrochanteric fractures are essentially the same as those seen with intertrochanteric fractures. The significant difference is an increased incidence of treatment failures in the case of subtrochanteric fractures.

Avulsion Fractures

Greater trochanter avulsions are due to abrupt contractions of those muscles attaching to the greater trochanter. This fracture occurs in the elderly patient but is uncommon unless associated with an intertrochanteric fracture.[176] Undisplaced fractures may be difficult to detect on the AP view. Oblique views and, occasionally, tomography may be necessary to demonstrate the fracture.

Lesser trochanteric avulsions are due to iliopsoas contractions and more commonly occur in young athletes.[174] Rogers stated that avulsion fractures of the lesser trochanter in adults are uncommon unless there is underlying pathology.[196]

Treatment of Trochanteric Fractures

As in femoral neck fractures, the treatment of trochanteric fractures also depends on their stability. Type 1 and 2 intertrochanteric fractures are reasonably stable, with good cortical support medially acting as a buttress. Thus, they can be treated in a variety of ways and simply held by internal fixation until union occurs. The sliding nail-plate or screw-plate is quite sufficient for most of these fractures (Fig. 4–94). Fixed nail-plates without the sliding component should not be used (Fig. 4–91), for stresses at the angle of the nail plate are considerable, especially if some absorption occurs at the fracture site. Heyse-Moore and colleagues compared the Richards screw-plate with the Jewett nail-plate in a large series of intertrochanteric fractures and found the Richards screw-plate superior, as it resulted in considerably less complications.[183] Ender pinning is also excellent and diminishes surgical time, blood loss, and the incidence of infection.[178]

In the more unstable fracture (usually four-part fractures with no medial stability), one must be especially cautious in selecting the type of internal fixation. The ordinary nail-plate will invariably fail. A sliding screw-plate can be successful provided that the distal fragment is displaced medially. This method has been demonstrated by Dimon and Hughston.[177] In this case medial displacement will relieve the lateral tension forces. A valgus position of the proximal fragment will act in the same way and can be achieved by an additional osteotomy. The latter was recommended by Sarmiento and Williams.[198]

Ender nailing can also be used in the unstable intertrochanteric fracture if a reduction of the fracture in valgus is first obtained (Fig. 4–95). Often an additional pin in the greater trochanter is helpful for control of position.[178] Significant complications may occur, however, and the operation is not an easy one. Experience leads to skill in placing Ender rods, and careful monitoring with an image intensifier in two planes will minimize the risk of complications. Ender nails seldom migrate proximally. If they do, they can be extracted from their entrance point above the knee. Pain about the knee is more common and may occur from distal migration of the nails. It can be relieved by removing them. Union is usually obtained with Ender fixation. An

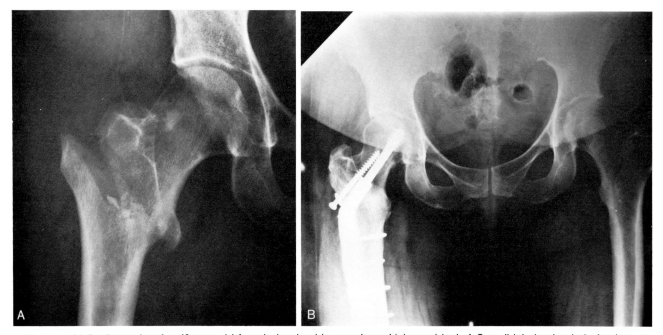

Figure 4–94. Radiographs of a 43-year-old female involved in a motor vehicle accident. *A,* Type II intertrochanteric fracture on admission. *B,* Appearance 3 years after open reduction and internal fixation with a Richards sliding nail-plate and supplementary screw. Excellent function.

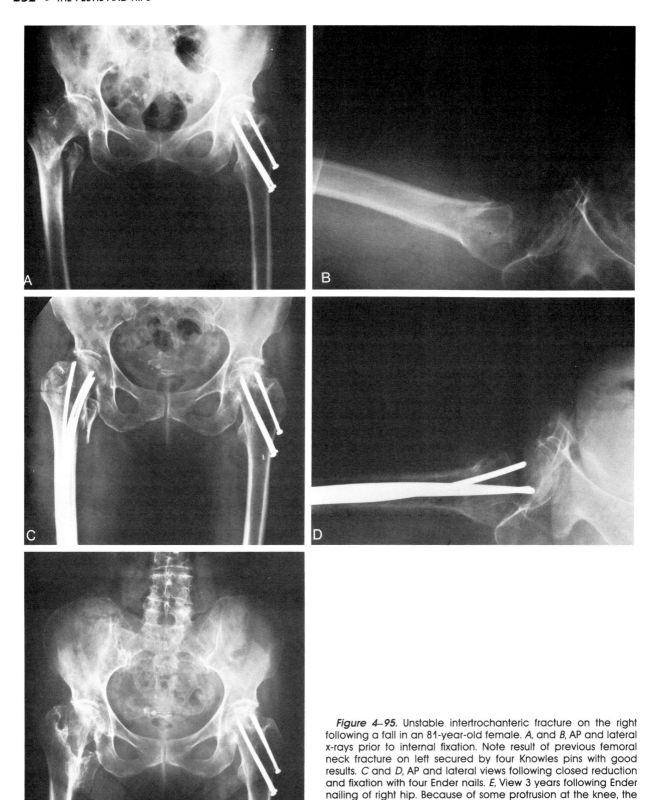

Figure 4–95. Unstable intertrochanteric fracture on the right following a fall in an 81-year-old female. *A,* and *B,* AP and lateral x-rays prior to internal fixation. Note result of previous femoral neck fracture on left secured by four Knowles pins with good results. *C* and *D,* AP and lateral views following closed reduction and fixation with four Ender nails. *E,* View 3 years following Ender nailing of right hip. Because of some protrusion at the knee, the pins were removed 1 year after insertion. Fractures healed in almost anatomic position.

external rotation deformity may occur; it can be minimized by reduction and nailing with the distal fragment in relative internal rotation.

A badly comminuted intertrochanteric fracture in an older, debilitated patient who must be rapidly mobilized may be treated with a primary trochanteric prosthesis of the Leinbach type. The indications are quite limited; but in the octogenarian with a comminuted fracture and marked osteoporosis, an endoprosthesis may be the proper choice.[189] For

THE PELVIS AND HIPS • 253

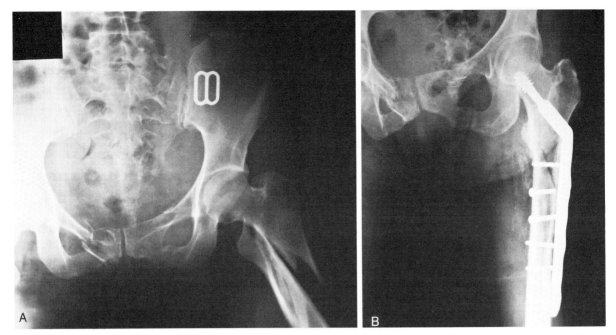

Figure 4–96. Radiographs of a 45-year-old female involved in a motor vehicle accident with multiple fractures, including pelvis, forearm, ankle, and tibia and fibula on the ipsilateral side. A long Richards screw-plate with interfragmentary fixation with two screws was elected for the femur. *A*, Appearance of the upper femur following fracture. *B*, Appearance 3 months following internal fixation. Union eventuated in excellent position.

these unstable four-part fractures in the osteoporotic patient, even methyl methacrylate reinforcement can be used in conjunction with some type of blade or nail-plate fixation.[199]

The subtrochanteric fracture requires different treatment. Because of the differences in stress at this level, lateral nail plating or sliding screw plating is seldom indicated. An exception is the very long comminuted fracture with a high degree of instability. Here a long ASIF nail-plate with additional bone grafting and cerclage wires or transfixion screws may salvage this type of fracture (Fig. 4–96).

Most subtrochanteric fractures are ideally treated with the Zickel nail.[202] While mastering the technique of the Zickel nail is difficult, its superiority for this purpose has been proved with time and use.[203] Ender nails are a useful alternative, especially in the patient who is a poor operative risk.

Pathologic fractures occur rather frequently in the area of the trochanter and should receive special attention.[191, 204] The addition of methyl methacrylate as an adjunct in the management of pathologic fractures was reported in a combined study from several orthopedic centers.[182] The acrylic is used, of course, in conjunction with internal fixation, the type depending on the lesion and its level (Fig. 4–97). Included in this study were 63 patients who were treated for fractures of the femoral head and neck and 109 patients treated for trochanteric and subtrochanteric fractures. Bony union after irradiation is actually enhanced by the use of acrylic.

Treatment of avulsion fractures is usually conservative. Surgical intervention is not indicated unless the fragment is displaced more than 2 cm.[176]

HIP ARTHROGRAPHY IN THE ADULT

Arthrography provides valuable information in patients with pain, clicking, locking, and other symptoms related to the hip. The study should be tailored to the clinical symptoms of each patient. Variable imaging techniques such as tomography, computed tomography, single versus double contrast, and anesthetic injection must be considered to obtain optimum information. When properly performed, the articular cartilage, capsule, and synovium can be accurately assessed with arthrography.[207, 208, 212, 213, 217, 218]

Indications for hip arthrography vary with the age of the patient. In children arthrography is most frequently performed to evaluate septic arthritis, congenital hip dysplasia, and Legg-Calvé-Perthes disease.[207, 208, 212] Arthrography in adults is usually performed to evaluate arthritides (e.g., rheumatoid arthritis, pigmented villonodular synovitis, osteoarthritis), infection, and intra-articular loose bodies.[207] In our practice the study is frequently performed to evaluate acetabular labral tears. A less common indication is evaluation of enlarged iliopsoas bursae.[220] Table 4–22 summarizes the indications for conventional arthrography at the Mayo Clinic. Subtraction arthrography is discussed later in this chapter.

Arthrographic Technique

Prior to performing arthrography all radiographic studies (routine films, isotope scans, CT scans, etc.)

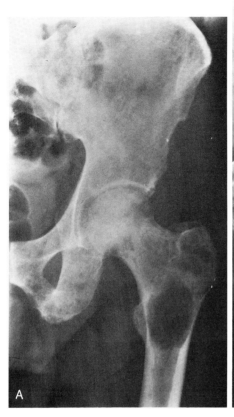
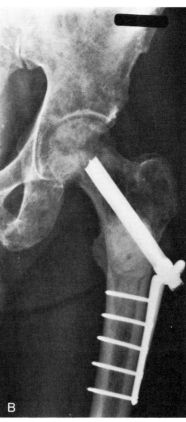

Figure 4–97. Radiographs of a 66-year-old male with multiple myeloma. Lytic lesions present throughout the skeleton but especially in the intertrochanteric area where fractures appear imminent. *A,* Appearance at time of internal fixation. *B,* Methacrylate packed into the large cavity opposite the lesser trochanter followed by McLaughlin nail-plate. The McLaughlin nail-plate provided adequate stability by the addition of the methacrylate.

should be thoroughly reviewed and the clinical findings discussed with the referring physician. These steps assist in determining the proper method of injection, appropriate contrast material, and filming technique that will best demonstrate the suspected pathology. Though allergic reactions during arthrography are rare,[207] a history of significant allergy to a contrast medium may require a difficult approach to the examination. If previous reactions were mild (i.e., hives, with no respiratory or vascular symptoms), premedication with diphen-

TABLE 4–22. Adult Hip Arthrography: Indications and Techniques

Indication	Technique
Arthritis	Routine views,
Osteoarthritis	single-contrast
Rheumatoid arthritis	
Septic arthritis	
Pimented villonodular	Tomography
synovitis	
Loose Bodies	Tomography
Osteoarthritis	
Trauma	
Synovial chondromatosis	Tomography and
	double-contrast
Osteonecrosis	Tomography
Acetabular labral tears	Routine (multiple
	obliques); CT
	with air alone or
	double-contrast
Iliopsoas bursal enlargement	Routine

hydramine (Benadryl) or chlorpheniramine (Chlor-Trimeton) may be all that is necessary. If a severe reaction occurred, the examination should not be performed. If necessary, injection of air followed with CT or tomography may be useful in patients with significant histories of allergic reaction. Bleeding is rarely reported with arthrography. Gelman stated that patients with clotting disorders or with platelet counts of less than 50,000 per ml may have bleeding problems during the procedure.[206]

Arthrography requires high-quality fluoroscopic equipment with easy access to the patient (see Introduction to Arthrography in Chapter 1). With the patient supine the injection site is prepared using sterile technique. An AP scout film is routinely obtained prior to injection (unless a hip series has just been performed on the same table). Scout films prior to the injection help prevent unnecessary repeat injections, which is significant in that repeating films will often result in a suboptimal study.

The injection site is determined by the appearance of the hip and the location of the femoral artery. The femoral artery, which must be palpated prior to injection, generally runs medial to the femoral neck. In patients with significant deformities of the hip as a result of previous surgery or trauma, however, the relationship of the neck to the femoral artery may vary. In making the injection we generally use an anterior approach, with the needle directed vertically just lateral to the midline at the junction of the head and neck (Fig. 4–98*A*). The

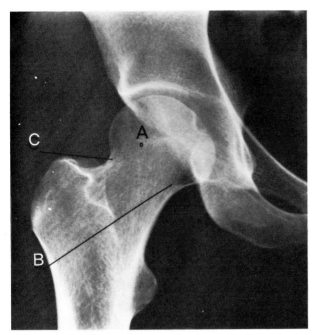

Figure 4–98. AP view of the hip demonstrating injection approaches. A, vertical; B, anterolateral; C, lateral.

anesthetic needle is positioned over the area, and the skin is infiltrated to form a wheal. After anesthetizing the superficial soft tissues, a 22-gauge, 3½-inch needle is advanced vertically until it makes contact with the femoral neck. The patient is then instructed to flex the hip slightly. This assures that the bevel of the needle is within the joint capsule. Larger needles (18 gauge) may be required in patients with suspected pyogenic arthritis. This will make aspiration of purulent material less difficult. Alternate approaches, such as the anterolateral (Fig. 4–98B) and lateral (Figure 4–98C), may be used if the clinical situation dictates.[213]

Needle position can be confirmed by (1) aspiration of synovial fluid, (2) injection of a small amount of contrast medium (0.5 ml), (3) injection of air, or (4) injection of 5 to 10 ml of sterile saline and reaspiration of the fluid. In the latter situation unaspirated saline may dilute the contrast medium. Though the incidence is rare, air embolism has been reported with air arthrography.[215] Therefore, we prefer to use a small test injection if no synovial fluid can be aspirated. Aspiration of the joint or saline flush with aspiration is usually performed if synovial fluid analysis for crystals, rheumatoid factor, immunoglobulins, or infection is indicated. Care must be taken not to inject large amounts of contrast medium prior to aspiration for culture purposes, as the contrast medium is a bacteriostatic agent.[207]

The choice of contrast agent and filming technique varies with the clinical situation (Table 4–22). In routine situations 6 ml or more of contrast medium (meglumine such as Hypaque-M-60) is injected. If too much contrast medium is injected, subtle changes will be obscured. Epinephrine is occasionally mixed with the contrast medium if tomography is contemplated. Use of epinephrine allows the contrast medium to remain in the joint for longer periods, resulting in improved film quality.[211, 219] In certain cases, double contrast technique (4 ml of contrast material plus 10 ml or more of air) is used. Other cases call for use of air alone.

Following the injection of the contrast agent or agents, the hip is exercised and observed fluoroscopically. Any painful motions, clicking, or position changes of intra-articular bodies can be observed. Patients are positioned fluoroscopically for filming. This technique provides added information and ensures proper positioning. Films are taken in internal and external rotation and in lateral and oblique projections. Depending upon the information obtained fluoroscopically, further views following exercise or additional oblique views are also obtained. If necessary, computed tomography or tomography may be obtained. This requires additional planning on the part of the arthrographer. If tomography is contemplated, the injection is usually made on the tomography table to reduce the time required to obtain the films.

Following the arthrogram bupivacaine (Marcaine) or a combination of bupivacaine and betamethasone (Celestone) is often injected. This is helpful in patients without definitive arthrographic findings. The injection helps determine whether the pain is intra-articular and in this way facilitates treatment programs in many cases. Betamethasone is not used if surgery is contemplated or if infection is suspected. The medication is not injected with the contrast medium, as dilution of the contrast medium would result in suboptimal arthrography.

Arthrographic Demonstration of Normal Anatomy

The normal arthrogram demonstrates the articular cartilage, labrum, capsular configuration, and synovial characteristics of the hip joint (Fig. 4–99).[206–208, 211, 213, 217, 218] The margins of the capsule extend from the acetabular rim to the base of the femoral neck. There are four recesses (Fig. 4–99). Proximally the superior articular recess extends above the cartilaginous labrum. Inferiorly the inferior recess outlines the inferior labrum. The superior recess colli lies above the femoral neck, and the inferior recess colli is found at the lower margin of the neck.[218] The distal insertion of the capsule is irregular and should not be mistaken for synovial inflammation. The acetabular labrum is difficult to visualize in its entirety. Oblique views demonstrate the labrum to best advantage (Fig. 4–99B). A constant extrinsic defect is seen below the femoral head owing to the transverse ligament. With the patient in the supine position, the posterior labrum may be seen as a straight line along the upper portion of

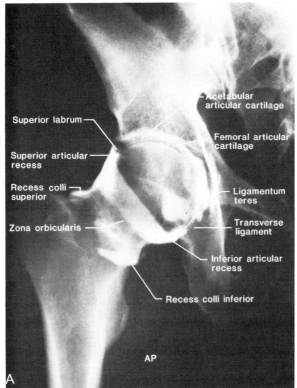
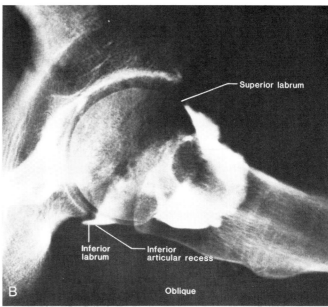

Figure 4-99. Normal hip arthrogram with anatomy labeled. *A*, AP view. *B*, oblique view.

the neck. Inferior to the labral line is the orbicular zone, which is caused by thickened ligamentous fibers encircling the capsule. The articular cartilage on the femoral head is well demonstrated and is usually thicker than the acetabular articular surface.[208] Medially the acetabular fossa is well demonstrated, but in normal patients the ligamentum teres is usually not visualized.[207, 208] Communication of the capsule with the iliopsoas bursa occurs in 15 to 20 percent of patients owing to a defect between the iliofemoral and pubofemoral ligaments.[208, 220]

Indications for Hip Arthrography

Arthritis

Arthrographic evaluation of patients with inflammatory joint diseases allows one to obtain anatomic and laboratory information. Synovial fluid should always be aspirated. If no fluid can be obtained, a saline flush (nonbacteriostatic sterile saline) with reaspiration can provide information regarding infection. Fluid analysis will vary depending upon the clinical situation (crystals in suspected gout or pseudogout; rheumatoid factor, differential count, and Gram stain in cases of suspected infection; immunoglobulins in chondrolysis). Grossly bloody fluid may indicate pigmented villonodular synovitis.[210, 216]

Evaluation of the articular cartilage is usually adequate with conventional film techniques. Tomography is useful in patients with abnormal routine radiographs or when subtle findings are sus-

pected. For example, in patients with chondrolysis tomography will assist in detection of the subtle erosions in the articular cartilage.[210, 216] Double-contrast technique may provide additional anatomic information.

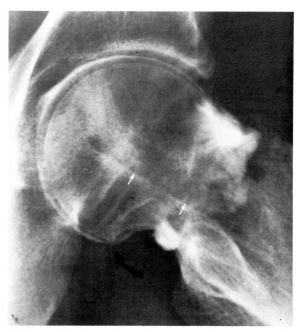

Figure 4-100. Painful hip with decreased range of motion following previous surgery. The femoral screw had been removed *(white arrows)*. The oblique view demonstrates reduction in the size of the recesses due to early capsulitis. A small bony spur is visible on the inferior margin of the head *(curved arrow)*. Capsular volume is 5 ml.

The configuration of the capsule (Fig. 4–99) is also easily defined arthrographically. The normal hip should accommodate at least 10 ml of fluid.[214] In patients with long-standing inflammatory arthritis the capsule may decrease in size with loss of the normal recesses (Fig. 4–100). Symptoms similar to adhesive capsulitis in the shoulder may develop. Injection of contrast material may be very difficult in patients with advanced capsulitis.[208] Identification of communicating sinus tracts or abcess cavities is also important. This finding may be present in infectious arthritis.

Synovial evaluation is usually adequate with routine arthrographic techniques. In patients with suspected pigmented villonodular synovitis double-contrast technique, with or without tomography, may be necessary to detect subtle granular changes in the synovium.[207] In later stages large lucent defects may be difficult to differentiate from synovial chondromatosis. A bloody synovial aspirate and erosive changes in the femur or acetabulum may be present with pigmented villonodular synovitis. Large areas of synovial proliferation may also be evident in rheumatoid arthritis and chronic infections.[207] Lymphatic filling may be present with any chronic inflammatory arthritis.[208]

Loose Bodies

Arthrography is frequently useful in identification of intra-articular osteocartilaginous bodies. On occasion subtle areas of calcification or more obvious calcifications may be evident on the plain films (Fig. 4–101). Arthrography will confirm the location of these densities. The most common cause of intraarticular loose bodies is degenerative arthritis.[207] Fragments of cartilage are nourished by synovial

fluid and may actually increase in size over a period of time.[207, 208]

Patients with osteonecrosis, Legg-Calvé-Perthes disease, osteochondritis dissecans, and previous fracture-dislocations of the hip may require arthrography to evaluate the articular surface. The position of the fragment (loose or covered by articular cartilage) can be assessed. Tomography is often necessary in these patients (Fig. 4–102).

A less common condition, synovial chondromatosis, may also cause loose bodies within the joint space (Fig. 4–103). This condition is due to synovial metaplasia and results in fine synovial irregularity. These areas of proliferation are released into the joint space and usually grow to significant size before symptoms develop. Calcification of these chondral bodies may occur.[207]

Acetabular Labral Tears

Evaluation of suspected acetabular labral tears is one of the most frequent indications for hip arthrography in our practice. Patients with tears in the labrum present with pain, clicking, especially with flexion and external rotation of the hip, and decreased range of motion. Routine radiographs are of little value. Conventional arthrography (Fig. 4–104) allows partial evaluation of the labrum, though the anterior and posterior portions are difficult to visualize. In this case fluoroscopically positioned oblique views in the frog-leg position allow evaluation of a large portion of the labrum. Tomography is also useful in studying the inferior portions. However, early experience indicates that these methods are not sufficiently accurate and that CT with air or double-contrast technique may prove to be the most valuable method for evaluation of

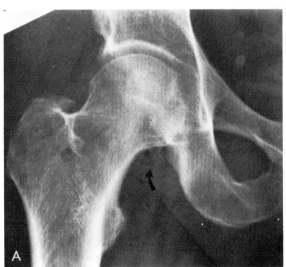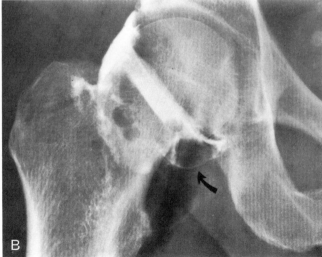

Figure 4–101. Male patient with right hip pain and clicking. The AP view *(A)* demonstrates a faint density inferior to the femoral head *(curved arrow).* The arthrogram *(B)* confirms the intra-articular location of this loose body.

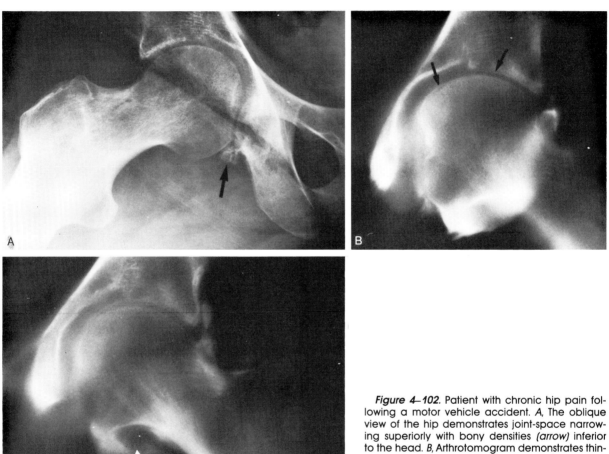

Figure 4–102. Patient with chronic hip pain following a motor vehicle accident. *A,* The oblique view of the hip demonstrates joint-space narrowing superiorly with bony densities *(arrow)* inferior to the head. *B,* Arthrotomogram demonstrates thinning of the articular cartilage with subchondral lucency *(arrows)* and irregularity of the femoral head below the fovea. The capsular volume is also reduced. *C,* Arthrotomogram demonstrates cartilaginous body inferior to the femoral head *(arrow)*. This may have originated from the femoral head defect.

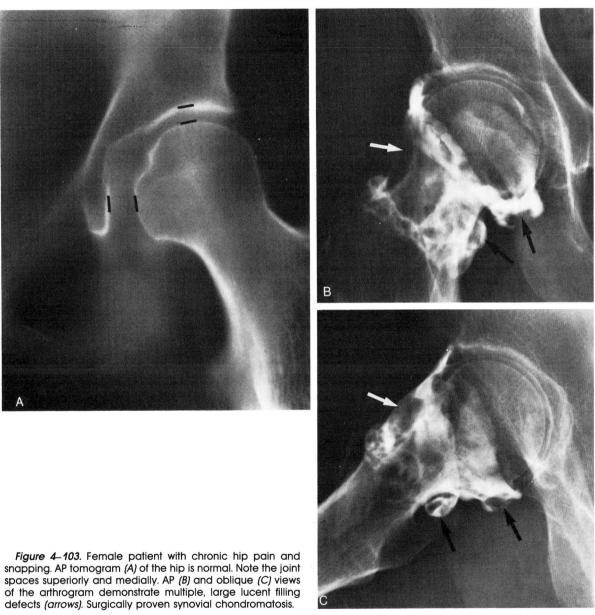

Figure 4-103. Female patient with chronic hip pain and snapping. AP tomogram *(A)* of the hip is normal. Note the joint spaces superiorly and medially. AP *(B)* and oblique *(C)* views of the arthrogram demonstrate multiple, large lucent filling defects *(arrows)*. Surgically proven synovial chondromatosis.

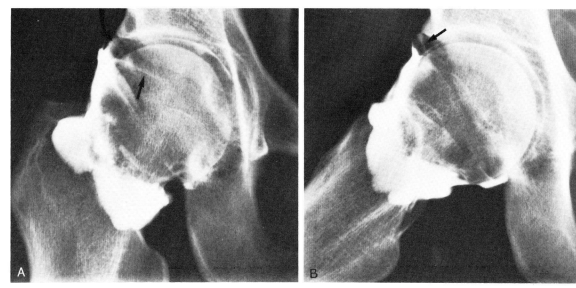

Figure 4-104. Patient with suspected acetabular labral tear. The AP view *(A)* demonstrates a faint area of contrast in the superior labrum *(curved arrow)* with a linear cleft of contrast *(arrow)* over the upper femoral head. The oblique view *(B)* clearly demonstrates the tear *(arrow)*.

the labrum (Fig. 4–105). To date, it appears that magnetic resonance imaging does not provide sufficient resolution for labral evaluation.

Enlarged Iliopsoas Bursa

As mentioned earlier, the joint capsule communicates with the iliopsoas bursa in 15 to 20 percent of patients.[205, 220] In long-standing inflammatory arthritis this communication may enlarge, resulting in an inguinal mass (Fig. 4–106).[207, 208, 220] If the bursa extends cephalad, compression of the femoral vessels, bladder, and colon may occur.[220] A triad of findings may suggest the diagnosis. These features include (1) a mass in the inguinal region, (2) pressure effects on the bladder, colon, or femoral vessels, and (3) radiographic evidence of arthritic changes in the hip. Associated arthritic conditions include osteoarthritis, rheumatoid arthritis, pig-

mented villonodular synovitis, and synovial chondromatosis.[220]

RADIOGRAPHIC EVALUATION OF JOINT REPLACEMENT

Joint replacement procedures have expanded greatly in recent years. About 75,000 hip replacements are performed in this country each year (with 300,000 to 400,000 worldwide).[240, 244, 246] There have been numerous articles concerning both early[231] and long-term follow-up of patients with hip arthroplas-

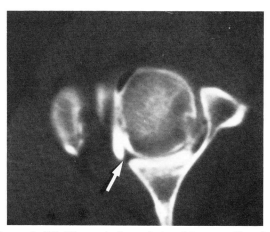

Figure 4-105. CT scan in the anterior oblique position demonstrating the posterior acetabular labrum *(arrow)*.

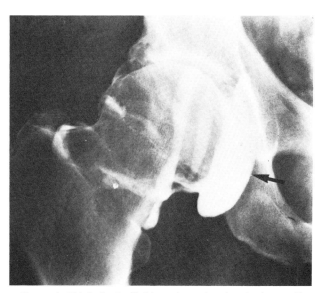

Figure 4-106. Patient with hip pain and an inguinal mass. The arthrogram demonstrates an enlarged iliopsoas bursa *(arrow)*. Osteoarthritis is also evident with cartilage thinning superiorly.

TABLE 4–23. Complications Associated with Total Hip Arthroplasties

Surgical		Medical	
Complication	*Incidence (%)*	*Complication*	*Incidence (%)*
Early			
Dislocation	2–3.9[223, 231, 260]	Cardiac	1.7
Infection	0.6–1.3[231]	Myocardial infarction	
Sciatic Nerve Palsy	0.5[231]	Arrhythmias	
		Cardiac heart failure	
Late			
		Pneumonitis	1.7
Loose femoral component	5–40[223, 238, 256, 257]	Phlebitis	3.4
Loose acetabular component	6.5–29[256, 257]	Pulmonary emboli	2.2
Infection	1.2–2[223, 231, 242]	Renal failure	0.8
Non-union greater trochanter	1–5[223, 231, 258]	Urinary tract infection	11.9
Bursitis	10[246]	Gout or pseudogout	0.7
Fracture cement	8[223, 237]	Mortality (cardiovascular)	0.4
Fracture femoral component	23–67[225]		
Heterotopic bone			
Moderate	33		
Severe	4.7[223]		
Methacrylate entrapment	—		
Fracture acetabular cup	—[229]		
Foreign body entrapment, cement and wire	0.06[256]		
Wire fracture	21[223]		
Acetabular wear	5[223]		
Calcar resorption	16[223]		

ties.[223, 255, 257, 259, 260] Although initial results are usually excellent, follow-up analysis has led to recognition of significant problems. Table 4–23 lists the surgical and medical complications in order of frequency. Loosening of the components and infection are the most significant complications.[223, 244, 255, 257] Sutherland followed 100 patients for a 10-year period and noted a 29 percent incidence of acetabular component loosening and a 40 percent incidence of loosening for the femoral component.[257] Beckenbaugh noted acetabular loosening in 6.5 percent of patients at 5 years.[223] Stauffer, following these same patients, noted loosening in 11.3 percent at 10 years.[255] Similarly, the incidence of femoral component loosening was 24 percent at 5 years and 29.9 percent at 10 years.

Infection occurs much less frequently than loosening, though the two can occur simultaneously.[223, 246] Murry reported the incidence of loosening in infected hips to vary from 50 to 92 percent.[248] The incidence of infection has been reported to be 1.2 to 2 percent in long-term follow-up series.[223, 242]

Dislocation usually occurs in the early postoperative period and is one of the more significant early complications. In Coventry's study 54 to 60 dislocations (in 2012 patients, or 2.9 percent) occurred within 3 months following surgery.[231] Factors responsible for dislocation include (1) improper positioning of the components,[231] (2) persistent hematoma in the pseudocapsule,[243] (3) avulsion of the greater trochanter,[247] and (4) movement during recovery from anesthesia. Woo reported that dislocations were more common in patients who had undergone re-operation and were treated with posterior surgical approaches.[260] The overall incidence of dislocation is 2 to 3.9 percent.[223, 231, 260]

Sciatic nerve palsy occurs in only about 0.5 percent of patients. This complication may be due to surgical injury or methacrylate compression of the nerve root.[231] Other complications, all less significant than loosening or infection, include non-union of the greater trochanter, heterotopic bone formation, and foreign body entrapment (Table 4–23). Coventry noted medical complications in 25 percent of patients following surgery (Table 4–23).[231] Most of these problems were not particularly troublesome. However, cardiovascular problems can be significant.

Radiographic assessment of patients with total hip arthroplasty is most often performed to evaluate loosening or infection. However, other causes of joint pain must be kept in mind if the examination is to be properly conducted. Routine radiographs,[246, 249] serial films, subtraction arthrography,[233, 238, 246] and radionuclide scans[238, 250] are all useful when properly applied.

Routine Radiography

Routine AP and lateral radiographs provide significant information concerning component position and potential complications. Plain film findings also assist in determining which further studies may be most helpful.

Multiple measurements can be made using the AP radiograph of the pelvis. This view should be obtained with standard technique (beam centered

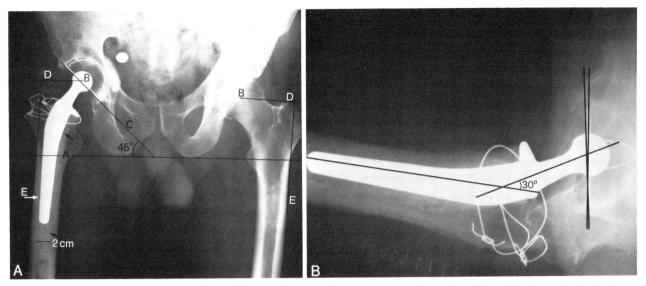

Figure 4-107. AP radiograph of the pelvis and hips showing normal measurements. *A,* AP view. (1) Acetabular angle. Angle formed by *lines A* (drawn at margins of ischial tuberosity) and *C* (line extended from marker ring). This angle should be 45°. (2) Lateral trochanteric position. *B,* center of femoral head; *D,* superior aspect of greater trochanter. Pre- and postoperative distances are measured, and a positive or negative change can be detected. Normally, the tip of the greater trochanter is on a line perpendicular to the center of the femoral head and perpendicular to the long axis of the femur (line E). Vertical trochanteric position. Measured from the ischial line (line A) to the superior aspect of the greater trochanter (D) via the femoral line (line E). (3) Cement should extend 2 cm below the tip of the femoral component *(lower arrow),* filling the medullary position of the shaft. The superomedial and inferolateral adjacencies *(arrows)* are most critical. *B,* Lateral view. Cross-table technique. The intersection of lines drawn along the shaft and neck portions of the component result in a 30° angle in this patient. Transferring this data to Figure 4–3 and Table 4–24 provides the angle of anteversion of the femoral component. The acetabular position is measured using a line along the marker ring and a line perpendicular to the film base. The component in this case is anteverted 3°.

just above the symphysis with the feet internally rotated and the patellas directed anteriorly; see Routine Radiography of the Pelvis and Hips earlier in this chapter). Reference points have been discussed by Gore[241] and Fackler.[236] The films should be studied both before and after surgery, comparing serial films. Reference points (Fig. 4–107A) are the center of the femoral heads (normal or femoral component) *(B),* a horizontal line drawn at the inferior margins of the ischial tuberosities *(A),* and a line parallel to the lateral cortex of the femoral shaft *(E).* A line drawn along the marker ring *(C)* of the acetabular component will intersect the ischial line. The angle should be 45° if the acetabular component is properly positioned.[231, 236, 246] A line

from the center of the femoral head crosses the tip of the greater trochanter, but following osteotomy of the greater trochanter this may not be the case (Fig. 4–107A, right hip). Comparison of pre- and postoperative films will allow one to assess the position change by subtracting the vertical change in distance between the ischial and trochanteric lines.[236, 241]

Evaluation of the cement technique and position of the femoral component has prognostic importance. This evaluation can be accomplished on routine radiographs only if the methyl methacrylate is impregnated with barium. Barium causes the cement to be opaque or white on the radiograph and allows one to differentiate the metal, cement, and

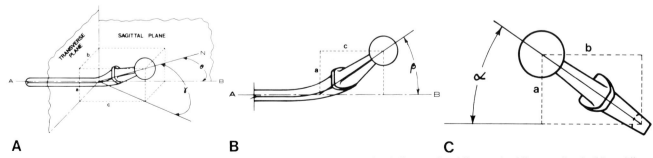

Figure 4-108. Femoral component in coronal, axial, and sagittal planes. *A,* γ is the angle of the neck of the prosthesis *(N)* and the coronal plane. θ is the angle between N and line AB. *B,* β is the angle measured on the radiograph (30°) and represents the sagittal projection of γ. *C,* is the angle of anteversion or γ in the axial plane. (From Ghelman, B.: Three methods for determining anteversion and retroversion of a total hip prosthesis. A. J. R. *133:*1127, 1979. © American Roentgen Ray Society.)

TABLE 4–24. Determination of True Angle of Anteversion*

Angle Beta (°)	Neck–Shaft Angle (°)				
	145	140	135	130	125
0	0	0	0	0	0
2	3	2½	2	2	1
4	6	5	4	3½	3
6	9	7	6	5	4
8	12	10	8	7	6
10	15	12	10	9	7
12	17	15	12	10	9
15	22	19	15	13	11
20	31	26	21	18	15
25	42	34	27	23	19
30	56	43	35	29	24
35	90	57	44	36	30
40	—	90	57	45	36
45	—	—	90	57	45

*From Ghelman, B.: Three methods for determining anteversion and retroversion of a total hip prosthesis. A.J.R. 133:1127, 1979.

bone. The femoral component should be in neutral position. Varus position predisposes to loosening.[223, 231, 246] Beckenbaugh has stated that ideally the cement should be concentrated in the upper medial and distal lateral aspects of the femoral component.[223] All of the medullary cancellous bone should be removed prior to cementing, and the cement should extend at least 2 cm beyond the femoral component (Fig. 4–107A). Newer methods pressurize the cement for better penetration into the bony trabeculae.

Ghelman describes three methods for determining the degree of anteversion or retroversion of the femoral components.[239] These methods are simple to perform and require only that the femur be parallel to the radiographic table. The first method involves the cross-table lateral view of the hip (Fig.

4–107B). This positioning requires that the patient be supine on the table with the involved hip closest to the film. The beam is horizontal. The angle of the head and neck of the femoral component is obtained as depicted in Figure 4–107B. This datum can then be applied to Figure 4–108 and Table 4–24 to determine the degree of anteversion (Fig. 4–109). This method is the most accurate.[239] The second method involves beam angle and distortion; and the third method is performed fluoroscopically, changing the tube angle until the neck is seen perpendicularly. The latter method is best suited to the T-28 prosthesis because of the prominent projection at the base of the neck.

The position of the acetabular component should also be assessed on the lateral view. Ideally the component should be in neutral to 15° of anteversion. This measurement is made by drawing a line along the marker ring of the acetabular component and measuring the angle formed by a line perpendicular to the base of the film (Figure 4–107B).[231, 246]

Obviously measurements may vary depending upon the experience of the examiner and the radiographic technique. However, the above measurements should be properly applied, as significant prognostic information can be obtained.

Radiographic Evaluation of Joint Replacement Complications

Radiographic assessment of total hip arthroplasties and resurfacing arthroplasties can be accomplished with routine films (serial films being most helpful), subtraction arthrography, and radionuclide scans.

Plain Film Evaluation

The applications of normal measurements on the AP and lateral views have been discussed and should be used in carefully evaluating potential

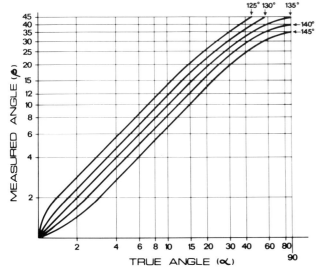

Figure 4–109. Measured angle (β) allows determination of the angle of anteversion (α) on horizontal axis. Diagonal lines are corrected for neck shaft angle. (From Ghelman, B.: Three methods for determining anteversion and retroversion of a total hip prosthesis. A. J. R. 133:1127, 1979. © American Roentgen Ray Society.)

TABLE 4–25. Plain Film Findings of Loosening and Infection[246]

Femur	Acetabulum
Varus migration	Change in position
Settling (subsidence)	Protrusion
	Tilt or cephalad migration
Cement fracture	> 1 cm lucency at bone-cement interface
Smooth endosteal resorption (usually lateral)	Fracture cement
Component fracture	Fracture acetabular component
Bone-cement lucency >1 mm or progression on serial films	
Voids in cement involving > 50% of cement area.	

complications, such as loosening and infection. Accuracy in duplicating pre- and postoperative techniques is critical.

Component Loosening. Table 4–25 summarizes the plain film findings associated with component loosening. Accuracy in predicting loosening of the components is greater for the femoral (85 percent) than for the acetabular component (69 percent).[246, 252] When dealing with the acetabular component, false negative interpretations are more common than false positive, and an error rate of 28 percent is reported in plain film evaluation of acetabular loosening.[246, 252] The error rate is significantly lower with plain film evaluation of the femoral component (15 percent).[252] With regard to femoral component loosening, the most reliable factor is varus migration. Another indication of loosening is lucency at the metal-cement or bone-cement interface superolaterally (Fig. 4–110).[223, 246, 257] Lucency at the bone-metal interface is most reliable as an indication of loosening if progressive widening is evident on serial films. However, a lucent zone at the bone-cement interface of greater than 1 mm is also generally considered diagnostic of loosening.[246] Dussault reported 100 percent accuracy in predicting loosening when progressive widening could be demonstrated on serial films.[235]

Widening of greater than 2 mm at the bone-cement interface is only slightly less accurate, with 89 percent accuracy reported by Dussault[235] and 93 percent reported by Lyons.[246] The significance of the lucent area at the bone-cement interface varies according to the degree of widening. Thus, extension of the zone over a greater area of the component without increasing width is not significant. Hendrix noted a lucent zone at the bone-cement interface in 75 percent of cases.[245] Linear extension occurred in 90 percent with no change in width or evidence of loosening. Goldring and colleagues noted membrane formation along the bone-cement interface in 20 patients with component loosening.[240] The membrane had synovial histochemical characteristics and levels of prostaglandin E_2 and collagenase that may explain the progressive lucency noted radiographically. Smooth endosteal resorption at the distal lateral aspect of the femoral

Figure 4–110. A, AP view of right total hip replacement with loose femoral component. There is resorption in the calcar region *(curved arrow)* and lucency at the metal-cement interface *(small black arrow)* indicating varus migration. Lucency is also evident at the bone-cement interface in Zone I of the acetabular component *(white arrow).* B, Loose femoral component. Considerable lucency is evident along the bone-cement interface of the femoral component with fracture of the cortex laterally. Varus migration and settling of the component has occurred. Note cement fracture distally *(arrow).*

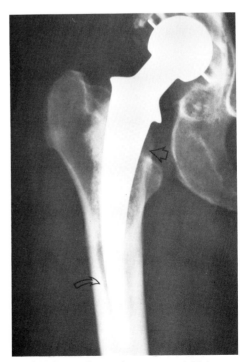

Figure 4–111. Loose femoral component. Note smooth endosteal resorption along the distal femoral component *(curved arrow)* and also lack of cement and calcar resorption superiorly *(open arrow).*

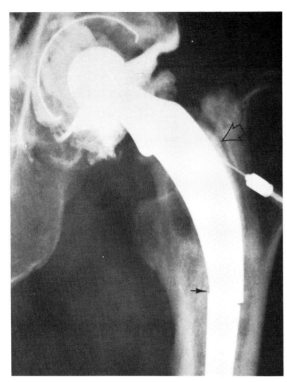

Figure 4–112. AP view of left total hip arthroplasty. Fracture of the femoral component at the junction of the medial and distal thirds *(small arrow)*. Note the varus migration with contrast at the metal-cement interface superiorly *(open arrow)*.

component is also commonly seen with loosening (Fig. 4–111).[246]

Fractures of the cement or even the femoral component (Fig. 4–112) also occur with loosening. Cement fractures most commonly occur along the margin of the distal third of the femoral component.[223, 246] Fractures of the femoral stem usually develop in the middle and upper third of the stem portion of the component. The fractures frequently occur in overweight patients, most commonly males, and in patients with improper positioning of the component.[225, 237]

Voids in the cement (Fig. 4–113) indicate difficulty in cement technique. If these changes are present in over 50 percent of the cement around the femoral component, loosening is also more common. This finding was evident in 91 percent of our patients with loosening of the femoral component.[246]

Evaluation of the acetabular component (Table 4–25) is more difficult. The acetabular region is divided into three zones according to the description of DeLee and Charnley.[232] The superior lateral aspect is Zone 1, the middle third of the acetabulum is Zone 2, and the inferior medial third is Zone 3 (Fig. 4–114). Lucent areas at the bone-cement interface are common in Zones 1 and 3 even in the early postoperative period (Fig. 4–110).[233, 253] DeLee and Charnley found radiographically detectable demarcation of the bone-cement interface in 69 percent of patients.[232] The lucent zone is rarely more than 1 mm in width and usually of no clinical signifi-

cance.[232, 253] Though lucent areas of greater than 2 mm are significant if they involve larger areas (at least two zones), change in the position of the acetabular component is the most reliable indication of loosening. In our experience change in the position of the acetabular component was not commonly detected. DeLee and Charnley reported motion of the acetabular component in 9.2 percent of their patients.[232] Anteversion and protrusion should be carefully checked.[246] Fractures in the cement or component rarely occur with loosening.[229, 231]

Infection and Joint-Related Symptoms. Infection is a significant problem, though fortunately the incidence is only 1.2 to 2 percent.[223, 242] Infection may involve the deep or superficial soft tissues. In the acute (first 12 weeks following surgery) and subacute (within the first year following surgery) phases the infection is usually related to the surgery. Later infections (more than 1 year after surgery) are probably hematogenous.[242] Patients with infection usually have an elevated S.E.D. rate.[223, 242] Plain film findings associated with infection include endosteal scalloping and laminated periosteal new bone formation (Fig. 4–115). In our experience, laminated periosteal new bone was evident in 71 percent and endosteal scalloping in 91 percent of patients with surgically documented infection.[246]

Pain and other joint-related symptoms may be encountered in patients without loosening or infection. Non-union of the greater trochanter occurs in 3 to 5 percent of patients.[223, 253] This may be evident on routine films (Fig. 4–116). Fracture of the wires

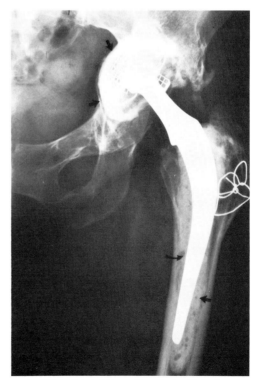

Figure 4–113. Left total hip arthroplasty. Note the numerous voids (lucent areas) in the cement *(arrows)*. There is also lucency at the bone-cement interface in Zones II and III of the acetabular component. Both components were loose.

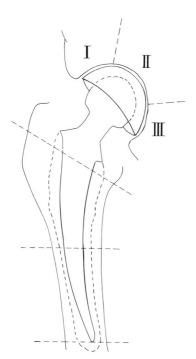

Figure 4–114. Zones for evaluation of femoral and acetabular component. The acetabular component is divided into three zones. The femoral component is divided into zones by a trochanteric *(upper line)* and mid-femoral line. (From Lyons, C. W., Berquist, T. H., Lyons, J. C., et al.: Evaluation of radiographic findings in painful hip arthroplasties. Clin. Orthop. May, 1985.)

is not clinically significant, unless accompanied by pseudarthrosis, and is usually related to metal fatigue.[247] Beckenbaugh noted wire fractures in 21 percent of 333 patients 5 years after surgery.[223]

Heterotopic bone formation occurs frequently. The incidence has been reported to be as high as 61 percent.[253] The frequency of this finding increases following re-operation, but even in these cases heterotopic bone formation occurs in significant amounts only in 3 to 4.7 percent of patients.[223, 253] Resorption of the calcar (see Fig. 4–110) may also be evident in up to 16 percent of patients but is of little significance.[223] Wear in the acetabular cup may be evident but is difficult to measure with clinical radiographs because of its lack of geometric consistency.[223, 228, 229, 234] If one measures the superior and the medial joint areas and then divides the difference by 2, the degree of wear can be roughly determined (Fig. 4–117).[228] Other potential problems such as foreign body entrapment (usually methyl methacrylate) and intra-articular wire fragments may also be noted on plain films. Vakili reported three cases of foreign bodies trapped in the acetabular region of the joint.[259] Two were cement fragments and one was a wire fragment. This is very uncommon (0.06 percent of 4,500 cases) but may result in increased and irregular wear of the acetabular component. Arthrography is usually required for confirmation of these findings (see Fig. 4–116*B*).

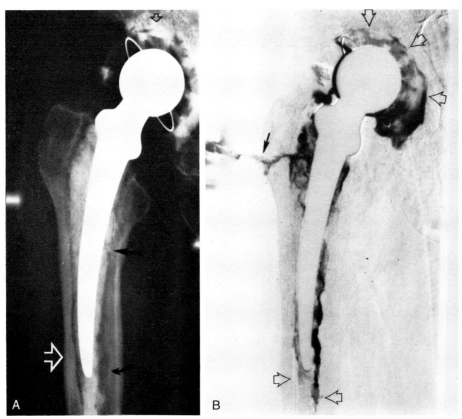

Figure 4–115. A, AP radiograph of a right total hip arthroplasty. Note endosteal scalloping *(medial black arrows)* and periosteal reaction (lower open arrow). Slight lucency in zone I of the acetabular component *(upper open arrow). B,* Subtraction arthrogram demonstrates loosening of both components *(open arrows)* with irregular extravasation around the component. A sinus tract is present laterally *(black arrow).* Both components were loose and infection was also present.

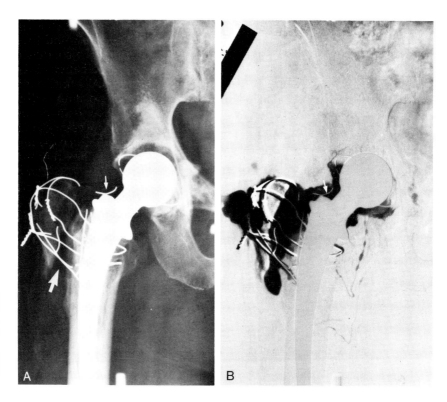

Figure 4-116. A, Routine radiograph showing fracture of wires with separation of the greater trochanter *(large white arrow)*. A wire fragment is projected near the femoral neck *(small arrow)*. B, Subtraction arthrogram reveals non-union with a trochanteric bursa and the wire fragment in the pseudocapsule.

Evaluation with Subtraction Arthrography

Subtraction arthrography offers the greatest versatility in evaluation of hip arthroplasties. Accuracy in detection of loosening of the components is reported to be as high as 96 percent.[246] Arthrography combined with aspiration is 94 percent accurate in detecting infections.[246] Other causes of pain such as non-union of the trochanter, bursitis, and intra-articular foreign bodies can also be assessed. Intra-articular anesthetic injection can be very useful in questionable cases. This assists in determining if the symptoms are intra-articular.

Attention to technique is essential if subtraction arthrography is to yield the maximum amount of information. One must carefully review the clinical setting. What are the patient's symptoms? What time interval has elapsed since surgery? Has the patient had a previous revision of the involved joint? These questions all play a role in planning the procedure and in interpreting the radiographic findings. Review of all available radiographs is also essential. Changes may suggest loosening of the components. Heterotopic bone formation may be extensive, requiring an alternate approach to the pseudocapsule during placement of the needle.

With the patient supine on the radiographic table, the area over the hip is prepared using sterile technique. The anterior vertical approach is most often used (Fig. 4–118). The femoral artery usually lies medial to the neck of the femoral component. The artery must be localized prior to needle placement. If the artery takes a more lateral course, the needle must be inserted more laterally and angled toward the neck of the femoral component. A

syringe with a 25-gauge needle is used for the local anesthetic. The tip of the needle is positioned over the base of the neck of the femoral component and a wheal is made in the skin. Various marking devices have been described (Stoker, for example,

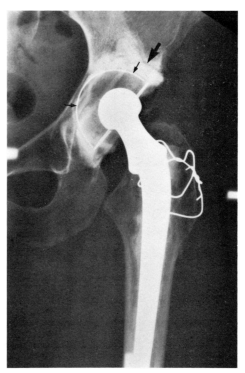

Figure 4-117. AP radiograph showing slight wear of the upper acetabular cup. Note difference in distance *(arrows)* medially and superiorly.

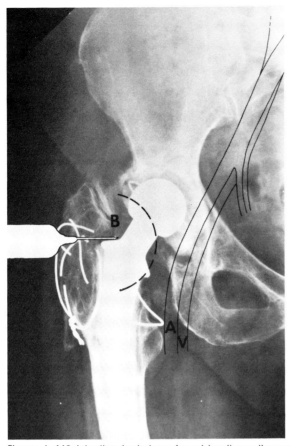

Figure 4–118. Injection technique for subtraction arthrography. The femoral artery must be palpated. A vertical approach along the lateral margin is most often used unless heterotopic bone is present. (Injection Zone B.) (From Lyons, C. W., Berquist, T. H., Lyons, J. C., et al.: Evaluation of radiographic findings in painful hip arthroplasties. Clin. Orthop. May, 1985.)

described a T-shaped metal marker[256]), but we have not found these devices necessary. The soft tissues are also anesthetized to the depth of the needle. A 22-gauge, 3½-inch needle is then advanced vertically until a metal grating is felt. This assures proper position within the pseudocapsule. If heterotopic bone is encountered a different course may be necessary (a lateral or anterolateral approach).

Once the needle is positioned, the patient is asked to flex the hip. This assists in properly positioning the needle bevel entirely within the pseudocapsule.[249] Following needle placement, the joint is aspirated and the fluid is sent for culture and bacterial sensitivity. Occasionally other studies of the synovial fluid may also be required. If no fluid can be aspirated, the joint is flushed with nonbacteriostatic sterile saline and the aspirate sent for culture.[224] At this point the patient must be comfortably immobilized to obtain proper subtraction films. This may be accomplished by using traction,[221, 252] sandbags, or other props that prevent motion of the extremity being examined. We have found that resting the extremity against a wedge or sandbag is the most comfortable for the patient and reduces the incidence of misregistration with subtraction (see Introduction to Arthrography in Chapter 1 for details on the principles of subtraction).

With the extremity immobilized, a mask film is taken. The joint is then injected with contrast medium. The pseudocapsule must be fully distended in order to obtain accurate studies. Filling is complete when the patient complains of mild discomfort or lymphatic filling is noted fluoroscopically. The injection should be monitored fluoroscopically and a second film obtained following the injection. This

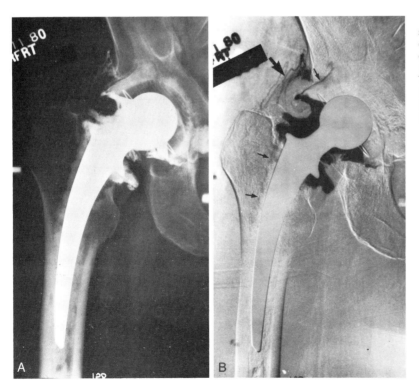

Figure 4–119. Arthrogram *(A)* and subtraction study *(B)* demonstrate contrast at the bone-cement interface below the level of the trochanteric line *(lower arrows)* and in Zone 1 *(upper arrow)* of the acetabular component. The latter finding is common and usually not indicative of loosening. Note nonspecific lymphatic filling *(large arrow)*. The femoral component was loose.

allows the subtraction film to be made. Following the second film, the needle may be removed and the extremity exercised. Lateral, internal and external rotation, frog-leg oblique, and traction views are then obtained. In certain cases changes may be seen fluoroscopically or on the pre-injection films. Further exercise may be required to document these subtle changes. In patients with questionable findings, injection of anesthetic may be helpful to confirm intra-articular pathology. Local anesthetic may also be used to assist patients with pain secondary to bursitis or other problems not related to loosening or infection.

Component Loosening. Subtraction arthrography is useful for the evaluation of femoral component loosening. For purposes of evaluation, the femoral component can be divided into zones (see Fig. 4–114). Two lines are drawn, one through the intertrochanteric region and a second through the midshaft of the component. Loosening is accurately diagnosed with conventional components if contrast medium penetrates the bone-cement interface to at least the intertrochanteric line (Fig. 4–119). If this penetration is asymmetrical or less extensive, loosening is unlikely. In the case of a long-stem component, contrast material must penetrate beyond the midshaft line to be significant. Even with this criterion, two false positive arthrograms in our department were noted with long-stem femoral components. In one the contrast material penetrated the bone-cement interface about the entire component. Lyons noted that penetration of the metal-cement interface was significant regardless of the depth (Fig. 4–120).[246] This occurs most frequently along the upper lateral component, indicat-

ing varus migration. Pseudocapsule size is also important. With large pseudocapsules the degree of penetration need not be as marked. Large capsules decompress the joint, making it more difficult to evaluate loosening accurately.[251] Post-exercise films improve the accuracy of detection in these patients, and patients with large pseudocapsules are more likely to have component loosening.[243] While the accuracy of subtraction arthrography in detecting femoral component loosening has been reported to be from 58 to 91 percent,[248, 251] in our experience the accuracy is 96 percent.

Loosening of the acetabular component is more difficult to detect accurately. Fibrous tissue at the margin of the cement may allow contrast agents to penetrate, giving the radiographic appearance of loosening in asymptomatic patients.[226, 227, 248] This may also represent preclinical loosening. The size of the pseudocapsule is very important in assessing acetabular loosening. Lyons and Berquist categorized pseudocapsules as small if the volume was 10 ml or less, medium if the volume was between 10 and 20 ml, and large if the capsule accepted more than 20 ml of contrast material.[246] Judging size from the radiographic appearance is less accurate, but a rough idea can be obtained with two views of the hip. In patients with small capsules (Fig. 4–121), the contrast can be forced around the acetabular component, mimicking loosening. To be significant, contrast medium must encircle the entire component, and the appearance should be irregular and wider than 1 mm. Even with careful attention to the pseudocapsule size, accuracy in demonstrating acetabular component loosening was only 82 percent. With moderate or large capsules contrast ma-

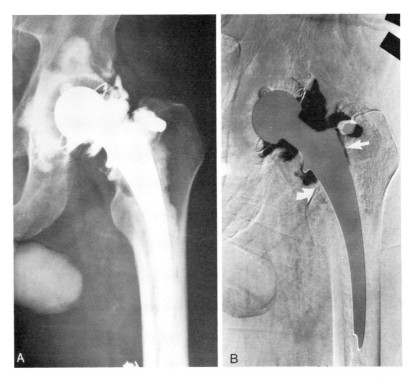

Figure 4–120. Conventional *(A)* and subtraction *(B)* arthrograms with loose femoral component. Note contrast at the metal-cement interface laterally *(arrows).* Calcar endosteal resorption medially.

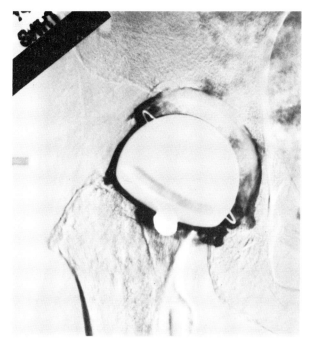

Figure 4–121. Subtraction arthrogram with resurfacing arthroplasty (pseudocapsule 10-cc). There is contrast in the bone cement interfaces in all zones except a portion of Zone II. The areas filled are irregular and wide, especially in Zone III. The component was loose.

terial must be present in the bone-cement interface in at least two zones (Fig. 4–122). Contrast extension into Zone 1 or Zone 3 alone was never significant.[246]

Resurfacing arthroplasties can also be evaluated arthrographically. The acetabular component should be approached in the same manner as in total joint replacements.[222] The femoral component

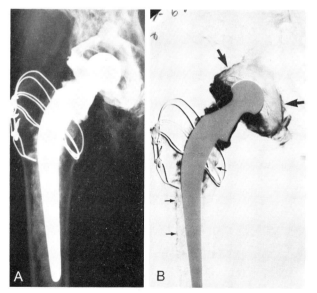

Figure 4–122. Routine (A) and subtraction arthrograms (B) in a patient with loosening of both components (pseudocapsule 20+ ml). Note contrast in Zones I and III of the acetabular component (irregular filling, large arrows). Arthrograms demonstrate Paget's disease involving the innominate bone.

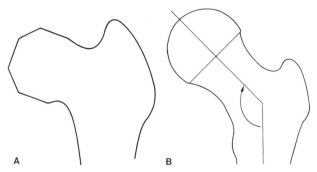

Figure 4–123. Surface replacement arthroplasty. A, Reshaping of the femoral head is performed during surgery. The head will conform to the shape of the femoral cup. B, The cup is placed over the head and cemented with methacrylate. A base-line angle using a line from the femoral shaft and a line bisecting the base of the cup can be used to evaluate subsequent position changes. (From Bassett, L. W., et al.: Radiology of failed surface replacement total hip arthroplasty. A. J. R. 139:1083, 1982.)

is difficult to evaluate, as the bone-cement interface is obscured by the metal (Fig. 4–123). Change in position on serial radiographs is the most helpful sign for the indication of femoral component loosening (Fig. 4–124).[222]

Infection and Joint Related Symptoms. Infection can be accurately assessed with subtraction arthrography coupled with aspiration of the joint and culture studies. Its accuracy when combined with these two steps was 94 percent in our series of surgically confirmed infections.[246] Arthrographic findings include large irregular pseudocapsules, sinus tracts (Fig. 4–115B), and outpouchings from the pseudocapsule (Fig. 4–125). Brown described pseudocapsular extensions as the most common finding with infection.[224] Lymphatic filling has also been described in association with infection.[230, 235] In our experience such filling is a nonspecific finding more closely related to filling pressure than to inflammation or infection.

Arthrography may also demonstrate changes, other than infection or loosening, which may explain the patient's symptoms. These include non-union of the trochanter (Fig. 4–116), bursitis (Fig. 4–126),[246, 250] and foreign-body localization (Fig. 4–116). Bursitis (a large trochanteric bursa with point tenderness) was evident in 10 percent of patients presenting with hip pain. Patients generally respond to bupivacaine (Marcaine) injection to localize the site of pathology. Large pseudocapsules may be associated with loosening or dislocation.[250] Another important feature is a normal arthrogram with negative cultures. The accuracy of these techniques (96 percent and 94 percent, respectively) assist in preventing unnecessary re-operation.

Evaluation with Radionuclide Scans

Radioisotope scans may be positive for up to 8 months following total joint replacement.[236, 241] It is generally accepted that increased uptake beyond 10

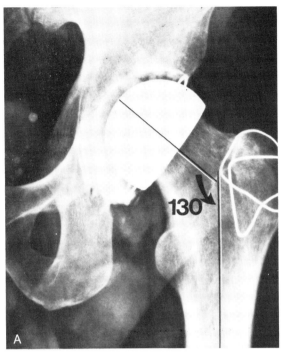

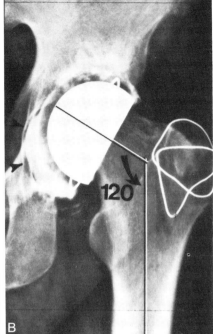

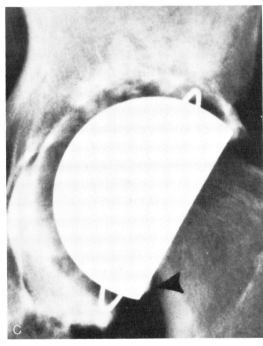

Figure 4–124. A, Post-operatively the angle is 130°. *B,* Two years later the angle has changed 10° to 120°. *C,* A fragment of methacrylate has migrated to the inferior margin of the cup *(arrow).* (From Bassett, L. W., et al.: Radiology of failed surface replacement total hip arthroplasty. A. J. R. *139:*1083, 1982.)

months is abnormal. Isotope studies have been reported to be accurate in detecting infection and loosening.[238, 245, 246, 258]

Accuracy in detecting femoral component loosening may approach that of arthrography. Uptake is considered indicative of loosening if accumulation is increased medially, laterally, and in the tip of the femoral component (Fig. 4–127).[258] If the bone scan is normal, most authors feel there is little chance that loosening is present. Tehranzadeh reported accurate diagnosis of femoral component loosening in 100 percent of cases (21 patients).[258] Scans were performed with Tc-99m.

Accuracy in detection of acetabular loosening is not as great. The joint regions normally demonstrate increased uptake, making diagnosis more difficult. Isotope scans detected loosening in 77 percent of our patients.

Gallium scans may be helpful in detection of infection (Fig. 4–128). The degree of specificity (67 percent) in our practice indicates the need for aspiration in most cases. Indium-111–labeled white blood cells may provide more specificity than gallium. Indium is particularly useful in acute infections.[254] Gallium may be more sensitive in chronic infection but lacks the specificity of indium.

Other causes of increased uptake may also be apparent and, in certain cases, misleading. These

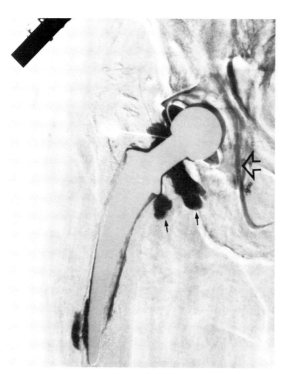

Figure 4–125

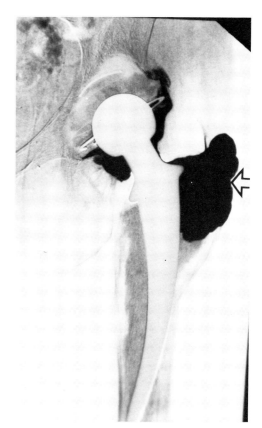

Figure 4–126

Figure 4–125. Subtraction arthrogram in a patient with loosening of the femoral component and infection. Note the pocketing medially *(arrows)*. Slight motion resulted in misregistration of the subtraction *(open arrow)*.

Figure 4–126. Subtraction arthrogram. No evidence of loosening. There is a large trochanteric bursa *(arrow)*.

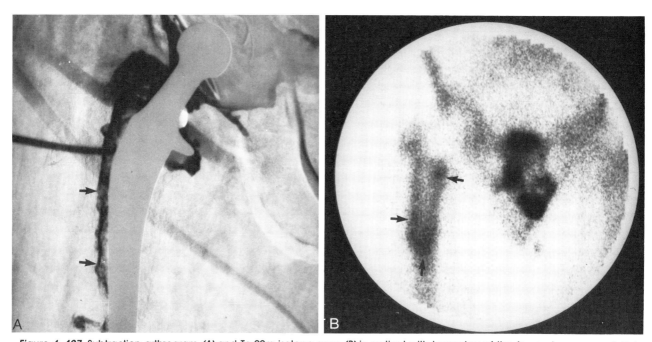

Figure 4–127. Subtraction arthrogram *(A)* and Tc-99m isotope scan *(B)* in patient with loosening of the femoral component. Note contrast along femoral component *(arrows)* on the arthrogram and increased uptake medially, laterally, and at the tip of the component *(arrows)* on the scan.

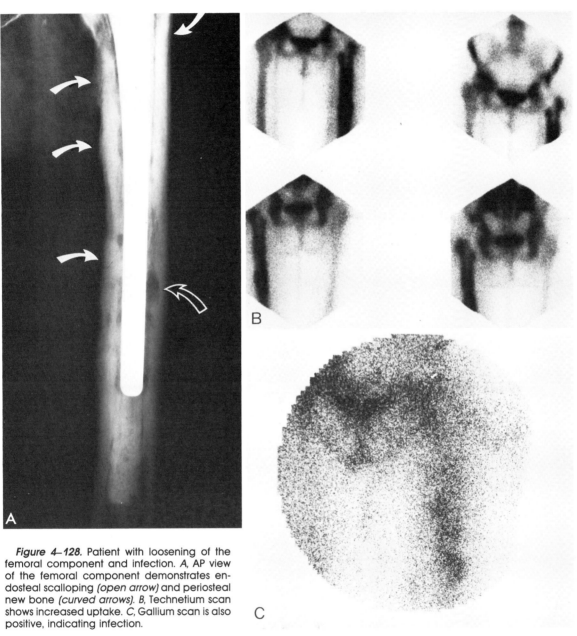

Figure 4–128. Patient with loosening of the femoral component and infection. *A,* AP view of the femoral component demonstrates endosteal scalloping *(open arrow)* and periosteal new bone *(curved arrows). B,* Technetium scan shows increased uptake. *C,* Gallium scan is also positive, indicating infection.

TABLE 4–26. Accuracy of Radiographic Techniques in Evaluation of Joint Replacement Loosening*246

Technique	Femoral Loosening	Acetabular Loosening	Infection
Routine	84	69	—
Isotope	89% (Tc-99m)	77% (Tc-99m)	77% (Ga)
Subtraction	96%	96%	94% (with aspiration)

*Loosening + infection in 50 to 92% of cases246

include Paget's disease, heterotopic bone formation, protrusio acetabuli, and stress fractures of the pubic rami.

Summary

Radiographic evaluation of joint replacements requires close communication between the radiologist and referring physician. Routine films, radioisotope scans, and subtraction arthrography (including aspiration and injection of the pseudocapsule) may be indicated in different clinical situations. Table 4–26 summarizes the accuracy of these modalities.

Most patients present with pain. One must exclude loosening, infection, and other problems described earlier. The arthrogram is most useful in defining anatomy and most causes of hip pain. Culture studies and diagnostic injections add to the versatility of subtraction arthrography and increase its accuracy.

Table 4–27 suggests possible approaches to evaluation of patients with painful hip arthroplasty. The diagnostic approach depends upon the clinical findings and features noted on the routine radiographs. But our discussion has also shown that features of loosening may not be evident on routine films even though components are loose.

If plain films are negative, a Tc-99m scan can be obtained. If this is negative, loosening is unlikely.258 If pain persists or if the scan if positive, an arthrogram should be performed. Pain may be secondary to bursitis rather than loosening, and the arthrogram will assist in diagnosis and treatment.

When films suggest loosening, arthrography is the procedure of choice to confirm the diagnosis and to exclude infection. If the arthrogram is negative but the plain film findings suggest loosening, further exercise and repeat films may result in a more definitive study. Penetration of contrast material around the components is especially difficult to obtain with large pseudocapsules, and further exercise will often result in detection of loosening on the arthrogram. Injection of the joint with bupivacaine (Marcaine) is also helpful in equivocal cases. A positive response indicates intra-articular pathology.

Occasionally patients with features suggestive of infection have negative cultures. In these situations the aspiration may be repeated, or indium and gallium scans may be obtained in an attempt to localize the infection.

TABLE 4–27. Diagnostic Approach to Painful Joint Replacement

REFERENCES

Anatomy

1. Armbuster, T. G., Guerra, J., Resnick, D., et al.: The adult hip: An anatomic study. Radiology 128:1, 1978.
2. Brooke, R.: The sacroiliac joint. J. Anat. 58:299, 1924.
3. Clark, S. S., and Prudencio, R. F.: Lower urinary tract injury associated with pelvic fracture: Diagnosis and management. Surg. Clin. North Am. 52:183, 1972.
4. Francis, C. C.: The Human Pelvis. St. Louis, C. V. Mosby Co., 1952.
5. Grant, J. C. B.: Grant's Atlas of Anatomy. 5th Ed. Baltimore, Williams and Wilkins, 1962.
6. Gray, H., and Goss, C. M.: Anatomy of the Human Body. Philadelphia, Lea and Febiger, 1966.
7. Guerra, J., Armbuster, T. G., Resnick, D., et al.: The adult hip: An anatomic study. Part II: Soft tissue landmarks. Radiology 128:11, 1978.
8. Hollinshead, W. H.: Anatomy for Surgeons. 3rd Ed. Philadelphia, Lea and Febiger, 1982.
9. Kane, W. J.: Fractures of the pelvis. In Rockwood, C. A., and Green, D. P.: Fractures. Philadelphia, J. B. Lippincott Co., 1975.
10. Lang, E. K.: The role of angiography in trauma. Radiol. Clin. North Am. 14:353, 1976.
11. Levin, P.: The coccyx—Its derangements and their treatment. Surg. Gynecol. Obstet. 45:705, 1927.
12. Lewis, M. S., and Norman, A.: The earliest signs of postoperative hip infection. Radiology 104:309, 1972.
13. Miller, W. E.: Massive hemorrhage in fractures of the pelvis. South. Med. J. 56:933, 1963.
14. Motsay, G. J., Manlove, C., and Perry, J. F.: Major venous injury in pelvic fractures. J. Trauma 9:343, 1969.
15. Reichman, S.: Roentgen soft tissue appearances in hip disease. Acta Radiol. Diagn. 6:167, 1967.
16. Resnick, D., and Niwayama, G.: Anatomy of the individual joints. In Resnick, D., and Niwayama, G.: Diagnosis of Bone and Joint Disorders. Philadelphia, W. B. Saunders Co., 1981.
17. Reuter, S. R., and Redman, H. C.: Gastrointestinal Angiography. Philadelphia, W. B. Saunders Co., 1977.
18. Ring, E. J., Athanasoulis, C., Waltman, A. C., et al.: Arteriographic management of hemorrhage following pelvic trauma. Radiology 109:65, 1973.
19. Ring, E. J., Waltman, A. C., and Athanasoulis, C.: Angiography in pelvic trauma. Surg. Gynecol. Obstet. 139:375, 1974.
20. Rowe, C. R., and Lowell, J. D.: Prognosis of fractures of the acetabulum. J. Bone Joint Surg. 43A:30, 1961.
21. Sclafani, S. J. R., and Becker, J. A.: Traumatic presacral hemorrhage: Angiographic diagnosis and therapy. A. J. R. 138:123, 1982.
22. Thaggard, A. III, Harle, T. S., and Carlson, V.: Fractures and dislocations of the bony pelvis and hips. Semin. Roentgenol. 13:117, 1978.
23. Truex, R. C., and Carpenter, M. B.: Strong and Elwyns Human Neuroanatomy. Baltimore, Williams and Wilkins Co., 1964.

Routine Radiography of the Pelvis and Hips

24. Armbuster, T. G., Guerra, J., Resnick, D., et al.: The adult hip: An anatomic study. Radiology 128:1, 1978.
25. Ballinger, P. W.: Merrill's Atlas of Radiographic Positions and Radiologic Procedures. 5th Ed. St. Louis, C. V. Mosby Co., 1982.
26. Berkebile, R. D., Fisher, D. L., and Albrecht, L. F.: The gull-wing sign: Value of the lateral view of the pelvis in fracture-dislocations of the acetabular rim and posterior dislocation of the femoral head. Radiology 84:937, 1965.
27. Bernau, A., and Berquist, T. H.: Orthopaedic Positioning in Diagnostic Radiology. Baltimore, Urban and Schwarzenberg, 1983.
28. Danelius, G., and Miller, L.: Lateral view of the hip. X-ray Technol. 9:176, 1938.

29. Friedman, L. J.: Lateral roentgen ray study of the hip joint. Radiology 27:240, 1936.
30. Harris, J. H., Loh, C. K., Perlman, H. C., et al.: The roentgen diagnosis of pelvic extraperitoneal effusion. Radiology 125:343, 1977.
31. Hickey, P. M.: Value of the lateral view of the hip. A. J. R. 3:308, 1916.
32. Janes, L.: Lateral roentgenography of the neck of the femur. A. J. R. 33:504, 1935.
33. Johnson, C. R.: A new method for roentgen examination of the upper femur. J. Bone Joint Surg. 30:859, 1932.
34. Judet, R., Judet, J., and Letournel, E.: Fractures of the acetabulum: Classification and surgical approaches to open reduction. J. Bone Joint Surg. 46A:1615, 1964.
35. Kalman, M. A.: Radiology of soft tissue shadows in the pelvis: Another look. A. J. R. 130:293, 1978.
36. Lauenstein, C.: Das Rontgenbild einer Luxatio femores infraglenoidales. Fortschr. Roentgenstr. 3:186, 1900.
37. Leonard, R. D., and George, A. W.: Cassette with a convex curve. A. J. R. 28:261, 1932.
38. Letournel, E.: Acetabular fractures: Classification and management. Clin. Orthop. 151:81, 1980.
39. Lorenz: Die rontgenographische Darstellung des subskapularen Raumes und des Schenkelhalses im Querschnitt. Forschr. Roentgenstr. 25:342, 1918.
40. Pennal, G. F., Tile, M., Waddell, J. P., et al.: Pelvic disruption: Assessment and classification. Clin. Orthop. 151:12, 1980.
41. Phillips, H. B.: New roentgen demonstration of the neck of the femur. Am. J. Surg. 5:392, 1928.
42. Schultz, R. J.: The Language of Fractures. Baltimore, Williams and Wilkins, 1972.
43. Taylor, R.: Modified AP projection of the anterior bones of the pelvis. Radiogr. Clin. Photo. 17:67, 1941.
44. Teufel, S.: Eine gezielte Aufsichtsaufnahme der Hüftgelenkspfanne. Röntgenpraxis 10:398, 1938.
45. Tile, M.: Pelvic fractures: Open vs non-operative treatment. Orthop. Clin. North Am. 11:423, 1980.
46. Tile, M.: Fractures of the acetabulum. Orthop. Clin. North Am. 11:481, 1980.

Pelvic Fractures

47. Bassett, L. W., Gold, R. H., and Epstein, H. C.: Anterior hip dislocation: Atypical superolateral displacement of the femoral head. A. J. R. 141:385, 1983.
48. Bavendam, F. A., and Nedelman, S. H.: Some considerations in roentgenology of fractures and dislocations. Semin. Roentgenol. 1:407, 1966.
49. Bonnin, J. G.: Sacral fractures and injury to the cauda equina. J. Bone Joint Surg. 27:113, 1945.
50. Bowerman, J. W.: Radiology and Injury in Sport. New York, Appleton-Century-Crofts, 1977.
51. Brosman, S. A., and Paul, J. G.: Trauma of the bladder. Surg. Gynecol. Obstet. 143:605, 1976.
52. Buchanan, T. I.: Bowel entrapment by pelvic fracture fragments: A case report and review of the literature. Clin. Orthop. 147:164, 1980.
53. Clark, S. S., and Prudencio, R. F.: Lower urinary tract injury associated with pelvic fractures. Surg. Clin. North Am. 52:183, 1972.
54. Colapinto, V.: Trauma of the pelvis: Urethral injury. Clin. Orthop. 151:46, 1980.
55. Colapinto, V., and McCallum, R. W.: Injury to the male posterior urethra in fractures of the pelvis: A new classification. J. Urol. 118:575, 1977.
56. Connally, W. B., and Hedberg, E. A.: Fractures and dislocations of the pelvis. J. Trauma. 9:104, 1969.
57. Cooke, C. P., Levinsohn, E. M., and Baker, B. E.: Septic hip in pelvic fracture with urologic injury. Clin. Orthop. 147:253, 1980.
58. Coventry, M. B.: The treatment of fracture-dislocations of the hip by total hip arthroplasty. J. Bone Joint Surg. 56A:1128, 1974.
59. Dunn, W., and Morris, H. D.: Fractures and dislocations of the pelvis. J. Bone Joint Surg. 50A:1639, 1968.

60. Dunn, W. A., and Russo, C. L.: Central acetabular fractures. J. Trauma *13*:695, 1975.

61. Duverney, J. G.: Traite des maladies des os. Vol. 1. Paris, De Bure l'Aine, 1751.

62. Eichenholtz, S. N., and Stark, R. M.: Central acetabular fractures: A review of 35 cases. J. Bone Joint Surg. *46A*:695, 1964.

63. Furey, W. W.: Fractures of the pelvis with special reference to associated fractures of the sacrum. A. J. R. *47*:89, 1942.

64. Harley, J. D., Mack, L. A., and Winquist, R. A.: CT of acetabular fractures: Comparison with conventional radiography. A. J. R. *138*:413, 1982.

65. Harris, J. J., and Harris, W. H.: The Radiology of Emergency Medicine. Baltimore, Williams and Wilkins, 1975.

66. Hartmann, K.: Blasen- und Harnröhrenverletzungen bei Beckenbrüchen. Arch. klin. Chir. *282*:943, 1955.

67. Holdsworth, E. W.: Dislocations and fracture-dislocations of the pelvis. J. Bone Joint Surg. *30B*:461, 1948.

68. Howard, F. M., and Meaney, R. P.: Stress fractures of the pelvis during pregnancy. J. Bone Joint Surg. *43A*:538, 1961.

69. Jackson, H., Kam, J., Harris, J. H., et al.: The sacral arcuate lines in upper sacral fractures. Radiology *145*:35, 1982.

70. Judet, R., Judet, J., and Letournel, E.: Fractures of the acetabulum: Classification and surgical approaches to reduction. J. Bone Joint Surg. *46A*:1615, 1964.

71. Kessler, F. B., and Driscoll, R.: Bilateral anterior inferior iliac spine avulsions. J. Trauma *3*:129, 1963.

72. Key, J. A., and Conwell, H. E.: Management of Fractures, Dislocations, and Sprains, St. Louis, C. V. Mosby Co., 1951.

73. Knight, R. A., and Smith, H.: Central acetabular fractures. J. Bone Joint Surg. *40A*:1, 1958.

74. Kvarstein, B., Riska, E. B., Slatis, P.: Pelvic fractures. Ann. Chir. Gynaecol. *70*:256, 1981.

75. Lansinger, O.: Fractures of the acetabulum: A clinical, radiological, and experimental study. Acta Orthop. Scand. *165*:1, 1977.

76. Letournel, E.: Surgical repair of acetabular fractures more than three weeks after injury, apart from total hip arthroplasty. Int. Orthop. *2*:305, 1979.

77. Letournel, E.: Acetabular fractures: Classification and management. Clin. Orthop. *151*:81, 1980.

78. Levine, J. I., and Crampton, R. S.: Major abdominal injury associated with pelvic fractures. Surg. Gynecol. Obstet. *116*:223, 1963.

79. Looser, K. J., and Crombie, H. D.: Pelvic fracture: An anatomic guide to the severity of injury. A review of 100 cases. Am. J. Surg. *132*:638, 1976.

80. Mack, L. A., Harley, D., and Winquist, R. A.: CT of acetabular fractures: Analysis of fracture patterns. A. J. R. *138*:12, 1980.

81. Margolies, M. N., Ring, E. J., Waltman, A. C., et al.: Arteriography in the management of hemorrhage from pelvic fractures. N. Engl. J. Med. *287*:317, 1972.

82. McAvay, J. M., and Cook, J. H.: A treatment plan for rapid assessment of the patient with massive blood loss and pelvic fractures. Arch. Surg. *113*:986, 1978.

83. McMurtry, R., Walton, D., Dickinson, D., et al.: Pelvic disruption in the polytraumatized patient. A management protocol. Clin. Orthop. *151*:22, 1980.

84. Mucha, P., and Farnell, M. B.: Analysis of pelvic fracture management. J. Trauma *24*:379, 1984.

85. O'Keefe, T. J.: Retroperitoneal abscess: A potentially fatal complication of closed fracture of the pelvis. J. Bone Joint Surg. *60*:1117, 1978.

86. Paster, S. B., Van Houten, F. X., and Adams, D. F.: Percutaneous balloon catheter. A technique for control of arterial hemorrhage caused by pelvic fractures. JAMA *23*:573, 1974.

87. Patterson, F. P., and Morton, K. S.: Neurological complications of fractures and dislocations of the pelvis. Surg. Gynecol. Obstet. *112*:702, 1961.

88. Pearson, J. R., and Hagedorn, E. J.: Fractures of the pelvis involving the floor of the acetabulum. J. Bone Joint Surg. *44B*:550, 1962.

89. Peltier, L. F.: Complications associated with fractures of the pelvis. J. Bone Joint Surg. *47A*:1060, 1965.

90. Pennal, G. F., Tile, M., Waddell, J. P., et al.: Pelvic disruption: Assessment and classification. Clin. Orthop. *151*:12, 1980.

91. Perry, J. F.: Pelvic open fractures. Clin. Orthop. *151*:41, 1980.

92. Rankin, L. M.: Fractures of the pelvis. Ann. Surg. *106*:226, 1937.

93. Ring, E. J., Athanasoulis, C., Waltman, A. C., et al.: Arteriography in management of hemorrhage from pelvic fractures. Radiology *109*:65, 1973.

94. Rockwood, C. A., and Green, C. P.: Fractures. Philadelphia, J. B. Lippincott Co., 1975.

95. Rogers, L. F.: Radiology of Skeletal Trauma. New York, Churchill Livingstone, 1982.

96. Rothenberger, D. A., Kellam, J., McGonigal, D.: Open pelvic fractures: A lethal injury. J. Trauma. *18*:184, 1978.

97. Rowe, C. R., and Lowell, J. D.: Prognosis of fractures of the acetabulum. J. Bone Joint Surg. *43A*:30, 1961.

98. Sampson, J., and Berquist, T. H.: Pelvic fractures: A review of 750 cases. Presentation, American Roentgen Ray Society, Las Vegas, Nevada, 1981.

99. Sampson, J., and Berquist, T. H.: Pelvic fractures. A review of 669 cases. Publication pending a larger series than presentation.

100. Sandler, C. M., Harris, J. H., Corriere, J. N., et al.: Posterior urethral injury after pelvic fracture. A. J. R. *137*:1233, 1981.

101. Sandler, C. M., Phillips, J. M., Harris, J. D., et al.: Radiology of the bladder and urethra in blunt pelvic trauma. Radiol. Clin. North Am. *19*:195, 1981.

102. Sauser, D. D., Billemoria, P. E., Rouse, G. A., et al.: CT evaluation of hip trauma. A. J. R. *138*:269, 1980.

103. Sclafani, S. J. A., and Becker, J. A.: Traumatic presacral hemorrhage: Angiographic diagnosis and therapy. A. J. R. *138*:123, 1982.

104. Sheldon, G. F., and Winestock, D. P.: Hemorrhage from open pelvic fracture controlled intraoperatively with balloon catheter. J. Trauma. *18*:68, 1978.

105. Silakovich, W., and Love, L.: Stress fracture of the pubic ramus. J. Bone Joint Surg. *36A*:573, 1954.

106. Slatis, P., and Karaharjn, E.: External fixation of unstable pelvic fractures with trapezoid compression frame. J. Bone Joint Surg. *63B*:2, 1981.

107. Stewart, M. J., Milford, L. W.: Fracture-dislocation of the hip. An end result study. J. Bone Joint Surg. *36A*:315, 1954.

108. Taylor, R. G.: Pelvic dislocation. Brit. J. Surg. *30*:126, 1942.

109. Thaggard, A. III, Harle, T. S., and Carlson, V.: Fractures and dislocations of the bony pelvis and hip. Semin. Roentgenol. *13*:117, 1978.

110. Thompson, K. R., and Goldin, A. R.: Angiographic technique in interventional radiology. Radiol. Clin. North Am. *17*:375, 1980.

111. Tile, M.: Fractures of the acetabulum. Orthop. Clin. North Am. *11*:481, 1980.

112. Tile, M.: Pelvic fractures: Operative vs. non-operative treatment. Orthop. Clin. North Am. *11*:423, 1980.

113. Urist, M. R.: Fractures of the acetabulum: The nature of traumatic lesions. Treatment and 2-year end results. Ann. Surg. *127*:1150, 1948.

114. Watson-Jones, R.: Dislocations and fracture-dislocations of the pelvis. Brit. J. Surg. *25*:773, 1938.

115. Weil, G. C., Price, E. M., Rusbridge, H. W.: The diagnosis and treatment of fractures of the pelvis and their complications. Am. J. Surg. *44*:108, 1939.

116. Wild, J. J., Hanson, G. J., Jr., Tullos, H. L.: Unstable fractures of the pelvis treated by external fixation. J. Bone Joint Surg. *64A*:1010, 1982.

117. Zorn, G.: Beckenbrüche mit Harnröhrenverletzungen ihre Behandlung und Ergebnisse. Beitr. klin. Chir. *201*:147, 1960.

Dislocations and Fracture-Dislocations of the Hip

118. Armstrong, J. R.: Traumatic dislocation of the hip joint. J. Bone Joint Surg. *30B*:430, 1948.

119. Brav, E. A.: Traumatic dislocation of the hip. Army expe-

rience and results over a 12-year period. J. Bone Joint Surg. *44A*:1115, 1962.

120. Chakrabort, S., and Miller, I. M.: Dislocation of the hip associated with fracture of the femoral head. Injury 7:134, 1975.
121. Clawson, R. K., and Melcher, P. J.: Fractures and dislocations of the hip. *In* Rockwood, C. A., and Green, C. P.: Fractures. Philadelphia, J. B. Lippincott, 1975.
122. Dehne, E., and Immerman, E. W.: Dislocation of the hip combined with fracture of the shaft of the femur on the same side. J. Bone Joint Surg. *33A*:731, 1951.
123. DeLee, J. C., Evans, J. A., and Thomas, J.: Anterior dislocation of the hip associated with femoral head fractures. J. Bone Joint Surg. *62A*:960, 1980.
124. Dussault, R. G., Beauregard, G., Fauteaux, P., et al.: Femoral head fracture following anterior hip dislocation. Radiology *135*:627, 1980.
125. Ehtisham, S. M. A.: Traumatic dislocation of the hip joint with fracture of the femoral shaft on the same side. J. Trauma *16*:196, 1976.
126. Epstein, H. C.: Posterior fracture-dislocation of the hip—comparison of open and closed methods of treatment in certain types. J. Bone Joint Surg. *43A*:1079, 1961.
127. Epstein, H. C.: Posterior fracture-dislocation of the hip. J. Bone Joint Surg. *56A*:1103, 1974.
128. Epstein, H. C.: Traumatic dislocation of the hip. Clin. Orthop. *92*:116, 1973.
129. Ghormley, R. K., and Sullivan, R.: Traumatic dislocation of the hip. Am. J. Surg. *85*:298, 1953.
130. Helal, B., and Skevis, X.: Concealed traumatic dislocation of the hip. Proc. Roy. Soc. Med. (Orthop. Sec.) *59*:119, 1966.
131. Pipkin, G.: Treatment of Grade IV fracture-dislocations of the hip. J. Bone Joint Surg. *39A*:1027, 1957.
132. Reigstad, A.: Traumatic dislocation of the hip. J. Trauma *20*:603, 1980.
133. Roeder, L. F., and DeLee, J. C.: Femoral head fractures associated with posterior hip dislocation. Clin. Orthop. *147*:121, 1980.
134. Rogers, L. F.: Radiology of Skeletal Trauma. New York, Churchhill Livingstone, 1982.
135. Rosenthal, R. E., and Coker, W. L.: Fracture-dislocations of the hip: An epidemiological review. J. Trauma *19*:572, 1979.
136. Scadden, W. J., and Dennyson, W. G.: Unreduced obturator dislocation of the hip: A case report. S. Afr. Med. J. *53*:601, 1978.
137. Scham, S. M., and Fry, L. R.: Traumatic anterior dislocation of the hip with fracture of the femoral head. A case report. Clin. Orthop. *62*:133, 1969.
138. Smith, G. R., and Loop, J. W.: Radiological classification of posterior hip dislocation. Radiology *119*:569, 1976.
139. Stewart, M. J., Milford, L. W.: Fracture-dislocations of the hip. J. Bone Joint Surg. *36A*:315, 1954.
140. Thaggard, A. III, Harle, T. S., Carlson, V.: Fractures and dislocations of the boney pelvis and hips. Semin. Roentgenol. *13*:117, 1978.
141. Thompson, V. P., and Epstein, H. C.: Traumatic dislocation of the hip. J. Bone Joint Surg. *33A*:747, 1951.
142. Urist, M. R.: Fracture-dislocation of the hip joint. J. Bone Joint Surg. *30A*:699, 1948.

Femoral Neck Fractures

143. Ambrose, G. B., Garcia, A., and Neer, C. S.: Displaced intracapsular fractures of the neck of the femur. J. Trauma *3*:361, 1963.
144. Arnoldi, C. C., Lemperg, R. K.: Fractures of the femoral neck. Clin. Orthop. *129*:217, 1977.
145. Asnis, S. E., Shoji, H., Bohne, W. H. O.: Scintimetric evaluation of complications of femoral neck fractures. Clin. Orthop. *121*:149, 1976.
146. Banks, H. H.: Factors influencing the results in fractures of the femoral neck. J. Bone Joint Surg. *44A*:931, 1962.
147. Barnes, R., Brown, J., Garden, R. S., et al.: Subcapital fractures of the femur. A prospective review. J. Bone Joint Surg. *58B*:2, 1976.
148. Bayliss, A. P., and Davidson, J. K.: Traumatic osteonecrosis of the head of the femur following intracapsular fractures: Incidence and earliest radiographic features. Clin. Radiol. *28*:407, 1977.
149. Bobechko, W. P., and Harris, W. R.: The radiographic density of avascular bone. J. Bone Joint Surg. *42B*:626, 1960.
150. Bowerman, J.: Radiology and Injury in Sports. New York, Appleton-Century-Crofts, 1977.
151. Coats, R. L., and Armour, P.: Treatment of subcapital femoral fractures by total hip replacement. Injury *11*:132, 1979.
152. De Haas, W., and Macnab, I.: Fractures of the neck of the femur. S. Afr. Med. J. *30*:1005, 1956.
153. Dunn, W. L., Wahner, H. W., and Riggs, B. L.: Measurement of bone mineral content in human vertebra and hip by dual-photon absorptiometry. Radiology *136*:485, 1980.
154. Ficat, P., and Arlet, J.: Diagnostic de l'ostéo-necrose fémorocapitale primitive au stade I (stade pré-radiologique). Rev. Chir. Orthop. *54*:637, 1968.
155. Garden, R. S.: Stability and union of subcapital fractures of the femur. J. Bone Joint Surg. *46B*:630, 1964.
156. Garden, R. S.: Reduction and fixation of subcapital fractures of the femur. Clin. Orthop. North Am. *5*:683, 1974.
157. Griffiths, W. E. G., Swanson, S. A., and Freeman, M. A. R.: Experimental fatigue fractures of the femoral neck. J. Bone Joint Surg. *54B*:136, 1971.
158. Hanson, B. A., and Solgaard, S.: Impacted fractures of the femoral neck treated by early mobilization and weight-bearing. Acta Orthop. Scand. *49*:180, 1978.
159. Hungerford, D. S.: Pathogenic consideration in ischemic necrosis of bone. Can. J. Surg. *24*:583, 1981.
160. Jeffrey, C. C.: Spontaneous fracture of the femoral neck. Orthop. Clin. North Am. *5*:713, 1974.
161. Meyers, M. H.: Impacted and undisplaced femoral neck fractures. The Hip. Proceedings of the Tenth Open Scientific Meeting of the Hip Society. St. Louis, C. V. Mosby Co., 1982.
162. Moon, K. L., Genant, H. K., Helms, C. A., et al.: Musculoskeletal applications of nuclear magnetic resonance. Radiology *147*:161, 1983.
163. Norman, A., and Bullough, P.: The radiolucent crescent sign. An early diagnostic sign of necrosis of the femoral head. Bull. Hosp. Jt. Dis. Orthop. Inst. *24*:99, 1963.
164. Pauwell, F.: Der Schenkelausbruch: ein mechanishes Problem. Grundlagen des heilungsvorganges Prognose und kausale Therapie. Stuttgart, Ferdinande Enke, 1935.
165. Phemister, D. B.: Bone growth and repair. Ann. Surg. *102*:261, 1935.
166. Rubin, R., Trent, P., Arnold, W., et al.: Knowles pinning of experimental femoral neck fractures: Biomechanical study. J. Trauma *21*:1036, 1981.
167. Salvati, E. A., and Wilson, P. D.: Long-term results of the femoral-head replacement. J. Bone Joint Surg. *55A*:516, 1973.
168. Scheck, M.: Intracapsular fractures of the femoral neck. Comminution of the posterior cortex as a cause of unstable fracture. J. Bone Joint Surg. *41A*:1187, 1959.
169. Schultz, R. J.: The Language of Fractures. Baltimore, Williams and Wilkins, 1972.
170. Sikorski, J. M., and Barrington, R.: Internal fixation versus hemiarthroplasty for the displaced subcapital fracture of the femur: A prospective, randomized study. J. Bone Joint Surg. *63B*:356, 1981.
171. Smith, K., Bonfiglio, M., and Montgomery, W.: Nontraumatic necrosis of the femoral head treated with tibial bone grafting: Follow-up note. J. Bone Joint Surg. *62A*:845, 1980.
172. Söreide, O., Mölster, A., and Raugstad, T. S.: Internal fixation versus primary prosthetic replacement in acute femoral neck fractures: A prospective, randomized clinical study. Br. J. Surg. *66*:56, 1979.

173. Stevens, J., Freeman, P. A., Nordin, B. E. C., et al.: The incidence of osteoporosis in patients with femoral neck fractures. J. Bone Joint Surg. *44B*:520, 1962.

Trochanteric Fractures

174. Bowerman, J.: Radiology and Injury in Sport. New York, Appleton-Century-Crofts, 1977.
175. Boyd, H. B., and Griffin, L. L.: Classification and treatment of trochanteric fractures. Arch. Surg. *58*:853, 1949.
176. Clawson, D. K., and Melcher, P. J.: Fractures and dislocations of the hip. *In* Rockwood, C. A., and Green, D. P.: Fractures. Philadelphia, J. B. Lippincott, 1975.
177. Dimon, J. H., and Hughston, J. C.: Unstable intertrochanteric fractures of the hip. J. Bone Joint Surg. *49A*:440, 1967.
178. Ender, H. G.: Treatment of trochanteric and subtrochanteric fractures of the femur with Ender pins. The Hip. Proceedings of the Sixth Open Scientific Meeting of the Hip Society. St. Louis, C. V. Mosby Co., 1978.
179. Evans, E. M.: The treatment of trochanteric fractures of the femur. J. Bone Joint Surg. *31B*:190, 1949.
180. Fielding, J. W.: Subtrochanteric fractures. Clin. Orthop. *92*:86, 1973.
181. Hafner, R. H. V.: Trochanteric fractures of the femur. J. Bone Joint Surg. *33B*:513, 1951.
182. Harrington, K., Sim, F. H., Enis, J. E., et al.: Methyl methacrylate as adjunct in internal fixation of pathologic fractures: Experience in 375 cases. J. Bone Joint Surg. *58A*:1047, 1976.
183. Hyse-Moore, G. H., MacEachern, A. G., and Evans, D. C.: Treatment of intertrochanteric fractures of the femur. A comparison of the Richards screw-plate with the Jewett nail-plate. J. Bone Joint Surg. *65B*:262, 1983.
184. Jensen, J. S.: Classification of trochanteric fractures. Acta. Orthop. Scand. *51*:803, 1980.
185. Jensen, J. S., and Michaelsen, M.: Trochanteric fractures treated with McLaughlin osteosynthesis. Acta. Orthop. Scand. *46*:795, 1975.
186. Kock, J. C.: The laws of bone architecture. Am. J. Anat. *21*:177, 1917.
187. Kuderna, H., Böhler, N., Collon, D. J.: Treatment of intertrochanteric and subtrochanteric fractures of the femur by the Ender method. J. Bone Joint Surg. *58A*:604, 1976.
188. Kyle, R. F., Gustilo, R. B., and Premer, R. F.: Analysis of 622 intertrochanteric hip fractures. J. Bone Joint Surg. *61A*:216, 1979.
189. Lord, G., Marotte, J. H., Blantard, J. P., et al.: Head and neck arthroplasty in treatment of intertrochanteric fractures after age 70. Rev. Chir. Orthop. *63*:135, 1977.
190. May, J. M. B., and Chacha, P. B.: Displacement of trochanteric fractures and their influence on reduction. J. Bone Joint Surg. *50B*:318, 1968.
191. Mickelson, M. R., and Bonfiglio, M.: Pathologic fractures of the proximal part of the femur treated by Zickel nail fixation. J. Bone Joint Surg. *58A*:1067, 1976.
192. Mulholland, R. C., and Gunn, D. R.: Sliding screw-plate fixation of intertrochanteric femoral fractures. J. Trauma *12*:581, 1972.
193. Naimark, A., Kossoff, J., and Schepsis, A.: Intertrochanteric fractures: Current concepts on an old subject. A. J. R. *133*:889, 1979.
194. Pankovich, A. M., and Tarabishy, I.: Ender nailing of intertrochanteric and subtrochanteric fractures of the femur: Complications, failures, and errors. J. Bone Joint Surg. *62A*:635, 1980.
195. Rasmussen, K.: McLaughlin osteosynthesis in trochanteric fractures. Acta Chir. Scand. *108*:246, 1953.
196. Rogers, L. F.: Radiology of Skeletal Trauma. New York, Churchill Livingstone, 1982.
197. Rybicki, E. F., Simonen, F. A., and Weis, E. G., Jr.: On the mathematical analysis of stress in the human femur. J. Biomech. *5*:203, 1972.
198. Sarmiento, A., and Williams, E. M.: Unstable trochanteric fracture: Treatment with valgus osteotomy and I-beam nail-plate: Preliminary report of 100 cases. J. Bone Joint Surg. *52A*:1309, 1970.
199. Schatzker, J., Ha'eri, J. B., Chapman, M.: Methyl methacrylate as adjunct in internal fixation of intertrochanteric fractures of the femur. J. Trauma *18*:732, 1978.
200. Seinsheimer, F.: Subtrochanteric fractures of the femur. J. Bone Joint Surg. *60A*:300, 1978.
201. Wade, P. A., Campbell, R. D., Kerin, R. J.: Management of intertrochanteric fractures of the femur. Am. J. Surg. *97*:634, 1959.
202. Whatley, J. R., Garland, D. E., Whitecloud, T. III, et al.: Subtrochanteric fracture of the femur: Treatment with ASIF blade-plate fixation. South. Med. J. *71*:1372, 1978.
203. Zickel, R. E., Bercik, M. J., and Licciardi, L. M.: A continuing study on the use of the Zickel intramedullary appliances in fractures and lesions of the proximal femur. The Hip. Proceedings of the Sixth Open Scientific Meeting of the Hip Society. St. Louis, C. V. Mosby Co., 1978.
204. Zickel, R. E., and Mouradin, W. H.: Intramedullary fixation of pathologic fractures in lesions of the subtrochanteric region of the femur. J. Bone Joint Surg. *58A*:1061, 1976.

Hip Arthrography in the Adult

205. Chandler, B.: The iliopsoas bursa in man. Anat. Rec. *58*:235, 1934.
206. Gelman, M.: Arthrography of the adult hip. *In* Dalinka, M. K. (ed.): Arthrography. New York, Springer-Verlag, 1980.
207. Ghelman, B., and Freiberger, R. H.: The adult hip. *In* Freiberger, R. H., and Kaye, J. J. (eds.): Arthrography. New York, Appleton-Century-Crofts, 1979.
208. Goldman, A. B.: Arthrography of the hip joint. CRC Crit. Rev. Diagn. Imaging *13*:111, 1980.
209. Goldman, A.B., Hallel, T., Salvati, E. M., et al.: Osteochondritis dissecans complicating Legg-Calvé-Perthes disease. Radiology *121*:561, 1976.
210. Goldman, A. B., Schneider, R., and Martel, W.: Acute chondrolysis complicating slipped capital femoral epiphysis. A. J. R. *130*:945, 1978.
211. Hall, F.: Epinephrine-enhanced knee arthrography. Radiology *111*:215, 1974.
212. Hublein, G. W., Greene, G. S., and Conforti, V. P.: Hip joint arthrography. A. J. R. *68*:736, 1952.
213. Kevin, A., and Levine, J.: A technique for arthrography of the hip. A. J. R. *68*:107, 1952.
214. Lequesne, M., Becker, J., Bard, M., et al.: Capsular constriction of the hip: Arthrographic and clinical considerations. Skeletal Radiol. *6*:1, 1981.
215. McCauley, R. G. K., Wunderlich, B. K., and Zimbler, S.: Air embolism as a complication of hip arthrography. Skeletal Radiol. *6*:11, 1981.
216. Moule, N. J., and Golding, J. R.: Idiopathic chondrolysis of the hip. Clin. Radiol. *25*:247, 1974.
217. Razzano, C. D., Nelson, C. L., and Wilds, A. H.: Arthrography of the adult hip. Clin. Orthop. *99*:86, 1974.
218. Resnick, D., and Niwayama, G.: Diagnosis of Bone and Joint Disorders. Philadelphia, W. B. Saunders Co., 1981.
219. Spataro, R. F.: Epinephrine enhanced knee arthrography. Invest. Radiol. *13*:286, 1978.
220. Warren, R., Kaye, J. J., and Salvati, E. A.: Arthrographic demonstration of an enlarged iliopsoas bursa complicating osteoarthritis of the hip. J. Bone Joint Surg. *57A*:413, 1975.

Radiographic Evaluation of Joint Replacement

221. Anderson, L. S., and Staple, T. W.: Arthrography of total hip replacement using subtraction technique. J. Can. Assoc. Radiol. *109*:470, 1973.
222. Bassett, L. W., Gold, R. H., and Hedley, A. K.: Radiology of failed surface replacement total hip arthroplasty. A. J. R. *139*:1083, 1982.
223. Beckenbaugh, R. D., and Ilstrup, D. M.: Total hip arthroplasty: A review of 333 cases with long follow-up. J. Bone Joint Surg. *60A*:306. 1978.
224. Brown, C. S., and Kneckenbacker, W. J.: Radiologic studies

in the investigation of the causes of total hip replacement failures. J. Can. Assoc. Radiol. 24:245, 1973.

225. Chao, E. Y. S., and Coventry, M. B.: Fracture of the femoral component after total hip arthroplasty. J. Bone Joint Surg. 63A:1078, 1981.

226. Charnley, J.: A biomechanical analysis of use of cement to anchor the femoral head prosthesis. J. Bone Joint Surg. 47B:354, 1965.

227. Charnley, J.: The reaction of bone to self-curing acrylate cement. J. Bone Joint Surg. 52B:340, 1970.

228. Clarke, I. C., Black, K., Rennie, C., et al.: Can wear of total hip arthroplasties be assessed from radiographs? Clin. Orthop. 121:126, 1976.

229. Collins, D. N., Chetta, S. G., and Nelson, C. L.: Fractures of the acetabular cup: A case report. J. Bone Joint Surg. 64A:939, 1982.

230. Coren, G. S., Curtis, J., and Dalinka, M.: Lymphatic filling visualized during hip arthrography. Radiology 115:621, 1975.

231. Coventry, M. B., Beckenbaugh, R. D., Nolan, D. R., et al.: 2,012 total hip arthroplasties: A study of postoperative course and early complications. J. Bone Joint Surg. 56A:273, 1974.

232. DeLee, J. G., and Charnley, J.: Radiographic demarcation of cemented sockets in total hip replacement. Clin. Orthop. 121:20, 1976.

233. Dolinskas, C., Campbell, R. E., and Rothman, R. H.: The painful Charnley total hip replacement. A. J. R. 121:61, 1974.

234. Dowling, J. M., Atkinson, J. R., Dowson, D., et al.: The characteristics of acetabular cups worn in the human body. J. Bone Joint Surg. 60B:375, 1978.

235. Dussault, R. G., Goldman, A. B., and Ghelman, B.: Radiologic diagnosis of loosening and infection in hip prosthesis. J. Can. Assoc. Radiol. 28:119, 1977.

236. Fackler, C. D., and Poss, R.: Dislocation in total hip arthroplasty. Clin. Orthop. 151:169, 1980.

237. Galante, J. O.: Causes of fracture of the femoral component in total hip replacement. J. Bone Joint Surg. 62A:670, 1980.

238. Gelman, M. I., Coleman, R. E., Stevens, P. M., et al.: Radiographic, radionuclide imaging, and arthrography in evaluation of total hip and total knee replaclement. Radiology 128:677, 1978.

239. Ghelman, B.: Three methods for determining anteversion and retroversion of total hip prosthesis. A. J. R. 133:1127, 1979.

240. Goldring, S. R., Schiller, A. L., Roelke, M., et al.: The synovial-like membrane at the bone-cement interface in loose total hip replacements and its proposed role in bone lysis. J. Bone Joint Surg. 65A:575, 1983.

241. Gore, D. R., Murry, M. P., Gardener, C. M., et al.: Roentgen measurements after Muller total hip replacement. J. Bone Joint Surg. 59A:948, 1977.

242. Gristina, A. G., and Kolkin, J.: Current concepts review: Total joint replacement and sepsis. J. Bone Joint Surg. 64A:128, 1983.

243. Hankey, S., McCall, I. W., Park, W. M., et al.: Technical problems in arthrography of the painful hip arthroplasty. Clin. Radiol. 30:653, 1979.

244. Harris, W. H.: Total joint replacement. N. Engl. J. Med. 297:650, 1977.

245. Hendrix, R. W., and Anderson, T. M.: Arthrographic and radiologic evaluation of prosthetic joints. Radiol. Clin. North Am. 19:349, 1981.

246. Lyons, C., Berquist, T. H., Lyons, J. C., et al.: Evaluation of radiographic findings in painful hip arthroplasties. Clin. Orthop. May, 1985.

247. Mullins, M. F., Sutton, R. N., and Lodwick, G. S.: Complications of total hip replacement A. J. R. 121:55, 1974.

248. Murry, W. R., and Rodrigo, J. J.: Arthrography for assessment of pain after total hip replacement. J. Bone Joint Surg. 57A:1060, 1975.

249. Phillips, W. C., and Kattapuram, S. V.: Prosthetic hip replacement: Plain films and arthrography for component loosening. A. J. R. 138:677, 1982.

250. Reing, C. M., Richin, P. F., and Kenmore, P. I.: Differential bone-scanning in the evaluation of painful total joint replacement. J. Bone Joint Surg. 61A:933, 1979.

251. Salenius, P., and Vanka, E.: Arthrography of the hip in diagnosis of postoperative conditions after total hip replacement. Ann. Chir. Gyn. 68:121, 1979.

252. Salvati, E. A., and Freiberger, R. H: Arthrography for complications of total hip replacement. J. Bone Joint Surg. 53A:701, 1971.

253. Salvati, E. A., Im, V. C., Aglietti, P., et al.: Radiology of total hip replacement. Clin. Orthop. 121:74, 1976.

254. Sfakianakis, G. N., Al-Sheikh, W., Heal, A., et al.: Comparison of scintigraphy with In-111 leukocytes in diagnosis of occult sepsis. J. Nucl. Med. 23:618, 1982.

255. Stauffer, R.: 10-year follow-up study of total hip replacement with particular reference to component loosening. J. Bone Joint Surg. 64A:983, 1982.

256. Stoker, D. J.: A simple technique of joint puncture following hip arthroplasty. Radiology 136:234, 1980.

257. Sutherland, C. J., Wilde, A. H., Borden, L. S., et al.: A 10-year follow-up of 100 consecutive Muller curved-stem total hip replacement arthroplasties. J. Bone Joint Surg. 64A:970, 1982.

258. Tehranzadeh, J., Schneider, R., and Freiberger, R. H.: Radiological evaluation of painful total hip replacement. Radiology 141:355, 1981.

259. Vakili, F., Salvati, E. A., and Warren, R. F.: Entrapped foreign body within the acetabular cup in total hip replacement. Clin. Orthop. 150:159, 1980.

260. Woo, R. Y. G., and Morrey, B. F.: Dislocations after total hip arthroplasty. J. Bone Joint Surg. 64A:1295, 1982.

5

FEMORAL SHAFT FRACTURES

C. E. BENDER • D. C. CAMPBELL, II

The femur is the longest, largest, and strongest bone in the body. Because of its length, width, and role as a primary weight-bearing bone, it must tolerate the extremes of axial loading and angulatory stresses. Massive musculature envelopes the femur. This musculature provides abundant blood supply to the bone, which also allows great potential for healing. Thus, the most significant problem relating to femoral shaft fractures is not healing, but resto-

ration of bone length and alignment so that the femoral shaft will tolerate the functional stresses demanded of it.[7]

ANATOMY

The shaft of the femur is tubular in shape (Fig. 5–1). It is generally smooth, except for the linea

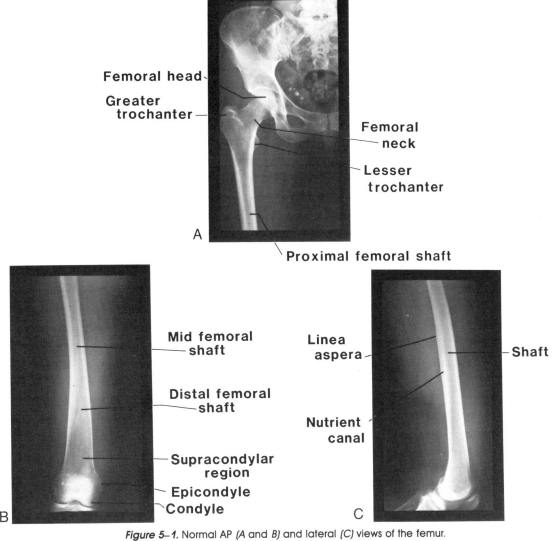

Figure 5–1. Normal AP *(A and B)* and lateral *(C)* views of the femur.

aspera, which is a prominent posterior longitudinal ridge extending from the intertrochanteric crest inferiorly to the middle half of the femur, where it diverges into a medial and lateral lip to become the respective supracondylar lines. The pectineal line extends from the lesser trochanter between the gluteal tuberosity and upper medial lip of linea aspera inferiorly to blend with this lip or the middle part of the linea.[4] The body of the femoral shaft is slightly bowed anteriorly (Fig. 5–1C). In standing position, the femoral shaft normally inclines medially about 10°. Structurally, the femur can resist angulating forces. But as a tubular structure its design is not the best for resisting torsional forces.

Massive muscle groups surround the femoral shaft (Fig. 5–2). Hip flexors, extensors, and abductors and knee flexor and extensor groups provide a bulk of soft tissue protection.

Blood supply to the femoral shaft is through metaphyseal, periosteal, and endosteal vessels. The very rich periosteal blood supply is from the large surrounding muscles and is interrupted only in injuries in which extensive stripping has occurred. The nutrient arteries are perforating vessels that originate from the profunda femoris artery. The perforating branches encircle the femur posteriorly

and perforate the muscle attachments adjacent to the linea aspera. Usually, there are four perforating branches. The lower part of the femur is supplied by a long descending branch of the nutrient artery in the intramedullary canal.[4] The main femoral artery, which is located medially to the shaft, perforates the adductor hiatus. With distal skeletal injury, this may be the site of vascular injury.

The sciatic nerve, well cushioned medially and posteriorly in the thigh, is rarely injured at the shaft level.

CLASSIFICATION AND MECHANISM OF INJURY

Major external violence, as encountered in trauma from motor vehicle accidents, is the usual mechanism of injury. Young adults and children are predominantly injured. The metaphyseal areas in the younger population are wider and dissipate stress better than the diaphysis. Thus, fracture of the femoral shaft is more likely to occur. However, in aging bones or in patients with metabolic bone disease, the metaphyseal areas are more brittle and more susceptible to fracture than the diaphysis. Because severe violence is often involved in the

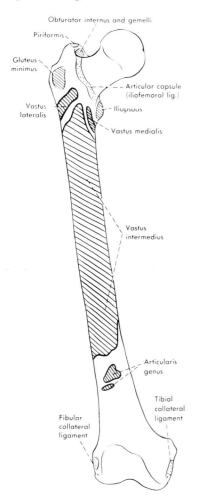

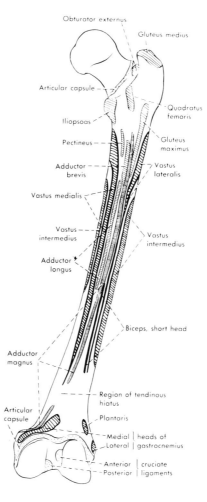

Figure 5–2. A, Anterior muscle attachments of femur. B, Posterior muscle attachments. (From Hollinshead, W. H.: Anatomy for Surgeons. 3rd Ed. Philadelphia, Harper and Row, 1982.)

A

B

production of femoral shaft fractures, significant soft tissue damage usually occurs as well.

Fractures may be either open or closed. Open fractures suggest greater injury to both bone and soft tissues. Open fractures may result from external damage to the soft tissues or from extrusion of fracture fragments from the inside outward. Simple fractures may be transverse, oblique, or spiral. With greater injury force, segmental or comminuted fractures may occur. Occasionally, linear cracks along the shaft may be present that are not visible radiographically. These are important to recognize if internal fixation is contemplated.[7] If such cracks go undetected, the simple fracture may be converted to a comminuted type secondary to shattering of bone during attempts at fixation.

Fractures of the femoral shaft may also be classified according to the type of force that produced the fracture. Angulation forces produce transverse fractures, transverse fractures with butterfly fragments, and segmental fractures; torsional forces produce oblique and spiral oblique fractures; impaction forces produce comminuted or segmental fractures; and penetrating forces may result in bone loss.[8]

Finally, fractures may be classified according to location. Fractures of the middle third of the shaft are most common. At this level, overriding of fracture fragments and shortening of the limb usually result. The displacement of the fracture may be the result of muscle pull. The proximal fragment may be rotated outward because of the forces of gravity and external rotator muscles.[4] In fractures of the upper third, the proximal fragment tends to be flexed by the iliopsoas, abducted by the gluteus medius and gluteus maximus, and externally rotated by the short rotators and the forces of gravity. The distal fragment may be adducted by the pull of the adductor muscles. In fractures of the lower third of the shaft, shortening and displacement can occur. Posterior displacement of the distal fragment occurs because of the action of the gastrocnemius, popliteus, and plantaris muscles. Injury to the popliteal vessels may occur.

RADIOGRAPHIC TECHNIQUE

The clinical diagnosis of femoral shaft fractures is usually quite easy. Angular deformity, shortening, and pain are readily apparent. An expanding thigh is a sign of hemorrhage and should alert physicians to the possibility of shock.

Standardized views of the femoral shaft include AP and lateral projections (Fig. 5–3; see Fig. 5–1), using Potter-Bucky technique. It is mandatory that the adjacent hip and knee joints be included on the films because of the significant incidence of associated ipsilateral injuries.

The AP view of the femur (Fig. 5–3A) is obtained with the patient supine, legs extended. The unaffected leg should be slightly abducted. The foot is

internally rotated approximately 15° in order to position the patella anteriorly and to minimize anteversion of the femoral neck. The central x-ray beam is directed vertically to the midpoint of the cassette. Soft tissues of the thigh must be included on the film. In this way subcutaneous air or hematomas are readily detected. With larger patients, it is necessary to radiograph the upper and lower femurs separately. The central beam is directed perpendicularly to the film in each case.

The lateral view is obtained with the patient turned onto the affected side. The uppermost knee is flexed and placed on a large pad in front of the involved extremity. The pelvis is then adjusted for a true lateral position. The involved dependent knee is slightly flexed. The central beam is directed perpendicularly to the midpoint of the film. A severely injured patient is not moved because of the danger of fracture displacement. A grid-front cassette is then placed along the medial or lateral aspect of the thigh and knee, with the central beam directed horizontally and perpendicularly to the cassette. Only the knee is usually included on this film. Proximal femur evaluation is performed with lateral hip views. X-rays examination of the hip is essential; dislocation and acetabular fractures may be present.

A lead apron is used for gonadal shielding.

Because of the severity of injury or its association with multiple skeletal injuries, true AP and lateral views often cannot be obtained. Careful attention to the position of the bony landmarks of the hip and knee and width of the cortex of the opposing fracture fragments will alert the physician to rotational deformity.

TREATMENT METHODS

Fracture of the femoral shaft is often the result of major violence. Additional bony injuries to the patient often occur and must also be treated. Any patient with a fracture of the femoral shaft is a potential candidate for shock. Immediate treatment of this complication must be carried out as the clinical situation indicates. Prompt splinting will reduce bleeding, additional soft tissue injury, and pain.

The basic principles in treatment of femoral shaft fractures are restoration of position and alignment, maintenance of length, immobilization until bone union occurs, and restoration of normal function after union. Apposition of bone fragments is required for union and acceptable alignment is necessary to minimize disabling deformities. Shortening of ¼ inch is well tolerated without hip or knee disability; shortening of greater than 1½ inches should be considered unacceptable.

While all agree that definitive treatment should begin as soon as possible for bone union to occur, the management of femoral shaft fractures is complex and remains controversial. Historically, fracture management has evolved from traction, body

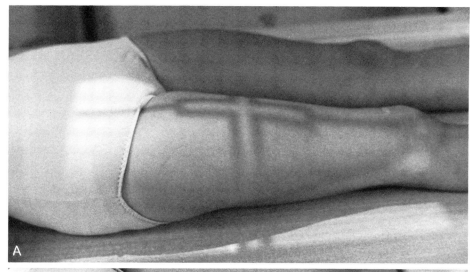

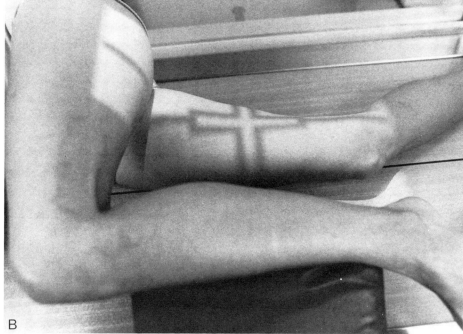

Figure 5–3. Patient positioned for AP *(A)* and lateral *(B)* views of the femur.

casts, and bracing in the first three decades of the century to the wide use of internal fixation and back again to nonoperative management of cases in which operative complications present significant risk.[10] Moreover, no single treatment applies to all fractures at the same anatomic level. Important considerations before institution of therapy include severity or comminution of fracture, soft tissue damage, and the patient's age, medical and physical condition, occupation, and associated injuries. In this survey various methods of treatment of femoral shaft fractures will be discussed.

Traction and Casting

Over 500 years ago, skin traction was used as the primary treatment method. During the American Civil War, adhesive plaster was used for traction, which became known as Buck's extension. Today, traction splinting is best used in the emergency treatment of femoral shaft fractures. The current application consists of traction applied to the foot and ankle with countertraction in the groin.

Skeletal traction is useful for the primary immobilization of a fracture of the femoral shaft when an operation must be delayed because of severity of injury and additional trauma.[8] This is the method of choice for highly comminuted fractures in which the surgeon cannot obtain good fixation and immobilization. Usually, a traction pin is placed either through the proximal tibia about 2 inches below the joint line or through the distal femur at the level of the adductor tubercle (Fig. 5–4). Suspension of the involved extremity with the knee flexed demands careful consideration and care. The position with

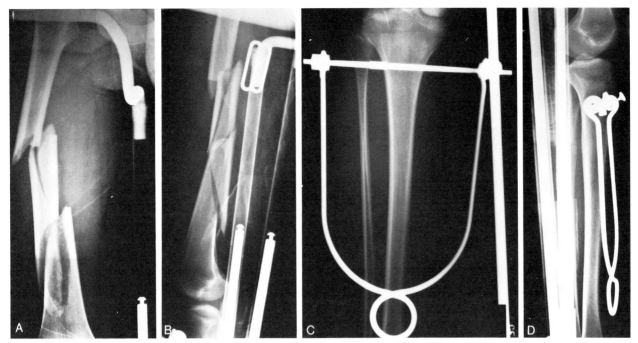

Figure 5–4. AP *(A)* and lateral *(B)* views of a comminuted femoral shaft fracture. AP *(C)* and lateral *(D)* views with traction pin in proximal tibia.

the knee flexed is a more comfortable position and more adequately reduces muscle forces, allowing easier alignment of the fracture.[1] Skeletal traction is indicated for oblique and transverse fractures when conditions preclude operation.

There are many disadvantages to skeletal traction. Prolonged bedrest and convalescence are required. With excessive traction, distraction may contribute to delayed union or non-union. With traction, the incidence of malunion, delayed union, and non-union is greater than with internal fixation. Pin tract infections may occur. Decubitus ulcers and other complications related to the immobilization of the patient also often occur. Hospitalization is usually prolonged when compared with treatments using cast bracing or internal fixation.[8]

Treatment of femoral shaft fractures with skeletal traction requires periodic radiographic evaluation. Careful portable AP and lateral films should be obtained frequently during the early course of treatment. Angulation, rotation, distraction, and over-riding of fracture fragments must be corrected. Errors can be avoided by standardizing the AP and lateral views with each patient.

Treatment of fractures of the femoral shaft by casting is one of the oldest forms of therapy; in certain patients, it is even mandatory and probably lifesaving. Immobilization in a cast is indicated in uncontrollable patients (i.e., patients with head injury) and in patients with severe wounds and severe infections of the back and buttocks.[8]

Disadvantages of cast treatment include discomfort, prolonged immobilization and convalescence,

joint stiffness, muscle atrophy, and increased possibility of delayed union, non-union, and malunion.

The cast brace technique (Fig. 5–5) avoids some of these disadvantages. Although favored by many orthopedists, its use remains controversial. Advantages of this treatment include early knee motion and ambulation and avoidance of surgical complications. Frequent radiographic follow-up is necessary in order to avoid unacceptable results. Preliminary skeletal traction is also controversial, but it is generally recommended for unstable fractures. Cast brace treatment is most useful for fractures at or distal to the midshaft level. The purpose of the cast brace is to provide a total contact capsule about the thigh, allowing the muscles to exert a hydrodynamic stabilizing effect on the fracture.[7] Suspension of the cast brace is obtained by casting the foot and leg and incorporating polycentric joints at the level of the knee. A skeletal traction pin inserted for preliminary traction may be incorporated into the cast during the early period. Correction of angular malalignment can be obtained by wedging the cast in the early period. The length of time required in the cast brace is usually 8 to 10 weeks.

Internal Fixation

Internal fixation is also a primary means of treatment of femoral shaft fractures. Various methods of internal fixation include use of intramedullary nail, occasionally supplemented with wires, screws, or, rarely, plates; use of dual plates placed at right

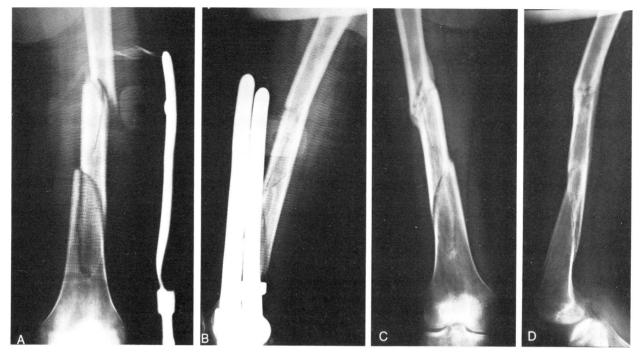

Figure 5–5. Cast-bracing seen on AP *(A)* and lateral *(B)* views (same patient as in Fig. 5–4). AP *(C)* and lateral *(D)* views 4 months after injury demonstrating healing.

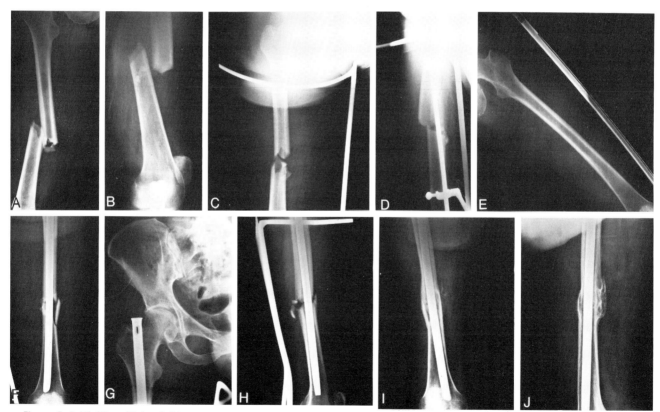

Figure 5–6. AP *(A)* and lateral *(B)* views of a comminuted fracture of the midshaft with overriding and rotation of fracture. Skeletal traction *(C and D)* shows improved alignment but a gap between the fragments. *(E)* Pre-operative film measuring intramedullary rod with normal intramedullary canal. Immediate postoperative films to check rod placement *(F, G, H)*. Twenty months following surgery the fracture is united *(I and J)*.

angles to each other on the femoral shaft; and bone grafting. Occasionally, a bone graft may be fixed to the femoral shaft with screws or wire. When considering internal fixation, the orthopedic surgeon must evaluate the geometry of the fracture and then choose a method appropriate for that particular fracture.

The Küntscher intramedullary nail (Fig. 5–6) is best designed for fractures of the middle shaft. With this device stresses are shared by both the appliance and the bone. The cross-sectional design of the Küntscher nail is a hollow cloverleaf pattern. This allows the nail to be compressed in the narrowest portion of the intramedullary canal. Other rods are available with cross-sectional shapes of diamonds, flanges, or squares and are thought to have improved mechanical qualities and provide better control of rotation.[10] These devices have also been experimentally shown not to engage and compress the entire endosteal ring, thus allowing endosteal revascularization.[6] The interlocking nail is a modification of the hollow intramedullary nail and is becoming popular. It permits fixation of the proxi-

mal or distal fracture fragment, or both at once, by placing a transverse screw through the bone and through the nail itself (Fig. 5–7). This technique reduces rotation at the fracture site and also controls shortening. It is possible, therefore, to use the technique of intramedullary nail fixation in fractures that would otherwise be too comminuted for this method.

Other intramedullary devices include flexible round Rush pins and Ender nails (Fig. 5–8). These devices are inserted without reaming and therefore produce less endosteal damage.

Each method has advantages and drawbacks. Intramedullary nailing is the procedure of choice in certain fractures of the middle three fifths of the femoral shaft. This is especially true in closed fractures with fracture surfaces that permit interlocking of the fracture fragments, thus preventing rotation following reduction. Often these fractures can be reduced closed, and the intramedullary rod can be inserted through a small incision at the greater trochanter. Fractures of the proximal or distal femoral shaft may require additional postoperative ex-

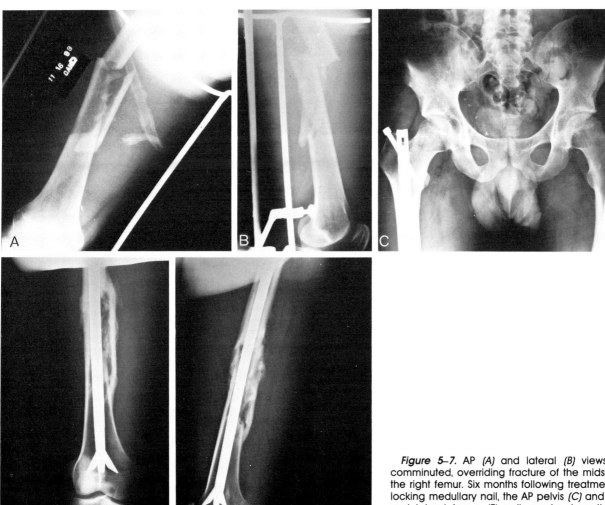

Figure 5–7. AP *(A)* and lateral *(B)* views of a comminuted, overriding fracture of the midshaft of the right femur. Six months following treatment with locking medullary nail, the AP pelvis *(C)* and AP *(D)* and lateral femur *(E)* radiographs show that the fracture has healed. Note that there is also a medullary rod on the left from an earlier fracture.

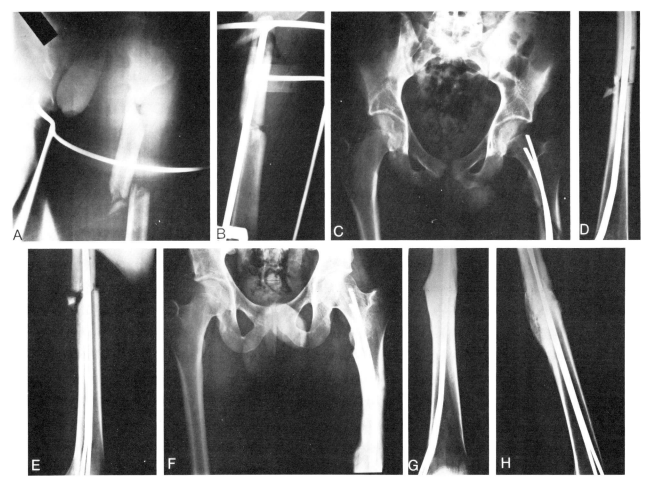

Figure 5–8. AP *(A)* and lateral *(B)* views of a comminuted fracture of the proximal femur in traction. AP *(C and D)* and lateral *(E)* views following Ender rodding. AP *(F and G)* and lateral *(H)* views 1 year following surgery show that the fracture has healed.

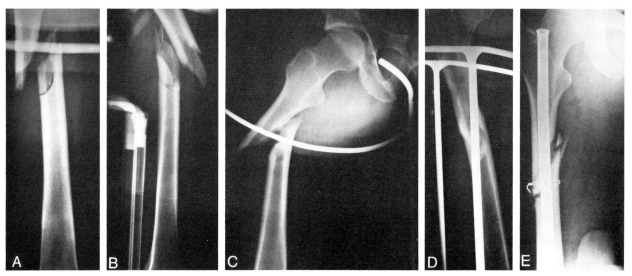

Figure 5–9. Initial AP *(A)* and lateral *(B)* views of an oblique fracture of the proximal femoral shaft with angulation and displacement. Three days later AP *(C)* and lateral *(D)* views show lack of reduction with abduction of the proximal fragment. The fracture was reduced with an intramedullary rod and cerclage wire *(E)*.

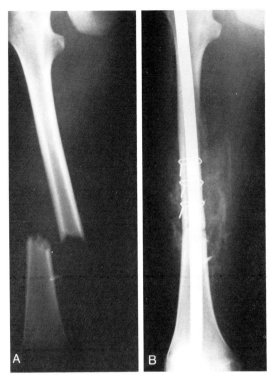

Figure 5–10. A, Transverse fracture of the distal shaft of the right femur. B, Note the thinning of the medial cortex, caused by eccentric reaming of the medullary canal. Cerclage wires were required to improve stability.

to attain rigid immobilization. Wire fixation has limitations; it affords limited stability and may loosen in the postoperative period. Also, if the type of metal used in the wire differs from that used in the nail, electrolysis may occur. Interfragmentary fixation with screws may increase stability. Although plates can be added to attempt further stabilization, the combination of intramedullary rodding and plating will disrupt both periosteal and endosteal circulation, increasing the risk of delayed union or non-union.[5]

The advantages of intramedullary nailing, especially with closed technique, include the relatively small incision, preservation of the soft tissue envelope, early periosteal callus, early weight-bearing and ambulation, decreased joint stiffness, reduced risk of infection, and shorter hospitalization.

Complications of intramedullary nailing include osteomyelitis or other infection, fat embolism, distraction of the fracture fragments with malunion or non-union, mechanical failure of the fixation device, neurovascular injury, and amputation. Other complications are those of any surgical treatment, including hemorrhage, thrombophlebitis, pulmonary embolism, and death. The technique of intramedullary nailing is demanding and requires the use of a fracture table with appropriate intra-operative x-ray equipment. Ideally, fluoroscopy should be available during the procedure to assess the position of the fracture fragments, reaming instruments, and fixation device. Careful monitoring will avoid technical errors. Eccentric reaming of the canal may destabilize the fracture (Fig. 5–10). Too large a nail may split the femoral shaft, while a nail that is too small may allow rotation of the fragments. Too long

ternal immobilization. Comminution and obliquity of the fracture are relative contraindications to intramedullary nail fixation. Additional fixation with wire (Fig. 5–9), screws, or plates may be necessary

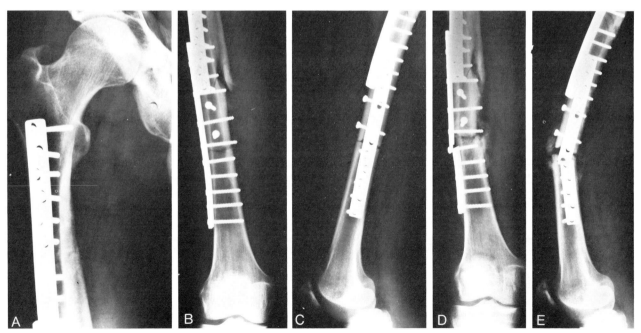

Figure 5–11. Comminuted fracture of the femoral shaft with two plates and segmental screws demonstrated on the AP (A and B) and lateral (C) views. AP (D) and lateral (E) views 3 months after surgery demonstrate fracture of the lower plate with anterior angulation of the lower fracture.

a nail may enter the knee joint. If the nail is too short, fixation will be suboptimal.

Plate fixation (Fig. 5–11) as a primary method of femoral shaft fracture treatment remains controversial.[7] Most advocates include as indications for its use unusual comminution or location of fractures, making intramedullary nailing impractical. Plating does permit anatomic reconstruction of bone, but at the same time a large operative wound is necessary. Bone fragments may be devitalized, increasing the risk of infection and delayed healing. The plate also functions as a load-bearing device and is thus susceptible to fatigue and fracture (Fig. 5–11). Intramedullary fixation, a load-bearing system, allows maximal bone impact and minimal stress on the device.[9] In rare cases it may be judged that plate fixation is the best method of treatment but that a single plate will be inadequate. In such a case, double plates may be utilized, positioned parallel to one another. These plates are oriented approximately 90° apart on the circumference of the femoral shaft. If double plates are used, they should not be of the same length in order to avoid stress concentration at the ends of the plates. In some patients, bone quality may be so poor that the purchase of the screws in the bone is inadequate. In these cases it may be helpful to utilize methyl methacrylate bone cement, which is injected into the screw holes, to better anchor the screws (Fig. 5–12). Femoral

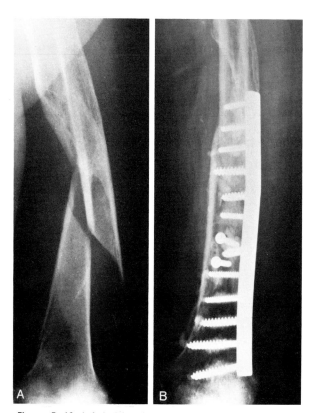

Figure 5–12. A, Spiral fracture of the distal femoral shaft with an old fracture deformity proximally. B, Fixation with interfragmentary lag screws and plate and screws. Methyl methacrylate cement was used to enhance fixation.

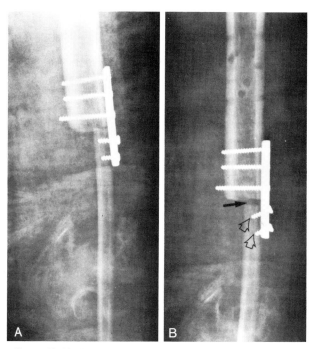

Figure 5–13. A, High-velocity injury resulted in distal femoral shaft loss. Lower extremity length is maintained by fibular graft with proximal internal fixation. B, Five days later separation of proximal graft occurred (black arrow). Note shift of distal two plate screws (open arrows).

fractures treated by plating usually require special protective measures following surgery. These may consist of casts, braces, and restricted weight-bearing.

Bone grafts (Fig. 5–13) play a role in fracture treatment. The goal of bone grafting is to expedite union and to decrease the incidence of non-union. Autogenous bone grafts are more desirable than homogeneous grafts. Autogenous corticocancellous bone may be particularly useful.

Complications

All methods of treatment of femoral shaft fractures carry the risk of major complications. These include infection and refracture. Refracture occurs in approximately 6 percent of femoral fractures treated by closed methods and in 1 percent of those treated by open methods. Such fractures usually consist of simple stress fractures without displacement. Treatment with protected weight-bearing and support using a cast brace or other device is usually sufficient. In addition, fixation devices may undergo bending, migration, or breakage.

Vascular injuries may occur at the time of fracture or during treatment. Thrombosis, laceration, false aneurysm formation, and arteriovenous fistula formation are potential complications. Arterial injuries are more common in fractures of the distal third of the shaft and in the supracondylar region.

Nerve injury is quite rare at the time of initial injury because of the protective role that the large

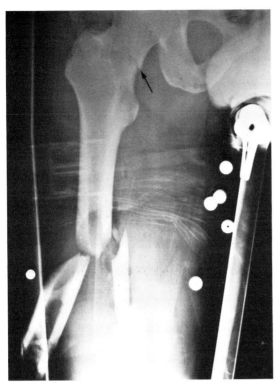

Figure 5-14. AP view of the femur with a comminuted midshaft fracture. Note the minimally displaced femoral neck fracture (arrow).

muscle mass provides. Most frequently, the peroneal nerve is injured as a result of prolonged or poorly monitored traction. Damage may occur to this nerve at the head of the fibula.

Non-union of the femoral shaft occurs in 1 percent of cases.[2] Factors influencing non-union include inadequate fixation, insufficient immobilization, excessive traction with distraction, and wound infection following internal fixation.[7] Treatment requires proper immobilization and therefore consists of intramedullary rodding or plating, often with bone grafting. Electrical stimulation is a controversial but increasingly common adjunct to treatment of fracture non-unions.

Malunion is more common than non-union. Because of unequal muscle forces, there is a tendency for angulation. Malunion is often associated with skeletal traction and plaster cast treatment of these fractures.

Delayed union is not uncommon in uncomplicated fracture management. Persistent bone pain and tenderness are the mainstay of clinical diagnosis. Radiographically the diagnosis is usually obvious. Treatment usually consists of improved external support and ambulatory care.

A serious complication of femoral shaft fractures is the unrecognized injury to the ipsilateral hip (Fig. 5-14) and knee. These injuries are usually rare, but early detection and treatment are important for best

recovery. They are usually associated with severe trauma, such as in motor vehicle accidents. The mechanism of injury is thought to be a longitudinal compressive force applied to a flexed abduction femur with the knee also flexed.

Ipsilateral hip dislocation is usually posterior. This may be accompanied by acetabular fracture as well. Early recognition favors reduction and decreases the incidence of avascular necrosis of the femoral head.

Concomitant fracture of the ipsilateral hip and knee can also occur without femoral shaft fractures and can easily be overlooked at the time of injury. Separate AP and lateral radiographs of the hip and knee should be obtained in any patient who has localized pain as well as in the critically injured patient. Thorough repeated examination of the entire patient is the best method for detecting associated injuries.

The incidence of bilateral femoral fractures is 7 percent.[1] Treatment is controversial and more difficult than for isolated femoral shaft fractures. In general, intramedullary fixation is more strongly indicated in such cases.

Various techniques for management of femoral shaft fractures have been discussed. The type of fracture, condition of the patient, and physician's preference determine the method of choice in management. Careful radiographic evaluation of the fracture initially and throughout the treatment period is very important in achieving optimal fracture healing.

REFERENCES

1. Beam, H. P., Jr., and Seligson, D.: Nine cases of bilateral femoral shaft fractures. A composite view. J. Trauma 20:399, 1980.
2. Carr, C. R., and Wingo, C. H.: Fractures of the femoral diaphysis. A retrospective study of the results and costs of treatment by intramedullary nailing and by traction and a spica cast. J. Bone Joint Surg. 55A:690, 1973.
3. Eriksson, E., and Hovelius, L.: Ender nailing in fractures of the diaphysis of the femur. J. Bone Joint Surg. 61A:1175, 1979.
4. Hollinshead, W. H.: Anatomy for Surgeons. Vol. 3: The Back and Limbs. 3rd Ed. New York, Harper & Row, 1982.
5. Rand, J. A., An, K. N., Chau, E. Y. S., et al.: A comparison of the effect of open intramedullary nailing and compression-plate fixation on fracture-site blood flow and fracture union. J. Bone Joint Surg. 63A:427, 1981.
6. Rhinelander, F. W.: Effect of medullary nailing on normal blood supply of the diaphyseal cortex. Instr. Course Lect. 22:161, 1973.
7. Rockwood, C. A., and Green, D. P.: Fractures. Philadelphia, J. B. Lippincott Co., 1984.
8. Taylor, L. W.: Principles of treatment of fracture and non-union of the shaft of the femur. J. Bone Joint Surg. 45A:191, 1963.
9. Winquist, R. A., and Hansen, S. T.: Segmental fractures of the femur treated by closed intramedullary nailing. J. Bone Joint Surg. 60A:934, 1978.
10. Zickel, R. E.: Fractures of the adult femur excluding femoral head and neck. Clin. Orthop. 147:93, 1980.

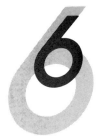

THE KNEE

JAMES A. RAND • *THOMAS H. BERQUIST*

The knee is anatomically and functionally complex and subjected to tremendous forces during normal activity. The ability of the knee to continue to function satisfactorily as a stable, pain-free, mobile support depends upon the integrity of its dynamic and static restraints. The complex kinematics of the knee are still incompletely understood. A knowledge of the anatomy and mechanics of the knee is essential for an understanding of the response of the knee to soft tissue or bony injury and prosthetic replacement.

ANATOMY AND BIOMECHANICS OF THE KNEE

The anatomy of the knee may be divided into static and dynamic anatomic restraints that guide normal motion and prevent abnormal motion (Table 6–1). The static restraints consist of the bony architecture, menisci, and ligaments. The dynamic restraints include the musculotendinous units and the stabilizing effect of joint load.

Bone

The bony architecture of the knee is unique and accounts for some of the complexity of knee motion. The anterior aspect of the femoral condyles is oval, providing increased stability in extension, while the posterior aspect is spherical, providing increased motion and rotation in flexion. The surface area of the medial femoral condyle is greater than that of the lateral condyle, reflecting the importance of the medial femoral condyle in load transmission across the knee. In the sagittal plane, the femoral condyle is eccentric, producing a "cam-like" mechanism that aids in maintaining collateral ligament tightness in extension and laxity in flexion. The tibial plateaus vary in shape, with the medial plateau being concave on its weight-bearing surface and the lateral

TABLE 6–1. Restraints of Knee Motion

Static	Dynamic
Bony architecture	Musculotendinous units
Menisci	Joint load
Ligaments	

tibial plateau slightly convex. This anatomic difference is important for the so-called "screw-home" mechanism of knee motion. The intercondylar eminence between the tibial plateaus provides both a mechanical block to translation and a place for cruciate ligament attachment. The degree of conformity between the tibia and femur is not exact and is improved considerably by the presence of the menisci. The patella is a sesamoid bone in the extensor mechanism. It is roughly triangular and ends in a rounded point on its anteroinferior margin, so that its anterior height exceeds its posterior height.[52] The articular surface is divided into medial and lateral facets by a vertical ridge. A second vertical ridge near the medial border isolates the odd facet. The patella may be divided into Wiberg types.[68] Type I has equal sized medial and lateral facets. Type II has a smaller medial facet. Type III has a very small medial facet that is convex with a broad concave lateral facet. Type II is the most frequent type, occurring in 57 percent of knees.[52]

The degree of conformity between the patella and femur is poor, especially when the multiple anatomic variations of the patella are considered. The patella functions to improve the lever arm of the extensor mechanism and helps to protect the femoral articular surface from direct trauma.

Meniscus

The importance of the menisci in joint function and the adverse consequences of meniscal excision are now well recognized. The lateral meniscus is small in diameter, circular, and wider and thicker than the medial meniscus.[5] The medial meniscus is thinner, narrower, and more semicircular and transcribes a larger circle than the lateral meniscus. The medial meniscus is firmly attached to the capsule of the knee by fibrous tissue. The lateral meniscus has a less firm attachment and is separated from the fibular collateral ligament and posterolateral capsule by the popliteus tendon. A ligament of Wrisberg may attach the lateral meniscus to the medial condyle of the femur but is sometimes absent. In fact, a ligament of Wrisberg (posterior meniscofemoral) or Humphry (anterior meniscofemoral) is absent in 30 percent of knees.[20]

The medial meniscus is attached anteriorly to the anterior intercondylar fossa of the tibia and is anterior to the anterior cruciate ligament.[21] The posterior attachment of the medial meniscus is fixed to the posterior intercondylar fossa of the tibia. The anterior attachment of the lateral meniscus is to the intercondylar eminence of the tibia and is lateral and posterior to the anterior cruciate ligament. The posterior attachment of the lateral meniscus is posterior to the intercondylar eminence of the tibia. The transverse ligament may connect the anterior margin of the two menisci. Abnormal menisci may be present, such as a discoid lateral meniscus. The vascular supply to the menisci is from branches of the middle genicular and the medial and lateral genicular arteries.[53] Only the outer 30 percent of the meniscus has a vascular supply and is capable of a healing response. The remainder of the meniscus relies upon diffusion from the synovial fluid. Both menisci slide posteriorly with knee flexion.[5]

The functions of the menisci include lubrication, force transmission, stability, articular cartilage nutrition, and shock absorption. In 1936 King showed that the extent of degeneration of articular cartilage in the canine knee correlated with the segment of the meniscus removed and was greatest following complete meniscectomy.[36] Claims have also been made for the menisci as important guides for the rotation of the tibia on the femur.[25] Thus meniscal injuries may affect the synchronous motion between the tibia and femur, leading to areas of articular cartilage erosion.

The menisci also aid in the distribution of load across the knee. The area of load bearing in the knee is increased from 2 cm^2 on each condyle in the absence of the menisci to 6 cm^2 in the presence of menisci.[64] At a 1000 N load the menisci transmit 45 percent of the load across the knee.[58] Meniscectomy alters presure distribution to a highly nonuniform state, with high stress gradients and large deformations of the cartilage.[58] The medial meniscus may carry 50 percent and the lateral meniscus 70 percent of the joint load.[55] At a 1000 N load the menisci occupy 70 percent of the total contact area, and excision of the menisci doubles peak pressure from 3 MPa to 6 MPa.[17] The lateral meniscus contributes more to weight-bearing in the lateral compartment than does the medial meniscus in the medial compartment.[17] Meniscal excision decreases the area for load transmission by approximately 50 percent.[42] Meniscectomy may result in a three-fold increase in stress across the joint.[37] The effect of partial meniscectomy on load-bearing of the meniscus has been studied by Burke and colleagues.[7] Partial meniscectomy does not affect load-bearing function in the peripheral rim of the meniscus and allows a more normal pressure distribution than total meniscectomy.[7]

The medial meniscus contributes to anteroposterior stability of the knee. The importance of the medial meniscus for this stability has been investi-gated by Levy and colleagues.[38] If the anterior cruciate is intact, medial meniscectomy does not affect the anteroposterior displacement of the knee or its coupled rotation. However, if the anterior cruciate is sectioned, loss of the medial meniscus significantly increases anteroposterior knee laxity and results in a loss of the coupled internal rotation associated with anterior tibial displacement.[38] Removal of both menisci with all ligaments intact results in 2 mm of increased laxity in the anteroposterior plane at 45° to 90° of flexion.[44]

The clinical correlation of this biomechanical information has been well documented. In 1948 Fairbank presented the classical roentgenographic findings following a meniscectomy: (1) an anteroposterior ridge, (2) generalized flattening of the femoral condyle, (3) narrowing of the joint space, and (4) squaring of the tibial margin[13] (Fig. 6–1). Thirty years following meniscectomy only 38 percent of the patients had a normal symptom-free knee.[61] The best long-term result occurs after a partial meniscectomy for a bucket-handle tear, with 67 percent having excellent results.[61] At 17.5 years following meniscectomy, 39.4 percent of the knees were found to have degenerative arthritis.[31] Therefore, meniscectomy is not an innocuous procedure and should be performed only when necessary. When feasible, partial meniscectomy is preferable to total meniscectomy.

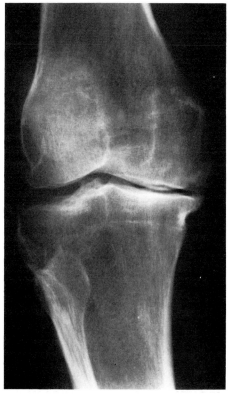

Figure 6–1. Fairbank's changes affecting the medial compartment of the right knee of a 40-year-old man 15 years following medial meniscectomy.

Ligaments

The ligamentous restraints for the knee may be considered with respect to their anatomic location. Thus, they can be classified as either medial or posteromedial, lateral or posterolateral, anterior or central.

Medial Ligamentous Structures

The medial ligamentous structures are complex, and their functional importance is controversial. Warren and Marshall have divided the medial capsular structures into three layers, from superficial to deep.[65] Layer I consists of the deep fascia. Layer II is composed of the superficial medial collateral ligament. Layer III consists of the joint capsule deep to the medial ligament. Layer I, the deep fascia, serves as a support for the muscle bellies and neurovascular structures. The sartorius muscle inserts into this layer. Layer I merges with Layer II 1 to 2 cm anterior to the superficial medial ligament[65] (Fig. 6–2). The tendons of the gracilis and semitendinosus lie between Layers I and II.

The superficial medial ligament lies in Layer II and is composed of two parts. The anterior portion of this ligament consists of long parallel fibers of 11 cm by 1.5 cm.[66] The anterior fibers are attached to the medial femoral condyle just distal to the adductor tubercle and are located around the axis of flexion of the knee. The tibial insertion of these fibers is in the anteromedial aspect of the tibia 4.6 cm distal to the joint line.[5] The posterior or oblique fibers of the superficial medial ligament have the same femoral attachment as the anterior parallel fibers but are triangular in shape, with the apex extending posteriorly along the joint line.[5, 66] Other authors have felt that these posterior oblique fibers are part of the deeper posterior oblique ligament.[27, 29] The maximum length of the superficial medial ligament is seen at 45° of flexion, when it is increased 1.75 mm over its resting length.[3, 66] During extension the superficial medial ligament moves anteriorly, while in flexion it moves posteriorly.[5] The posterior border of the superficial medial ligament is tightest in extension and becomes slack at 30° of flexion, allowing normal rotation of the tibia on the femur.[3, 60] In extreme flexion, the posterior border of the ligament slips under the anterior border near its femoral attachment.[3]

Layers II and III join posteriorly to form the posteromedial capsule and are joined by the tendon sheath of the semimembranosus.[65] Layer II splits at the anterior margin of the superficial medial ligament. The anterior fibers of the split join with Layer I, forming the parapatellar retinacular fibers.[65] Layer III, on the other hand, is the true capsule of the knee.[66] The anterior portion of the capsule is thin but may be important in preventing lateral patellar subluxation and anteromedial rotatory instability.[60] Layer III is thickened beneath the superficial medial ligament and has been referred to as the deep medial ligament or middle capsular ligament.[65] The deep medial ligament is attached to the medial femoral epicondyle anterior to the superficial ligament and is strongly attached to the outer margin of the medial meniscus.[60] It extends distally as the coronary ligament to attach to the tibia just below the articular margin.

The posteromedial capsule has been termed the posterior oblique ligament. It extends from the posterior margin of the superficial medial ligament anteriorly to the insertion of the direct head of the semimembranosus posteriorly[27, 29, 60] and from the adductor tubercle proximally to the tibia distally.[29] The posterior oblique ligament has a firm attachment to the medial meniscus and the posteromedial corner of the knee.[29] The distal attachment consists of three arms: (1) the central or tibial arm, which attaches to the margin of the articular surface and is central to the upper edge of the semimembranous tendon; (2) the superior or capsular arm, which is continuous with the posterior capsule and the proximal part of the oblique popliteal ligament; and (3) the inferior or distal arm, which attaches distally to the sheath of the semimembranosus and tibia[29] (Fig. 6–3). The posterior oblique ligament is relaxed at 60° of flexion. This ligament has been felt to be essential for static medial capsular stability.

The parallel anterior fibers of the superficial medial ligament are the primary stabilizers of the medial side of the knee to valgus stress.[66] Isolated section of the deep medial capsular ligament and posterior oblique ligament alone does not allow medial joint space opening.[66] Division of the super-

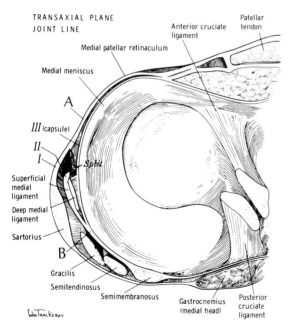

Figure 6–2. Layers of the medial aspect of the knee. (From Warren, F., and Marshall, J.: The supporting structures and layers on the medial side of the knee. J. Bone Joint Surg. *61A*:56, 1979.)

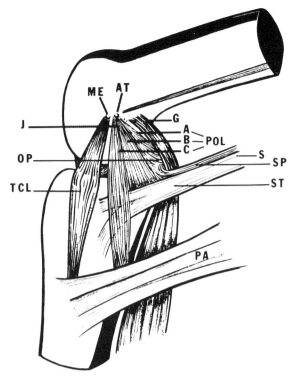

Figure 6–3. The three arms of the posterior oblique ligament (POL). (From Hughston, J., and Eilers, A.: The role of the posterior oblique ligament in repairs of acute medial (collateral) ligament tears of the knee. J. Bone Joint Surg. *55A*:923, 1973.)

ficial medial ligament results in a 2° increase in external rotation in extension and a two-fold increase in external rotation at 90° of flexion. The superficial medial ligament provides 57.4 percent of the restraint to valgus stress at 5° of flexion and 78.2 percent at 25° of flexion.[23] The anterior and middle parts of the medial capsule provide only 4 to 8 percent of the restraint to valgus stress. The posteromedial capsule provides 17.5 percent of the restraint to valgus stress.

Lateral Ligamentous Structures

The lateral aspect of the knee contains many important stabilizing structures. These structures may be considered from anterior to posterior or from superficial to deep layers. The anterior third consists of the capsular ligament, which extends posteriorly from the lateral border of the patellar tendon and patella to the anterior border of the iliotibial band, and is reinforced by the lateral retinaculum from the quadriceps mechanism.[28] The middle third is composed of the iliotibial band and the capsular ligament deep to it and extends posteriorly as far as the fibular collateral ligament.[28] Both the iliotibial tract, which provides static support, and the iliotibial band, which provides dynamic support, reinforce the middle third capsular liagment.[28] The middle third of the lateral capsule extends from the lateral epicondyle of the femur to the tibial joint line, providing static support at 30° of flexion. Finally, the posterior third consists of the capsular and noncapsular ligaments that compose the arcuate complex.[28] The arcuate complex is composed of the fibular collateral ligament, the arcuate ligament, and the aponeurosis of the popliteus muscle.

The lateral aspect of the knee consists of three layers (Figs. 6–4 and 6–5).[54] The superficial layer, or Layer I, consists of the iliotibial tract and its expansion anteriorly and the superficial portion of the biceps and its expansion posteriorly. The peroneal nerve lies on the posterior aspect of the biceps tendon.

Layer II is formed by the retinaculum of the quadriceps and is incomplete.[54] It is composed of two patellofemoral ligaments. The proximal ligament joins the terminal fibers of the lateral intramuscular system. The distal ligament ends posteriorly on the fibula or posterolateral capsular reinforcements provided by the lateral head of the gastrocnemius on the femoral condyle.[54] The proximal patellofemoral ligament travels in Layer II

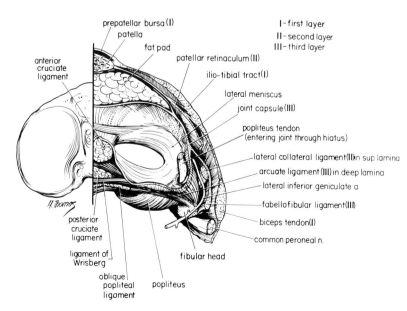

Figure 6–4. The three layers of the lateral aspect of the knee. (From Seebacher, J., Inglis, A., Marshall, J. L., et al.: The structure of the posterolateral aspect of the knee. J. Bone Joint Surg. *64A*:536, 1982.)

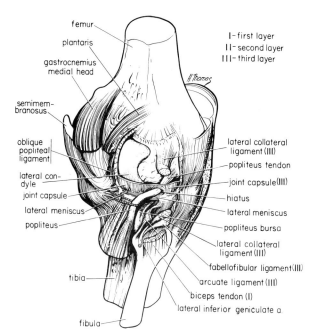

Figure 6-5. The structure of the posterolateral aspect of the knee. (From Seebacher, J., Inglis, A., Marshall, J. L., et al.: The structure of the posterolateral aspect of the knee. J. Bone Joint Surg. *64A*:536, 1982.)

obliquely from the patella, attaching to the margin of the lateral meniscus, and terminates on Gerdy's tubercle. The fibular collateral ligament lies in Layer II and extends from the posterior lateral femoral condyle proximal to the groove of the popliteus to the lateral side of the head of the fibula anterior to the styloid process.[21, 54]

Layer III is the lateral joint capsule.[54] The capsular attachment to the outer edge of the lateral meniscus is the coronary ligament and contains a hiatus for the popliteus tendon. Posterior to the overlying iliotibial tract the capsule divides into two laminae.[54] The superficial lamina encompasses the fibular collateral ligament and ends posteriorly at the fabellofibular ligament. The deep lamina forms the coronary ligament and terminates posteriorly at the arcuate ligament. The Y-shaped arcuate ligament spans the junction between the popliteus muscle and its tendon and extends from the fibula to the femur.[54] The inferior lateral genicular vessels pass between these two laminae. The arcuate and fabellofibular ligaments insert on the apex of the fibular styloid process. They ascend to the lateral head of the gastrocnemius, where they join the posterior termination of the oblique popliteal ligament. The arcuate ligament fans out over the musculotendinous portion of the popliteus muscle and adheres to it.[54]

Three anatomic variations in the posterolateral aspect of the knee have been identified.[54] In 13 percent of knees, the arcuate ligament alone reinforces the capsule. In 20 percent of knees, the fabellofibular ligament alone reinforces the capsule. In 67 percent of knees, both the arcuate and fabellofibular ligaments reinforce the posterolateral cap-

sule. Seebacher and colleagues noted that the size of the fabella correlated with these anatomic variations.[54] If the fabella was large, there was no arcuate ligament, but the fabellofibular ligament was also large. Conversely, when the fabella was absent, only the arcuate ligament was present.

Biomechanical studies of the importance of the lateral stabilizers have been performed.[23] The lateral collateral ligament is the primary restraint to varus stress, providing 55 to 69 percent of the restraint. The entire lateral capsule provides only 8 to 17 percent of the restraint to varus stress.

Cruciate Ligaments

The cruciate ligaments are one of the key aspects of the functional anatomy of the knee. Injuries to the cruciate ligaments are frequent clinical problems resulting in significant morbidity. The anterior cruciate ligament has its femoral attachment on the posterior aspect of the medial surface of the lateral femoral condyle.[2, 20] The tibial attachment of the anterior cruciate ligament is to a fossa anterior and lateral to the anterior tibial spine. Fascicles from the anterior cruciate ligament may blend with the anterior and posterior attachments of the lateral meniscus.[2, 20] The anterior cruciate ligament does not attach to the tip or upper part of the anterior surface of the anterior tibial spine.[20] The tibial attachment is wider and stronger than the femoral attachment.[2, 20]

The fascicles of the anterior cruciate ligament create a slight outward spiral as they cross the joint. These fascicles have been divided into an anteromedial band and a posterolateral bulk.[2, 20] The anteromedial band originates at the proximal aspect of the femoral attachment and inserts at the anteromedial aspect of the tibial attachment. The anteromedial band becomes tense in flexion as the anterior cruciate ligament twists on itself, while the posterolateral bulk becomes loose (Fig. 6–6).[2, 19, 20] In exten-

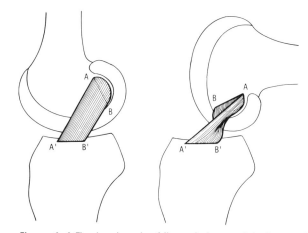

Figure 6-6. The two bands of the anterior cruciate ligament and their differential tensions during flexion and extension of the knee. (From Girgis, F., and Marshall, J.: The cruciate ligaments of the knee joint. Clin. Orthop. *106*:216, 1975.)

sion, the posterolateral bulk becomes tight while the anteromedial band becomes lax.[2, 19] A positive anterior drawer test indicates a tear of the antero-medial band.[19] The posterolateral band is a secondary restraint and the medial collateral ligament a tertiary restraint to the anterior drawer test.[19] The anterior cruciate ligament limits external and internal rotation in extension. It is actually a continuum of fascicles, a different portion of which is taut throughout the range of motion.[2]

The posterior cruciate ligament is attached to the anterior portion of the intercondylar aspect of the medial femoral condyle. The tibial attachment of the posterior cruciate ligament is to a depression behind the intraarticular upper surface of the tibia.[20] The posterior cruciate ligament sends a slip to blend with the posterior horn of the lateral meniscus. The fibers of the posterior cruciate ligament are attached in a lateromedial direction on the tibia and in an anteroposterior direction on the femur.[20] The posterior cruciate ligament may be divided into an anterior portion that forms the bulk of the ligament and a smaller posterior part.[20] The posterior fibers are loose in flexion while the bulk is taut (Fig. 6–7). In extension, the posterior fibers become taut while the anterior fibers relax.

The transitional zone between cruciate ligament and bone is mediated by a transitional zone of fibrocartilage and mineralized fibrocartilage that allows for a graduated change in stiffness and stress concentration at the attachment site.[2, 48] The femoral attachment of both cruciate ligaments and the tibial attachment of the posterior cruciate ligament are behind the axis of flexion of the knee.[20] The location of the cruciate attachment sites combined with the cam-shaped femoral condyle results in the differential tightening of portions of each cruciate ligament with flexion-extension motion.[20] The eccentric cruciate ligament attachments result in their being wound in flexion and unwound in extension with respect to each other.

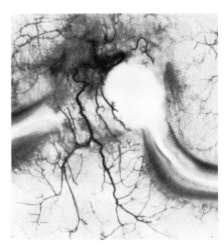

Figure 6–8. The vascular supply to the anterior cruciate ligaments. (From Scapinelli, R.: Studies on the vasculature of the human knee joint. Acta Anat. 70:305, 1968.)

The vascular supply to the cruciate ligaments is derived from branches of the middle genicular artery, which also supplies the synovial membrane and posterior capsule.[53] The largest branch is the tibial intercondylar artery[33, 53] (Figs. 6–8 and 6–9). The anterior cruciate ligament is covered by a synovial fold, the ligamentum mucosum, which contains many of the small vascular branches.[2] A few small branches from the lateral inferior genicular artery may contribute to this vascular plexus. The vessels are oriented in a longitudinal manner parallel to the fibers of the ligament. The vascular supply to the anterior cruciate ligament is predominantly of soft tissue origin without a significant contribution from the osseous junctions.[2, 53] The

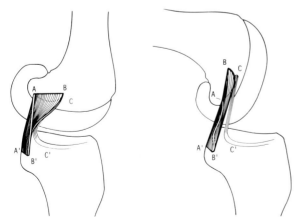

Figure 6–7. The two bands of the posterior cruciate ligament and their differential tensions during flexion and extension of the knee. (From Girgis, F., and Marshall, J.: The cruciate ligaments of the knee joint. Clin. Orthop. 106:216, 1975.)

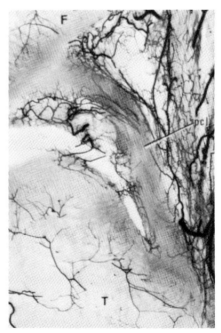

Figure 6–9. The vascular supply to the posterior cruciate ligament. (From Scapinelli, R.: Studies on the vasculature of the human knee joint. Acta Anat. 70:305, 1968.)

posterior cruciate ligament receives arteries originating from the infrapatellar fat pad entering along the anterior synovial fold.[1] A few vessels enter the proximal part of the ligament from a posterior direction along the intercondylar notch. The posterior cruciate ligament has a greater number of intrinsic vessels than the anterior cruciate ligament.[1] The central portion of the cruciate ligaments is less well vascularized than the proximal and distal parts.[1] Although the vasculature appears important for cruciate ligament nutrition, diffusion of nutrients may also play a role, especially if the vasculature is disrupted.[67]

The nerve supply to the anterior cruciate ligament derives from branches of the tibial nerve that penetrate the joint capsule posteriorly.[2] Most of the fibers are related to vasomotor control, but some may have a proprioceptive function.[2, 33]

The cruciate ligaments together provide 13 to 14 percent of the restraining moment to valgus stress.[23] At 25° of flexion the posterior cruciate ligament provides 75 percent of the restraint to valgus stress provided by the two cruciate ligaments.[23] The cruciates provide 12 to 22 percent of the restraint to varus stress.[23] Therefore, the cruciate ligaments are secondary restraints to medial and lateral opening of the knee upon stress. The tensile strength of the anterior cruciate ligament is 600 ± 132 N, while that of the posterior cruciate ligament is 450 ± 12 N.[10] Other authors have suggested that the anterior cruciate ligament can withstand loads of 1000 to 1,730 N prior to microscopic failure.[8, 9, 22, 48] The tensile strength of the human anterior cruciate ligament decreases with age.[48] Since ligaments are viscoelastic, the rate of loading determines the mode of failure. Under high loading rates for the anterior cruciate ligament, primary ligamentous disruption occurs; under low loading rates, tibial avulsion fractures are more frequent.[47] The strain to maximum load for the anterior cruciate ligament is 20 to 30 percent.[33] When ligamentous failure occurs, the ligament undergoes 57 to 100 percent elongation prior to loss of continuity.[47] Ligament failure results in serial failure throughout the entire ligament prior to final separation, giving a "mop-end" appearance.[33, 47]

Functionally, the cruciate ligaments in conjunction with the collateral ligaments help control lateral rotation of the tibia on the femur.[5] The anterior cruciate ligament acts as a check against external rotation in flexion but does not limit internal rotation.[20] The anterior cruciate ligament prevents anterior displacement of the tibia on the femur, especially in extension.[5] Severance of the anterior cruciate ligament results in hyperextension, increased external rotation of 6 to 12°, increased internal rotation of 2° to 8°, and increased anterior drawer in extension and to a lesser extent in flexion as well.[20] Loss of the posterior cruciate ligament results in instability in flexion, with a 3° increase in medial and an 8° increase in lateral rotation, as well as posterior displacement of the tibia on the femur in flexion.[20]

Anterior Ligamentous Structures

The anterior aspect of the knee consists primarily of the extensor mechanism of the knee. The four-part structure of the quadriceps is well known. The rectus femoris becomes tendinous 5 to 8 cm proximal to the patella.[52] The rectus fibers fan out over the patella and are continuous with the patellar tendon. The vastus medialis has two components.[52] The proximal fibers are long while the distal fibers are oblique in orientation. Some of the fibers insert into the patella while others contribute to the medial retinaculum. The vastus lateralis becomes tendinous 2.8 cm proximal to the patella.[52] The medial fibers of the vastus lateralis insert into the patella, while the lateral fibers contribute to the lateral retinaculum. The vastus intermedius lies deep to the other muscle groups and sends fibers into the superior border of the patella.[52] There is a blending of the tendinous fibers at the insertion of the various muscle groups into the patella, creating a complex structure.

The fascia lata spreads to create a superficial interlocking layer with the quadriceps complex, contributing to the patellar retinacula.[52] The patellofemoral ligaments are thickenings of the joint capsule that connect the patella to the femoral epicondyles. The most common is the lateral epicondylopatellar ligament of Kaplan. Actually two lateral patellofemoral ligaments are frequently present.[52] The proximal ligament terminates on the lateral intermuscular system. The distal one ends on the fabella and posterolateral capsule. On the medial side, a patellofemoral ligament runs deep to the vastus medialis and attaches near the femoral attachment of the medial superficial ligament.[65]

The patellar ligament is flat and receives fibers from the central portion of the rectus femoris.[52] The patellar ligament extends from the inferior surface of the patella to the tibial tubercle and fascial expansions of the iliotibial tract on the anterior surface of the tibia. The average length of the patellar ligament is 4.6 cm.

Reider and colleagues also noted a correlation between the patellar shape and the width of the lateral patellofemoral ligament.[52] The closer the patellar profile to that of Wiberg Type III, the broader was the lateral patellofemoral ligament. The larger the patellar ligament, the smaller the size of the medial patellofemoral ligament. These findings on radiographs may be helpful in assessing the potential for lateral patellar subluxation.

Muscle

The quadriceps mechanism is an important dynamic stabilizer of the knee, and its anatomy has been described. Other important dynamic stabilizers exist. On the lateral aspect of the knee, the iliotibial tract, as described earlier, provides passive ligament tension and also transmits active muscle forces. The popliteus muscle is important in the screw-home mechanism of the knee. Activity in the popliteus muscle coincides with internal rotation of the tibia on the femur.[40] The popliteus muscle extends from the lateral femoral epicondyle to the proximal posterior medial tibia proximal to the popliteal line.[21] The biceps femoris, which attaches to the fibular head, is an important dynamic restraint on the lateral aspect of the knee.[27, 28] Studies of the contributions of these dynamic stabilizers to lateral knee stability in cadavers have shown minimal restraint but probably do not reflect the *in vivo* situation.[23]

On the medial aspect of the knee, the semimembranosus is an important dynamic stabilizer.[65] There are five sites of attachment of the semimembranosus[65] (Fig. 6–10). The semimembranosus inserts into the posteromedial corner of the tibia below the joint line. A second bony insertion lies anteriorly on the medial aspect of the tibia below the joint line deep to the superficial medial ligament. The semimembranosus tendon sheath sends an extension into the posterior capsule, which forms the oblique popliteal ligament. The oblique popliteal ligament supports the posterior aspect of the knee and inserts into the medial aspect of the lateral femoral condyle. Two additional insertions include

one into the posteromedial capsule and another distal to the tibia posterior to the oblique portion of the superficial medial ligament. Through its multiple sites of attachment, the semimembranosus provides a dynamic reinforcement for the posterior medial aspect of the knee.[27, 29, 60] It is an internal rotator of the tibia and supports the knee against valgus thrust as well as anteromedial tibial displacement.[60] The medial and lateral heads of the gastrocnemius reinforce their respective corners of the knee.[27]

The pes anserinus muscles, the sartorius, gracilis, and semitendinosus muscles, flex the knee and hold the tibia within a normal range of external rotation on the femur.[60] These muscles attach to the anteromedial tibia below the joint line and the fascia of the leg. Even after transplantation, the pes muscles continue to function primarily as flexors, although their rotational activity is increased.[49] The contribution to rotational force provided by the pes muscles is 34 percent for the sartorius, 40 percent for the gracilis, and 26 percent for the semitendinosus.[49] However, the long-term effectiveness of pes transfer is questionable when done as the sole treatment of anteromedial instability.[16]

Few studies have been performed on the *in vivo* effect of the musculature as dynamic stabilizers. The effective stiffness of the medial ligamentous complex may be increased by 108 percent by the pes anserinus and by 164 percent by the quadriceps femoris muscle groups.[51] The maximum amount of tibial torque that can be sustained without injury to the knee ligaments may be effectively doubled by maximum muscle resistance.[57]

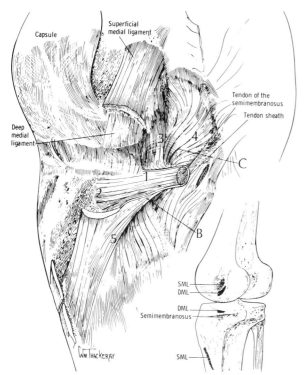

Figure 6–10. The five sites of attachment of the semimembranous muscle on the posteromedial aspect of the knee. (From Warren, F., and Marshall, J.: The supporting structures and layers on the medial side of the knee. J. Bone Joint Surg. *61A:56,* 1979.)

Vascular Supply

The vascular supply about the knee is provided by five major groups of vessels: the supreme genicular, the medial and lateral superior genicular, the medial and lateral inferior genicular, the middle genicular, and the anterior and posterior tibial recurrent arteries.[53] The supreme genicular arises from the femoral artery and divides into three branches: the saphenous, the muscular articular, and the deep oblique. The saphenous branch is subcutaneous. The muscular branch supplies part of the vastus medialis and contributes to the parapatellar plexus. The deep oblique branch supplies muscles along the medial aspect of the femoral shaft and the anterior and medial aspects of the distal femur. The medial and lateral superior genicular arteries are branches from the popliteal artery and contribute to the "rete articulare genu" and the epiphyseal circulation. The medial and lateral inferior genicular arteries arise from the popliteal artery and lie deep to the collateral ligaments. The middle genicular arises from the popliteal artery and supplies the cruciate ligaments, the distal femoral, and the proximal tibial epiphyses. The anterior and posterior tibial recurrent arteries arise from the anterior tibial artery and supply the anterior aspect of the knee, the superior tibiofibular joint, and the lateral condyle of the tibia. The patella is supplied by midpatellar vessels penetrating the middle third of its anterior surface and by polar vessels entering the apex behind the patellar ligament. Therefore, the majority of the vascular supply to the patella is in its inferior half, making the proximal half of the patella susceptible to ischemia following fracture.[53]

Biomechanics

The complexity of knee motion and the extent of force transmisison across the knee underscore the importance of a thorough understanding of knee mechanics for appropriate management of knee disorders. The functional importance of the various static stabilizers is summarized in Table 6–2.

The forces acting across the knee during normal walking include a direct compression force, a mediolateral shear force, and an anteroposterior shear force that is resisted by the cruciate ligaments.[45] These forces are generated by the effect of gravity and muscular action. The joint forces occurring during normal walking are 2 to 4 times body weight, with a mean of 3.03 times body weight.[45, 46] There are three peaks of loading during the gait cycle. These correspond to muscle activity in the hamstrings, quadriceps femoris, and gastrocnemius.[45] The peak force is during the late-stance phase associated with contraction of the gastrocnemius.[14] A force equal to body weight is present in the late swing phase, corresponding to contraction of the hamstrings as they decelerate the knee.[14] The maximum forces developed in the quadriceps are 167 lb, in the hamstrings 270, and in the gastrocnemius 234.[46]

Forces acting on the cruciate ligaments range as high as 112 lb, with the posterior cruciate ligament carrying two thirds of the load.[46] Forces acting in the medial collateral ligament are small, with a maximum value of 29 lb. However, forces carried by the lateral collateral ligament are as high as 148 lb and act to prevent adduction of the knee during stance phase. The maximum shear force developed during walking is 0.26 times body weight.[46] In stance phase, during normal walking with the knee between 0° and 30° of flexion, the femorotibial force peaks at 3 times body weight.[6] Upon arising from a chair or ascending or descending a slope or stairs, forces of several times body weight occur with knee flexion angles of 60° or more. Patellofemoral forces are also quite high with increasing knee flexion. During stance phase, the greater part of the load is transmitted by the medial condyles, while in swing phase the load acts mainly on the lateral condyles.[46]

The stress (force per unit area) depends upon the load and the contact area for force transmission. The medial compartment contact area is 1.6 times greater than the lateral compartment contact area and is present through the first 35° of flexion.[35] The mean area of contact on the medial plateau is 4.68

TABLE 6–2. Ligamentous Restraints*

Author	Stress	Primary Stabilizer	Secondary Stabilizer
Butler	Anterior	ACL 85–87%	ITB 25% Middle medial capsule 22% Middle lateral capsule 21% MCL 16% LCL 12%
Markolf	Anterior	ACL	ACL and PCL Menisci MCL and LCL
Fukubayashi	Anterior	ACL	
Crowninshield	Anterior	ACL	Middle medial capsule MCL and LCL Posteromedial capsule
Butler	Posterior	PCL 90–94%	Posterolateral capsule and popliteus 58% MCL 16% Posterior medial capsule 7% LCL 6% Middle medial capsule 6%
Markolf	Posterior	PCL	ACL and PCL Menisci MCL and LCL
Fukubayashi	Posterior	PCL	
Crowninshield	Posterior	PCL	MCL and LCL Posteromedial capsule Middle medial capsule
Grood	Valgus	MCL 57–78%	ACL and PCL 13–15% Anterior and middle medial capsule 4–8% Posteromedial capsule 4–17%
Warren	Valgus	MCL	Middle medial capsule
Markolf	Valgus	MCL	ACL and PCL Menisci
Crowninshield	Valgus	MCL	Middle medial capsule Posterior medial capsule
Grood	Varus	LCL 55–69%	ACL and PCL 12–22% Anterior and middle lateral capsule 4% Posterolateral capsule 5–13% ITB 5–10%
Markolf	Varus	LCL	ACL and PCL Menisci
Crowninshield	Varus	LCL	
Markolf	Rotation	MCL	ACL and PCL
Warren	Rotation	MCL	
Crowninshield	Rotation	MCL	ACL and PCL Posteromedial capsule LCL
Lipke	Internal rotation	ACL	Posterolateral capsule LCL

*ACL, anterior cruciate ligament; PCL, posterior cruciate ligament; MCL, medial collateral ligament; LCL, lateral collateral ligament; ITB, iliotibial band. Numbers indicate percentage of stability contributed by the ligament or ligament group.

cm² and on the lateral plateau 2.97 cm². With increasing knee flexion, these contact areas decrease in area and move posteriorly on the tibial plateaus.[35] The menisci appear to contribute to the static loading.[35] At small loads, contact occurs on the lateral and posterior borders of the menisci and on a small area of the medial aspect of the tibial spine.[6] With increasing loads, the contact area spreads to both meniscal surfaces and exposed articular cartilage. With no applied load, the area of contact is 50 percent of the lateral meniscus, 55 percent of the medial meniscus, and 12 percent of the exposed cartilage on the medial tibial plateau.[6] With 150 kg of applied load, the average area of contact is 65 percent of the lateral meniscus, 67 percent of the medial meniscus, 38 percent of the lateral exposed cartilage, and 43 percent of the medial exposed cartilage.[6] Excision of the menisci decreases the areas of contact by approximately 50 percent.[42]

The effects of joint deformities on force transmission across the knee have been studied. Perry examined the effect of knee flexion on the quadriceps force required to stabilize the knee.[50] She concluded that the quadriceps force required to stabilize the flexed knee is proportional to the load on the femoral head and the angle of knee flexion. For each degree of flexion, the required force increased an average of 6 percent of the load on the femoral head. For a 70 kg man, quadriceps tension rises from 187 N at 5° of flexion to 1375 N at 30°.[50] The compression forces on the patella also depend on the angle of knee flexion.

Any change in the direction of the patellofemoral reaction force carried by an abnormal patellar position will provide abnormal stresses in the joint.[12] In knee flexion, the patellofemoral reaction force can exceed the tibiofemoral reaction force. The patella displaces the extensor tendon forward away from the point of contact between the tibia and femur. Patellectomy may result in a 14 percent increase in tibiofemoral reaction force and a 250 percent increase in tangential force in the tibiofemoral joint.[12] These findings emphasize the functional impairment induced by a knee flexion contracture or loss of the patella.

The effects of varus and valgus changes in axial alignment of the knee on force transmission have also been investigated. The normal angle between the femur and tibia on AP radiographs is 7° ± 2°.[12] This angle is the anatomic axis. The mechanical axis of the knee is a line drawn from the center of the femoral head to the center of the ankle. The mechanical axis normally falls within the center of the knee on weight-bearing stance. A variation of 4° in the anatomic axis can change the line of force transmission across the joint to the outer one third of a compartment, and a variation of 10° can place the line of force transmission beyond the articular surface.[12] A high correlation exists between the mechanical and anatomic axis when the mechanical axis falls within the knee.[30] However, when the mechanical axis falls outside the joint, there is a wide range of tibiofemoral angles.[30] The line of action of the resultant force across the knee varies during gait.[42] The resultant force depends upon the power of the lateral muscles, body weight, varus or valgus deformity, and the center of gravity of the body.[42] The line of action of the resultant force may be displaced medially by weakening of the lateral muscles, by an increase in body weight, by a varus deformity, or by permanent displacement of the center of gravity of the body to the side opposite the loaded knee.[42]

Comparative evaluation of static radiographs and dynamic gait analysis has revealed a discrepancy in calculating force transmission across the knee.[30] For varus deformities, the load on the medial tibial plateau rapidly approaches 100 percent of the total load on the joint. However, for valgus deformities, there is no significant correlation between the mechanical axis and the dynamic force transmission across the joint. The discrepancy can be explained by the normal horizontally-directed medial shear force that develops on weight-bearing.[30] A similar lack of correlation between the angular deformity of the knee and the force distribution across the joint upon gait analysis has been noted by Harrington.[24] The center of pressure in the knee varies with the gait cycle and is not directly related to the magnitude of angulation of the joint. The inclination of the tibia in the coronal plane also affects the magnitude of the abducting-adducting moments on the knee.[24]

Joint load is an important mechanism for knee stability. Application of a tibiofemoral contact force increases anteroposterior, mediolateral, varus-valgus, and torsional stiffness with a corresponding decrease in laxity.[43] Joint load is an important protective mechanism that avoids ligament strain.[43] The compression load is generated by body weight and muscle action.[26, 43] These findings emphasize the importance of the dynamic stabilizers in maintaining joint stability. The most important factor in reducing laxity under load is the conformity of the condylar surfaces.[26]

The complex kinematics of knee motion are continually being studied. During knee flexion-extension, rotation in a horizontal plane occurs, ranging from 4° to 13°.[14] External rotation of the tibia occurs during knee extension and reaches a peak value just before heel strike.[14] The rotatory motion of the knee with flexion and extension has been termed the "screw-home" mechanism. The rotatory motion is synchronous with a coupling of extension and lateral tibial rotation or flexion and medial rotation.[25] The axis of rotation for this rotatory motion is the medial intercondylar tubercle of the tibial plateau.[56] Integrity of the anterior cruciate ligament is essential for control of this rotatory motion. Pathologic lesions, such as meniscus tears, disrupt the normal synchronous movement.[25]

A coupled motion of tibial rotation and anteroposterior motion of the knee also exists. Upon anterior displacement of the tibia, there is a coupled internal rotation, while on posterior displacement there is an associated external rotation.[18, 62, 63] The rotation averages 7°.[62] Sectioning of the anterior cruciate ligament eliminates the coupled internal rotation, while sectioning of the posterior cruciate ligament eliminates the coupled external rotation.[18] These findings emphasize the importance of the cruciate ligaments for normal knee kinematics.

The axis of rotation of the knee for flexion-extension is not static but changes on knee motion. In the normal knee, the instant center of rotation lies within the femoral condyle, indicating a sliding mechanism for knee motion.[4] The total translational movement of the instantaneous center axis is about 10 mm.[4] The cruciate ligaments have little effect on the location of the instantaneous center of rotation, which depends more upon the geometry of the bones and perhaps the collateral ligaments.[4]

The kinematics of the knee are complex and require the coordinated function of the bony architecture, ligamentous guides, and muscular function for satisfactory synchronous movement. Derangements in knee mechanics may lead to articular surface damage and degenerative arthritis.

ROUTINE RADIOGRAPHIC TECHNIQUES

AP and lateral radiographs fulfill the minimum requirement for examination of the knee following trauma. In addition we routinely obtain both oblique views.

AP View

The AP view is obtained with the patient supine, the leg extended, and the patella positioned ante-riorly.[69, 70] The cassette should be centered about 1 cm below the apex of the patella (palpable) (Fig. 6–11A). The central beam may be angled slightly to the head (5°) or perpendicular to the cassette. This view (Fig. 6–11B) demonstrates the medial and lateral compartments. Upright standing views are required for accurate evaluation of the joint space. The patella can be seen extending just above the intercondylar area of the femur. The tibial spines are clearly demonstrated.

Lateral View

The lateral view may be obtained using routine positioning or with cross-table technique. In most situations the lateral projection is obtained by positioning the patient on his side with the involved knee adjacent to the table top (Fig. 6–12A). The knee should be flexed about 30°. This permits more accurate assessment of the patellofemoral space and patellar position. The 8 × 10 inch cassette is centered under the joint with the beam angled 5° to the head.[70] This prevents the magnified medial condyle from obscuring the joint space.[69]

This view (Fig. 6–12B) allows one to assess the patella, patellofemoral space, tibial plateau, and upper fibula. Effusions may also be detected on the lateral view. Detection of effusions on the lateral view is approximately 77 percent accurate.[72] In the

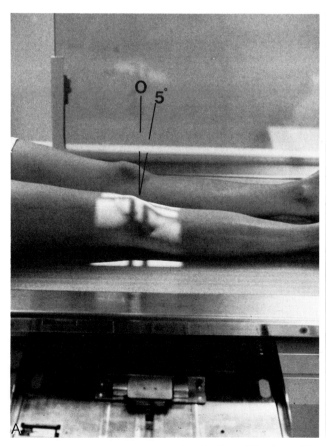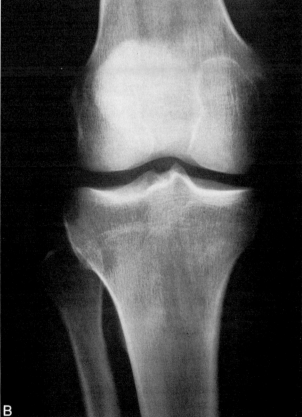

Figure 6–11. A, Patient positioned for AP view of the knee. The central beam *(broken lines)* is centered 1 cm below the apex of the patella and is perpendicular (0°) or angled (5°) to the head. *B,* Normal AP view of the knee demonstrating the distal femur and upper tibia and fibula.

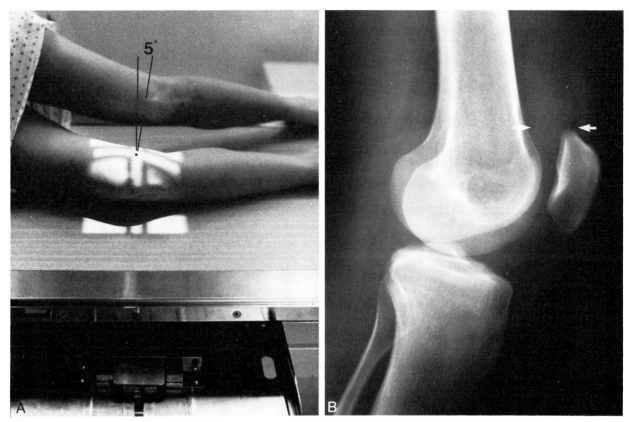

Figure 6–12. *A,* Patient positioned for routine lateral view of the right knee. The knee is flexed about 30°. The central beam *(broken lines)* is angled 5° toward the head and centered on the joint space which is just inferior to the apex of the patella. *B,* Lateral view of the knee demonstrating an effusion in the suprapatellar bursa *(arrows).*

presence of an effusion the posterior quadriceps tendon may be indistinct, the suprapatellar and prefemoral fat pads may be separated by 5 mm or more (Fig. 6–12*B*), or a suprapatellar soft tissue density larger than 10 mm may appear.[72, 73] The patella may also be displaced more anteriorly in relationship to the femur. An uncommon sign is

displacement of the fabella. This displacement requires a large effusion.[72]

An alternative method for the lateral view, the cross-table technique (Fig. 6–13*A*), is useful in patients who cannot be moved or in patients with subtle fractures. The cassette is positioned perpendicularly to the table and may be held between the

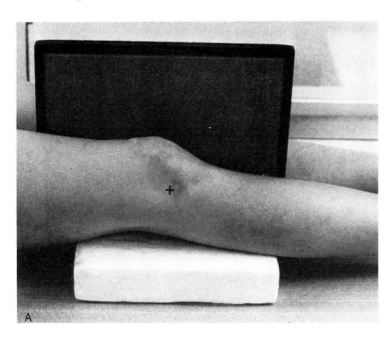

Figure 6–13. *A,* Patient positioned for cross-table lateral view of the knee. A small cushion under the knee will ensure that the entire structure is included on the film. The beam is centered on the joint (+) and is perpendicular to the cassette.

Illustration continued on opposite page

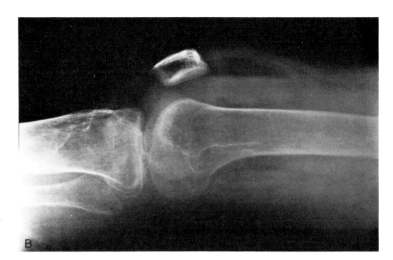

Figure 6–13 Continued. B, Cross-table lateral view of the knee demonstrating a lipohemarthrosis due to a subtle intra-articular fracture.

knees for support. A small cushion under the knee will ensure that the entire structure is included in the film. The beam is centered on the joint and directed perpendicular to the cassette. This view will demonstrate a lipohemarthrosis, which may be the only indication of an intra-articular fracture (Fig. 6–13B).

Oblique Views

Both oblique views can be obtained with the patient supine. For the internal oblique view the leg is internally rotated about 45° (Fig. 6–14A). The

cassette is centered under the joint space with the central beam perpendicular to the cassette. This view provides excellent detail of the upper fibula and tibiofibular articulation. The lateral femoral condyle is also seen to better advantage (Fig. 6–14B).

The external oblique is obtained using the same parameters but with the leg rotated externally 45° (Fig. 6–15A). The fibula is projected behind the upper tibia. The medial tibial plateau and femoral condyle are clearly demonstrated (Fig. 6–15B).

These four views (AP, lateral, and both obliques) are usually sufficient for evaluation of the acutely injured patient. However, the clinical setting may

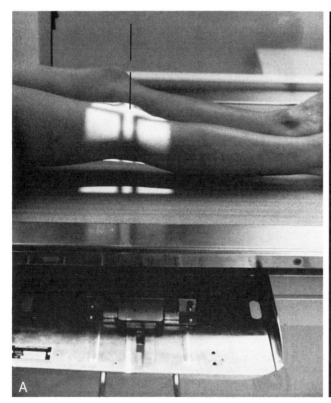
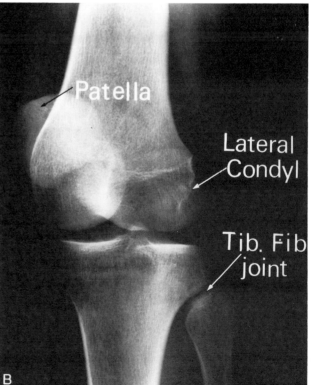

Figure 6–14. A, Patient positioned for the internal oblique view. The leg is internally rotated about 45°. The beam is perpendicular to the joint. *B,* Internal oblique view demonstrating the tibiofibular articulation and lateral femoral condyle.

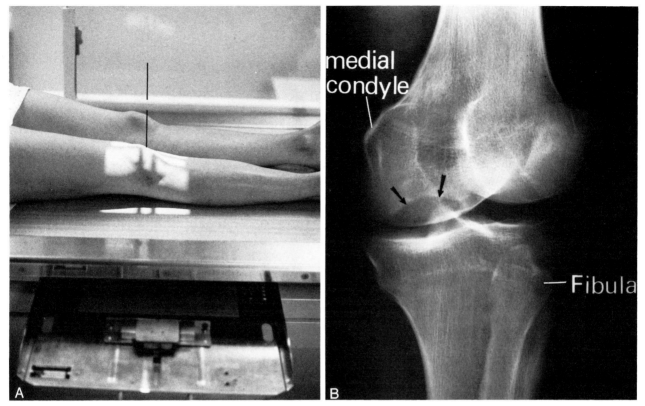

Figure 6-15. *A,* Patient positioned for the external oblique view. The leg is externally rotated about 45°. *B,* The radiograph demonstrates the medial structures more clearly. Note the large osteochondral defect in the medial condyle *(arrows).*

dictate that views of the patella or intercondylar notch be obtained.

Notch View

This view is obtained with the patient prone on the table. The knee is flexed 40° and supported on a bolster (Fig. 6–16A). The 8 × 10 cassette is placed under the knee with the tube centered on the cassette and angled 40° toward the feet. Simultaneous views of both knees can also be obtained.

This view is particularly useful in evaluating patients with osteochondritis dissecans, in visualizing the tibial spines, and in detecting osteochondral

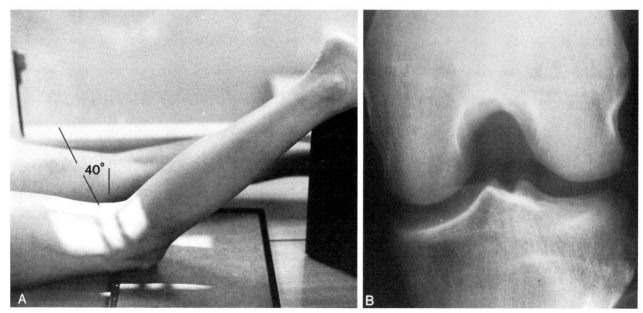

Figure 6-16. *A,* Patient positioned for notch view of the knee. The lower leg is supported by a cushioned prop. The tube is angled 40° toward the feet. *B,* Normal notch view of the knee.

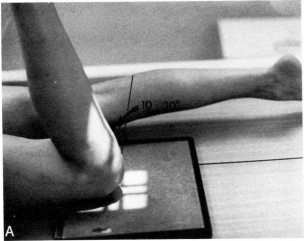

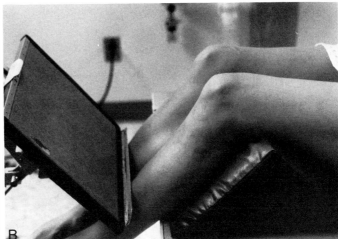

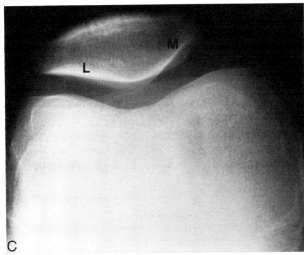

Figure 6–17. Patient positioning for the patellar views. *A,* Settegast technique with the patient prone and the knee flexed. The tube is angled 10° to 20° to the head and centered on the anterior aspect of the knee. *B,* Merchant view with the legs flexed 45° and the beam centered on the cassette and angled 30° to the horizontal. *C,* Patellar view demonstrating the medial *(M)* and lateral *(L)* facets and relationship to the femoral condyles.

fragments in the joint space (Fig. 6–16*B*).[69, 71] An alternative method has been described by Holmblad.[74]

Patellar Views

Tangential views of the patella are frequently required to evaluate position, fractures, and the patellofemoral joint space (Fig. 6–17*C*). Numerous techniques have been described for patellar evaluation. These will be discussed more fully later in this chapter. The two most commonly used techniques at our institution are the Merchant[79] and Settegast[80] methods.

The Settegast technique is performed with the patient prone. The involved knee is flexed 90° with the cassette centered under the knee. The beam is angled about 10° to 20°, so that it is perpendicular to the patellofemoral joint (Fig. 6–17*A*).

Consistency is obtained more readily with the Merchant view (Fig. 6–17*B*). The knees are flexed 45° over the table with the cassette perpendicular to the legs. The beam is angled 30° to the horizontal and centered on the cassette.[69, 70, 79] The resulting view clearly demonstrates the patella and patellofemoral relationship.

Stress Views

Initial assessment of suspected ligament injury can be accomplished with stress views. Accuracy of stress views depends upon the experience of the examining physician and the patient's symptoms. Pain and swelling make it difficult to perform this technique in the acutely injured knee. Acute injuries usually require anesthetic injection, general anesthesia, or spinal anesthesia. The examination is most commonly performed manually by fixing the extremity with a bolster or strap and applying force in the opposite direction. Jacobsen[76, 77] has devised an instrument (gonylaxometer) to obtain more accurate measurements. However, this instrument is not universally available.

Positioning of the joint for both mediolateral and AP instability is best done fluoroscopically. This allows proper angulation of the tube to ensure that the beam is tangential to the joint surfaces.

The measurement can be calculated from the films using the normal knee for comparison. In the normal knee, minimal motion is possible with stress. On the AP view lines are constructed along the inferior margin of the femoral condyles and lower cortical margins of the tibial plateaus. The angle

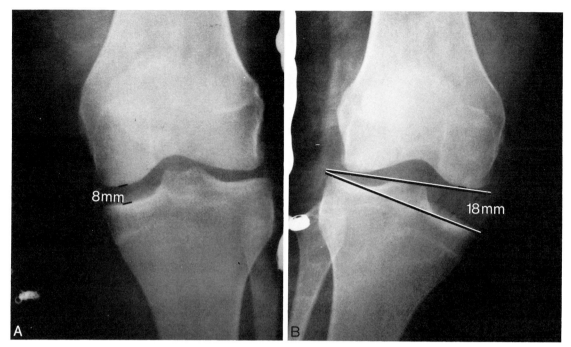

Figure 6–18. Radiographs of young athlete with suspected medial collateral ligament tear and internal derangement. *A,* Stress view of the normal left knee demonstrates joint space of 8 mm. Note the double line of the tibial plateau medially. The lower cortical margin *(line)* was chosen. *B,* Stress view on the right demonstrates a joint space opening of 18 mm confirming the suspected ligament damage. The angle formed by the tibial and condylar lines could also be used.

formed by these lines, as well as the vertical distance in the joint space, is then measured during varus and valgus stress (Fig. 6–18).[77] The femoral line is not difficult to evaluate; however, variation in the tibial plateaus can create confusion.[76, 77] The most inferior cortical line should be used.[76]

Measuring AP instability is much more difficult using radiographic techniques. Positioning is more difficult, and consistency in measurement is difficult to obtain.[77] Clinical examination is probably as accurate in most situations of suspected capsular or cruciate ligament injury. If AP stress views are to

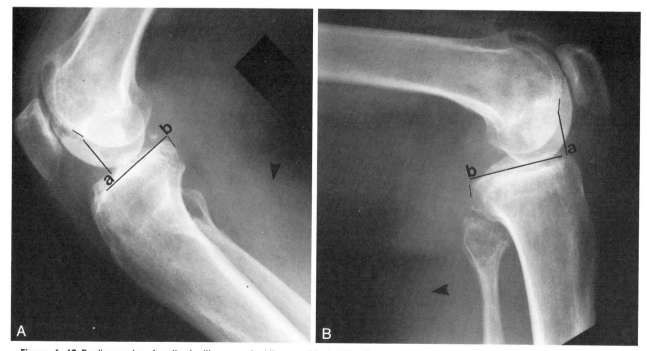

Figure 6–19. Radiographs of patient with suspected ligament instability. The anterior and posterior stress views were performed. *A,* Anterior stress on the tibia. The knee is not in a true lateral position. Note the overlap of the medial and lateral *(line)* femoral condyles. This reduces measurement accuracy. The tibial surface *(line)* and posterior margin are labeled and the distance (*a* to *b*) can be calculated and compared with the neutral radiograph. *B,* Posterior stress view. Again there is not true alignment. The distance (*a* to *b*) is increased compared with the anterior stress view.

be performed, the knee is flexed 90° with anterior and posterior forces applied to the tibia just below the knee. Lateral views should be obtained on both the injured and uninvolved knee during these maneuvers. Jacobsen[77] has described this technique in detail. The most important factor is consistency in noting anatomic landmarks. We choose to use the posterior tibial margin (Fig. 6–19) and anterior condylar margin for measuring. The point at which the condylar line is perpendicular to the tibial line is used for the anterior measurement. Measurement differences of greater than 3 mm between the normal and abnormal knee suggest ligament injury (see Fig. 6–49).

There are numerous routine views that have not been discussed. Some of these will be discussed later in this chapter as they apply to specific clinical situations. Other radiographic techniques (tomography, CT, MRI, etc.) will also be included.

PATELLAR DISORDERS

Disorders of the patellofemoral joint are frequent clinical problems. Patellofemoral arthralgia, instability, and fractures are frequent. A knowledge of the anatomy, biomechanics, and techniques of radiographic study of the patellofemoral joint is necessary to diagnose and treat these problems.

Anatomy

Although the anatomy of the patellofemoral joint has been discussed earlier in this chapter, a review of some of the pertinent aspects of anatomy is essential in order to comprehend many patellar problems. The triangular patella is divided on its articular surface by a vertical median ridge into medial and lateral facets. A small vertical ridge divides the medial facet from the most medial odd facet. The medial facet is convex while the lateral facet is concave. The thickest articular cartilage, which may measure up to 4 to 5 mm in thickness, is present on the median ridge.[93] The trochlear surface of the femur may be divided into convex medial and lateral facets. The lateral trochlear facet is larger and extends more proximally than the medial facet.[136] The superior aspect of the lateral trochlear facet has a smooth transition with the anterior femoral cortex, while the superior medial trochlear facet has a prominent bony and cartilaginous ridge from 3 to 8 mm in height.[127]

The stabilizers of the patella are both static and dynamic. The static stabilizers on the medial side are the patellofemoral ligament superiorly and the meniscopatellar ligament inferiorly.[93] The lateral static stabilizers are the patellofemoral ligament superiorly and the meniscopatellar ligament inferiorly. The fascia lata also has an attachment laterally to the patella. As the lateral stabilizers are denser than the medial stabilizers, there is greater strength on the lateral side. The dynamic stabilizers consist

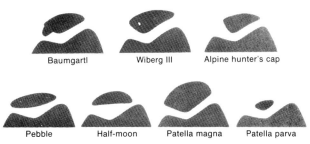

Figure 6–20. Variations in patellar shape. (From Ficat, R. P., and Hungerford, D. S.: Disorders of the Patellofemoral Joint. Baltimore, Williams and Wilkins, 1977. © 1977, the Williams and Wilkins Co., Baltimore.)

of the four components of the quadriceps muscle. The patellar ligament extends from the inferior part of the patella to the tibial tubercle and has a slight lateral orientation.

The vascular supply to the patella is extensive. An anastomotic circle of vessels surrounds the patella.[134] The main vessels contributing to the anastomosis are the supreme genicular, medial superior genicular, medial inferior genicular, lateral superior genicular, lateral inferior genicular, and anterior tibial recurrent arteries. The intra-osseous arteries are composed of two main systems.[134] One system is the midpatellar vessels, which enter vascular foramina on the middle anterior surface. The second system enters from the infrapatellar anastomosis behind the patellar ligament. Therefore, the proximal part of the patella may be susceptible to ischemic changes following fracture.

A variety of patellar shapes may be present as well as varying configurations of the trochlea (Fig. 6–20). The dysplasias may be a potential source of confusion to the examining physician and in some instances may be pathologic (Fig. 6–21). Wiberg reported on the major patellar types.[136] In Type I the medial and lateral patellar facets are equal in

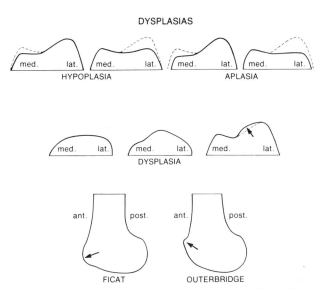

Figure 6–21. Variations in trochlear appearance. (From Ficat, R. P., and Hungerford, D. S.: Disorders of the Patellofemoral Joint. Baltimore, Williams and Wilkins, 1977. © 1977, the Williams and Wilkins Co., Baltimore.)

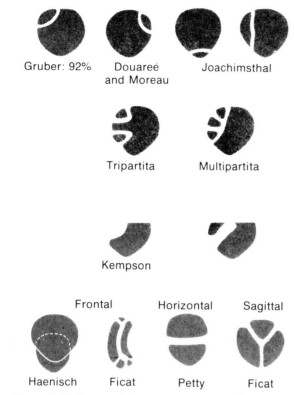

Gruber: 92%   Douareé   Joachimsthal
               and Moreau

Tripartita   Multipartita

Kempson

Frontal   Horizontal   Sagittal

Haenisch   Ficat   Petty   Ficat

Figure 6–22. Fragmentation of the patella. (From Ficat, R. P., and Hungerford, D. S.: Disorders of the Patellofemoral Joint. Baltimore, Williams and Wilkins, 1977. © 1977, the Williams and Wilkins Co., Baltimore.)

size. In Type II the medial facet is slightly smaller than the lateral facet. In Type III the medial patellar facet is very small, and there may be hypoplasia of the medial trochlear facet of the femur. A Wiberg Type II patella is the most frequent type.[94] Aplasia and hypoplasia (patella parva) of the patella may occur but are usually associated with other lesions or systemic syndromes.[94] The flattened patella or hemipatella with one facet (alpine hunter's cap) is frequently associated with symptoms of patellar instability.[94] Patellar fragmentation (Fig. 6–22) is a common finding, with a bipartite patella being present in 0.05 to 1.66 percent of knees.[94] A bipartite patella may be distinguished from a fracture by (1) a clearly defined radiolucency with rounded margins separating the fragments, (2) sclerosis of the margins, and (3) bilaterality of the lesion.

Biomechanics

In the extended position, the patella lies above the trochlear surface of the femur and rests on a layer of subsynovial fat.[136] In this position the patella lies laterally in 87 percent of knees, with contact being made between the crest of the patella or lateral facet and lateral trochlear facet.[91] Contact between the patella and trochlea occurs at 10° to 20° of flexion and involves the inferior aspect of the patella (Fig. 6–23).[97, 102] In 20° to 30° of flexion, only

29 percent of patellas are centered in the trochlear groove.[91] With increasing flexion, the area of contact moves proximally on the patella, and only the articular surface of the patella contacts the trochlea between 30° and 80° of flexion.[97, 102] With increasing flexion, the patella also becomes more centered in the trochlear groove, and 96 percent of the patella is centered with 90° of flexion.[91] Beyond 80° to 90° of knee flexion, the patellar tendon begins to articulate with the femur.[97, 102] Beyond 90° of flexion, the medial patellar facet lies within the intercondylar notch of the femur.[97, 102] At 135° of flexion, the odd facet begins to articulate with the medial femoral condyle.[97] The lack of contact on the odd facet except at maximal knee flexion may account for areas of chondromalacia frequently seen in this location.[96, 97] Osteochondritis dissecans of the medial femoral condyle may be related to trauma from contact of the patella in this area upon maximal knee flexion.[96] The size of the contact area between the patella and femur ranges from a low of 2 cm² at 30° to 3.5 to 6.0 cm² at 90° of knee flexion.[93, 102] The greater contact area with increased flexion aids in the distribution of patellofemoral forces over a broad area.[102]

The screw-home mechanism of the knee with external rotation of the tibia in the terminal 30° of extension rotates the tibia laterally. This external rotation produces a valgus vector between the quadriceps tendon and the patellar ligament, the Q-angle.[102] This valgus vector tends toward lateral displacement of the patella and must be resisted by the static and dynamic medial stabilizers, which consist of the vastus medialis, medial retinaculum, and the bony architecture of the femur and patella.[102] As knee flexion progresses, the patella is drawn from its superior lateral position onto the

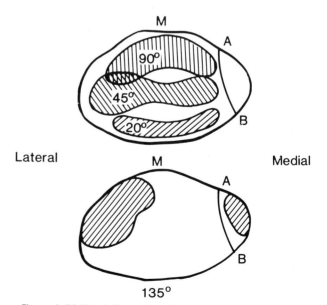

Figure 6–23. Patellofemoral contact apex in different degrees of knee flexion. (After Ficat, R. P., and Hungerford, D. S.: Disorders of the Patellofemoral Joint. Baltimore, Williams and Wilkins, 1977. © 1977, the Williams and Wilkins Co., Baltimore.)

trochlear surface of the femur and gradually into the intercondylar notch, resulting in a C-shaped tracking that is open laterally.[102]

The patella facilitates knee extension by increasing the distance between the extensor mechanism and the rotational axis of the femur.[93, 102] The patella also centralizes the action of the quadriceps muscle, allowing transmission of its force around an angle during knee flexion with minimal loss due to friction.[102] Additionally the patella protects the underlying surfaces of the femoral condyles.[102] The viscoelastic articular cartilage allows some deformation under load, which in turn allows better force distribution to a larger area.[102]

In full extension, the patella is responsible for almost 30 percent of the quadriceps moment arm.[108] Following patellectomy, a 15 to 30 percent increase in quadriceps force is necessary to obtain full extension.[108] Loss of the patellar lever arm results in increased compression forces between the femur and tibia.[120] Patellectomy results in a decrease in stance-phase flexion and decreased flexion with ascending or descending stairs.[109] An alteration in the path of the instant center also occurs following patellectomy.[109] Patellofemoral compression forces are substantial and result from muscle activity about the knee during knee flexion. Two factors increase these forces with increasing knee flexion: (1) an increase in the moment arm of the flexor, and (2) an increase in the resultant normal vector to the patellofemoral contact surface.[93, 102] The patellofemoral reaction force is approximately 0.5 times body weight for level walking and 3.3 times body weight during stair climbing.[132] Patellofemoral forces increase from near 0 in full extension to 2.0 times body weight at 60° of knee flexion.[131] The increased patellofemoral forces correspond to an increase in the quadriceps force needed to stabilize the knee with increasing knee flexion.[131] During deep knee bends, a patellofemoral reaction force of up to 7.8 times body weight may be generated.[121] Contact stresses of up to 35 to 40 psi have been measured on the patellofemoral joint.[92] Between 13 and 30 percent of the patellar surface bears joint loads of between 421 and 3420 N, resulting in stress values equal to or in excess of tibiofemoral stresses.[121]

Elevation of the tibial tuberosity has been utilized as a technique to increase the moment arm for the extensor mechanism and thus decrease patellofemoral stress.[92, 108, 120, 189] An anterior displacement of 2 cm reduces patellar compression forces by 50 percent.[119, 120] Experimentally, an elevation of the tibial tuberosity by 1.3 cm results in an 83.5 percent reduction in average stress.[92] Following patellectomy, a 1.5 cm elevation of the tibial tuberosity will restore the normal extensor moment arm.[108]

Examination

Evaluation of the patellofemoral joint must include both a careful physical examination and ap-

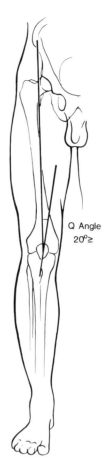

Figure 6–24. Method of measurement of the "Q-angle."

proximate radiographs. The problems to be detected are those of instability and degeneration of the articular cartilage. Therefore, examination must be directed at associated abnormal anatomy, patellar position, stability, motion, crepitus, and effusion. Alignment of the patella in extension and flexion should be evaluated as well as the pattern of patellar tracking during motion. A lateral subluxing patella often may be seen to lie more laterally than normal in the flexed position.[101] The Q-angle (Fig. 6–24) may also reveal significant information. It is measured clinically by drawing a line from the tibial tuberosity to the center of the patella and a second line along the direction of the quadriceps mechanism. The normal Q-angle is 14°, with greater than 20° considered abnormal.[81, 104] An increased Q-angle has been associated with patellar instability and degenerative changes. Evaluation of the hip for excess femoral anteversion and the tibia for external torsion should also be performed, as both these anatomic changes will lead to an increase in the Q-angle.[83, 106]

Other anatomic problems that have been associated with instability include a deficient or high-riding vastus medialis obliquus, contracted iliotibial band, excess valgus alignment of the knee, and a deficient lateral femoral condyle.[83] The "apprehension test" consists of lateral displacement of the patella in both extension and in 20° to 30° of flexion

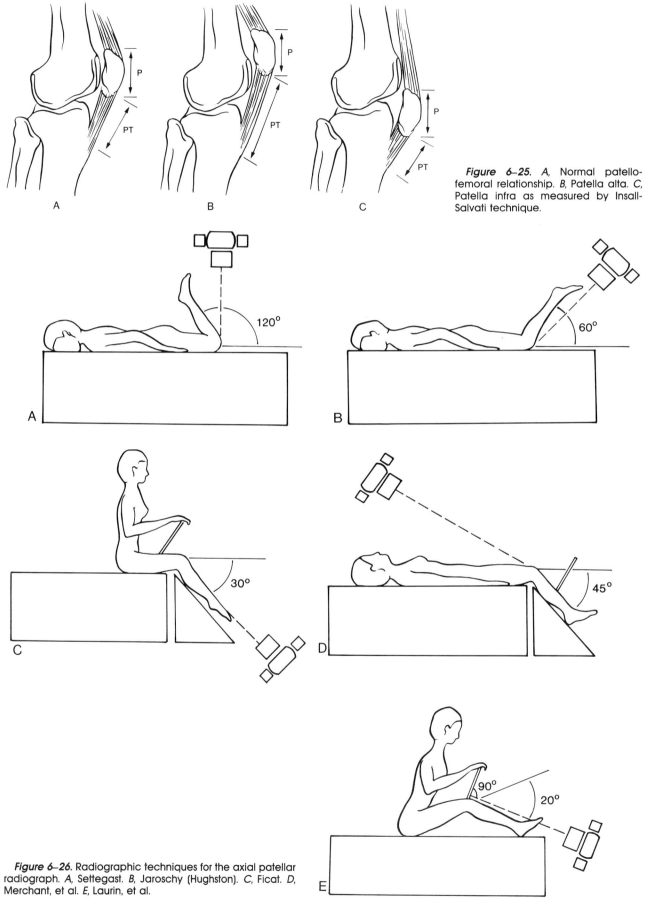

Figure 6–25. A, Normal patellofemoral relationship. B, Patella alta. C, Patella infra as measured by Insall-Salvati technique.

Figure 6–26. Radiographic techniques for the axial patellar radiograph. A, Settegast. B, Jaroschy (Hughston). C, Ficat. D, Merchant, et al. E, Laurin, et al.

with the quadriceps relaxed.[101, 102, 103] If there is laxity of the medial restraints and subluxation of the patella, the patient's symptoms of instability are reproduced. Patellofemoral crepitation should be sought as evidence of degenerative changes in the articular cartilage. Palpation of the patella during active flexion and extension of the knee may reveal crepitus. Passive proximal distal and medial lateral movement of the patella while a compression force is applied may reveal crepitation.[101] Subluxation of the patella in a medial and lateral direction with palpation of the facets for tenderness is also helpful but not specific, as synovial tissue is also examined. Atrophy of the vastus medialis may be seen on visual examination with the quadriceps contracted and should be compared with the contralateral limb.[101, 106] Measurement of the thigh circumference of both limbs should be performed at a fixed distance above the adductor tubercle. The presence or absence of knee effusion and especially a hemarthrosis following an acute injury should also be evaluated.

Radiographs taken of the patellofemoral joint must include AP, lateral, and axial patellar views. The lateral radiograph should be taken in 30° of flexion to place the patellar tendon under tension[93] (see Fig. 6–12). Additional lateral views in 60° and 90° of flexion may be useful to evaluate the patellofemoral joint space at different areas of contact.[93] The lateral radiograph is also useful in assessing the height of the patella relative to the joint line. A high-riding patella, or patella alta, is associated with recurrent lateral subluxation, dislocation, and chondromalacia.[93, 104, 105] A low-riding patella, or patella infra (patella baja), is usually seen postoperatively following excessive distal transfer of the tibial tuberosity, but it may also be seen in achondroplasia.[93]

Patella alta may be assessed according to three measurements: the Insall-Salvati index, the Blackburne index, or Blumensaat's line.[85, 105, 130] In Blumensaat's method, the lower pole of the patella should lie superior to a line projected along the ventral aspect of the intercondylar notch. This technique is usually unreliable.[85, 105, 130] The Insall-Salvati index (Fig. 6–25C) is determined by the ratio of the length of the patellar tendon to the length of the patella.[105] The value for this ratio is 1.02 ± 0.13 (mean and standard deviation).[81, 105] Any deviation of more than 20 percent is abnormal.[105] In Blackburne's technique the ratio of the articular length of the patella to the height of the lower pole of the articular cartilage above the tibial plateau is measured.[85] The normal value is defined as 0.8 (0.54 to 1.06, 0.95 ± 0.13), and patella alta is present when the ratio is greater than 1.0.[85] There is little correlation between the techniques for measuring patella alta.[130] The most widely used technique is that of Insall and Salvati.

Axial views of the patellofemoral joint are used to view the joint line without distortion, to assess the configuration of the patella and trochlea, and to indicate the relationship of the patella to the femur. A variety of techniques have been utilized with varying degrees of knee flexion (Fig. 6–26). The traditional "skyline" view as described by Settegast has the knee in acute flexion, but this view does not visualize patellofemoral relationships in the area where patellar subluxation and dislocation most frequently occur (Fig. 6–26A). Since instability of the patella occurs close to full extension, other radiographic techniques have been advocated. The Jaroschy or Hughston view is taken with the knee in 50° to 60° of flexion and with the x-ray tube angled 45° from the vertical (Fig. 6–26B).[101] Wiberg recommended 40° of knee flexion and Brattstrom 90°.[87, 136] Ficat recommended views in 30°, 60°, and 90° of knee flexion to evaluate subluxation as well as successive areas of patellofemoral contact at the inferior, middle, and superior thirds (Figs. 6–26C and 6–27).[93, 94] The two most useful techniques currently being used are those of Merchant and Laurin.[116, 124] In the Merchant technique, the knee is flexed 45°, and the x-ray beam is oriented 30° from the horizontal, providing a beam to femur angle of 30° (Fig. 6–26D).[124] In the Laurin technique, the knees are flexed 20° to 30°, and the x-ray beam is directed cephalad from below parallel to the anterior surface of the tibia (Fig. 6–26E).[116]

Using these special axial views, a variety of measurements of the trochlea, patella, and patellofemoral congruence may be made. The sulcus angle (Fig. 6–28) is defined as the angle formed by the highest point on the medial and lateral femoral condyles and the lowest point in the intercondylar sulcus. The normal sulcus angle is 141° to 142°,[87] 138° ± 6°,[124] or 137°.[81] A higher value for the sulcus angle is indicative of dysplasia and a tendency to

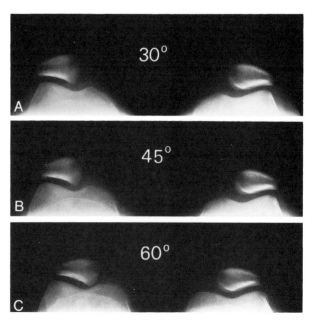

Figure 6–27. Axial views of the patella in varying degrees of knee flexion in the same patient. *A,* 30°. *B,* 45°. *C,* 60°.

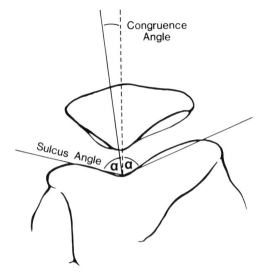

Figure 6–28. Sulcus and congruence angles.

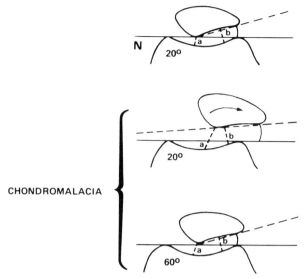

Figure 6–30. Patellofemoral index. (From Laurin, C. A., Dussault, R., and Levesque, H. P.: The Tangential x-Ray investigation of the patellofemoral joint: x-Ray technique, diagnostic criteria, and interpretation. Clin. Orthop. 144:16, 1979.)

sublux.[110] The congruence angle (Fig. 6–28) is formed by a line bisecting the sulcus angle and a second line projected from the apex of the sulcus angle through the lowest point on the articular ridge of the patella.[124] If the apex of the patellar articular ridge is lateral to the zero line it is positive, and if medial it is negative. The normal congruence angle is −6°,[124] or −8° ± 6°.[81] It is 23° in knees with recurrent dislocation.[124] The lateral patellofemoral angle is defined by two lines: (1) a line joining the summits of the femoral condyles, which is a function of the femoral sulcus and is related to the stabilizing role of the lateral femoral condyle, and (2) a line through the limits of the lateral patellar facet (Fig. 6–29).[115, 116] The lateral patellofemoral angle is open laterally in 97 percent of normal knees, while it is parallel in 80 percent and open medially in 20 percent of knees with subluxation of the patella.[116] The patellofemoral index is the ratio between the thickness of the medial patellofemoral interspace and that of the lateral patellofemoral interspace (Fig. 6–30).[115] The lateral patellofemoral interspace corresponds to the shortest distance between the lateral patellar facet and the articular surface of the lateral femoral condyle. The medial patellofemoral interspace is measured by calculating the shortest distance between the lateral limit of the

medial patellar facet and the medial femoral condyle. The normal patellofemoral index is 1.6 or less.[115] An increased patellofemoral index is present in 97 percent of patients with chondromalacia patellae.[115]

Lateral patellar displacement may be assessed by drawing a line perpendicular to the line joining the summits of the femoral condyles. The perpendicular line originates at the margin of the articular cartilage of the medial femoral condyle (Fig. 6–31).[115] In 97 percent of normal cases, the medial edge of the patella is medial to this line and in 3 percent it is lateral to the line by only 1 mm.[115] In subluxing patellae, the medial edge of the patella touches or is lateral to this line in 53 percent.[116] In the case of lateral subluxation, the importance of a relaxed extensor mechanism during the axial radiograph has been emphasized by Laurin,[115] but Sikorski[135] has recommended a vigorous quadriceps contraction to visualize lateral subluxation more effectively. Some variation in the measured parameters of patellar position also exists based upon sex[81] and should not be confused with subluxation. Lateral patellar rotation with quadriceps contraction may be estimated from the ratio of the lateral to medial

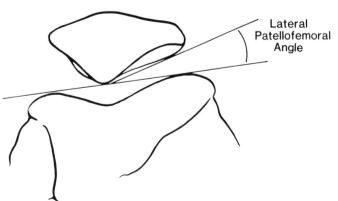

Figure 6–29. Lateral patellofemoral angle.

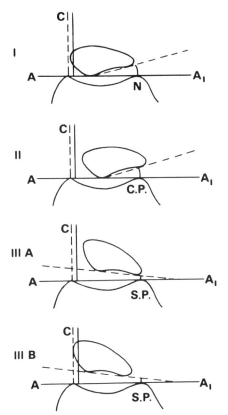

Figure 6–31. Technique of assessment of lateral patellar displacement. (From Laurin, C. A., Dussault, R., and Levesque, H. P.: The Tangential x-Ray investigation of the patellofemoral joint: x-Ray technique, diagnostic criteria, and interpretation. Clin. Orthop. *144*:16, 1979.)

patellar facets. An increased patellar rotation may correlate with chondromalacia.[135]

Axial radiographs of the patella will visualize osteochondral fractures of the lateral femoral condyle associated with recurrent patellar dislocation as well as marginal fractures of the medial aspect of the patella.[95] Calcification in the medial patellar retinaculum without a fracture is also indicative of a previous patellar dislocation with tearing of the medial retinaculum (Fig. 6–32).

Other techniques have also been used for the evaluation of the patella. Computed tomography has been used to evaluate patellar subluxation.[111] Arthrography has been advocated as an additional diagnostic modality for evaluation of the patellofemoral joint.[93, 94] Injection of contrast material can

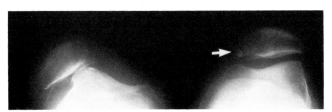

Figure 6–32. Axial view revealing severe subluxation of the right patella and medial calcification of the left patella indicative of a previous dislocation.

be used to evaluate the integrity of the articular cartilage of the patella when combined with axial radiographs taken in 30°, 45°, 60°, and 90° of flexion.[93] The diagnosis of chondromalacia of the patella using arthrography has been reported to be as high as 90 percent.[100] However, arthroscopy has been stated to be a more efficient technique for evaluation of small areas of chondromalacia on the medial facet of the patella.[93]

Patellofemoral Pain Syndromes

The clinical syndromes related to the patellofemoral joint are those related to pain and instability. The term "chondromalacia patellae" was initially used by Aleman in 1928 to describe episodes of crepitus and synovitis associated with softening and fissuring of the articular surface of the patella.[82] Aleman recognized that in a series of 220 patients undergoing arthrotomy, one third of the knees had abnormal articular cartilage on the patella without symptoms referable to the patellofemoral joint. Unfortunately, the term "chondromalacia patellae" has been used for a variety of disorders varying from pathologic studies to reviews of clinical symptomatology without any pathologic confirmation. To avoid this confusion, the term patellofemoral pain syndrome, as recommended by other authors,[93, 94, 96, 110] is best utilized for the description of the patient with patellofemoral pain without instability. The term chondromalacia is best restricted to cases involving description of a pathologic entity.

Patellofemoral arthralgia or pain in the anterior aspect of the knee presents with retropatellar pain associated with sitting and ascending or descending stairs and crepitation.[93, 107] Symptoms of giving way, pseudolocking, and swelling are frequent.[107] On physical examination there is patellofemoral crepitation, pain on compression of the patella, facet tenderness, effusion, and perhaps abnormal patellar tracking.[93, 107] The differential diagnosis includes prepatellar bursitis, painful retropatellar fat pad, pes anserinus bursitis, plica syndrome, meniscal lesions, generalized synovitis, and ligamentous instability.[93, 98] The "excessive lateral pressure syndrome" is a clinical radiologic entity characterized by pain and radiographic evidence of tilting of the patella laterally without lateral subluxation.[93] Physical examination reveals a tight lateral retinaculum. Radiographs reveal (1) narrowing of cartilage, (2) increased density in the subchondral bone layer, with a change in alignment of the trabeculae from their normal orientation perpendicular to the equator of the patella to a position perpendicular to the lateral facet, and (3) a tight and thickened lateral retinaculum.[93]

The pathologic changes of chondromalacia patellae frequently accompany the clinical syndromes of anterior knee pain. The pathologic changes may be classified in several manners. Outerbridge classified the changes in the articular cartilage into four

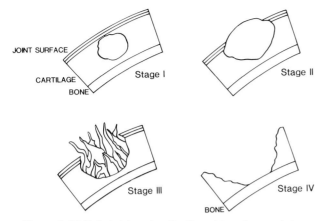

Figure 6–33. Outerbridge classification of four stages of chondromalacia.

grades: (1) softening and swelling of the articular cartilage, (2) fragmentation and fissuring in an area 0.5 inch or less, (3) fragmentation and fissuring in an area greater than 0.5 inch in diameter, and (4) erosion of cartilage down to bone (Fig. 6–33).[127] An arthroscopic grading system for chondromalacia has also been suggested.[107] These arthroscopic grades include (1) early fibrillation or softening of the articular cartilage, involving one or more facets of the patella without involvement of the femur; (2) fragmentation or erosion of the articular surface that is limited to the patella; and (3) articular cartilage changes involving the femur as well as the patella. Goodfellow and colleagues have suggested that there are two distinct pathologic processes affecting the patella: basal degeneration and surface degeneration.[96] Surface degeneration is present in youth, becomes more frequent with age, and primarily affects the odd facet.[96] This process is not associated with patellofemoral pain in youth but may lead to degenerative arthritis in later years. Basal degeneration is a fasciculation of collagen in the middle and deep zones of cartilage that later affects the surface.[96] Basal degeneration affects the ridge separating the medial from the odd facet and is associated with patellofemoral pain in the young individual.[96] It may be divided into three stages: (1) fasciculation of the deep collagen layers with an intact surface, (2) blister formation, and (3) fasciculation extending through the surface of the articular cartilage. Basal degeneration may be the result of excessive pressure and trauma to the patella in this area.[96]

Chondromalacia may also be classified by its anatomical location. Five groups have been established.[94] Group 1 involves the lateral patellar facet, usually just lateral to the median ridge. Group 2 involves the medial facet, usually the odd facet. Group 3 is central chondromalacia affecting the median ridge and extending onto both facets. Group 4 is bipolar chondromalacia involving the central portion of the two facets separated by a normal median ridge. Group 5 is global or total chondromalacia involving the totality of both facets.

The etiology of chondromalacia and patellofemoral pain has remained controversial. Chondromalacia patellae may be related to biomechanical or biochemical causes.[107] Biomechanical causes can be divided into acute and chronic problems. Acute problems include dislocation, direct trauma, and fracture. Chronic problems include recurrent subluxation, patellar malalignment, excessive lateral pressure syndromes, and meniscal injury leading to loss of synchronous joint motion.[107] Biochemical causes include (1) diseases affecting articular cartilage, such as rheumatoid arthritis, recurrent hemarthrosis, alkaptonuria, crystal synovitis, sepsis, and adhesions; (2) iatrogenic factors resulting from intraarticular steroids or prolonged immobilization; and (3) degenerative factors, such as primary osteoarthritis.[107] Another etiologic classification system has established six major categories: (1) trauma; (2) dislocation; (3) malalignment with patellar subluxation; (4) normal alignment with osteochondral ridge; (5) increased cartilage vulnerability, as is typical following surgery or immobilization; and (6) occupational hazards.[129] The importance of a prominent osteochondral ridge on the medial aspect of the trochlear surface of the femur, which results in shearing forces on the patella at 15° to 30° of flexion, has been emphasized by Outerbridge[127, 128, 129] but not by other authors. Ficat and colleagues have suggested that chondromalacia involving the lateral facet of the patella is a manifestation of the excessive lateral pressure syndrome.[94] Central chondromalacia may be a manifestation of excessive pressure related to anatomic abnormalities.[93] Chondromalacia of the medial patellar facet may relate to incongruity in the trochlea or patellar facets, leading to increased stress.[94, 127, 128, 129, 136] Laurin and colleagues have stated that chondromalacia patellae results from malalignment leading to excessive pressure on the lateral facet and that hypopressure on the medial facet results in chondromalacia in that area (Fig. 6–34).[116]

Radiologic evaluation of patients with patellofemoral pain and chondromalacia has been performed by several investigators. In one series of 83 knees, only 40 showed an abnormal Q-angle and only 24 showed patella alta.[104] In a series of 71 knees with

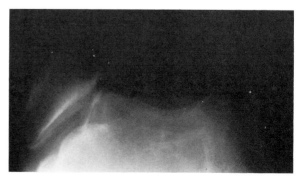

Figure 6–34. Chronic recurrent lateral patellar dislocation occurring with repetitive knee flexion over a 1-year period resulting in severe chondromalacia.

chondromalacia, patella alta was seen in 38 percent and Haglund's excavation in 56 percent.[130] Compared with control knees, the findings were statistically significant.[130] Other radiologic changes such as subchondral sclerosis, osteophytes, lateralization of trabeculae, internal decalcification, or Wiberg patella type were not significantly different.[130] The lateral patellofemoral angle opens laterally in 90 percent of knees with chondromalacia patellae and in 97 percent of normal knees.[115] In 53 patients, the Q-angle was increased to 20°, patella alta measured 1.08, and the congruence angle was −2°, all of which were statistically significant when compared with control values.[81]

Treatment of the patient with patellofemoral pain depends upon recognition of the etiologic factor or factors responsible for the disorder. A nonoperative regimen may be utilized initially. This consists of modification in activity to avoid repetitive knee flexion, especially under load, and may also include isometric quadriceps strengthening, salicylates, and crutches with immobilization for acute episodes of synovitis.[90, 110, 129, 137] In a series of 100 knees with patellofemoral pain, arthroscopic visualization of the articular surface of the patella, and nonoperative treatment, all patients with a normal articular surface became asymptomatic. Of the patients with synovitis and fibrillation of the patella but without femoral changes, 75 percent became asymptomatic. However, only 18 percent of patients with changes involving the patella and femur became asymptomatic.[137]

These results indicate that the presence of pathologic changes on the joint surface correlates with a less satisfactory prognosis and that caution should be used in applying pathological terms such as chondromalacia to the patellofemoral pain syndrome. In a series of 75 athletes with a clinical diagnosis of patellofemoral pain, 66 percent were able to return to unrestricted activity and 23 percent to restricted athletics when treated with a four-phase program consisting of (1) symptomatic control, (2) isometric quadriceps and hamstring exercises, (3) a graduated running program, and (4) a maintenance program.[90] Therefore, a nonoperative treatment regimen should be the initial form of therapy for the patient with patellofemoral pain.

Surgical treatment of the patient with patellofemoral pain should be considered only after a failure of at least 6 months of nonoperative treatment. The operative treatment options include lateral retinacular release, proximal realignment, distal realignment, tibial tubercle elevation, chondrectomy (shaving), facetectomy, medial ridge excision from the trochlear surface of the femur, and patellectomy.[110, 129] Lateral retinacular release has a minimum morbidity and may be performed arthroscopically. The best results with this technique correlate with absence of patella alta, a normal sulcus angle, and a Q-angle of 20° or less.[110] In a series of 60 knees with Outerbridge Grade 1 or 2 chondromalacia treated by lateral retinacular release, 87 percent

satisfactory results were present at 1 year but decreased to 37 percent at 3 years.[126] In a short-term follow-up of 6 months, 76 percent of 174 knees with a patellar compression syndrome were improved following lateral retinacular release.[93] In a series of patients with patellar compression syndrome treated by lateral retinacular release, 28 of 31 were improved at an average of 18 months following surgery.[112] Although localized excision of areas of abnormal cartilage to subchondral bone, with drilling of the subchondral bone, has been found to result in pain relief in 18 of 23 knees,[96] longer follow-up is needed to assess this mode of therapy. Shaving of the patella is unreliable, leading to only 43 percent satisfactory results.[84] In a series of 184 knees with chondromalacia patellae treated by a variety of techniques and monitored with a 4-year follow-up, satisfactory results were obtained in 67 percent of 71 knees treated by trephine combined with drilling, in 61 percent of 57 treated by facetectomy, in 57 percent of 35 treated by shaving, and in only 19 percent of 12 treated by a combined procedure.[122] Worse results have been reported with en bloc excision of articular cartilage when compared with knees in which the articular cartilage is intact and has been treated with realignment procedures.[104] An 83 percent satisfactory result has been obtained in 53 knees treated by proximal realignment compared with 56 percent of 34 knees treated by distal realignment procedures.[104] Relief of patellofemoral pain following proximal realignment correlates with correction of the congruence angle more than with the grades of chondromalacia.[103] Satisfactory results have been obtained in 37 of 39 knees treated by elevation of the tibial tuberosity at 4.7 years of follow-up.[119] Patellectomy remains the ultimate salvage technique for the knee in which other modes of therapy have failed. Patellectomy will provide 83 percent satisfactory results but will result in significant quadriceps weakness.[84]

Patellar Instability

Patellar subluxation and dislocation represent problems related to more extensive extensor malalignment than that present with chondromalacia. Subluxation and dislocation may follow a significant traumatic incident, or malalignment and trauma may both be etiologic factors. Many authors have stated that recurrent patellar subluxation and dislocation have predisposing congenital components.[83, 87, 101, 113] In one series, 73 percent of the knees with subluxation of the patella had at least one congenital deficiency.[101] The importance of superimposed trauma has been debated. Heywood found a history of major trauma in only 5 percent of 90 knees.[99] In a series of athletes, 72 percent reported a traumatic onset of symptoms.[101] Although the patella may be dislocated by a direct blow to the medial aspect of the knee, an indirect mechanism of injury is more frequent.[83, 101] The normal Q-angle results in a lateral vector to the extensor mechanism that tends to displace the patella laterally.[93] The patella subluxes or dislocates when a strong quadriceps contraction is combined with external rotation of the tibia, genu valgum, and slight knee flexion, such as during a cutting maneuver.[83, 101] Dislocation results during the acceleration phase of activity, when the quadriceps is contracting and the extremity is weight-bearing.[83]

Recurrent patellar subluxation may be considered to be of two types, major or minor.[93] In a major subluxation, the patella tracks laterally over the trochlear facet and returns to the patellofemoral groove with an audible snap on the beginning of knee flexion.[93] In a minor subluxation, the patella deviates laterally without clinically apparent relocation.[93] Acute patellar dislocation is usually lateral but may be medial, intra-articular, or superior.[113]

The pathologic changes associated with recurrent dislocation or subluxation include damage to the articular cartilage and the soft tissues. Tearing of the medial retinaculum either from damage to the medial border of the patella or from rupture of the origin of the vastus medialis obliquus may occur.[83] Tears of the medial capsule of the knee, the cruciate ligaments, and the menisci may also occur and must be carefully sought.[83] A hemarthrosis is a frequent finding. The pathologic changes that appear in the articular cartilage are a result of trauma to the medial patellar facet and lateral trochlear facet during relocation of the patella.[99] Trauma may lead to such pathologic changes as chondromalacia, osteochondritis dissecans, osteochondral fracture, loose bodies, and late patellofemoral arthritis.[99]

A variety of factors predisposing to chondromalacia and the patellar pain syndrome have been reviewed. These same anatomic abnormalities have been implicated in the pathogenesis of recurrent subluxation and dislocation.[83, 93, 101, 112, 113] The physical examination and history of symptoms are critical in the recognition of these abnormalities and have been reviewed earlier. An electromyographic study of recurrent patellar subluxation has revealed diminished activity in the vastus medialis muscle, especially at 30° of flexion. This diminished activity is felt to be secondary to static alterations of the extensor mechanism.[118] Radiographic findings are useful in diagnosis and merit review. In Hughston's experience, the more frequent abnormalities visualized include tilting or subluxation of the patella and a relatively low lateral femoral condyle visualized on the axial view.[101] Femoral dysplasia with a shallow sulcus was a frequent finding in another series.[87] A lateral patellofemoral angle that opened medially (40 percent) or in which the lines were parallel (60 percent) was found in a series of recurrent patellar subluxations compared with the normal angle, which is open laterally in 97 percent of knees.[116] A radiographic study of recurrent patellar dislocations revealed an abnormal sulcus angle in 60 percent, Wiberg type III patella in 45 percent, patellar subluxation in the axial view in 100 percent, patella alta in 49 percent, and an abnormal Q-angle

in 52 percent of knees.[112] However, no single factor or combination of factors leads to an increased frequency of redislocation when compared with other knees that present only one abnormality.[112] In a series of 37 knees with recurrent lateral subluxation, the Q-angle was not significantly different from controls, but patella alta (1.23), sulcus angle (147° 30′), and congruence angle (16°) were different from controls.[81] Soft tissue calcification along the medial border of the patella related to ossification of the torn medial retinaculum also often indicates previous dislocation.[93, 123]

The natural history of the untreated patellar subluxation or dislocation is controversial. In Heywood's series, 15 percent had complete cessation of symptoms after physical therapy with development of the quadriceps.[99] Crosby and Insall found that dislocation became less frequent with advancing age.[89] There was little evidence of osteoarthritis, with 65 percent of patients having satisfactory results after nonoperative treatment. The risk of recurrent dislocation is significantly less in patients older than 20 years of age compared with those less than 20 years of age at the time of the initial dislocation.[112] In a series of 50 knees with a single patellar dislocation followed for 5 years, 44 percent developed at least one recurrent dislocation, and 27 percent had symptoms severe enough to merit late reconstruction.[88] In contrast, other authors have felt that all recurrent subluxation will proceed to cartilage damage and patellofemoral arthritis as well as possible dislocation.[93] Therefore, operative treatment may be indicated.

A multitude of operative procedures have been described for patellar subluxation and dislocation. These can be divided into seven major types: (1) capsulorrhaphy, (2) fascioplasty, (3) osteotomy, (4) patellectomy, (5) patellar ligament procedures, (6) myotendinous procedures, and (7) combined procedures.[93] In deciding which procedure or procedures are indicated, the possible components of the malalignment must be evaluated and treatment directed at the abnormal components.[110] The four components to be evaluated are tight lateral structures, lax medial structures, an increased Q-angle, and patella alta.[110] The extent of damage to the articular surface must also be assessed. Acute surgical repair of a dislocation with correction of any underlying pathology has been advocated.[86] Of 17 knees treated by acute repair, there were no recurrent dislocations but 12 knees remained painful.[86] Lateral retinacular release has the lowest morbidity of all the surgical options. Arthroscopic lateral release has given 86 percent satisfactory results at 1 year and 74 percent satisfactory results at 40 to 58 months.[125] Poor results with this technique correlate with failure to maintain quadriceps strength.[125] Proximal realignment of the extensor mechanism yields 75 percent satisfactory results, with no evidence of osteoarthritis at 8 years of follow-up.[89] In contrast, distal realignment yields 59 percent satisfactory results, with evidence of degenerative changes in 22 of 31 knees.[89]

In summary, patellar problems are a frequent clinical problem. A careful distinction between clinical symptoms and pathologic changes in the articular cartilage must be made. A detailed history, physical examination, and radiologic study is necessary to define the problem. Treatment must be directed at any underlying anatomic abnormalities.

FRACTURES ABOUT THE KNEE

Fractures about the knee have a variable presentation. Injury may occur to the distal femur, proximal tibia, or patella. Fracture may be extensive or may involve only small osteocartilaginous fragments. A recognition of the fracture types and assessment of the results of treatment are essential to obtain satisfactory results.

Osteochondral Fractures

Fractures involving the joint surface may result from direct blows or indirect injuries. Recognition of these lesions may be difficult, and careful interpretation of the clinical presentation and high-quality radiographs are essential to define the lesion. One of the most frequent areas of injury involves the patella and is associated with patellar dislocation. As the patella dislocates laterally, damage to the lateral patellar facet and lateral trochlear facet of the femur may occur from shearing forces.[168] Upon reduction of the dislocation, the patella strikes the prominent edge of the lateral femoral condyle, resulting in cartilaginous injury or osteocartilaginous fractures of the medial patellar facet as well as the trochlear surface of the femur (Fig. 6–35).[168] Fractures complicate 5 to 28 percent of all acute patellar dislocations.[184] Treatment of these injuries is by excision or replacement of the articular fragments depending upon size, combined with repair of the acute dislocation.[184]

Fractures involving the weight-bearing surface of the joint may be exogenous, resulting from direct injury, or endogenous. The latter involve combined rotatory and compression forces.[165] In the case of exogenous fractures, the applied forces include compaction, due to direct force applied vertically; shearing, due to rotatory or translational forces; or avulsion, due to the pull of ligamentous attachment.[175] Exogenous shearing forces result in peripheral chondral fractures, while endogenous forces result in centrally located lesions.[165] The clinical diagnosis of these injuries is difficult, with the lesion remaining unsuspected in one third of knees.[167] The clinical presentation is usually a rotatory stress accompanied by a snap and an acute onset of swelling with hemarthrosis.[165, 167, 174] The differential diagnosis must include meniscal and/or ligamentous injury.

Radiographically, the displaced fragment may be difficult to visualize. High-quality radiographs are required, including AP, lateral, tunnel, and axial

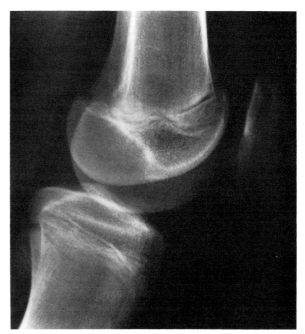

Figure 6–35. Osteochondral fracture of the patella.

views.[165, 167] The defect in the femoral condyle is difficult to visualize initially but becomes sclerotic with passage of time.[167] Early treatment is indicated. Replacement of the fragment and fixation are indicated if it is large, on the weight-bearing surface, and accessible.[165, 167, 174] Either Smillie nails or bone pegs may be utilized for fixation.[162] If the fragment is small (Fig. 6–36) or only cartilaginous, the frag-

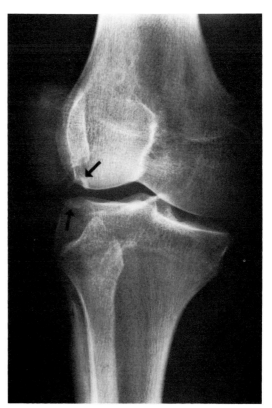

Figure 6–36. Osteochondral fracture of the lateral femoral condyle. Defect *(upper arrow)* and displaced fragment *(lower arrow)*.

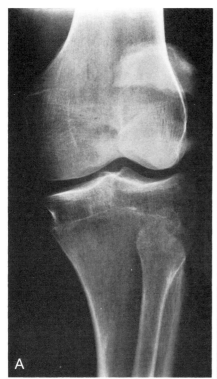
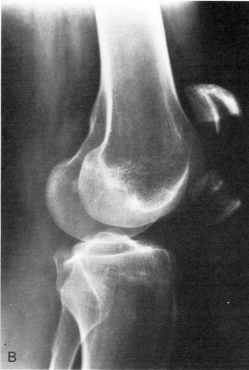

Figure 6–37. AP *(A)* and lateral *(B)* views of a displaced transverse patellar fracture resulting from indirect violence.

ment may be removed and the bed trephined.[174] Early active motion is essential for nourishment of the articular cartilage.[167, 174]

Patellar Fractures

Fractures of the patella are frequent injuries, comprising 1 percent of all injuries.[144] The subcutaneous position of the patella at the anterior aspect of the knee places it in a vulnerable position for direct trauma. The most frequent modes of injury in a series of 422 patellar fractures were motor vehicle accidents in 28 percent, falls on level ground in 54 percent, falls from a height in 14 percent, and other means of direct trauma in 4 percent.[144] Indirect violence owing to quadriceps force on a semiflexed knee may also result in a patellar fracture.[144] Considerable separation of the fracture fragments most frequently accompanies indirect violence (Fig. 6–37).[144]

Patellar fractures may be classified into several types: transverse or oblique, which compose 34 percent; comminuted or stellate, which compose 16 percent; longitudinal fractures, which compose 28 percent; apical and basal fractures, which compose 28 percent, and frontal plane fractures.[144] The position of the knee at the time of injury as well as the mechanism of injury influences the type of fracture that occurs. Indirect violence results in a transverse fracture, while direct violence usually results in a comminuted fracture but may also result in other fracture types as well (Fig. 6–38).[144] Careful attention should be directed to assessment of the degree of fracture surface separation, as wide sep-

aration indicates significant tearing of the patellar retinacula.

Patellar fractures affect all age groups, and a slight male predominance has been noted. In addition to a history of the mechanism of injury a careful physical examination is essential. Palpation for separation of the patellar fragments and the extent of hemarthrosis should be performed. Recognition of

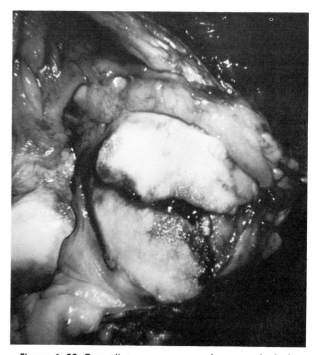

Figure 6–38. Operative appearance of a comminuted patellar fracture following direct violence.

the extent of injury to the soft tissues is important, whether the fracture is open or closed. Active extension of the knee to 0 degrees by the patient is the most useful technique for assessment of associated damage to the retinacula. Complete knee extension is not possible in the presence of a complete tear of the retinacula.[144] Concomitant injuries are frequent and are present in at least 15 percent of patients.[144]

Accurate assessment of the fracture requires excellent-quality radiographs including AP, lateral, and axial views. The axial view is important in assessment of the degree of incongruence of the articular surface, which is the key to decisions regarding the mode of treatment. These same views are essential in the evaluation of treatment. Particular attention must be given to the degree of fracture fragment separation, the accuracy of restoration of articular surface congruency, and the extent of comminution.

The principles of treatment include (1) anatomic fracture reduction, (2) maintenance of reduction until union, (3) repair of the soft tissues, and (4) restoration of the functional integrity of the joint.[144] The options for treatment are nonoperative or operative. Operative treatment may consist of reduction and internal fixation of all fragments, partial patellectomy with repair of the extensor mechanism, or total patellectomy. The generally accepted criterion for nonoperative treatment is a fracture separation of no greater than 2 to 3 mm with minimal incongruency of the articular surface.[144] For nonoperative treatment to be successful, the patellar retinacula must be intact. The preservation of extension capability is present in 39 percent of fractures.[144] Once the fracture surface separation reaches 4 mm, loss of active quadriceps function occurs.

In one study nonoperative treatment of 287 fractures in 282 patients was utilized for fractures with less than 3 mm articular surface displacement and less than 4 mm diastasis.[144] Treatment consisted of a cylinder cast for 4 weeks. Nonunion occurred in 4 fractures. At a mean follow-up of 8.9 years, the result was satisfactory in 99 percent.[144] Boström recommends nonoperative treatment for fractures in which extension capacity is preserved, the diastasis is 3 to 4 mm or less, and the step in the articular surface is 2 to 3 mm or less.[144]

Accordingly, operative treatment is recommended for fractures with loss of active extension of the knee, a diastasis of more than 3 to 4 mm, and a step in the articular surface of more than 2 to 3 mm.[144] Operative treatment that included osteosynthesis (75 cases), partial patellectomy (28 cases), or total patellectomy (5 cases) in 108 knees achieved 79 percent satisfactory results at 8.9 years of follow-up.[144] In the case of the most severe fractures, satisfactory results were obtained in 81 percent following osteosynthesis and in 82 percent following partial patellectomy, but in only one of five treated by total patellectomy.[144]

The results of treatment correlate with the degree of separation of fracture fragments. Satisfactory results were obtained in 98 percent of cases if only slight diastasis was present. Results were satisfactory in only 80 percent, however, with diastasis greater than 4 mm and tears of the patellar retinacula.[144] Osteoarthritis of the patellofemoral articulation did not correlate with enlargement of the patella or with a step in the articular surface of greater than 1 mm.[144] In a 10 to 30 year follow-up, patellar enlargement did correlate, but the extent of the step in the articular surface did not correlate with osteoarthritis.[194] Osteoarthritis of the patellofemoral joint was present in 70 percent of the fractured joints and in only 31 percent of contralateral uninjured knees.[194] Osteoarthritis of the patellofemoral joint was observed in 22 percent of the knees at 8.9 years of follow-up.[144] Osteoarthritis correlated with the severity of injury, as it was present in 42 percent of comminuted fractures and in only 19 percent of the other fracture types.[144]

The technique of internal fixation of the patella and the mechanical stability of the repair have been studied.[196] A comparison between circumferential wiring, Magnusson wiring, and modified tension-band wiring revealed improved stability with the Magnusson or modified tension-band techniques (Fig. 6–39).[196] The retinacular repair also contributed to the stability of the repair.

Partial patellectomy with retention of one major fragment has been advocated for comminuted patellar fractures.[139] The adverse consequences of total patellectomy from a biomechanical standpoint have already been reviewed in the section of this chapter on the patella. The decision regarding the portion of the patella to be removed is based upon the degree of comminution and location of the major fragment. Frequently, the comminution is distal and fragments can be removed with preservation of the proximal fragment.[139] In this case the patellar ligament is repaired and attached to the articular edge of the patella to prevent tilting or instability of the patella. In a series of 58 displaced fractures of the patella treated by partial patellectomy, none required subsequent patellectomy or chondroplasty of the patella at a 4 year follow-up.[139] Partial patellectomy has also been advocated for displaced longitudinal fractures of the patella.[139]

In considering partial patellectomy, a knowledge of the blood supply to the patella is important. The two sources of intra-osseous arterial supply are through midpatellar vessels entering anteriorly and polar vessels entering inferiorly behind the patellar ligament.[186] In traverse fractures of the midpatella, the superior fragment is easily isolated from the blood supply. This accounts for the 25 percent incidence of partial avascular necrosis seen in a series of 162 of these fractures (Fig. 6–40).[186] These findings have led to the recommendation that the distal one half of the patella should be preserved.[186]

Total patellectomy has been utilized in the management of severe comminuted fractures. A long-

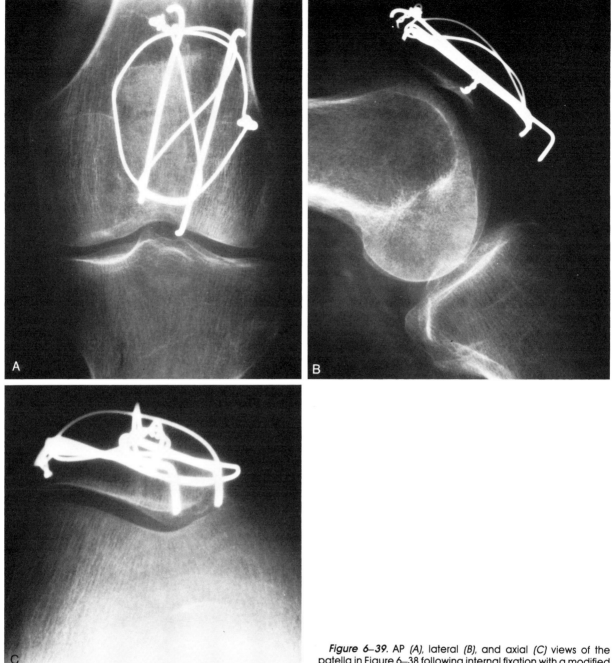

Figure 6–39. AP *(A)*, lateral *(B)*, and axial *(C)* views of the patella in Figure 6–38 following internal fixation with a modified tension band technique and circlage wire.

term follow-up (4 to 13 years) of 31 patients treated by patellectomy for fractures revealed 22 percent excellent, 39 percent good, and 39 percent poor results.[197] In this series of 31 patients, no evidence of osteoarthritis was found, and there was no correlation between symptoms and calcification in the patellar tendon. Maximal recovery of knee function following patellectomy required up to 3 years.[197]

Supracondylar Fractures of the Femur

A supracondylar fracture of the femur is a fracture involving the distal 9 cm of the femur measured from the articular surface of the femoral condyles.[153]

An intra-articular fracture of the femoral condyle may accompany the diaphyseal or metaphyseal component.[153] Other authors have stated that a supracondylar fracture may involve up to the distal 15 cm of the femur.[188]

The average age of the patient affected by supracondylar fractures is variable but has been taken to be 40 years,[195] 54,[188] 47,[169] and 54,[156] with a range from 16 to 101 in various series. There is no sex predilection. The extent of trauma necessary to induce a fracture decreases with age, as the frequency of osteoporosis increases. Associated local injuries are frequent. In a series of 83 supracondylar femur fractures, there were 2 ipsilateral tibial pla-

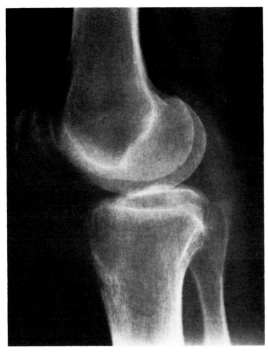

Figure 6–40. Avascular necrosis of the proximal pole of the patella following a transverse fracture.

teau fractures and 5 major knee ligamentous injuries that compromised the results of fracture treatment.[188]

A variety of classification schemes have been utilized for supracondylar femur fractures. Schatzker and colleagues have divided the fractures into three types: Type I, simple; Type II, comminution without joint involvement; and Type III, fracture with involvement of the articular surface.[188] Healy and Brooker suggested four groups: (1) simple intra-articular, (2) simple extra-articular, (3) complex intra-articular, and (4) complex extra-articular.[156] A simple fracture was defined as nondisplaced, while a complex fracture was defined as having a displacement greater than 1 to 2 mm, angulation, comminution, or a combination of these factors.

The most widely utilized classification is that of Neer and colleagues, with Type I defined as minimal displacement (31 percent), Type IIA as medial displacement of the condyles (29 percent), Type IIB as lateral displacement of the condyles (21 percent), and Type III as conjoined supracondylar and shaft fractures (19 percent) (Fig. 6–41).[173] The mechanism of injury was trivial trauma in 45 percent and included all Type I and 15 percent of 25 Type IIA injuries.[173] Type I fractures result from trauma to the flexed knee with osteoporotic bone. Type IIA fractures result from a violent force applied to the anterolateral side of the flexed knee, while Type IIB result from a force to the lateral side of the extended knee or the medial side of a flexed knee. Type III fractures result from extensive violence to the anterior aspect of the flexed knee.

A more recent classification is that of Seinsheimer, with 4 types recognized (Fig. 6–42).[192] Type I is nondisplaced with less than 2 mm displacement of the fragments. Type II involves the distal metaphysis without extension into the intercondylar notch or femoral condyles and has two subtypes: (a) two-part fractures and (b) comminuted fractures (Fig. 6–43B). Type III involves the intercondylar notch, in which one or both condyles are separate fragments, and has three subtypes: (a) the medial condyle is separated, (b) the lateral condyle is separated, and (c) both condyles are separated. Type IV involves the articular surface of the femoral condyle and has two subtypes: (a) a fracture through the lateral condyle (two-part or comminuted) and (b) more complex comminuted fractures involving one femoral condyle and the intercondylar notch, both femoral condyles, or all three.

Treatment of supracondylar fractures of the femur may be nonoperative, involving combinations of traction and cast immobilization, or operative. Treatment may be complicated by the fact that the adductors, quadriceps, hamstrings, and gastrocnemius muscles pull the distal fragment into flexion, adduction, and shortening, while the hip externally rotates and may lead to a fracture deformity of varus and internal rotation.[173, 195] Nonoperative treatment with traction thus encounters four major problems. These include excessive flexion of the knee, varus and internal rotation of the distal frag-

Figure 6–41. Classification of supracondylar femur fractures. (From Neer, C. S., Grantham, A., and Sheldon, M. L.: Supracondylar fracture of the adult femur. A study of one hundred and ten cases. J. Bone Joint Surg. *49A*:591, 1967.)

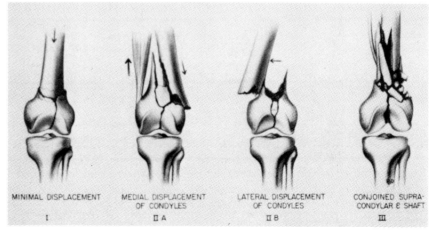

MINIMAL DISPLACEMENT   MEDIAL DISPLACEMENT OF CONDYLES   LATERAL DISPLACEMENT OF CONDYLES   CONJOINED SUPRACONDYLAR & SHAFT

I   II A   II B   III

TYPE 2

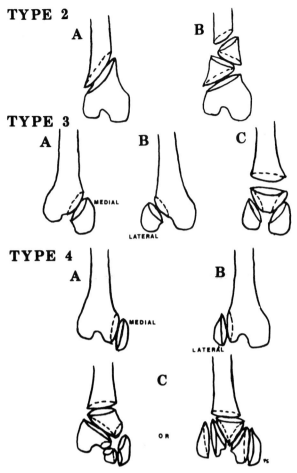

TYPE 3

TYPE 4

Figure 6–42. Classification of supracondylar femur fractures. (From Seinsheimer, F.: Fractures of the distal femur. Clin. Orthop. *153*:169, 1980.)

ment relative to the external rotation of the hip, inconsistent radiographs that are not corrected for the rotated position of the limb in traction, and prolonged immobilization of the knee.[173] In a series of 77 fractures followed for a mean of 5.6 years, satisfactory results were obtained in 15 of 29 treated operatively compared with 43 of 48 nonoperatively.[173] Inadequate fixation in osteoporotic bone, which necessitated prolonged immobilization, was the major reason for poor results in the operatively treated group. In a series of fractures followed for at least 1 year, satisfactory results were obtained in 67 percent of 144 nonoperatively compared with 54 percent of 69 treated by open reduction and internal fixation.[195] Delayed union or non-union occurred in 20 of the 69 fractures treated operatively compared with 14 of 144 treated nonoperatively.[195] A survey of orthopedic surgeons in 1972 suggested 61 percent favoring closed over open treatment.[183] The major reason for closed treatment giving preferable results in early series was inadequate implants and techniques to allow early motion of the knee. Traction followed by a cast brace has been utilized in 150 distal femoral fractures, with union occurring within 15 weeks and no non-unions.[170] However, 30 percent of these patients had less than 90° of knee flexion. A recent comparative study of open and closed treatment of 98 fractures, however, revealed satisfactory results in 38 of 47 treated operatively compared with 18 of 51 treated nonoperatively.[156] Satisfactory results were obtained with closed treatment in the nondisplaced fractures, while superior results were obtained by internal fixation compared with nonoperative treatment in the case of complex fractures.

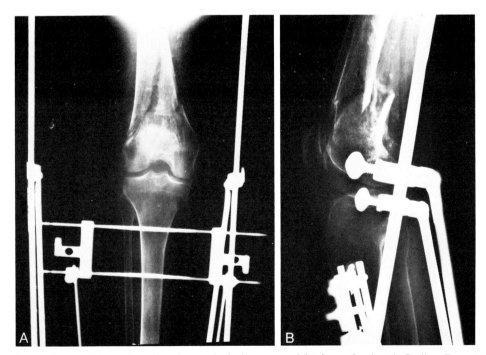

Figure 6–43. AP *(A)* and lateral *(B)* radiographs of comminuted supracondylar femur fracture in fixation. There is residual flexion of the distal fragment due to the pull of the gastrocnemius muscle. This would be a Type IIB in Seinsheimer's classification.

Part of the recent success of open methods is due to a variety of newer implants developed for internal fixation of supracondylar fractures of the femur. One involves an intramedullary device with screw fixation of the condyles.[163, 200] Using the Zickel supracondylar device in 15 patients, union occurred by 14 weeks, with one non-union.[200] However, 6 patients required a cast brace for additional support following surgery. In a series of 27 fractures treated with the Zickel device, union occurred in 16 weeks, with 88 percent satisfactory results.[163] However, complications occurred in 31 percent, and 50 percent required additional operative procedures, usually for removal of the fixation device.[167] Another implant, the angled blade plate, was used in 15 fractures, none of which were comminuted, and union occurred in 14.[175] However, there were 4 infections, and 5 knees had less than 90° of knee flexion. In another series of 71 fractures, in which 49 were available for follow-up, 24 were treated with a supracondylar blade plate. This method achieved a satisfactory result in 75.5 percent compared with 12 of 25 treated nonoperatively.[187] In another series, 49 of 83 fractures treated with a blade plate were available for follow-up. Of 17 fractures treated without technical error, 71 percent had satisfactory results; satisfactory results were seen in only 21 percent of 18 fractures with technical errors of fixation.[188] Fourteen fractures were treated nonoperatively, but the results of treatment were not analyzed.[188] Eighty percent satisfactory results have been obtained in 30 fractures treated with a blade plate, with union at 16 weeks and a 6.6 percent incidence of infection.[169] In another series of 26 supracondylar femur fractures treated with a blade plate, union was obtained within 16 weeks; these showed no infection and an average knee motion of 120°.[153]

The technical errors related to internal fixation that may lead to poor results include incomplete reduction, failure to achieve interfragmental compression, failure to use bone grafts to correct defects, incorrect use of acrylic cement, too long an implant, and incorrect implant positioning.[189]

Indications for open reduction and internal fixation of supracondylar femoral fractures include open intra-articular fractures with displacement, associated neurovascular injuries, associated ipsilateral fractures of the tibia or tibial plateau, multiple trauma,[69, 189] and a fractured patella in which rigid fixation will allow early knee motion. Relative contraindications to internal fixation include a severely comminuted fracture or osteoporotic bone in an elderly patient.[189]

Therefore, well performed internal fixation of supracondylar fractures of the femur with careful restoration of the articular surface and early knee motion will provide excellent results. However, internal fixation is technically difficult; and if poorly performed, it will lead to worse results than nonoperative treatment. Additionally, it carries the risk of infection.

Fractures of the Tibial Condyles

Fractures of the tibial condyles represent problems in management. Treatment is controversial. The objective of treatment is to obtain a stable, painless, mobile joint and to delay the onset of arthrosis. This etiology of these injuries is variable, but they are frequently related to motor vehicle accidents (54 percent) and falls (46 percent). Any age group may be affected, but these fractures occur most frequently in the sixth decade. The sexes are affected equally.

The diagnosis of the fracture is based upon the history of injury and physical examination of knee effusion, tenderness, range of motion, and stability. Routine radiographs in an AP plane will demonstrate the fracture, but these are inadequate to determine the extent of displacement of all fragments. Moore has recommended a tibial plateau radiograph, which allows more accurate estimation of the extent of condylar depression.[171] The normal articular surface of the tibia forms an angle of 76° with the line of the tibial crest (i.e., posterior slope). Therefore, in the tibial plateau view, the radiographic beam must be angled at 105° to the tibial crest to be parallel to the articular surface of the tibia.[171] Tomography has been recommended to evaluate the amount of articular surface depression or displacement, the site of the fracture, and the extent of comminution.[151, 189] Tomography is especially useful in differentiating split-depression fractures from fractures in which depression of the articular surface alone is present (Fig. 6–44).[151] Tomography led to more accurate reclassification of 13 of 21 such fractures when compared with classification drawn from plain radiographs.[151] The amount of depression is quantitated by measuring the distance from the remaining intact articular surface or an extension of the other tibial condyle to the point of maximum depression.[189] Arthrotomography using double-contrast techniques is also useful in assessing the degree of incongruity of the articular surface following fracture union.[138] Therefore, radiography should be utilized to assess the extent of the fracture, the degree of comminution, the depth of articular surface depression, and the extent of lateral displacement or condylar widening.

Patients with a tibial condylar fracture should be evaluated for associated injuries as well. Neurovascular injuries may accompany these fractures. Peroneal palsy was present in 6 of 260 fractures in one study[180] and has been found to occur in 1 to 5 percent of all cases.[147] Fractures of the fibular head are relatively common, and peroneal nerve injury may accompany this bony lesion.[147] One contusion of the popliteal artery leading to a compartment syndrome occurred in a series of 260 fractures.[180] The possibility of other fractures, such as a fracture of the femoral condyle, should also be considered.

The most frequent associated injuries are to the menisci and ligaments of the knee. In a series of 291 tibial condylar fractures, ligamentous insuffi-

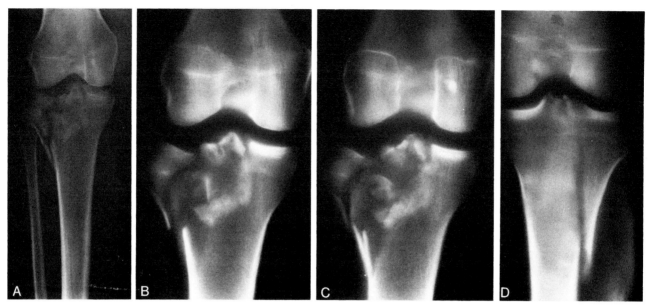

Figure 6–44. AP radiograph *(A)* and AP tomograms *(B* and *C)* of a split depression lateral tibial plateau fracture. AP tomogram *(D)* of the pure split type without displacement, which should be compared with the split depression type.

ciency was the primary reason for an unacceptable result in 4.5 percent.[142] In a series of 91 fractures treated operatively, 33 ligamentous injuries were repaired.[199] Tears of the medial collateral ligament were the most frequent (13 of 16) and occurred in conjunction with fractures of the lateral condyle.[199] Repair of the cruciate ligaments was performed in 13 of 24 knees.[199] Enlargement of the medial joint space on valgus stress roentgenograms is a sign of collateral ligament insufficiency.[193, 199] The presence of a capsular rupture on an arthrogram has been helpful in identifying ligamentous injuries.[193] In a follow-up study of 196 knees, 20 percent were noted to be unstable as a result of ligamentous insufficiency.[199] In one series a rupture of the medial collateral ligament always accompanied a fracture of the lateral tibial plateau and proximal fibula.[193] In another series of 260 fractures, rupture of the anterior cruciate ligament was present in 5.4 percent, rupture of the medial collateral ligament in 3.8 percent, and rupture of the posterior cruciate or lateral collateral ligament in 0.4 percent. In contrast to other authors, Rasmussen stated that although ligamentous injuries may contribute to instability, they are of minor consequence compared with the fracture and may be ignored.[180] He feels that stress roentgenograms are of little therapeutic benefit. In contrast, Schatzker and colleagues believe that stress views are valuable in determining whether instability is due to fracture or ligamentous tear.[189] In another series of 208 fractures, ligamentous calcification was noted in 16 percent at follow-up.[172] Comparison for laxity between the injured and noninjured knee on stress radiographs at follow-up revealed no significant differences in laxity.

Meniscus tears, the other most frequent injury associated with tibial condylar fractures, were present in 19 of 110 fractures, of which 7 were peripheral and could be repaired.[145] In another series, 14 pe-

ripheral meniscus tears were repaired in a series of 94 fractures.[189] A torn meniscus was seen in 44 of 91 fractures.[142] Meniscus injuries have been reported in up to 50 percent of fractures at arthrotomy.[182] The results of 35 meniscectomies associated with 200 fractures revealed worse results in the knees treated with meniscectomy.[149]

A variety of classification schemes have been suggested for tibial condylar fractures. These various classifications make comparison between series difficult. Porter chose to classify fractures as either split, bicondylar, or crush types.[177] Burri suggests a classification including nondisplaced fractures of the condyles, mono- and bicondylar displaced-depression fractures, fractures with impaction, combination fractures, and comminuted fractures.[147] Schatzker and colleagues suggest that Type I include pure cleavage fractures, Type 2 cleavage fractures combined with depression, Type 3 pure central depression fractures, Type 4 fractures of the medial condyle, Type 5 bicondylar fractures, and Type 6 tibial plateau fractures with dissociation of the tibial metaphysis and diaphysis.[189] Schulak and Gunn suggest an alternative classification, with Type I including minimally displaced fractures, Type II displaced lateral plateau fractures, Type III displaced medial plateau fractures, and Type IV displaced bicondylar fractures.[190] Type II divides into three categories: local or total depression, split, and mixed. Type III also divides into total and split depression categories. The most widely utilized classification, however, is that of Hohl and Luck as modified by Hohl (Fig. 6–45).[159, 160] Type I is undisplaced and constitutes 24 percent; Type II is central depression and constitutes 26 percent; Type III is split depression and constitutes 26 percent; Type IV is total depression and constitutes 11 percent; Type V is split and constitutes 3 percent; Type VI is comminuted and constitutes 10 percent. The

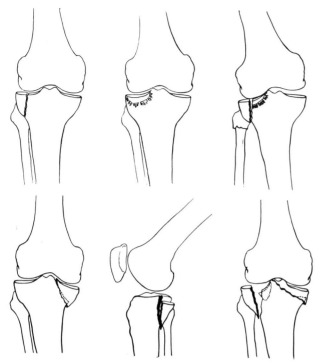

Figure 6–45. Classification of tibial plateau fractures. (From Hohl, M.: Tibial condylar fractures. J. Bone Joint Surg. *49A:*1455, 1967.)

frequency of the various types is outlined in Table 6–3.

The mechanism of injury of the various fracture types has been reviewed by several authors. Schulak and Gunn have provided an excellent review (Fig. 6–46).[190] One factor affecting the type of fracture is the point of the impact; this in turn determines the size of the fragment.[180] The extent of crushing depends upon the age of the patient, the resistance of the subchondral bone, the amount of knee flexion, and the magnitude of the axial force.[180] The majority of these fractures are produced by the prominent anterior part of the lateral femoral condyle being driven like a wedge into the underlying tibial plateau.[180] The frequent lateral plateau fractures result from combined abduction and compression forces.[140]

A wide variety of the therapeutic modalities have been utilized in the management of these injuries. Two philosophies of treatment have emerged: (1) nonoperative treatment with early knee motion to mold the displaced fragments into acceptable positions, and (2) operative reduction of the fracture with various types of internal fixation. The objective of any treatment method is to provide a mobile,

painless, stable, well-aligned knee with function as close to normal as possible. The choice of treatment will be influenced by the age, general health, and ambulatory status of the patient as well as by associated injuries, the extent of fracture displacement, and the experience of the surgeon.

Nonoperative treatment generally consists of an initial period of traction followed by cast immobilization. Apley has advocated closed reduction followed by early motion of the knee in skeletal traction.[140] In a 5-year follow-up study of 27 of 48 tibial condylar fractures treated by traction (69 percent of which were displaced fractures), satisfactory results were obtained in 21 knees.[140] Early motion serves to restore movement and power, molds the fractured tibial condyle to the shape of the femoral condyle, and promotes healing.[140, 141] Mobilization in a cast brace following an early period in traction has resulted in a decreased hospitalization time and satisfactory results.[146, 185, 191] In the case of unstable fractures, internal fixation should be utilized prior to application of the cast brace.[146, 191] In a series of 29 fractures treated with a cast brace (of which 7 received some internal fixation), 26 had satisfactory results, with progression of deformity in only 1 knee.[191] In a series of 30 fractures of which 5 received internal fixation treated by a cast brace, there was no progression of deformity.[146] However, an experimental study of tibial condylar fractures fixed with a cast brace revealed that fractures with an associated fracture of the fibular head or with concurrent medial condylar fractures were not suitable for this technique, as collapse will occur.[185] Cast-brace treatment should be reserved for fractures with minimal displacement involving the lateral plateau and in which the fibular head is intact; alternatively, it may

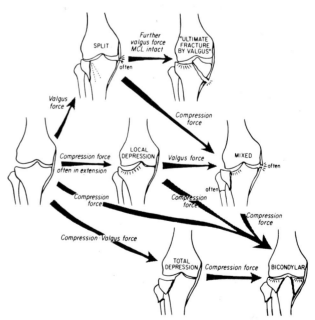

Figure 6–46. Mechanisms of injury producing the various types of fractures of the tibial plateau. (From Schulak, D. J. and Genn, D. R.: Fractures of the tibial plateau. A review of the literature. Clin. Orthop. *109:*167, 1975.)

TABLE 6–3. Frequency of Tibial Condylar Fractures (%)

Author	No.	Type I	Type II	Type III	Type IV	Type V	Type VI
Hohl	805	24	26	26	11	3	10
Dovey	261	18	14	40	5	2	21
Lucht	109	28	23	17	11	4	17
Bakalim	197	18	45	0	11	10	16
Bowes	110	48	12	13	5	2	20

be used as a supplementary treatment following internal fixation.[146, 185, 191] Closed reduction followed by a hip spica cast has been utilized in the management of 61 displaced fractures of the tibial plateau.[150] At 3.8 years of follow-up, 85 percent satisfactory results were achieved. The initial displacement correlated inversely with the end result, and the poorest results were seen in the split depression fractures.[150] Nonoperative treatment has also been recommended for management of central compression fractures in which the knee in extension is stable under stress.[181] A 4- to 9-year follow-up of 40 displaced fractures treated by cast immobilization revealed satisfactory results in 30 of 32 knees.[181] Roentgenographic evidence of moderate arthrosis was noted in only 2 knees. Closed reduction followed by limited fixation with a wire loop combined with cast immobilization has been utilized for bicondylar plateau fractures.[155] In a 6- to 12-year follow-up of 12 knees, satisfactory results were present in 10 knees with no loss of fracture reduction.

The decision regarding operative treatment and the factors affecting the long-term results have been reviewed by many authors. However, data on operative vs. nonoperative treatment of comparable groups of patients with similar fractures is not available. Generally, the more severe the injury, the more frequently surgical treatment is utilized. A review of various authors' indications for operative treatment and their results will aid in evaluation of these treatment modalities.

The factors that result in permanent disability after fracture are limited motion, instability, angular deformity, lack of full extension, pain, traumatic arthritis, and muscle weakness.[159] Limited motion relates to prolonged immobilization. Instability results from either residual depression of the articular surface, ligamentous laxity, degenerative changes, or a combination of these factors. Angular deformity results from incomplete fracture reduction, collapse of the fracture during healing, or degenerative change. Lack of full extension follows from prolonged immobilization with the knee held in flexion or from the posterior capsular contracture associated with fractures involving the posterior tibial condyles. Traumatic arthritis relates to the degree of malalignment, the accuracy of reduction, and the extent of articular cartilage damage.

Rasmussen has stated that the presence of lateral instability in extension is an indication for operative treatment.[178–180] Instability depends more upon the localization and extent of compression than upon its depth.[178–180] Anteriorly located compression makes the knee unstable in full extension, while posterior compression results in instability in slight flexion.[178] Only the fractures that produce instability in extension require operative treatment.[178–180]

In a series of 192 fractures, Rasmussen found that instability in extension was present in 46 percent.[179] A 10° increase in lateral deviation upon clinical testing compared with the normal side was taken as a sign of instability requiring surgical treatment.[180] The frequency of instability according to fracture type in 260 fractures was 70 percent of 66 split depression fractures, 24 percent of 80 local compression fractures, 45 percent of 29 medial condyle fractures, and 52 percent of 48 bicondylar fractures.[180] Of 260 fractures in which 44 percent were treated operatively, follow-up was obtained in 78 percent at a mean of 7.3 years following fracture.[180] Using instability as the criterion for surgery, 87 percent had satisfactory results at follow-up. There was a lack of correlation between the functional and anatomic results. Of the 202 patients followed, 21 percent had roentgenographic evidence of arthrosis. Arthrosis was present in 42 percent of the bicondylar fractures compared with 16 percent of the lateral and 21 percent of the medial condyle fractures.[179, 180] Arthrosis also correlated with axial alignment. It was present in 79 percent of the patients with varus alignment and in 31 percent with excess valgus alignment greater than 10°, but arthrosis was found in only 13 percent of the knees with normal alignment.[179, 180] Arthrosis was found in 46 percent of the knees with instability in extension compared with 14 percent with instability in 20° of flexion or the 18 percent associated with normal stability.[179, 180] Condylar widening greater than 5 mm appeared to correlate with osteoarthritis.[179] The presence of osteoarthritis correlated with a poor clinical result.[180]

In a series of 200 fractures followed for 1.5 to 10 years, of which 62 were treated surgically, the split depression fractures had better results with nonoperative care, while the bicondylar fractures had similar results regardless of the method of treatment.[149] In local compression fractures, the result correlated with the amount of depression. Acceptable results were present in 94 percent of the fractures with less than 3 mm of depression but in only 50 percent of fractures with more than 10 mm of depression.[149] Regardless of the fracture type or method of treatment, improved results were seen with early motion.[149] A residual valgus deformity of greater than 10° was present in 4 percent and correlated with a poor result. Instability in full extension was present in 7.5 percent of the knees but did not influence the clinical result. Although the radiographs may reveal significant bony depression, fibrocartilage was found to fill the defect in 2 knees.

A comparative study of operative reduction versus nonoperative treatment with either traction or cast immobilization was performed in 39 patients who had local depression fractures exceeding 10 mm.[177] At 6 years of follow-up, 10 of 10 treated by nonoperative means compared with 4 of 20 treated operatively had unacceptable results.[177] Therefore, operative treatment was recommended for fractures with greater than 10 mm of depression.

Another study assessed treatment modalities in a series of 109 fractures in which 53 percent were treated and followed for an average of 5.75 years.[166]

Nonoperative treatment provided satisfactory results for fractures that were depressed less than 10 mm. All patients with depression greater than 10 mm were treated operatively, with 79 percent satisfactory functional results but only 58 percent acceptable anatomic results. Improved results were seen with knee motion begun prior to the eighth week. Acceptable results were seen in 90 percent of these knees compared with 71 percent in which motion was begun at a later date.[166]

The results of treatment correlate with the fracture type. One study established this correlation in a series of 197 fractures followed for a mean of 4.5 years.[142] Nonoperative treatment provided satisfactory results in 35 of 36 undisplaced fractures. In local depression fractures, satisfactory results were obtained in 30 of 39 treated nonoperatively compared with 29 of 50 treated operatively. The results correlated with the accuracy of reduction. Results were acceptable in 47 of 62 fractures with less than 5 mm of residual depression compared with 13 of 27 with more than 5 mm of residual depression. A satisfactory result was obtained in 12 of 18 total depression fractures with less than 5 mm of depression compared with 1 of 3 with depression greater than 5 mm. Of 19 split fractures, all had acceptable results, and the result did not correlate with the extent of residual widening. Finally, of 31 bicondylar fractures, acceptable results were obtained in 21 and correlated with the accuracy of reduction.

Hohl has reported on an extensive series of 917 tibial plateau fractures and has suggested a treatment regimen based upon fracture types.[157–160] For undisplaced fractures, a soft dressing followed by protected weight-bearing until bone union occurs gives generally satisfactory results. Immobilization should not exceed 3 weeks to avoid adhesion formation. Local depression fractures with less than 5 mm of depression may be treated nonoperatively, while depression of greater than 5 to 8 mm requires operative reduction to avoid valgus deformity and instability. The prognosis for local depression fractures depends upon accuracy of reduction and maintenance of the articular surface as well as integrity of the soft tissues.[159] The results for split depression fractures correlate with the quality of reduction. Poor results are obtained if more than 11 mm of residual depression is present.[157–160] Reduction may be more adequately obtained with operative techniques than with nonoperative methods. For total condylar depression, reduction may be obtained by traction or operative techniques, but operative treatment is superior.[157–160] Although split fractures often lead to poor results, the best results are obtained with operative treatment. Comminuted fractures appear best treated by manipulation and traction, possibly aided by limited open reduction.[157–160] The results following treatment utilizing this approach correlated with several factors. Fractures with less than 4 mm of depression had better results than those with greater depression.[158] Residual condylar widening of greater than 4 mm was associated with less satisfactory results. Instability

was present in 30 percent of knees with less than 7 mm of depression compared with 46 percent of knees with greater amounts of depression. The frequency of degenerative change increased with the extent of angular deformity. Degenerative change appeared in 46 percent with no deformity and in 84 percent if the deformity was greater than 15°.[158] Early motion within 2 weeks of injury provides improved results compared with later mobilization of the knee.[158]

Utilizing the principles of restoration of articular congruity, limb alignment, and early motion, acceptable results were obtained in 84 percent of 110 fractures.[145] Anatomic reduction did not always lead to an acceptable result if knee motion was delayed.[145]

Operative methods of treatment are being more widely utilized as surgical techniques and implants improve.[147, 189] In one study, satisfactory results at 28 months of follow-up were present in 78 percent of surgically treated fractures compared with 58 percent of the nonoperative group.[189] Schatzker and colleagues recommended anatomic reduction, bone grafting as necessary, and internal fixation followed by early motion as the most appropriate form of management for displaced fractures.[189] They stated that the articular defect does not fill with articular cartilage and remains incongruous. Surgical experience is also relatively important in the operative management of tibial plateau fractures. In a series of 278 fractures treated operatively, good results were obtained in 66 percent by less experienced surgeons compared with 76 percent by more experienced surgeons.[147] Burri and colleagues recommended operative treatment for all fractures with depression, displacement, or impaction and suggested use of a buttress plate (Fig. 6–47).[147]

In summary, fractures of the tibial condyle merit careful evaluation to determine the fracture type,

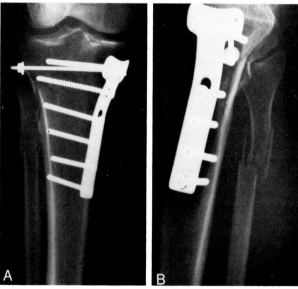

Figure 6–47. AP (A) and lateral (B) radiographs of a local condylar depression type fracture of the lateral tibial plateau treated with a buttress plate. There is still an area of residual depression of the articular surface.

mechanism of injury, and extent of articular surface displacement. Associated injuries of the soft tissues, especially ligaments and menisci, must be sought and treated. The best results correlate with reduction of the fracture and correction of articular surface incongruity, instability, and axial alignment of the knee. The treatment choice should allow early knee motion.

Ipsilateral Fractures of the Femur and Tibia

Ipsilateral fractures of the femur and tibia present problems in management related to loss of stabilization of the knee and difficulty in rehabilitation. This injury has been termed the "floating knee."[143] High-velocity trauma is required to inflict these injuries, and floating knee occurs most frequently in motor vehicle accidents.[143, 154, 161, 164, 176] Associated injuries frequently involve other organ systems and additional skeletal trauma, both of which should be carefully sought.[143, 154, 161, 164, 176] Severe abdominal and thoracic injuries are present in 20 percent of cases.[154, 161, 176] The mortality rate in these patients is 4 to 13 percent.[152, 154] The fractures are frequently open (59 percent in a series of 222 fractures).[152] Neurovascular injuries are present in 7 percent and knee ligamentous injuries in 8 percent.[152] Ligament injuries about the knee are frequently difficult to diagnose initially because of the instability of the fractures; accordingly, they are seen five times more frequently at follow-up than at the time of injury.[152] Men are affected more frequently than women, and the patients are generally in the second to fourth decades of life.[143, 152, 154, 161, 164, 176]

Two classifications have been utilized for these fractures. Blake and McBryde classified Type 1 as the case in which the knee is isolated completely from either shaft fracture.[143] In type 2A, the injury extends into the knee joint, while in Type 2B the injury involves the hip or ankle joints. Fraser and colleagues classified 222 cases as follows: Type 1, 71 percent, a shaft fracture of the tibia and femur without extension into the knee; Type 2A, 16.5 percent, fracture into the tibial plateau; Type 2B, 4.5 percent, fracture intra-articularly in the distal femur; and Type 2C, 8 percent, articular fractures on both sides of the knee (Fig. 6–48).[152]

Treatment of these fractures may consist of non-operative management of both fractures, operative treatment of one fracture, or operative treatment of both fractures. In one study nonoperative management of both fractures consisting of traction for the femur and a cast for the tibia was utilized in 24 cases.[198] Delayed union of the tibia occurred in 6 fractures and non-union in 2, while delayed union of the femur occurred in 3 fractures. Only 9 of 24 cases obtained full knee motion. A selected series of 15 cases treated initially in traction followed by a cast brace revealed healing of the femoral fracture by 15 weeks in all fractures, but 6 tibial fractures required secondary procedures for delayed union.[148]

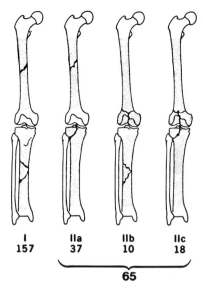

Figure 6–48. Classification of ipsilateral fractures of the femur and tibia. (From Fraser, R. D., Hunter, C. A., and Waddeld, J. P.: Ipsilateral fracture of the femur and tibia. J. Bone Joint Surg. 60B:510, 1978.)

In a report of 20 ipsilateral fractures of the femur and tibia, 9 femoral fractures and 2 tibial fractures received internal fixation.[176] The average healing time for both fractures when the femur was treated operatively but the tibia nonoperatively was 14 weeks; the average healing time was 22.5 weeks when both fractures were treated nonoperatively. In a series of 37 cases, 11 femoral and 0 tibial fractures were treated operatively, while 26 cases with combined femoral and tibial fractures were treated nonoperatively.[143] Delayed union or non-union occurred in 13 femurs and 20 tibias. Of the 26 cases with both fractures, 13 required delayed surgical procedures. Knee motion of 90° or more was obtained in 20 knees. Significant functional disability was present at follow-up in 60 to 70 percent of the patients. In a series of 52 cases, 26 femoral fractures and 29 tibial fractures received nonoperative treatment.[154] Three femoral fractures developed non-union (1 with nonoperative treatment), and 10 tibias had delayed union (8 with nonoperative treatment). Infection occurred in 5 tibial and 1 femoral fracture, 3 of which had operative treatment. Gillquist and colleagues thus recommended internal fixation of both fractures.[154] In a later series of 21 cases using internal fixation for 16 femoral and 13 tibial fractures, there were no problems with femoral union and 2 cases of delayed union of the tibia.[161] Excellent results were obtained in 16 femoral and 17 tibial fractures.[161]

A comparison of operative treatment of both fractures in 14 cases, operative treatment of only 1 fracture in 3 cases, and nonoperative treatment of both fractures in 15 cases was performed.[164] Clinical union was obtained by 25 weeks in the first group, by 23 weeks in the second group, and by 34.8 weeks in the third group. Satisfactory results were obtained in 12 of 14 treated operatively, 0 of 3 treated by fixation of one fracture, and 4 of 10 treated nonoperatively. In a series of 222 cases, 35 percent required late operation for delayed union, non-union, osteomyelitis, refracture, or malunion regardless of treatment type.[152] The 222 cases were divided into three treatment groups: Group I included 27 cases in which both fractures were internally fixed, Group II included 92 cases in which only one fracture was fixed, and Group III included 91 cases in which both fractures were treated nonoperatively. Satisfactory results were obtained in 30 percent of Group I, 36 percent of Group II, and 23 percent of Group III. Infection occurred in 30 percent of Group I compared with 11 percent in Group II and 8 percent in Group III. Fraser and colleagues recommended internal fixation of the femur followed by cast-brace treatment of the tibial fracture.[152]

In conclusion, careful attention to the types of fracture, degree of displacement, and adequacy of reduction is essential in treating fractures about the knee. A treatment program should be directed toward early mobilization of the knee, accurate reduction of the articular surface, and axial alignment of the limb. A treatment modality that meets these objectives with the lowest complication rate, whether operative, nonoperative, or some combination of the two, should be selected.

LIGAMENTOUS INJURIES OF THE KNEE

Injuries to the ligaments of the knee are frequent clinical problems. Injuries may occur by direct trauma but most frequently result from indirect mechanisms. The early diagnosis of these injuries requires a high index of suspicion. The morbidity following injury is variable and relates to the extent of the initial injury, the mode of treatment, the functional demands of the patient, and any subsequent injuries. A knowledge of the natural history of ligamentous injuries, the techniques of diagnosis, and the classification of these injuries is essential before deciding upon treatment. A large number of reconstructive techniques are currently being utilized for chronic and in some instances acute injuries. Long-term results of these techniques will need to be obtained prior to assessment of their efficacy, especially in the prevention of arthrosis. Therefore, a detailed review of these reconstructive techniques will not be included in this discussion.

Natural History

Injury to the anterior cruciate ligament is one of the most frequent knee ligamentous injuries and is present in 70 percent of the knees with an acute hemarthrosis (see the discussion of arthroscopy later in this chapter). Unfortunately, few studies have focused upon the natural history of these lesions. Other associated knee ligamentous injuries

are variable. In addition, methods of treatment and the functional demands of different patients also vary. Thus a homogeneous group of patients is difficult to obtain.

Feagin and colleagues have presented the results obtained in primary repair of acute tears of the anterior cruciate ligament.[206–208] Primary repair of the torn anterior cruciate ligament was performed in 64 cases.[207] At a 2-year follow-up of 30 patients, 25 had satisfactory results.[207, 208] However, at 5 years (32 cases), 71 percent had pain, 66 percent stiffness, 94 percent instability, and 53 percent a significant reinjury.[207, 209] The conclusion from these studies was that "incompetence of the anterior cruciate ligament leads to progressive deterioration of function of the knee."[208] McDaniel and Dameron studied 53 knees with documented anterior cruciate ligament tears at an average of 10 years after injury.[232] Seventy-two percent of the patients returned to sports, and 47 percent felt that they had no restrictions because of the knee. Factors associated with improved results were adequate muscle rehabilitation, stability with anterior and rotatory stress, and return to unrestricted sports. Poorer results were associated with medial and lateral meniscectomy, thigh atrophy, restricted sports, and instability with anterior and rotatory stresses. Twenty-eight of the 53 knees showed evidence of arthrosis with Fairbank's signs, but 9 knees had not had a meniscectomy.

Noyes and colleagues studied 103 patients with chronic laxity of the anterior cruciate ligament without other associated major ligamentous injuries at a mean of 5.5 years of follow-up.[239] Subjective disability was noted by 31 percent for walking, 44 percent for activities of daily living, and 74 percent for sports activities.[238] If a meniscectomy had been performed, there was a two- to fourfold increase in symptoms of pain and swelling.[239] At 5.5 years 21 percent of the knees, and at 11.2 years 44 percent, had roentgenographic evidence of arthrosis, even those without meniscectomy.[239] Kennedy reported on 31 untreated tears of the anterior cruciate ligament followed at 44 months and found that 77 percent had a satisfactory result.[226] The greater the anterior instability, the poorer the result.[225] In 10 of 50 knees with a documented anterior cruciate ligament tear, a meniscectomy was performed, but no poor results occurred and there was no progressive instability.[225] Fetto and Marshall reported 223 knees with anterior cruciate ligament insufficiency with 2 to 3 years of follow-up.[210] Of 176 knees that did not undergo early surgery, there were 68 isolated anterior cruciate ligament injuries and 108 with lesions of other ligaments, frequently the medial collateral ligament. There was significant deterioration in function over time for both isolated anterior cruciate ligament and mixed ligamentous lesions. At 2 years, only 15 percent of the knees were minimally symptomatic. Sixty-six of 78 knees had evidence of arthrosis on roentgenograms. At 5 years of follow-up only 15 percent of untreated knees were rated as better than poor. Arnold and colleagues reported 105 untreated tears of the anterior cruciate ligament followed at 4.3 years.[201] On a rating scale of 100 points, the mean score of these patients was 55. Radiograpic evidence of arthrosis was present in 29 percent of the knees. Balkfors studied 383 knees with a variety of ligamentous injuries at a minimum of 5 years after injury.[203] The most frequent injury was an isolated anterior cruciate ligament tear (39 percent) or an anterior cruciate plus medial collateral ligament tear (30 percent). Of 183 anterior cruciate ligament injuries of which 86 had primary repair, 30 percent had subjective symptoms, 40 percent noted instability, and 35 percent avoided athletics. There were no differences between the repair and nonrepair groups. Of 165 injuries of the anterior cruciate ligament of which 125 were complete and 40 partial tears, gonarthrosis was seen in 15 complete tears but in 0 partial tears. A roentgenographic review of 368 knees revealed osteophytes in 33 percent and gonarthrosis in 7 percent.[203] Twenty-two of the 26 knees with gonarthrosis had had a meniscectomy.[203] Balkfors concluded that gonarthrosis is increased by a factor of 10 in patients with knee ligament injuries.[203]

Diagnosis

The diagnosis of acute knee ligamentous injuries may be difficult but must be carefully sought. The most frequent injury involves the anterior cruciate ligament, but a variety of ligamentous injuries may occur (Table 6–4). Even with a careful search, ligamentous stretching and a change in the biomechanical function of a ligament may occur without obvious visual signs of failure, making diagnosis difficult. Following failure of a primary ligamentous stabilizer of the knee, progressive stretching and failure with time may occur in the secondary stabilizers, changing the pattern of knee instability.

Assessment of an acute knee injury requires a careful history and physical examination. The acute anterior cruciate ligament injury presents with a characteristic history and physical examination. The most common mechanism of injury is indirect (78 percent), with deceleration and a rapid change in direction ("cutting") being frequent.[209, 239] Two common mechanisms of indirect injury have been reported. One is sudden external rotation of the tibia on the femur combined with knee flexion and a valgus force.[208, 210, 225] Injury to the medial collateral ligament and medial meniscus are common in this type.[210] The other frequent indirect mechanism is hyperextension of the knee with the leg in internal rotation.[201, 210, 225] A less common mechanism is hyperflexion.[210] Finally, forced internal rotation of the tibia on the femur may also tear the anterior cruciate ligament, as will an anteriorly directed force applied to the posterior surface of the tibia while in 90° of flexion.[225]

Other characteristic aspects of the history of the injury have been reported. The sites of anterior cruciate injury were midsubstance in 72 percent, proximal end in 18 percent, distal end in 4 percent, and unrecorded in 6 percent in a series of 50 knees.[225] Patients report hearing or feeling a "pop" at the moment of injury with a frequency of 34 percent,[210] 65 percent,[239] or 86.7 percent.[201] Inability to bear weight on the affected knee immediately following injury is frequent, reaching 77 percent in one series.[201] Acute knee swelling within 12 hours is common and represents a hemarthrosis.[209, 239] The combination of a pop at the time of injury, the inability to continue participation in athletics, and gross swelling of the knee that is maximal within 12 hours of injury gives a diagnostic accuracy of 85 percent for an acute tear of the anterior cruciate ligament.[208]

The physical examination at the time of the initial injury may be difficult because of pain and guarding by the patient. In one series, only 6.8 percent of the anterior cruciate ligament tears were diagnosed at the time of the original injury.[239] The physical examination reveals evidence of increased anterior laxity on drawer examination in 93.7 percent (Fig. 6–49).[209] However, other authors have found the anterior drawer sign without anesthesia to be present in only 10 percent.[205] The Lachman test performed in 20° to 30° of flexion is more reliable than the anterior drawer; it is positive without anesthesia in 85 percent and with anesthesia in 100 percent.[205] Associated injuries to the medial and lateral ligamentous structures as well as to the meniscus should be sought. Examination under general anesthesia to eliminate muscle spasm and guarding is necessary if a hemarthrosis has accumulated by the time the patient is seen.

TABLE 6–4. Frequency of Ligamentous Injuries in 389 Knees (After Balkfors[203])*

Ligament	No.	Percent of Total Knee Injuries
ACL	151	39
ACL and MCL	118	30
ACL and PCL Medial capsule	1	0
MCL	47	12
Posterior medial capsule	12	3
ACL and LCL	7	2
LCL	2	1
PCL	19	5
MCL and PCL	8	2
MCL, ACL, and PCL	17	4
MCL, ACL, PCL, and LCL	1	0
MCL, PCL, and LCL	1	0
ACL and PCL	2	1
ACL, PCL, and LCL	3	1
Total	389	100

*ACL, anterior cruciate ligament; PCL, posterior cruciate ligament; MCL, medial collateral ligament; LCL, lateral collateral ligament.

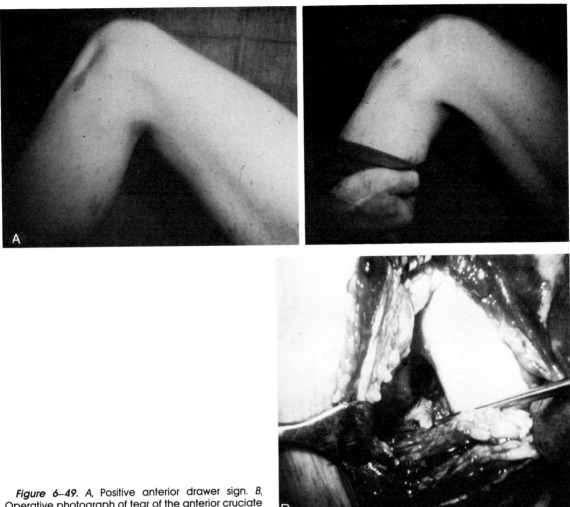

Figure 6–49. A, Positive anterior drawer sign. *B,* Operative photograph of tear of the anterior cruciate ligament.

Arthroscopy is an essential part of evaluation of the acutely injured knee and is discussed in more detail later in the section on knee arthroscopy and arthrography. Arthrography has been recommended for the evaluation of the acutely injured knee.[208, 228] An arthrogram will detect capsular tears, may reveal meniscal injuries, and may aid in the definition of anterior cruciate ligament tears.[228] Using a single-contrast arthrogram for acute knee injuries, injury to the anterior cruciate ligament was documented in 44 of 47 cases of surgically confirmed ruptures.[228] During arthrography, horizontal cross-table and fluoroscopic views are useful in the evaluation of the anterior cruciate ligament.[243] The knee should be flexed 45° to 70° and stressed with an anterior drawer.[243] An intact anterior cruciate ligament appears straight, while a torn ligament appears acutely angled; a torn ligament with intact synovium appears as a wavy edge, and an attenuated but intact ligament has an anteriorly concave appearance.[243] Computed tomography may have some value, but knee positioning is difficult.[243]

Routine radiography remains important in the evaluation of knee ligamentous injuries. A joint effusion on the lateral view appears as an ovoid soft tissue density in the retropatellar region (see Fig. 6–12B).[243] Avulsion fractures of either end of the anterior cruciate ligament may be seen on the lateral or tunnel view (Figs. 6–50 and 6–51). An avulsed fragment from the lateral tibial plateau, the lateral capsular sign or Segond fracture, has a high correlation with injury to the anterior cruciate ligament (Fig. 6–52).[231, 243, 249] The lateral capsular sign represents an avulsion of the tibial attachment of the middle one third of the lateral capsular ligament.[249] If positive, the sign implies a reparable disruption of the middle one third of the lateral capsule and a tear of the anterior cruciate.[249] This sign is infrequent, however, being present in only 3 of 50 knees with tears of the anterior cruciate ligament.[231] Notches may be present on the lateral femoral condyle seen on the lateral or internal oblique roentgenogram (Fig. 6–53; see also Fig. 6–14). These result from chronic anterior subluxation of the lateral femoral condyle into the tibia, leading to impingement.[201, 231] Stress roentgenograms are also helpful (Figs. 6–54 and 6–55; see also Figs. 6–18 and 6–19).

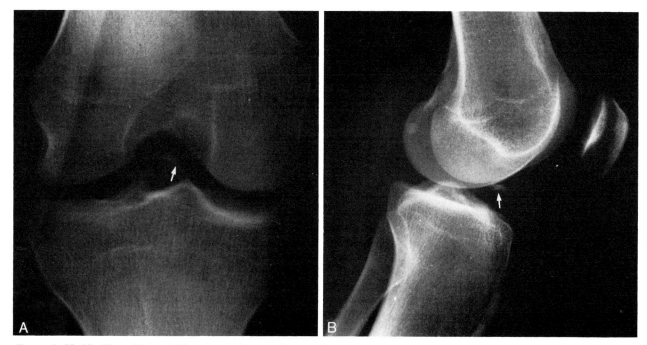

Figure 6–50. AP *(A)* and lateral *(B)* radiographs revealing avulsion fracture *(arrows)*, indicating a tear of the anterior cruciate ligament.

Types of Instability

An understanding of the types of instabilities of the knee and the specific tests for each instability is essential for patient management. Instability may be either straight or single-plane, rotary, or combined.[211] One-plane instability may be either medial, lateral, anterior, or posterior.[211] Rotatory instability may be anteromedial, anterolateral, posteromedial, or posterolateral.[211] The presence of posteromedial rotatory instability is controversial.[218] Combined instabilities may be anteromedial-anterolateral, anterolateral-posterolateral, or anteromedial-posteromedial.[211] The instabilities are classified by the di-

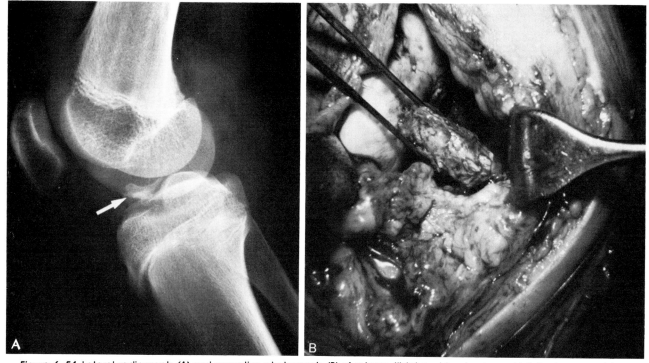

Figure 6–51. Lateral radiograph *(A)* and operative photograph *(B)* of a large tibial avulsion fracture which had occurred 3 years previously. The anterior cruciate ligament was partially attached to this fragment.

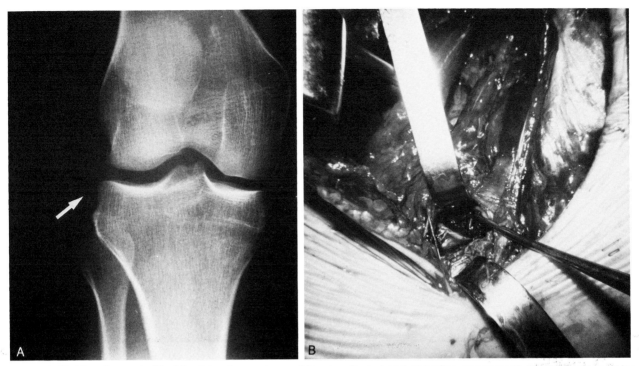

Figure 6–52. AP radiograph *(A)* of the lateral capsular avulsion sign *(arrow)* and operative appearance *(B)* of disruption of the middle third lateral capsular ligament at the tip of the probe.

rection of movement of the tibia relative to the femur upon a specific stress. A single-plane instability means that the posterior cruciate ligament is torn and, therefore, that the axis of rotation has been lost.[218] Upon stress, the tibia does not rotate but the knee joint opens in a way similar to a door.[221] In contrast, in a rotatory instability the posterior cruciate ligament is intact and provides an axis for rotatory movement.[221]

The magnitude of the force, the position of the knee, the state of muscle tone, the quality of the bone, the degree of fixation of the foot, and the

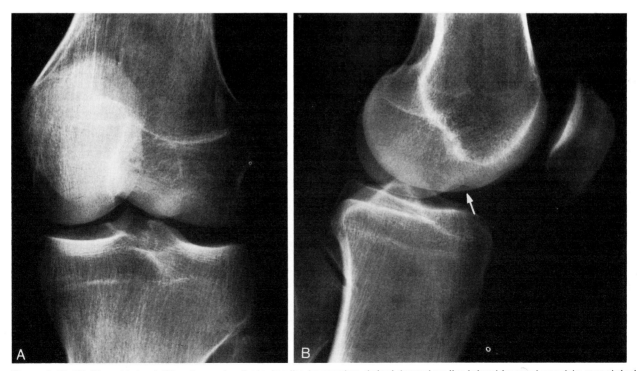

Figure 6–53. AP *(A)* and lateral *(B)* radiographs displaying the impression defect *(arrow)* on the lateral femoral condyle associated with chronic anterolateral rotatory instability.

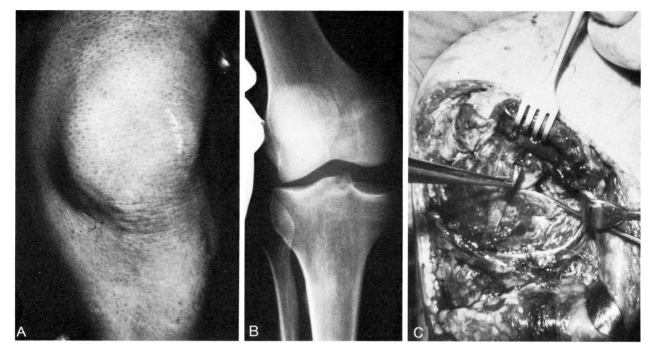

Figure 6–54. Complete medial capsular disruption. *A,* Clinical appearance under stress. *B,* AP stress radiograph. *C,* Operative photograph. The superficial medial ligament is illustrated by the forceps and the tear of the posteromedial capsule by the probe.

extent of body load all affect the magnitude and type of injury. The extent of ligamentous tearing or sprain may be classified.[218] An injury with a minimum number of fibers torn and localized tenderness but no instability is a Grade 1 sprain. A disruption of more fibers associated with tenderness but no instability is a Grade 2 sprain. Complete disruption of the ligament with resultant instability is a Grade 3 sprain. The degree of instability may also be classified by the amount of joint surface separation

upon stress.[218] A 1+ instability involves up to 5 mm of opening, a 2+ instability involves 5 to 10 mm of opening, and a 3+ instability involves 10 mm or more opening upon stress. Since individuals vary in their extent of ligamentous laxity, it is essential to compare the injured to the noninjured side.

A variety of clinical signs and tests are utilized in the evaluation of individuals with knee instabilities. A review of the injured structures and the findings

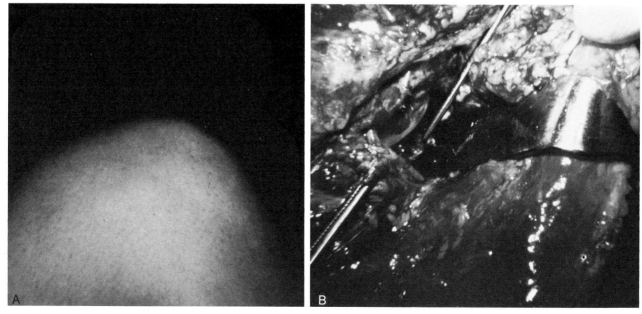

Figure 6–55. *A,* Posterior sag of the tibia on the femur associated with an acute tear of the posterior cruciate ligament. *B,* Operative photograph of acute posterior cruciate ligament tear indicated by probe.

associated with each pattern of instability will aid in the comprehension of both the examination and the instability.

Straight or Single-Plane Instability

A straight or single-plane medial instability indicates a tear of the medial compartment ligaments combined with a tear of the posterior cruciate ligament. The injured structures may include the middle third medial capsular ligament, the superficial medial ligament, the posteromedial capsular ligament, and both cruciate ligaments.[211, 218] An opening of the knee medially upon valgus stress with the knee in full extension will occur (Fig. 6–54).[218] A Grade 1 or 2 sprain of the middle third capsular ligament and superficial medial ligament will be stable to valgus stress in extension but may show severe instability in 30° of flexion.[211] A straight lateral instability results from a tear of the lateral compartment ligaments combined with a tear of the posterior cruciate ligament.[219] The injured structures may include the middle third lateral capsular ligament, the fibular collateral ligament, the arcuate-popliteus complex, both cruciates, the biceps tendon, the iliotibial tract, and the peroneal nerve.[211]

Physical examination reveals instability upon varus stress with the knee in full extension.[219] Instability to varus stress at 30° but stability at 0° is indicative of a sprain of the middle third lateral capsular ligament.[211] A lateral capsular avulsion sign may accompany these injuries, resulting in straight lateral instability.[211] A straight anterior instability results from a tear of both cruciate ligaments.[218] Upon anterior drawer testing there is equal forward translation of both tibial condyles.[218] An apparent straight anterior drawer test may occur in the presence of a combined anteromedial and anterolateral rotatory instability.[218] A straight posterior instability results from a tear of the posterior cruciate combined with the posteromedial (posterior oblique) capsular ligament and the arcuate complex.[218] A positive posterior drawer sign is evident when the tibial condyles subluxate equal amounts posteriorly.[218] A combined posterolateral and posteromedial rotatory instability may give a similar drawer sign.[211]

Rotatory Instability

An anteromedial rotatory instability demonstrates medial laxity and anterior displacement of the medial tibial condyle on the femur upon anterior drawer testing.[211] Injury may involve the medial compartment ligaments, including the middle third medial capsular ligament, superficial medial ligament, posteromedial capsule (posterior oblique), anterior cruciate ligament, and frequently peripheral detachment of the medial meniscus.[218, 245]

The basic lesion necessary for an anteromedial rotatory instability is a rupture of the medial capsular ligament; this rupture allows abnormal external rotation of the tibia.[245] The mechanism of injury that results in an isolated lesion of the medial capsular ligament is a valgus external rotation stress applied to the knee in a position of 90° of flexion.[245] The anterior medial capsule is most frequently injured with the knee flexed 90°, the middle portion with the knee flexed between 30° and 90°, and the posterior portion with the knee close to full extension.[245] The sequence of injury begins with rupture of the medial capsular ligament, proceeds to rupture of the superficial medial ligament, and ends with rupture of the anterior cruciate ligament.[245] Peripheral tears of the medial meniscus are frequently present in fresh injuries, while posterior horn tears of the medial meniscus are present in chronic injuries related to repetitive impingement.[245] In a series of 24 acute injuries, the middle portion of the medial capsule was torn in 24, a peripheral tear of the medial meniscus was present in 23, and an anterior cruciate ligament tear appeared in only 5 knees.[245] In a series of 45 knees, the same authors found a deficient anterior cruciate ligament in all knees and laxity of the arcuate ligament complex and injury to the lateral meniscus in 44 knees.

Physical findings include a positive valgus stress test at 30° of flexion and a positive anterior drawer test performed with the tibia in 15° to 30° of external rotation.[245] An abduction or valgus stress test that is negative at 0° but positive at 30° of flexion indicates a tear of the medial compartment ligaments.[218] The extent of displacement during the anterior drawer test correlates with the extent of injury, with a positive 1+ test indicating injury to the capsule alone and a positive 3+ test indicating capsular, collateral, and anterior cruciate ligament injury.[245]

An anterolateral rotatory instability of the knee reveals anterior and lateral subluxation of the tibia on the femur as the knee approaches extension.[211] Injury may involve the middle third lateral capsular ligament, arcuate ligament, anterior cruciate ligament, and frequently the posterior horn of the lateral meniscus.[218, 219]

A biomechanical study of knee ligamentous structures revealed increases in external rotation and anterior drawer testing with injury to the anterior cruciate ligament alone.[229] The internal rotation was increased by sectioning of the lateral collateral ligament or posterolateral complex. If the anterior cruciate was intact, sectioning of the posterolateral ligament alone did not increase internal rotation. In contrast, Hughston believes that the key element for anterolateral rotatory instability is a tear of the middle third lateral capsular ligament.[219] In chronic anterolateral rotatory instability, laxity of the posterolateral capsule was combined with a tear of the anterior cruciate in 45 of 45 knees.[204] The lateral meniscus invariably had peripheral detachment or a posterior horn tear related to chronic impingement during subluxation of the tibia. In a series of 36 knees with acute anterolateral rotatory instability, the middle third lateral capsular ligament was torn in 21 cases; the lateral capsule in 16; the anterior

TABLE 6–5. Tests for Anterolateral Rotatory Instability

Test	Author	Technique	Mechanics
Pivot shift	Galway & McIntosh	Supine valgus stress, foot in internal rotation, knee in extension	Sudden reduction at 30° during flexion
Jerk	Hughston	Supine valgus stress, foot in internal rotation, knee in 90° flexion	Subluxation maximal at 30° during extension, then reduction upon further extension
Flexion-rotation drawer	Noyes	Supine, knee in 20°–30° of flexion, downward drawer, free femoral rotation	Reduction with further knee flexion
A.L.R.I. test	Slocum	Lateral decubitus position on opposite side, 30°–50° posterior rotation of pelvis, knee in 10° of flexion, foot supported on table	Reduction at 25°–45° upon knee flexion
Losee	Losee	Supine knee and hip in 45° flexion, external rotation, valgus stress	Subluxation followed by reduction upon extension

cruciate ligament in 4; the anterior cruciate ligament, lateral capsule, and iliotibial tract in 3; and the anterior cruciate combined with iliotibial tract in 2.[235] The mechanism of injury is usually indirect, with rotation without contact in 10 of 14 cases. Direct trauma was noted in 4 of 14 acute injuries. Deceleration with cutting away from the supporting foot combined with knee flexion has been felt to be the most frequent mechanism of injury.[244]

Physical examination reveals a positive anterior drawer test, with the tibia in neutral or slight internal rotation showing increased forward displacement of the lateral tibial condyle.[219] A variety of specialized tests have been devised to reproduce the anterior subluxation of the lateral tibial plateau or its reduction. The tests for anterolateral rotatory instability include the pivot shift, jerk, flexion-rotation drawer, Slocum, and Losee tests (Table 6–5).[213, 214, 219, 230, 231, 236] All of these tests are designed to identify anterior subluxation of the lateral tibial plateau on the lateral femoral condyle with the knee in mild flexion and reduction of the subluxation at 30° to 40° of flexion.[213, 214, 230, 231, 244] The iliotibial tract causes the subluxation of the tibia to reduce upon flexion.[215]

An experimental study was performed to determine the structural defects and mechanics of the pivot shift.[209] Sectioning of the anterior cruciate ligament alone induced a positive pivot shift in 89 percent of the knees tested. Sectioning of this ligament alone induced both components of the pivot shift, the increased anterior displacement of the tibia and the increased internal rotation. Sectioning of the iliotibial band, lateral collateral ligament, or popliteus singly or in combination will not induce a pivot shift in the presence of an intact anterior cruciate ligament. Lateral meniscectomy will eliminate the pivot shift. The pivot shift results in the lateral meniscus being forced posteriorly, followed by a sudden anterior subluxation of the tibia and lateral meniscus beneath the lateral femoral condyle, resulting in widening of the lateral compartment. When the knee is in 0° to 20° of flexion, the instant center of rotation is displaced anteriorly.[246]

At 20° to 40° of flexion the instant center of rotation suddenly displaces posteriorly. The "crossover" test consists of immobilization of the foot of the affected extremity with the patient instructed to rotate his body, crossing the unaffected leg over the fixed foot.[201] A sensation that the knee will give way is a positive sign of pivot shift.

In addition to the physical examination and history of the knee giving way, especially on cutting, radiographs are valuable in diagnosis. The lateral capsular sign was present in 3 of 36 knees in one series[204] and in 3 of 50 knees in another.[235] A notch in the lateral femoral condyle is frequently visible[201, 239] and was present in 14 of 15 knees in another series.[230] Arthrography may diagnose tears of the lateral meniscus as well as tears of the anterior cruciate ligament.[204, 243]

Posterolateral rotatory instability is present when there is increased external rotation of the tibia in a posterolateral direction. This instability results from a tear of the arcuate complex.[219] Biomechanical studies have shown that sectioning of the posterolateral complex and the lateral collateral ligament results in significantly increased external rotation.[229] Additional sectioning of the anterior cruciate ligament results in only a small increase in external rotation. The injured structures include the arcuate-popliteus complex (arcuate ligament, fibular collateral ligament, popliteus muscle, and gastrocnemius muscle), the biceps femoris, the lateral capsular ligament, and perhaps the posterior cruciate ligament.[202, 211] In a series of 17 knees, the popliteus musculotendinous unit was torn in 16, the arcuate ligament in 17, the fibular collateral ligament in 10, the gastrocnemius in 4, the biceps femoris in 8, and the iliotibial tract in 2.[202] The peroneal nerve was injured in 2, the anterior cruciate ligament in 11, and the lateral meniscus in 4 of the 17 knees.

The mechanism of injury in posterolateral rotatory instability is direct trauma to the proximal medial tibia, resulting in hyperextension or an indirect mechanism of hyperextension and external rotation.[202] The physical findings in acute injuries include tenderness and induration over the arcuate complex and positive results in several specific tests. The adduction or varus stress test performed at 30° of flexion is frequently positive (11 of 12) but is not diagnostic.[202] A positive posterolateral drawer test or external rotation recurvatum test, on the other hand, is diagnostic of posterolateral rotatory instability.[202, 219, 227] The external rotation recurvatum test is produced by holding the leg by the toes with the knee extended. Recurvatum and apparent varus occurs as the tibia rotates posteriorly.[218, 219, 222] The posterolateral drawer test is a posterior drawer test performed with the tibia in neutral, internal, and external rotation.[222] The posterior drawer test in internal rotation must be negative to indicate a functioning posterior cruciate ligament.[222] An increased posterior drawer in 15° of external rotation compared with neutral rotation with further posterior displacement of the lateral rather than medial tibial plateau is considered positive.[222] In the reverse pivot shift, the posterior subluxation of the lateral tibial plateau reduces as the flexed knee is extended and the tibia is externally rotated.[224]

Posteromedial rotatory instability is controversial. Hughston and colleagues claim that posteromedial rotatory instability does not exist, because an intact posterior cruciate ligament would prevent posteromedial subluxation of the tibia, and an absent posterior cruciate ligament would in any case eliminate the rotatory component, making a straight posterior instability.[218] A posteromedial instability results from tears of the superficial medial ligament, the medial capsular ligament, the posterior oblique ligament, and the anterior cruciate ligament.[227] Disruption of these ligaments allows a posteromedial sag. The mechanism of injury is a hyperextension and valgus force.[227] Physical examination reveals the posteromedial sag of the tibia, minor hyperextension, and medial opening of the joint space on valgus stress of the extended knee.[227]

Combined Instability

Combined rotatory instabilities may occur, the most frequent being a combined anterolateral and posterolateral or anteromedial and anterolateral.[218] A long-standing anteromedial rotatory instability may progress to combined anteromedial-anterolateral instability from repetitive stress to the secondary stabilizers. In this combined instability, the anterior drawer sign performed in neutral may appear to displace directly forward, indicating a straight anterior instability.[218] However, specific tests for each type of instability will be present and tests for the posterior cruciate ligament will indicate its integrity. Combined anterolateral-posterolateral rotatory instability may result from the same injury, with severe damage to the lateral joint ligaments and anterior cruciate ligament. Physical examination will reveal positive tests for both types of instability. In a series of 17 knees with posterolateral rotatory instability, 6 had a combined anterolateral-posterolateral, 3 a combined anteromedial-antero-lateral-posterolateral, and 1 a combined anteromedial-posterolateral rotatory instability.[202]

Posterior cruciate ligament injuries leading to a straight posterior instability are less frequent lesions than those involving the anterior cruciate ligament. In the presence of a posterior cruciate ligament tear, all instabilities become straight because the tibia no longer rotates on the femur about a central axis.[221] Gallie and LeMesurier in 1927 stated that with a torn posterior cruciate ligament "the patient is almost invariably left with a knee in which the femur dislocates violently and painfully forward, whenever weight is borne on the flexed limb."[212]

The mechanism of injury to the posterior cruciate ligament is violent trauma, with either posterior displacement of the tibia on the femur when the knee is in flexion or hyperextension.[225, 233] Motor vehicle accidents, falls, and sports injuries are the most frequent etiologies.[221, 233, 247] Associated ligamentous injuries are frequent. In a series of 32 acute injuries, 26 had injury to the medial compartment, 2 to the lateral compartment, and 1 to both the medial and lateral compartments.[221] Other frequent injuries are to the anterior cruciate ligament and posterior horn of the medial or lateral meniscus.[221, 247] Physical examination may reveal abrasions or lacerations over the proximal tibia (13 of 21 knees).[247] Additional physical findings include tenderness in the popliteal fossa and hemarthrosis.[247] The posterior drawer sign with the tibia in internal rotation is positive in the knee with a chronic deficiency in the posterior cruciate ligament, but it may be negative in an acute injury if the arcuate complex is not injured (see Fig. 6–55).[218] The posterior drawer test was negative in 20 of 29 knees with an acute posterior cruciate ligament tear.[221] A positive abduction or adduction stress with the knee in 0° is a reliable sign of a tear of the posterior cruciate ligament.[218] In 26 knees with acute injuries of the posterior cruciate ligament and medial compartment, the abduction stress test in full extension was negative in only one knee under anesthesia.[221] In contrast, the adduction stress test at 0° was negative in all patients with a torn posterior cruciate except for the 3 knees with lateral compartmental injury.[221] The anterior drawer test with the knee in full internal rotation was negative in only 4 of 30 acute posterior cruciate ligament tears.[221] In 7 knees with an intact anterior cruciate but torn posterior cruciate ligament, a positive anterior drawer test was present in external rotation. Genu recurvatum may accompany this injury.[247] Radiographic findings may or may not be present. Failure of the ligament may occur at either its femoral or tibial attachment or its midsubstance. In 29 knees the location of the tear was at the femoral attachment in 16, at the tibial attachment in 8, and midsubstance in 5.[221] An avulsion fracture frequently accompanies only avulsion of the tibial attachment and may present as only a small flake of bone in the intracondylar notch.[225, 233, 247, 248]

Treatment of the torn posterior cruciate ligament

may be operative or nonoperative with cast immobilization. Nonoperative treatment of 5 knees with avulsion fractures of the tibial end of the posterior cruciate ligament resulted in 2 non-unions with poor results.[247] In another series of 6 tibial avulsions, 4 of 5 displaced fractures progressed to non-union and functional disability.[233] Therefore, surgical repair of the torn posterior cruciate ligament and repair of associated injuries is recommended by most authors.[221, 225, 233, 247, 248] Open reduction and internal fixation is indicated for fractures with 0.3 cm separation or 0.5 cm upward displacement with or without rotation from the tibial base.[247] Surgery is also indicated for comminuted fractures with large, rotated fragments.[247] Internal fixation of 6 fractures resulted in union in 5, with satisfactory results in these cases.[233] In a series of 26 acute posterior cruciate ligament tears followed for an average of 9 years following repair, patients reported 25 good and 1 fair result.[221] Objective examination of 20 of the 25 knees revealed 13 good, 4 fair, and 3 poor results.[221] Therefore, early diagnosis and treatment of injuries of the posterior cruciate give satisfactory results.

Treatment

The treatment of injuries to the major ligamentous structures of the knee is controversial. The options include nonoperative treatment with later reconstruction if needed or early surgical repair. Early surgical repair may be combined with reconstructive techniques to augment the strength of severely injured ligamentous structures.

In 1917 Hey Groves stated that "ruptures of the crucial ligaments are now much more frequently recognized than formerly . . . [an injury] which produces permanent total disablement for active pursuits. . . ."[217] Hey Groves recognized the phenomenon of the pivot shift and described a reconstructive technique for the cruciate ligaments using the iliotibial band.[216] Palmer contributed much to the diagnosis and function of the knee ligaments and recommended early repair.[242] O'Donoghue recommended early surgical repair within 2 weeks of injury and claimed that better results would be obtained with early repair than with late reconstruction.[241] Although these and many other reports have recommended early treatment, some selected lesions continue to receive nonoperative management.

Nonoperative care must be considered in view of the natural history of the lesions being treated, the extent of instability, and the activity level and goals of the patient. Primary repair of an "isolated" midsubstance tear of the anterior cruciate ligament has revealed a high incidence of instability at 5 years.[208] Therefore, many surgeons consider this lesion to be unsuitable for primary repair and recommend either nonoperative care or primary reconstruction.[239] Nonoperative treatment consisting of a vig-

orous physical therapy program has been utilized in 24 knees with an anterior cruciate ligament tear.[215] Although 59 percent of the patients returned to sports, 13 of 22 knees showed some degenerative changes on radiographs, and 42 percent required a meniscectomy. The best results were obtained with a hamstring-quadriceps strength ratio that was equal.[215] In a series of 84 knees with chronic anterior cruciate ligament laxity treated with a vigorous rehabilitation program and followed for 3 years, one third of the knees improved but remained somewhat symptomatic, one third became worse with increasing symptoms, and 18 of the knees required reconstruction.[238] Therefore, 43 percent of the 84 knees benefited from the rehabilitation program. However, it was not possible to predict which knee would or would not improve with physical therapy.[238] Therefore, Noyes and colleagues recommended an initial nonoperative approach to the knee with a chronic anterior cruciate ligament deficiency.

Bracing may be combined with a muscle rehabilitation program to control rotatory stresses (Fig. 6–56). A brace will aid in the control of rotatory instabilities of the knee.[234] Nonoperative treatment with a cast brace has been utilized in highly selected patients for medial collateral ligament injuries. In a prospective randomized study of isolated complete medial collateral ligament injuries treated either by surgery or a cast brace, the results at 2 to 3 years of follow-up were similar. Therefore, selected patients with either acute ligament injuries or chronic instabilities may be treated nonsurgically with satisfactory results, but extreme care in patient selection appears essential.

The long-term results of acute repair for rotatory instabilities have been reported by few authors. Hughston and colleagues reported on a series of 93 of 154 knees treated with primary repair of acute anteromedial rotatory instability with a follow-up of 7.9 years.[220] Satisfactory results were obtained in 89 percent subjectively but in only 73 percent objectively.[220] Nine knees required subsequent reconstructive surgery. Meniscectomy had an adverse effect; no knee with a meniscectomy revealed excellent results, and the overall results were decreased 5 percent by a meniscectomy.[220] There were no significant differences among the knees with or without a functioning anterior cruciate ligament.[220] Hughston and colleagues concluded that the key to a satisfactory result was preservation of the medial meniscus and repair of the posterior oblique ligament. Norwood and colleagues reported the results of acute repair of 21 of 36 knees with acute anterolateral rotatory instability followed at 5.4 years.[235] Satisfactory results were obtained in 16 of the 21 knees. Resection of the anterior cruciate ligament did not adversely affect the results. Finally, Baker and colleagues reported results obtained with 17 knees treated for acute posterolateral rotatory instability followed at 4.5 years.[202] Satisfactory results were obtained in 85 percent subjectively and in 77 percent objectively.

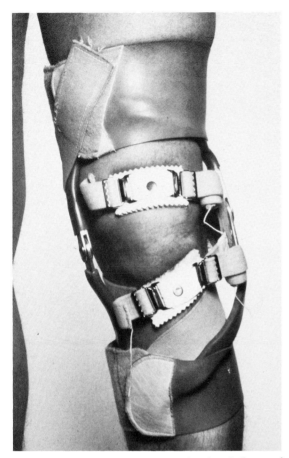

Figure 6–56. Lennox-Hill brace utilized for chronic ligamentous instability.

Although early surgical repair of all injured structures may give a high proportion of satisfactory results, some individuals will present late with chronic instability. A multitude of reconstructive procedures have been advocated for each of the various instabilities. However, a detailed description of these reconstructive procedures and their results is beyond the scope of this review. The indication for anterior cruciate ligament reconstruction has been aptly stated by O'Donoghue: "instability sufficiently severe to interfere with the person's normal everyday living."[241] The reconstructive procedures may be considered extra-articular, intra-articular, or combined. The extra-articular reconstruction attempts to reinforce the secondary stabilizers of the knee and partially to substitute their function for that of the anterior cruciate ligament. In contrast, the intra-articular reconstruction attempts to reproduce normal anterior cruciate ligament function but does not address the problem of the damaged secondary stabilizers. With either of these approaches, the reconstruction is forced to bear the load that is normally shared by the anterior cruciate ligament and secondary stabilizers. In contrast, the combined procedure attempts to reinforce the secondary stabilizers as well as to reconstruct the function of the anterior cruciate ligament, allowing load sharing among the reconstructed struc-

tures. Although some extra-articular reconstructions have been found to fail with time, the long-term results of many of the reconstructive procedures are not yet available. Many important factors go into patient selection and choice of a reconstruction. The demands of the individual, the ability to cooperate in a prolonged rehabilitation program, and the patient's comprehension of long-term limitations are essential. The surgical technique must consider the strength of the graft utilized, its vascularity, the time of beginning rehabilitation and motion, and the duration of time needed for obtaining maximal strength and integrity of the graft.[237]

In summary, the early diagnosis and treatment of injuries to the ligaments of the knee will optimize the treatment options available. In the presence of significant instability in the active individual, early repair of all injured structures will give satisfactory results. Late reconstructions may provide an alternative mode of salvage in those individuals for whom a late diagnosis is made, but further data are necessary to determine optimal techniques.

KNEE ARTHROSCOPY AND ARTHROGRAPHY

The evaluation and management of knee disorders has been greatly aided by the development of arthrography and arthroscopy. These techniques are useful in the evaluation of menisci, cruciate ligaments, articular cartilage, synovial diseases, loose bodies, intra-articular fractures, and patellar alignment. A review of the role of these modalities and their accuracy is valuable for the attending physician.

Accuracy of arthrography is greater than 90 percent in experienced hands.[260, 276, 354, 373] When it is combined with arthroscopy, these complementary techniques provide a diagnostic accuracy of 97 percent.[269]

The most common indication for knee arthrography is evaluation of the menisci. Nicholas[342] reported accurate evaluation of medial meniscal tears in 99.7 percent and in 93 percent for the lateral meniscus. Extrameniscal anatomy can also be effectively evaluated.[269, 281, 288, 308, 353, 368] Table 6–6 summarizes the indications and techniques used for knee arthrography.

TABLE 6–6. Indications and Approach to Knee Arthrography

Indication	Technique
Meniscal tears	Single- or double-contrast
Cruciate ligament	Double-contrast (tomography, xeroradiography), CT, MRI
Articular cartilage	Double-contrast ± tomography, CT
Synovitis	Double-contrast
Loose bodies	Single-contrast ± tomography
Chondromalacia	Double-contrast, axial views, CT
Popliteal cysts	Single- or double-contrast
Plicae	Double-contrast and CT, tomography, special views
Extra-articular	Double-contrast ± CT

The complexity of examining the extrameniscal portions of the knee (cruciate ligaments, collateral ligament, and plicae) necessitates good communication between the referring physician and radiologist. Special views, choice of contrast material, and the possible use of CT or MRI in conjunction with the arthrography may be necessary.

Arthrographic Technique

As demonstrated in Table 6–6, the approach to knee arthrography varies considerably with the clinical indication. Review of the clinical data, radiographs, isotope scans, and CT studies should be accomplished prior to the arthrogram. This will allow proper planning of the arthrographic technique.

The equipment and arthrogram tray are important and have been discussed in Chapter 1 (Introduction to Arthrography). The most frequently used positive contrast agents are diatrizoate meglumine (Hypaque-M-60 and Renografin-M-60).[269, 288] Contrast material is rapidly absorbed and diluted, which necessitates rapid filming. Delays of 5 to 10 min may result in suboptimal studies. Metrizamide (Amipaque) and Dimer-X have been investigated as potential arthrographic contrast media. They provide the advantage of prolonged concentration in the joint, allowing more time for filming.[288, 323] Epinephrine (0.3 ml of 1:1000) may also be added to the contrast material. This results in reduced fluid accumulation in the joint, higher iodine concentrations, and more time for filming.[269, 288, 300, 367] This is especially helpful if additional special views, tomography, or CT will be performed with the arthrogram.

Air or CO_2 may be used alone or in conjunction with positive contrast material.[294, 316, 340, 358] Air is more readily available than CO_2 and causes less pain following the arthrogram.[294] CO_2 is more rapidly absorbed and consequently reduces the chance of air embolus.[358] But air embolism is extremely rare;[269] we have not experienced air embolism or infection using room air. Room air will remain in the joint for several days and patients should be informed that the joint may be "noisy" until the air is absorbed.

When the contrast medium and film techniques have been chosen, the patient is positioned on the radiography table. The patient should be supine with the involved knee closest to the examiner. The knee is prepared using sterile technique.[301] A cushion may be positioned under the knee for comfort and to assist with aspiration.[328] The injection may be performed using a medial or lateral approach. This decision depends on the site of the suspected lesion and skin condition. Areas of cutaneous inflammation should obviously be avoided. Though the medial patellofemoral joint is slightly wider than the lateral, the lateral approach is more frequently chosen.[269, 288, 301] There is less soft tissue laterally, and in our practice the lesion is usually on the medial side.

Numerous injection techniques have been described both with and without local anesthetic.[269, 300, 301, 303, 373] The injection depends on the clinical setting. In the acutely injured or painful knee, aspiration and anesthetic injection may be required prior to the arthrogram. This will allow adequate stressing of the joint during the arthrogram. In the usual situation local anesthetic with a single-syringe injection technique is used. The patient's leg is internally rotated. This allows free movement of the patella and permits a superior angle for the needle as it enters the joint. The needle should enter the joint at the midpoint of the patella. The local anesthetic is injected in the skin inferior to the point at which the needle will enter the joint (Fig. 6–57). The soft tissues are infiltrated

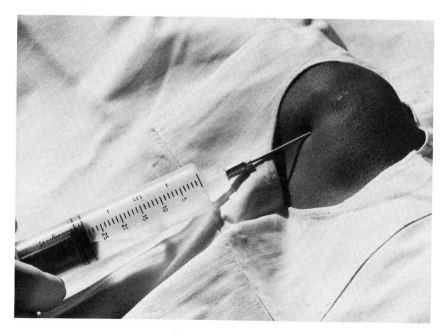

Figure 6–57. Needle placement for knee arthrography. The needle is angled superiorly to enter the joint inferior to the midpatella. This position keeps the air in the distal portion of the syringe, allowing the intra-articular position to be easily checked. Note contrast medium in the dependent portion of the syringe.

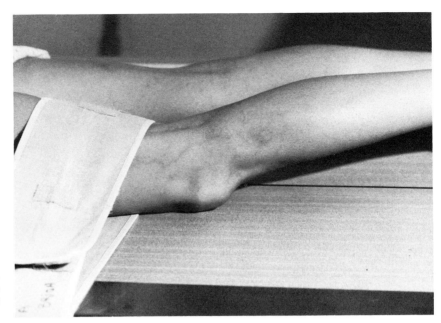

Figure 6–58. Patient positioned for examination of the medial meniscus. Adjustable strap allows the knee to be easily stressed.

slightly as the needle is advanced into the joint. Proper needle position is noted if the anesthetic meets no resistance or if fluid can be aspirated from the joint. If fluid is present, it should be aspirated as completely as possible. This is facilitated by the knee pad. In some cases gravity will allow better evacuation, as aspiration may be hindered by synovium drawn against the needle tip. A catheter with side holes has also been used for more complete aspiration.[328] Examination of the fluid may be very helpful. Microscopic analysis for crystals, Gram stain, culture, etc., may be indicated. Wear particles, for example, have been described in patients with osteoarthritis, chondromalacia, and meniscal tears.[365] The presence of blood in the fluid may indicate a ligament tear, peripheral meniscal separation, or, rarely, synovial hemangioma.[269, 288, 332, 353]

The presence or absence of fluid in the joint has some bearing on the amount of contrast material injected. If the joint is "dry," 3 to 5 ml of contrast material is used with about 20 to 40 ml of air. If a large effusion is evacuated, 5 to 7 ml of contrast material or even slightly more may be used. In certain cases single-contrast may be used instead of the preferred double-contrast technique. If significant allergy to iodine is present, air alone may be injected.

With the standard double-contrast technique the anesthetic needle is left in position and a 20 to 25 ml syringe, with 5 ml of contrast material and 20 ml of air, is attached to the needle. The upward angle of the needle results in the air filling the distal portion of the syringe. Gentle pressure on the barrel of the syringe will meet no resistance if the needle is within the joint capsule. Once this is confirmed, the contents of the syringe can be injected with one gentle motion. The syringe can be refilled with air and an additional 20+ ml injected. Following removal of the needle the joint is slowly exercised with the patient on the table. By rotating the patient to the right and left the contrast can be uniformly distributed in the medial and lateral compartments. The patient may also be exercised in the upright position (walking, etc.), but this may result in excess air bubble formation. The possibility of syncopal episodes can also be avoided by exercising the knee on the table.[269, 301]

Filming of the medial and lateral menisci should be performed fluoroscopically using a stress device (Fig. 6–58). Nine to twelve images of each meniscus should be obtained. We routinely examine the medial meniscus in both the prone and supine position (double-contrast technique), as subtle tears are more easily detected.[361] If indicated, the lateral meniscus may be similarly studied. Following fluoroscopic filming, overhead films are obtained in the AP and lateral projections. A stress lateral should be obtained for evaluation of the anterior cruciate ligament (Fig. 6–59).[277, 288, 354, 359] Notch views and patellar views may also be indicated. If indicated (Table 6–6), CT, MRI, or tomography may be required for complete evaluation.

We do not routinely reaspirate the joint following the procedure. If significant discomfort is present, reaspiration may be useful. Patient activity following the examination may be restricted for 24 hours.[301] However, in most cases normal activity is allowed.

Normal Arthrographic Anatomy

The anatomy of the knee has been described earlier in this chapter. Certain points bear repeating in describing the normal arthrographic anatomy. The normal medial meniscus is C-shaped (Fig. 6–60C). The transverse length is greater posteriorly (average 14 mm) than anteriorly (average 6 mm).[330] The meniscus is firmly attached to the capsule and deep portion of the medial collateral ligament. This reduces mobility and results in an increased inci-

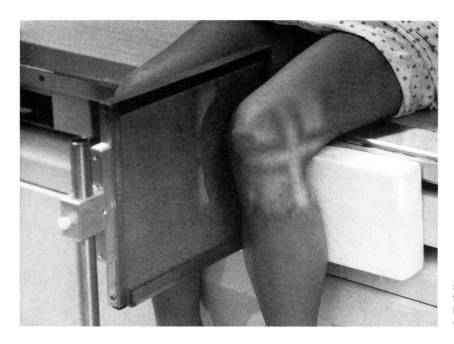

Figure 6–59. Patient positioned for the stress lateral view. The knee is flexed over the bolster. Cassette position is maintained by the patient. This permits consistency for examination of the cruciate ligaments.

dence of tears compared with the lateral meniscus.[269, 288] Anteriorly the medial meniscus is attached to the tibia anterior to the anterior cruciate ligament attachment. Posteriorly the medial meniscus attaches to the tibia midway between the lateral meniscus and the posterior cruciate ligament attachment.

The lateral meniscus is smaller, more circular, and more equal in width (Fig. 6–60C) than the medial meniscus. The anterior two thirds of the meniscus is attached to the coronary ligament. Posteriorly the popliteus tendon with its synovial sheath passes through the joint capsule. This results in incomplete attachment of the meniscus posteriorly. In some cases the popliteus muscle may partially attach to the lateral meniscus posteriorly.[307]

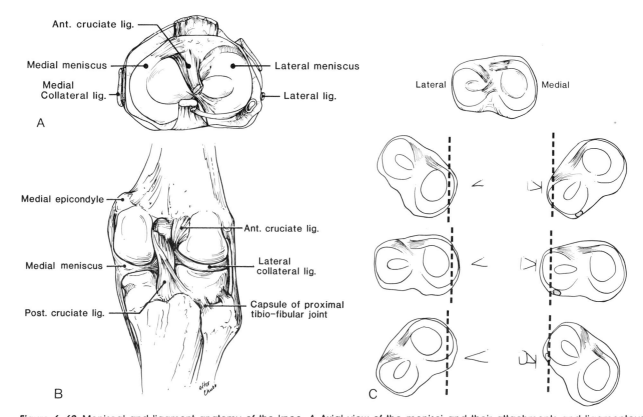

Figure 6–60. Meniscal and ligament anatomy of the knee. *A,* Axial view of the menisci and their attachments and ligamentous relationships. *B,* Posterior view of the knee, demonstrating the collateral ligaments and posterior cruciate ligament. *C,* Illustration of axial and tangential views of the anterior mid- and posterior portions of the medial and lateral meniscus.

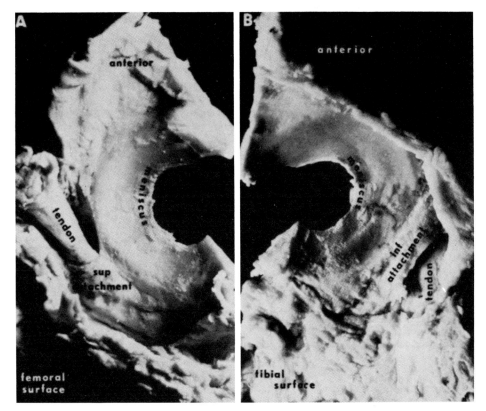

Figure 6–61. Anatomy of the posterior horn of the lateral meniscus. A, Lateral meniscus viewed from the femoral surface. The superior attachment covers the tendon except where it exits the tunnel superiorly. B, Tibial surface of the lateral meniscus. The inferior attachment is interrupted where the popliteus tendon enters the tunnel. (From Wickstrom, K. T., et al.: Roentgen anatomy of the posterior horn of the lateral meniscus. Radiology 116:617, 1975.)

The lateral wall of the tendon is attached to the joint capsule in most cases. Therefore contrast medium will not completely surround the tendon.[377] The meniscus maintains superior and inferior attachments except where the tendon enters the joint inferiorly and exits superiorly (Fig. 6–61).[376] Failure to visualize these attachments or changes in the normal configuration of the tunnel may be associated with meniscal tears (Fig. 6–62).[288, 321, 377]

The cruciate ligaments are extrasynovial and intracapsular. They are best demonstrated on the stressed lateral view and notch views (see Figs. 6–66 and 6–67B). The anterior cruciate ligament arises between the anterior horns of the menisci in the anterior intercondylar fossa. The ligament angles superiorly to insert into the medial aspect of the lateral femoral condyle.[270] The posterior cruciate ligament attaches to the posterior intercondylar portion of the tibia and courses anteriorly to insert into the lateral aspect of the medial femoral condyle. Brody and colleagues studied the cruciate ligaments in 167 patients.[258] The apical angle formed by the cruciate ligaments and the fact that the anterior cruciate inserts into the tibia approximately 8 mm posterior to the anterior tibial margin assist in differentiating the anterior cruciate ligament from the infrapatellar plica. The normal infrapatellar plica inserts more anteriorly than the anterior cruciate ligament. The angle formed with the posterior cru-

ciate ligament was 90° or more in 76 percent of cases. The normal apical angle formed by the cruciate ligaments is never greater than 90°.[258]

As mentioned above, the deep fibers of the medial collateral ligaments are attached to the capsule and medial meniscus. The superficial fibers arise below the adductor tubercle and insert near the upper tibial metaphysis. The lateral collateral ligament is not associated with the joint capsule in the manner of the medial collateral ligament. Its origin is the lateral femoral condyle, and it inserts into the superior aspect of the fibular head (Figs. 6–60 and 6–63).[269, 288]

The articular cartilage on the femoral condyles, tibia, and patella is well demonstrated with double-contrast technique (Figs. 6–64 and 6–65). The cartilage should be smooth and 2 to 4 mm thick.[269] Subtle changes in the articular cartilage or menisci may be overlooked if too much contrast material is injected.

The joint capsule is large and normally freely communicates with the suprapatellar (quadriceps) bursa (Fig. 6–63B). The gastrocnemio-semimembranous bursa communicates with the joint in 50 percent of patients.[286] The proximal tibiofibular joint may communicate with the joint capsule in up to 10 percent of patients.[356] The normal arthrographic views are demonstrated in Figures 6–64 through 6–68.

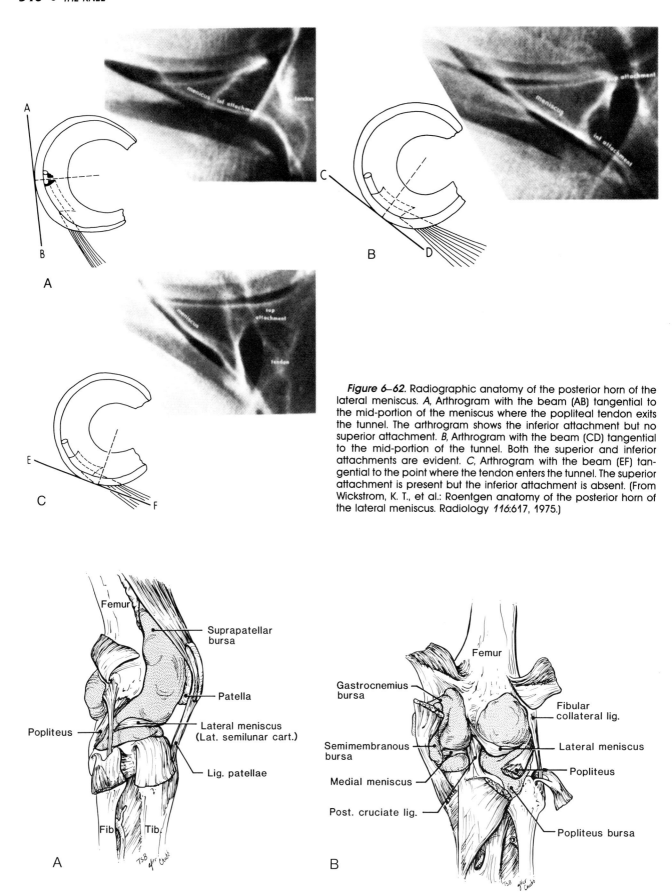

Figure 6–62. Radiographic anatomy of the posterior horn of the lateral meniscus. *A,* Arthrogram with the beam (AB) tangential to the mid-portion of the meniscus where the popliteal tendon exits the tunnel. The arthrogram shows the inferior attachment but no superior attachment. *B,* Arthrogram with the beam (CD) tangential to the mid-portion of the tunnel. Both the superior and inferior attachments are evident. *C,* Arthrogram with the beam (EF) tangential to the point where the tendon enters the tunnel. The superior attachment is present but the inferior attachment is absent. (From Wickstrom, K. T., et al.: Roentgen anatomy of the posterior horn of the lateral meniscus. Radiology *116*:617, 1975.)

Figure 6–63. Illustrations of the distended knee joint. *A,* Lateral view demonstrating the suprapatellar (quadriceps) bursa, posterior recess, and popliteus tendon. *B,* Posterior view demonstrating the semimembranous bursa and popliteus bursa.

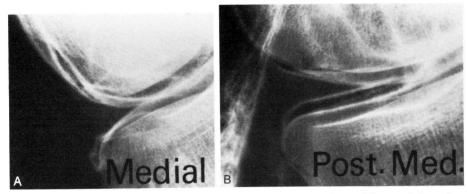

Figure 6-64. Normal medial meniscus with double contrast technique. *A*, Anterior horn of the medial meniscus. Note the normal inferior recess. *B*, Posterior medial meniscus. Note the size difference between the anterior and posterior horns. There is contrast in the semimembranous bursa posteriorly but the meniscus is not obscured.

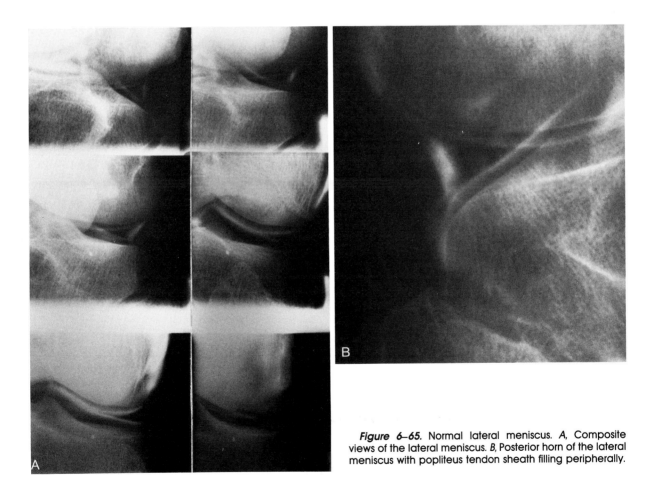

Figure 6-65. Normal lateral meniscus. *A*, Composite views of the lateral meniscus. *B*, Posterior horn of the lateral meniscus with popliteus tendon sheath filling peripherally.

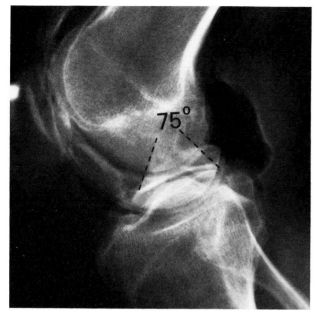

Figure 6–66. Double contrast lateral view. The angle formed by the anterior and posterior cruciates is 75°. Note the distance from the anterior insertion to the anterior tibial margin (white bands).

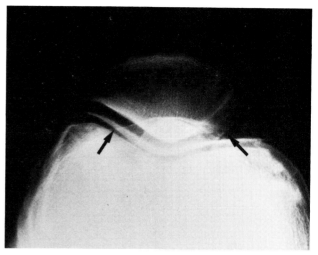

Figure 6–68. Axial view of the patella following double contrast arthrogram. The articular cartilage on the femoral condyles and patella is clearly demonstrated *(arrows)*.

Arthrographic Evaluation of Knee Abnormalities

Meniscal Abnormalities

Knee arthrography is most commonly performed to evaluate the menisci. Tegtmeyer evaluated double- and single-contrast technique in 951 patients and felt that both were equally effective in detecting meniscal tears.[373] Double-contrast technique, however, offers better anatomic detail of the menisci, articular cartilage, and cruciate ligaments.[373] Therefore a more complete examination is usually ob-

tained. Also, prone and supine films with double-contrast techniques increase the detection rate of subtle tears.[361]

Meniscal Tears. Arthrography is extremely accurate in detecting meniscal tears. Most tears occur medially owing to the lack of mobility of the medial meniscus. Brown reported lateral meniscal tears in 37 percent of patients and tears in both menisci in 9 percent of cases.[260] Nicholas reported 99.7 percent accuracy in detection of medial meniscal tears and 93 percent accuracy for lateral tears using double-contrast technique.[342] The accuracy is definitely related to the experience of the examiner.

Arthrography is accurate in defining the location of the tear. This is the most important factor for the orthopedic surgeon. However, exact description of the tear is often difficult arthrographically, though certain descriptive terms are well accepted. Tears

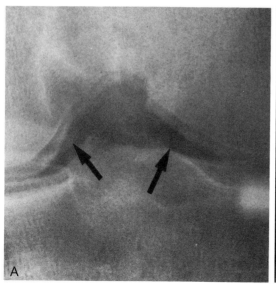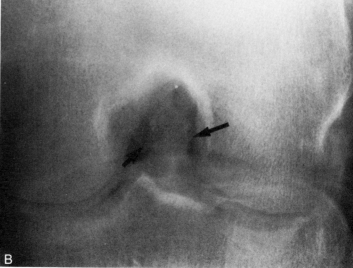

Figure 6–67. Notch views taken following double contrast arthrogram. *A*, Normal articular cartilage on the femoral condyles *(arrows)*. *B*, Changing the angle slightly results in visualization of the cruciate ligaments *(arrows)*.

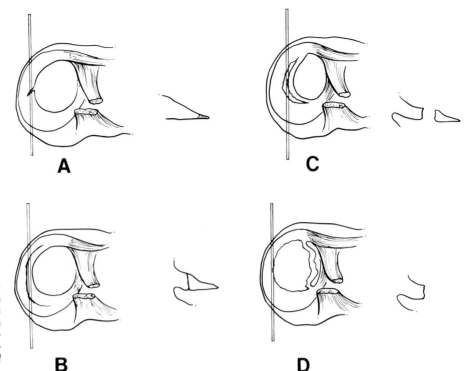

Figure 6–69. Illustration demonstrating the appearance of the meniscus from above and tangentially as seen by the fluoroscopist. *A,* Radial tear in the body of the meniscus. *B,* Undisplaced vertical tear. *C* and *D,* Bucket-handle tears with varying degrees of separation.

are commonly described as vertical, horizontal, radial, complex, and partial or complete. The appearance of the tear depends upon the positioning of the meniscus in the radiographic beam (Fig. 6–69). A vertical tear divides the triangular meniscus into central and peripheral segments (Fig. 6–70). If the anterior and posterior horn remain intact, this tear is termed a bucket-handle tear. With bucket-handle tears the inner fragment may be displaced into the

intercondylar region. Radial tears are vertical tears in the inner margin of the meniscus. Arthrographically these are often subtle and usually present with an area of contrast density on the inner margin of the meniscus (Fig. 6–71). Horizontal tears begin medially and usually do not extend to the periphery of the meniscus (Fig. 6–72). Peripheral meniscal cysts may be associated with these tears.

Peripheral tears usually originate from the inferior

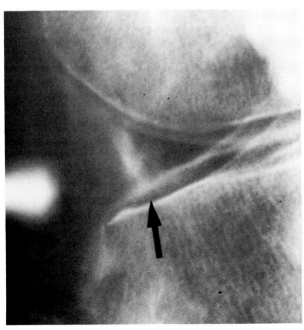

Figure 6–70. Vertical tear of the meniscus. There is a vertical contrast collection *(arrow)* in the medial meniscus.

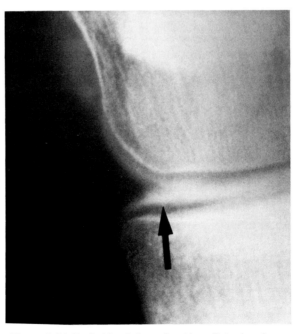

Figure 6–71. Central (radial) meniscal tear. There is enhanced contrast appearance at the inner apex of the meniscus *(arrow)* with loss of the normal triangular configuration.

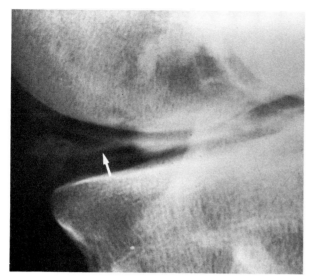

Figure 6–72. Arthrogram demonstrating a horizontal tear *(white arrow)* in the posterior horn of the medial meniscus.

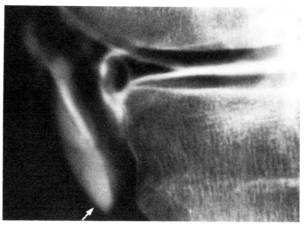

Figure 6–73. Complex peripheral tear in the medial meniscus. Note the collection of contrast material medially *(arrow)* due to an associated medial collateral ligament tear.

tibial surface.[269] These tears may be partial or complete. The outer one third of the meniscus has a rich blood supply and therefore healing may occur. The medial two thirds of the meniscus relies on synovial fluid for nourishment. Complex tears are demonstrated by extensive involvement and multidirection disruption (Fig. 6–73).

Detection of lateral meniscal tears is somewhat more difficult than detection of medial tears. The posterior anatomy (Figs. 6–61 and 6–62) and the slightly increased difficulty in obtaining true tangential positioning is responsible. Subtle changes in the popliteus tendon sheath may be useful. If the normal oval or rectangular shape is not present, a lateral meniscus tear should be suspected.[289] Pavlov and Goldman noted changes in the popliteus tendon in 58 patients.[351] In 47 patients the bursa was narrowed or compressed. Forty-five patients (78 percent) had torn menisci. Discoid menisci were present in 4 patients (7 percent). When the popliteus bursa was absent the lateral meniscus was torn in 64 percent.

Postoperative evaluation of the menisci may be difficult. One cannot be certain if tears are new or represent posterior horn remnants not completely removed at the time of surgery. Degenerative changes in the articular cartilage are common following meniscectomy (Fig. 6–74).[269, 273]

Discoid Menisci. Discoid menisci are abnormally broad and disk-shaped. The lateral meniscus is

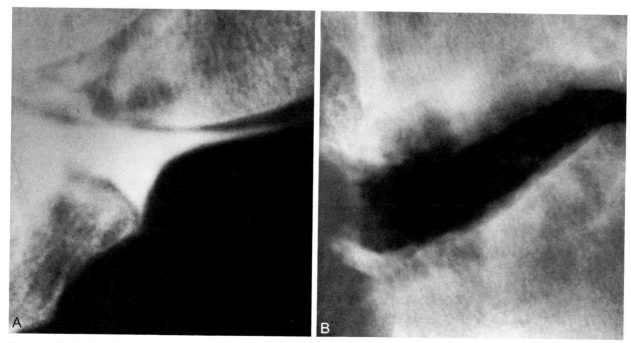

Figure 6–74. Post-meniscectomy arthrograms. *A,* Patient with recent medial meniscectomy and persistent pain. The arthrogram shows no remaining meniscus anteriorly. *B,* Later changes may result in extensive cartilage loss, synovitis, and subchondral bony erosion.

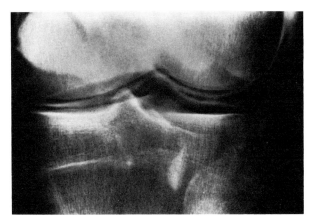

Figure 6–75. Discoid lateral meniscus with multiple vertical tears.

more commonly involved than the medial meniscus. Because of their configuration, the meniscus extends further between the femoral condyle and tibial plateau and is more susceptible to tearing (Fig. 6–75).[269, 288, 298] The etiology is uncertain. Some authors feel this is a congenital defect; however, the consensus is that the presence of discoid menisci is a developmental defect due to abnormal peripheral attachments.[269, 288, 326]

The majority of discoid menisci produce symptoms during childhood. Thus, the condition should be suspected in children with symptoms of internal derangement.[288]

Hall detected 27 discoid lateral menisci in reviewing 985 knee arthrograms (incidence 2.7 percent).[298] The majority (19 of 27, or 70 percent) were typical

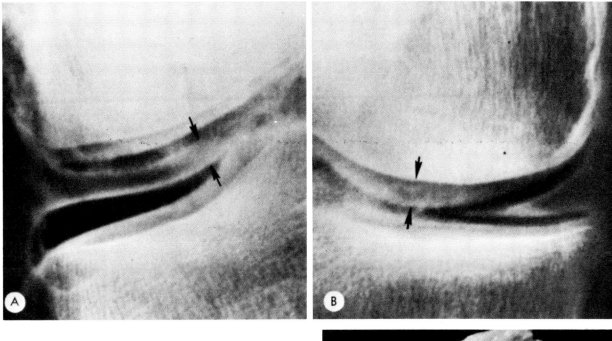

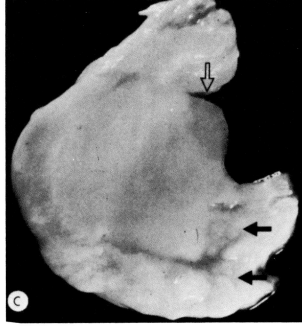

Figure 6–76. Slab type of discoid lateral menisci. *A,* The meniscus extends farther into the joint space and has fairly uniform width. The medial margins *(arrows)* are often indistinct. *B,* The articular cartilage is thicker on the medial femoral condyle than on the lateral condyle shown in *A. C,* Specimen of slab-type meniscus. Surgical markers *(lower arrows).* The tear *(open arrow)* was not detected arthrographically. (From Hall, F. M.: Arthrography of the discoid lateral meniscus. A. J. R. *128*:993, 1977.)

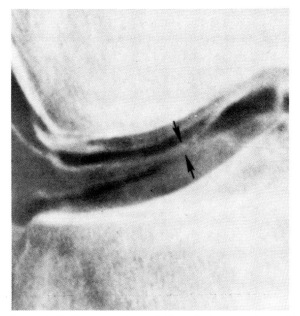

Figure 6–77. Biconcave type of discoid lateral meniscus with central thickening *(arrows)*. (From Hall, F. M.: Arthrography of the discoid lateral meniscus. A. J. R. *128*:993, 1977.)

disk-shaped menisci. The remaining menisci presented different shapes. Hall classified discoid lateral menisci into six types.[298] These menisci had the following characteristics:

Type 1, Slab type. Thick rounded slab with parallel superior and inferior surfaces (Fig. 6–76).

Type 2, Biconcave type. Slab-like with a thin central portion (Fig. 6–77).

Type 3, Wedge type. Often smaller than the slab type. Appearance is that of an elongated triangular meniscus.

Type 4, Assymetric. Anterior horn larger than the posterior horn (Fig. 6–78).

Type 5, Forme Fruste. Between normal and slab-type.

Type 6, Grossly torn. Menisci fall into one of the first five types but with extensive tears.

No discoid medial menisci were noted in Hall's series of 985 arthrograms.[298]

Degenerative Meniscal Lesions. The menisci are composed of fibrocartilage made up of collagen and noncollagen proteins. With age the ratio of collagen to noncollagen protein decreases. This occurs more commonly in the medial meniscus, resulting in less degenerative change in the lateral menisci.[315] Noble and Hamblein noted degenerative tears in 60 percent of the menisci in 100 cadavers.[343] The average age was 65 years.

The arthrographic findings include fraying, increased contrast coating due to the irregular surface, and partial horizontal tears (Fig. 6–79).

Ossicles in the menisci have also been reported.[255, 364] Patients usually present with a painful knee. The etiology is unclear but may be due to recurrent trauma or heterotopic bone formation.[255] Ossicles can be differentiated from loose bodies by their intrameniscal location. This finding may occur in either meniscus, and an associated tear is often present.

Schuldt and Wolfe noted meniscal cysts in 50 of 2,522 arthrograms.[364] The lateral meniscus was involved twice as frequently as the medial meniscus.

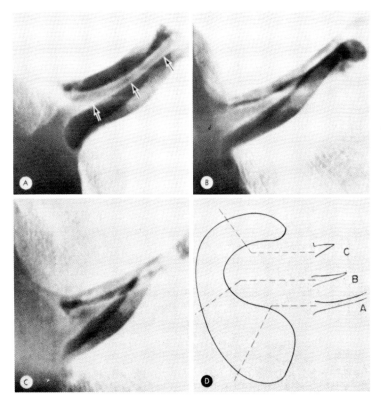

Figure 6–78. Discoid meniscus with asymmetric anterior horn enlargement. *A,* Enlarged anterior horn *(arrows)* which extends into the joint space. *B,* The midportion of the meniscus is only minimally elongated. *C,* The posterior horn appears more normal except for failure to visualize the popliteal tendon. *D,* Diagram of the meniscus seen from above. Tangential views: anterior, A; mid-body, B; and posterior, C. (From Hall, F. M.: Arthrography of the discoid lateral meniscus. A. J. R. *128*:993, 1977.)

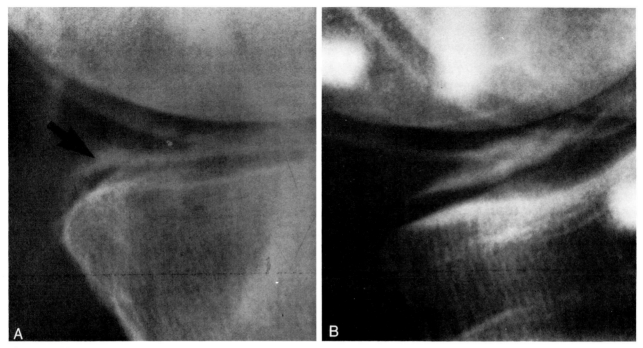

Figure 6–79. Degenerative changes in the menisci. *A,* Early degenerative change in the medial meniscus with increased contrast absorption inferiorly *(arrow).* *B,* Enhanced absorption along the central margins of the meniscus with a subtle horizontal tear.

Patients presented with a palpable mass in most cases. In all cases horizontal tears were present that allowed arthrographic communication with the cyst (Fig. 6–80). Arthrography will not demonstrate the cyst if a communicating tear is not present.[288]

Ligament Abnormalities

Multiple techniques are available for evaluation of the cruciate ligaments (Table 6–6). Pavlov utilizes

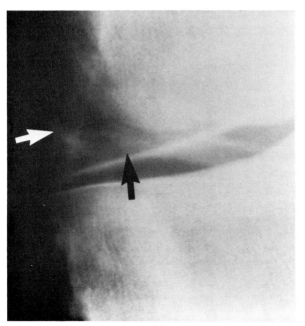

Figure 6–80. Meniscal cyst. Arthrogram demonstrates a horizontal tear *(black arrow)* filling a cystic structure peripherally *(white arrow).*

double-contrast technique with a stressed lateral view (see Fig. 6–59).[354] We find this technique is most practical and reproducible. Lateral tomography is also useful in selected cases.[250] Dalinka reports 90 percent accuracy using this technique.[271] Xeroradiographs may be useful but are not always available; they also increase radiation dose to the patient.[295] (See Xeroradiography section, Chapter 1.) Computed tomography and magnetic resonance imaging may also prove useful in cruciate ligament injury (Fig. 6–81).[255, 352]

Tears of the anterior cruciate ligament are much more common than posterior cruciate ligament tears.[269, 288] Associated meniscal tears and collateral ligament tears are common.[288] Pavlov reported medial meniscal tears in 63 percent of anterior cruciate ligament tears.[354]

When arthrography with the stressed lateral view is used, accuracy in detection of cruciate ligament injury approaches 95 percent.[354] Blood in the aspirate may also be associated with a ligament tear.[353] Identification of the cruciate ligament may be difficult in patients with large effusions owing to lack of coating. The ligament inserts into the tibia more posteriorly than the infrapatellar synovial fold. These structures should not be confused (Fig. 6–82).[270] The normal anterior cruciate ligament is straight and forms an angle of less than 90° with the posterior cruciate at the femoral attachment.[258] The anterior cruciate ligament is torn if the ligament is absent or has a wavy or irregular appearance.[354] If the ligament is stretched or lax, a concave upper margin will be evident. The infrapatellar plicae has been reported to be more apparent when the anterior cruciate ligament is torn.

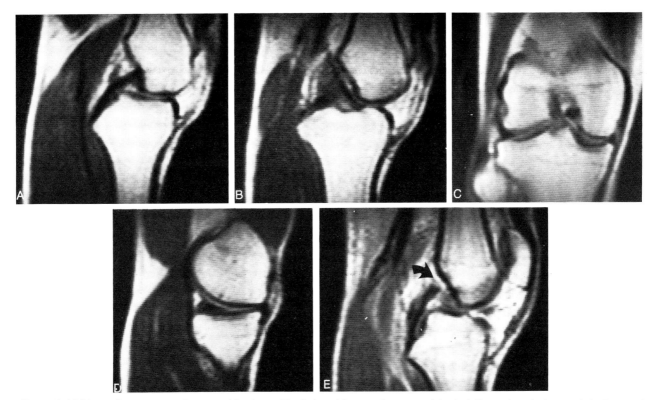

Figure 6–81. Magnetic resonance images of the knee. Menisci and ligaments appear black. *A,* Normal posterior cruciate ligament. *B,* Normal anterior cruciate ligament. The knee must be rotated 15° to 20° to include the entire ligament because of its oblique course. *C,* Coronal view of the knee showing normal menisci (black). *D,* Sagittal view of the normal posteromedial meniscus. *E,* Sagittal view demonstrating a tear *(arrow)* in the upper posterior cruciate ligament.

Arthrography may also be useful in studying the medial collateral ligament. The deep fibers of the medial collateral ligament blend with the capsule. Therefore, disruption of this ligament will result in extravasation of contrast medium at the site of the defect (see Fig. 6–73).[353] Tears in the medial meniscus and anterior cruciate ligament are often associated. Examination should be performed within 48 hours of the injury.[288] Small tears may seal after this time interval.

If only the deep fibers are torn, the contrast medium will outline the superficial fibers. If only the superficial fibers are torn, no contrast medium will leave the normal capsule. When both deep and superficial fibers are torn, the extravasation appears more extensive, with irregular margins.

Since the lateral collateral ligament does not blend with the capsule, arthrography is of little value. Stress views will demonstrate widening of the lateral joint space.[256, 288, 353]

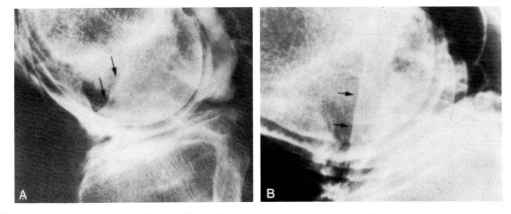

Figure 6–82. Lateral stress views of the knee with double contrast arthrography. *A,* Infrapatellar synovial plicae *(arrows)* with a concave upper margin and inserting more anteriorly than the normal anterior cruciate ligament. *B,* Normal anterior cruciate ligament with straight upper margin inserting just anteriorly to the tibial spine. (From Brody, G. A., et al.: Plica synovialis infrapatellaris: Arthrographic sign of anterior cruciate ligament disruption. A. J. R. *140:*767, 1983.)

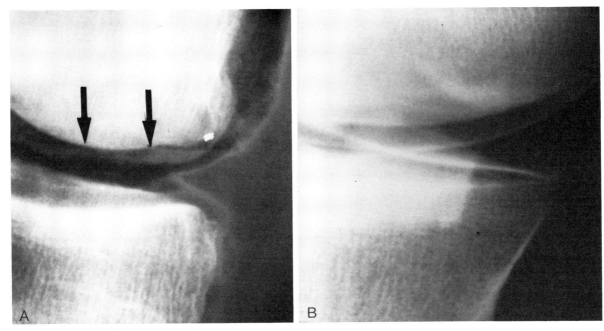

Figure 6–83. Arthrograms of patient with chronic medial compartment pain. *A,* The meniscus is normal. The femoral articular cartilage is thin, irregular, and increased in density. Changes are due to degenerative arthritis. *B,* Normal femoral articular cartilage for comparison. The contrast medium has the normal thin-coated appearance.

Disruption of the quadriceps tendon can rarely be detected arthrographically.[322] Contrast medium will extravasate from the suprapatellar region. This is usually a clinical diagnosis. MRI is more useful in evaluating the quadriceps tendon and patellar ligament.

Articular Abnormalities

Evaluation of the articular cartilage is better accomplished with double-contrast technique. In selected cases tomography or CT may also be useful.

The tibial and femoral cartilage is particularly well demonstrated in the meniscal regions, though notch and axial views increase the detail of the femoral and patellar cartilage (see Fig. 6–67 and 6–68).

Changes in the articular cartilage may be seen with degenerative arthritis and other arthritides, osteochondritis dissecans, chondral fractures, and chondromalacia.

Degenerative changes in the cartilage may be seen with chronic meniscal injury or degenerative arthritis. The articular surface appears irregular and fissured, with increased contrast enhancement due to the increased absorption of contrast medium (Figs. 6–83 and 6–84).[269]

Osteochondritis dissecans is common in young adults. This condition usually involves the lateral surface of the medial femoral condyle. The patella and lateral condyle may also be involved. This condition is thought to occur following acute or chronic trauma.[288] Changes may be bilateral and are more common in males.[269, 288] Arthrography is useful in evaluating the position of the fragment and the appearance of the articular cartilage. Arthrographic

demonstration of intact cartilage over the fragment may lead to conservative management.

Chondromalacia of the patella is a common cause of knee pain in young adults. Locking and instability may occasionally be present, causing difficulty in differentiating it from other causes of internal derangement. The exact etiology of chondromalacia is uncertain.[269] Arthrography is of little value in early detection. Swelling of the articular cartilage occurs initially. This is not detectable on the arthrogram. Later subchondral sclerosis, fissures, and increased contrast absorption occur. Double-contrast arthrography with axial views and lateral views with internal and external rotation[288] may detect these changes. Horn described 90 percent accuracy in detection of chondromalacia arthrographically.[312]

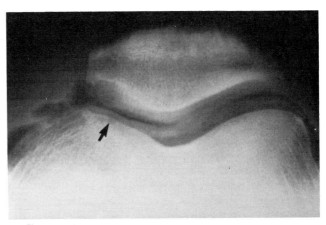

Figure 6–84. Arthrogram of patient with patellofemoral pain. Axial view of the double contrast arthrogram demonstrates cartilage loss on the medial femoral condyle and patellar facet *(arrow).*

More importantly, exclusion of other intra-articular pathology is important. Up to 15 percent of patients with chondromalacia have associated meniscal tears.[316] The combination of arthrography and a CT scan performed with the knee flexed 15° may provide the best detail.[256] This is useful only in selected cases. Other structures, especially the menisci, are not as well demonstrated with CT. Currently, magnetic resonance imaging is not helpful in evaluating the articular cartilage, though MRI can easily detect subchondral bony changes.

Intra-articular loose bodies may result from degenerative disease, trauma, or synovial chondromatosis. Arthrographic detection may be difficult owing to the multiple compartments and size of the capsule. If double-contrast technique is used, air bubbles can be mistaken for chondral bodies. Careful exercise will reduce the number of air bubbles. In our experience, single-contrast technique with tomography may be the most reliable method.

Synovial Abnormalities

Arthrographically detectable synovial changes include synovitis (pigmented villonodular synovitis, proliferative synovitis of rheumatoid arthritis), synovial chondromatosis, neoplasms, and cysts.[269, 288, 304, 332, 368] Double-contrast technique provides the best detail. The normal synovium is smooth and finely coated with contrast material.

Proliferation of the synovium may result from almost any chronic inflammatory condition (rheumatoid arthritis, degenerative arthritis, tuberculo-sis, etc.). Differentiation on the arthrographic appearance alone may be difficult. Examination of plain films may suggest the diagnosis. In certain cases the chondral bodies are calcified or ossified, assisting with the diagnosis. Also, careful evaluation of the synovial fluid may be useful. Synovial fluid may be bloody with synovial hemangiomas[269, 288, 332] or dark (xanthochromic) with pigmented villonodular synovitis.[304]

Patients with pigmented villonodular synovitis are usually young adults with chronic knee pain and swelling. Routine radiographs may be normal or demonstrate soft tissue masses and subchondral erosions.[304] Arthrographically diffuse or localized nodular changes in the synovium may be apparent. The diffuse changes may be difficult to differentiate from the synovitis seen in rheumatoid arthritis or synovial chondromatosis. The latter condition is uncommon, with the synovial fluid normal and routine x-rays usually unremarkable. With synovial chondromatosis the synovial changes are often fine and granular (which also assist in the differential diagnosis).[355]

Uncommon synovial masses include hemangiomas and synovial fat proliferation.[269, 332, 368] Hemangiomas may cause intra-articular bleeding, resulting in changes similar to hemophilia. Cutaneous hemangiomas are often associated.[269]

Synovial cysts or bursa enlargements are not uncommon. The popliteal cyst develops as an enlargement of the gastrocnemio-semimembranous bursa. The cyst usually forms as the result of chronic inflammation.[288, 309] Rarely cysts may form anteriorly

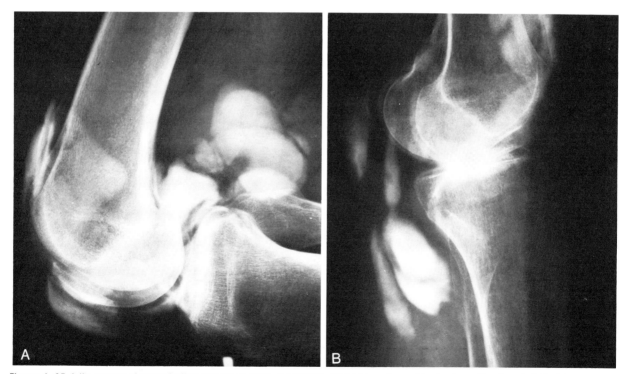

Figure 6–85. Arthrograms demonstrating popliteal cysts. *A,* Patient with knee pain and typical popliteal cyst. *B,* Upright lateral view in a patient with rheumatoid arthritis. The joint space is narrowed. There is a dissecting popliteal cyst, which was evident only following repeat exercise and upright technique.

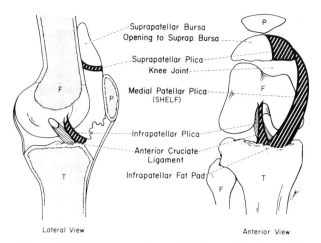

Figure 6–86. Illustration of synovial plicae of the knee. (From Patel, D.: Arthroscopy of the plicae—synovial folds and their significance. A. J. Sports Med. 6:217, 1978.)

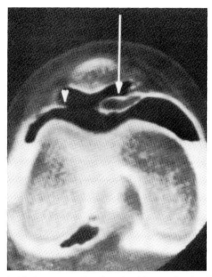

Figure 6–88. CT scan following double contrast arthrography demonstrating a thickened mediopatellar plica *(long white arrow)* and a small nonthickened lateral plica *(small arrow).* (From Boven, F., et al.: Synovial plicae of the knee on computed tomography. Radiology, *147*:805, 1983.)

and superiorly.[366] Meniscal tears are also frequently present in association with popliteal cysts.[260] Single- or double-contrast technique can be used to demonstrate these abnormalities. Post-exercise and upright views may be required to demonstrate dissecting cysts (Fig. 6–85). Ultrasound is also an accurate method of diagnosing popliteal cysts, especially in symptomatic patients.[309]

Synovial plicae have become increasingly important with the advent of arthroscopy. These plicae are embryonic remnants that may be present in the normal knee. The most common plicae are the suprapatellar, mediopatellar, and infrapatellar (Fig. 6–86). These may be present in 20 to 60 percent of normal knees.[252, 257, 282] If these plicae become inflamed, they appear white and thick arthroscopi-

cally and may be symptomatic. Patients often complain of medial knee pain with exercise.[257] Symptoms are usually related to trauma and may be difficult to differentiate from other intra-articular pathology.

Arthrographically the plicae are best seen with double-contrast technique. The lateral projection will demonstrate the suprapatellar plica (Fig. 6–87). This appears as a band running obliquely from the anterior to posterior portions of the suprapatellar bursa. The infrapatellar plica may be confused with the anterior cruciate ligament (Fig. 6–82A). However, as previously mentioned, the ligament inserts more posteriorly on the tibia.[257, 258] The medial plica is not often seen.

CT has been useful in determining the thickness of plicae and therefore has allowed recognition of some degree of correlation between this thickness and the patient's symptoms (Fig. 6–88).[257]

If a plica persists in its entirety, the joint will lose its normal configuration. Persistence of the entire suprapatellar plicae may result in detectable arthrographic changes (Fig. 6–89).[282] In this situation the patient often presents with a suprapatellar soft tissue mass.[256, 257]

Pitfalls in Knee Arthrography

Most errors in knee arthrography are related to misinterpretation of normal structures or faulty technique. Complications with the technique are rare.

Proper injection technique is critical. Contrast medium should not be injected in the region of suspected pathology. Extravasation may lead to findings simulating collateral ligament tears or ob-

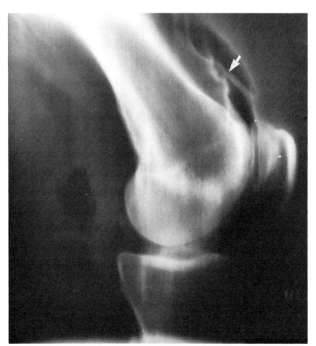

Figure 6–87. Double contrast arthrotomogram demonstrating the suprapatellar plicae *(arrow).*

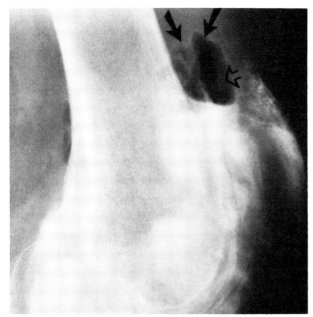

Figure 6–89. Persistent suprapatellar plicae with synovial thickening *(arrows)* and abnormally short suprapatellar bursa.

scure the anatomy of interest. Too much contrast material can obscure subtle changes or pool in the inner condylar region, simulating a loose body.[302]

With double-contrast technique the patient must be exercised slowly to avoid excess air bubble formation. Air bubbles may simulate chondral bodies. Exercise must be sufficient to coat the menisci. If the undersurface of the menisci is not thoroughly coated, the area should be reexamined. Freiberger

noted lack of inferior coating in association with meniscal tears.[288]

Errors in positioning are common if one is not an experienced arthrographer. Tangential positioning of the menisci may be difficult, especially in the case of the lateral meniscus. Also improper distraction of the joint may cause buckling of the meniscus or anatomic distortion, mimicking a tear (Fig. 6–90).[299] An overlying semimembranous bursa may obscure the midportion of the medial meniscus, making evaluation more difficult (Fig. 6–91).

Normal anatomy may also be confused with pathology. The anterior portions of the menisci lose their normal triangular configuration near the insertion. If films are taken in this position, the meniscus may appear torn (Fig. 6–92). Synovial folds and fat may also be superimposed on the anterior menisci, mimicking tears.[302]

Meniscal recesses are common inferiorly in the anterior lateral meniscus and superiorly in the posterior medial meniscus.[303] Recesses in other locations most likely represent partial peripheral tears (Fig. 6–93).[302, 303] These tears may heal with conservative treatment, as reepithelialization can occur peripherally.[303]

Errors in interpretation due to the above problems or misinterpretation are not uncommon. Walt found a 50 percent reporting error rate in patients in whom the arthrographic and surgical findings did not correlate.[375] For example, oblique bucket-handle tears may look normal if the central fragment is totally detached.[300]

Significant complications following knee arthrography, on the other hand, are rare. Contrast me-

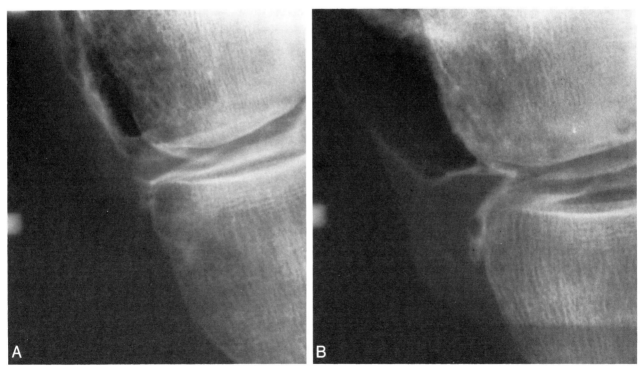

Figure 6–90. Anterior horn of the medial meniscus. *A,* Initial view appears abnormal owing to insufficient distraction of the joint and improper positioning. *B,* Repositioning demonstrates a normal meniscus.

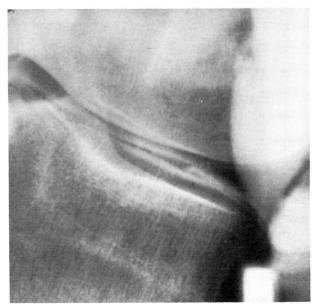

Figure 6-91. Arthrogram of the mid-portion of the medial meniscus. An enlarged semimembranous bursa obscures the peripheral portion of the meniscus.

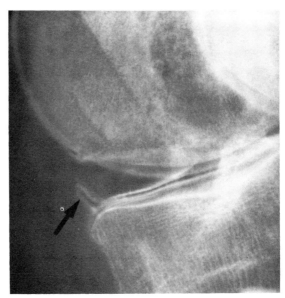

Figure 6-93. Partial peripheral tear in the posterior medial meniscus. There is a long, densely coated cleft in the inferior posterior portion of the medial meniscus *(arrows)* owing to a partial tear.

dium reactions (usually urticaria) occur in 1 to 2 percent of patients.[269, 288] Occasionally painful synovitis with effusion may occur within 24 hours of the injection. This occurs in about 1 percent of patients.[250] More rarely this may require removal of the fluid.

Infections are also rare.[357] In a combined series of 33,000 cases only 2 infections were reported.[269, 288, 342]

Air embolism (1 case) and pneumomediastinum (1 case) have been reported following double-contrast technique.[269]

Arthrography Following Knee Arthroplasty

Arthrography also provides significant information in evaluation of loosening and infection following total knee arthroplasty. The technique differs from conventional arthrography. Subtraction technique is useful owing to the presence of metal- and barium-impregnated methacrylate. (See Chapter 1, Arthrography—Subtraction Technique.)

Technique

With the patient in the supine position the leg to be examined is immobilized. This can be accomplished with sandbags or other props. The knee is prepared and draped using sterile technique. In most situations the needle (22-gauge 1½ inch) is inserted into the patellofemoral space as with conventional arthrography. If the patella has been removed, the needle is placed in the lateral tibiofemoral compartment. The joint should be aspirated and the aspirate sent for culture studies. If no fluid can be obtained, the joint should be flushed with nonbacteriostatic sterile saline and the aspirate sent for cultures. Following the aspiration an AP film is obtained to serve as the subtraction mark.

The joint is then injected with contrast material (Hypaque-M-60) until complete filling has been obtained. This usually requires at least 20 ml of contrast material. Lymphatic filling, resistance, and slight patient discomfort are useful in determining when the joint is adequately distended. A second film is obtained prior to removing the needle (re-

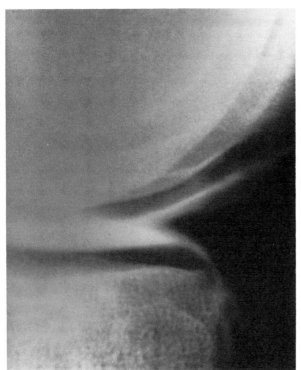

Figure 6-92. Film taken of the anterior horn of the medial meniscus in an almost lateral position. The inner margin is not sharp. The triangular appearance is lost near the insertion of the meniscus anteriorly. This is not abnormal.

moving the needle first may result in patient movement). This serves as the subtraction film. The needle is then removed and the joint exercised under fluoroscopic guidance. Films are obtained in the AP, lateral, and oblique positions as well as with traction.

In patients with equivocal arthrographic findings injection of bupivacaine (Marcaine) may be helpful. Reduction in the pain is indicative of intra-articular pathology.

Arthrographic Findings

Normally the contrast material fills the medial, lateral, and suprapatellar compartments. Loosening of the tibial component occurs more frequently than loosening of the femoral component.[363] Contrast medium may extend around the bone-cement interface at the periphery of the tibial component. This is usually not significant.[333, 363] Contrast medium

that extends beyond 2 cm or below the tibial component, on the other hand, indicates loosening.

With most types of knee prostheses the femoral component is not easily evaluated on the AP subtraction view (Fig. 6–94). The lateral and oblique views may be more helpful. Isotope studies may also be useful in evaluation of the femoral component. Infection may cause capsular irregularity, sinus tracts, or outpouching of the capsule. Periosteal new bone formation and endosteal scalloping occur less frequently with infected knee arthroplasties than with infected hip arthroplasties.

Arthrography in evaluation of knee arthroplasty is less accurate than arthrographic evaluation of hip arthroplasties. Hunter reported correlation with surgical findings in 67 percent of knee arthroplasties.[313] This is at least partially due to the size of the joint. Large pseudocapsules in the hip may also cause problems. This causes more difficulty in accurately filling the bone-cement interface.

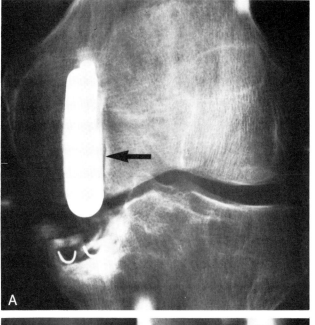

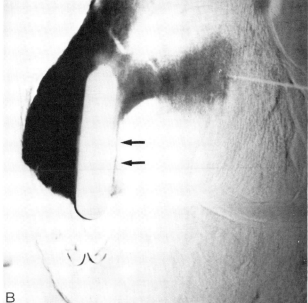

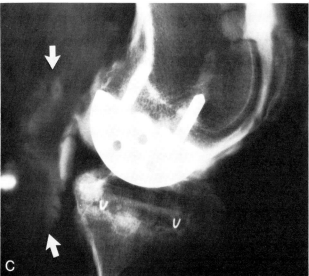

Figure 6–94. Male patient with pain following medial compartment arthroplasty. A, Routine AP view demonstrates lucency at the bone-cement interface lateral to the femoral component (arrow). B, Subtraction arthrogram demonstrates contrast medium along the lateral margin of the component (arrows). It is diifficult to determine the true extent of extravasation owing to the overlying contrast material. C, Lateral view following complete joint distension demonstrates a large popliteal cyst (arrows). The femoral component is difficult to evaluate. The tibial component is well-seated.

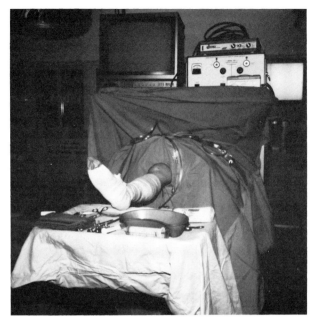

Figure 6–95. Routine preparation and equipment for arthroscopy.

Arthrography may also be useful in evaluation of the position of cement and bone fragments about the joint.

Arthroscopy

Arthroscopy of the knee was first performed by Takagi in 1918.[371] Early use of the arthroscope in the United States was primarily related to management of tuberculosis of the knee.[261, 285] Watanabe developed the first clinically practical arthroscope and published an *Atlas of Arthroscopy* in 1957.[374] Subsequently, much activity has revolved about the development and teaching of diagnostic and arthroscopic surgical techniques (Fig. 6–95).

The initial indications for diagnostic arthroscopy included diagnosis of meniscal lesions or defects of articular cartilage, synovial biopsy, follow-up of surgically treated patients, and visualization of pa-

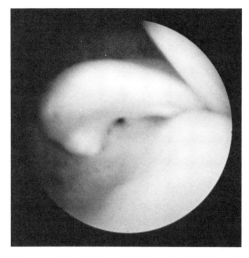

Figure 6–96. Flap tear of the posterior horn of the medial meniscus, which has displaced into the posterior medial compartment as visualized from the posteromedial portal.

tellofemoral relationships.[264] Contraindications to arthroscopy included adjacent sepsis and ankylosis of the joint. In an early report on the value of arthroscopy in 60 knees, Casscells found that the arthroscopic diagnosis was correct in 80 percent of cases, with 6 false positive and 6 false negative results.[264]

The accuracy of arthroscopy in the diagnosis of intra-articular lesions and especially in comparison to arthrography have been more recently addressed by several authors (Table 6–7).[263, 268, 274, 291, 311, 319, 325, 335, 345] The areas that are difficult to visualize arthroscopically are the posterior horns of the menisci, especially the medial meniscus in a knee with tight ligaments.[319] The retropatellar fat pad is also difficult to assess arthroscopically. The posteromedial portal (Fig. 6–96), patellar tendon portal (Fig. 6–97), and midpatellar lateral portal have allowed improved visualization of the posterior cruciate ligament, the

TABLE 6–7. Accuracy of Arthrography and Arthroscopy in Diagnosis of Intra-Articular Lesions

Author	Year	Clinical	Arthroscopy	Arthrography
Nicholas	1970	80.	—	97.5
Jackson	1972	68.5	88	68.2*
DeHaven	1975	72	94	78
McGinty	1976	—	89.8	50
Hirschowitz	1976	72	94	77
Gillquist	1978	—	91	27*
Gilles	1979	85	68	83
Korn	1979	—	98	94
Carruthers	1980	—	96	—
Ireland	1980	—	84	86
Curran	1980	71	97	52
Casscells	1980	70	95	—
Crabtree	1981	—	93	94

*Single contrast

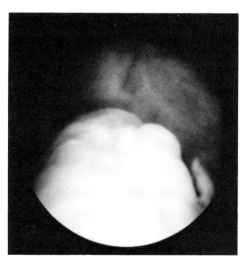

Figure 6–97. Loose body in the posterolateral compartment as visualized through the intercondylar notch with the arthroscope in the patellar tendon portal.

peripheral attachments of the menisci, and the anterior aspects of the joint. Arthroscopy, on the other hand, appears to be more accurate than arthrography in the diagnosis of patellar problems, tears of the anterior cruciate ligament, and tears of the lateral meniscus.[280]

Arthroscopic evaluation of 614 knees resulted in avoidance of open operation in 32 percent, a change in the planned operation in 27 percent, and an important change in 41 percent.[275] In some cases arthroscopy is superior to arthrography. Thus, tears of the lateral meniscus are difficult to evaluate arthrographically because of the popliteus tendon hiatus. Also, the accuracy of arthrography in the evaluation of lateral meniscus tears has been as low as 36 percent,[265] 57 percent[345] or 88 percent[327] in various series. If arthroscopy and arthrography are combined, the accuracy of diagnosis increases to 98 percent.[317] Therefore, these two techniques should be considered complementary. Clinical diagnosis is frequently inaccurate because of failure to appreciate associated pathology that may be better defined arthroscopically.[325]

Arthroscopic Evaluation

Arthroscopy has proved to be a useful tool in the evaluation of acute knee injuries and should be combined with a careful examination of ligamentous stability under anesthesia. A potential candidate for arthroscopy is the individual who presents with a history of a valgus, varus or rotational stress, a rapid deceleration injury to the knee, an audible pop, and the rapid onset of a hemarthrosis, all of which indicate significant injury.[278, 292, 346, 347] In such cases tears of the anterior cruciate ligament (Fig. 6–98) are frequent, appearing in 50 to 72 percent of the knees.[278, 292, 346] Other frequent lesions include meniscus injuries, especially at the posterior periph-

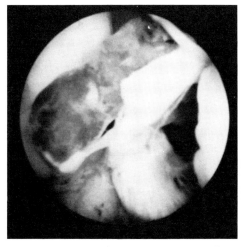

Figure 6–98. Acute tear of the anterior cruciate ligament in a patient with an acute hemarthrosis. (From Rand, J. A.: The role of arthroscopy in the management of knee injuries in the athlete. Mayo Clin. Proc. 59:77, 1984.)

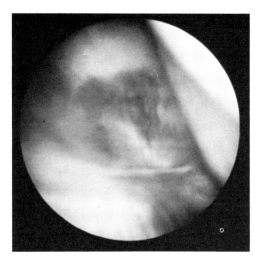

Figure 6–99. Acute hemorrhage in the medial capsule of the knee following a valgus stress indicating portal capsular tearing. (From Rand, J. A.: The role of arthroscopy in the management of knee injuries in the athlete. Mayo Clin. Proc. 59:77, 1984.)

eral detachment (57 to 62 percent); osteochondral fractures (6 to 20 percent); and posterior cruciate ligament tears (3 percent).[278, 346] Minor ligamentous tears without laxity may be diagnosed in 41 percent by the presence of capsular hemorrhage (Fig. 6–99).[346] Examination under anesthesia combined with arthroscopy yields useful information in these acute knee injuries in 68 percent,[291] 86 percent,[278] or 94 percent[345] of the knees. Arthroscopy is not recommended in the evaluation of the patient with severe ligamentous injury and extensive capsular disruption, as saline may extravasate into the calf, leading to a potential compartment syndrome.[272] Combined with examination of ligamentous stability under anesthesia, arthroscopy is also useful in the management of knees chronically deficient with regard to the anterior cruciate ligament.[272, 277] Finally, some patients may benefit from removal of loose bodies or large anterior cruciate stubs that cause impingement. Partial meniscectomy may also be recommended for meniscal tears in the presence of chronic anterior cruciate ligament insufficiency.[272] In these cases arthroscopy may assess the extent of arthrosis affecting the joint surface.[272] Following adequate assessment of the degree of instability and correction of intra-articular pathology, a more accurate assessment of the results of a rehabilitation program or the need for ligamentous reconstruction may be made.

The recognition of "new" pathologic lesions that may mimick lesions of menisci have become recognized through arthroscopy. The medial fibrous plica is an example (Fig. 6–100).

Plicae or synovial folds were recognized as early as 1939 by Iino.[314] Three synovial folds exist within the knee: the plica synovialis suprapatellaris, the plica synovialis mediopatellaris, and the plica synovialis infrapatellaris (see Figure 6–86).[350] A lateral plica may also be present.[320] The suprapatellar plica

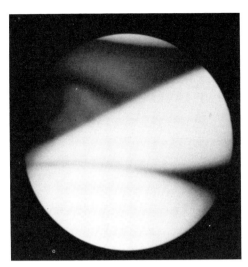

Figure 6–100. Medial fibrous plica lying between the patella superiorly and the medial femoral condyle inferiorly. (From Rand, J. A.: The Role of arthroscopy in the management of knee injuries in the athlete. Mayo Clin. Proc. *59:*77, 1984.)

is present in 20 percent of knees and represents a remnant of an embryologic septum that divides the knee.[350] The suprapatellar plica is usually asymptomatic. The infrapatellar plica or ligamentum mucosum covers the anterior cruciate ligament.[350] This structure may cause confusion in the interpretation of arthrograms that appear similar to the anterior cruciate ligament. The ligamentum mucosum is an asymptomatic structure. The medial synovial plica or shelf is present in 18.9[350] to 60 percent[320] of knees.

In some individuals this latter membrane may become thickened and fibrous, presumably following local trauma. The plica may then impinge on the anteromedial femoral condyle at 30° to 45° of knee flexion, resulting in pain and snapping. Patel has noted a 60 percent incidence of chondromalacia of the medial facet of the patella and a 40 percent incidence of chondromalacia of the medial femoral condyle adjacent to symptomatic medial plicae.[350] A pathologic plica that is symptomatic is present in only 17 percent of knees that have a medial plica.[320] Resection of the plica may be performed arthroscopically, with relief of symptoms in 70 to 93 percent of patients.[259, 320, 341]

Arthroscopy has been applied to injuries of the menisci as well as problems associated with meniscal surgery. The functional importance of the menisci has been previously discussed. All menisci regardless of injury or degenerative changes transmit load.[306] A partial meniscectomy will decrease load transmission by the meniscus from 85 to 25 percent medially or 75 to 50 percent laterally.[306] Therefore, from a mechanical standpoint partial meniscectomy appears preferable to total meniscectomy. Clinical studies of arthrotomy and partial meniscectomy have found improved results with preservation of a portion of the meniscus.[262, 336, 372] For bucket-handle tears of the meniscus, excellent

or good results were obtained in 83 percent for partial meniscectomy compared with 72 percent for total meniscectomy.[372] Partial meniscectomy results in a shorter rehabilitation time and four-fold decrease in postoperative complications compared with total meniscectomy.[336]

Arthroscopic surgical techniques also allow a selective approach to meniscal lesions. A carefully controlled partial meniscectomy may be performed for a variety of lesions, leaving a stable, contoured, and intact peripheral rim (Fig. 6–101). The long-term results of arthroscopic partial meniscectomy support this technique. A 6-year follow-up of 208 bucket-handle tears excised arthroscopically revealed a low morbidity and no evidence of progressive degenerative arthritis.[349] A 5-year follow-up of 131 arthroscopic partial meniscectomies revealed 85 percent good to excellent results.[344] Ninety percent excellent or good results in 95 patients with 3 years of follow-up has also been reported.[344] Finally, one study reported a success rate of 87 percent for partial meniscectomy in 125 patients followed for 2 years.[293] Arthroscopic meniscectomy offers the advantages of selective partial meniscectomy, early rehabilitation, and few complications.[318]

Arthroscopic evaluation may also be applied to the identification and management of peripheral tears of the meniscus that may be salvaged by peripheral reattachment. Peripheral detachment of the meniscus most frequently occurs in either an anterior central location or posterior peripheral location (Fig. 6–102). Successful repair has been accomplished in 21 of 22 knees with anterior central detachment.[370] Posterior peripheral detachments may be salvaged with only an 8 to 9 percent incidence of retear.[279] Arthroscopy allows evaluation of the integrity of the body of the meniscus, the extent of the tear, and the possibility of associated lesions,

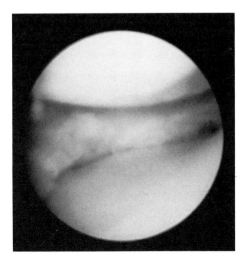

Figure 6–101. Peripheral rim of the medial meniscus following arthroscopic partial medial meniscectomy. (From Rand, J. A.: The role of arthroscopy in the management of knee injuries in the athlete. Mayo Clin. Proc. *59:*77, 1984.)

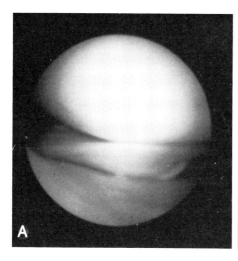 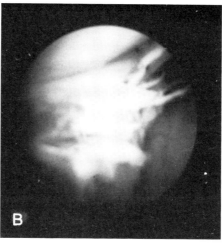

Figure 6–102. Posterior peripheral detachment of the medial meniscus as visualized arthroscopically. *A,* Appearance visualized anteriorly with traction applied by a probe. *B,* Appearance via posteromedial portal. (From Rand, J. A.: The role of arthroscopy in the management of knee injuries in the athlete. Mayo Clin. Proc. *59:*77, 1984.)

such as a torn anterior cruciate ligament. In some instances, arthroscopic repair of the peripheral tear is feasible.

Arthroscopy has proved valuable in the management of other knee disorders. Loose bodies are a frequent cause of knee symptoms and mimic a torn meniscus. Loose bodies may or may not be radioopaque, making radiographic localization difficult in some cases. In one series, only 38 of 50 loose bodies removed were visible on radiographs.[275] Loose bodies may be multiple in 30 percent of the knees.[275] Loose bodies arise from osteochondral fractures (Fig. 6–103), synovial chondromatosis, osteochondritis dissecans, and osteoarthritis (Fig. 6–104). Other lesions that present in a similar manner include foreign bodies, fragments of menisci, and local benign synovial tumors (Fig. 6–105). Common locations for loose bodies include the supra-

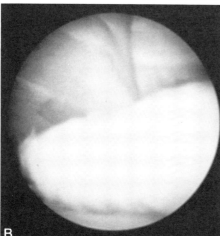

Figure 6–103. A, Arthroscopic appearance of an old osteochondral fracture of the patella. *B,* Appearance of loose body in the suprapatellar pouch. (From Rand, J. A.: The role of arthroscopy in the management of knee injuries in the athlete. Mayo Clin. Proc. *59:*77, 1984.)

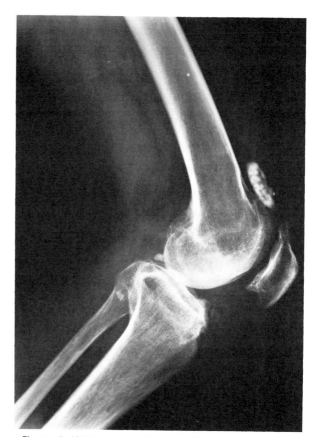

Figure 6–104. Lateral radiograph showing the typical appearance of loose bodies associated with osteoarthritis.

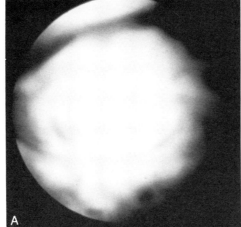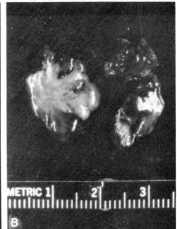

Figure 6–105. Arthroscopic appearance of a localized pigmental villonodular synovitis attached to the anteromedial joint capsule. *A,* Arthroscopic appearance. *B,* Gross pathology.

patellar pouch, especially behind a suprapatellar plica; the intercondylar notch; popliteus tunnel; posteromedial and posterolateral compartments; and the area beneath the posterior horn of the lateral meniscus.[275] The arthroscope allows a thorough evaluation of all of these areas with minimal morbidity. The etiology of the loose bodies may be determined by direct inspection of the joint surface and synovium.

Osteochondritis dissecans in the adult is a difficult lesion to manage (Fig. 6–106). In a long-term study with an average 33-year follow-up, only 10 of 48 patients with adult-onset osteochondritis dissecans did not show evidence of gonarthrosis. In these patients, the gonarthrosis begins 10 years earlier than primary gonarthrosis and more com-

monly involves all three articulations of the knee.[331] The etiology of the disorder remains controversial and includes direct or indirect trauma, ischemia, abnormal ossification, and genetic factors.[266] Radiographic evaluation should include AP, lateral, and tunnel views for visualization.[266, 296] Tomograms are very useful in the assessment of healing (Fig. 6–107). The classic location is the posterolateral aspect of the medial femoral condyle.

Arthroscopy offers evaluation of the degree of irregularity of the surface, treatment with a decreased rehabilitation time, and fewer complications than open surgery.[296] The primary objective of treatment is to save or improve the articular surface with healing of the defect and thus to avoid arthrosis.[296] Lesions may be classified on the basis of

Figure 6–106. A, Tunnel radiograph of osteochondritis dissecans of the medial femoral condyles of a 21-year-old man. *B,* Arthroscopic appearance of fragmentation of the articular cartilage overlying the lesion. *C,* Arthroscopic appearance of lesion with loose body.

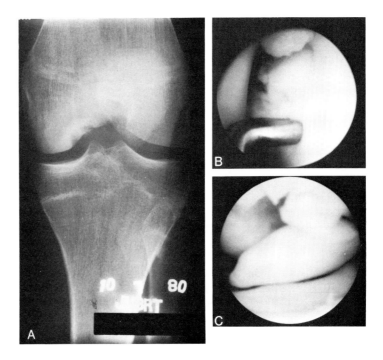

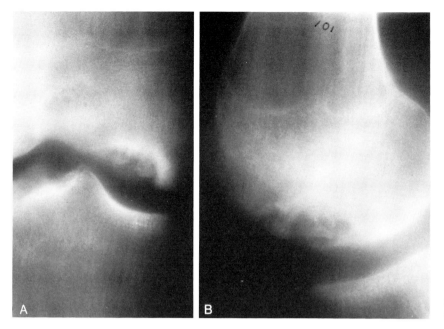

Figure 6–107. AP *(A)* and lateral *(B)* to-mograms showing healing osteochondritis dissecans.

their arthroscopic appearance into the following types: intact, early separation, partially detached, and crater with loose bodies.[296] Lesions should be classified according to location. Lesions of the medial femoral condyle are classified as central, centrolateral, and inferocentral, while those of the lateral femoral condyle are inferocentral, lateral, or anterior.[296] Surgical intervention is indicated for patients over the age of 12 with lesions greater than 1 cm in size located in the weight-bearing area.[296] The type of treatment depends upon the stage of the lesion and varies from drilling of intact lesions to trimming the bed and removal of a loose fragment.[296] Of 49 knees treated arthroscopically, 44 healed in an average time of 5 months.[296]

Arthroscopic techniques have been applied to the management of synovial disorders. Crystalline synovitis associated with chondrocalcinosis may be improved by arthroscopic lavage and debridement (Fig. 6–108).[348] An improvement in symptoms occurred in 16 of 17 knees treated by arthroscopic means.[348] Synovectomy of the knee may be performed arthroscopically in the management of the

rheumatoid patient who is unresponsive to non-operative management.[253, 310] In 33 knees treated with arthroscopic synovectomy with a mean follow-up of 44 months, 70 percent were symptomatically improved.[253]

Arthroscopy has also been applied to the evaluation and management of patellar disorders. The advantages of arthroscopic visualization of patellofemoral relationships include the ability to follow dynamic changes on flexion-extension of the knee. The position of the apex of the patella relative to the intercondylar notch gives valuable information concerning patellar tracking.[283, 362] A study of incremental patellar tracking with knee flexion revealed slight patellar subluxation of 0°, subluxation with patellofemoral contact at 20°, and centering of the patella in the trochlear groove of the femur by 40° to 60° of flexion.[283] These arthroscopic findings aid in the interpretation of radiographs of the patellofemoral joint made in varying degrees of knee flexion. Arthroscopy allows visualization of the articular surface of the patella and the extent of chondromalacia (Fig. 6–109). Debridement of the

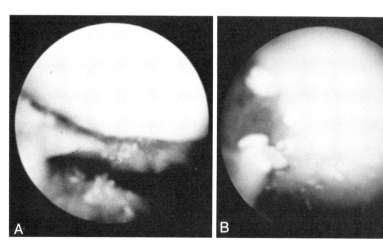

Figure 6–108. A, Arthroscopic appearance of chondrocalcinosis of the menisci. *B,* Chondrocalcinosis in the articular cartilage.

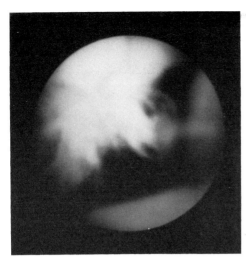

Figure 6–109. Arthroscopic appearance of chondromalacia of the patella. (From Rand, J. A.: The role of arthroscopy in the management of knee injuries in the athlete. Mayo Clin. Proc. *59:*77, 1984.)

patella may be performed. Lateral retinacular release may be performed under arthroscopic control in management of patellar chondromalacia or malalignment.[339, 362, 368]

Arthroscopy is currently being applied to the management of a variety of other knee disorders. Degenerative joint disease may be improved by arthroscopic lavage and debridement (Fig. 6–110). Exposed areas of bone may be drilled to encourage fibrocartilaginous ingrowth. Recently, a technique of abrasion arthroplasty has been applied to areas of exposed bone for this purpose.[324] A superficial debridement of dead and sclerotic bone to a depth of 1 mm is performed until active bleeding is identified. Two-year results have revealed that 75 per cent of the patients improved, with some evidence of an increasing joint space on radiographs.[324]

In summary, arthrography and arthroscopy are complementary in the evaluation of knee disorders. Arthroscopy allows the surgical management of a

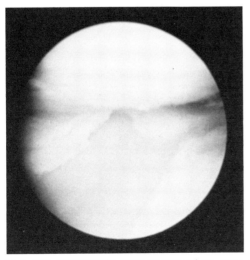

Figure 6–110. Arthroscopic appearance of an area of exposed bone on the medial tibial plateau and femoral condyle in a patient with osteoarthritis.

variety of lesions with less morbidity than arthrotomy. However, experience is extremely important with either technique in order to obtain optimal information and results.

TOTAL KNEE ARTHROPLASTY

Total knee arthroplasty is an accepted method for treatment of the knee with severe arthrosis. A wide variety of prosthetic designs and techniques are available. The results of total knee arthroplasty vary with the pathology, prosthesis utilized, and surgical technique. An understanding of the biomechanics of knee replacement, prosthetic choices available, results of prosthetic replacement, and proper component positioning are necessary for optimal patient management.

Biomechanics

Normal knee mechanics have been reviewed in an earlier section of this chapter. To review, the normal knee is a modified hinge joint with one degree of freedom, three constraint forces, and two moments. Three types of motion are possible: sliding, spinning, and rolling. Sliding motion has no change in the point of contact of the moving body and represents pure translation. The instantaneous center of rotation is at infinity. This type of motion results in high friction and wear. Spinning motion has no change in the contact point of the fixed body. The instantaneous center of rotation is at the center of the moving object. Spinning motion results in moderate friction and wear. In rolling motion, the areas of contact of the two moving surfaces are the same length. The instantaneous center of rotation is at the point of contact. Rolling motion offers the least friction and wear of the three types.

Normal knee motion is a combination of rolling and spinning motion, resulting in moderate frictional forces. Prosthetic design may mimic combinations of these motions or simulate normal knee motion, depending upon the extent of constraint of the prosthesis. The unconstrained prosthesis that only attempts resurfacing, such as the polycentric prosthesis, allows a combination of rolling and spinning motion similar to the normal knee. The semiconstrained prostheses, such as the geometric, allow spinning motion only, as do such fully constrained hinges as the Guepar prosthesis.

There are advantages and disadvantages to the use of unconstrained, semiconstrained, or constrained prostheses. Prosthesis choice must include decisions regarding which surfaces to replace, whether or not to substitute for ligament function, how to balance motion and stability, and how to protect the bone-cement interface from excessive stress to minimize loosening. Obviously, these are complex goals and are in some measure mutually exclusive. The needs of each patient vary, and

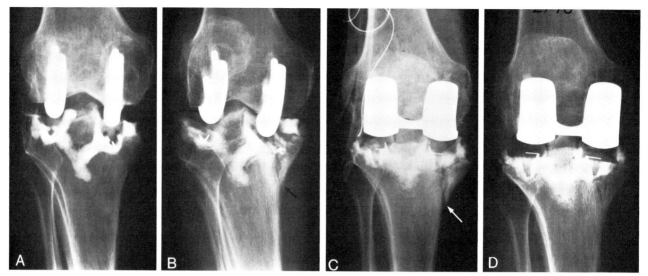

Figure 6–111. A, AP radiograph of polycentric prosthesis. B, Stress fracture of medial tibial plateau. C, Revision to a geometric prosthesis at the time of fracture. D, Six months following revision with union of the fracture. (From Rand, J. A., and Coventry, M. B.: Stress fractures of the tibia following total knee arthroplasty. J. Bone Joint Surg. 62A:226, 1980.)

therefore one prosthetic design is not optimal for all patients. Optimal prosthetic design should replace diseased or worn articular surfaces while retaining functioning ligamentous and muscular restraints.[387] The components should allow distraction, sliding, and rolling motion; avoid shear stress and allow only compressive stress to the bone; preserve all soft tissues and restore them to their normal tension; and maintain a large enough area of contact to avoid damage to the prosthetic components.[387]

Attempts to resurface the bone with small components that are totally unconstrained allow normal motion of the knee and minimize shear on the bone-cement interface but place large compressive stresses on the prosthesis and underlying bone.[408] The increased stresses may lead to prosthetic failure or fracture of the cancellous bone.[409] If the components bear load through large areas of contact, they must be of a conforming design, which results in large shear and tension stresses being transmitted to the bone-cement interface.[387] Therefore, a compromise in design must be accepted. Some incongruity of component design with increased stress on the components is necessary if the advantages of unconstrained movement with decreased stress on the bone-cement interface are to be realized.[387] If the prosthesis substitutes for ligamentous function so that tensile loads are not borne by the soft tissues, the shear and tension is necessarily transmitted to the bone-cement interface, resulting in loosening.[387] This mechanism explains the high failure rate of the constrained hinge prosthesis. Therefore, there must be a balance between stability and loosening of the prosthesis.

The choice of prosthetic design must consider the needs of the patient for normal function. Knee motion of 100° to 110° of flexion is necessary for arising from a chair or descending stairs.[399] Approx-

imately 7° of abduction-adduction occurs during walking, which distributes force across the tibial plateau.[399] Thirteen degrees of rotation are used in level walking.[399]

Gait analysis following total knee arthroplasty has recorded significant deviation from normal, reflecting altered kinematics. Abnormalities that have been noted include a shorter than normal stride length, reduced midstance knee flexion, and abnormal patterns of external flexion-extension movement of the knee.[378] However, total knee arthroplasty may provide excellent function in a highly selected group of patients with monarticular disease.[416] In a series of 12 patients studied at 2 years following duopatellar total knee arthroplasty, gait velocity; stride length; arc of motion of the hip, knee, and ankle; phasic muscle activity; and mechanical work performed were similar to controls.[416] However, these patients spent 30 percent more time in double-limb stance than controls.[416] The most unconstrained prostheses with cruciate ligament retention allow greater knee motion and improved function during stair climbing than the more constrained implants.[378]

The importance of maintenance or removal of the cruciate ligaments in total knee arthroplasty has been controversial. The decision regarding the cruciate ligaments must correspond to the choice of the design of the prosthesis. If a conforming prosthetic design is utilized and the cruciate ligaments are retained, flexion of the knee is restricted owing to large constraint forces that are developed in the posterior cruciate ligament.[400] Further flexion can only be obtained at the expense of distraction between the components.[400] Low conformity of components allows anteroposterior displacements to accompany a full range of flexion, with normal forces in the posterior cruciate ligament.[400] A kinematic prosthetic design with low conformity of the components thus allows improved motion with an intact posterior cruciate ligament.[400] Therefore, if cruciate ligament retention is felt to be desirable by the surgeon, a low-conformity prosthesis should be utilized.[400, 418] Conversely, if a high-conformity prosthesis is to be utilized, the cruciate ligament should be sacrificed. A partially conforming prosthesis with partial ligament function appears to be a satisfactory compromise between stability, motion, and stress at the bone-cement interface.[418]

Tibial component loosening is believed to result from high stress levels at the bone-cement interface. Several studies of prosthetic design have attempted to minimize these forces and protect against loos-

ening. Addition of an intramedullary central peg to the tibial component aids in fixation and decreases stresses on the cancellous bone.[381, 402, 418, 420] However, an excessively long stem may result in stress shielding of the proximal tibial bone and osteopenia.[413] A long intramedullary stem would be beneficial in the presence of bone deficiency to minimize load on the weak area.[413] The addition of a metal tray to the tibial component reduces stress on the proximal tibial cancellous bone by 16 to 39 percent relative to a polyethylene component.[381] Metal components are less likely to allow cement fracture, result in lower cancellous bone stresses than polyethylene components, and are therefore

Figure 6–112. AP *(A)* and lateral *(B)* view of various semiconstrained and unconstrained prostheses. Left to right, top: kinematic condylar, cruciate condylar, anametric, Townley-Botham; bottom: porous-coated anatomic, polycentric.

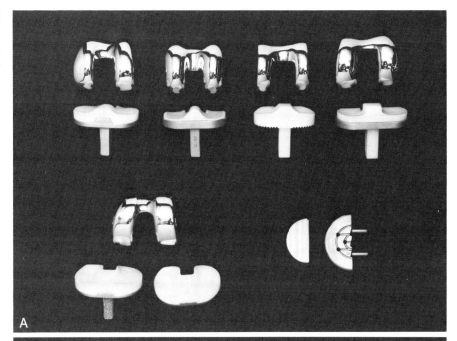

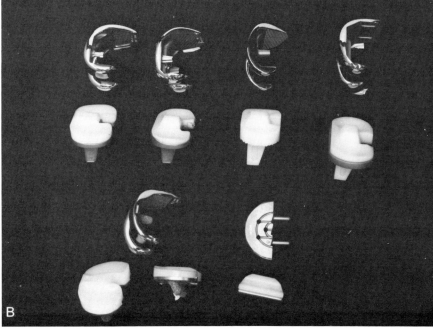

preferable.[381, 402, 420] Separate component designs for each compartment lead to increased bone-cement stresses and result in higher shear stresses than one-piece designs.[381, 402, 420] Direct transfer of the load to the cortical shell is preferable to loading on cancellous bone alone and may be best obtained with a metal-backed tibial component that contacts the tibial cortex.[381, 413]

Therefore, the choice of the prosthetic design for total knee arthroplasty should depend upon the quality of the ligaments in the affected knee; appraisal of these ligaments should figure in the decision concerning constraint. The least constrained prosthesis possible should be chosen to minimize bone-cement stresses, but the prosthesis must also be matched to the ligamentous constraints. A metal-backed tibial component with a central intramedullary peg large enough to contact the cortical rim of the tibia should be chosen. Rigidly constrained devices that do not allow rotation should be avoided.

Prosthetic Choices

A variety of prosthetic choices are available, and the number of potential prostheses is increasing. A review of all of the prostheses in use, however, would be difficult and not useful. The available prostheses may be divided into several main groups, and examples of commonly used prostheses that are typical of each group will be presented. The prostheses may be classified according to the extent of constraint to movement. Prostheses may be unconstrained, with retention of both cruciate ligaments; semiconstrained, with or without retention of only the posterior cruciate;

moderately constrained, with sacrifice of both cruciate ligaments and insertion of a central post between the femoral and tibial components; or constrained, either allowing rotation or relying upon a fixed hinge.

The classic example of the unconstrained prosthesis is the polycentric prosthesis, which consisted of four components that resurfaced the femur and tibia (Fig. 6–111). This very unconstrained design depended upon intact and functioning ligamentous restraints. The Cloutier knee is currently more frequently used as an unconstrained prosthesis. The semiconstrained prosthesis that has been most widely utilized is the total condylar prosthesis, with or without posterior cruciate retention (Fig. 6–112). The kinematic condylar, Townley, and PCA prostheses are similar but constrain movement slightly less (Fig. 6–112). The moderately constrained prostheses sacrifice both cruciate ligaments and utilize a central peg between the components for improved stability. Examples are the posterior stabilized total condylar and kinematic stabilizer prostheses (Figs. 6–113 and 6–114). The constrained implants are of two types. The older implants consisted of a fixed hinge that did not allow rotation owing to a fixed axis of rotation. The implants were large and sacrificed excessive bone. The metal on metal-bearing implants led to metallic debris in the knee. Examples of this type were the Guepar and Walldius hinges (Fig. 6–115). The newer constrained prostheses allow rotation and distraction between the components. An example is the kinematic rotating hinge (Fig. 6–113). The indications for this type of prosthesis include severe loss of bone stock and deficient collateral ligaments.[419] Satisfactory early results have been reported using the kinematic rotating hinge in 22 knees.[419]

A separate group of arthroplasties that span these

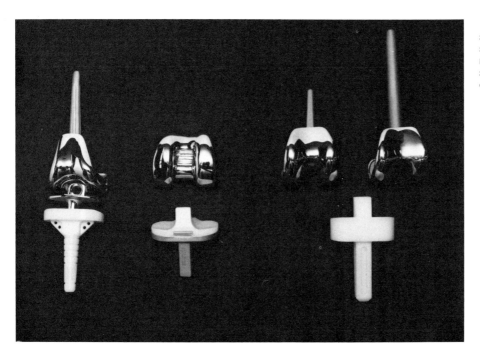

Figure 6–113. AP view of constrained and moderately constrained prostheses. Left to right: kinematic rotating hinge, kinematic stabilizer, total condylar III, total condylar III with augmented stem.

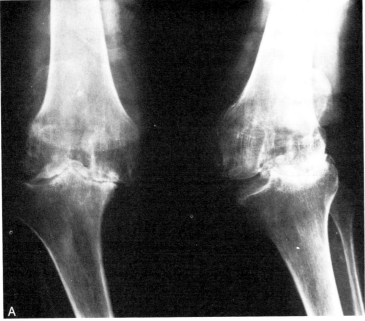
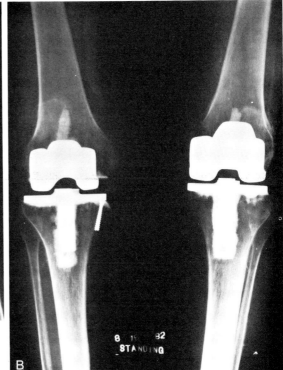

Figure 6–114. A, AP radiograph showing severe osteoarthritis. B, AP radiograph following bilateral kinematic stabilizer prosthesis.

types of prostheses may be considered. These are the revision prostheses. The revision prostheses share the need to bypass weak areas of cortical and cancellous bone in the tibia and femur and therefore have intramedullary stems for this purpose. Three of the widely used prostheses are the PCA revision, kinematic stabilizer revision, and the total condylar III prosthesis (Figs. 6–116 and 6–117). The least constrained is the PCA revision, and the most constrained is the total condylar III prosthesis. Variants of these prostheses are available with distal and posterior femoral augmentation to compensate for bone loss (Fig. 6–116). Femoral augmentation allows maintenance of the center of rotation of the knee in the correct location and allows balancing of

ligament tension in flexion and extension. Custom components are available with areas of metal build-up to aid in stress transfer to the remaining femoral cortex for difficult revisions (Fig. 6–118).[381]

The wide variety of prosthetic choices available for total knee arthroplasty presents a difficult decision for the surgeon. Which prosthesis is best? Which prosthesis should be utilized for which patient? Should some prostheses be avoided? What is the potential for salvage if infection occurs? What type of fixation of the components should be utilized? Unfortunately these questions are difficult to answer. A review of several prostheses that have been utilized in the past presents some information that helps to answer these questions.

Text continued on page 376

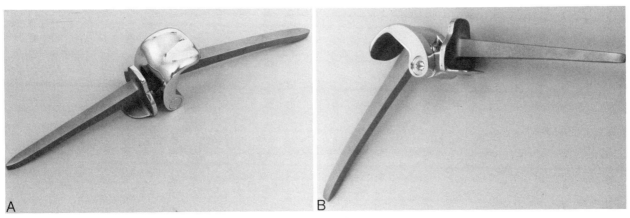

Figure 6–115. AP *(A)* and lateral *(B)* view of fully constrained Guepar hinge.

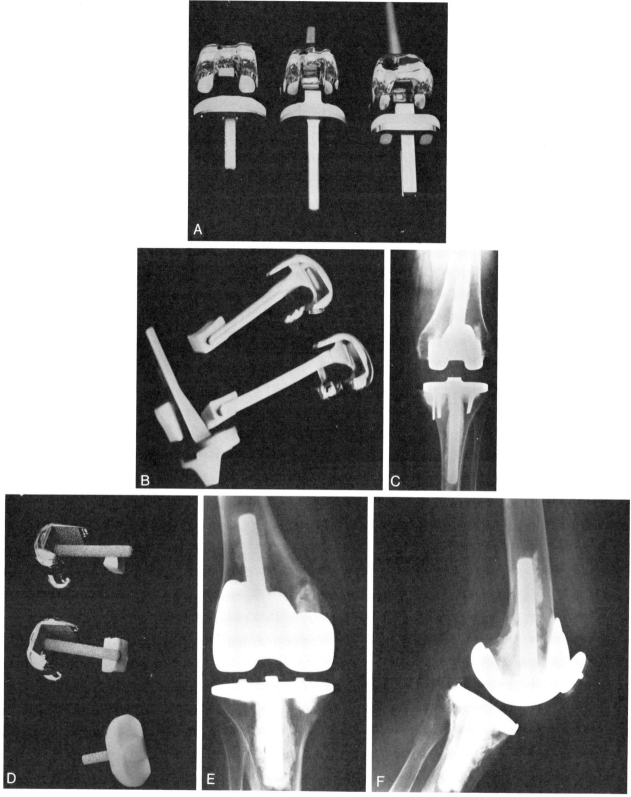

Figure 6–116. *A*, Revision prostheses. Left to right: PCA revision, kinematic stabilizer revision, total condylar III augmented revision prothesis. *B* and *C*, Kinematic stabilizer. *D, E,* and *F*, PCA revision.

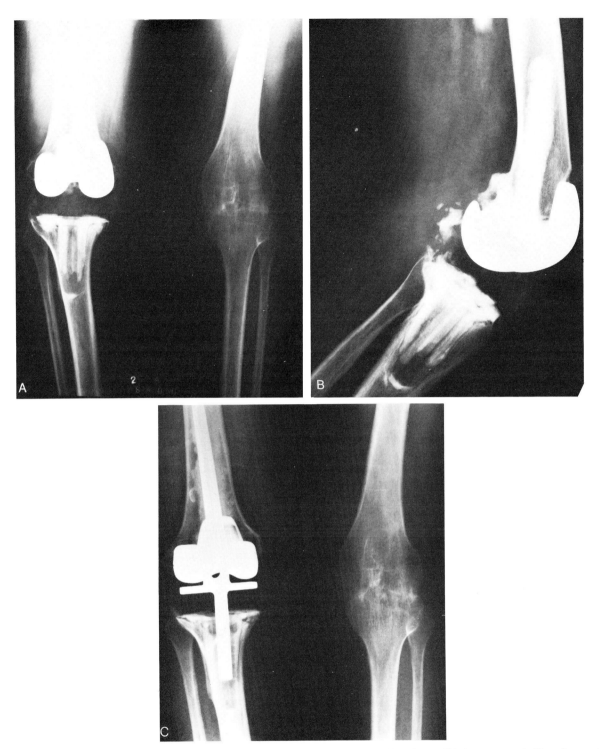

Figure 6–117. AP *(A)* and lateral *(B)* radiographs of total condyle III prosthesis with a loose tibial component. AP radiograph *(C)* following revision to a kinematic rotating hinge prosthesis.

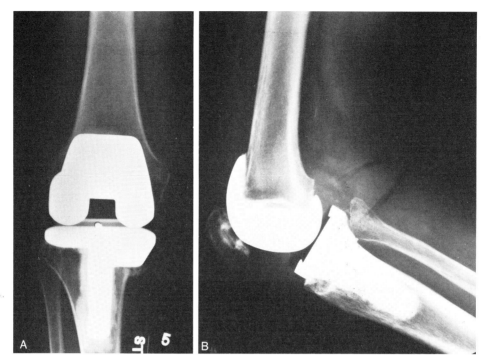

Figure 6–118. AP *(A)* and lateral *(B)* radiographs showing augmented tibial component of a modified Insall-Burstein prosthesis for use with tibial bone loss.

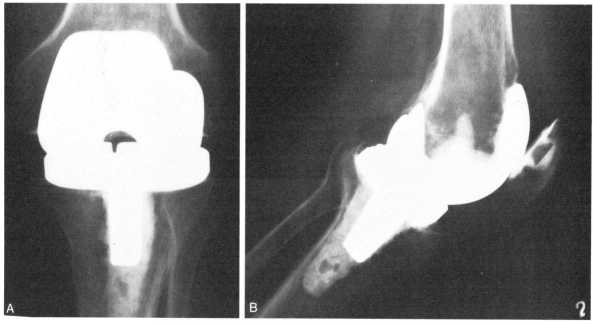

Figure 6–119. AP *(A)* and lateral *(B)* radiographs of a total condylar prosthesis.

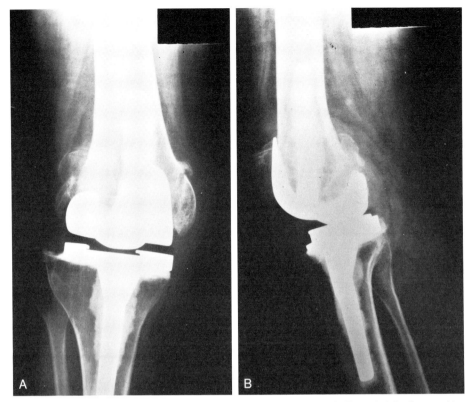

Figure 6–120. AP *(A)* and lateral *(B)* radiographs of a variable axis prosthesis. There is infection and loosening.

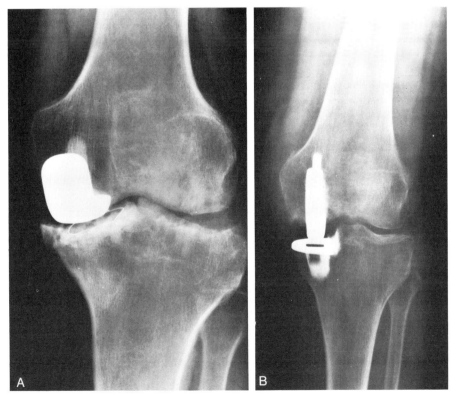

Figure 6–121. A, AP radiograph of unicompartmental Marmor prosthesis. B, AP radiograph of unicompartmental polycentric total knee.

The rigid hinge prostheses were the earliest design. Only flexion-extension motion was allowed, and no attempt was made to simulate normal knee kinematics. The concept of the Guepar hinge prosthesis was a simple design for individuals who would require only a minimum amount of use.[404] Unfortunately, the metal on metal-bearing surfaces led to wear debris in the joint, and constraint led to loosening of the prosthesis and cement. The Walldius prosthesis was a hinged prosthesis originally designed to be used without cement, although many were cemented.[396] Fully constrained hinges were rarely satisfactory for long periods of time, and even in early series these prostheses showed an unacceptable infection rate of 5 to 7.5 percent.[385, 396, 404] The infection rate associated with the Shier hinge has been as high as 12.5 percent.[379]

The use of an unconstrained prosthesis was initially advocated by Gunston in the design of the polycentric prosthesis (see Fig. 6–111A).[388] The concept of the prosthesis was to allow normal knee motion. In an early review of the 565 prostheses, the infection rate was 2.3 percent, but problems with instability and bone fracture occurred in an additional 3.4 percent.[407] A 10-year follow-up of this arthroplasty has revealed a 41.6 percent success rate in 209 knees, with failures due to instability in 12.9 percent, loosening in 7.2 percent, and infection in 3.3 percent.[401] The geometric prosthesis preserved both cruciate ligaments but had constraint designed into the femoral and tibial components to provide additional stability.[383, 384] Failures occurred with both the geometric and polycentric components owing to design problems that led to stress concentration in the proximal tibia.[406, 409] The stress concentration led to loosening and bone fracture (see Fig. 6–111).

The total condylar knee prosthesis is an improved semiconstrained design that allows patellar resurfacing (Fig. 6–119). The prosthesis may be utilized for a wide range of deformities when combined with appropriate soft tissue balancing.[393, 395] At a 3- to 5-year follow-up of 220 knees, 90 percent were good to excellent.[395] Complications of infection were present in 1.4 percent, and instability appeared in 1.9 percent.[395] At a mean of 6.6 years of follow-up of 100 knees in 79 patients with osteoarthritis, there were satisfactory results in 91 knees.[393] Nine prostheses required revision, only 2 of which were for loosening.[393] A modification of this prosthesis with a central peg to compensate for the posterior cruciate ligament had revealed 88 percent good or excellent results in 119 cases at 2 to 4 years of follow-up.[394]

The variable axis knee was designed to provide rotational motion but also provided anteroposterior and mediolateral stability by a nonlinked central ball and socket configuration (Fig. 6–120). The addition of intramedullary stems allowed proximal stress transfer. In a review of 52 knees followed for a minimum of 2 years, 79 percent good or excellent results were reported.[405] The spherocentric prosthesis was designed as an intrinsically stable, linked prosthesis that was capable of triaxial rotation.[398] Of 82 knees followed from 2 to 6 years, infection occurred in 4 percent and loosening in 5 percent.[398]

Unicompartmental replacement has been advocated for the older patient with medial or lateral compartment disease. Advantages of unicompartmental replacement include preservation of bone stock, cruciate ligaments, the patellofemoral joint, and the opposite normal compartment.[415] Complications related to this technique include loosening and progression of disease in an unresurfaced compartment.[397] With this technique satisfactory results have been obtained in 89 percent of 184 knees[397] and in 92 percent of 114 knees[415] (Fig. 6–121).

One of the major complications of total knee arthroplasty has been prosthetic loosening at the bone-cement or prosthesis-cement interface (Fig. 6–122). Newer prosthetic designs are being utilized without cement to achieve biologic fixation by bony ingrowth or bony interlock. One approach is the ICLH prosthesis, which achieves fixation by polyethylene pegs on the tibial component; this results in an interference fit in the cancellous bone (Fig. 6–123).[382, 386] Bone does not grow into this type of prosthesis; rather, a fibrous interface forms between the prosthesis and bone.[382] Results with an uncemented tibial component of the ICLH design with 2 years of follow-up in 52 patients have been satisfactory in 51, with no evidence of loosening.[386] The other approach to biologic fixation has been to encourage bony ingrowth into a porous-coated metal surface on the components. Relative contrain-

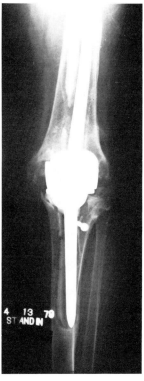

Figure 6–122. AP radiograph of loose Guepar prosthesis.

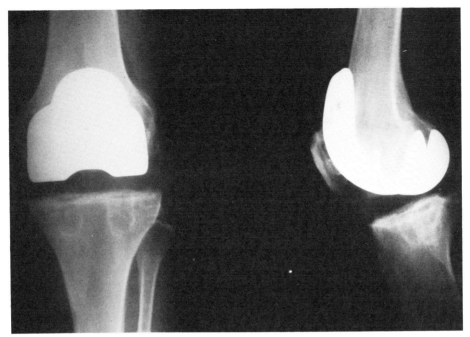

Figure 6–123. AP (left) and lateral (right) radiographs of ICLH prosthesis inserted without cement.

dications to porous ingrowth fixation include deficient bone that is osteosclerotic, osteoporotic, or missing, or poor surgical technique that does not allow immediate stability of the implant.[391] Satisfactory results without loosening have been reported for 16 PCA knees followed for a minimum of 6 months.[391] At an average of 1 year of follow-up of 26 knees with the PCA prosthesis, good or excellent results were present in 93.5 percent, with no evi-

dence of interface failure between the prosthesis and cement.[390] The advantages of fixation without cement are decreased surgical time, lack of acrylic debris that may induce wear, and maximal bone stock if revision is subsequently required.[390, 391] The PCA prosthesis is one example of this type of design (Fig. 6–124). Early results with both types of fixation appear promising but require exacting technique for proper insertion.

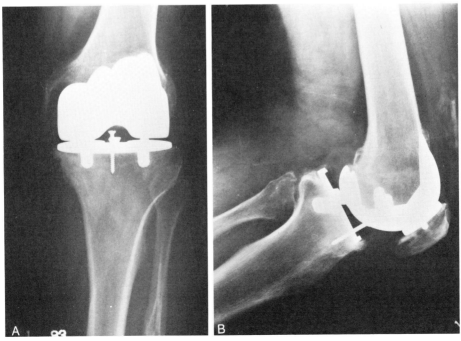

Figure 6–124. AP *(A)* and lateral *(B)* radiographs of an uncemented PCA total knee at 1 year.

Techniques

Surgical technique is as important or more important than prosthetic selection for prosthetic function. The basic principles of insertion are correct axial alignment, soft tissue balance that confers stability, and proper component orientation. A positive correlation exists between proper roentgenographic positioning of a prosthesis and clinical findings in the patient.[403] Correct axial alignment is the key to appropriate force balance between the medial and lateral compartments of the knee. Loss of stance-phase flexion-extension, flexion deformity, and either varus or valgus deformity increase the force per unit area applied to the prosthetic im-

plant.[399] Using the ICLH prosthesis, a 91 percent failure rate was noted for knees aligned in varus compared with 11 percent failure for knees in valgus.[380] A significant correlation has been noted between loosening and a postoperative alignment of less than 7° of valgus for the spherocentric prosthesis.[398] Failure to correct axial alignment has also been noted to correlate with fatigue fracture of the tibia and component loosening.[409]

The ideal placement for the tibial component in a total condylar knee arthroplasty is 90° ± 5° to the long axis of the tibial shaft on both the AP and lateral roentgenograms.[393, 395] Correct placement of the femoral component is 5° to 7° ± 5° of valgus on the AP roentgenogram and 90° ± 5° on the lateral

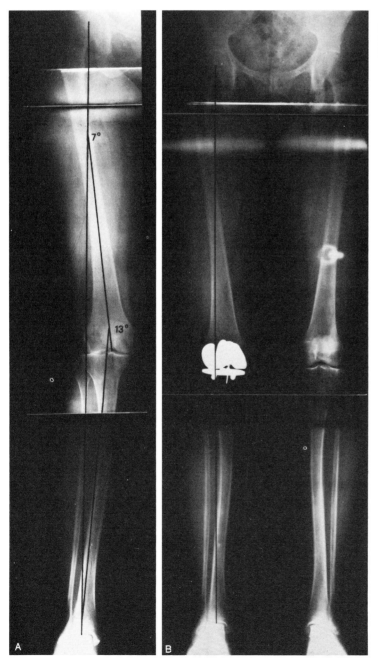

Figure 6–125. A, Full-length radiograph to determine the mechanical axis preoperatively. B, Radiograph postoperatively after insertion of an uncemented PCA prosthesis.

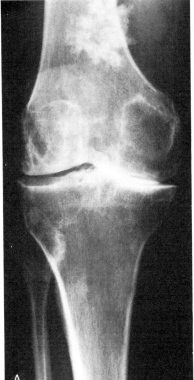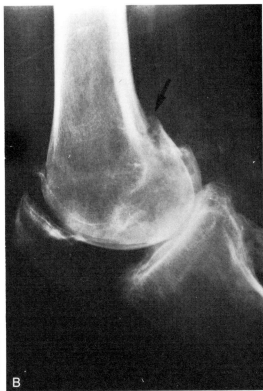

Figure 6–126. AP *(A)* and lateral *(B)* radiographs of a patient with osteoarthritis. Note the fracture in the lateral femoral condyle posteriorly *(arrow)*.

roentgenogram.[393, 395] For the PCA prosthesis, a 3° varus cut on the tibia in the AP roentgenogram has been recommended.[390, 391] The varus cut maintains the tibial component's perpendicular orientation to the mechanical axis of the limb, since the ankles are closer together than the knees.[390, 391] A full-length standing AP roentgenogram is necessary to define the mechanical axis and to decide upon the degree of valgus placement of the femoral component, for these depend upon the width of the pelvis (Fig. 6–125).

Lucent lines are commonly present following total knee arthroplasty. A 22 percent incidence of incomplete radiolucent lines about either component has been reported following total condylar prosthetic replacement.[393, 395] At a mean of 6.6 years of follow-up, 41 percent of a series of 100 total condylar knees had some radiolucency, but none were complete or circumferential lines.[393] The radiolucency was present by the end of the first year, and in 81 percent there was no further change.[393] A 32 percent incidence of incomplete tibial lucent lines has been found about a slightly more constrained posterior stabilized condylar prosthesis.[394] The presence of an incomplete lucent line at the bone-cement interface does not signify clinical failure of the arthroplasty.[412] Criteria for definitive diagnosis of loosening are (1) serial roentgenograms showing a definite change in position of the prosthesis relative to the bone, (2) stress roentgenograms revealing motion between the prosthesis and bone, and (3) motion detected at subsequent surgery.[398] Lucent lines are a common finding following revision of a total knee arthro-

plasty, appearing in up to 84 percent of patients.[389] But lucent lines do not appear to correlate with the clinical result of the patient.[411]

Preoperative evaluation of the patient for total knee arthroplasty should include standing AP views to assess axial alignment, extent of compartmental involvement, and evidence of subluxation indicating instability; lateral views to assess possible bone loss (Fig. 6–126); and patellar views to evaluate patellar alignment and the patellofemoral joint space. Tc-99m bone scanning is helpful in evaluating the extent of compartmental involvement in difficult cases (Fig. 6–127).[417] Computed tomography and tomograms may be useful in assessing the quality of bone stock in post-traumatic situations and in obtaining bony dimensions for custom prostheses.[414]

Radiographic Study of Total Knee Arthroplasties

The radiographic study of a total knee arthroplasty should evaluate component position, axial alignment, loosening, patellar position, stability, possible infection, integrity of the components, cement debris, and bony integrity.[414] The minimal radiographs should include a standing AP x-ray to evaluate axial alignment, component position, and tibial loosening; a lateral view to assess component alignment and femoral loosening; and a patellar view at 30° to 45° of flexion to evaluate patellar alignment and loosening. Additional radiographs

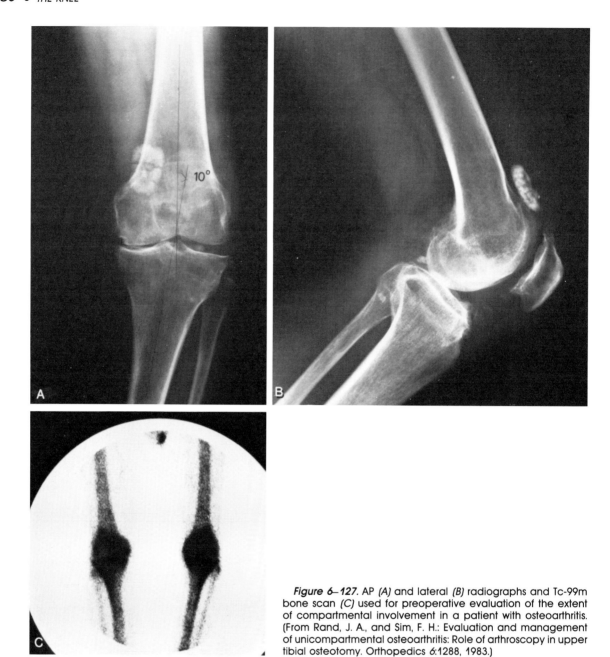

Figure 6–127. AP *(A)* and lateral *(B)* radiographs and Tc-99m bone scan *(C)* used for preoperative evaluation of the extent of compartmental involvement in a patient with osteoarthritis. (From Rand, J. A., and Sim, F. H.: Evaluation and management of unicompartmental osteoarthritis: Role of arthroscopy in upper tibial osteotomy. Orthopedics 6:1288, 1983.)

Figure 6–128. AP *(A)* and lateral *(B)* fluoroscopic views of PCA bone ingrowth prosthesis. Fluoroscopy allows exact bone radiographs to assess the bone-prosthesis interface.

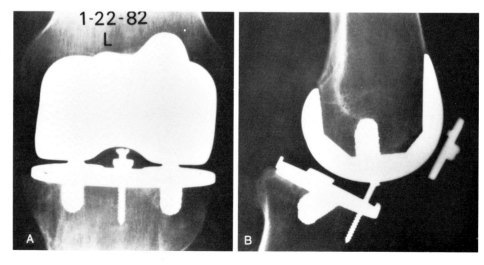

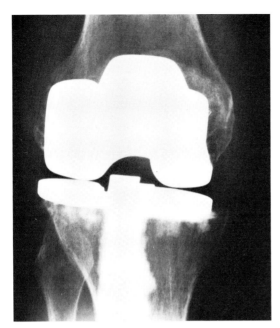

Figure 6–129. AP radiograph of kinematic condylar prosthesis with slight lateral position of the tibial component. The tibial cut is in slight varus.

may be obtained, including a full-length standing AP view of both lower extremities for the mechanical axis (Fig. 6–127); fluoroscopic views for evaluation of lucent lines or bony ingrowth (Fig. 6–128); and stress views for defining instability. These radiographs will usually suffice for most purposes.

Component position should be carefully assessed in relation to the femur and tibia. Appropriate angulation of the components as well as anteroposterior and mediolateral placement should be studied. Translation of the components medially or laterally should be avoided to prevent excessive stress in one compartment (Fig. 6–129). Notching of the anterior femoral cortex may lead to supracondylar fracture (Fig. 6–130), or excessive tibial component angulation combined with varus may lead to stress fracture of the medial tibial plateau (see Fig. 6–114).[409] Instability is often evident on routine radiographs as widening of the joint space (Fig. 6–131). Fracture of a component may easily be seen (Fig. 6–132).

Lucent lines should be sought and reported regarding width, location, and extent (Fig. 6–133). A complete lucent line greater than 2 mm in width or a progressive increase in size of a lucent line on serial radiographs is usually indicative of loosening.[410] Sclerosis of the bone adjacent to the lucent line often indicates a repair process and stabilization of the underlying bone.[410] An irregular or indistinct border between the cancellous bone and the lucent line is more likely to be indicative of loosening.[410] Arthrography may be helpful in the assessment of loosening in selected cases but is usually not necessary.[414]

Evaluation of infection is difficult on the basis of radiographs. A clinical history suggestive of infection, such as excessive prolonged pain, drainage, fever, or a postoperative hematoma, is helpful in

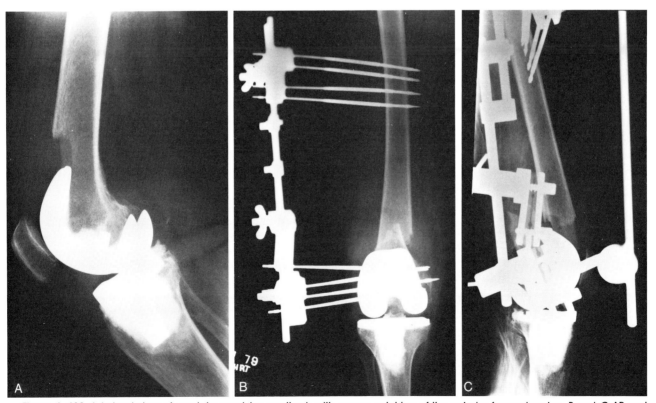

Figure 6–130. A, Lateral view of cruciate condylar prosthesis with severe notching of the anterior femoral cortex. B and C, AP and lateral radiographs showing subsequent supracondylar femoral fracture being treated with a Hoffman external fixation device.

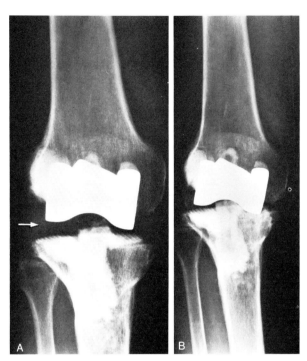

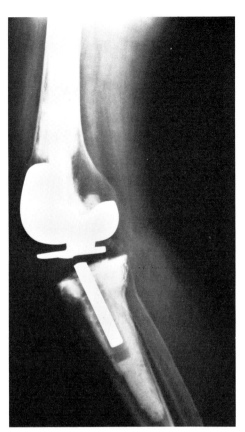

Figure 6–131. A, AP radiograph of anametric prosthesis with poor soft tissue balance as evidenced by widening of the lateral joint space (arrow). B, Two years later there has been subsidence of the tibial component and recurrent varus deformity.

Figure 6–132. Fracture of the stem of a kinematic rotating hinge prosthesis of the original design. The design has subsequently been modified.

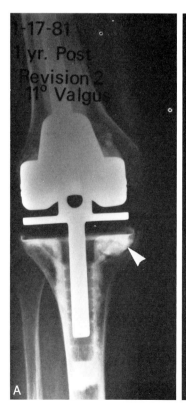

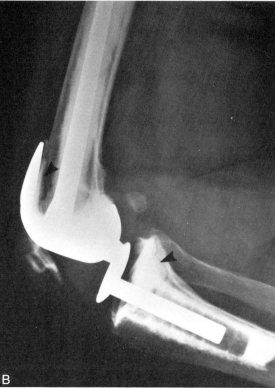

Figure 6–133. AP (A) and lateral (B) radiographs showing incomplete lucent lines about a kinematic rotating hinge prosthesis used for revision.

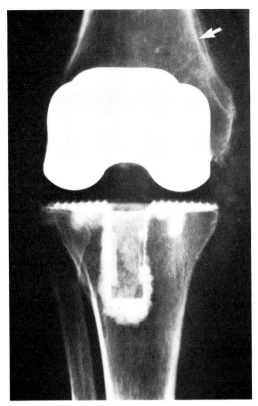

Figure 6–134. AP radiograph of long-standing infection of a total condylar prosthesis. There is periosteal new bone formation on the medial aspect of the femur.

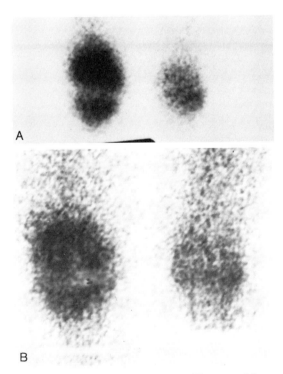

Figure 6–135. Tc-99m *(A)* and gallium *(B)* scans of the prosthesis in Figure 6–134. There is increased uptake about the infected implant.

assessment. Radiographs may reveal periosteal new bone formation in long-standing cases of infection (Fig. 6–134). Aspiration of the knee may or may not be helpful.[410] Differential Tc-99m and gallium bone scans may be a useful adjunct in difficult cases (Fig. 6–135).[410] The gallium scan should show increased uptake relative to the Tc-99m scan to be considered positive. Bone scanning is not a useful criterion by itself for assessment of loosening.[392]

In conclusion, a thorough knowledge of the biomechanics of the normal knee and the mechanics of the various types of prosthetic replacements available is central to an appropriate matching of the prosthesis to the patient's needs. An understanding of proper component insertion with careful technique will aid in minimizing prosthetic failure and the need for revision. Careful preoperative and postoperative assessments of the knee are essential for evaluation of the success of the procedure.

REFERENCES

Anatomy and Biomechanics of the Knee

1. Alm, A., Ekstrom, H., Gillquist, J., et al.: The anterior cruciate ligament. Acta Chir. Scand. (Suppl.) *445*:3, 1974.
2. Arnoczky, S.: Anatomy of the anterior cruciate ligament. Clin. Orthop. *172*:19, 1983.
3. Bartel, D. L., Marshall, J. L., Schieck, R. A., et al.: Surgical repositioning of the medial collateral ligament. J. Bone Joint Surg. *59A*:107, 1977.
4. Blacharski, P. A., and Somerset, J. H.: A three dimensional study of the kinematics of the human knee. J. Biomech. *8*:375, 1975.
5. Brantigan, O. C., and Voshell, A. F.: The mechanics of the ligaments and menisci of the knee joint. J. Bone Joint Surg. *23*:44, 1941.
6. Bullough, P. G., and Walker, P. S.: The distribution of load through the knee joint and its possible significance to the observed patterns of articular cartilage breakdown. Bull. Hosp. J. Dis. *37*:110, 1976.
7. Burke, D. L., Ahmed, A. M., and Miller J.: A biomechanical study of partial and total medial meniscectomy of the knee. Orthop. Trans. *1*:130, 1977–1978.
8. Butler, D. L., Noyes, F. R., and Grood, E. S.: Ligamentous restraints to anterior-posterior drawer in the human knee. J. Bone Joint Surg. *62A*:259, 1980.
9. Butler, D. L., Noyes, F. R., Grood, E. S., et al.: Mechanical properties of transplants for the anterior cruciate ligament. Orthop. Trans. *3*:180, 1979.
10. Clancy, W. G., Narechania, R. G., Rosenberg, T. D., et al.: Anterior and posterior cruciate ligament reconstruction in rhesus monkeys. J. Bone Joint Surg. *63A*:1270, 1981.
11. Crowinshield, R., Pope, M. H., and Johnson, R. J.: An analytical model of the knee. J. Biomech. *9*:397, 1976.
12. Denham, R. R., and Bishop, R. E. D.: Mechanics of the knee and problems in reconstructive surgery. J. Bone Joint Surg. *60B*:345, 1978.
13. Fairbank, T. J.: Knee joint changes after meniscectomy. J. Bone Joint Surg. *30B*:664, 1948.
14. Frankel, V. H.: Biomechanics of the knee. Orthop. Clin. North Am. *2*:175, 1971.
15. Frankel, V. H., Burstein, A. H., and Brooks, D. B.: Biomechanics of internal derangement of the knee. J. Bone Joint Surg. *53A*:945, 1971.
16. Freeman, B. L., Beaty, J. H., and Haynes, D. B.: The pes anserinus transfer. J. Bone Joint Surg. *64A*:202, 1982.
17. Fukubayashi, T., and Kurosawa, H.: The contact area and

pressure distribution pattern of the knee. Acta Orthop. Scand. 51:871, 1980.

18. Fukubayashi, T., and Torzilli, P.: An *in vitro* biomechanical evaluation of anterior-posterior motion of the knee. J. Bone Joint Surg. 64A:258, 1982.

19. Furman, W., Marshall, J., and Girgis, F. G.: The anterior cruciate ligament. J. Bone Joint Surg. 58A:179, 1976.

20. Girgis, F., and Marshall, J.: The cruciate ligaments of the knee joint. Clin. Orthop. 106:216, 1975.

21. Gray, H., and Goss, C. M.: Anatomy of the Human Body. 28th Ed. Philadelphia, Lea and Febiger, 1972.

22. Grood, E., and Noyes, F.: Cruciate ligament prosthesis: Strength, creep and fatigue properties. J. Bone Joint Surg. 58A:1083, 1976.

23. Grood, E., Noyes, F., Butler, D. L., et al.: Ligamentous and capsular restraints preventing straight medial and lateral laxity in intact human cadaver knees. J. Bone Joint Surg. 63A:1257, 1981.

24. Harrington, I.: Static and dynamic loading patterns in knee joints with deformities. J. Bone Joint Surg. 65A:247, 1983.

25. Helfet, A.: Mechanism of derangements of the medial semilunar cartilage and their management. J. Bone Joint Surg. 41B:319, 1959.

26. Hsieh, H., and Walker, P.: Stabilizing mechanisms of the loaded and unloaded knee joint. J. Bone Joint Surg. 58A:87, 1976.

27. Hughston, J., Andrews, J., Cross, M., et al.: Classification of knee ligament instabilities. Part I. The medial compartment and cruciate ligaments. J. Bone Joint Surg. 58A:159, 1976.

28. Hughston, J., Andrews, J., Cross, M., et al.: Classification of knee ligament instabilities. Part II. The lateral compartment. J. Bone Joint Surg., 58A:173, 1976.

29. Hughston, J., and Eilers, A.: The role of the posterior oblique ligament in repairs of acute medial (collateral) ligament tears of the knee. J. Bone Joint Surg. 55A:923, 1973.

30. Johnson, F., Leitl, S., and Waugh, W.: The distribution of load across the knee. J. Bone Joint Surg. 62B:346, 1980.

31. Johnson, R., Kettelkamp, D., Clark, W., et al.: Factors affecting late results after meniscectomy. J. Bone Joint Surg. 56A:719, 1974.

32. Kennedy, J., Hawkins, R., Willis, R. B., et al.: Tension studies of human knee ligaments. J. Bone Joint Surg. 58A:350, 1976.

33. Kennedy, J., Weinberg, H., and Wilson, A.: The anatomy and function of the anterior cruciate ligament. J. Bone Joint Surg. 56A:223, 1974.

34. Kettelkamp, D., and Chao, E.: A method for quantitative analysis of medial and lateral compression forces at the knee during standing. Clin. Orthop. 183:202, 1972.

35. Kettelkamp, D., and Jacobs, A.: Tibiofemoral contact area—determination and implications. J. Bone Joint Surg. 54A:349, 1972.

36. King, D.: The function of the semilunar cartilages. J. Bone Joint Surg. 18:1069, 1936.

37. Krause, W., Pope, M., Johnson, R. J., et al.: Mechanical changes in the knee after meniscectomy. J. Bone Joint Surg., 58A:599, 1976.

38. Levy, M., Torzilli, P., and Warren, R.: The effect of medial meniscectomy on anterior-posterior motion of the knee. J. Bone Joint Surg. 64A:883, 1982.

39. Lipke, J., Janecki, C., Nelson, C., et al.: The role of incompetence of the anterior cruciate and lateral ligaments in anterolateral and anteromedial instability. J. Bone Joint Surg. 63A:954, 1981.

40. Mann, R. A., and Hagy, J. L.: The popliteus muscle. J. Bone Joint Surg. 59A:924, 1977.

41. Maquet, P.: The biomechanics of the knee and the surgical possibilities of healing osteoarthritic knee joints. Clin. Orthop. 146:102, 1980.

42. Maquet, P., Van de Berg, A., and Simonet, J.: Femorotibial weight-bearing areas. J. Bone Joint Surg. 57A:766, 1975.

43. Markolf, K., Bargar, W., Shoemaker, S. C., et al.: The role of joint load in knee stability. J. Bone Joint Surg. 63A:570, 1981.

44. Markolf, K., Mensch, J., and Amstutz, H.: Stiffness and laxity of the knee—The contributions of the supporting structures. J. Bone Joint Surg. 58A:583, 1976.

45. Morrison, J. B.: Bioengineering analysis of force actions transmitted to the knee joint. Biomed. Engineering 3:164, 1968.

46. Morrison, J. B.: The mechanics of the knee joint in relation to normal walking. J. Biomech. 3:51, 1970.

47. Noyes, F., DeLucas, J., and Torvik, P.: Biomechanics of anterior cruciate ligament failure: An analysis of strain rate sensitivity and mechanism of failure in primates. J. Bone Joint Surg. 56A:236, 1974.

48. Noyes, F., and Grood, E.: The strength of the anterior cruciate ligament in humans and rhesus monkeys. J. Bone Joint Surg. 58A:1074, 1976.

49. Noyes, F., and Sonstegard, D.: Biomechanical function of the pes anserinus at the knee and the effect of its transplantation. J. Bone Joint Surg. 55A:1225, 1973.

50. Perry, J., Antonelli, D., and Ford, W.: Analysis of knee joint forces during flexed knee stance. J. Bone Joint Surg. 57A:961, 1975.

51. Pope, M., Johnson, R., and Brown, D.: The role of the musculature in injuries to the medial collateral ligament. J. Bone Joint Surg. 61A:398, 1979.

52. Reider, B., Marshall, J., Koslin, B., et al.: The anterior aspect of the knee joint. J. Bone Joint Surg. 63A:351, 1981.

53. Scapinelli, R.: Studies on the vasculature of the human knee joint. Acta Anat. 70:305, 1968.

54. Seebacher, J., Inglis, A., Marshall, J., et al.: The structure of the posterolateral aspect of the knee. J. Bone Joint Surg. 64A:536, 1982.

55. Seedhom, B., Dowson, D., and Wright, V.: Functions of the menisci: A preliminary study. J. Bone Joint Surg. 56B:381, 1974.

56. Shaw, J., and Murray, D.: The longitudinal axis of the knee and the role of the cruciate ligaments in controlling transverse rotation. J. Bone Joint Surg. 56A:1603, 1976.

57. Shoemaker, S., and Markolf, K.: *In vivo* rotatory knee stability. J. Bone Joint Surg. 64A:208, 1982.

58. Shrive, N., Phil, D., O'Connor, J. J., et al.: Load bearing in the knee joint. Clin. Orthop. 131:279, 1978.

59. Sim, F. H.: Complications and late results of meniscectomy. AAOS Symp. on Athlete's Knee, 1978.

60. Slocum, D., Larson, R., and James, S.: Late reconstruction of ligamentous injuries of the medial compartment of the knee. Clin. Orthop. 100:23, 1974.

61. Tapper, E., and Hoover, N.: Late results after meniscectomy. J. Bone Joint Surg. 51A:547, 1969.

62. Torzilli, P., Greenburg, R., and Insall, J.: An *in vivo* biomechanical evaluation of anterior-posterior motion of the knee. J. Bone Joint Surg. 63A:960, 1981.

63. Trent, P., Walker, P., and Wolf, B.: Ligament length patterns, strength, and rotation axes of the knee joint. Clin. Orthop. 117:263, 1976.

64. Walker, P., and Erkman, M.: The role of the menisci in force transmission across the knee. Clin. Orthop. 109:184, 1975.

65. Warren, F., and Marshall, J.: The supporting structures and layers on the medial side of the knee. J. Bone Joint Surg. 61A:56, 1979.

66. Warren, F., Marshall, J., and Girgis, F.: The prime static stabilizer of the medial side of the knees. J. Bone Joint Surg., 56A:665, 1974.

67. Whiteside, L., and Sweeney, R.: Nutrient pathways of the cruciate ligaments. J. Bone Joint Surg., 62A:1176, 1980.

68. Wiberg, G.: Roentgenographic and anatomic studies on the femoropatellar joint, with special reference to chondromalacia patellae. Acta Orthop. Scand. 12:319, 1941.

Routine Radiographic Techniques

69. Ballinger, P. W.: Merrill's Atlas of Roentgenographic Positions and Standard Radiologic Procedures. 5th Ed. St. Louis, C. V. Mosby, 1982.

70. Bernau, A., and Berquist, T. H.: Orthopedic Positioning in Diagnostic Radiology. Baltimore, Urban & Schwarzenberg, 1983.

71. Camp, J. D., and Coventry, M. B.: Use of special views in roentgenography of the knee joint. US Naval Med. Bull. *42:*56, 1944.

72. Englestad, B. L., Friedman, E. M., and Murphy, W. A.: Diagnosis of joint effusion on lateral and axial projections of the knee. Invest. Radiol. *16:*188, 1981.

73. Hall, F. M.: Radiographic diagnosis and accuracy in knee joint effusions. Radiology *115:*45, 1975.

74. Holmblad, E. C.: Postero-anterior x-ray view of the knee in flexion. JAMA *109:*1196, 1937.

75. Hughston, J. C.: Subluxation of the patella. J. Bone Joint Surg. *50A:*1003, 1968.

76. Jacobsen, K.: Radiologic technique for measuring instability in the knee joint. Acta Radiol. (Diagn.) *18:*113, 1977.

77. Jacobsen, K.: Stress radiographical assessment of antero-posterior, medial, and lateral instability of the knee joint. Acta Orthop. Scand. *47:*355, 1976.

78. Kimberlin, G. E.: Radiological assessment of the patello-femoral articulation and subluxation of the patella. Radiol. Technol. *45:*129, 1975.

79. Merchant, A. C., Mercar, R. L., Jacobsen, R. H., et al.: Roentgenographic analysis of the patellofemoral congru-ence. J. Bone Joint Surg., *56:*1391, 1974.

80. Settegast, H.: Typische Roentgenobilder von normalen menschen. Lehmanns Med. Atlanton *5:*211, 1921.

Patellar Disorders

81. Aglietti, P., Insall, J. N., and Cerulli, G.: Patellar pain and incongruence. I. Measurements of incongruence. Clin. Or-thop. *176:*217, 1983.

82. Aleman, O.: Chondromalacia post-traumatica patellae. Acta Chir. Scand. *63:*149, 1928.

83. Bassett, F. H. II: Acute dislocation of the patella, osteo-chondral fractures, and injuries of the extensor mechanism of the knee. Instr. Course Lect. *25:*40, 1976.

84. Bentley, G.: Chondromalacia patellae. J. Bone Joint Surg. *52A:*221, 1970.

85. Blackburne, J. S., and Peel, J. E.: A new method of meas-uring patella weight. J. Bone Joint Surg. *59B:*241, 1977.

86. Boring, T. N., and O'Donoghue, D. H.: Acute patellar dislocation: Results of immediate surgical repair. Clin. Or-thop. *136:*182, 1978.

87. Brattstrom, H.: Shape of intercondylar groove normally and in dislocation of the patella. Acta Orthop. Scand. (Suppl.) *68:*134, 1964.

88. Cofield, R. H., and Bryan, R. S.: Acute dislocation of the patella: Results of conservative treatment. J. Trauma *17:*526, 1977.

89. Crosby, E. B., and Insall, J.: Recurrent dislocation of the patella. J. Bone Joint Surg., *58A:*9, 1976.

90. DeHaven, K. E., Dolan, W. A., and Mayer, P. J.: Chondro-malacia patellae in athletes: Clinical presentation and con-servative management. Am. J. Sports Med. *7:*5, 1979.

91. Delgado-Martins, H.: A study of the position of the patella using computerized tomography. J. Bone Joint Surg., *61B:*443, 1976.

92. Ferguson, A. B., Brown, T. D., Fu, F. H., et al.: Relief of patellofemoral contact stress by anterior displacement of the tibial tubercle. J. Bone Joint Surg. *61A:*159, 1979.

93. Ficat, R. P., and Hungerford, D. S.: Disorders of the Patellofemoral Joint. Baltimore, Williams and Wilkins, 1977.

94. Ficat, R. P., Philippe, J., and Hungerford, D. S.: Chondro-malacia patellae: A system of classification. Clin. Orthop. *144:*55, 1979.

95. Freiberger, R. H., and Kozier, L. M.: Fracture of the medial margin of the patella: A finding diagnostic of lateral dislo-cation. Radiology *88:*902, 1967.

96. Goodfellow, J. W., Hungerford, D. S., and Woods, C.: Patellofemoral joint mechanics and pathology. II. Chon-dromalacia patellae. J. Bone Joint Surg. *58B:*291, 1976.

97. Goodfellow, J. W., Hungerford, D. S., and Zindel, M.: Patellofemoral mechanics and pathology: I. Functional anat-omy of the patellofemoral joint. J. Bone Joint Surg. *58B:*287, 1976.

98. Gruber, M. A.: The conservative treatment of chondroma-lacia patellae. Orthop. Clin. North Am. *10:*105, 1979.

99. Heywood, A. W. B.: Recurrent dislocation of the patella. J. Bone Joint Surg. *43B:*508, 1961.

100. Horns, J. W.: The diagnosis of chondromalacia by double contrast arthrography of the knee. J. Bone Joint Surg. *59A:*119, 1977.

101. Hughston, J. C.: Subluxation of the patella. J. Bone Joint Surg. *50A:*1003, 1968.

102. Hungerford, D. S., and Barry, M.: Biomechanics of the patellofemoral joint. Clin. Orthop. *144:*9, 1979.

103. Insall, J. N., Aglietti, P., and Tria, A. J.: Patellar pain and incongruence. II. Clinical application. Clin. Orthop. *176:*225, 1983.

104. Insall, J. N., Falvo, K. A., and Wise, D. N.: Chondromalacia patellae. J. Bone Joint Surg. *58A:*1, 1976.

105. Insall, J. N., and Salvati, E.: Patella position in the normal knee joint. Radiology *101:*101, 1971.

106. Jackson, R. W.: Examination of the patella. Instr. Course Lect. *25:*31, 1976.

107. Jackson, R. W.: Etiology of chondromalacia patellae. Instr. Course Lect. *25:*36, 1976.

108. Kaufer, H.: Mechanical function of the patella. J. Bone Joint Surg. *53A:*1551, 1971.

109. Kaufer, H.: Patellar biomechanics. Clin. Orthop. *144:*51, 1979.

110. Kettelkamp, D. B.: Management of patellar malalignment. J. Bone Joint Surg. *63A:*1334, 1981.

111. Kettelkamp, D. B., and DeRosa, G. P.: Biomechanics and functional rehabilitation of the patellofemoral joint. Instr. Course Lect. *25:*27, 1976.

112. Larsen, E., and Lauridsen, F.: Conservative treatment of patellar dislocations. Influence of evident factors on the tendency to redislocate and the therapeutic result. Clin. Orthop. *171:*131, 1982.

113. Larson, R. L.: Subluxation-dislocation of the patella. *In* Kennedy, J. C. (ed.): The Injured Adolescent Knee. Balti-more, Williams and Wilkins, 1979.

114. Larson, R. L., Cabaud, H. E., Slocum, D. B., et al.: The patellar compression syndrome: Surgical treatment by lat-eral release. Clin. Orthop. *134:*158, 1978.

115. Laurin, C. A., Dussault, R., and Levesque, H. P.: The tangential x-ray investigation of the patellofemoral joint: X-ray technique, diagnostic criteria, and interpretation. Clin. Orthop. *144:*16, 1979.

116. Laurin, C. A., Levesque, H. P., Dussault, R., et al.: The abnormal lateral patellofemoral angle. J. Bone Joint Surg. *60A:*55, 1978.

117. Leach, R. E.: Malalignment syndrome of the patella. Instr. Course Lect. *25:*49, 1976.

118. Mariani, P. P., and Caruso, J.: Electromyographic investi-gation of subluxation of the patella. J. Bone Joint Surg. *61B:*169, 1979.

119. Maquet, P.: Advancement of the tibial tuberosity. Clin. Orthop. *115:*225, 1976.

120. Maquet, P.: Mechanics and osteoarthritis of the patello-femoral joint. Clin. Orthop. *144:*70, 1979.

121. Matthews, L. S., Sonstegard, D. A., and Henke, J. E.: Load bearing characteristics of the patellofemoral joint. Acta Orthop. Scand. *48:*511, 1977.

122. McCarroll, J. R., O'Donoghue, D. M., and Grana, W. A.: The surgical treatment of chondromalacia of the patella. Clin. Orthop. *175:*130, 1983.

123. McDougall, A., and Brown, D.: Radiological sign of recur-rent dislocation of the patella. J. Bone Joint Surg. *50B:*841, 1968.

124. Merchant, A. C., Mercer, R. L., Jacobsen, R. M., et al.: Roentgenographic analysis of patellofemoral congruence. J. Bone Joint Surg. *56A:*1391, 1974.

125. Metcalf, R. W.: An arthroscopic method for lateral release of the subluxing or dislocating patella. Clin. Orthop. *167:*9, 1982.

126. Osborne, A. H., and Fulford, P. C.: Lateral release for chondromalacia patellae. J. Bone Joint Surg. *64B:*202, 1982.

127. Outerbridge, R. E.: The etiology of chondromalacia patellae. J. Bone Joint Surg. *43B:*752, 1961.

128. Outerbridge, R. E.: Further studies on the etiology of chondromalacia patellae. J. Bone Joint Surg. *46B:*179, 1964.

129. Outerbridge, R. E., and Dunlop, J. A. Y.: The problem of chondromalacia patellae. Clin. Orthop. *110*:177, 1975.
130. Perrild, C., Hejgaard, N., and Rosenklint, A.: Chondromalacia patellae: A radiographic study of the patellofemoral joint. Acta Orthop. Scand. *53*:131, 1982.
131. Perry, J., Antonelli, D., and Ford, W.: Analysis of knee joint forces during flexed knee stance. J. Bone Joint Surg. *57A*:961, 1975.
132. Reilly, D. T., and Martins, M.: Experimental analysis of quadriceps muscle force and patellofemoral joint reaction force for various activities. Acta Orthop. Scand. *43*:126, 1972.
133. Satku, K., Bose, K., and Seaw, M.: Habitual subluxation of the patella on extension of the knee. J. Western Pacific Orthop. Assn. *19*:17, 1983.
134. Scapinelli, R.: Blood supply of the human patella. Its relation to ischemic necrosis after fracture. J. Bone Joint Surg. *49B*:563, 1967.
135. Sikorski, J. M.: The importance of femoral rotation in chondromalacia patellae as shown by serial radiography. J. Bone Joint Surg. *61B*:435, 1979.
136. Wiberg, G.: Roentgenographic and anatomic studies of the femoropatellar joint, with special reference to chondromalacia patellae. Acta Orthop. Scand. *12*:319, 1941.
137. Wissinger, H. A.: Chondromalacia patellae: A nonoperative treatment program. Orthopedics *5*:315, 1982.

Fractures About the Knee

138. Anderson, P. W., Harley, J. B., and Maslin, P. V.: Arthrographic evaluation of problems with united tibial plateau fractures. Radiology *119*:75, 1976.
139. Andrews, J. R., and Hughston, J. C.: Treatment of patella fractures by partial patellectomy. South. Med. J. *70*:809, 1977.
140. Apley, A. G.: Fractures of the lateral tibial condyle treated by skeletal traction and early mobilization. J. Bone Joint Surg. *38B*:699, 1956.
141. Apley, A. G.: Fractures of the tibial plateau. Orthop. Clin. North Am. *10*:61, 1979.
142. Bakalim, G., and Wilppula, F.: Fractures of the tibial condyles. Acta Orthop. Scand. *44*:311, 1973.
143. Blake, R., and McBryde, A.: The floating knee: Ipsilateral fractures of the tibia and femur. South. Med. J. *68*:13, 1975.
144. Boström, A.: Fracture of the patella. A study of 422 patellar fractures. Acta Orthop. Scand. (Suppl.) *143*:1, 1972.
145. Bowes, D. N., and Hohl, M.: Tibial condylar fractures: Evaluation of treatment and outcome. Clin. Orthop. *171*:104, 1982.
146. Brown, G. A., and Sprague, B. L.: Cast brace treatment of plateau and bicondylar fractures of the proximal tibia. Clin. Orthop. *119*:184, 1976.
147. Burri, C., Bartzke, G., Coldewey, J., et al.: Fractures of the tibial plateau. Clin. Orthop. *138*:84, 1979.
148. DeLee, J. C.: Ipsilateral fracture of the femur and tibia treated in a quadrilateral cast brace. Clin. Orthop. *142*:115, 1979.
149. Dovey, H., and Heerford, J.: Tibial condyle fractures: A follow-up of 200 cases. Acta Chir. Scand. *137*:521, 1971.
150. Drennan, D. B., Locher, F. C., and Maylahn, D. J.: Fractures of the tibial plateau. Treatment by closed reduction and spica cast. J. Bone Joint Surg. *61A*:989, 1979.
151. Elstrom, J., Pankovich, A. M., Sassoon, H., et al.: The use of tomography in assessment of fractures of the tibial plateau. J. Bone Joint Surg. *58A*:551, 1976.
152. Fraser, R. D., Hunter, G. A., and Waddel, J. P.: Ipsilateral fracture of the femur and tibia. J. Bone Joint Surg. *60B*:510, 1978.
153. Giles, J. B., DeLee, J. C., Heckman, J. D., et al.: Supracondylar-intercondylar fractures of the femur treated with a supracondylar plate and lag screw. J. Bone Joint Surg. *64A*:864, 1982.
154. Gillquist, J., Rieger, A., Sjodahl, R., et al.: Multiple fractures of a single leg. Acta Chir. Scand. *139*:167, 1973.
155. Gottfries, A., Hagert, C. G., and Sorensen, S. E.: T and Y fractures of the tibial condyles. Injury *3*:56, 1971.
156. Healy, W. L., and Brooker, A. F.: Distal femoral fractures. Comparison of open and closed methods of treatment. Clin. Orthop. *174*:166, 1983.
157. Hohl, M.: Treatment methods in tibial condylar fractures. South. Med. J. *68*:985, 1975.
158. Hohl, M.: Tibial condylar fractures: Long-term follow-up. Tex. Med. *70*:46, 1974.
159. Hohl, M.: Tibial condylar fractures. J. Bone Joint Surg. *49A*:1455, 1967.
160. Hohl, M., and Luck, J. V.: Fractures of the tibial condyle. A clinical and experimental study. J. Bone Joint Surg. *38A*:1001, 1956.
161. Hojer, H., Gillquist, J., and Liljedahl, S. O.: Combined fractures of the femoral and tibial shafts in the same limb. Injury *8*:206, 1977.
162. Johnson, E. W., and McLeod, J. L.: Osteochondral fragments of the distal end of the femur fixed with bone pegs. J. Bone Joint Surg. *59A*:677, 1977.
163. Joseph, F. R.: Evaluation of the Zickel supracondylar fixation device. Clin. Orthop. *169*:190, 1982.
164. Karlstrom, G., and Olerud, S.: Ipsilateral fracture of the femur and tibia. J. Bone Joint Surg. *59A*:240, 1977.
165. Kennedy, J. C., Grainger, R. W., and McGraw, R. W.: Osteochondral fractures of the femoral condyle. J. Bone Joint Surg. *48B*:436, 1966.
166. Lucht, V., and Pilgaard, S.: Fractures of the tibial condyles. Acta Orthop. Scand. *42*:366, 1971.
167. Mathewson, M. H., and Dandy, D. J.: Osteochondral fractures of the lateral femoral condyle. A result of indirect violence to the knee. J. Bone Joint Surg. *60B*:199, 1978.
168. Milgram, J. E.: Tangential osteochondral fracture of the patella. J. Bone Joint Surg. *25*:271, 1943.
169. Mize, R. D., Bucholz, R. W., and Gregor, D. P.: Surgical treatment of displaced comminuted fractures of the distal end of the femur. J. Bone Joint Surg. *64A*:871, 1982.
170. Mooney, V., Nickel, V. L., Harvey, J. P., et al.: Cast-brace treatment for fractures of the distal part of the femur. J. Bone Joint Surg. *52A*:1563, 1970.
171. Moore, T. M., and Harvey, J. P.: Roentgenographic measurement of tibial plateau depression due to fracture. J. Bone Joint Surg. *56A*:155, 1974.
172. Moore, T. M., Meyers, M. H., and Harvey, J. P.: Collateral ligament laxity of the knee: Long-term comparison between plateau fractures and normal. J. Bone Joint Surg. *58A*:594, 1976.
173. Neer, C. S., Grantham, A., and Sheldon, M. L.: Supracondylar fracture of the adult femur. A study of one hundred and ten cases. J. Bone Joint Surg. *49A*:591, 1967.
174. O'Donoghue, D. M.: Chondral and osteochondral fractures. J. Trauma *6*:469, 1966.
175. Olerud, S.: Operative treatment of supracondylar-condylar fractures of the femur. J. Bone Joint Surg. *54A*:1015, 1972.
176. Omer, G. E., Moll, J. H., and Bacon, W. L.: Combined fractures of the femur and tibia in a single extremity. J. Trauma *8*:1026, 1968.
177. Porter, B. B.: Crush fractures of the lateral tibial table. Factors influencing the prognosis. J. Bone Joint Surg. *52B*:676, 1970.
178. Rasmussen, P. S.: Lateral condylar fracture of the tibia. Acta Orthop. Scand. *42*:429, 1971.
179. Rasmussen, P. S.: Tibial condylar fractures as a cause of degenerative arthritis. Acta Orthop. Scand. *43*:566, 1972.
180. Rasmussen, P. S.: Tibial condylar fractures. Impairment of knee joint stability as an indication for surgical treatment. J. Bone Joint Surg. *55A*:1331, 1973.
181. Rasmussen, P. S., and Sorensen, S. E.: Tibial condylar fractures. Nonoperative treatment of lateral compression fractures without impairment of knee joint stability. Injury *4*:265, 1973.
182. Reibel, D., and Wade, P.: Fractures of the tibial plateau. J. Trauma *2*:337, 1962.
183. Riggins, R. S., Garrick, J. G., and Lipscomb, P. R.: Supracondylar fractures at the femur. Clin. Orthop. *82*:32, 1972.
184. Rorabeck, C. H., and Bobechko, W. P.: Acute dislocation of the patella with osteochondral fracture. J. Bone Joint Surg. *58B*:237, 1976.

185. Sarminento, A., Kinman, P. B., and Latta, L. L.: Fractures of the proximal tibia and tibial condyles: A clinical laboratory comparative study. Clin. Orthop. *145*:136, 1979.

186. Scapinelli, R.: Blood supply of the human patella. Its relation to ischemic necrosis after fracture. J. Bone Joint Surg. *49B*:563, 1967.

187. Schatzker, J., Horne, G., and Waddel, J.: The Toronto experience with the supracondylar fracture of the femur: 1966–1972. Injury *6*:113, 1975.

188. Schatzker, J., and Lambert, D. C.: Supracondylar fractures of the femur. Clin. Orthop. *138*:77, 1979.

189. Schatzker, J., McBroom, R., and Bruce, D.: The tibial plateau fracture. The Toronto experience: 1968–1975. Clin. Orthop. *138*:94, 1979.

190. Schulak, D. J., and Gunn, D. R.: Fractures of the tibial plateau. A review of the literature. Clin. Orthop. *109*:167, 1975.

191. Scotland, T., and Wardlaw, D.: The use of cast-bracing as treatment for fractures of the tibial plateau. J. Bone Joint Surg. *63B*:575, 1981.

192. Seinsheimer, F.: Fractures of the distal femur. Clin. Orthop. *153*:169, 1980.

193. Shelton, M. L., Neer, C. S., and Grantham, S. A.: Occult knee ligament ruptures associated with fractures. J. Trauma *11*:853, 1971.

194. Sorensen, K. H.: The late prognosis after fracture of the patella. Acta Orth. Scand. *34*:198, 1964.

195. Stewart, M. J., Sisk, T. D., and Wallace, S. L.: Fractures of the distal third of the femur. A comparison of methods of treatment. J. Bone Joint Surg. *48A*:784, 1966.

196. Weber, M. J., Janecki, J., McLeod, P., et al.: Efficacy of various forms of fixation of transverse fractures of the patella. J. Bone Joint Surg. *62A*:215, 1980.

197. Wilkinson, J.: Fracture of the patella treated by total excision. A long-term follow-up. J. Bone Joint Surg. *59B*:352, 1977.

198. Winston, M. E.: The results of conservative treatment of fractures of the femur and tibia in the same limb. Surg. Gynecol. Obstet. *134*:985, 1972.

199. Wilppula, E., and Bakalim, G.: Ligamentous tear concomitant with tibial condylar fracture. Acta Orthop. Scand. *43*:292, 1972.

200. Zickel, R. E., Fieti, V. G., Lawsing, J. F., et al.: A new intramedullary fixation device for the distal third of the femur. Clin. Orthop. *125*:185, 1977.

Ligamentous Injuries of the Knee

201. Arnold, J. A., Coker, T. P., Heaton, L. M., et al.: Natural history of anterior cruciate tears. Am. J. Sports Med. *7*:305, 1979.

202. Baker, C. L., Norwood, L. A., and Hughston, J. C.: Acute posterolateral rotatory instability of the knee. J. Bone Joint Surg. *65A*:614, 1983.

203. Balkfors, B.: The course of knee-ligament injuries. Acta Orthop. Scand. (Suppl.) *198*:1, 1982.

204. Cabaud, H. E., and Slocum, D. B.: The diagnosis of chronic antero-lateral rotatory instability of the knee. Am. J. Sports Med. *5*:99, 1977.

205. DeHaven, K. E.: Arthroscopy in the diagnosis and management of anterior cruciate ligament deficient knee. Clin. Orthop. *172*:52, 1983.

206. Feagin, J. A.: The syndrome of the torn anterior cruciate ligament. Orthop. Clin. North Am. *10*:81, 1979.

207. Feagin, J. A., Abbott, H. G., and Rokous, J. R.: The isolated tear of the anterior cruciate ligament. J. Bone Joint Surg. *54A*:1340, 1972.

208. Feagin, J. A., and Curl, W. W.: Isolated tear of the anterior cruciate ligament: 5-year follow-up study. Am. J. Sports Med. *4*:95, 1976.

209. Fetto, J. F., and Marshall, J. L.: Injury to the anterior cruciate ligament producing the pivot-shift sign. J. Bone Joint Surg. *61A*:710, 1979.

210. Fetto, J. F., and Marshall, J. L.: The natural history and diagnosis of anterior cruciate ligament insufficiency. Clin. Orthop. *147*:29, 1980.

211. Fowler, P. J.: The classification and early diagnosis of knee joint instability. Clin. Orthop. *147*:15, 1980.

212. Gallie, W. E., and LeMesurier, A. B.: The repair of injuries to the posterior cruciate ligament of the knee joint. Am. Surg. *85*:592, 1927.

213. Galway, R. D., Beaupre, A., and McIntosh, D. L.: Pivot shift: A clinical sign of symptomatic anterior cruciate insufficiency. J. Bone Joint Surg. *54B*:763–764, 1972.

214. Galway, H. R., and McIntosh, D. L.: The lateral pivot shift: A symptom and sign of anterior cruciate insufficiency. Clin. Orthop. *147*:45, 1980.

215. Giove, T. P., Miller, S. J., Kent, B. E., et al.: Non-operative treatment of the torn anterior cruciate ligament. J. Bone Joint Surg. *56A*:184, 1983.

216. Hey Groves, E. W.: The crucial ligaments of the knee joint: Their function, rupture and the operative treatment of the same. Br. J. Surg. *7*:505, 1920.

217. Hey Groves, E. W.: Operation for the repair of the crucial ligaments. Lancet *2*:674–675, 1917.

218. Hughston, J. C., Andrews, J. R., Cross, M. J., et al.: Classification of knee ligament instabilities. Part I. The medial compartment and cruciate ligaments. J. Bone Joint Surg. *58A*:159, 1976.

219. Hughston, J. C., Andrews, J. R., Cross, M. J., et al.: Classification of knee ligament instabilities. Part II. The lateral compartment. J. Bone Joint Surg. *58A*:173, 1976.

220. Hughston, J. C., and Barret, G. R.: Acute anteriomedial rotatory instability. Long-term results of surgical repair. J. Bone Joint Surg. *56A*:145, 1983.

221. Hughston, J. C., Bowden, J. A., Andrews, J. R., et al.: Acute tears of the posterior cruciate ligament. J. Bone Joint Surg. *62A*:438, 1980.

222. Hughston, J. C., and Norwood, L. A.: The posterolateral drawer test and external rotational recurvatum test for posterolateral rotatory instability of the knee. Clin. Orthop., *147*:82, 1980.

223. Indelicato, P. A.: Nonoperative treatment of complete tears of the medial collateral ligament of the knee. J. Bone Joint Surg. *65A*:323, 1983.

224. Jakob, R. P., Hassler, H., and Staeubli, H. V.: Observations on rotatory instability of the lateral compartment of the knee. Acta Orthop. Scand. (Suppl.)*191*:1, 1981.

225. Kennedy, J. C., and Grainger, R. W.: The posterior cruciate ligament. J. Trauma *7*:367, 1967.

226. Kennedy, J. C., Weinberg, H., and Wilson, A.: The anatomy and function of the anterior cruciate ligament. J. Bone Joint Surg. *56A*:223, 1974.

227. Larson, R. L.: Physical examination in the diagnosis of rotatory instability. Clin. Orthop. *172*:38, 1983.

228. Liljedahl, S., Lindvall, N., and Wetterfors, J.: Early diagnosis and treatment of acute ruptures of the anterior cruciate ligament. J. Bone Joint Surg. *47A*:1503, 1965.

229. Lipke, J., Janecki, C. J., Nelson, C. L., et al.: The role of incompetence of the anterior cruciate and lateral ligaments in anterolateral and anteromedial instability. J. Bone Joint Surg. *63A*:954, 1981.

230. Losee, R. E.: Concepts of the pivot shift. Clin. Orthop. *172*:45, 1985.

231. Losee, R. E., Johnson, T. R., and Southwick, W. O.: Anterior subluxation of the lateral tibial plateau. J. Bone Joint Surg. *60A*:1015, 1978.

232. McDaniel, W. J., and Dameron, J. B.: Untreated ruptures of the anterior cruciate ligament. J. Bone Joint Surg. *62A*:696, 1980.

233. Meyers, M. H.: Isolated avulsion of the tibial attachment of the posterior cruciate ligament of the knee. J. Bone Joint Surg. *57A*:669, 1975.

234. Nicholas, J. A.: Bracing the anterior cruciate ligament deficient knee using the Lenox Hill derotation brace. Clin. Orthop. *172*:137, 1983.

235. Norwood, L. A., Andrews, J. R., Meisterling, R. C., et al.: Acute anterolateral rotatory instability of the knee. J. Bone Joint Surg. *61A*:704, 1979.

236. Noyes, F. R., Bassett, R. W., Grood, E. S., et al.: Arthroscopy in acute traumatic hemarthrosis of the knee. J. Bone Joint Surg. *62A*:687, 1980.

237. Noyes, F. R., Butler, D. L., Paulos, L. E., et al.: Intra-articular cruciate reconstruction. I. Perspectives on graft strength, vascularization, and immediate motion after replacement. Clin. Orthop. *173*:71, 1983.

238. Noyes, F. R., Matthews, D. S., Mooar, P. A., et al.: The symptomatic anterior cruciate deficient knee. Part II: The results of rehabilitation, activity modification, and counseling on functional disability. J. Bone Joint Surg. *65A*:163, 1983.

239. Noyes, F. R., Mooar, P. A., Matthews, D. S., et al.: The symptomatic anterior cruciate deficient knee. Part I: The long-term functional disability in athletically active individuals. J. Bone Joint Surg. *65A*:154, 1983.

240. O'Donoghue, D. H.: An analysis of end results of surgical treatment of major injuries to the ligaments of the knee. J. Bone Joint Surg. *37A*:1, 1955.

241. O'Donoghue, D. H.: A method for replacement of the anterior cruciate ligament of the knee. J. Bone Joint Surg. *45A*:905, 1963.

242. Palmer, I.: Injuries to the cruciate ligaments of the knee joint as a surgical problem. Wiederherstellungschirurgie und Traumatologie *4*:181, 1957.

243. Pavlov, H.: The radiographic diagnosis of the anterior cruciate ligament deficient knee. Clin. Orthop. *172*:57, 1983.

244. Slocum, D. B., James, J. L., Larson, R. L., et al.: Clinical test for anterolateral rotatory instability of the knee. Clin. Orthop. *118*:63, 1976.

245. Slocum, D. B., and Larson, R. L.: Rotatory instability of the knee. J. Bone Joint Surg. *50A*:212, 1968.

246. Tamea, C. D., and Hening, C. E.: Pathomechanics of the pivot shift maneuver. An instant center analysis. Am. J. Sports Med. *9*:31, 1981.

247. Torisu, T.: Isolated avulsion fracture of the tibial attachment of the posterior cruciate ligament. J. Bone Joint Surg. *59A*:68, 1977.

248. Trickey, E. L.: Rupture of the posterior cruciate ligament of the knee. J. Bone Joint Surg. *50B*:334, 1968.

249. Woods, G. W., Stanley, R. F., and Tullos, H. S.: Lateral capsular sign: X-ray clue to a significant knee instability. Am. J. Sports Med. *7*:27, 1979.

Knee Arthroscopy and Arthrography

250. Anderson, P. W., Harley, J. D., and Mosler, R. T.: Arthrographic evaluation of problems with ununited tibial plateau fractures. Radiology *119*:75, 1976.

251. Anitrella, L. J., and Arcomano, J. P.: Knee arthrogram recorded on high detailed film screen combination. Radiology *132*:743, 1979.

252. Apple, J. S., Martinez, S., Hardaker, W. T., et al.: Synovial plicae of the knee. Skeletal Radiol. *7*:257, 1982.

253. Aritomi, H., and Yamamoto, M.: A method of arthroscopic surgery. Clinical evaluation of synovectomy with the electric resectoscope and removal of loose bodies in the knee joint. Orthop. Clin. North Am. *10*:565, 1979.

254. Berquist, T. H.: NMR imaging: Preliminary experience in orthopedic radiology. Magnetic Resonance Imaging *2*:41, 1984.

255. Bernstein, R. M., Folsson, H. E., Spitzer, R. M., et al.: Ossicle of the meniscus. A.J.R. *127*:785, 1976.

256. Boven, F., Bellemans, M. A., Geurts, J., et al.: A comparative study of the patellofemoral joint on axial roentgenograms, axial arthrogram, and CT following arthrography. Skeletal Radiol. *8*:179, 1982.

257. Boven, F., De Boeck, M., and Polvliege, R.: Synovial plicae of the knee on CT. Radiology *147*:805, 1983.

258. Brody, G. A., Pavlov, H., Warren, R. F., et al.: Plica synovialis intrapatellaris: Arthrographic significance of anterior cruciate ligament disruption. A.J.R. *140*:767, 1983.

259. Broukhim, B., Fox, J. M., Blazina, M. E., et al.: The synovial shelf syndrome. Clin. Orthop. *142*:135, 1979.

260. Brown, E. W., Allman, F. L., and Eaton, S. B.: Knee arthrography. A comparison of radiographic and surgical findings in 295 cases. Am. J. Sports Med. *6*:165, 1978.

261. Burman, M. S.: Arthroscopy or the direct visualization of joints. An experimental cadaver study. J. Bone Joint Surg. *13*:669, 1931.

262. Cargill, A. O. R., and Jackson, J. P.: Bucket-handle tear of the medial meniscus. A case for conservative surgery. J. Bone Joint Surg. *58A*:248, 1976.

263. Carruthers, C. C., and Kennedy, M.: Knee arthroscopy: A follow-up of patients initially not recommended for further surgery. Clin. Orthop. *147*:275, 1980.

264. Casscells, S. W.: Arthroscopy of the knee joint. A review of 150 cases. J. Bone Joint Surg. *53A*:287, 1971.

265. Casscells, S. W.: The place of arthroscopy in the diagnosis and treatment of internal derangement of the knee. Clin. Orthop. *151*:135, 1980.

266. Clanton, T. O., and DeLee, J. C.: Osteochondritis dissecans. History, pathophysiology and current treatment concepts. Clin. Orthop. *167*:50, 1982.

267. Crabtree, S. D., Bedford, A. F., and Edgar, M. A.: The value of arthrography and arthroscopy in association with a sports injury clinic: A prospective and comparative study of 182 patients. Injury *13*:220, 1981.

268. Curran, W. P. Jr., and Woodward, P.: Arthroscopy: Its role in diagnosis and treatment of athletic knee injuries. Am. J. Sports Med. *8*:415, 1980.

269. Dalinka, M. K.: Arthrography. New York, Springer-Verlag, 1980.

270. Dalinka, M. K., and Garofola, J.: The infrapatellar synovial fold: A cause for confusion in the evaluation of the anterior cruciate ligament. A.J.R. *127*:589, 1976.

271. Dalinka, M. K., Gohel, V. K., and Rancer, L.: Tomography in evaluation of the anterior cruciate ligament. Radiology *108*:31, 1973.

272. Dandy, D. J., Flanagan, J. P., and Stenmeyer, V.: Arthroscopy and the management of the ruptured anterior cruciate ligament. Clin. Orthop. *167*:43, 1983.

273. Dandy, D. J., and Jackson, R. W.: The diagnosis of problems after meniscectomy. J. Bone Joint Surg. *57B*:349, 1975.

274. Dandy, D. J., and Jackson, R. W.: The impact of arthroscopy on the management of disorders of the knee. J. Bone Joint Surg. *57B*:346, 1975.

275. Dandy, D. J., and O'Carroll, P. F.: The removal of loose bodies from the knee under arthroscopic control. J. Bone Joint Surg. *64B*:473, 1982.

276. Debnam, J. W., and Staple, T. W.: Arthrography of the knee after meniscectomy. Radiology *113*:67, 1974.

277. DeHaven, K. E.: Arthroscopy in the diagnosis and management of the anterior cruciate ligament deficient knee. Clin. Orthop. *172*:52, 1983.

278. DeHaven, K. E.: Diagnosis of acute knee injuries with hemarthrosis. Am. J. Sports Med. *8*:9, 1980.

279. DeHaven, K. E.: Peripheral meniscus repair. An alternative to meniscectomy. Orthop. Trans. *5*:399, 1981.

280. DeHaven, K. E., and Collins, H. R.: Diagnosis of internal derangement of the knee. J. Bone Joint Surg. *57A*:802, 1975.

281. DeSmet, A. A., and Neff, J. R.: Knee arthrography for preoperative evaluation of juxta-articular masses. Radiology *143*:663, 1982.

282. Deutsch, A. L., Resnick, D., Dalinka, M. K., et al.: Synovial plicae of the knee. Radiology *141*:627, 1981.

283. Dunbar, W. H.: Incremental patellar tracking: A simple method of evaluation. Arthroscopy Association of North America. Chicago, 1982.

284. Ficat, R. P., Philippe, J., and Hungerford, D. S.: Chondromalacia patellae: A system of classification. Clin. Orthop. *144*:55, 1979.

285. Finkelstein, H., and Mayer, L.: The arthroscope: A new method of examining joints. J. Bone Joint Surg. *13*:583, 1931.

286. Foote, G. A.: Delayed films in double-contrast knee arthrography. Australas. Radiol. *22*:273, 1978.

287. Frede, T. E., and Lee, J. K.: The "overturned" lateral view on arthrography of the knee. Radiology *134*:249, 1980.

288. Freiberger, R. H., and Kaye, J. J.: Arthrography. New York, Appleton-Century-Crofts, 1979.

289. Ghelman, M. I., and Dunn, H. K.: Radiology of the knee in joint replacement. A.J.R. *127*:447, 1979.

290. Gilles, H., and Seligson, D.: Precision in the diagnosis of meniscal lesions: A comparison of clinical evaluation, arthrography, and arthroscopy. J. Bone Joint Surg. *61A*:343, 1979.

291. Gillquist, J., and Hagberg, G.: Findings of arthroscopy and arthrography in knee injuries. Acta Orthop. Scand. *49*:398, 1978.

292. Gillquist, J., Hagberg, G., and Oretorp, N.: Arthroscopy in acute injuries of the knee joint. Acta Orthop. Scand. *48*:190, 1977.

293. Gillquist, J., and Oretorp, N.: Arthroscopic partial meniscectomy, technique, and long-term results. Clin. Orthop. *167*:29, 1982.

294. Goldberg, R. P., Hall, F. M., and Wyshak, G.: Pain in knee arthrography: Comparison of air vs. CO_2 and reaspiration vs. no reaspiration. A.J.R. *136*:377, 1981.

295. Griffiths, H. J., and D'Orsi, C. J.: Use of xeroradiography in cruciate ligament injury. A.J.R. *121*:94, 1974.

296. Guhl, J. F.: Arthroscopic treatment of osteochondritis dissecans: A preliminary report. Orthop. Clin. North Am. *10*:671, 1979.

297. Guhl, J. F.: Arthroscopic treatment of osteochondritis dissecans. Clin. Orthop. *167*:65, 1982.

298. Hall, F. M.: Arthrography of the discoid lateral meniscus. A.J.R. *128*:993, 1977.

299. Hall, F. M.: Buckled meniscus. Radiology *126*:89, 1978.

300. Hall, F. M.: Further pitfalls in knee arthrography. J. Can. Assoc. Radiol. *29*:179, 1978.

301. Hall, F. M.: Methodology in knee arthrography. Radiol. Clin. North Am. *19*:269, 1981.

302. Hall, F. M.: Pitfalls in knee arthrography. Radiology *118*:55, 1976.

303. Hall, F. M.: Pitfalls in the assessment of menisci by knee arthrography. Radiol. Clin. North Am. *19*:305, 1981.

304. Halpern, A. A., Donovan, T. L., Horowitz, B., et al.: Arthrographic demonstration of pigmented villonodular synovitis of the knee. Clin. Orthop. *132*:193, 1978.

305. Hamburg, P., Gillquist, J., and Lysholm, J.: Suture of new and old peripheral meniscus tears. J. Bone Joint Surg. *65A*:193, 1983.

306. Hargreaves, D. J., and Seedhom, B. B.: On the bucket-handle tear: Partial or total meniscectomy? A quantitative study. J. Bone Joint Surg. *61B*:381, 1979.

307. Harley, J. D.: An anatomic arthrographic study of the relationship of the lateral meniscus and popliteus tendon. A.J.R. *128*:181, 1977.

308. Hermann, J., Alvarez, E., and Lavine, L. S.: Value of knee arthrography in non-meniscal damage. NY State J. Med. *77*:916, 1977.

309. Hermann, J., Yeh, H., Lehr-Janus, C., et al.: Diagnosis of popliteal cyst: Double-contrast arthrography and sonography. A.J.R. *137*:369, 1981.

310. Highgenboten, C. L.: Arthroscopic synovectomy. Orthop. Clin. North Am. *13*:399, 1982.

311. Hirschowitz, D.: Clinical assessment, arthrography, arthroscopy, and arthrotomy in the diagnosis of internal derangement of the knee. J. Bone Joint Surg. *58B*:367, 1976.

312. Horns, J. W.: The diagnosis of chondromalacia by double-contrast arthrography of the knee. J. Bone Joint Surg. *59A*:119, 1977.

313. Hunter, J. C., Hattner, R. S., Murray, W. R., et al.: Loosening of the total knee arthroplasty: Detection by radionuclear bone scanning. A.J.R. *135*:131, 1980.

314. Iino, S.: Normal arthroscopic findings of the knee in adult cadavers. J. Jap. Orthop. Assoc. *14*:467, 1939.

315. Ingman, A. M., Ghosh, P., and Taylor, T. K. F.: Variations of collagenous and non-collagenous proteins of human knee meniscus with age and degeneration. Gerontology *20*:212, 1974.

316. Insall, J., Falvo, K. A., and Wise, D. W.: Chondromalacia patella. J. Bone Joint Surg. *58A*:1, 1976.

317. Ireland, J., Trickey, E. L., and Stoker, D. J.: Arthroscopy and arthrography of the knee. J. Bone Joint Surg. *62B*:3, 1980.

318. Jackson, R. W.: Current concepts review. Arthroscopic surgery. J. Bone Joint Surg. *65A*:416, 1983.

319. Jackson, R. W., and Abe, I.: The role of arthroscopy in the management of disorders of the knee. J. Bone Joint Surg. *54B*:310, 1972.

320. Jackson, R. W., Marshall, D. J., and Fujisawa, Y.: The

321. Jelaso, D. V.: The fascicles of the lateral meniscus: An anatomic-arthrographic correlation. Radiology *114*:335, 1975.

322. Jelaso, D. V., and Morris, G. A.: Rupture of the quadriceps tendon: Diagnosis by arthrography. Radiology *116*:621, 1975.

323. Johanson, J. J., Lilleas, F. G., and Nordshus, T.: Arthrography of the knee joint with Amipaque. Acta Radiol. (Diagn.) *18*:523, 1977.

324. Johnson, L. L.: Arthroscopic abrasion arthroplasty. 50th Annual Meeting, American Academy of Orthopedic Surgeons. Anaheim, CA, 1983.

325. Johnson, L. L.: Impact of diagnostic arthroscopy on the clinical judgment of an experienced arthroscopist. Clin. Orthop. *167*:75, 1982.

326. Kaplan, E. B.: Discoid lateral meniscus of the knee joint. J. Bone Joint Surg. *39A*:77, 1957.

327. Korn, M. W., Spitzer, R. M., and Robinson, K. E.: Correlations of arthrography with arthroscopy. Orthop. Clin. North Am. *10*:535, 1979.

328. Kyo, R. L., and Bigongiari, L. R.: A modern catheter needle for knee arthrography. Radiology *132*:743, 1979.

329. Levinsohn, E. M., and Baker, B. E.: Pre-arthrotomy diagnostic evaluation of the knee. A review of 100 cases diagnosed by arthrography and arthroscopy. A.J.R. *134*:107, 1980.

330. Lindblom, K.: The arthrographic appearance of the ligaments of the knee joint. Acta Radiol. (Suppl.) *74*, 1984.

331. Linden, B.: Osteochondritis dissecans of the femoral condyle: A long-term follow-up study. J. Bone Joint Surg. *59A*:769, 1977.

332. Linson, M. A., and Posner, I. F.: Synovial hemarthrosis as a cause of recurrent knee effusion. JAMA *242*:2214, 1979.

333. Major, M., Johnson, R. P., Carrera, E., et al.: Arthrographic pseudoloosening of Marmar TKA in hemophilic arthropathy. Clin. Orthop. *160*:114, 1981.

334. McGinty, J. B.: Arthroscopic removal of loose bodies. Orthop. Clin. North Am. *13*:173, 1976.

335. McGinty, J. B., and Freedman, P. A.: Arthroscopy of the knee. Clin. Orthop. *121*:173, 1976.

336. McGinty, J. B., Geuss, L. F., and Marvin, R. A.: Partial or total meniscectomy: A comparative analysis. J. Bone Joint Surg. *59A*:763, 1977.

337. Metcalf, R. W.: An arthroscopic method for lateral release of the subluxing or dislocating patella. Clin. Orthop. *167*:9, 1982.

338. Metcalf, R. W., Coward, D. B., and Rosenberg, T. D.: Arthroscopic partial meniscectomy: A five year follow-up study. 50th Annual Meeting, American Academy of Orthopedic Surgeons. Anaheim, CA, 1983.

339. Miller, G. K., Dickerson, J. M., Fox, J. M., et al.: The use of electrosurgery for arthroscopic subcutaneous lateral release. Orthopedics *5*:309, 1982.

340. Mink, J. H., and Dickerson, R.: Air or CO_2 for knee arthrography? A.J.R. *134*:991, 1980.

341. Mital, M. A., and Hayden, J.: Pain in the knee in children: The medial plica shelf syndrome. Orthop. Clin. North Am. *10*:713, 1979.

342. Nicholas, J. A., Freiberger, R. H., and Killoran, P. J.: Double-contrast arthrography of the knee. J. Bone Joint Surg. *52A*:203, 1970.

343. Noble, J., and Hamblen, D. L.: The pathology of the degenerative meniscus of the knee. J. Bone Joint Surg. *52A*:203, 1970.

344. Northmore-Ball, M. D., and Dandy, D. J.: Long-term results of arthroscopic partial meniscectomy. Clin. Orthop. *167*:34, 1982.

345. Norwood, L. A., Shields, C. L., Jr., Russo, J., et al.: Arthroscopy of the lateral meniscus in knees with normal arthrograms. Am. J. Sports Med. *5*:271, 1977.

346. Noyes, F. R., Bassett, R. W., Grood, E. S., et al.: Arthroscopy in acute traumatic hemarthrosis of the knee. J. Bone Joint Surg. *62A*:687, 1980.

347. O'Connor, R. L.: Arthroscopy in the diagnosis and treat-

ment of acute ligament injuries of the knee. J. Bone Joint Surg. *56A*:333, 1974.

348. O'Connor, R. L.: The arthroscope in the management of crystal induced synovitis of the knee. J. Bone Joint Surg. *55A*:1443, 1973.

349. O'Connor, R. L., Shahriaree, H., Sprague, N., et al.: Six years follow-up on arthroscopic excision of bucket-handle tears. Orthop. Trans. *5*:401, 1981.

350. Patel, D.: Arthroscopy of the plicae-synovial folds and their significance. Am. J. Sports Med. *6*:217, 1978.

351. Pavlov, H., and Goldman, A. B.: The popliteus bursa: An indicator of subtle pathology. A.J.R. *134*:313, 1979.

352. Pavlov, H., Hirschy, J. C., and Torg, J. S.: CT of the cruciate ligament. Radiology, *132*:389, 1979.

353. Pavlov, H., and Schneider, R.: Extrameniscal abnormalities as diagnosed by knee arthrography. Radiol. Clin. North Am. *19*:287, 1981.

354. Pavlov, H., Warren, R. F., Sherman, M. T., et al.: The accuracy of double-contrast arthrographic evaluation of the anterior cruciate ligament. J. Bone Joint Surg. *65A*:175, 1983.

355. Prager, R. J., and Mall, J. C.: Arthrographic diagnosis of synovial chondromatosis. A.J.R. *127*:344, 1976.

356. Resnick, D., Newell, J. D., Guerra, J., Jr., et al.: Proximal tibiofibular joint: Anatomic pathological-radiographic correlation. A.J.R. *131*:133, 1978.

357. Robinson, S. C.: *Bacillus cereus* septic arthritis following arthrography. Clin. Orthop. *145*:237, 1979.

358. Roebuck, E. J.: Double-contrast knee arthrography. Some new points of technology including the use of Dimer X. Clin. Radiol. *28*:47, 1977.

359. Rosenthal, D. I., Murray, W. T., Jauernek, R. R., et al.: Stressing the knee joint for arthrography. Radiology *134*:250, 1980.

360. Sadler, R. B., Jigarjian, A., Picchione, P. V., et al.: Pseudomasses on the supra-patellar pouch at arthrography. J. Can. Assoc. Radiol. *31*:251, 1980.

361. Salazar, J. E., Sebes, J. I., and Scott, R. L.: The supine view in double-contrast knee arthrography. A.J.R. *141*:585, 1983.

362. Schneider, D.: Arthroscopy and arthroscopic surgery in patellar problems. Orthop. Clin. North Am. *13*:407, 1982.

363. Schneider, R., Freiberger, R., Ghelman, B., et al.: Radiologic evaluation of painful joint prosthesis. Clin. Orthop. *170*:156, 1982.

364. Schuldt, D. R., and Wolfe, R. D.: Clinical and arthrographical findings in meniscal lesions. Radiology *134*:49, 1980.

365. Sedwick, W. J., et al.: Wear particles: Their value in knee arthrography. Radiology *136*:11, 1980.

366. Seidl, G., Scherak, O., and Hofner, W.: Antefemoral dissecting cysts in rheumatoid arthritis. Radiology *133*:343, 1979.

367. Spataro, R. F., Katzberg, R. W., Burgener, F. A., et al.: Epinephrine enhanced knee arthrography. Invest. Radiol. *13*:286, 1978.

368. Staple, T. W.: Extrameniscal lesions demonstrated by double-contrast arthrography of the knee. Radiology *102*:311, 1972.

369. Stoker, D. J., Renston, P., and Fulton, A.: The value of arthrography of internal derangement of the knee: The first 1,000 are the worst. Clin. Radiol. *32*:557, 1981.

370. Stone, R. G.: Peripheral detachment of the menisci of the knee: A preliminary report. Orthop. Clin. North Am. *10*:643, 1979.

371. Takagi, K.: Arthroscope. Clin. Orthop. *167*:6, 1982.

372. Tapper, E. M., and Hoover, N. W.: Late results after meniscectomy. J. Bone Joint Surg. *51A*:517, 1969.

373. Tegtmeyer, C. J., McCue, F. C., Higgins, S. M., et al.: Arthrography of the knee: A comparative study of the accuracy of single- and double-contrast techniques. Radiology *132*:37, 1979.

374. Watanabe, M., Takeda, S., and Ikeuchi, H.: Atlas of Arthroscopy. 3rd Ed. Tokyo, Igaku Shoin, 1978.

375. Watt, I., and Tasker, T.: Pitfalls in double-contrast knee arthrography. Br. J. Radiol. *53*:754, 1980.

376. Whipple, T. L., and Bassett, F. H. III.: Arthroscopic examination of the knee. Polypuncture technique with percuta-

377. Wickstrom, K. T., Spitzer, R. M., and Olsson, H. E.: Roentgen anatomy of the posterior horn of the lateral meniscus. Radiology *116*:617, 1975.

Total Knee Arthroplasty

378. Andriacchi, T. P., Galante, J. O., and Fermier, R. W.: The influence of total knee-replacement design on walking and stair-climbing. J. Bone Joint Surg. *64A*:1328, 1982.

379. Arden, G. P.: Total knee replacements. Clin. Orthop. *94*:92, 1973.

380. Bargren, J., Blaha, J., and Freeman, M. A. R.: Alignment in total knee arthroplasty. Clin. Orthop. *173*:178, 1983.

381. Bartel, D., Burstein, A., Santavicca, E., et al.: Performance of the tibial component in total knee replacement. J. Bone Joint Surg. *64A*:1026, 1982.

382. Blaha, J., Insler, H., Freeman, M., et al.: The fixation of a proximal tibial polyethylene prosthesis without cement. J. Bone Joint Surg. *64B*:326, 1982.

383. Coventry, M. B., Finerman, G. A., Riley, L. H., et al.: A new geometric knee for total knee arthroplasty. Clin. Orthop. *83*:157, 1972.

384. Coventry, M. B., Upshaw, J. E., Riley, L. H., et al.: Geometric total knee arthroplasty. Clin. Orthop. *94*:171, 1973.

385. Deburge A., Guepar: Guepar hinge prosthesis. Clin. Orthop. *120*:47, 1976.

386. Freeman, M. A., Blaha, J., Bradley, G., et al.: Cementless fixation of ICLH tibial component. Clin. Orthop. *13*:141, 1982.

387. Goodfellow, J., and O'Connor, J.: The mechanics of the knee and prosthesis design. J. Bone Joint Surg. *64B*:358, 1978.

388. Gunston, F.: Polycentric knee arthroplasty. J. Bone Joint Surg. *53B*:272, 1971.

389. Hood, R. W., and Insall, J. N.: Total knee revision arthroplasty: Indication, surgical technique, and results. Orthop. Trans. *5*:412, 1981.

390. Hungerford, D., Kenna, R., and Krackow, K.: The porous-coated anatomic total knee. Orthop. Clin. North Am. *13*:103, 1982.

391. Hungerford, D. S., and Kenna, R. V.: Preliminary experience with a total knee prosthesis with porous coating used without cement. Clin. Orthop. *176*:95, 1983.

392. Hunter, J. C., Hathner, R. S., Murray, W. R., et al.: Loosening of the total knee arthroplasty: Detection by radionuclide bone scanning. A.J.R. *135*:131, 1980.

393. Insall, J. N., Hood, R. W., Flaun, L. B., et al.: The total condylar knee prosthesis in gonarthrosis. J. Bone Joint Surg. *65A*:619, 1983.

394. Insall, J., Lachiewicz, P., and Burstein, A.: The posterior stabilized condylar prosthesis: A modification of the total condylar design. J. Bone Surg. *61A*:1317, 1982.

395. Insall, J., Scott, N., and Ranawat, C.: The total condylar knee prosthesis. J. Bone Joint Surg. *61A*:173, 1979.

396. Jones, G.: Total knee replacement—The Walldius hinge. Clin. Orthop. *94*:50, 1973.

397. Jones, W., Bryan, R., Peterson, L., et al.: Unicompartmental arthroplasty using polycentric and geometric hemicomponents. J. Bone Joint Surg. *63A*:943, 1981.

398. Kaufer, H., and Matthews, L.: Spherocentric arthroplasty of the knee. J. Bone Joint Surg. *63A*:545, 1981.

399. Kettelkamp, D., and Nasca, R.: Biomechanics and knee replacement arthroplasty. Clin. Orthop. *94*:8, 1973.

400. Lew, W., and Lewis, J.: The effect of knee prosthesis geometry on cruciate ligament mechanics during flexion. J. Bone Joint Surg. *64A*:734, 1982.

401. Lewallen, D. G.: Polycentric total knee arthroplasty: A ten-year follow-up study. 50th Annual Meeting, Academy of Orthopedic Surgeons. Anaheim, CA, 1983.

402. Lewis, J., Askew, M., Jaycox, D.: A comparative evaluation of tibial component designs of total knee prosthesis. J. Bone Joint Surg. *64A*:129, 1982.

403. Lotke, P., and Ecker, M.: Influence of positioning of pros-

thesis in total knee replacement. J. Bone Joint Surg. *59A*:77, 1977.

404. Mazas, F.: Guepar total knee prosthesis. Clin. Orthop. *94*:211, 1973.
405. Murray, D., and Webster, D.: The variable axis knee prosthesis. J. Bone Joint Surg. *63A*:687, 1981.
406. Nogi, J., Caldwell, J., Jauzlarich, J., et al.: Load testing of geometric and polycentric total knee replacements. Clin. Orthop. *114*:235, 1976.
407. Peterson, L., Bryan, R., and Combs, J.: Polycentric knee arthroplasty. Instr. Course Lect. *23*:6, 1974.
408. Radin, E.: Biomechanics of the knee joint. Orthop. Clin. North Am. *4*:539, 1973.
409. Rand, J. A.: Stress fractures after total knee arthroplasty. J. Bone Joint Surg. *62A*:226, 1980.
410. Rand, J. A., and Bryan, R.: Revision after total knee arthroplasty. Orthop. Clin. North Am. *13*:201, 1982.
411. Rand, J. A., and Bryan, R. S.: Revision total knee arthroplasty. 50th Annual Meeting, American Academy of Orthopedic Surgeons. Anaheim, CA, 1983.
412. Reckling, F., Asher, M., and Dillon, W.: A longitudinal study of the radiolucent line at the bone-cement interface following total joint replacement procedures. J. Bone Joint Surg. *59A*:355, 1977.
413. Reilly, D., Walker, P. S., Ben-Dov, M., et al.: Effects of

tibial components on load transfer in the upper tibia. Clin. Orthop. *165*:273, 1982.
414. Schneider, R., Hood, R., and Ranawat, C.: Radiologic evaluation of knee arthroplasty. Orthop. Clin. North Am. *13*:225, 1982.
415. Scott, R., and Santore, R.: Unicondylar unicompartmental replacement for osteoarthritis of the knee. J. Bone Joint Surg. *63A*:536, 1981.
416. Simon, S. R., Trieshmann, H. W., Burdett, R. C., et al.: Quantitative gait analysis after total knee arthroplasty for monarticular degenerative arthritis. J. Bone Joint Surg. *65A*:605, 1983.
417. Thomas, R., Resnick, D., Alazarkis, N., et al.: Compartmental evaluation of osteoarthritis of the knee: A comparative study of available diagnostic modalities. Radiology *116*:515, 1975.
418. Walker, P., and Hsieh, H.: Conformity in condylar replacement knee prostheses. J. Bone Joint Surg. *59B*:222, 1977.
419. Walker, P., Emerson, R., Potter, T., et al.: The kinematic rotating hinge: Biomechanics and clinical application. Orthop. Clin. North Am. *13*:187, 1982.
420. Walker, P., Green, D., Reilly, D., et al.: Fixation of tibial components of knee prostheses. J. Bone Joint Surg. *63A*:258, 1981.

FRACTURES OF THE SHAFTS OF THE TIBIA AND FIBULA

CLAIRE E. BENDER • *DONALD C. CAMPBELL*

Fractures of the shafts of the tibia and fibula are the most common long bone fractures. This chapter will discuss tibial and fibular shaft fractures. Treatment of tibial and fibular fractures is similar and, therefore, reference will primarily be made to the tibia.

ANATOMY

The anatomy of the body or shaft of the tibia (Figs. 7–1 to 7–3) is straightforward. The body has three borders: anterior, medial, and interosseous. It also has three surfaces: medial, posterior, and lateral. The anterior border and medial surface are predominately subcutaneous. Special markings include the tibial tuberosity located on the upper anterior border and the soleal line on the upper posterior surface. The tuberosity is the attachment of the ligamentum patellae. The soleal line is the tibial origin of the soleus muscle. There are no special markings on the medial or lateral surfaces of the tibial body.

The body of the fibular shaft is long and slender. It also has interosseous, anterior, and posterior borders and medial, lateral, and posterior surfaces. The anatomy is difficult to identify because the borders and surfaces spiral laterally and caudally. In addition, there is a prominent medial crest on the midposterior surface of the bone, thus dividing the bone into four possible surfaces.[11]

The tibia and fibula are joined by the tibiofibular synovial joint, the interosseous membrane, and the tibiofibular syndesmosis. The tibiofibular synovial joint is between the head of the fibula and the posterolateral part of the lower surface of the tibial condyle.

The interosseous membrane is composed of strong fibers that pass laterally and caudally from the interosseous crest to the fibular crest. The interosseous ligament is the thickest part of the membrane; it lies between the lower ends of the tibia

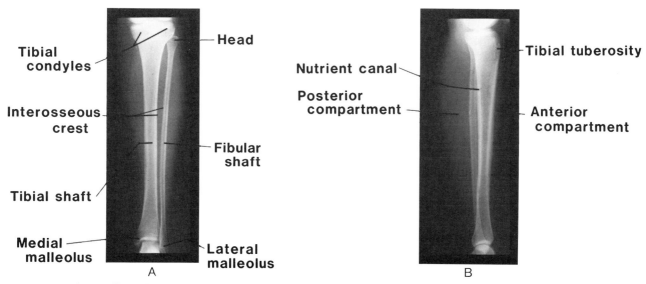

Figure 7–1. *A,* Normal AP radiograph of the tibia and fibula. *B,* Normal lateral radiograph.

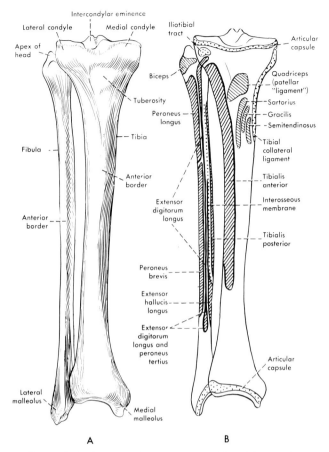

Figure 7–2. Musculoskeletal anatomy of the tibia and fibula. *A,* Anterior bony anatomy. *B,* Anterior muscular insertions and origins. (From Hollinshead, W. H.: Anatomy for Surgeons, Vol. 3: The Back and Limbs. 3rd Ed. New York, Harper & Row, 1982.)

and fibula. The anterior tibial vessels pass just above the interosseous membrane through a small aperture. Inferiorly there is a smaller aperture for the perforating branch of the peroneal artery.

The tibiofibular syndesmosis is between the lower ends of the tibia and fibula. It may be converted into a synovial joint by a diverticulum from the talocrural joint.[11] The tibiofibular syndesmosis, the lower thickened part of the interosseous membrane, and the anterior and posterior tibiofibular ligaments comprise the inferior transverse ligament.

Muscles of the lower leg are divided into antero-lateral and posterior groups (Figs. 7–2 and 7–3). The posterior, or calf muscles, are within two compartments. The transverse crural septum, or deep transverse faciae of the leg, separates the superficial and deep compartments. The gastrocnemius, soleus, and plantaris form the superficial group; the popliteus, flexor hallucis longus, flexor digitorum longus, and tibialis posterior occupy the deep compartment and arise in part from the covering fascia.[11]

The anterolateral muscles of the leg consist of the lateral compartment group—the peroneus longus and peroneus brevis—and the anterior compartment group—the tibialis anterior, extensor digitorum longus, and extensor hallucis longus.

Major vessels (Fig. 7–4) and nerves of the calf arise from parent structures in the popliteal space. Major popliteal arterial branches include the anterior tibial, posterior tibial, and peroneal arteries. A variety of branching patterns is possible. The most common pattern will be described. The origin of the anterior tibial artery is at the level of the popliteus muscle. Accompanied by the anterior tibial vein, it passes laterally and forward between the lower border of the popliteus and the upper border of the tibialis posterior to pass above the upper margin of the interosseous membrane and enter the anterior aspect of the leg.

The posterior tibial artery (accompanied by the vein) continues inferiorly deep to the soleus and then penetrates the deep transverse fascia of the leg. It then continues medially downward in a fascial canal with the tibialis posterior and flexor digitorum longus. Most of the posterior tibial artery branches supply blood to muscle.

The peroneal artery branches approximately 1 inch below the origin of the posterior tibial artery. Beneath the soleus, it is accompanied by two veins. The peroneal artery passes obliquely downward and laterally across the upper posterior surface of the tibialis posterior muscle and enters a canal

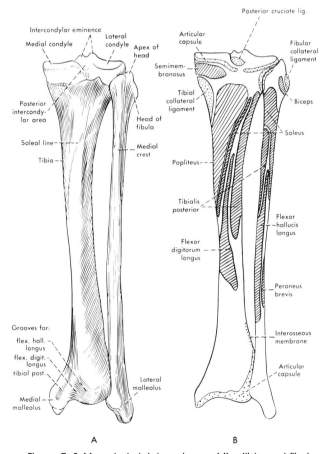

Figure 7–3. Musculoskeletal anatomy of the tibia and fibula. *A,* Posterior bony anatomy. *B,* Posterior muscle origins and insertions. (From Hollinshead, W. H.: Anatomy for Surgeons, Vol. 3: The Back and Limbs. 3rd Ed. New York, Harper & Row, 1982.)

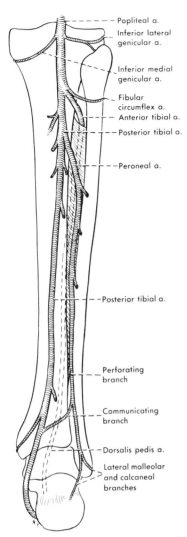

Figure 7–4. Illustration of major arterial supply of the tibia and fibula. (From Hollinshead, W. H.: Anatomy for Surgeons, Vol. 3: The Back and Limbs. 3rd Ed. New York, Harper & Row, 1982.)

Image labels: Popliteal a.; Inferior lateral genicular a.; Inferior medial genicular a.; Fibular circumflex a.; Anterior tibial a.; Posterior tibial a.; Peroneal a.; Posterior tibial a.; Perforating branch; Communicating branch; Dorsalis pedis a.; Lateral malleolar and calcaneal branches

formed by the fibula anterolaterally, tibialis posterior anteromedially, and flexor hallucis longus from behind.[11] As it passes downward, some of its branches pass through the interosseous membrane to supply the anterior muscle group.

Three blood-supply systems nourish the tibia: the nutrient artery, the periosteal system, and the epiphyseal-metaphyseal system. The major blood supply to the tibial shaft is the nutrient artery, which arises close to the upper end of the posterior tibial artery at the junction of the upper and middle thirds of the shaft. It enters the tibia posteriorly and has a rather long oblique intracortical course. When it reaches the intramedullary space, it divides into ascending and descending branches, which form a dense network of vessels. These vessels supply approximately two thirds of the cortex of the tibial shaft.[15]

The periosteal vessels originate from the anterior tibial artery or vessels of the interosseous membrane. These vessels run transversely to the long axis of the tibia. Abundant anastomoses exist between these transverse branches and with adjacent muscle arteries.[12]

It is the periosteal vessels that are of major importance in fracture healing. Because they run transversely, they are not interrupted as compared with the nutrient vessels.

The fibula is similarly supplied by the nutrient artery, periosteal system, and epiphyseal-metaphyseal system. The nutrient artery typically originates from the proximal peroneal artery.

Major nerves in the leg include the tibial and peroneal nerves. The tibial nerve passes through the popliteal fossa lying lateral to the popliteal vessels. It then passes behind them to their medial side as the popliteal vessels enter beneath the soleus muscle. The nerve continues downward with the posterior tibial vessels on the tibialis posterior muscle, then on the posterior aspect of the tibia, and then disappears in the neurovascular compartment of the flexor retinaculum.

The common peroneal nerve is located subcutaneously just behind the head of the fibula, where it is extremely vulnerable to injury. It then courses laterally and forward around the neck of the fibula deep to the peroneus longus. At this level, it divides into the superficial and deep peroneal nerves. The superficial peroneal nerve runs downward, paralleling the fibula, and supplies the peroneus longus and brevis. The deep peroneal nerve continues forward to penetrate the anterior intermuscular septum to reach the anterior compartment. It courses downward with the tibial vessels.

The leg is divided into three compartments.[16] The anterior compartment contains the tibialis anterior, extensor digitorum longus, extensor hallucis longus, and peroneus tertius muscles, the anterior tibial artery, and the deep peroneal nerve. These are enveloped by a relatively tight compartment composed of the tibia medially, fibula laterally, interosseous membrane posteriorly, and the tough anterior fascia. The lateral compartment contains the peroneus longus and brevis muscles. These muscles tend to protect the fibular shaft. The posterior compartment contains the gastrocnemius, soleus, tibialis posterior, flexor hallucis longus and flexor digitorum longus muscles, posterior tibial and peroneal arteries, and posterior tibial nerve. This compartment is larger and more elastic than the anterior compartment.

MECHANISM OF INJURY AND CLASSIFICATION OF FRACTURES

Direct high-energy forces, such as those associated with motor vehicle accidents or gunshot wounds, can result in severe damage, with open wounds, skin loss, soft tissue damage, and tibial and fibular comminution. Fractures can be transverse, segmental, or comminuted. Indirect injuries usually result from falls or ski injuries in which the foot is fixed. Fractures of the tibia are usually oblique or spiral. The fibula can remain intact. Generally the greater the injury force, the greater the likelihood that both the tibia and fibula will be fractured.

Incomplete or simple fractures of the tibia or fibula may occur from a direct blow or fall. The radiographic appearance of these fractures should not be confused with nutrient canals. In the tibia, the vascular grooves have sclerotic margins and run obliquely and inferiorly in the proximal tibia.

Fractures are more common in the middle and distal thirds of the tibial shaft. Distal shaft fractures may extend into the tibial plafond. These may occur as a result of a fall from a height or from a blow on the anchored foot that forces the talus up into the tibial plafond.[16] Various types of ankle fractures can be associated with these injuries.

Various classification schemes have been developed for tibial fractures. The most useful scheme is that which aids the orthopedic surgeon in fracture management and prognosis. Fractures should be described according to (1) precise anatomic location, (2) pattern of the fracture line, (3) position of the fragments, (4) degree of comminution, and (5) whether the fracture is open or closed.

Ellis[8] proposed a classification of tibial fractures based on severity. A fracture of minor severity is undisplaced, not angulated, and involves only a minor degree of comminution or a minor open wound. Moderate severity is complete displacement or angulation, with a small degree of comminution or a minor open wound. Major severity involves a major comminution or a major open wound with total displacement of the fracture.

Nicoll's[14] classification was based on the most significant factors affecting union: (1) initial displacement, (2) comminution, and (3) associated soft tissue wounds, infections, and distraction. He then graded each of these parameters from moderate to severe or nil to slight. With this system he could reasonably predict the outcome of any type of fracture. In his series of 705 patients (674 treated conservatively), the incidence of delayed union or non-union varied from 9 percent in the most favorable type to 39 percent in the least favorable.

Because of the importance of soft tissues in the healing of open tibial fractures, Müller[13] has classified the severity of soft tissue damage. Grade I fractures are compounded from within, with minimal soft tissue damage. Grade II fractures are compounded from without; the soft tissue injury is much less than the degree of bone injury. Grade III fractures are comminuted, and skin and muscle damage is extensive.

RADIOGRAPHIC EVALUATION

Standard views of the shafts of the tibia and fibula include AP and lateral projections, with the patient supine. Adjacent knee and ankle joints must be included on films owing to the possibility of associated injuries (see Fig. 7–1). Unless the lower leg is quite long, the 17-inch long film will include both joints. With longer legs, it is possible to place the film diagonally using opposite corners. However, in some patients two films must be used; the longer film can be placed proximally (including the knee), and a smaller film can be used for the distal leg and ankle. Soft tissues of the leg are included on films in order to exclude injury.

The AP projection (Fig. 7–5) is obtained with the patella anterior and the foot slightly inverted. The central beam is perpendicular to the center of the cassette.

The lateral projection (Fig. 7–6) can be made with

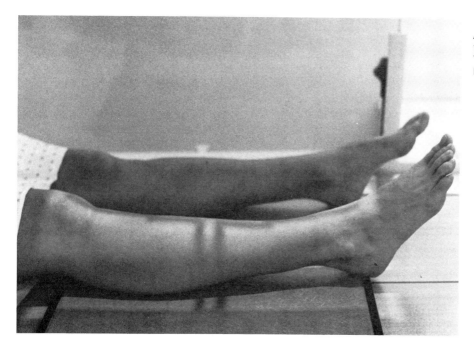

Figure 7–5. Patient positioned for AP view of the tibia and fibula. The foot is in slight internal rotation. The cone *(crossed light)* includes the knee and ankle.

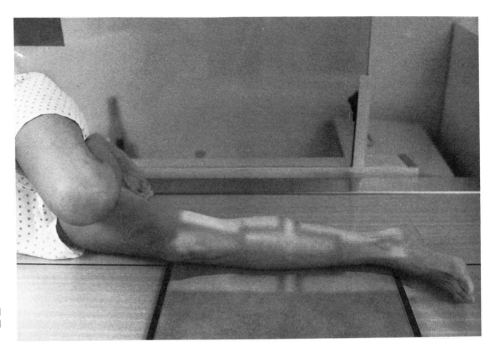

Figure 7-6. Patient positioned for lateral view of the tibia and fibula.

the patient turned on the affected side. The knee is slightly flexed. The unaffected side is placed in front of the involved side. If the patient cannot be turned, a cross-table projection is made by placing a nonopaque rigid support under the leg and then placing a cassette along the medial or lateral aspect of the leg.

Oblique projections can give additional information about fracture rotation and alignment.

In all projections, the central ray is directed vertically to the midpoint of the film.

Tomography and other techniques are rarely necessary for diagnosis, though stress fractures are an exception. Stress fractures are thoroughly discussed in Chapter 15.

MANAGEMENT OF FRACTURES

The literature is voluminous with regard to tibial and fibular shaft fracture management. With any fracture, the orthopedic surgeon will use the method of reduction and immobilization that has proved satisfactory in his or her experience.

The methods of fracture treatment are quite varied, and management choices have changed from decade to decade. In the 1930's and 1940's, closed methods were popular. Open reduction was more popular in the 1950's and 1960's. Presently, the method of choice is based upon the experience of the orthopedic surgeon.

Generally in fractures of both the tibial and fibular shafts, the management is the same. Fracture of the fibula contributes to increased instability of the tibial fracture. With an intact fibula, the displacement of the tibial fracture is usually less, and thus the prognosis is better.

Basic principles of fracture management include (1) maintenance or restoration of functional length, (2) restoration of normal weight-bearing alignment, (3) preservation of soft tissue, and (4) adjustment of treatment to the fracture.[3]

The goal of fracture management is acceptable reduction.[16] This means good alignment, no rotation, minimal shortening, and minor angulation in both the AP and lateral planes. Establishing good reduction improves the opportunity for better union. Because of the subcutaneous nature of much of the tibial shaft, only minimal displacement is acceptable. Displacement may be tolerated as long as rotation, shortening, and angulation are controlled. Rotation must be as nearly perfect as possible in order to maintain a functional extremity. If the opposite limb is normal, assessment of desired rotational position is noted by drawing a line from the normal anterior superior iliac spine through the midpatella down to the foot. This line should normally extend to the space between the first and second toes. In order to maintain normal weight-bearing stresses, the ankle and knee joint surfaces must be parallel.

Acceptable angulation is 5° in the AP and lateral planes (Fig. 7–7). However, with more exact reduction there will be less shortening and a better functional result.

Shortening of 5 to 7.5 mm is allowed in most fractures (see Fig. 7–11). In patients with extensive comminuted fractures or bone loss, more shortening may be tolerated. Distraction of fracture fragments is not acceptable. Five mm of distraction can lengthen the healing time of tibial fractures 4 to 8 months beyond the usual mean healing time of 4 months.[18]

Tibial fractures can be managed by closed or open

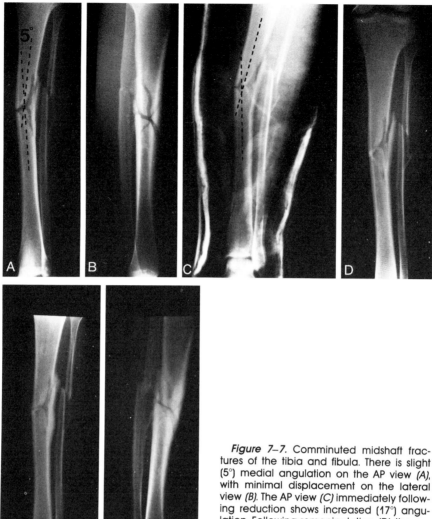

Figure 7–7. Comminuted midshaft fractures of the tibia and fibula. There is slight (5°) medial angulation on the AP view *(A)*, with minimal displacement on the lateral view *(B)*. The AP view *(C)* immediately following reduction shows increased (17°) angulation. Following remanipulation *(D)*, the angulation is reduced to less than 5°. AP *(E)* and lateral *(F)* views 3 months after reduction show healing with good callus.

reduction methods. Choice of method depends upon (1) the type of fracture, (2) the experience of the orthopedic surgeon, and (3) the medical condition of the patient. Most tibial fractures are managed by closed reduction and cast application.

A variety of casting techniques is possible. Long-leg casts are applied with some degree of knee flexion to allow weight-bearing and to relax the pull of the gastrocnemius. The foot is casted in neutral position.

The patellar-tendon-bearing (PTB) below-knee cast for tibial fractures was described by Sarmiento.[17] After initial long-leg cast management for several weeks (allowing edema to subside), the carefully molded cast around the tibial condyles and patella is applied. Sarmiento believes that careful molding decreases tibial rotation and allows progress with weight-bearing. Weight-bearing forces are placed on the tibial condyles, but the major distribution is placed on the soft tissues of the leg. With walking, body-weight forces are passed through the soft tissues, under compression, to the cast and then to the ground. Hydrostatic principles are utilized to provide reduced stress at the fracture site. Rigid immobilization is not provided by this cast, but rotation, shortening, and angulation are prevented. The intermittent compression of fracture fragments during weight-bearing is a positive factor in healing. The PTB cast also allows easier ambulation and sitting.

Follow-up of closed reduction consists of periodic radiographic evaluations to check for change in position of the fracture (Fig. 7–7). If the fracture position has changed since initial treatment, the orthopedic surgeon has several alternatives: (1) reduce the fracture and reapply a new cast, (2) utilize another reduction technique, or (3) wedge the cast. Cast wedging must be done carefully. The site of wedging is the fracture site itself, as performed by Watson-Jones,[20] or the intersection of the long axis of the two fragments, as performed by Böhler[1] and Charnley.[5] Metal markers can be placed on the cast site and confirmed with radiographs. Opening or closing wedges are used. Open wedging (Fig. 7–8) is preferred because it does not cause pressure on the underlying skin. The major disadvantage of the open wedge is a tendency toward fracture distraction.

Insertion of Steinmann pins above and below the fracture site is another method of treatment. With the patient under anesthesia, the pins are placed and the fracture is reduced. Plaster cast is then applied from the toes to the tibial tubercle, incorporating the pins in plaster. The cast is then extended to the thigh level. Pins are removed after 6 weeks. Weight-bearing is begun at the appropriate time, depending on the severity of the fracture and the extent of soft tissue injury.

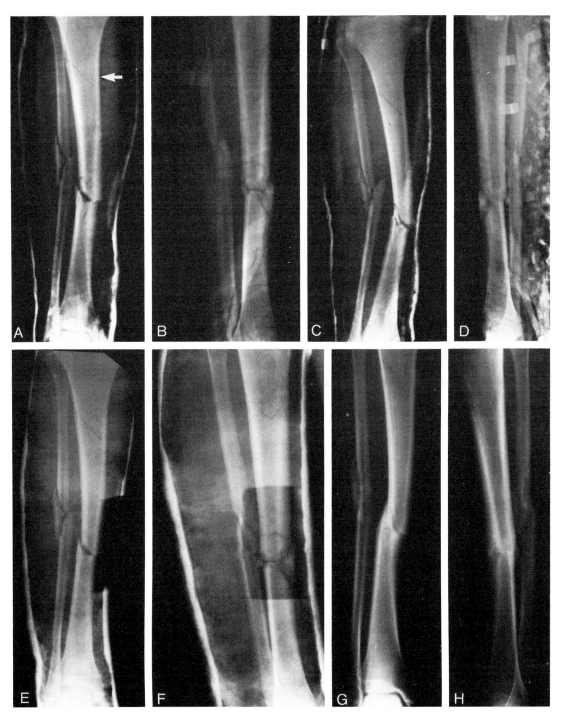

Figure 7–8. AP *(A)* and lateral *(B)* views of a comminuted fracture of the midtibia and fibula with an undisplaced upper tibial fracture *(arrow* in *A)*. There is minimal medial angulation. Follow-up AP *(C)* and lateral *(D)* views show increasing medial angulation. Open wedging was performed medially and the fracture realigned *(E* and *F)*. AP *(G)* and lateral *(H)* views 6 months after realignment show the fracture healed.

In severe unstable fractures, in which traditional closed reduction techniques do not establish stabilization and where internal fixation is likely to be hazardous, external fixation using the Hoffman apparatus provides a good treatment choice (Fig. 7–9). This device consists of heavy threaded pins carefully placed above and below the fracture with an adjustable frame that has four vertical supports to increase the rigidity of the fixation. The advantages of this device are controlled fracture reduction and accessibility of the wound for debridement and skin grafting. The Fischer apparatus provides similar advantages (Fig. 7–10).

Open reduction methods include compression plating, intramedullary nailing, and screw fixation. This has been one of the most controversial subjects in orthopedic surgery. Van der Linden[19] randomized 100 consecutive patients with displaced frac-

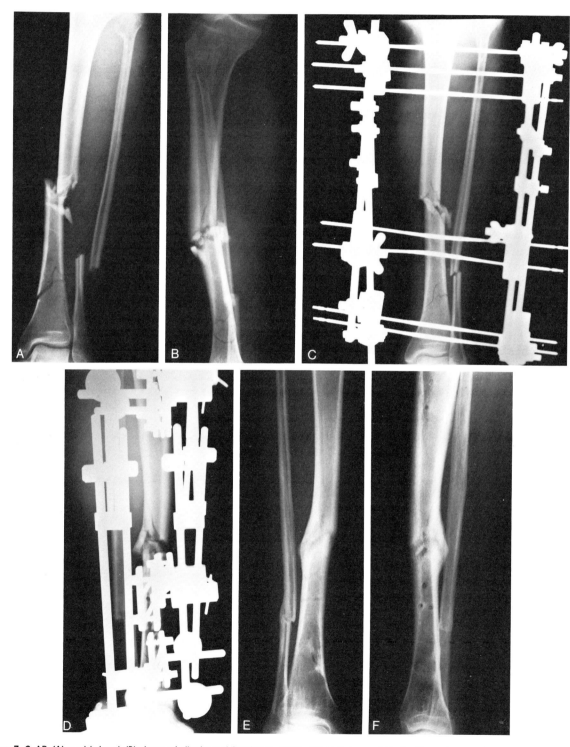

Figure 7–9. AP *(A)* and lateral *(B)* views of displaced fractures of the distal tibia and fibula. There is overriding and rotation of the fragments. Reduction was achieved with Hoffman fixation *(C* and *D).* Fracture was healed 1 year later *(E* and *F).*

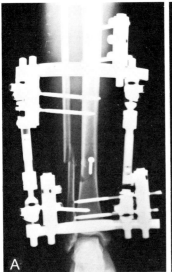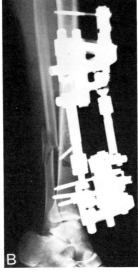

Figure 7–10. AP *(A)* and lateral *(B)* views of distal tibia and fibular fractures with Fischer fixation.

tures of the tibial shaft and established two groups, one treated with AO plate fixation and the other with conservative method (Fig. 7–11). Caution is emphasized in the use of this technique. Careful attention must be given to maintaining vascular integrity of the bone for good healing. Anatomic results were better and mean healing time was shorter with the AO plate group, but risk of infection was greater and duration of hospital stay was longer. Van der Linden's conclusions were that AO plate fixation was suitable for closed longitudinal fractures but not for open fractures. This aspect of tibial fracture treatment remains controversial. Gustilo and Anderson argue strongly against the use of internal fixation in open fractures,[9] while Chapman

believes it to be a very useful treatment in certain circumstances.[4] Other complications include fixation failure, implant failure, delayed union or non-union, and re-fracture.

Intramedullary nailing is used in (1) segmental tibial fractures, (2) angulated or displaced transverse or short oblique fractures of the middle third of the tibial shaft, and (3) non-united fractures (Fig. 7–12). Closed nailing techniques required a short incision at the level of the tibial tubercle. Use of an image intensifier is necessary in order to reduce the fracture properly and to guide the reamers and the intramedullary nail. In this way the periosteal blood supply is not disturbed, and the soft tissue vascularity is maintained. The nail interrupts the endosteal blood supply. Risk of infection is low with this closed technique. Open technique adds an incision at the fracture site. This may be required if closed reduction is not possible—that is, when soft tissues are interposed between the fracture fragments. Some intramedullary devices allow rotation to occur. Therefore, the use of some type of external support such as a brace or cast may be necessary until clinical union has started to progress.

A modification of the Küntscher intramedullary nail allows placement of bone screws transversely through the bone and nail. This can be done at one or both ends of the nail, in this way preventing distraction, overriding, or rotation at the fracture site (Fig. 7–13). Such a device allows the indications for intramedullary nailing to be expanded to include fractures more comminuted or more distal or proximal than was previously the case.

Fixation with multiple screws alone may be obtained in certain oblique fractures. This technique allows anatomic reduction and fixation with minimal soft tissue dissection. Casting or bracing is

Figure 7–11. AP *(A)* and lateral *(B)* views of overriding fractures of the distal tibia and fibula with several centimeters of shortening. Reduction *(C and D)* was accomplished with a seven-hole AO plate and screws.

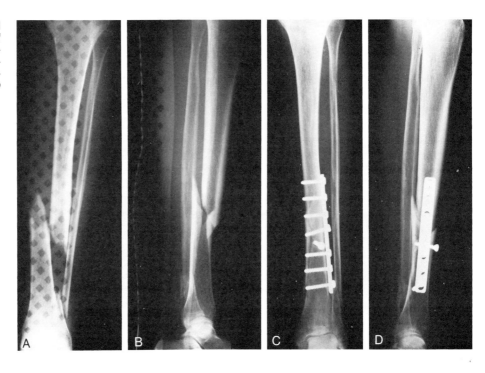

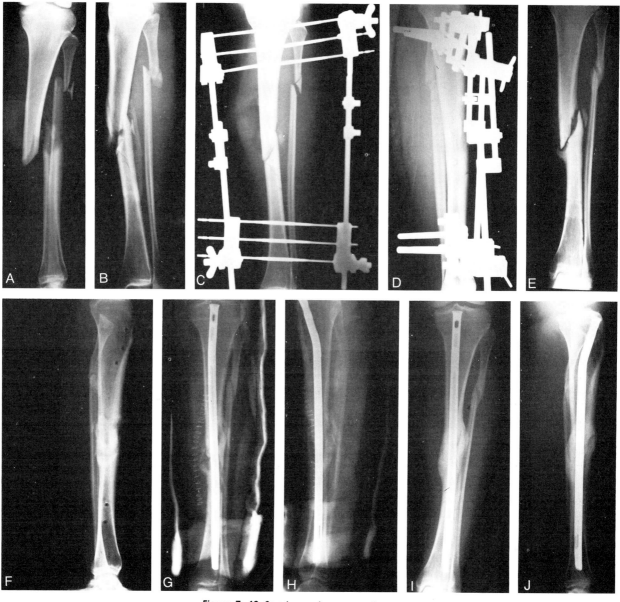

Figure 7-12. See legend on opposite page

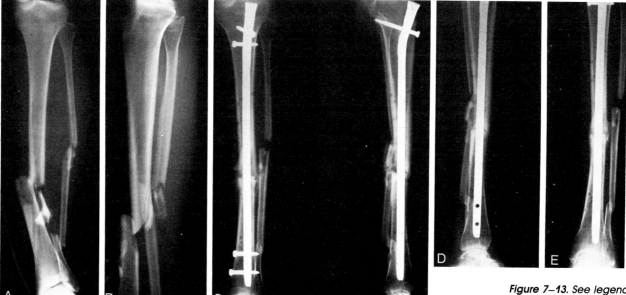

Figure 7-13. See legend
on opposite page

Figure 7–12. AP *(A)* and lateral *(B)* views of displaced bodily comminuted open tibial fracture. There is 90° rotation of the distal fragment. Note that the foot is directed laterally on the AP view *(A)* and anteriorly on the lateral view *(B)*. Initial reduction was accomplished with a Hoffman apparatus *(C* and *D)*. The fracture was not united at 4 months *(E* and *F)*. An intramedullary rod was used *(G* and *H)*, with healing 2 months later *(I* and *J)*.

Figure 7–13. AP *(A)* and lateral *(B)* views of an open comminuted fracture of the tibia with medial angulation. There are displaced mid- and distal fibular fractures. The fracture was fixed *(C)* with a locking medullary rod. AP *(D)* and lateral *(E)* views after healing of the tibial fracture. The lower locking screws have been removed and weight bearing is permitted.

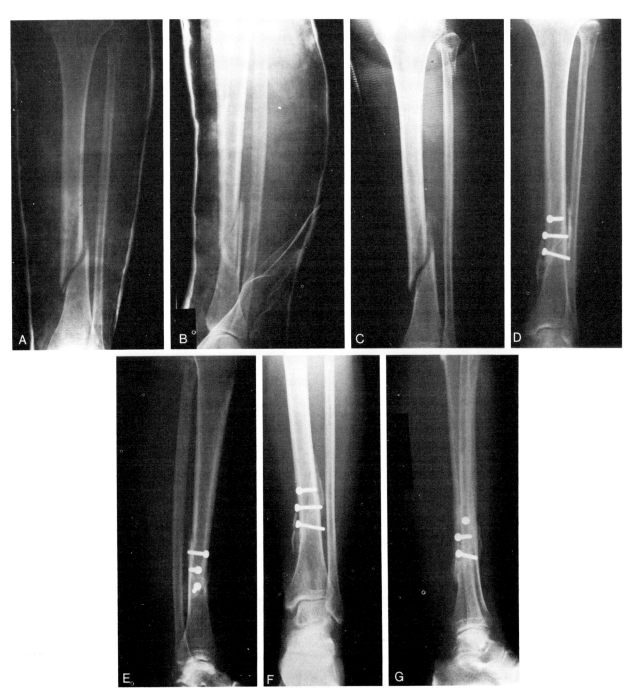

Figure 7–14. AP *(A)* and lateral *(B)* views of the tibia showing a distal spiral tibial fracture and proximal fibular fracture. (Both bones must always be entirely visualized.) Follow-up film in PTB cast at 3 months *(C)* shows minimal callus. Bone grafts and leg screws were used *(D* and *E)*, with healing *(F* and *G)* 5 months later.

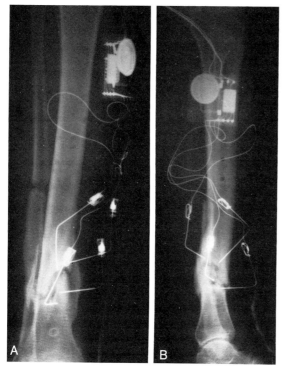

Figure 7–15. AP *(A)* and lateral *(B)* views of a distal tibial non-union with percutaneously placed electrodes.

absolutely necessary after such treatment. This technique combined with bone grafting may be useful for treatment of some cases of delayed union (Fig. 7–14).

Prognosis for fracture healing is based upon (1) type of fracture, (2) mechanism of injury, (3) soft tissue damage that includes open wounds, (4) infection, and (5) treatment. The treatment method of choice depends upon the orthopedic surgeon's experience and expertise. Generally uncomplicated tibial fractures heal in 10 to 13 weeks, but open comminuted fractures may take from 16 to 26 weeks. Delayed union is marked by absence of osseous union radiographically and presence of pain beyond the expected healing time. Non-union is diagnosed clinically by motion across the fracture site and radiographically by a persistent fracture line with sclerosed, flared margins (Fig. 7–15).

Fracture healing time is about the same for the proximal, middle, and distal thirds of the tibia.[14, 17] The presence or absence of a concomitant fibular fracture affects healing of the tibia. The intact fibula gives strut-like support to the tibia. However, it may also contribute to angular deformity of the tibia, and delayed union or non-union may result. Resection of a small segment of fibula may then be necessary for appropriate tibial healing.[16]

COMPLICATIONS

Delayed union is a common complication of tibial fractures and occurs in up to 15 percent of pa-

tients.[16, 17] Non-union is most commonly seen in severely displaced comminuted fractures with open wounds but can occur in any type of fracture, especially at the junction of the middle and distal thirds of the shaft. Treatment of non-united fractures includes bone grafts, fibular osteotomy, compression plating, intramedullary nailing, and electrical stimulation.

Electrical stimulation was first used in 1912 for fracture healing, but not until the 1970's did definite interest develop in the use of electrical stimulation.[2] Different systems have been developed: (1) constant direct current with percutaneous cathodes (Fig. 7–15), (2) constant direct current with implanted electrodes and power pack, and (3) the inductive coupling device. The success rate is about 80 to 85 percent for all three systems. All systems require good basic fracture management. Electricity must be concentrated at the non-union site. Three to 6 months are required for healing. Ineffective results occur when there is a large gap between fragments or pseudarthrosis. Actively draining osteomyelitis is a contraindication for the percutaneous or implanted electrodes.

Additional complications include malunion, extremity shortening, infection, skin loss, amputation, refracture, and neurovascular injuries.

Direct vascular injuries can be seen in severe, high-energy trauma. The most common injury site is the upper fourth of the tibia, where the anterior tibial artery passes forward through the interosseous membrane. Rare aneurysms of the proximal portion of the anterior and posterior tibial arteries have been described.[6, 7]

The anterior compartment syndrome results from increased pressure due to hemorrhage and edema following fracture. Venous flow is impeded, and eventually arterial supply is occluded. Muscle ischemia then occurs. Halpern[10] measured anterior compartment pressures in 20 patients and noted higher pressures when fractures occurred in the proximal third of the tibia, when the fracture was more than 50 percent displaced, and when the fracture resulted from high-energy trauma. Passive flexion of the toes that elicits pain in the anterior compartment region is the earliest sign. Weakness of the extensor hallucis longus and digitorum longus then occurs, with hypesthesia of the first web space being the last sign. Acutely, the dorsalis pedis pulse may not be absent, but in late stages it is lost. Compartment syndrome can also develop in the posterior and lateral compartments. Treatment involves immediate compartmental fasciotomy and stabilization of the fracture, usually with an external fixator.

Direct nerve injury as a result of fracture is uncommon. Nerve injury is most often due to pressure from the cast or soft tissue swelling where the peroneal nerve crosses the fibular neck.

Isolated fractures of the fibular shaft are uncommon; they usually occur from direct violence. Treatment consists of cast application for relief of pain.

REFERENCES

1. Böhler, L.: The Treatment of Fractures. 5th Ed. New York, Grune and Stratton, 1956–1958.
2. Brighton, C. T.: The treatment of non-unions with electricity. J. Bone Joint Surg. *63A*:847, 1981.
3. Carpenter, E. B.: Management of fractures of the shaft of the tibia and fibula. J. Bone Joint Surg. *48A*:1640, 1966.
4. Chapman, M. W.: Immediate internal fixation in open fractures. Orthop. Clin. North Am. *11*:579, 1980.
5. Charnley, J.: The Closed Treatment of Common Fractures. 3rd Ed. Edinburgh, E. S. Livingstone, 1961.
6. Crellin, R. O., and Tsapogas, M. J. C.: Traumatic aneurysm of the anterior tibial artery. Report of a case. J. Bone Joint Surg. *45B*:142, 1963.
7. Dreyfus, U., and Fishman, J.: False aneurysm of the posterior tibial artery complicating fracture of the tibia and fibula. J. Trauma *20*:186, 1980.
8. Ellis, H.: Disabilities after tibial shaft fractures. J. Bone Joint Surg. *40B*:190, 1958.
9. Gustilo, R. B., and Anderson, J. T.: Prevention of infection in the treatment of 1025 open fractures of long bones. J. Bone Joint Surg. *58A*:453, 1976.
10. Halpern, A. A., and Nagel, D. A.: Anterior compartment pressures in patients with tibial fractures. J. Trauma *20*:786, 1980.
11. Hollinshead, W. H.: Anatomy for Surgeons. Vol. 3: The Back and Limbs. 3rd. Ed. Philadelphia, Harper and Row, 1978.
12. Jackson R. W., and MacNab, I.: Fractures of the shaft of the tibia. J. Surg. *97*:543, 1959. .
13. Müller, M. E., Allgower, M., and Willenegger, H.: Technique of Internal Fixation of Fractures. Revised for the American Edition by G. Segmuller, New York, Springer-Verlag, 1965.
14. Nicoll, E. A.: Fractures of the tibial shaft. J. Bone Joint Surg *46B*:373, 1964.
15. Rhinelander, E. W.: Tibial blood supply in relation to fracture healing. Clin. Orthop. *105*:34, 1974.
16. Rockwood, C. A., and Green, D. P.: Fractures, 2nd Ed. Philadelphia, J. B. Lippincott Co., 1984.
17. Sarmiento, A.: A functional below-the-knee cast for tibial fracture. J. Bone Joint Surg. *49A*:855, 1967.
18. Urist, M. R., Mazet, R. Jr., and McLean, F. C.: The pathogenesis and treatment of delayed union and non-union. A survey of eighty-five un-united fractures of the shaft of the tibia and one hundred control cases with similar injuries. J. Bone Joint Surg. *36A*:931, 1954.
19. van der Linden, W., and Larsson, K.: Plate fixation versus conservative treatment of tibial shaft fractures. J. Bone Joint Surg. *61A*:873, 1979.
20. Watson-Jones, R.: Fractures and Joint Injuries. 4th Ed. Baltimore, Williams and Wilkins, Vol. 1, 1952, 1955.

FOOT AND ANKLE

8

BERNARD F. MORREY • JOSEPH R. CASS • KENNETH A. JOHNSON
THOMAS H. BERQUIST

THE ANKLE AND SUBTALAR JOINT

GROSS ANATOMY

The ankle joint is composed of the distal tibia, distal fibula, and talus.

The distal tibia is composed of the metaphysis, which flares medially to form the medial malleolus. The tibial plafond is not flat but rather has gentle recesses medially and laterally. These curve anteriorly to posteriorly, forming the biconcave surface that articulates with the trochlear-shaped talar dome[1] (Fig. 8–1). Hyaline cartilage is continuous over the distal tibia and extends medially to cover the medial malleolus. Posteriorly the metaphysis extends distally to form the so-called posterior malleolus. Articular cartilage does not completely cover the entire posterior malleolus. This is important in assessing the significance of fractures and their radiographic appearance after reduction (Fig. 8–2).

Laterally the distal fibula forms the lateral malleolus, which, with its articular facet, completes the ankle mortise. The fibula extends more distally than the medial malleolus and is oriented more posteriorly than the medial malleolus. Although considerable individual variation exists, a line connecting the tip of the malleoli forms an angle of about 8° with the horizontal in the frontal plane (Fig. 8–3) and an angle of about 20° posteriorly in the transverse plane (Fig. 8–4). Therefore, the true mortise view taken in the frontal plane of the malleoli requires about 20° internal rotation of the foot.[4]

The talus is a complex bone with a trochlear-shaped dome to match the tibial plafond. It is about 2 to 3 mm wider anteriorly than posteriorly (Fig. 8–5).[3, 4] The head of the talus articulates with the navicular bone, which makes an angle of about 20° medially to the dome of the talus (Fig. 8–6).[6] The plantar aspect articulates with the calcaneus at the posterior middle and anterior facets. The radiographic appearance of the articular relationship between the talus and calcaneus is important clinically on both the AP and lateral projections. In the lateral plane, the talus makes an angle of approximately 50° with the long axis of the calcaneus (Fig. 8–7).[6, 5] In the AP plane a line between the long axis of the talus and the axis of the calcaneus forms an angle

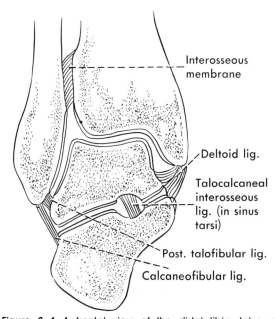

Figure 8–1. A frontal view of the distal tibia, talus, and calcaneus demonstrates the trochlear nature of the articular surface as well as the ring of ligamentous structures stabilizing the complex. The latter include medial and lateral collateral ligaments as well as the syndesmosis. (From Hollinshead, W. H.: Anatomy for Surgeons. Vol. 3: The Back and Limbs. 3rd Ed. New York, Harper & Row, 1982.)

Interosseous membrane

Deltoid lig.

Talocalcaneal interosseous lig. (in sinus tarsi)

Post. talofibular lig.

Calcaneofibular lig.

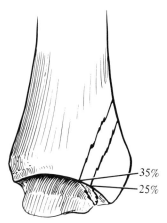

Figure 8–2. The posterior malleolus is posterior to the medial malleolus and assumes significance in assessment of ankle fractures. (From Hamilton, W. C.: Disorders of the Ankle. New York, Springer Verlag, 1984.)

35%
25%

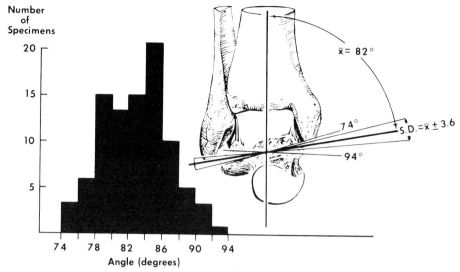

Figure 8–3. A line drawn between the tips of the malleoli in the coronal plane demonstrates a mean 8° tilt down from medial to lateral. (From Inman, V. T.: The Joints of the Ankle. Baltimore, Williams and Wilkins, 1976.)

of about 35° (Figs. 8–7 and 8–8).[6] In both measurements ±20° variation is seen,[6] and the values are less in the immature foot.[5]

Finally, the entire ankle complex is stabilized by the three ligaments closing the ring of the mortise: the deltoid, the lateral ligamentous complex, and the distal tibiofibular syndesmosis (see Fig. 8–1).[2, 3]

ROUTINE RADIOGRAPHIC TECHNIQUES

Ankle

Evaluation of the ankle requires AP, lateral, and mortise views. Following trauma an external oblique projection is also routinely obtained.[7–9, 19]

AP View

The patient is supine with the foot vertical and centered on an 8 × 10 cassette. The central beam is perpendicular to the cassette and centered on the ankle (tibiotalar) joint. The joint is 1 to 2 cm above the malleolar tips (Fig. 8–9A).[8, 9] The radiograph demonstrates the normal tibiotalar joint and medial mortise. The lateral mortise is not clearly seen, as the fibula overlaps the tibia and talus (Fig. 8–9B).

Lateral View

The patient is on his or her side with the ankle adjacent to the 8 × 10 cassette. The central beam is perpendicular to the cassette and centered 1 to 2 cm above the tip of the medial malleolus (palpable unless swelling is extensive) (Fig. 8–10). Alternate positions include the cross-table lateral and reverse

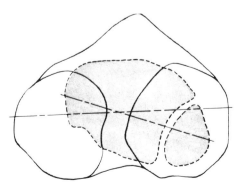

Figure 8–4. The fibula makes an angle of 20° to 30° with the coronal plane. The leg must be rotated this amount in order to obtain a true mortise view. (From Giannestras, N. J.: Foot Disorders. 2nd Ed. Philadelphia, Lea and Febiger, 1973.)

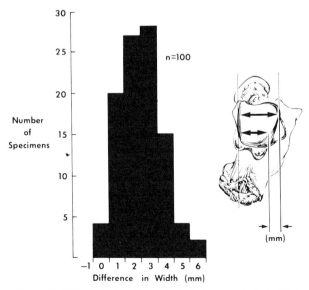

Figure 8–5. The talus is wider anteriorly than posteriorly. While considerable variation exists, this averages about 3 mm. (From Inman, V. T.: The Joints of the Ankle. Baltimore, Williams and Wilkins, 1976.)

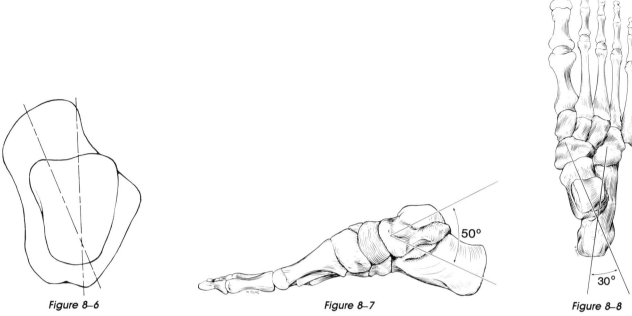

Figure 8–6   Figure 8–7   Figure 8–8

Figure 8–6. The head and neck of the talus make an angle of about 20° with the transverse axis of the trochlea. (From Giannestras, N. J.: Foot Disorders. 2nd Ed. Philadelphia, Lea and Febiger, 1973.)

Figure 8–7. The lateral talocalcaneal angle measures approximately 50°, although there is significant individual variation. (From Hollinshead, W. H.: Anatomy for Surgeons. Vol. 3: The Back and Limbs. 3rd Ed. New York, Harper & Row, 1982.)

Figure 8–8. The talocalcaneal angle viewed from the anterior posterior plane averages about 30°, again with significant individual variation. (From Hollinshead, W. H.: Anatomy for Surgeons. Vol. 3: The Back and Limbs. 3rd Ed. New York, Harper & Row, 1982.)

lateral (lateromedial view) views, with the medial malleolus adjacent to the cassette.[8, 9]

The lateral view demonstrates the AP dimensions of the tibiotalar joint and the posterior subtalar joint. The base of the 5th metatarsal is also included on most films. This is useful when an inversion injury causes a fracture of the base of the 5th metatarsal but the patient's clinical findings suggest

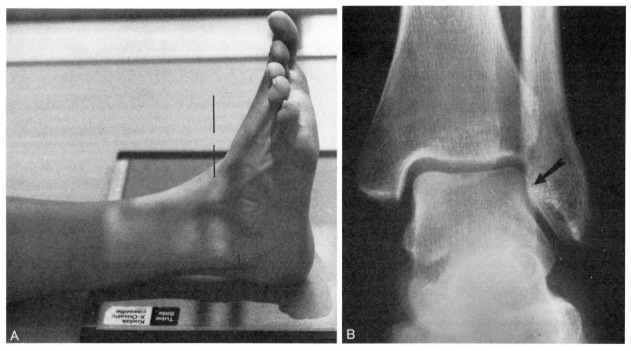

Figure 8–9. *A,* Patient positioned for AP view of the ankle. The tibiotalar joint is 1 to 2 cm above the medial malleolus *(line)*. *B,* AP radiograph. The tibia, talus, and fibula are demonstrated. The lateral portion of the mortise is difficult to evaluate owing to fibular overlap *(arrow).*

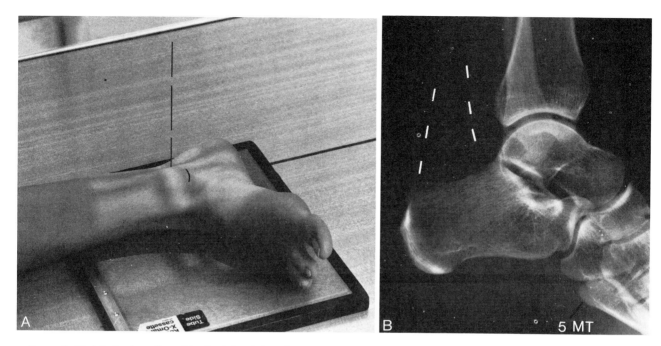

Figure 8–10. *A*, Patient positioned for the lateral view. The medial malleolus is usually palpable. *B*, Lateral radiograph of the ankle. The tibiotalar, posterior subtalar, talonavicular, and calcaneocuboid articulations are well seen. The pre-Achilles fat plane *(broken lines)* and 5th metatarsal should be evaluated.

an ankle injury. Soft tissue structures on the lateral view include the pre-Achilles fat pad (Fig. 8–11*B*). This is a large triangular fat collection anterior to the Achilles tendon. Hemorrhage in this region is due to Achilles injury. Significant ankle or calcaneal fractures will also cause distortion of this fat pad (Fig. 8–12).[23, 30]

Detection of fluid in the ankle is important. Effusions present with a "teardrop" shaped soft tissue mass anterior to the tibiotalar joint (Figs. 8–11 and 8–12). This results in elevation of the pretalar fat pad.[24] Less obvious changes may also be evident posteriorly. However, the anterior "teardrop" is the most consistent sign of effusion. An effusion may be the only sign of a subtle talar dome fracture. The presence of an effusion is evidence of an intact

capsule and ligaments (Fig. 8–12). In the immediate post-injury period this may be useful. However, small tears may seal, reducing the reliability of this sign after 48 hr.

Mortise View

On the AP view, the entire ankle mortise is not seen. The fibula overlaps the lateral joint space. By internally rotating the ankle 15° to 20°, however, the fibula is projected more laterally, allowing visualization of the entire ankle mortise.[7, 8, 12] The central beam is still perpendicular to the ankle joint (Fig. 8–13*A*). The radiograph (Fig. 8–13*B*) allows assessment of the entire joint space and distal talofibular articulation. In this position the posterior

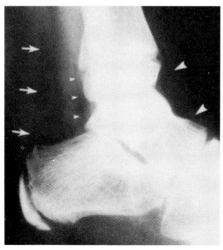

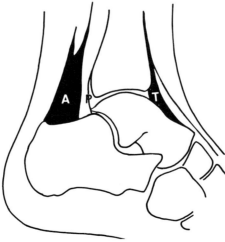

Figure 8–11. Lateral radiograph *(A)* and diagram *(B)* of the normal fat pads of the ankle: pretalar fat stripe *(large arrowheads,* T), posterior pericapsular fat stripe *(small arrowheads,* P) and pre-Achilles fat pad *(arrows,* A). (From Tobin, R., Dunbar, J. S., Towbin, J., et al.: Teardrop sign: Plain film recognition of ankle effusion. A. J. R., *134:*985, 1980.)

A   **B**

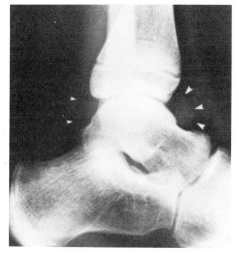
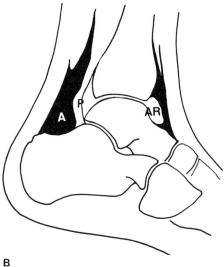

Figure 8–12. Lateral radiograph *(A)* and illustration *(B)* of ankle effusion. The effusion presents with an anterior soft tissue density *(large arrowheads, AR).* Less frequently posterior displacement of the pericapsular fat stripe *(small arrowheads, P)* is noted. The pre-Achilles fat pad is slightly compressed *(A).* (From Tobin, R., Dunbar, J. S., Towbin, J., et al.: Teardrop sign: Plain film recognition of ankle effusion. A. J. R., *134*:985, 1980.)

A   **B**

portion of the lateral talar facet is seen tangentially. The talar dome is better demonstrated.

Oblique Views

The oblique views of the ankle are obtained by rotating the foot 45° internally and 45° externally (Fig. 8–14).[9] The beam remains perpendicular to the cassette and is centered on the ankle joint. The radiographs demonstrate the fibula (internal oblique) and medial malleolus (external oblique) more completely (Fig. 8–14C). The external oblique is normally obtained as a part of our department's trauma series. In most cases the mortise view is

used in place of the internal oblique. Additional information regarding the hindfoot relationships can also be obtained using the oblique views.

Stress Views

Stress views may be useful in evaluating ligament injury following ankle sprains.[14, 15, 17, 18, 21, 25, 27, 28] Often the appearance of malleolar fractures will allow one to determine the degree of ligament injury.[15] However, if no fracture is evident or if findings are not conclusive, stress views may be indicated.[7, 9, 10, 16, 17]

In the immediate post-injury period, stress views

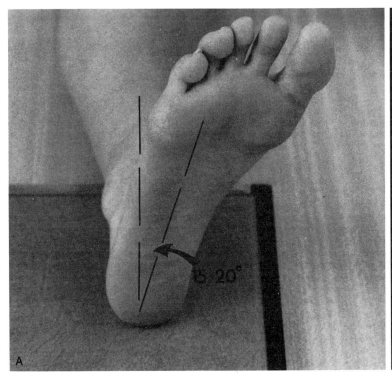
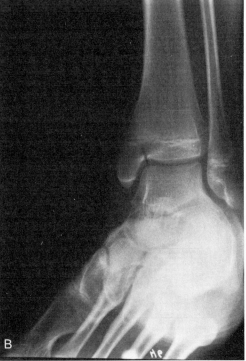

Figure 8–13. A, Patient positioned for mortise view. The foot is internally rotated 15° to 20°. *B,* Radiograph of mortise view. Note the steep oblique fracture medially. This is due to an inversion (supination) injury.

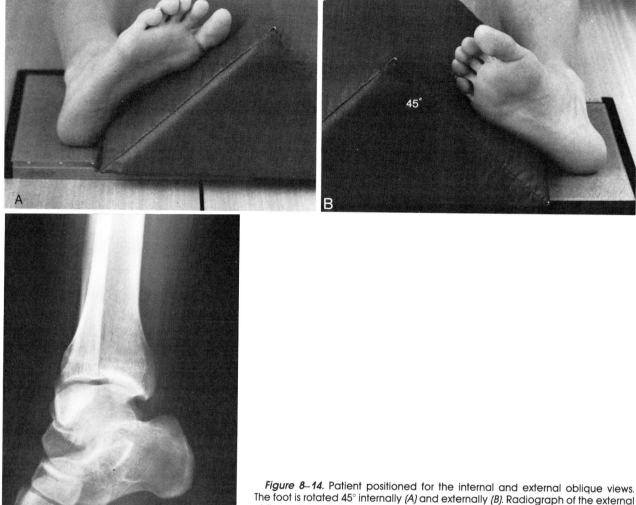

Figure 8–14. Patient positioned for the internal and external oblique views. The foot is rotated 45° internally (A) and externally (B). Radiograph of the external oblique view (C). The fibula is projected behind the tibia. The posterior margin of the medial malleolus is seen. The subtalar joint is not visible owing to overlapping of the talus and calcaneus.

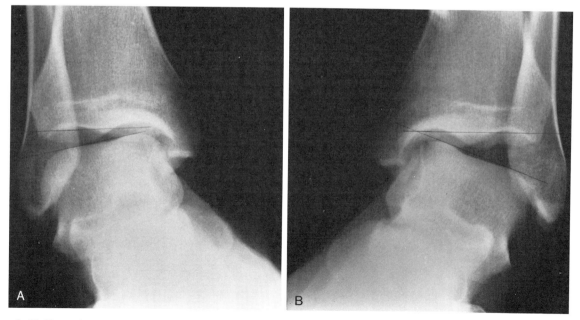

Figure 8–15. Stress views of the ankle. A, Normal ankle. There is minimal increase in the lateral tibiotalar joint with talar tilt of 5°. B, Injured ankle. Talar tilt is 20°, with widening of the tibiotalar joint indicating lateral ligament disruption.

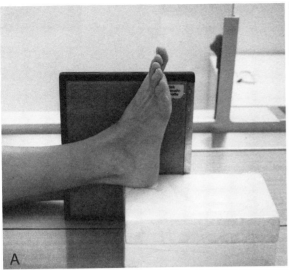

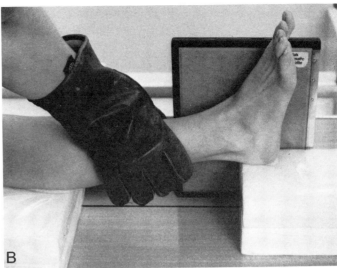

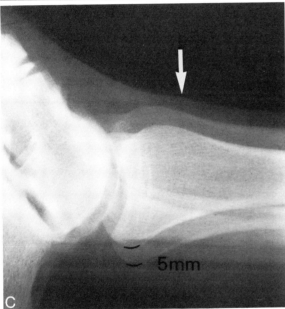

Figure 8–16. AP stress view. Patient positioned for stress view in neutral (A) and during stress (B). Double-exposed film before and during stress (C) allows motion to be easily measured. There is 5 mm of posterior displacement of the tibia on the talus.

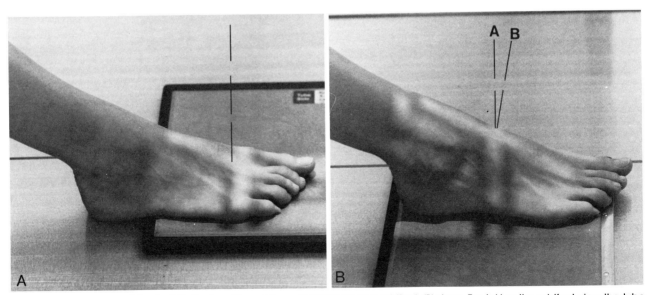

Figure 8–17. AP view of the foot. Patient positioned for metatarsal (A) and midfoot (B) views. For taking the midfoot view the tube can be perpendicular (A) or angled 10° (B).

may be difficult to perform owing to pain and swelling. For accurate results, injection of local anesthetic may be required. Positioning should be performed by an experienced physician. Stress views should be performed in the varus and valgus positions (Fig. 8–15), with the foot in the neutral and plantar flexed positions. Comparison with the uninjured side is essential. Olson[25] reported a normal talar tilt of up to 25° in the hypermobile asymptomatic ankle.

The distance from the lateral aspect of the talar dome to the lateral articular surface is measured during varus stress. The medial articular surfaces are measured with valgus stress. Several measuring techniques have been mentioned in the orthopedic literature.[12, 18, 21, 25, 27, 28] A difference of 3 mm between the injured and uninjured sides indicates ligament injury.[18, 21, 25] The angle of talar tilt can also be measured. If the angle of the injured ankle exceeds that of the normal ankle by 5°, injury is most likely present.[18, 21, 25] If the difference is 10°, a ligament tear is almost certainly present.[12, 21]

Lateral stress views can be obtained by placing the patient's leg on a support, so that the ankle and knee are level. This removes stress from the ankle. The cassette is positioned perpendicularly to the table, and a cross-table technique is used (Fig. 8–16A). After taking the initial film, stress is applied to the tibia just above the ankle (Fig. 8–16B). A second exposure is made on the same film (double

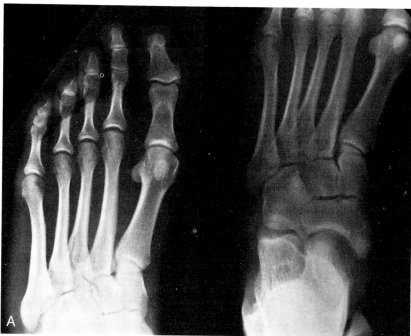

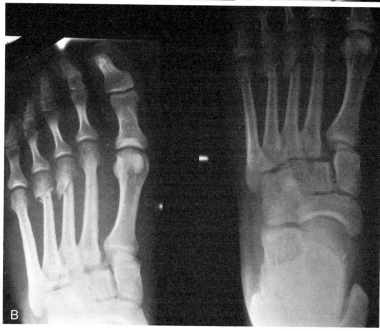

Figure 8–18. A, Normal AP view of the foot. B, Fractures of the distal 2nd to 4th metatarsals. Note the widening of the 1st and 2nd metatarsal bases and tarsometatarsal joints owing to fracture-dislocation.

exposure). This allows easy comparison and measurement (Fig. 8–16C).[21] The difference between the nonstressed and stressed position is measured on both ankles. If the injured side moves 2 mm more than the uninjured side, the drawer sign is considered positive.[21]

Foot

AP, lateral, and oblique views are routinely obtained in patients with foot trauma. Special localized views may be required in certain situations.

AP View

Two AP views of the foot are routinely obtained. This allows visualization of the metatarsals (forefoot) and tarsals (midfoot). The patient sits on the table with the knee flexed. The plantar surface of the foot is placed on an 8 × 10 inch cassette with the heel resting on the table (Figure 8–17A). The central beam is perpendicular to the cassette and is centered over the distal 3rd metatarsal.[8, 9] The midfoot view is obtained with the entire foot on the cassette and the central beam either perpendicular to the cassette or angled 10° toward the head. The latter technique allows better visualization of the tarsometatarsal joints.[8] In either case the beam is centered on the base of the metatarsals (3rd usually) (Fig. 8–17B).

The radiographs (Fig. 8–18) demonstrate the articular relationships of the tarsometatarsal and phalangeal joints. Care should be taken in evaluating the articular surfaces. They should be uniform and parallel, especially the tarsometatarsal joints. The space between the bases of the 1st and 2nd metatarsals should also be studied. Widening of this space (Fig. 8–18B) may be the only sign of subtle subluxation or dislocation.[17, 24]

Oblique View

Multiple techniques have been described for obtaining oblique views of the foot.[8] We routinely use the medial oblique projection. This involves elevating the lateral aspect of the foot 30° off the cassette. The leg and knee are rotated internally (Fig. 8–19A). This view separates the 3rd through 5th tarsometatarsal joints, which overlap on the AP view. The calcaneocuboid and talonavicular joints are also clearly seen (Fig. 8–19B).

Lateral View

The lateral view is most frequently taken with the patient on his or her side. The lateral aspect of the foot is placed against the cassette (8 × 10 or 10 × 12). The plantar surface of the foot should be parallel with the bottom of the cassette, if possible. The central beam is perpendicular to the cassette and is centered on the midfoot (Fig. 8–20A).

The radiograph shows overlapping of the metatarsal bases. The relationships of the mid- and hindfoot are well seen (Fig. 8–20B). Normally, a line drawn along the tuberosity and posterior facet forms a 20° to 40° angle (Böhler's angle) with a line from the posterior facet to the anterior superior calcaneus.[26, 29] This angle and calcaneal evaluation will be more accurate if the radiograph is centered

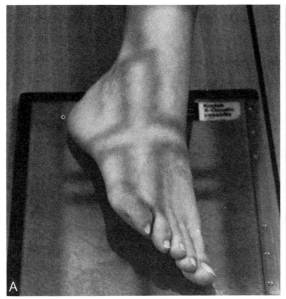
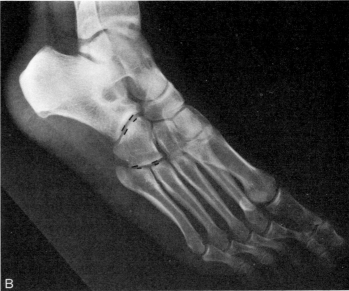

Figure 8–19. Oblique view of the foot. *A,* Patient positioned with the lateral aspect of the foot elevated and the beam centered on the midfoot. *B,* Radiograph demonstrating no overlap of the 3rd to 5th metatarsal bases and the calcaneocuboid and cubometatarsal joints *(lines).*

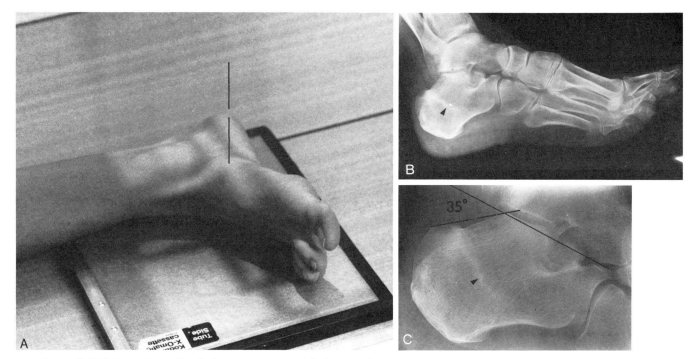

Figure 8–20. Lateral view of the foot and calcaneus. *A*, Patient positioned for lateral view. *B*, Lateral radiograph. Note trabecular condensation *(arrows)* in the calcaneus owing to a fracture. *C*, Radiograph centered on the calcaneus more clearly demonstrates the hindfoot. Note stress fracture *(arrow)* and normal Böhler's angle.

over the calcaneus rather than over the midfoot (Fig. 8–20C).

Special Views

The complex anatomy of the hindfoot articulations may require further views for more complete evaluation.[8, 9, 22]

Axial Calcaneal View

In addition to the lateral view described above, an axillary view of the calcaneus should be obtained in patients with suspected calcaneal fractures.

The patient is prone on the table. The ankle is supported with the 8 × 10 inch cassette flat against the foot. The cassette and holder (Fig. 8–21A) are perpendicular to the table. The central beam is

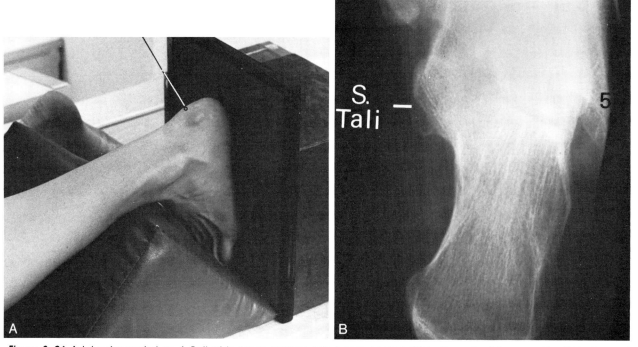

Figure 8–21. Axial calcaneal view. *A*, Patient in prone position with beam angled 40° to the axis of the cassette. *B*, Radiograph demonstrating axial view.

angled at 40° and is centered on the calcaneus. This view can also be taken in the upright position.[8]

The radiograph more clearly demonstrates the trochlear process, sustentaculum tali, and calcaneocuboid articulation (Fig. 8–21B).

Subtalar Views

Numerous techniques have been described for evaluation of the subtalar joint.[8–11, 16, 20] The oblique views are easily accomplished. The patient's foot is rotated medially or laterally (Fig. 8–22A and B). The hindfoot is centered on the cassette, with the beam centered on the malleolus (medial or lateral) and angled 10° to the head.

The radiographs (Fig. 8–22C and D) demonstrate the subtalar joint (lateral oblique) and sinus tarsi region (medial oblique). Variations in anatomy may cause difficulty in reproducing these views.[11] Tomography may be needed in these situations.

Sesamoid Views

Fractures of the sesamoid bones are uncommon. However, these structures are often not clearly seen on routine views. Sesamoid views can easily be obtained.[8, 9, 13] The patient is supine with the foot dorsiflexed (Fig. 8–23A). The beam is centered just plantar to the 1st metatarsal head and perpendicular to the cassette.

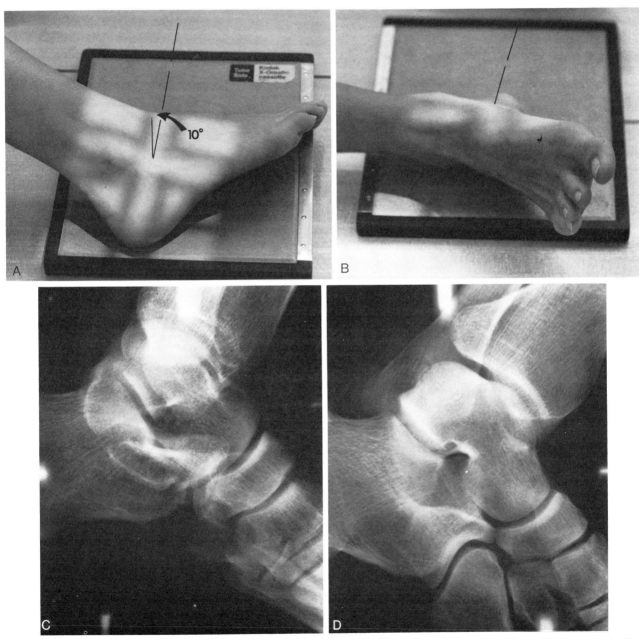

Figure 8–22. Subtalar views. Foot positioned for medial *(A)* and lateral *(B)* oblique views. The medial oblique *(C)* demonstrates the sinus tarsi region and the lateral *(D)* the posterior subtalar joint.

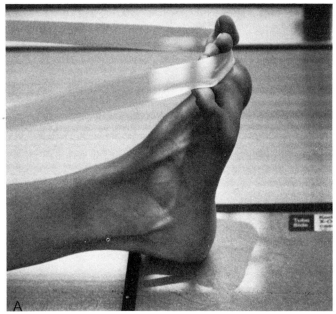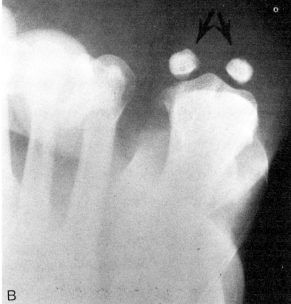

Figure 8–23. Sesamoid view. *A,* Patient supine with strap dorsiflexing the toes. *B,* Radiograph demonstrating the sesamoids of the great toe *(arrows).*

The radiograph projects the sesamoid bones away from the metatarsal, allowing fractures to be more readily identified (Fig. 8–23*B*).

ARTHROGRAPHY AND TENOGRAPHY OF THE FOOT AND ANKLE

Contrast injection of the articulations and tendons of the foot and ankle is a safe, valuable method of studying the ligaments, capsule, and articular anatomy.

Ankle Arthrography

Ankle arthrograms are most frequently performed in patients with suspected ligament tears. Goergen and Resnick reported that 95 percent of arthrograms are performed in patients with suspected ligament injury.[40] Arthrograms are less commonly performed to evaluate articular cartilage (talar dome fractures, osteochondritis dissecans)

TABLE 8–1. Ankle Arthrography: Techniques and Indications

Indication	Technique
Ligament injury	Single contrast, 6 to 8 ml
Articular evaluation	Double contrast
Osteochondritis dissecans	(1 ml iodinated contrast + 8
Talar dome fractures	ml air)
Loose bodies	Single or double contrast ± tomography
Arthritis	Double contrast
Capsulitis	Single contrast
Painful arthroplasty	Subtraction technique

and loose bodies.[39, 40, 46] Table 8–1 lists the indications for and technical variations used in ankle arthrography.

Technique

Radiographs (routine and stress views) should be evaluated prior to obtaining the arthrogram. Pertinent clinical information concerning the type of trauma and other indications for the arthrogram are important. Arthrographic technique varies acording to clinical indications (Table 8–1).

The patient is supine on the radiographic table. The anterior aspect of the ankle is prepared with sterile technique (5-minute povidone-iodine [Betadine] scrub). Prior to needle positioning, the dorsalis pedis pulse is palpated. The extensor tendons are usually easily located. In most situations the joint is entered anteriorly and medial to the dorsalis pedis artery (Fig. 8–24). If a medial ligament injury is suspected, a lateral approach may be used. The skin over the injection site is anesthetized with 1 percent lidocaine (Xylocaine) using a 25-gauge 1/2-inch needle. A 22-gauge 1 1/2-inch needle is used to perform the arthrogram. Once the needle has penetrated the skin, the ankle can be rotated into the lateral position. This allows one to judge the depth of the needle penetration. The joint is entered just inferior to the tibia. The needle should be directed slightly inferiorly to avoid the tibial lip.

When the needle is within the capsule, any fluid or blood should be aspirated. Appropriate laboratory studies should be obtained in patients with suspected infection or other arthritides. Contrast-material injection depends upon the clinical setting (Table 8–1). For patients with acute trauma, 6 to 8

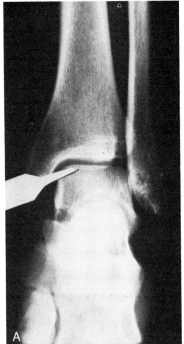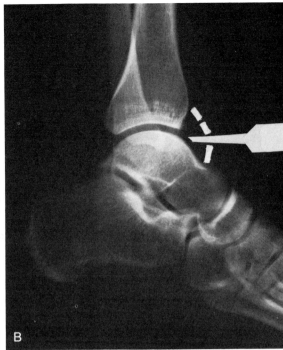

Figure 8–24. AP *(A)* and lateral *(B)* radiographs demonstrating the needle position for ankle arthrography.

ml of contrast material (meglumine diatrizoate) is injected. Mixing 2 to 4 ml of lidocaine with the contrast material may facilitate stress views.[10] If double-contrast technique is indicated, 1 ml of contrast medium combined with 6 to 8 ml of air is injected.[47] Rarely air alone may be used in patients with significant allergy to iodine. Occasionally 0.1 to 0.2 ml of 1:1000 epinephrine is injected with the contrast material. This is helpful if tomography or CT are to be used in conjunction with the arthrogram.[9, 10] (See Introduction to Arthrography in Chapter 1.)

Excessive amounts of contrast medium should be avoided, for this can obscure the internal structures of the ankle, especially the articular cartilage. Also, contrast material may extravasate along the needle

tract or actually leak out of the capsule. The latter is reported in older individuals.[40] These changes should not be confused with ligament injuries.

Following the injection, the ankle is exercised and observed fluoroscopically. Films are obtained in the AP, lateral, and oblique projections. If a ligament injury is suspected, stress views may also be taken. Vuust suggests the oblique axial view to improve detection of calcaneofibular ligament tears.[54]

Normal Arthrographic Anatomy

The anatomy of the ankle has been discussed in the first section of this chapter. Arthrographically, certain anatomic features are easily assessed.

The capsule of the anterior ankle extends from

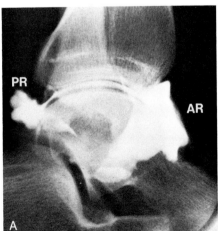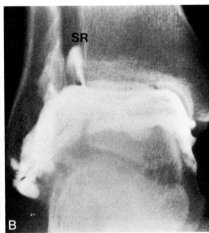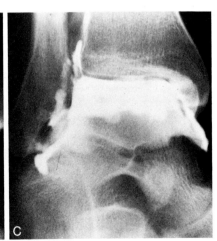

Figure 8–25. Normal ankle arthrogram. *A,* Lateral view. Anterior recess (AR) and posterior recess (PR). *B,* AP view. Syndesmotic recess (SR). Note the normal medial and lateral extent of the capsule with no contrast beyond the malleolar tips. *C,* Mortise view. The lateral and posterolateral aspects of the capsule are better demonstrated.

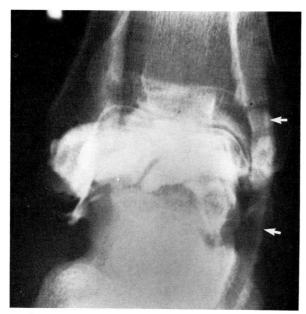

Figure 8–26. AP view demonstrating normal communication with the flexor tendons *(arrows)* medially.

the neck of the talus to a point 5 mm superior to the distal tibial margin. This anterior recess is best seen on the lateral view (Fig. 8–25). Posteriorly a second recess is also evident. This recess is more irregular and its size more variable compared with the anterior recess. Medially and laterally the capsule extends to the tips of the malleoli. The margins should be smooth.[39, 40, 46, 50]

Superiorly the capsule extends between the distal tibia and fibula (Fig. 8–25), forming a syndesmotic recess. Normally this is smooth and does not extend more than 2.5 cm above the joint space.[40, 43, 50]

In about 10 percent of patients the tibiotalar joint communicates with the posterior subtalar joint. Communication with the flexor tendons (flexor hallucis longus and flexor digitorum longus) along the medial aspect of the ankle is noted in about 20 percent of patients (Fig. 8–26).[40, 43, 50]

Abnormal Arthrograms

There is considerable controversy concerning the management of acute ankle injuries.[31, 32, 53] Both open and closed methods have been advocated. In young active individuals surgical reduction is more commonly performed. Certainly, inadequate management can lead to recurrent injury and instability.[31–33, 42, 48]

In the acute post-injury period arthrography is easily performed and more accurate than stress views.[49] Accuracy in assessing ligament injury decreases if the arthrogram is performed more than 72 hours following the injury. Ideally the test should be performed within 48 hours.[39, 40, 43]

The ligaments of the ankle are not directly visible arthrographically. The medial complex (deltoid ligament) is broad and triangular. The fibers pass from the medial malleolus to insert into the talus and calcaneus.[39, 40, 43, 50] Laterally there are three major ligaments. The anterior talofibular ligament extends from the lateral malleolus to the talus and blends with the anterior capsule.[39, 43] The calcaneofibular ligament is not intimately associated with the capsule. The posterior talofibular ligament extends posteriorly from the fibula to the talus.

The anterior talofibular ligament is most frequently disrupted. This is usually the result of an inversion injury. The capsule is also torn, allowing contrast material to extravasate laterally and ante-

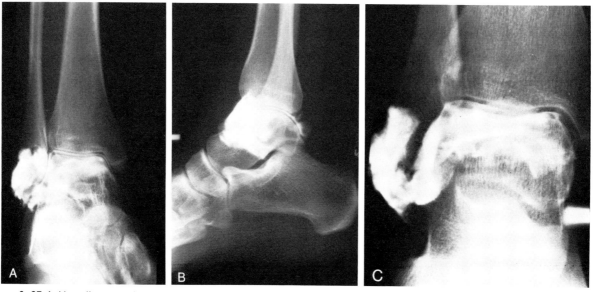

Figure 8–27. Ankle arthrogram in a patient with inversion sprain. AP *(A)* and lateral *(B)* views demonstrate extravasation of contrast medium laterally. The external oblique view *(C)* projects the contrast medium laterally, indicating that the extravasation is anterior to the fibula. This in turn indicates an anterior talofibular ligament tear.

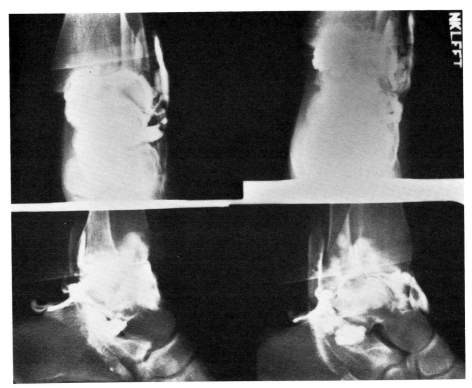

Figure 8–28. Ankle arthrogram (AP, lateral, and oblique views) in a patient with tears of the anterior talofibular and calcaneofibular ligaments. Note filling of the peroneal tendon sheaths.

rior to the distal fibula. The abnormality is best localized on the external oblique view. The contrast material will be projected lateral to the fibula if extravasation has occurred anteriorly. The lateral view is also useful (Fig. 8–27). Contrast medium may reach the tip of the lateral malleolus and extend superiorly.[40] Anterior talofibular ligament tears may seal within 48 hours. Thus, arthrograms performed more than 2 days after injury may appear negative.[39, 46, 47]

More significant ankle injuries may involve both the anterior talofibular and calcaneofibular ligaments. This injury classically results in filling of the peroneal tendon sheaths as well as capsular extravasation (Fig. 8–28).[36, 39, 40, 44, 46, 51]

Diagnosis of calcaneofibular ligament tears may be difficult. Spiegel and Staples reported 8 false negative arthrograms in 26 patients with surgically proven calcaneofibular ligament tears.[51]

Difficulty in diagnosis of calcaneofibular tears may be due to decompression of the capsule by the associated anterior talofibular ligament and capsular tear. The contrast material takes the path of least resistance.[36, 40, 51] Olson suggests that lack of resistance in filling the joint with massive extravasation indicates disruption of both ligaments.[46, 47] Pre-arthrographic injection of the joint with lidocaine followed by exercise and stress or repeated exercise views following the arthrogram may be helpful in more accurate assessment of the calcaneofibular ligament.

Extravasation of contrast material posterior and lateral to the malleolus may also indicate a tear even though the peroneal tendon sheaths are not filled.[44, 48] This finding is best seen on the internal oblique or axial oblique view.[54] Direct injection of the peroneal tendon sheath may provide the most accurate method of diagnosing calcaneofibular ligament tears.[31, 36, 40, 56] Isolated tears of the calcaneofibular ligament are rare. If peroneal tendon sheath filling occurs without an associated anterior talofi-

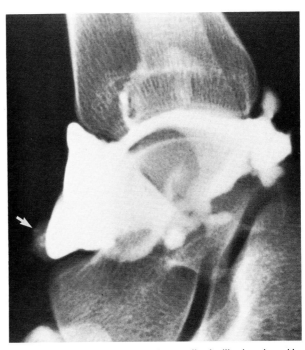

Figure 8–29. Ankle arthrogram in a patient with chronic ankle sprain. Note the old capsular injury *(arrow)* resulting in a well localized capsular diverticulum.

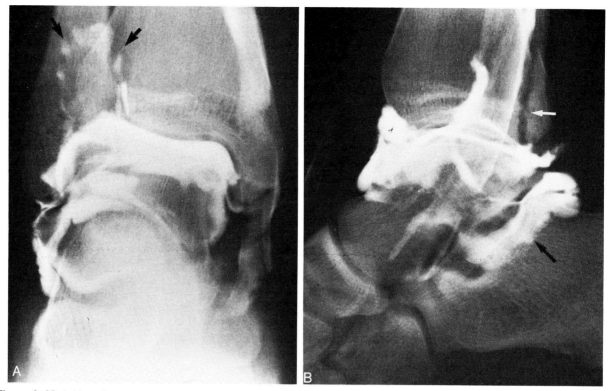

Figure 8–30. Ankle arthrogram following eversion (pronation) injury. The AP view *(A)* demonstrates disruption of the syndesmotic recess *(arrows).* The filling of the medial tendon sheath and posterior subtalar joint may occur normally. The medial contrast extravasation is partially obscured by the tendon sheaths. The lateral view *(B)* demonstrates a posterior tibial fracture *(white arrow)* and filling of the subtalar joint *(black arrow).*

bular ligament tear, one can assume that the injury is not acute.[39] Occasionally incomplete, old, or partially healed tears are noted. These injuries present with subtle irregularity of the capsule or ulcerlike projections (Fig. 8–29).

Tears of the posterior talofibular ligament are unusual and do not occur as isolated inju-

ries.[39, 40, 46, 47] Gross instability is usually evident clinically, obviating the need for arthrography.

Medial ligament injuries are less common and usually involve both the deltoid and syndesmosis of the distal tibia and fibula. The arthrogram will demonstrate extravasation around the tip of the medial malleolus and extension, disruption, or ir-

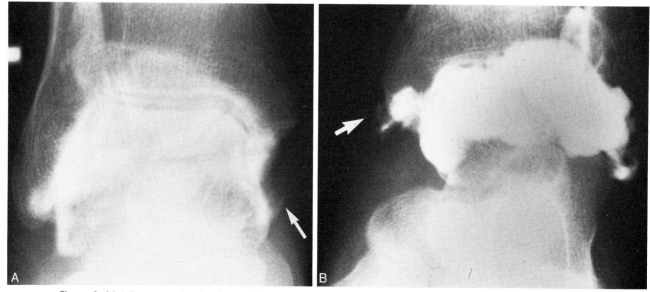

Figure 8–31. Arthrogram showing incomplete *(A)* and small complete *(B)* tears in the deltoid ligament *(arrows).*

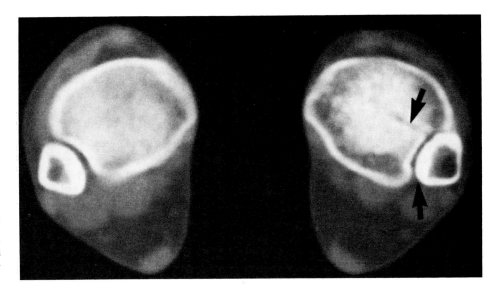

Figure 8–32. Patient with persistent pain following fracture-dislocation. The CT scan demonstrates stenosis of the distal tibiofibular joint *(arrows)* compared with the normal ankle. This would be more difficult to evaluate with arthrography alone.

regularity of the syndesmotic recess (Figs. 8–30 and 8–31). Rupture of the anterior talofibular ligament may be associated with syndesmotic tears.[46] The lateral view will demonstrate loss of the normal lucent zone anterior to the distal tibia. (Isolated complete tears of the anterior tibiofibular ligament are uncommon.)

Following treatment of ankle injuries, arthrogra-

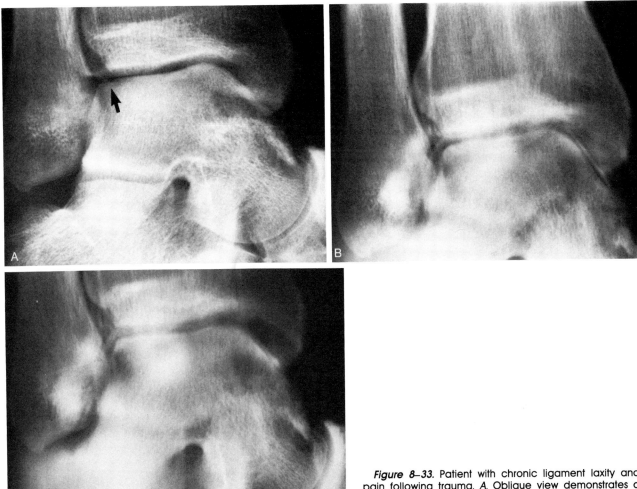

Figure 8–33. Patient with chronic ligament laxity and pain following trauma. *A,* Oblique view demonstrates a small talar dome fracture *(arrow).* Tomograms *(B* and *C)* with double-contrast arthrography demonstrate that the cartilage is intact. The fragment is not free in the joint.

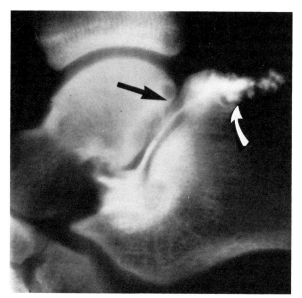

Figure 8–34. Arthrotomogram of the subtalar joint demonstrating subchondral erosions *(straight arrow)* and an enlarged posterior recess with synovitis *(curved arrow)*.

phy with or without computed tomography may be useful in evaluating patients with persistent pain or instability (Fig. 8–32).[35] Persistent instability, adhesive capsulitis, and other complications will be clearly demonstrated.

Arthrography is less commonly performed to evaluate subtle articular or synovial changes. Articular cartilage is best studied using double-contrast technique (see Table 8–1). The combination of re-

duced contrast medium and air provides better detail of the articular surface. This is particularly useful in evaluating osteochondral defects such as talar dome fractures and osteochondritis dissecans.[40, 46] Additional information is provided by using tomography in conjunction with the double-contrast technique (Fig. 8–33). Tomography should be performed in the AP and lateral projections. Subtle synovial changes and loose bodies can also be evaluated with arthrotomography.

Following trauma, persistent pain and decreased range of motion may indicate adhesive capsulitis. In this clinical setting, single-contrast technique is most useful. Injection may be more difficult owing to the constricted capsule.

Goergen and Resnick[40] describe the use of ankle arthrography in patients with arthritis, ganglia, and total joint replacement; but these are uncommon indications. Subtraction arthrography is less effective for the evaluation of arthroplasty in the ankle than in the hip. The surface area of the components is smaller, and overlying contrast material may obscure the bone-cement interface.

Arthrograms of the tarsal joint, subtalar joints, and foot are infrequently performed. The subtalar joint can be easily entered medially. Fluoroscopic guidance will allow a straight vertical approach into the posterior joint. The examination is most often performed in patients with persistent post-traumatic pain or to ensure proper needle position for aspiration or therapeutic injections. Tomography is useful in improving anatomic detail following the injection of contrast medium (Fig. 8–34).

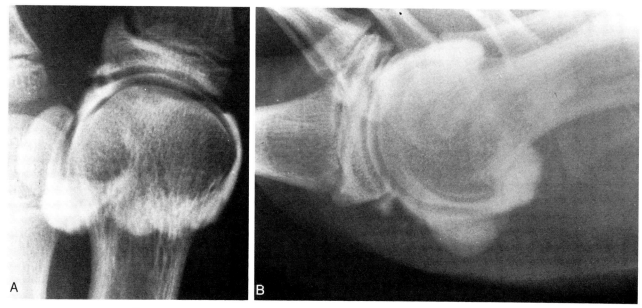

Figure 8–35. A and B, Normal arthrograms of the 1st metatarsophalangeal joint.

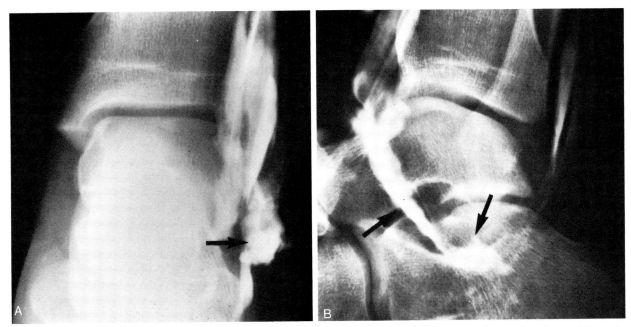

Figure 8–36. Normal peroneal tenogram. AP *(A)* and lateral *(B)* views. Note the subcutaneous extravasation *(arrows)*. There is no contrast medium in the joint space.

Injections of the metatarsophalangeal and intertarsal joints is easily accomplished using a dorsal approach (Fig. 8–35).

Peroneal Tenography

Peroneal tenography is most commonly performed to evaluate calcaneofibular ligament tears, suspected peroneal tendon subluxation, or peroneal tendinitis and entrapment.[31, 36, 38, 40, 45 52]

Technique

Examination of the lateral ankle usually allows palpation of the peroneal tendons just posterior and proximal to the lateral malleolus. Flexing and extending the everted foot is useful in localization,

Figure 8–37. Abnormal peroneal tenograms with contrast medium in the joint space.

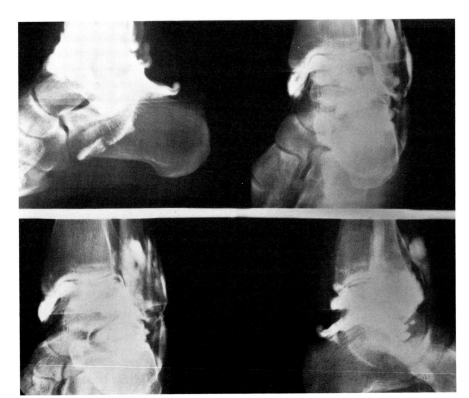

but such motion may be difficult acutely if extensive soft tissue swelling is present.

The patient should be in the lateral recumbent position, with the involved ankle supported by a cushion or towel and the medial surface nearest the table.[31] An Ace wrap or blood-pressure cup may be placed around the lower calf to prevent proximal filling of the muscle and tendons. The ankle is prepared using sterile technique. The skin over the

tendon and just above the posterior aspect of the lateral malleolus is infiltrated with 1 percent lidocaine (Xylocaine). A 22-gauge 1 1/2-inch needle is directed oblique (cephalad to caudad) into the tendon. The bevel of the needle should face down. The oblique needle position and inferiorly directed bevel reduce the incidence of extravasation. Resistance will be apparent when the needle enters the tendon.[40] A small test injection will outline the

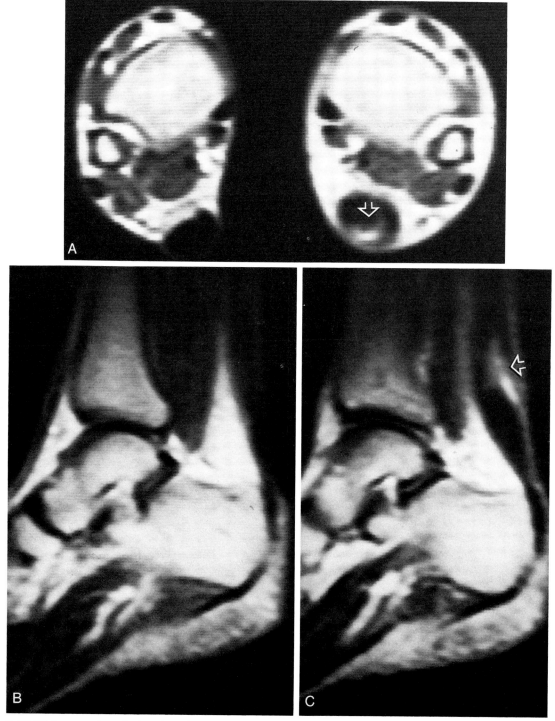

Figure 8–38. MR images of the foot and ankle. Axial views *(A)* through the Achilles tendons. Note the increased signal *(arrow)* due to tearing and hemorrhage. Sagittal views of the normal *(B)* and torn *(C)* Achilles tendon *(arrow* indicates tear).

tendon in the sheath if proper position is achieved. Five to 20 ml of contrast material may be required to fill the tendon sheaths. The injection must be fluoroscopically monitored. Extravasation may be technical rather than pathologic. This is difficult to determine without fluoroscopic control.

Following the injection the needle is removed, and the ankle is exercised fluoroscopically. Films are taken in the AP, lateral, and oblique projections.

Normal Tenographic Anatomy

The peroneus longus and brevis share a common tendon sheath from just above the lateral malleolus to just above the calcaneal trochlea. The sheaths separate at this point. The sheaths are covered by the inferior retinaculum at the midcalcaneal level.[37] The tendon sheath of the peroneus brevis inserts into the tuberosity of the 5th metatarsal. The tendon sheath of the peroneus longus may end inferiorly to the cuboid, forming a second sheath distal to the long plantar ligament. In certain cases the tendon sheath is continuous. The peroneus longus inserts into the base of the 1st metatarsal.[41] Normally contrast material will remain within the tendon sheath. The extent of distal filling is variable. However, both sheaths are usually clearly seen to the level of the calcaneocuboid joint. Beyond this point filling of the peroneus longus is usually incomplete.

In the normal setting (Fig. 8–36) the sheaths should be clearly outlined and smooth. Some subcutaneous extravasation may occur with overfilling. Contrast medium should not enter the joint space or stop at the calcaneal retinaculum.

Abnormal Tenograms

As noted previously, ankle arthrography may be inaccurate in the detection of calcaneofibular ligament tears. Tenography is considered more accurate. Black evaluated 106 patients.[31] Surgical confirmation in 30 patients correlated with the findings on the tenogram. Twenty-five patients had complete tears. Partial tears were noted in 5 cases. Evans noted only 1 false negative tenogram in 16 patients.[36] If the calcaneofibular ligament is torn, contrast material will enter the joint (Fig. 8–37). This communication may close after 3 to 7 days; therefore, the tenogram should be performed as soon as possible following the ankle injury.[31, 33, 43] Soft tissue extravasation or contrast material confined to the tendon sheath is considered normal.[36]

Peroneal tendinitis may occur following calcaneal fractures, ankle sprains, or lateral malleolar fractures.[37, 38] Tenography will demonstrate irregularity, stenosis, obstruction, or tendon rupture.[37, 38, 40] Following calcaneal fractures, bone spurs or fibrosis usually result in defects near the inferior calcaneal retinaculum.

Subluxation of the peroneal tendons is uncommon.[34, 45] The exact mechanism of injury is unclear.

Stover and Bryan felt that the injury resulted from inversion with the foot dorsiflexed.[52] Often the diagnosis can be made clinically. Patients complain of the ankle "giving way." Palpation and stressing of the ankle may allow the subluxation to be reproduced by the examining physician. Tenography with stress applied under fluoroscopic guidance is useful in more difficult cases. A small chip fracture of the lateral malleolus may also be present. This is best seen on the internal oblique view.[34]

A recent noninvasive imaging technique, magnetic resonance imaging, shows promise in evaluation of ligament and tendon injuries of the foot and ankle (Fig. 8–38). Further study is required to determine the accuracy of this technique in evaluating soft tissue trauma. (See Magnetic Resonance Imaging in Chapter 1.)

FRACTURES OF THE ANKLE

Several classifications describe the wide variety of ankle fracture patterns. These classifications may be grouped according to whether they emphasize the pathologic anatomy,[78] the mechanism of injury,[56, 65–68] the treatment,[63] or a combination of the three.

Pathologic Anatomy

As well described by Charnley,[61] fractures about the ankle are best considered by taking into account the ligamentous attachments of the fractured segments. This intimate relationship is quite important not only with respect to understanding what is fractured but also with regard to the mechanism of injury and even the treatment options.

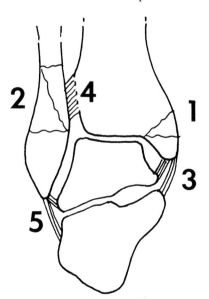

Figure 8–39. Schematic representation of the ring of soft tissue and articular surfaces resulting in ankle stability. The sites of disruptions are labeled 1 through 5.

The ankle can and should be thought of as a closed ringlike structure, as demonstrated in Figures 8–1 and 8–39. The distance of the medial malleolus to the talus, the talus to the plafond, and the lateral malleolus to the talus should essentially be the same. Means of measuring the tibiofibular distance at the syndesmosis have not been standardized, but the radiographic anatomy should be well understood (Fig. 8–40). Recently, Leeds and Ehrlich have emphasized the necessity of a careful and standardized assessment of the width of the syndesmosis to judge the adequacy of reduction.[69] By their criteria this distance measures 4.5 mm. If the distance exceeds that of the opposite ankle by more than 2 mm, the ankle is felt to be inadequately reduced.[69]

In general, five sites of disruption occur singularly or in combination (Fig. 8–39).

Beginning medially, the medial malleolus (Site 1) may be pulled or sheared off, depending upon the direction of the force (Figs. 8–41 and 8–42). Usually, this is not, therefore, a comminuted fragment. The deltoid ligament is not disrupted with the medial malleolar fracture but remains attached to the medial malleolus.

Fracture of the fibula (Site 2), beginning at the level of the plafond (Site 2A), occurs with tension, shear, or torsion. When this occurs, an associated injury of the medial malleolus or deltoid ligament must be excluded clinically and radiologically. With a direct blow or with some valgus stress loads, the fibula may fracture above the level of the syndesmosis (Site 2B) (Fig. 8–41). In this setting the frac-

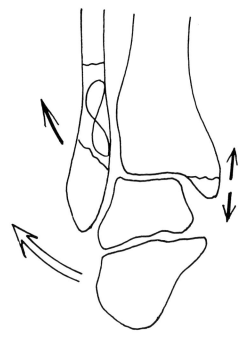

Figure 8–41. A valgus stress tends to cause a shearing injury of the lateral column and a tension injury on the medial side, either a rupture of the ligament or a medial malleolar transverse fracture.

ture is transverse or comminuted. An associated injury of the syndesmosis (Site 4) and sometimes the deltoid ligament (Site 3) should be assumed with this fracture, even if not obvious.

Isolated complete tears of the deltoid ligament (Site 3) are quite rare. An associated fracture of the lateral malleolus or a tear of the lateral ligaments and syndesmosis must be considered with this injury.

The syndesmosis (Site 4) may be torn in whole or in part by external rotation or valgus injuries.

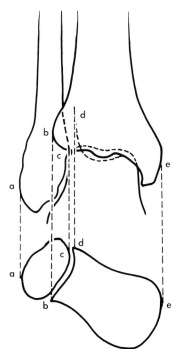

Figure 8–40. Diagrammatic representation of the radiographic shadows of the syndesmosis. (From Chapman, M. W.: Fractures and fracture-dislocations of the ankle and foot. *In* Mann, R. A. (ed.): DuVries' Surgery of the Foot. 4th Ed. St. Louis, C. V. Mosby Co., 1978.)

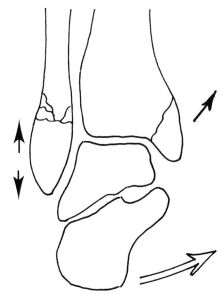

Figure 8–42. A varus stress results in a more transverse injury of the fibula and a shearing or oblique fracture of the medial malleolus.

External rotation may disrupt a portion of the syndesmosis. Fractures above or through the syndesmosis cannot occur without disruption at Sites 1, 2, or 3, either in bending or torsion. Finally, the syndesmosis is often at least partially torn with fractures of the fibula. Isolated disruption of the syndesmosis is possible but is rarely felt to be the primary pathologic event.

The lateral ankle ligaments (Site 5) are probably the most frequent site of trauma. This anatomic site is not a major concern with ankle fractures. Most often external rotation with or without varus stress causes an isolated ligament tear or a bimalleolar fracture. Clinically, residual lateral ligamentous instability after ankle fractures has not been appreciated in our practice.

More complex fracture patterns are seen with axial load, and all such fractures depend on the position of the foot at the time of loading.[68] The plantar flexed axially loaded foot accounts for the posterior malleolar component of the trimalleolar fracture. Assessment of the integrity of the plafond is of paramount importance. Damage to this structure as a result of compressive loads is probably the most significant pathologic feature of ankle trauma.[62, 71, 75]

Classification Systems

For any classification system to be of value, four requirements should be more or less satisfied: (1) the system is easy to understand and remember; (2) the classification allows a description and, therefore, a better understanding of the mechanism of injury; (3) the categorization aids in understanding the pathologic anatomy and thus possibly the treatment; (4) the system relates to the ultimate prognosis to be anticipated. It is appropriate to judge each of the more popular classification systems according to these standards.

Probably the most widely known classification system is that popularized by Lauge-Hansen.[67] The most commonly used is probably that of Weber.[78] These will be discussed in detail.

Lauge-Hansen Classification

The Lauge-Hansen classification is a more sophisticated version of an earlier scheme described by Ashhurst and Bromer.[56] This classification is the best known system of describing ankle fractures but is not routinely used. It is based on the position of the foot and the force directed against the foot at the time of injury.[65–68] The appearance of the fibular fracture allows one to define four categories of injury that provide accurate assessment of the mechanism of injury, fracture pattern, and ligament involvement (Table 8–2).[55, 56] As a further refinement, Arimoto and Forrester devised an algorithm based on the malleolar fractures, particularly the

TABLE 8–2. Lauge-Hansen Classification[55]

Pronation-abduction (see Fig. 8–43)
Stage I. Ruptured deltoid ligament or transverse medial malleolar fracture.
Stage II. Disruption of the distal tibiofibular ligaments (anterior and posterior).
Stage III. *Oblique fibular fracture at the joint level (best seen on AP view).
Pronation–lateral rotation (see Fig. 8–44)
Stage I. Rupture of the deltoid ligament or transverse medial malleolar fracture.
Stage II. Disruption of the anterior tibiofibular ligament and interosseous membrane.
Stage III. *Fibular fracture above the joint space (usually 6 cm or more above the joint line).
Stage IV. Posterior tibial chip fracture or rupture of posterior tibiofibular ligament.
Supination-adduction (see Fig. 8–45)
Stage I. Lateral ligament injury or *transverse lateral malleolar fracture below the ankle joint.
Stage II. Steep oblique fracture of the medial malleolus.
Supination–lateral rotation (see Fig. 8–46)
Stage I. Disruption of the anterior tibiofibular ligament.
Stage II. *Spiral fracture of the distal fibula near the joint (best seen on the lateral view).
Stage III. Rupture of the posterior tibiofibular ligament.
Stage IV. Transverse fracture of the medial malleolus.

*Fibular fracture appearance is key to determining mechanism of injury.

appearance of the fibula.[55] Use of this system allows an accurate description of the mechanism and degree of bone and soft tissue injury.

If the foot is in a pronated (eversion) position, abduction force at the talus produces medial traction and lateral compression. If the force is continued, the injury progresses from the medial to the lateral side of the ankle (Table 8–2) (Fig. 8–43).

If the talus is rotated laterally during pronation (eversion), the same medial stress is present. If the force is continued, the injury, which begins with a medial malleolar fracture or deltoid tear, progresses laterally in a circular fashion about the joint (Fig. 8–44). The fibular fracture is usually well above the joint space.[68]

Injuries with the foot in supination (inversion) combined with adduction force place traction on the fibula or lateral ligaments. The talus compresses the medial malleolus (Fig. 8–45) (Table 8–2). This results in lateral ligament injury or a transverse fracture of the fibula at or below the joint space. If a medial malleolar fracture occurs, it is oblique.

Supination of the foot with lateral rotation of the talus forces the distal fibula posteriorly.[55] Thus, the anterior tibiofibular ligament is injured initially. If the force continues, a circular pattern again develops (Fig. 8–46), progressing through the fibula (oblique fracture best seen on the lateral view), the posterior tibiofibular ligament, and finally the medial structures. This is the most common mechanism of injury and causes the typical bimalleolar fracture.[59, 60]

The accuracy of assessment of bone and soft tissue injury approaches 90 to 95 percent using the Lauge-Hansen system.[55]

Text continued on page 434

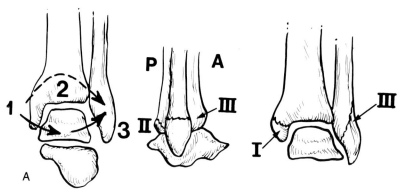

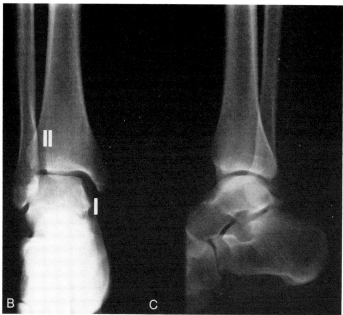

Figure 8–43. Pronation-abduction injury. Illustration of mechanism of injury (A). Stages of injury begin with medial malleolus or deltoid (I), and as the force continues the injury may progress to disruption of the distal tibiofibular ligament (II) and an oblique fibular fracture (III). PA (B) and lateral (C) views of a Stage II pronation-abduction injury. The medial ankle mortise is widened. There is no fibular fracture, but the talar shift indicates a second injury (distal tibiofibular ligaments).

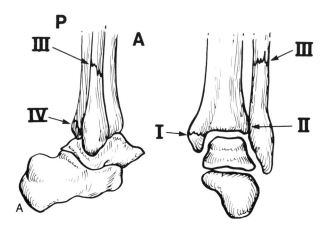

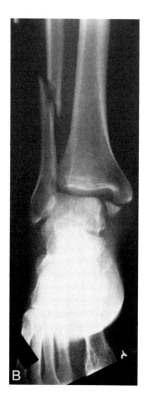

Figure 8–44. Pronation–lateral rotation injury. A, Diagram of mechanism of injury. The injury begins with the medial malleolus or deltoid ligament and progresses laterally around the joint, ending with fracture of the posterior tibia or posterior tibiofibular ligament tear. The fibular fracture (III) is well above the joint line. B, PA view of the ankle demonstrating a pronation–lateral rotation injury that has progressed to at least Stage III. Note high fibular fracture.

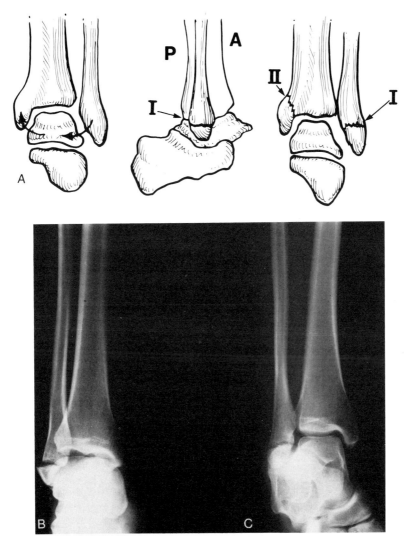

Figure 8–45. Supination-adduction injury. *A,* Diagram demonstrating transverse fracture of the fibula below the joint. If the force persists, a steep oblique medial malleolar fracture (Stage II) will occur. *B,* Supination-adduction Stage I. Transverse fibular fracture below the ankle joint.

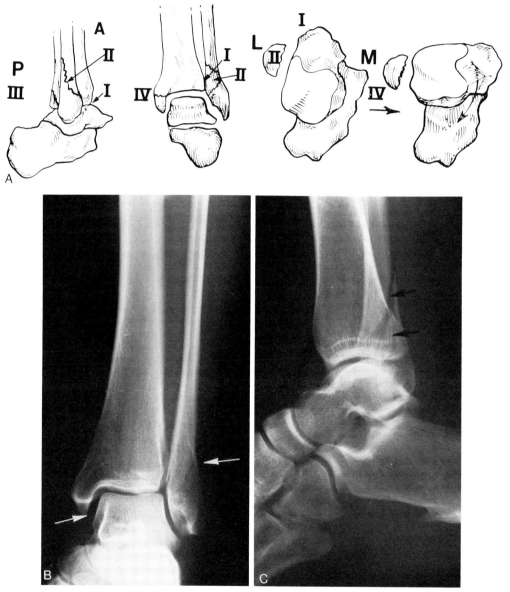

Figure 8–46. Supination–lateral rotation injury. *A*, Diagram of stages of injury beginning with the anterior tibiofibular ligament (I) and progressing to the medial malleolus (IV). Note circular progression. *B* and *C*, Supination–lateral rotation Stage IV injury with a spiral fibular fracture best seen on the lateral view *(C, upper arrow)*. There is a posterior tibial fracture *(lower arrow)* with widening medially *(upper arrow)* due to ligament disruption.

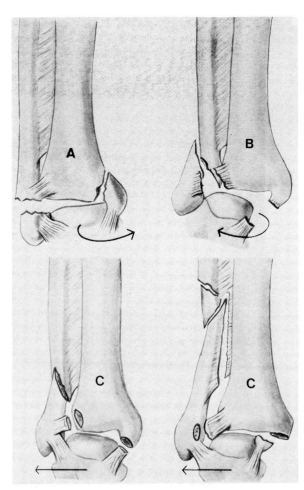

Figure 8–47. The Weber classification system relates the type of fracture to the syndesmosis. Type A is below the syndesmosis, Type B is through the syndesmosis, and Type C is through or above the distal tibiofibular syndesmosis. (From Mueller, M. E., Allgower, M., Schneider, R., et al.: Manual of Internal Fixation. New York, Springer Verlag, 1979.)

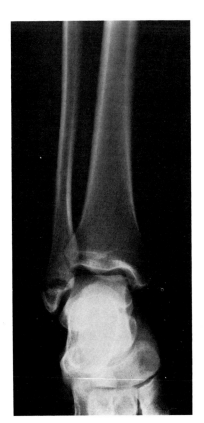

Figure 8–48. Fracture of the fibula at the level of the plafond, a Weber Type A fracture, is not common.

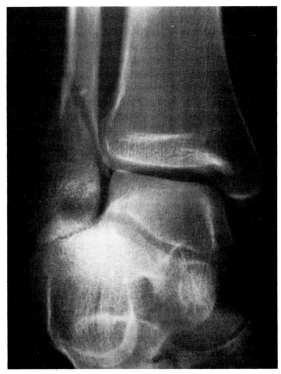

Figure 8–49. A 35-year-old female with a fracture across the syndesmosis of the lateral malleolus, a Weber Type B fracture.

Weber Classification

The Weber classification of ankle fractures is based upon the level of fibular involvement (Fig. 8–47).

Type A. An oblique or transverse fracture at or below the tibial plafond. The medial malleolus or deltoid ligament may be and often is involved, but the syndesmosis is intact (Fig. 8–48).

Type B. Fibular fracture at the level of the syndesmosis. The fracture often results from an external rotation or valgus stress, and the posterior syndesmosis is partially spared with the spiral fracture (Fig. 8–49). The medial malleolus or deltoid ligaments are injured and disrupted if significant displacement has occurred.

Type C. A posterolateral portion of the tibial articulation may be involved, occurring at the attachment of the syndesmosis (Subtype 1) (Fig. 8–50) or more proximally to include the interosseous membrane (Subtype 2) (Fig. 8–51). The medial malleolus sustains a transverse traction fracture or its equivalent, a deltoid ligament disruption. An associated avulsion fracture of the posterolateral tibial articulation is also common, which converts the injury to a trimalleolar fracture.

Authors' Preferred Classification

Because bone as a tissue fails primarily in shear,[58] which may appear clinically as a tension failure, we prefer to describe the fracture simply according to the mechanism of injury and its effect on the bone. The classification is therefore based on the orientation of the fracture line and the following principles. (1) If an oblique fracture line appears, a shearing fracture is present, indicating the direction of the applied force. (2) A transverse fracture line indicates a fracture that failed in tension. (3) The direction of torsional injuries can be identified according to the direction of the obliquity of the fracture line (Figs.

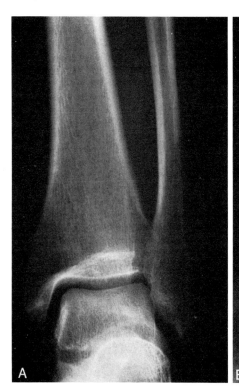
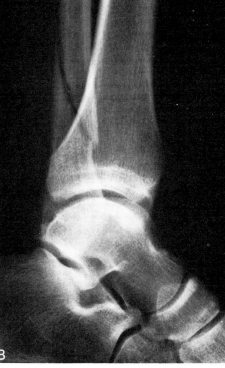

Figure 8–50. AP *(A)* and lateral *(B)* views of an essentially undisplaced rotational type of lateral malleolar fracture (Weber Type C fracture), which can be appreciated only on the lateral view. This fracture may be treated in a cast.

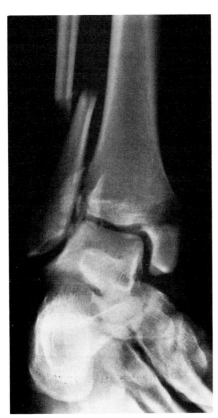

Figure 8–51. The more proximal fracture of the fibula is another variant of the Weber Type C fracture.

8–41 and 8–42). Theoretically, torsional fractures are oriented at a 45° angle with the long axis of the bone. (4) An axial blow causes fractures of the plafond, and plantar flexion of the foot is required

for fracture of the posterior malleolus. By noting the site of fracture and displacement, one can obtain an awareness of the soft tissue injury. Hence, we describe a fracture as a rotational, shearing, or tension injury of the specific bone. Once the fracture is described, we employ the Weber system to aid in deciding the appropriate treatment.

It is felt, therefore, that the fracture should be described in terms of the extent of injury. A detailed knowledge of bone and ligamentous anatomy and a classification system that helps the interpretation of the radiograph should be developed by all who assess the radiographic appearance or who care for patients with this fracture.

Prognosis

The prognosis is predicated on two general considerations: severity of the injury and adequacy of reduction.[62, 70, 75] The severity of the injury may also be estimated by the degree of displacement, the specific type of fracture, plafond involvement, documentation of cartilage loss, and the degree of soft tissue injury. Some have correlated a specific classification of a fracture with a poor prognosis.[64] We were unable to make this correlation consistently, however.[62] Probably the most important variable with respect to injury type is the amount of cartilage damage and the related but not necessarily commensurate fracture of the plafond.[59, 62, 70, 71, 77, 80] Pettrone and colleagues have also shown that statistically significant prognostic factors include age and restoration of the deltoid and syndesmosis ligaments. These are particularly important with respect to the anatomic reduction.[73]

Figure 8–52. A, A transverse medial malleolar fracture. This occurred with a nearly pure valgus stress to the ankle joint. The fracture must be treated with fixation because it is displaced more than 2 mm. *(B)* This fracture, displaced more than 2 mm, has progressed to a non-union.

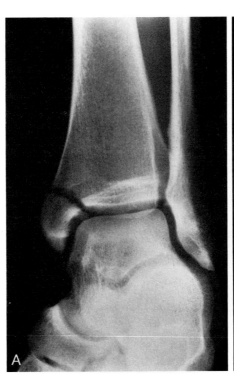
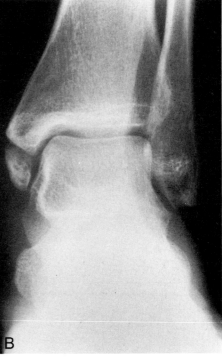

While the fracture type is clearly beyond the control of the treating physician, the adequacy of reduction is an important variable that reflects the quality of treatment. The theoretical sensitivity of incongruity due to talar displacement has been clearly shown by Ramsey and Hamilton, who have demonstrated a reduction of approximately 50 percent of the contact area with only a 2 mm lateral translation of the talus articulation.[74] This extreme sensitivity to translation is explained by the high degree of congruity of the joint, which is due to the trochlear nature of the articulation (Fig. 8–39). The

sensitivity of the surgical result as a function of lateral tibiotalar translation has been substantiated in the clinical literature.[62, 80] Thus, lateral translation of more than 1 mm is not generally felt to be desirable, and a perfect, or anatomic, reduction is preferable.[71, 75] This assessment of translation can only be made accurately, however, on the 20° internal rotation or true mortise radiograph.

On occasion, delay of treatment may be necessary because of an associated injury or a delay of presentation. In this circumstance, an anatomic or even acceptable reduction is more difficult to obtain,

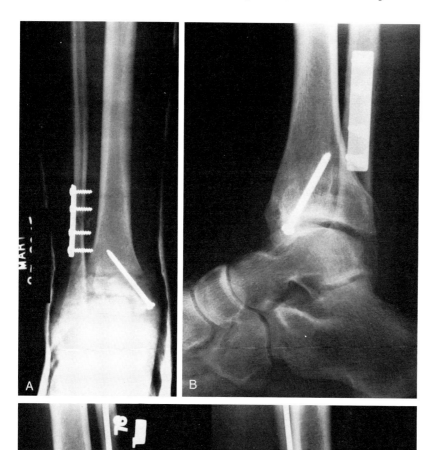

Figure 8–53. The bimalleolar fracture in Figure 8–51 was treated with a plate laterally and a screw medially, and the treatment resulted in an essentially anatomic reduction (A and B). This displaced fibular fracture was treated with a Rush rod (C).

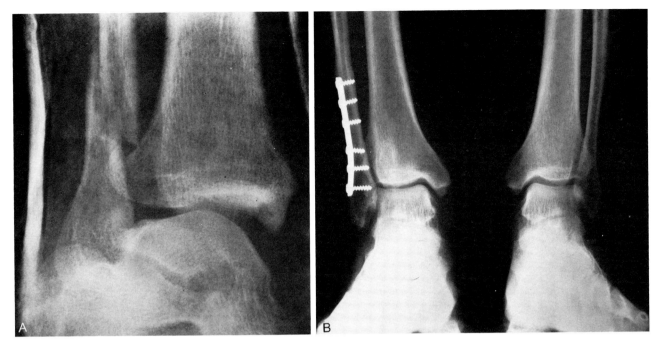

Figure 8–54. A Weber Type C fracture was displaced in plaster *(A)* but was stabilized by this reduction *(B)*, and the syndesmosis screw was not necessary.

though it is not necessarily impossible. This difficulty in achieving reduction is particularly noticeable on the lateral radiograph. The posterior malleolus is often observed to become rapidly osteoporotic, and a unsatisfactory delayed reduction is not uncommon.[62]

Finally, most of the recent literature emphasizes the mechanical importance of the fibula[76] and the necessity of both preserving or restoring the normal alignment and length of this bone and securing the fracture rigidly enough to allow early motion.[71, 72, 80] The goals are better met with open reduction and fixation of both sides of the fractured ankle.[73] It is important, therefore, to scrutinize the lateral radiograph for fibular angulatory alignment and the mortise view for fibular angulation and length. Axial rotation of the fibula, on the other hand, is rarely an identified clinical problem, possibly because axial rotation cannot be well documented with routine views. The CT scan, however, can quite accurately demonstrate this aspect of malalignment in selective cases.

Treatment

Treatment of the ankle fracture obviously depends upon the specific nature of the injury. The one common factor in all, however, is the goal of a perfect reduction of the articular surfaces. The standard treatment may be summarized as follows.

Single Malleolar Fracture, Undisplaced. This fracture will be treated as a function of the degree of displacement (Figs. 8–50 and 8–51). If less than 2 mm of displacement is evident, the ankle mortise will usually be intact. There will be no significant ligamentous injury, and the fracture will be treated by cast immobilization for a variable period of time, usually not less than 3 or more than 8 weeks. With adequate reduction non-union is uncommon.[79] Re-

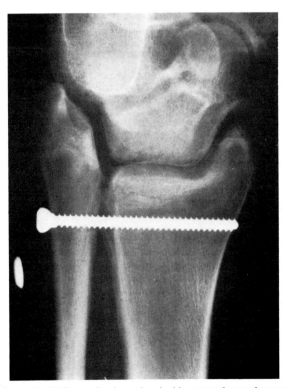

Figure 8–55. This patient was treated by a syndesmosis screw in order to stabilize the lateral malleolus until the syndesmosis had healed. This is a controversial procedure, and in general we do not prefer this particular technique.

sidual symptoms are uncommon with this treatment. Follow-up for the first several weeks with x-rays through plaster is appropriate to ensure that displacement does not occur.

Single Malleolar Fracture, Displaced. If the medial malleolus is displaced by 2 mm, internal fixation of the fragment, which is rarely comminuted, with the single malleolar screw is the treatment of choice (Fig. 8–52). After surgery, immobilization to allow healing of the soft tissue is maintained for approximately 2 weeks. Similarly, the lateral malleolus may be treated with a rod, screws, or a plate.[71, 72, 75, 79] The patient is then placed in an air splint or hinged orthosis and uses crutches as needed for an additional 6 to 10 weeks. In most instances, the fracture will heal in 3 months.

Bimalleolar Fracture. This fracture is generally displaced more than 1 mm, which precludes closed treatment (Fig. 8–53). In most instances the bimalleolar fracture will not be associated with significant comminution, and, therefore, the medial malleolus

is fixed with a malleolar screw. For the lateral malleolus, if a rotatory component is present or a long oblique fracture line has occurred, interfragmentary screws are used. For more transverse lesions we prefer the use of a plate, although a Rush rod may be used in these patients by those experienced with this technique (Fig. 8–53).

If the lateral malleolus is fractured through (Weber B) or, more particularly, if it is fractured above the syndesmosis (Weber C), careful restoration of this fracture fragment is necessary.[72, 80] If the fibular fracture can be reduced and fixed and the mortise thus reduced, we do not feel that a syndesmosis screw is necessary or even desirable despite significant initial displacement. If the lateral malleolus heals in an anatomic or near anatomic position, the syndesmosis will also heal adequately, and the syndesmosis screw is thus not needed for the stability of the system (Fig. 8–54).

The use of supplementary fixation is complicated by three factors. (1) Incorrect tightening of the screw

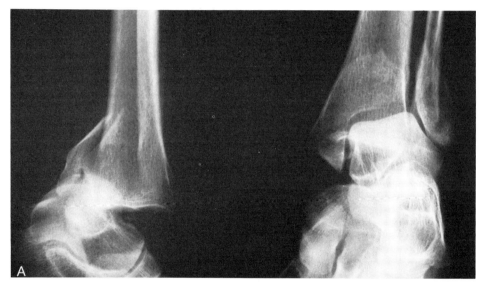
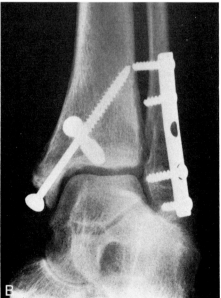
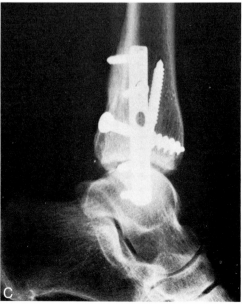

Figure 8–56. Trimalleolar fracture with intact plafond. Radiographs *(A)* show difficulty in determining size of posterior malleolus. AP *(B)* and lateral *(C)* views show anatomic reduction with plate and screw fixation.

with the ankle in plantar flexion may limit dorsiflexion, since the talar dome is wider anteriorly than posteriorly.[4] (2) Tilting of the distal fracture fragment may lead to malalignment of the ankle mortise with the fibula, the proximal portion of the distal fragment tilting medially and the distal fragment laterally. (3) If the screw is not removed, significant resorption may occur around the screw, resulting in pain. If a screw across the syndesmosis is used, it should be removed. This adds an additional, albeit anticipated, surgical procedure to the treatment plan (Fig. 8–55).

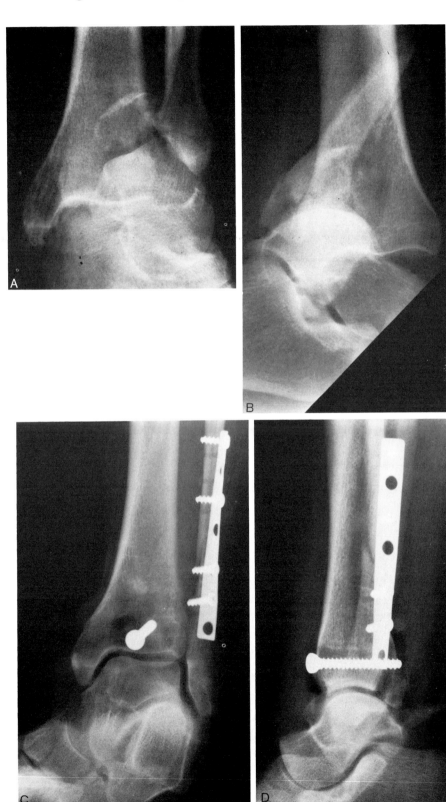

Figure 8–57. Trimalleolar fracture *(A and B)* with good reduction evident on AP view *(C)*. But note proximally displaced posterior malleolus *(D)*.

Trimalleolar Fracture. The medial and lateral malleolar fractures are managed as described above. The posterior malleolus is reduced and fixed if more than 25 percent of the articular surface is involved (Fig. 8–56). To evaluate this feature of the fracture properly, several views may be necessary, since displacement distorts the usual landmarks for the routine lateral radiograph (Fig. 8–56). It should be remembered that a good portion of the posterior malleolus does not involve hyaline cartilage; thus, near normal ankle function can be preserved even if this is left displaced. When fixation is required,

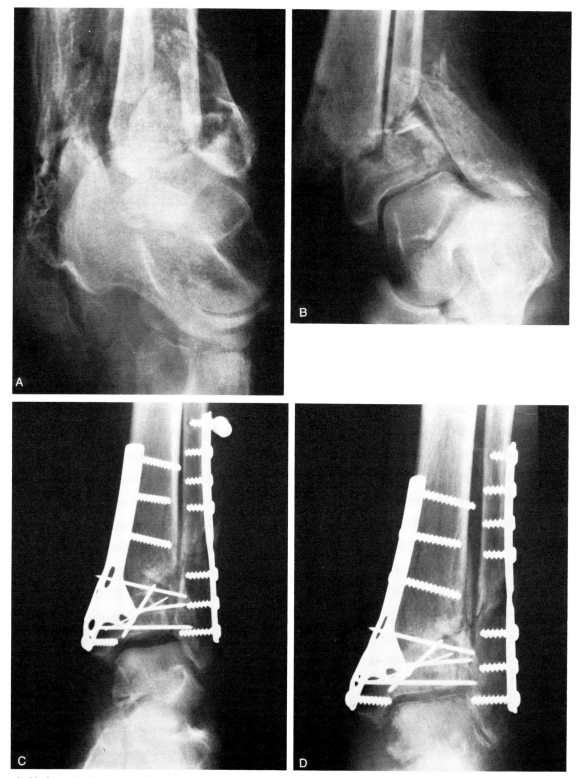

Figure 8–58. Comminuted plafond fracture *(A and B)* was treated by open reduction, internal fixation, and traction. The follow-up radiographs *(C and D)* reveal reasonably satisfactory results on the AP view. Notice widened joint space because of calcaneal traction in *C.*

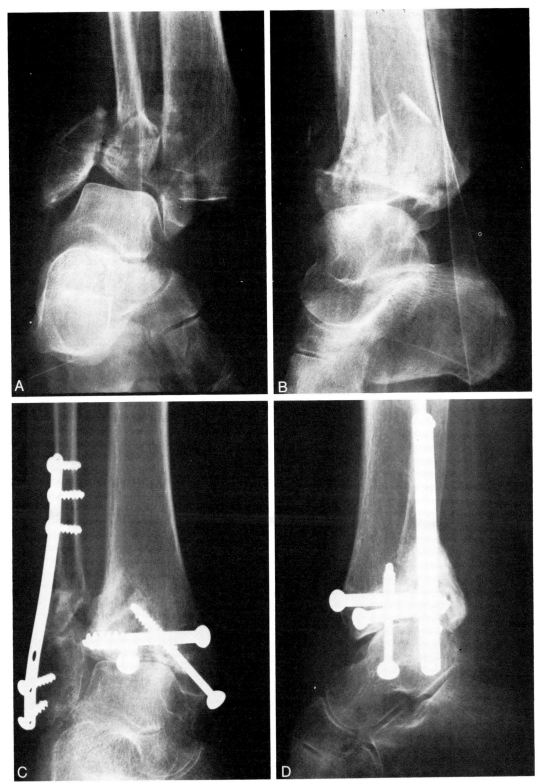

Figure 8–59. Plafond fracture *(A and B)* treated with open reduction and internal fixation *(C and D).* An adequate reduction was followed by a late arthrosis.

the technique is demanding, and an anatomic reduction is frequently not obtained (Fig. 8–57). It has not been determined whether absolute restoration of this particular fragment is necessary for normal function. The usual modality of the fixation is interfragmentary compression. Usually the fixation is

applied from the front, although occasionally a posterior exposure and approach is more convenient (Fig. 8–56).

Fracture of the Tibial Plafond. Plafond fractures are serious injuries. The articular cartilage may be so disrupted and fragmented that portions of the plafond are lost or missing; additionally, a loose fragment may result from inadequate healing. Thus, anatomic restoration as demonstrated by the radiograph may still be associated with significant cartilage damage. In such cases the damage is revealed only by follow-up radiographs showing arthrosis. The best treatment anatomically restores the fragments as best as possible with interfragmentary screws. If there is a component of the fracture involving the metaphysis, neutralization plates are likewise employed. For severely comminuted fractures, the distal tibia is bone grafted (Fig. 8–58).[75]

Comminuted Fractures. The standard of treatment at this time for displaced ankle fractures calls for rigid fixation and early mobilization.[71] The early mobilization, however, is allowed only if the surgeon feels that rigid fixation has been obtained. The badly comminuted fracture, which by its very nature may not be amenable to such a treatment modality, is treated by inserting a calcaneal pin; traction is applied for a variable period, usually about 2 weeks (Fig. 8–58). This may help preserve the ankle mortise and allow fibrous ingrowth that prevents or at least delays the appearance of post-traumatic arthritis.

Results

The results of treatment are directly correlated with the fracture type as well as the severity of the injury.[62, 64, 80] Again, plafond fractures and cartilage damage are the most significant variables. With bi- and trimalleolar fractures that do not involve sig-

nificant cartilage injury, rigid fixation and early mobilization in most instances is associated with greater than 80 percent satisfactory results. If one of the more serious prognostic factors obtains, then satisfactory results are seen in less than 50 percent. In fact, it is felt that with follow-up examination post-traumatic arthritis will be expected eventually in virtually all of these injuries (Fig. 8–59).

Complications

The most readily apparent radiographic complication of ankle fractures is the loss of reduction. Although usually seen with nonoperative treatment involving plaster casts (see Fig. 8–54), loss of reduction may occur in instances in which internal fixation has been employed.[57] Comminuted medial malleolar fractures are difficult to manage. Usually multiple pins or small screws are employed. The comminuted displaced fibula is likewise a difficult fracture to manage. Often only a marginally adequate reduction is possible in the presence of a comminuted lateral malleolus. Both the AP and lateral roentgenogram are necessary for a full evaluation of the adequacy and maintenance of the reduction.

An important feature of radiographic significance is the anterior or posterior translocated displacement of the talus. The mortise or AP view appears to show a narrowing of the ankle joint even early after injury, leading to the incorrect diagnosis of post-traumatic arthrosis. However, the lateral roentgenogram reveals subluxation of the talus, usually

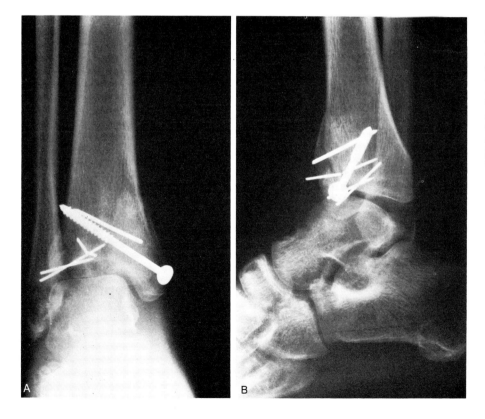

Figure 8–60. Mortise view of what appears to be post-traumatic arthrosis *(A)*, although this patient suffered plafond fracture only 6 weeks earlier. Lateral view *(B)* reveals an anterior subluxation of the talus, demonstrating that what appeared to be ankle arthrosis actually resulted from the subluxation. This case illustrates the fact that both AP and lateral views of fractures of the joint are minimal requirements for accurate assessment.

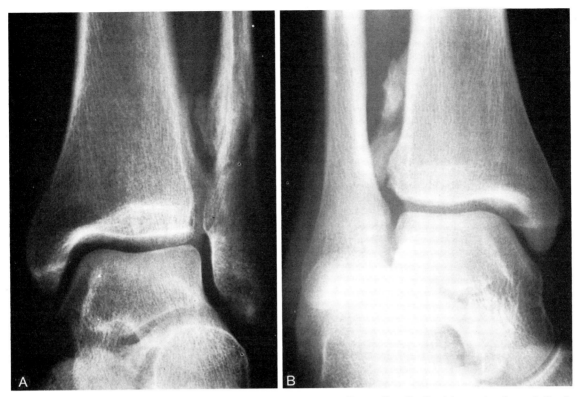

Figure 8–61. *A,* Patient with a Weber Type C injury of the lateral malleolus. Six months after the injury, extensive calcification of the syndesmosis has occurred, but the patient has no symptoms referable to this. *B,* Ossification of the synostosis can also occur after a soft tissue injury alone.

posteriorly, thus providing an explanation of the apparent narrowing seen on the AP radiograph (Fig. 8–60). Post-traumatic arthritis may have a similar roentgenographic appearance. The brief duration since the injury and the findings on the lateral radiograph should rule out any confusion of this malalignment with post-traumatic arthrosis.

Finally, with Weber B or C fractures, the syndesmosis may become calcified (Fig. 8–61). This has theoretical implications with respect to ankle me-

chanics but is of little clinical relevance even if apparent synostosis has occurred.

LIGAMENTOUS INJURIES

Soft tissue injuries are usually not amenable to ready or accurate diagnosis by radiographic techniques. Ankle ligamentous injury as associated with instability is, however, more clearly defined and

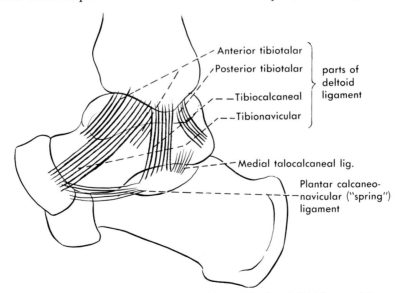

Figure 8–62. The ligamentous distribution of the medial aspect of the ankle, the deltoid ligament, is composed of superficial and deep fibers. This very strong ligament complex is rarely sprained, and medial instability is quite unusual. (From Hollinshead, W. E.: Anatomy for Surgeons, Vol. 3: The Back and Limbs. 3rd Ed. New York, Harper & Row, 1982.)

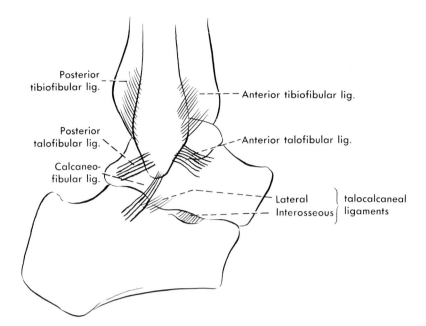

Figure 8–63. The lateral ligamentous complex is vulnerable to ankle sprain. Sprains most frequently involve the anterior talofibular ligament and, with severe injuries, the calcaneal fibular ligament. (From Hollinshead, W. E.: Anatomy for Surgeons, Vol. 3: The Back and Limbs. 3rd Ed. New York, Harper & Row, 1982.)

clarified by the several radiographic procedures discussed earlier.

Anatomy

The high degree of congruity of the ankle joint is well recognized and has been previously discussed. The nature of the motion and the lever arm provided by the foot can result in severe stresses placed on the articular system. These stresses, in turn, can disrupt the ligamentous and soft tissue supporting structures. Medially, the deltoid ligament is observed to be a thick strong structure originating from the tip of the medial malleolus and inserting

on the medial aspect of the talus below the articular surface in a fan-like manner (Fig. 8–62). As with the lateral ligamentous complex, three portions have been described: the anterior and posterior superficial deltoid ligaments and the intermediate deep deltoid or tibiotalar ligament. These structures, while identifiable in the dissection laboratory, are rarely observed clinically. They are visible only when the lateral malleolus has been fractured with lateral displacement of the talus and without medial malleolar fracture. The deltoid sprain as an isolated soft tissue injury is rare owing to the considerable strength of the ligament. Thus, complete disruption without fibular fracture is quite rare.[103]

The lateral stabilizing structures consist of three

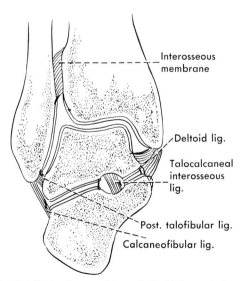

Figure 8–64. The position of the posterior talofibular ligament is such that it is rarely involved in ankle sprains. (From Hollinshead, W. E.: Anatomy for Surgeons, Vol. 3: The Back and Limbs. 3rd Ed. New York, Harper & Row, 1982.)

portions. The anterior talofibular ligament originates from the anterior aspect of the distal fibula and inserts on the lateral aspect of the talus just inferior and distal to the anterior lateral articulation (Fig. 8–63). The posterior talofibular ligament originates from the posterior distal aspect of the fibula and inserts on the posterior aspect of the talus (Fig. 8–64). The calcaneofibular ligament originates from the tip of the fibula and inserts onto the calcaneus. Thus, this particular ligament spans both the ankle and the subtalar joints (Fig. 8–63). As with many ligamentous structures of the body, these ligaments are sometimes rather difficult to isolate accurately, as they primarily represent a specialized thickening of the ankle articular capsule.[3]

The orientation of the lateral ligaments is of some importance in trying to understand the mechanism of ankle sprain and instability. The anterior fibular ligament is almost horizontal to the floor when the ankle is dorsiflexed. With the foot flat or in plantar flexion, it makes an angle of approximately 45° to the horizontal. This orientation is rather variable. However, recognition of this orientation does serve to emphasize the primary function of this ligament, which is to restrict internal rotation of the foot.[82, 85, 89, 100] The posterior talofibular ligament can be described as the mirror image of the anterior fibular ligament but oriented posteriorly. In general, the calcaneofibular ligament is vertically oriented with respect to the horizontal, assuming a slight anterior angulation with dorsiflexion and a posterior angulation with plantar flexion. Thus, in most of its functional range, this ligament tends to resist varus displacement or angulation of the ankle joint.[90]

Function

As mentioned earlier, a significant amount of variation exists with respect to the orientation of the ligamentous complex.[4] In general, the medial ligament simply consists of a fan-shaped thickening of the capsule. The orientation of its fibers appears to be less significant.

Laterally, however, the more horizontal orientation of the anterior talofibular ligament suggests its function. It resists internal rotation but offers less resistance to pure inversion.

The calcaneofibular ligament, on the other hand, offers relatively little resistance to internal rotation but does offer significant varus stability to this joint. However, the calcaneofibular ligament makes no contribution to subtalar joint stability, even though it does cross this joint. Brantigan and colleagues have suggested that chronic subtalar instability is more common than usually appreciated and is associated with lateral ankle sprains.[82] The difficulty of adequately imaging subtalar joints by radiographic methods, however, makes this claim still somewhat speculative, and the data have not been advanced in a way that accurately indicates the

incidence of subtalar instability. An important anatomic and radiographic feature of the calcaneofibular ligament is its intimate relationship with the peroneal tendon sheath. As stated earlier, if this ligament is torn, a communication exists between the joint and the peroneal sheath. Hence the rationale for the ankle arthrogram.

The posterior talofibular ligament is of relatively little importance clinically, but it does tend to resist external rotation of the ankle. The congruity of the ankle articulation itself also supports this function.[85]

Mechanism of Injury

Ankle sprains are caused by an inversion and internal rotation of the foot (Fig. 8–65). This occurs most often in some degree of ankle plantar flexion. The combined effect is to produce a supination force to the foot with the combined plantar flexion, inversion, and internal rotation. Many types of accidents can obviously produce a sprained ankle, but most severe injuries occur during sports, usually contact sports. However, the diagnosis has also been made as a result of patients "falling off their high-heeled shoes."

The mechanism of chronic instability or the precise pathologic anatomy is a more difficult matter, however. Although it has generally been assumed that chronic instability simply represents repeated sprains or twisting of the ankle, experimental and clinical data suggest that the perception of the chronic instability may, in fact, be due to a relocation of the ankle during heel strike from a slightly

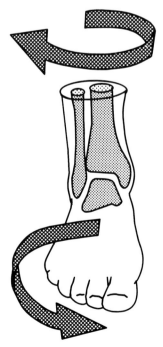

Figure 8–65. Sprains of the ankle result in a complex motion of both eversion and external rotation of the foot.

subluxed position that occurs in plantar flexion and external rotation during the swing-through phase of gait.[86] It is likely that elements of both are involved. Some individuals do sustain repeated inversion and twisting injuries of the hindfoot, resulting in chronic instability or recurrent sprains. However, the painful sensation of giving way may, in fact, be more indicative of the latter explanation. The sensation of giving way in this case would relate to the reduction of the slightly subluxed talotibial joint that occurs on heel strike. In this instance, the radiograph, even the stress view, may be deceptively negative.[109]

Classification and Pathologic Anatomy

The precise pathologic anatomy of the sprained ankle has not been scientifically confirmed, largely because minor injuries that result in a stable joint are not surgically explored. Thus, the pathologic evidence of injury is lacking. Experimental data confirm the clinical impression that the anterior talofibular ligament is the first to be disrupted.[90] More extensive internal rotation of the foot is then accompanied by an inversion stress on the talus and calcaneus. With this increased stress the calcaneofibular ligament tears, and the ankle becomes grossly unstable.[100, 106] The generally accepted clinical classification is as follows.

The patient with Grade I injury (mild sprain) will present with a painful ankle and will usually be able to ambulate with mild to moderate soft tissue swelling localized to the level of the lateral malleolus (Fig. 8–66). The patient is tender precisely over the anterior talofibular ligament but not over the region of the calcaneofibular or posterior talofibular ligaments. The radiograph shows increased soft tissue swelling but not more than a mild or moderate degree. Significantly, the ankle is stable on stress testing and radiograph. It is felt that this represents a simple stretching or partial tear of some of the fibers of the anterior talofibular ligament.

Grade II injury (moderate sprain) is the most difficult type of injury to diagnose accurately, since swelling is a highly unreliable sign of the nature or extent of pathology. Usually a significant and, in some instances, massive amount of swelling will develop. We have observed ecchymosis to be present a third of the way up the leg in a patient subsequently diagnosed with a Grade II sprain at follow-up (Fig. 8–67). The degree of swelling may, in fact, be greater than that associated with ankle fractures. Thus, this particular finding is of little benefit to the clinician or radiologist in helping to differentiate this sprain from a Grade III injury. Palpation demonstrates the precise and localized tenderness over the anterior talofibular ligament and may, on occasion, demonstrate mild discomfort over the calcaneofibular ligament. Inversion and internal rotation of the ankle does reproduce pain, but significantly the ankle appears stable on a stress

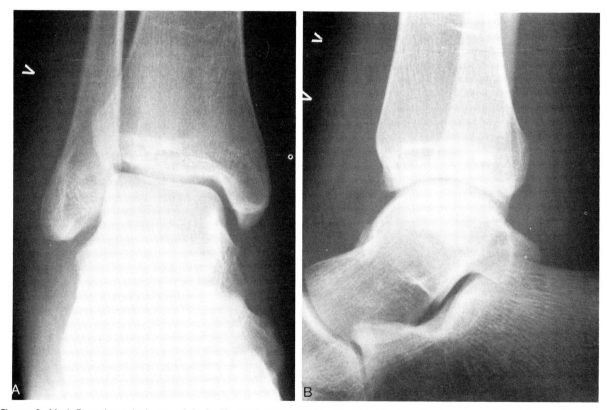

Figure 8–66. A, Type I sprain is associated with moderate swelling observed on the AP view *(arrow)*. B, If the swelling is more extensive, the lateral view also demonstrates this finding.

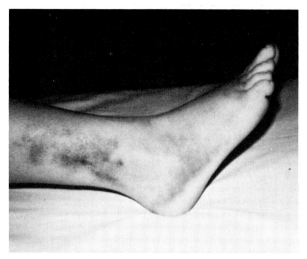

Figure 8–67. This patient had considerable ecchymosis over the lateral aspect of the ankle, yet the ankle was stable. This was a Type II injury.

roentgenogram. In this instance, the anterior talofibular ligament has been partially torn, while the calcaneofibular ligament has been strained or stretched. We should emphasize, again, that there is no demonstrable instability with the Grade II sprain regardless of the degree of soft tissue swelling.

In Grade III injury (severe sprain) the swelling is usually rather significant. When seen early, however, the swelling may be deceiving, since the hemorrhage occurring about the tear is dissipated

through the torn capsule. In fact, a Grade II sprain may commonly have a greater degree of swelling than the Grade III injury. The tenderness, however, not only is localized precisely over the anterior talofibular ligament but also appears at the tip of the fibula, at the calcaneofibular ligament. The posterior talofibular ligament is almost always spared in the ankle sprain.

The significant feature that distinguishes the Grade III, or severe sprain, from the Grade II sprain is the demonstration of ankle instability. This cannot be accurately assessed by the routine stress view taken in an emergency room. Ankle instability should be assessed by a stress radiograph but only after the ankle has been adequately anesthetized. We prefer to perform an intra-articular injection of 1 percent lidocaine (Xylocaine), placing approximately 15 ml into the joint. This will anesthetize the injury adequately, allowing one to obtain a stress view without a great deal of pain. Importantly, if no resistance is met upon this injection, significant capsular damage and hence instability should be suspected. The stress views should be performed with the ankle in about 10° of plantar flexion with as much varus tilt placed directly on the calcaneus as can be tolerated. The identical position and stress should be applied to the opposite ankle (Fig. 8–68).

Interpretation of the stress radiograph has generated a significant amount of controversy. This has been analyzed by many observers[89, 98, 108, 110] with data that are extremely difficult and frankly confusing (see earlier discussion). The best data are prob-

Figure 8–68. Bilateral stress views of a patient with a symptomatic left ankle. Notice the talar tilt is equal bilaterally. Thus, this is not considered an unstable joint in spite of the 10° talar tilt.

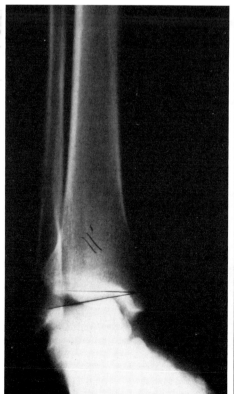
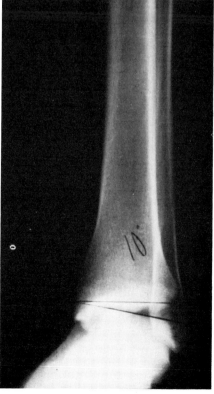

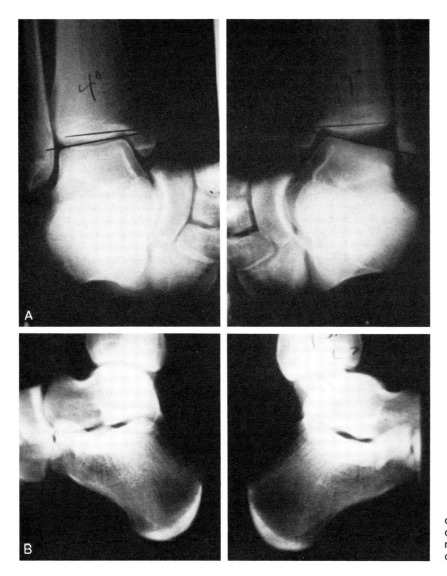

Figure 8–69. Stress view of a patient with a Type III injury. *A,* Notice the significant amount of talar tilt on the AP view. *B,* Also note the corresponding positive anterior drawer sign on the lateral view.

ably those of Cox, who has reported a prospective study of Annapolis midshipmen.[89] In this group 3° to 20° absolute talar tilt was observed. Thus, the tilt must be compared with that of the opposite ankle, and a difference of greater than 5° is presumptive evidence of a Grade III, or severe, sprain.

A supplementary test of instability includes the anterior drawer stress measurement from a lateral radiograph (see earlier discussion) (Fig. 8–69). Interpretation is somewhat more difficult owing to the fact that the landmarks are not as readily identified or measured.[108] Further, rotatory displacement may occur that is not completely demonstrated. It is generally felt that more than 2 mm of anterior translation of the talar dome from under the plafond compared with the normal opposite side is again evidence of ankle instability (Fig. 8–70). It should be noted from the discussion of anatomy that this test specifically stresses the anterior talofibular ligament. It is felt that the test cannot be positive without disruption of the calcaneofibular ligament as well.

Because of the high degree of individual variability and the difficulty of demonstrating with certainty a Grade III or unstable ankle in some instances, an arthrogram may be obtained. The rationale, technique, and interpretation of this study have already been described.

Routine Radiography

The routine radiographic views of an ankle that has sustained an acute ligamentous injury show soft tissue swelling but are invariably negative for

Figure 8–71. This patient sustained a significant ankle injury. *A,* Notice that the non-weight-bearing AP radiograph does show some slight widening of the lateral joint *(arrows). B,* This is a subtle clue to a possible significant disruption, which is verified here with the stress test.

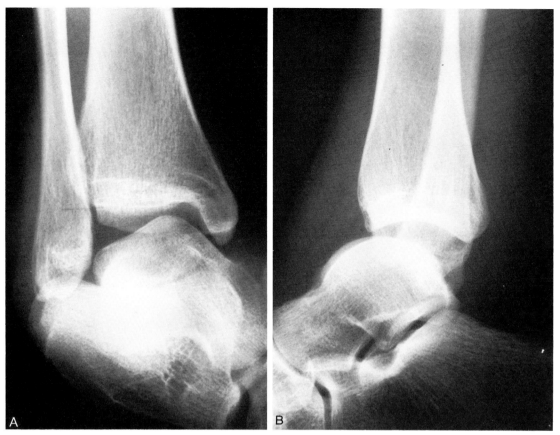

Figure 8–70. This patient had a significant injury with resulting instability, as demonstrated by both the varus tilt *(A)* and the anterior drawer signs *(B)*. This patient was casted for 8 weeks and went on to an uneventful recovery. The talar tilt was equal bilaterally at 3 months, and she was able to resume her activities as a professional ballet dancer.

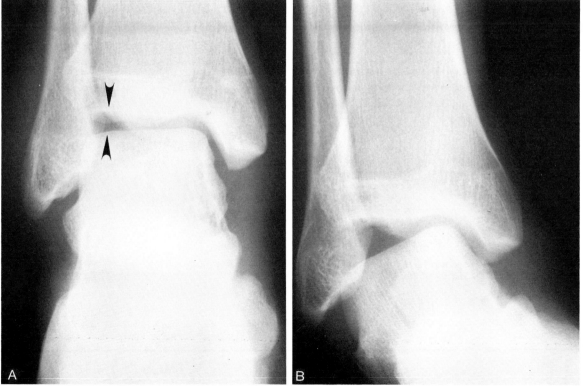

Figure 8–71. See legend on opposite page

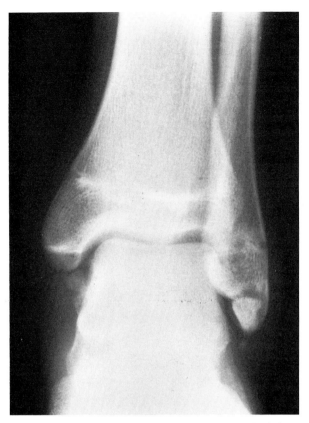

Figure 8–72. Chronic ankle sprains result in heterotopic bone formation about the tips of the malleoli in the substance of the ligaments. Note the presence of these signs on both the medial and lateral aspects of the ankle joint.

osseous injury. In a rare instance, talar tilt will be observed in the mortise view after a severe injury if the patient is supine and not weight-bearing (Fig. 8–71). For the individual with chronic instability, the radiographs will frequently reveal either talar tilt on the non-weight-bearing AP radiograph or calcification of the ligaments laterally or at the tip of the fibula. The presence of calcific or osseous densities usually helps to diagnose significant prior ankle injury and is not generally associated with the acute event (Fig. 8–72). No specific treatment is generally required. For the chronic sprain a stress device is used to impart a uniform load to the ankle, but this cannot be used in the acute setting (Fig. 8–73).

Treatment

The treatment of the more severe ankle sprain is somewhat controversial.[83, 84, 93, 101, 107, 109] Generally treatment is rendered according to the grade of injury.

Grade I sprains are usually treated with a simple Ace bandage, ice, elevation, and ambulation as tolerated. Crutches are not routinely necessary. Symptoms resolve within a week or 10 days, and the patient may return to activity or competition.

Grade II sprains are somewhat variable in their presentation as well as treatment. For the milder Grade II injuries, the joint is taped; crutches are

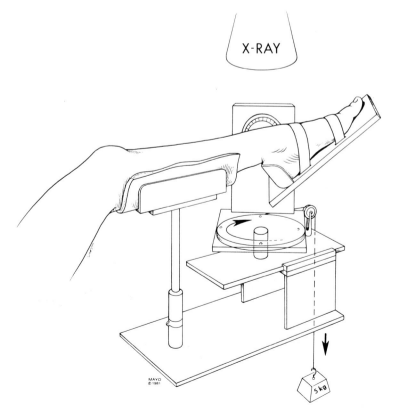

Figure 8–73. For a consistent assessment of chronic ankle instability, a standardized test is performed at our institution. The foot is dorsiflexed 10°, and a uniform weight is applied to the ankle in a varus manner.

X-RAY

MAYO
© 1981

5 kg

variably required. It has been demonstrated that the patient will return to normal activity more rapidly if an aggressive functional type of rehabilitation program is undertaken,[97] that is, one that emphasizes early motion and strengthening exercises. Greater controversy exists with regard to the more severe injuries. Some still strap the ankle with a severe Grade II injury; however, a short period of immobilization in a plaster cast or a compressive type of Robert Jones dressing is frequently employed. It should be recognized that the use of immobilization prolongs the rehabilitation.[97] Further, while taping the ankle does provide some stability, the effect is quickly lost due to stretching of the tape.[99] Crutches are universally used for the severe Grade II injury. Resolution of the symptoms is usually observed in 2 to 4 weeks, although occasionally the more severe sprain will require even longer rehabilitation. Peroneal tendon strengthening exercises are regularly recommended for the patient with this type of sprain.

Treatment of Grade III sprains is also controversial. Some recommend immediate surgery and repair of the torn ligaments,[81, 101, 111] while others recommend a nonoperative program.[93] This controversy has not been well resolved. A study performed at our institution, however, has indicated a near equal functional result in ankles immediately repaired compared with those reconstructed at a later date.[111] If a high level of competition is required or if the uncertainty of an initial treatment period cannot be tolerated, the injury is surgically repaired. Otherwise, casting is performed for approximately 4 to 6 weeks followed by air splint and peroneal strengthening exercises. In general, although estimates vary,[111] treatment in this manner provides 80

percent satisfactory results,[86] with a stable ankle demonstrated both subjectively and with the varus stress test. In the 20 percent who do have some residual instability, a small percentage may require reconstructive procedures, but once again it is felt that this can be offered with a high degree of reliability at a later date.

A variety of reconstructive procedures, usually using the peroneus brevis tendon, are universally reported to provide satisfactory results.[87, 92, 94, 96]

Complications

Complications of a sprained ankle include development of recurrent joint instability. This is uncommon unless the initial injury was a Grade III sprain. Even in this instance late instability develops in only approximately 20 percent of patients.[88, 91]

If the sprained ankle is improperly taped, blisters may develop. Removal of the tape can likewise cause gouging in the skin if it is done carelessly, if there is a significant amount of swelling, or if the tape has been applied too tightly. Studies have demonstrated that immediate repair of the ligament is regularly associated with paresthesias in about 5 percent of patients in the region of the incision, since the sural nerve and its branches are in the immediate vicinity of the pathology.[85] This is usually felt to be a minor problem. Recurrent sprain is a rare complication seen in virtually none of the individuals treated by immediate repair, but it has been reported in approximately 5 to 10 percent of the patients who have undergone a reconstructive procedure.[87, 92, 94, 96]

Late degenerative arthritis has been suspected

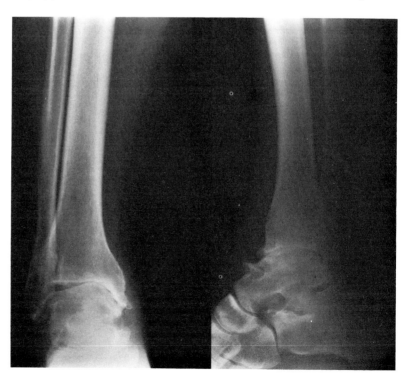

Figure 8–74. This man had a history of recurrent ankle sprains as a youth. At age 59 a significant amount of degenerative arthritis is present. Note the characteristic talar tilt.

with chronic, recurrent instability of the ankle but is difficult to prove. Some documentation of this association does exist,[95] and we have two patients requiring ankle arthrodesis after a long history of post-traumatic instability and arthritis without fracture (Fig. 8–74). Tibiotalar impingement has been implicated by O'Donoghue as evidence of chronic ankle instability.[103, 104] Peroneal nerve palsy has also been documented to occur with lateral ligament sprain,[75] but this is an uncommon event.

There are no specific complications referable to the diagnostic radiography.

THE TALUS*

ANATOMY

This irregular bone presents a complex three-dimensional anatomy that is difficult to appreciate from viewing two-dimensional radiographs (Fig. 8–75). A general description of the anatomy of the

---

*We gratefully acknowledge the contribution and assistance of Dr. Kenneth Pettine for the section on talar dome fractures.

talus is found at the beginning of this chapter. In addition to the dome of the talus, which articulates with the tibial plafond, three articular surfaces on the plantar aspect of this bone articulate with the calcaneus and compose the subtalar joint. These are the posterior, medial, and anterior subtalar joints (Fig. 8–76). The posterior facet is the largest and is often driven into the calcaneus with axial load, causing depressed calcaneal fractures. The middle facet is of functional significance, as this articulation is supported by the sustentaculum tali of the calcaneus and forms the anterior border of the sinus tarsi.[139]

Because greater than 50 percent of its surface is covered with articular cartilage, the vascular supply of the talus is limited. There are three basic sources of blood for the talus (Fig. 8–77). The first involves branches from the dorsalis pedis to the superior aspect of the talar neck. The second is the artery of the tarsal sinus, usually a branch of the peroneal artery. The third is the artery of the tarsal canal, a branch of the posterior tibial artery. These vessels form an anastomotic sling around the neck of the talus. There are smaller branches into the posterior tubercle of the talus and the medial walls of the deltoid ligament, but these vessels alone cannot support the nutritional requirements of the bone (Fig. 8–77).[124, 133]

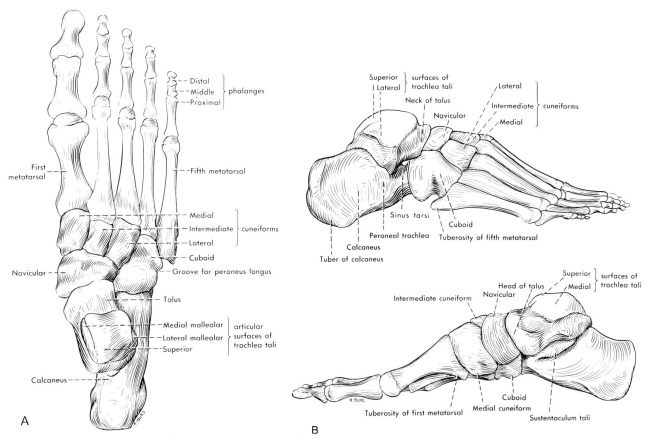

Figure 8–75. AP (A) and lateral (B) bony structure of the ankle demonstrates the complex geometry of the talus and its relationship to the calcaneus and also reveals why this bone is not adequately depicted by routine AP and lateral radiographs (From Hollinshead, W. H.: Anatomy for Surgeons. Vol. 3: The Back and Limbs. 3rd Ed. New York, Harper & Row, 1982.)

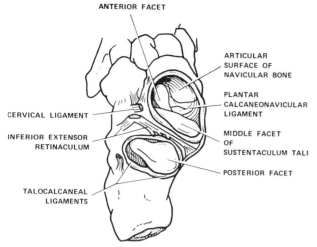

Figure 8–76. The anterior and middle subtalar joints are anterior to the sinus tarsi, with the medial subtalar joint resting on the sustentaculum tali. The large, posterior subtalar joint is crucial to the understanding of calcaneal fractures. (From Resnick, D.: Radiology of the talocalcaneal articulations. Radiology, *111*:581, 1974.)

FUNCTION

The talus articulates with both the ankle and the calcaneocubonavicular complex. There are no tendinous attachments to the talus. Therefore, motion of the talus itself is in response to action transmitted to the other articulations. This intercalary bone thus forms a component of the ankle joint, and as such it is subjected to large compressive stresses from above, in addition to plantar and dorsiflexion directed force. As a component of the subtalar articulation, it transmits these forces to the hindfoot. At the same time it must also rotate about the subtalar axis, which has a different orientation than the flexion axis of the ankle. Finally, as a component of the talonavicular joint, the head of the talus absorbs compressive and torsional stresses across the head and neck portions of the bone. Therefore, a compressive load to the talotibial joint may be transmitted as a rotational torque to the hindfoot or forefoot complex.

The combination of these axial loads and rotational torques applied at different positions and at different rates leads to a variety of talar and subtalar injuries. In this section fractures of the talus will be discussed, along with the subtalar and talonavicular dislocations and fracture-dislocations. As with any bony injury, although malunion or non-union can occur, the major complications after these injuries are post-traumatic arthroses of the ankle and subtalar joints and avascular necrosis of the talus.

FRACTURES OF THE TALUS

Transchondral Fractures

Transchondral fractures, osteochondral fractures, osteochondritis dissecans, and dome fractures of the talus are all names still used to describe similar lesions of the talus.[112, 114, 117, 141, 144] This fracture remains controversial, both in terms of the mechanism of injury and the optimal method of treatment.[133, 137, 147]

Historically, König in 1888 coined the term osteochondritis dissecans to describe loose bodies in joints that he felt were the result of spontaneous necrosis of subchondral bone.[128] Kappis in 1922 used

Figure 8–77. Arterial blood supply to the talus. Note the main sources of the blood to the talus: the branches through the dorsal aspect of the talar neck from the dorsalis pedis, the branches to the lateral aspect of the talus from the tarsal sinus branches, and the branches to the medial aspect of the talus from the artery of the tarsal canal. Notice also the small contributions from branches through the posterior tubercle and deltoid ligament attachments. (From Mulfinger, G. L., and Trueta, J.: The blood supply of the talus. J. Bone Joint Surg. *52B*:160, 1970.)

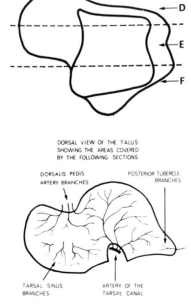

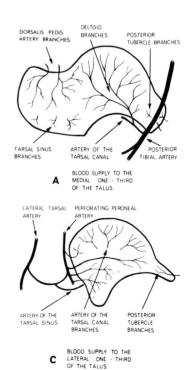

this term specifically to describe loose bodies in the ankle.[127] Rendu in 1932 used the term intra-articular fracture to describe the same lesion in the ankle.[138] The literature continues to use numerous terms to describe radiographically identical lesions. Berndt and Harty in 1959 felt that this lesion of the talus was unique and proposed a new term, transchondral fracture, "a name correct from both anatomical and etiologic points of view."[114]

A transchondral fracture is a fracture of a joint involving the articular cartilage and subchondral bone. The transchondral fracture differs from other small compression or chip fractures in several unique characteristics. First of all, it is difficult to recognize clinically and radiographically as a fracture, since it may occur as a result of trauma so trivial that it passes unnoticed and may contain little bone. Or its presence may be masked by more painful soft tissue injuries near the lesion. The avulsed segment of bone has no soft tissue attachments, no blood supply, and no nerve supply, and it is consequently painless and quite susceptible to the development of avascular aseptic necrosis.

Mechanism of Injury

The etiology of this lesion is controversial.[114, 115, 130, 140] Ischemic necrosis, abnormal patterns of vasculature, congenital factors, spontaneous necrosis, localized vascular damage following repeated minor trauma, and trauma in general all continue to be proposed as etiologic mechanisms.[112, 115, 130, 134] In our experience with 67 lesions, a definite history of trauma was reported in 90 percent.[137] Males are involved more frequently than females, with a 1.5:1 ratio.

Berndt and Harty are the only investigators to report on the duplication of transchondral fractures of the talus in cadavers.[114] Using amputated lower extremities, they stabilized the foot in a special wooden block and applied various types of pressure to duplicate lateral lesions in one cadaver and medial lesions in two (Fig. 8–78). A lateral lesion was created by forced inversion of the dorsiflexed ankle. Medial lesions were produced by forced inversion of the plantar flexed ankle with lateral rotation of the tibia on the talus.

Classification

The generally accepted classification of these fractures is that proposed by Berndt and Harty and relates to separation of the fragment (Fig. 8–79).

Stage I lesions involve a compression fracture of the talus before any ligaments are sprained or ruptured; thus, they are often painless.

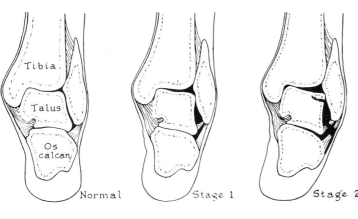

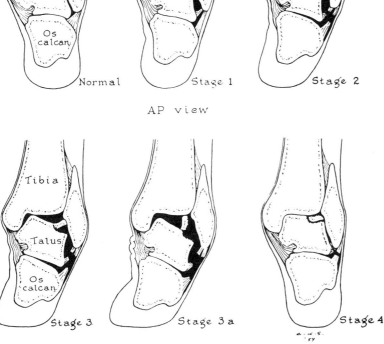

Figure 8–78. Representation of the mechanism of injury to account for both medial and lateral osteochondral fractures of the talus. (From Berndt, A., and Harty, M.: Transchondral fractures (osteochondritis dissecans) of the talus. J. Bone Joint Surg., *41A*:988, 1959.)

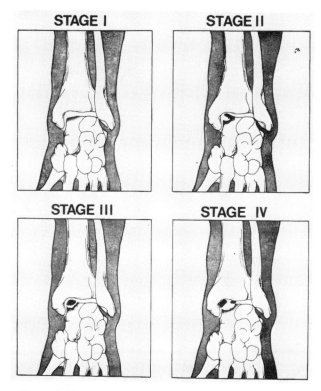

STAGE I **STAGE II**

STAGE III **STAGE IV**

Figure 8–79. Classification of the types or stages of osteochondral fractures of the dome of the talus. This classification is based on the extent of separation of the fragment. (From Canale, T., et al.: Osteochondral lesions of the talus. J. Bone Joint Surg., *62A:*97, 1980.)

Stage II lesions involve a partial osteochondral fracture.

Stage III lesions involve a complete nondisplaced osteochondral fracture.

Stage IV lesions involve a detached loose osteochondral fragment.

Stage II, III, and IV lesions are in themselves painless but are all accompanied by a painful sprain or rupture of the medial or lateral ligaments. Clinically lateral transchondral fractures are anterior and shallow wafer-life lesions. Medial transchondral fractures tend to be associated with a larger fragment of bone. The medial lesion is slightly less common (44 percent) than the lateral injury.[137]

Diagnosis

There are no pathognomonic symptoms for transchondral fractures of the talus. It is very difficult to make this diagnosis by physical examination alone. In the acute phase, symptoms are those of the accompanying sprain, with swelling, pain, ecchymosis, and limitation of motion about the ankle. These symptoms last from several weeks to several months, depending on the severity of the ligament injury. In the chronic phase, the symptoms continue longer than is expected of a ligament sprain. In a Stage IV lesion, there may be symptoms of locking because of the loose osteocartilaginous fragment.

Figure 8–80. A, Initial x-ray of a patient complaining of pain in the region of the ankle after a twisting injury. The initial film was read as negative. *B,* The radiograph 10 days later demonstrates the osteochondral defect of the lateral talar dome. *C,* Note the lack of positive findings on the lateral x-ray. *D,* The "true" mortise view also appears normal.

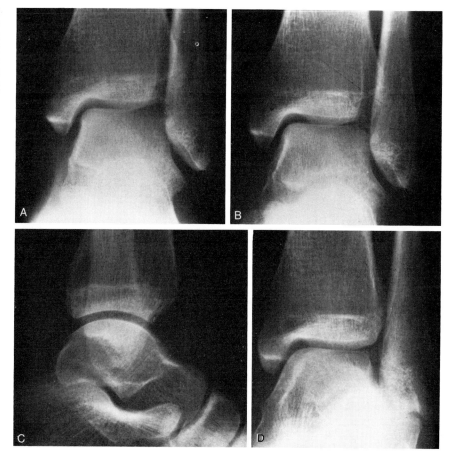

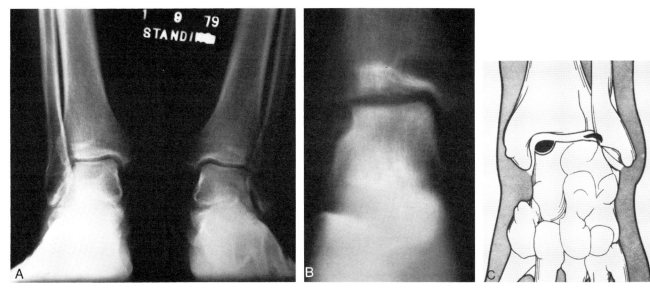

Figure 8–81. Although the mortise view appears normal *(A)*, a tomogram nicely demonstrates the location and size of the osteochondral fragment *(B).* This confirms the different morphology of the fragments *(C).* (From Canale, T., et al.: Osteochondral lesions of the talus. J. Bone Joint Surg., *62A:97, 1980.)*

Radiographic Diagnosis

Good quality x-rays are imperative in making the diagnosis of this fracture.[114] The initial radiographic study should consist of AP, lateral, and mortise views of the ankle. In some instances mortise views of the ankle in plantar flexion, neutral position, and dorsiflexion will reveal the lesion. To further complicate the diagnosis, initial x-rays can often be negative. After a week to 10 days, the necrotic areas of the fracture will be delineated, allowing the lesion to be identified on repeat roentgenograms (Fig. 8–80). Thus, it may be advisable to obtain repeat films in patients who complain of continual symptoms of "ankle sprain" without specific tenderness of the anterior talofibular ligament. Tomograms can be extremely helpful (Fig. 8–81). Naumetz[137] states that 20 percent of patients required tomograms to identify lesions that were undetectable on any routine x-ray. This observation is consistent with our experience. About 30 percent of the fractures were initially missed and diagnosed as "sprains."[134] Half of these ultimately required surgical excision. Obviously CT or MRI could also diagnose this lesion, though these modalities will require a precisely localized section.

Treatment

A review of the literature reveals disagreement over the optimal treatment for these lesions.[112, 121, 122, 130, 132, 144]

Transchondral fractures can heal like other fractures if they are reduced and immobilized until bone union has taken place. In a Stage IV lesion, the displaced bone cannot heal unless the fragment is replaced in its bed. In all but the Stage I lesion, the blood supply of the avulsed fragment is disrupted at the fracture line. The healing process will only occur by the ingrowth of capillaries across the fracture. The bone fragment remains in a condition of avascular aseptic necrosis until the arrival of a new blood supply. The cartilaginous portion, on the other hand, remains alive because of its low metabolic requirements and continuous nourishment from the synovial fluid. If a non-union of the fracture occurs, degenerative traumatic osteoarthritis is a common sequela. Canale[117] reported that 50

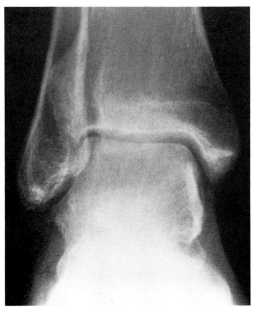

Figure 8–82. Mild degenerative arthritis (lateral narrowing) following excision of the lateral osteochondral fragment. Most literature suggests that patients do well following this procedure, but our experience indicates that there are significant residual symptoms in many patients.

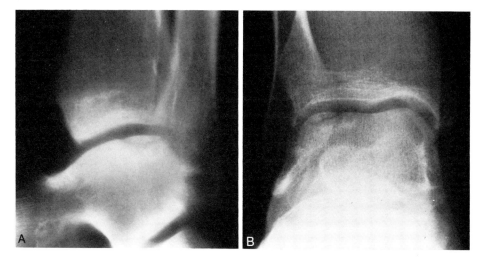

Figure 8–83. Lateral tomogram *(A)* of a lateral lesion shown in an initial radiograph *(B).* Note that the location of this lesion is anterior to the lateral malleolus, thus allowing excision through a simple arthrotomy.

percent of 28 patients had evidence of degenerative joint disease within an average 11.2-year follow-up (Fig. 8–82).

Stage I and II lesions should initially be treated nonoperatively, regardless of location, with a patellar-tendon-bearing (PTB) cast application. Stage III lesions of the medial talus should also be treated nonoperatively initially as described earlier.[117] If symptoms persist after adequate nonoperative treatment, then excision of the fragment in any of the above lesions is appropriate. Lateral Stage III lesions

and all Stage IV fractures should undergo immediate excision of the fragment with curettage and drilling of the base.[117] Unless removed, lateral lesions of the talus tend to be more symptomatic and also lead to more degenerative changes in the ankle. On the other hand, medial lesions tend to be less symptomatic, with less incidence of progression to degenerative changes. Lateral lesions tend to be anterior in position and can surgically be approached through an anterolateral approach, in this way avoiding osteotomy of the lateral malleolus

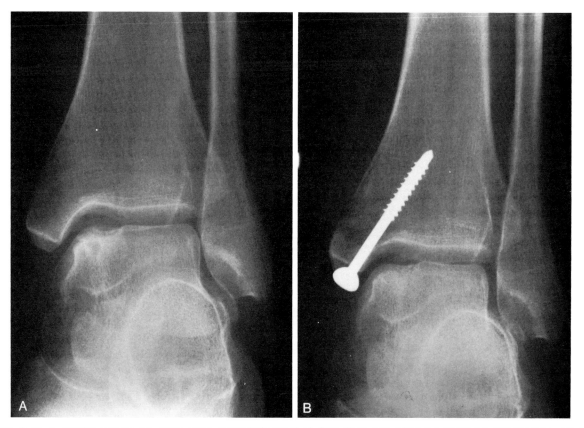

Figure 8–84. A, Medial lesions are often more posteriorly located. Thus, they can often be observed adequately only by an osteotomy of the medial malleolus. *B,* Radiograph shows the fixation of the osteotomy.

(Fig. 8–83). Medial lesions tend to be posterior in location, requiring osteotomy of the medial malleolus for adequate exposure (Fig. 8–84).

Results

A classification system for results has been established.[114] A result is good if the patient reports none or only slightly persistent symptoms. A fair result is one with symptoms somewhat improved but with some measure of disability. The result is considered poor if the symptoms continue unchanged, even though periods of freedom from pain are present at times. Based on this or a similar system, most studies of transchondral fractures report encouraging results.[112, 117]

Analysis of our 75 patients, however, reveals an outcome worse than the previous literature indicates. Using the Berndt and Harty classification of results, only 40 percent of patients are currently rated good, and 60 percent fall into the fair to poor categories. These patients are quite symptomatic, with pain, swelling, crepitus, and feelings of instability. Physical examination reveals decreased range of motion, and x-rays indicate degenerative changes in the ankle joint. Careful history reveals that these patients have slowly modified their lifestyle to accommodate their loss of ankle function.

Similarly, the symptoms in the untreated lesion are those of traumatic osteoarthritis. There is pain with motion or weight-bearing. There can be swelling, crepitus in the ankle with motion, symptoms of locking, loss of motion, and at times a feeling of instability with a tendency to recurrence of sprains. The duration of symptoms in the chronic phase appears to be indefinite unless surgical intervention is undertaken.

It is obvious, therefore, that early diagnosis and proper treatment of this intra-articular fracture are of extreme importance.

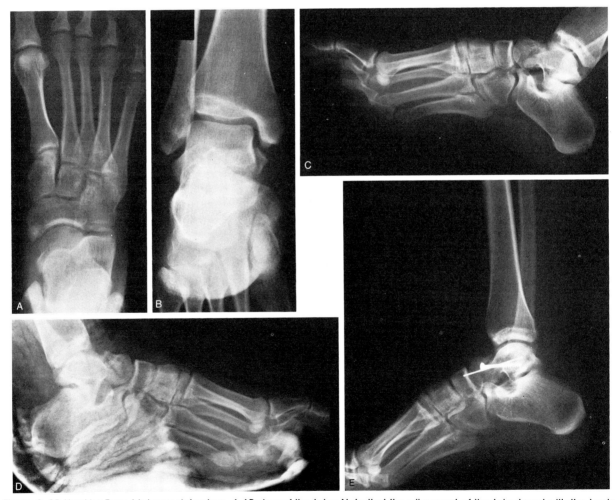

Figure 8–85. Hawkins Type I talar neck fracture. *A,* AP view of the talus. Note that the alignment of the talar head with the body of the talus is essentially normal. *B,* The AP view of the ankle shows that the tibiotalar mortise is not subluxed. *C,* The lateral view of the hindfoot demonstrates the fracture but shows that the subtalar joint is not subluxed. *D,* This fracture displaced somewhat as the ankle was brought to the neutral position. Therefore, it was felt to be appropriate to perform open reduction and to fix the injury internally. *E,* This was performed using the screw and pin as seen. Patient was treated in a non-weight-bearing cast for 4 weeks followed by a walking cast for 4 weeks, at which time the pin was removed; she gradually returned to her full activity level without residual symptoms.

Fractures of the Talar Neck

Mechanism of Injury

These injuries most typically occur from a fall from a height or when the foot strikes the floorboard in an automotive accident. The basic mechanism for these injuries is felt to be forced dorsiflexion of the talus against the anterior aspect of the tibia. Applied rotational forces can also accompany this stress and cause medial or lateral subtalar dislocations. Historically, these fractures are known as aviator's astragalus.[113]

Classification

Talar neck fractures have been divided into three major groups,[127, 138, 139] with one author adding a fourth subtype.[116] Basically, Type I injuries consist of isolated talar neck fractures without subtalar or ankle subluxation (Fig. 8–85). Type II are talar neck fractures associated with subtalar subluxation or

dislocation (Fig. 8–86). Type III injuries are talar neck fractures associated with both subtalar and ankle subluxation or dislocation (Fig. 8–87). Canale has added a fourth subtype, which has an additional component of dislocation or subluxation of the talar head from the talonavicular joint.[116]

The value of the classification is its predictive power with regard to the rate of avascular necrosis. Osteonecrosis of the body of the talus occurs rarely in Type I fractures, in 40 to 50 percent of the Type II fractures, and in nearly all of the Type III injuries.[116, 125, 129, 135, 136] There were only two Type IV fractures in Canale's series, one of which went on to osteonecrosis and one in which primary talectomy was performed. With nondisplaced fractures of the neck, it is felt that the anastomotic sling around the talus is left intact and thus that the blood supply to the body of the talus is adequate. With Type II fractures, it is felt that the dorsal neck vessels as well as the supply from the artery of the tarsal sinus are disrupted, leaving only one major

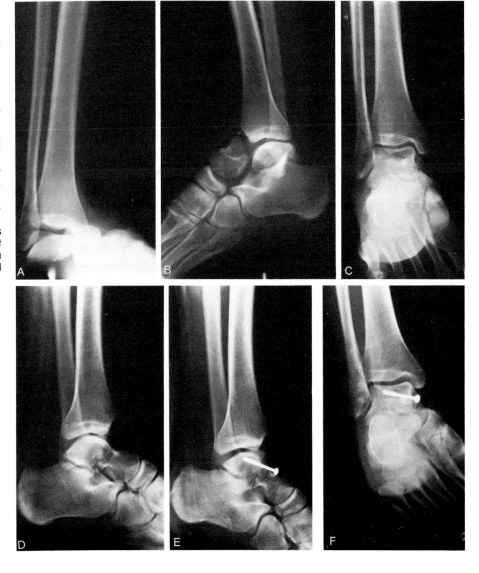

Figure 8–86. Hawkins Type II fracture-dislocation of the talar neck. *A,* On the initial AP view of the ankle one can see that the talus remains in the mortise, although there is a moderate amount of talar tilt. The talar head and calcaneus are subluxed medially. *B,* On the lateral view one can also see the displacement of the talar neck from the talar body and the subtalar joint. *C* and *D,* This injury was reduced through closed reduction, as one can see on the AP and lateral views of the ankle. It was felt necessary to further stabilize this, however, with the use of a screw across the fracture site. *E* and *F,* One can see from the two views taken that it is difficult to determine whether the talar head is adducted or abducted with respect to the talar body. This is where a true AP view of the talar neck would have been useful.

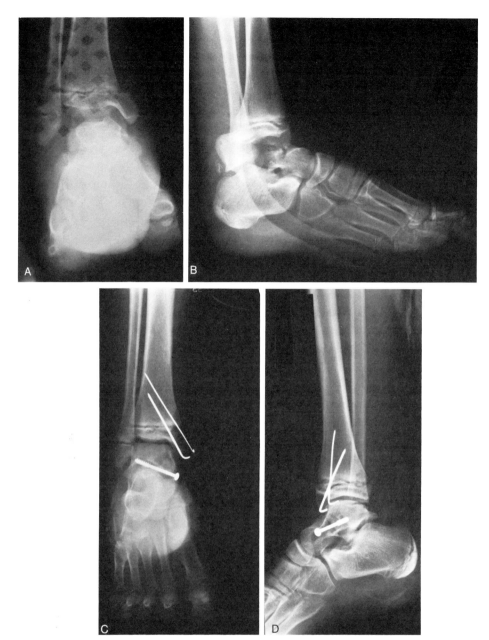

Figure 8-87. Hawkins Type III fracture-dislocation of the talar neck. This patient with open physes suffered a closed injury. *A,* One can see from the AP radiograph that the talar head remains articulated with the navicular, but the body of the talus has been extruded posteriorly. In the course of the injury both the talar mortise and the posterior facet of the calcaneus have been dislocated. *B,* The lateral view shows that the dislocation is posterior, and on the AP view a concomitant medial malleolar physeal injury is also seen, along with the posterior dislocation of the talar body. *C,* This injury was reduced closed. *D,* However, because of the remaining displacement, it was elected to fix the talar neck fracture internally and to apply open reduction and internal fixation to the malleolar fracture.

blood supply to the body. With Type III, all three vessels are disrupted.

Diagnosis

The initial physical examination should note in particular any gross deformities and also any skin compromise due to the deformity. Initial radiographic evaluation should include AP and lateral views of the ankle and also an AP radiograph of the foot. The technique as described by Canale and colleagues is useful.[116] Here the cassette is placed

directly under the foot, the ankle is placed in the maximum plantar flexed position, slight pronation is applied to the foot itself, and the tube is directed at a 75° angle from the horizontal. This view allows one to detect any valgus or varus deformity to the head or neck of the talus (Fig. 8–88).

After the initial radiographs have been evaluated and any injury classified, treatment can be initiated. If there is any soft tissue compromise because of underlying bony pressure, it is very important that emergency reduction be undertaken to prevent skin necrosis. If the vascular compromise is severe, one

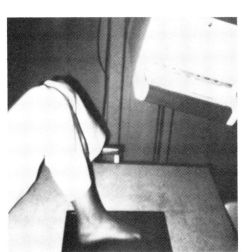
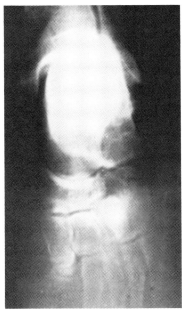

Figure 8–88. Positioning for AP view of the talar neck. The ankle is in a maximum plantarflexed position. The hindfoot is slightly pronated and the tube is directed at an angle 75° above the horizontal. Varus-valgus deformities of the talar neck can be detected by this view.

should not hesitate to reduce the malalignment immediately, prior to radiographic evaluation. These fractures can usually be reduced closed; but if it is necessary, open reduction must be undertaken. The goal is accurate reduction of both the dislocations and the neck fracture. If internal fixation is required, compression screws or K-wires across the fracture site can be used. The patient is then placed in a non-weight-bearing cast for a period of 4 to 8 weeks, followed by progressive weight-bearing with the ankle immobilized.

Results

At the time of the initial evaluation the fracture can be classified, but it is still difficult to determine

Figure 8–89. This is the same patient as in Figure 8–86. One can see the subchondral lucency present in the AP *(A)* and lateral *(B)* views of the ankle 8 weeks following treatment. This is the Hawkins' sign, which is helpful in determining the viability of the talar bone.

whether or not the body of the talus will go on to necrosis. At 4 to 8 weeks, however, Hawkins noticed a subchondral lucent area in the talus in those patients who were not developing necrosis (Fig. 8–89).[125] He felt that this was a sign of vascularity, as the bone was undergoing disuse osteopenia. Other authors have found that this radiographic sign does indeed have predictive value. However, if the sign is absent at 4 to 8 weeks, it is of less help, as not all of these will develop osteonecrosis (Fig. 8–90).[116, 129] Regarding other complications, infection occurs in up to 5 percent of these injuries, usually secondary to the degree of soft tissue trauma at the time of the initial injury. Malunion can occur. The two most common types of malunion are residual dorsiflexion of the distal fragment of

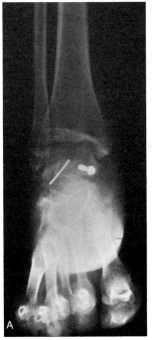
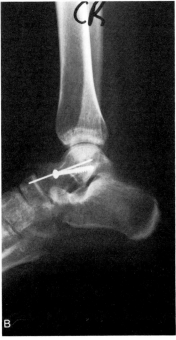

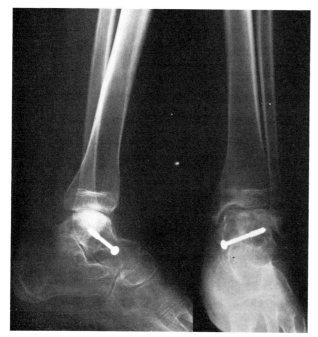

Figure 8–90. This is the same patient as in Figure 8–88. The patient went on to develop avascular necrosis of the dome of the talus. This was treated with a prolonged period of non-weight-bearing followed by a period of protected weight-bearing. The subchondral bone eventually reconstituted without collapse of the articular surface. Note the relatively increased radio-opacity of the bone in the dome of the talus along with the irregular areas of cystic and sclerotic changes in the subchondral region.

the talus and a varus position of the distal fragment. This latter type of malunion tends to occur in those treated with closed reduction. The incidence of post-traumatic arthrosis of the ankle or subtalar joints increases with increasing severity of the injury and also is obviously associated with osteonecrosis of the body of the talus. However, in one study Type I fractures of the neck of the talus were associated with ankle arthrosis in 15 percent and with subtalar arthrosis in 24 percent.[129] Non-union can occur in up to 4 percent of these patients.

Treatment of patients with these complications is difficult. Accurate and early reduction of the fractures is important. If osteonecrosis develops, prolonged periods of protective weight-bearing are indicated in the hope that the bone will revascularize before collapse occurs. If collapse should ensue and the patient is symptomatic, arthrodesis of the involved areas is probably the treatment of choice. Total ankle arthroplasty has not been successful in the treatment of this problem.

Fractures of the Talar Body

According to Coltart fractures of the body of the talus account for less than 0.1 percent of all fractures.[120] As with talar neck fractures, however, they can be associated with a high incidence of unsatisfactory results.

Classification

Because of the rarity of these injuries, large series are difficult to find. The largest series is that of Sneppen and colleagues, with 51 patients.[142] They divided these injuries into a type involving compression of the trochlea (which did not involve the subtalar joint), shear fractures either in the coronal or sagittal plane, posterior margin fractures, lateral process fractures, or crush injuries (Fig. 8–91).

Diagnosis

Radiographic evaluation of these patients should include standard ankle and feet views, as 17 of Sneppen's 51 patients had associated injuries of the foot and ankle. If those with serious injuries to the foot and ankle are also included, 28 of 62 had associated injuries, as 11 more patients had serious ankle injuries with associated talar body fractures. Tomography is useful in outlining the size of the

A. Compression fracture

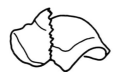

B. Coronal shearing fracture

C. Sagittal shearing fracture

Figure 8–91. Types of talar fractures. (From Sneppin, O., Christensen, S. B., Krogsoe, O., et al.: Fractures of the body of the talus. Acta Orthop. Scand. *48*:317, 1977.)

D. Fracture in the posterior tubercle

E. Fracture in the lateral tubercle

F. Crush fracture

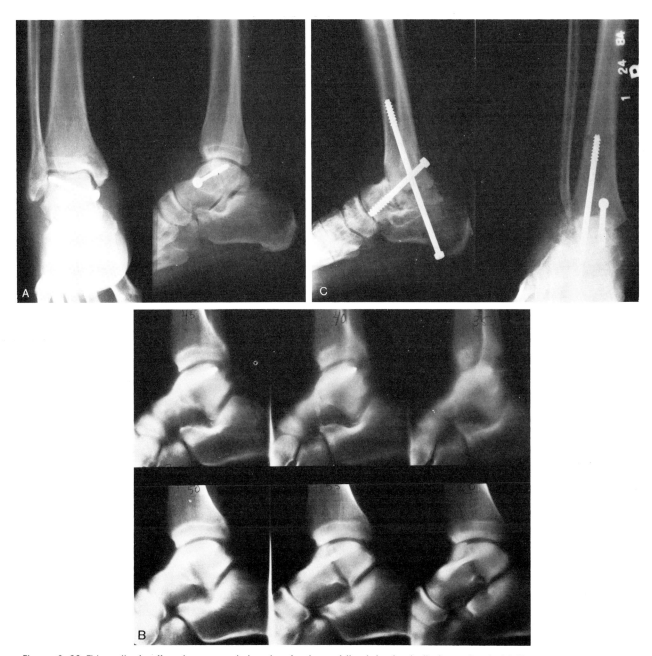

Figure 8–92. This patient suffered a coronal shearing fracture of the talar body that was treated initially by closed reduction, followed by an open reduction and pinning. At the time of his presentation, he was complaining of pain with ambulation and swelling. *A,* Initial AP and lateral views at the time of his presentation to our clinic showed increased radiodensity of the posterior aspect of the talus along with a fracture gap. *B,* Our recommendation at that time was that he have a tibiocalcaneal arthrodesis. He returned to his home physician, where an attempt at this was performed. Postoperatively, however, the arthrodesis failed to unite and he was left with a varus heel and a 30° plantarflexion deformity. *C,* He returned to our institution, where a modified Blair tibiotalar arthrodesis was performed with the insertion of autogenous bone grafts between the tibia and calcaneus. Postoperatively, he has done well. Ideally, with any sort of ankle or tibiocalcaneal arthrodesis, the foot should be at 90° with respect to the ankle and the heel in slight valgus. Also, from a biomechanical standpoint, one would like to position the tibia relatively anteriorly on the foot to decrease the dorsiflexion moment about the ankle during gait. However, with the tibiotalar, or modified Blair, arthrodesis this cannot be done, because the arthrodesis must be performed between the tibia and the remaining head of the talus. Thus, it is difficult to advance the tibia anteriorly.

fragments and the amount of displacement (Fig. 8–92).

Treatment

Following the precepts for care of all intra-articular injuries, treatment should be directed toward anatomic reduction of the fragments. Authors differ over the best approach, but most agree that an adequate visualization requires either a medial or lateral malleolar osteotomy. Although opponents of medial osteotomy claim that the talar blood supply is further disrupted by the interruption of the deltoid branch, a medial approach to the fragment may

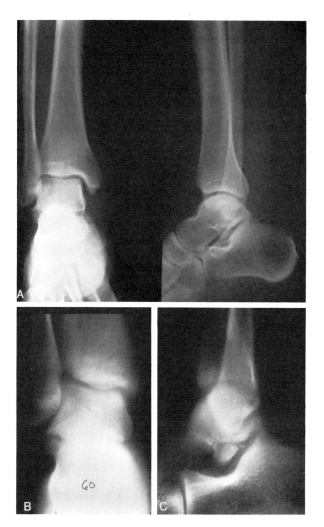

Figure 8–93. This patient suffered an inversion injury to his right ankle. A, Notice the minimally displaced fracture of the lateral process of his talus. B and C, AP and lateral tomograms confirm the fact that the fracture was minimally displaced, and the patient was treated in a short leg non-weight-bearing cast for 4 weeks followed by a weight-bearing cast for 3 weeks. The fracture healed without any residual symptoms. This fragment is covered with articular cartilage on its plantar surface. It may thus predispose one to premature degenerative changes in the subtalar facet if it is not accurately reduced.

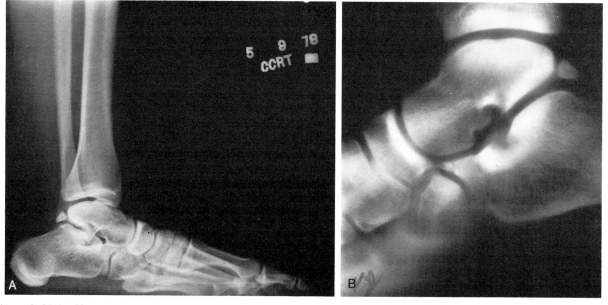

Figure 8–94. An 18-year-old active tennis player who complained of pain on the posterior aspect of the ankle. On examination she had tenderness in the posterior ankle region and pain with plantar flexion. The lateral radiograph of her foot (A) reveals an os trigonum, which on lateral tomography (B) demonstrates an area of adjacent sclerosis on the posterior aspect of the talus. Also, notice a non-united anterior process fracture of the calcaneus. The patient was not symptomatic in this area. A local anesthetic was injected under image intensifier control into the region of the os trigonum. The patient noted complete relief of her symptoms. Through a posterior approach this fragment was excised, and the patient's symptoms resolved.

be necessary, if indeed that is where the pathology exists. In spite of anatomic reduction, however, arthrosis may ensue, probably because of the amount of cartilage damaged by the injuring force.

Posterior marginal and lateral process fractures, if nondisplaced, can be treated by immobilization (Fig. 8–93). If the fracture is displaced, open reduction or excision of the fragment is indicated. Even though the fragments are relatively small and seemingly peripheral, they may develop complications. Both of these fragments have surfaces that are covered with articular cartilage and are, as such,

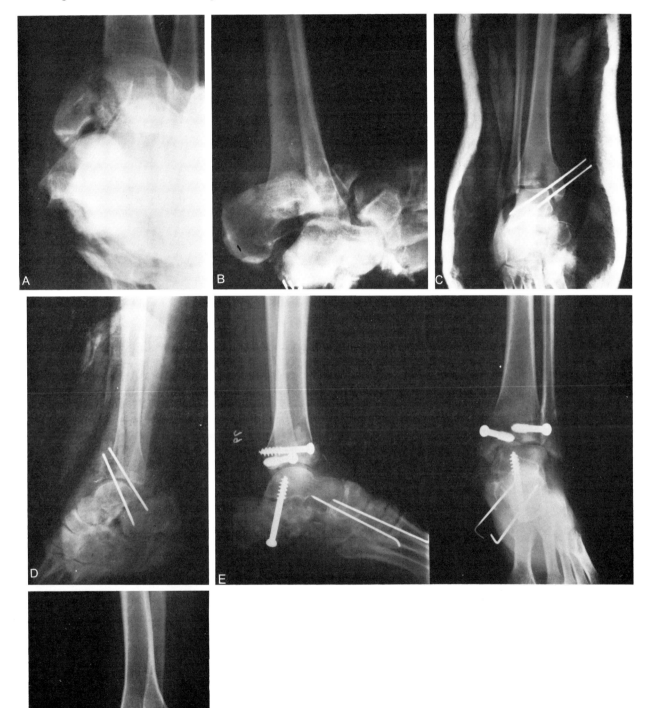

Figure 8–95. A and B, Radiographs of injury commonly seen with a total dislocation of the talus. Patient was treated with debridement and limited internal fixation while soft tissues healed. C and D, She then underwent a primary subtalar arthrodesis because of the degree of damage to the subtalar articulation. E and F, Because of excessive heel valgus, she later underwent a closing wedge osteotomy of the calcaneus; hence the presence of the staple in the calcaneus on last follow-up. Four years after the injury, she had mild pain and limited motion of the ankle but was functioning reasonably well. Interestingly, she did not develop overt osteonecrosis of the talus.

involved in the articulations of the talotibial and subtalar joints. Thus, because of the degree of force required to fracture these bones, significant cartilage damage may accompany the fracture. Of 20 patients in Sneppen's study with either of these injuries, 10 had radiographic evidence of osteoarthritis.[142]

A posterior margin injury may also occur as a result of fatigue fracture. Although other etiologies are possible, repetitive stress is felt to be one mechanism of injury. These patients present with a chronic history of pain in the posterior ankle region, particularly with forced plantar flexion. There may be some doubt as to the diagnosis. Tomography and radioisotope scanning may be useful. Excision of the fragment is worthwhile (Fig. 8–94).

Of the 51 patients followed by Sneppen, 39 had some difficulties. Eight developed avascular necrosis; 28 developed arthrosis. One third of the patients with initial displacement were left with a malunion.[142]

If arthrosis or avascular necrosis of the talus ensues after any of these injuries, arthrodesis of the involved articulations is the treatment of choice at this time. If there is extensive collapse of the talus, the only alternative may be tibiocalcaneal fusion or perhaps a variation of the tibiotalar neck (Blair) fusion (Fig. 8–92).

Subtalar and Talar Dislocation

Dislocation of the subtalar joint without fracture rarely occurs.[118, 126, 131] These dislocations are classified as either medial or lateral. The medial dislocation is thought to be due to an inversion force, and the lateral dislocation is thought to be due to an eversion force. By definition, the medial dislocation means that the foot is medially displaced with respect to the ankle; the lateral dislocation implies the opposite. The talus remains in the ankle mortise, but the talonavicular and talocalcaneal articulations are disrupted. The proper radiographic assessment of this region of the foot can be extremely difficult. Review of the intimate relationship between the subtalar and Chopart's joints is necessary to diagnose pathology in this region accurately.[139]

Medial dislocations, in general, have a better prognosis. Associated regional fractures occur less frequently. Most authors feel that the associated soft tissue damage is also less severe. On the other hand, lateral dislocations, although much less common, are associated with extensive medial soft tissue disruption, often including the deltoid ligament, posterior tibial tendon, and long-toe flexor tendons. Also, they have a higher incidence of associated fractures.

Evaluation should include assessment of the skin and the neurovascular status of the foot. Appropriate radiographs should be taken, including standard ankle and foot views. One should observe closely for possible associated injuries.

Treatment begins with reduction. Open reduction is rarely necessary. After reduction these injuries are usually stable and can be treated with immobilization. In a series of 30 cases, 2 needed open reduction.[118] The long-term outlook is better for medial than for lateral dislocations. Avascular necrosis can develop, although this is infrequent. Osteoarthritis is also a problem. In the same series of patients, 19 had degenerative changes in the subtalar joint; and of these, 6 had pantalar arthrosis.

Total dislocation of the talus occurs infrequently.[119, 123] As would be expected, reduction is difficult to accomplish closed, and most, if not all, require open reduction. In spite of reduction, vascular damage is extensive, and nearly all of these patients develop avascular necrosis. Furthermore, because the force required to cause these injuries is large, the soft tissue damage is extensive (Fig. 8–95). In Detenbeck's series of 9 patients, 7 injuries were reduced openly.[123] Infection developed in 8 of 9 of these injuries. Primary talectomy and tibiocalcaneal fusion have been suggested as the most appropriate treatment. Other treatments emphasize reduction and immobilization in the hope of salvaging some part of the talus. Fortunately, these injuries are relatively uncommon.

NAVICULAR FRACTURES

Injuries to the navicular bone can be divided into three groups: acute fractures, stress fractures, and dislocations of Chopart's joint.

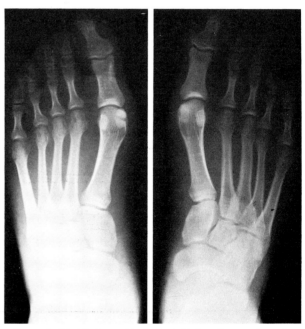

Figure 8–96. AP view of both feet. Notice the small avulsion fracture off the distal medial aspect of the navicular on the left. This patient was treated by cast immobilization, and the injury healed without sequelae.

Acute Fractures of the Navicular Bone

Fractures of the navicular bone have been divided into three types: cortical avulsions (usually dorsal lip), fractures of the body, and tuberosity fractures.[145] Avulsion fractures account for nearly half of the injuries (Fig. 8–96). The exact mechanism of each of these injuries is unclear, but acute fractures are thought to be the result of either twisting or longitudinal compression along the line of the medial border of the foot. These injuries are difficult to define radiographically, and a high index of suspicion must be maintained. In the same study quoted above, the radiographs were erroneously reported as normal in 8 of 67 injuries, and in 9 no radiographs were taken. Appropriate radiographs include AP, lateral, and oblique views of the foot,

and also an AP view of the navicular bone itself. Tomograms may be necessary to define the position of the fragments. Associated fractures are common in this injury also. Thirty-one of the 67 patients in the study had associated fractures (Fig. 8–97).

If the fragments are nondisplaced, casting, with the patient non-weight-bearing initially, is the treatment of choice. If the fragments are displaced, open reduction and internal fixation with either wires or screws is indicated.

Unlike talar fractures, in which avascular necrosis is common, navicular fractures are not usually associated with avascular necrosis. However, anatomic reduction should be sought, as post-traumatic arthrosis is not uncommon. If this ensues, arthrodesis of the involved bones is the appropriate treatment.

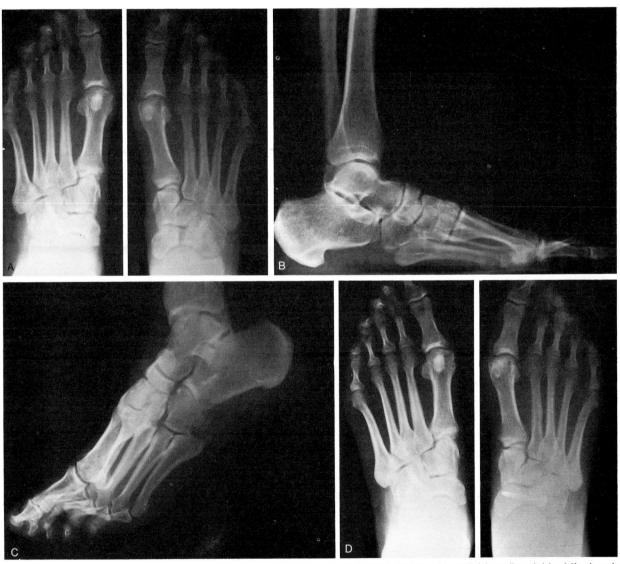

Figure 8–97. This 62-year-old man presented first to our institution with a 1-month history of a painful swollen right midfoot region. He was referred here with a probable diagnosis of inflammatory arthropathy. Although AP *(A)* and lateral *(B)* radiographs of his feet were reported as unremarkable, the fracture of the navicular on the right AP view is apparent on close inspection. The fracture is not visible on the oblique view *(C)*. The patient was treated with reduction, autogenous bone grafting, and internal fixation of the fractured navicular, with resolution of his symptoms *(D)*.

Stress Fractures

Stress fractures may also occur in the navicular bone, as is the case in all bones.[146, 148] Typically stress fractures are oriented in a sagittal plane and can involve one or both cortices. They are, however, easily missed. Nine of 21 injuries were missed in one series.[148] The authors reporting on this series suggested that the use of an AP view of the navicular and tomography would be helpful. Tc-99m scanning is also helpful, if necessary.[146]

Treatment of nondisplaced stress fractures is by cast and non-weight-bearing for 6 to 8 weeks. If the stress fracture is displaced, open reduction with or without supplemental bone grafting is the treatment of choice. Torg and colleagues undertook a vascular study of the navicular and found that although medial and lateral areas were well supplied via the soft tissue attachment, the central third was relatively avascular.[148] It was in this location that stress fractures occurred, but actual avascular necrosis was rare.

If appropriately treated, the outlook for these stress fractures is good. Only 4 of 21 were symptomatic. In these 4 the fracture had failed to unite or had recurred. The authors cautioned that when the appropriate diagnosis is made, treatment is simple and effective.

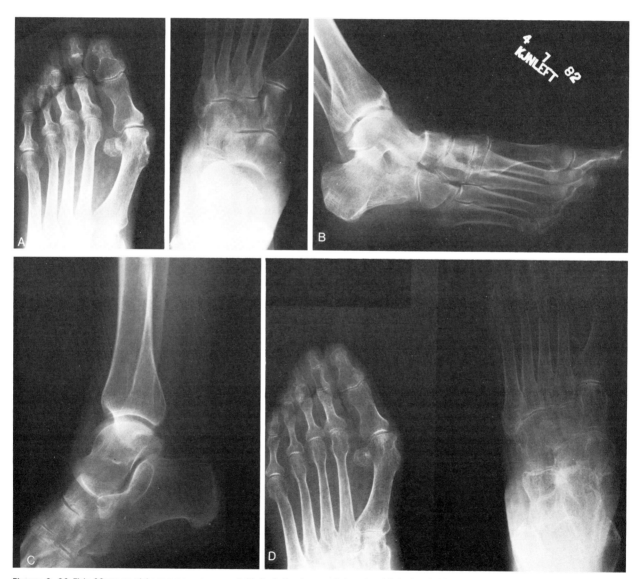

Figure 8–98. This 80-year-old woman was seen initially following an injury in which she twisted her ankle. She was evaluated in an emergency room, where the AP *(A)*, lateral *(B)*, and oblique *(C)* views were taken and reported as normal. She was followed for 6 months, during which time she complained of persistent pain and swelling in the midfoot region. It was finally discovered that she had suffered a swivel dislocation of the talonavicular joint. This was present on the initial radiographs. One can notice on the AP view that the talar head is absent from the navicular fossa. On the lateral and oblique views there is overlap of the talus with the navicular, suggesting that it is not properly articulated. Also, on the AP view there is a fracture of the talar head with the medial portion sheared off proximally. She was treated with reduction and talonavicular arthrodesis *(D)*, with resolution of her symptoms.

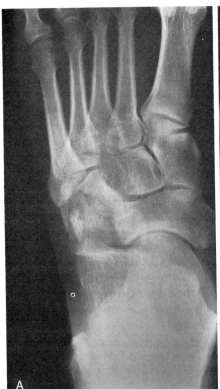
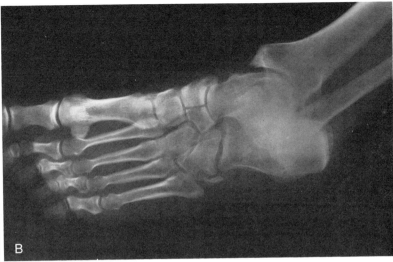
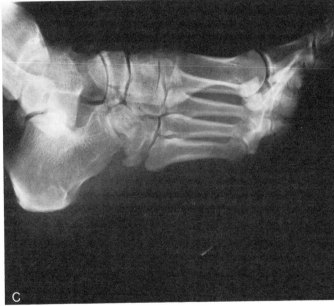
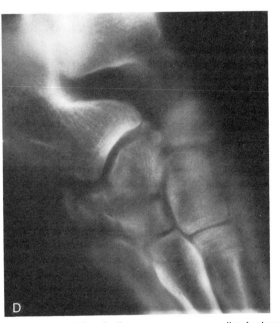

Figure 8–99. This man suffered a crushing injury to his left foot. At the time of presentation to the emergency room, the foot was markedly swollen. The AP view of the foot *(A)* reveals a comminuted fracture of the cuboid; there is no fracture of the navicular apparent. However, with the oblique film *(B)* one can plainly see a fracture of the navicular with minimal displacement. It is also visible on the rotated lateral view of the foot *(C)*. Lateral tomography was performed to delineate the extent of cuboid disruption *(D)*. One can see that it is quite comminuted, but its articular surface with the calcaneus as well as with the 4th and 5th metatarsals is reasonably well maintained. He was treated in a short leg cast, non-weight-bearing, for a period of 4 weeks followed by a period of weight-bearing in a cast for 4 more weeks. His fracture healed, and he returned to full employment.

Dislocations of Chopart's Joint

Aside from isolated case reports, there is only one large series dedicated to this problem. Main and Jowett reviewed 71 injuries.[147] These injuries were first classified as fracture-sprains (avulsion injuries), fracture-subluxations, or dislocations, and swivel dislocations. They were also subclassified according to the type of force responsible for the injury.

As with navicular fractures, a high index of suspicion is necessary to detect these dislocations.

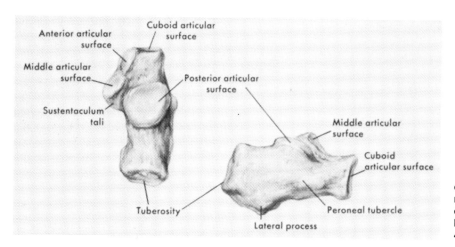

Figure 8–100. Anterior and lateral anatomy of the calcaneus. (From Chapman, M. W.: Fractures and fracture-dislocations of the ankle and foot. In Mann, R. A. (ed.): DuVries' Surgery of the Foot. 4th Ed. St. Louis, C. V. Mosby Co., 1978.)

Thirty of 71 of these injuries were initially missed in this series. Routine AP, lateral, and oblique views are necessary. Also, a view of the foot perpendicular to the plane of the metatarsals and centered on the navicular bone is recommended.

In this series, fracture-sprains consisted of flake fractures of the talus, navicular, calcaneus, or cuboid, though location of the avulsion depended on the direction of the deforming force. Fracture-subluxations or dislocations occurred at Chopart's joint, both at the talonavicular and calcaneocuboid joints. The authors also defined an injury known as a swivel dislocation, in which only the talonavicular joint is grossly disrupted (Fig. 8–98).[147] In this injury the calcaneocuboid joint is intact, as is the interosseous talocalcaneal ligament. The posterior facet of the subtalar joint is subluxated but not dislocated. This can occur with the talus medial to the calcaneus, as with an eversion force injury, or with it lateral to the calcaneus, as with an inversion force. In the eversion force injury, or lateral force swivel injury, an accompanying "nutcracker" injury to the cuboid may be present (Fig. 8–99), but this injury is rare.

Treatment of these injuries consists of reduction and immobilization. If necessary, surgery is indicated to ensure an anatomic reduction of the navicular fragments or to hold an unstable reduction. Late complications are mainly due to post-traumatic degenerative disease and are best treated with arthrodesis of the involved joints.

THE CALCANEUS*

ANATOMY

The calcaneus is the largest tarsal bone. Its irregular shape causes difficulty in obtaining a clear

*The authors gratefully acknowledge the assistance of Drs. K. Wiedman and K. Disler in preparing this section.

image of the three-dimensional anatomy of the bone (Fig. 8–100). There are three articular surfaces on the superior aspect. These accommodate the posterior, mid-, and anterior articular facets of the talus, forming the subtalar joint (Fig. 8–101). The middle articulation is supported by the sustentaculum tali of the calcaneus, which assumes particular importance with respect to reduction following fracture of the calcaneus.[179, 192, 193] The posterior articulation is convex and ovoid in the posteromedial to anterolateral directions. Laterally, the articulation goes from posterior superior to anterior inferior and forms the posterior border of the sinus tarsi.[187] The midportion of the bone consists of the middle articular facet, which rests on the sustentaculum tali and supports the undersurface of the talus. The bone is subtended medially and anteriorly by the sinus tarsi, which runs in the same orientation as the posterior facet. The middle articular facet forms the anterior border of the sinus tarsi and is continuous with the anterior facet (Fig. 8–101).[150]

On the medial surface below the sustentaculum tali, there is a groove for the extensor hallucis longus. The tuberosity of the calcaneus is the dominant projection at the back of the inferior surface (Fig. 8–102). This forms a part of the so-called tuberosity (Böhler's) angle, which averages about 30° and is an important anatomic landmark to assess the severity of injury and adequacy of reduction when this bone is fractured in its midportion.

CALCANEAL FRACTURES

Fractures of the calcaneus account for about 2 percent of all fractures[158, 191] and are the most common of any of the fractures of the bones in the foot,[163] accounting for about 60 percent of such fractures. Males are involved in these fractures much more frequently than females.

Classification of Calcaneal Fractures

Fractures of the calcaneus may vary in significance from the avulsion type to the incapacitating

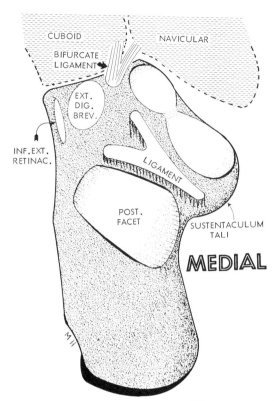

Figure 8–101. Anatomic relationship of the components of the subtalar joint. (From Harty, M.: Anatomic considerations in injuries of the calcaneus. Orthop. Clin. North Am. *4*:179, 1973.)

TABLE 8–3. Essex-Lopresti Classification of Calcaneal Fractures

I. Not involving subtalar joint
  A. Tuberosity fracture
    1. Beak type
    2. Avulsion medial border
    3. Vertical
    4. Horizontal
  B. Involving calcaneocuboid joint
    1. Parrot-nose type
    2. Vertical
II. Involving subtalar joint
  A. Without displacement
  B. With displacement
    1. Tongue type
    2. Central depression of joint
    3. Sustentaculum tali alone
  C. With gross comminution
    1. Severe tongue and joint depression
    2. Dislocation of subtalar joint

"blow-out" fracture. A general classification of the various fractures of the calcaneus was proposed by Cotton and Wilson in 1908.[160] The most revered of all general classifications of calcaneal fractures is probably that proposed by Rowe in 1963 (Fig. 8–103).[189] This classification is actually a synthesis of earlier attempts by Böhler (1931),[155] Warrick and Bremmer (1953),[196] and Watson-Jones (1955).[197]

The avulsion fractures comprise the Rowe Type I and II fractures. The Type I fracture is usually due to a twisting injury; the Type II injury, the so-called beak fracture, represents an avulsion of the posterior calcaneus by the Achilles tendon. The significance of Type I and II fractures varies considerably. The anterior process avulsion may involve the calcaneocuboid joint and thus may represent a rather significant injury. Large displacements with the beak fracture may also require special attention and even, in some instances, surgical reduction.

Clearly, the most important clinical problem is the adequate recognition of the extent and treatment of fractures involving the midportion or articular aspects of this bone.

The Rowe classification is less popular than that proposed by Essex-Lopresti to describe intra-articular fractures or fractures that involve the body of this bone. The scheme proposed by Essex-Lopresti (Table 8–3) divides the fractures into two large categories: those that involve the subtalar joint and those that do not, with prognostic significance attributed to the various types.[164] Essex-Lopresti ob-

Figure 8–102. Böhler's tuber angle averages about 30° and is an important landmark to assess the adequacy of reduction of calcaneal fractures. (From Harty, M.: Anatomic considerations in injuries of the calcaneus. Orthop. Clin. North Am. *4*:180, 1973.)

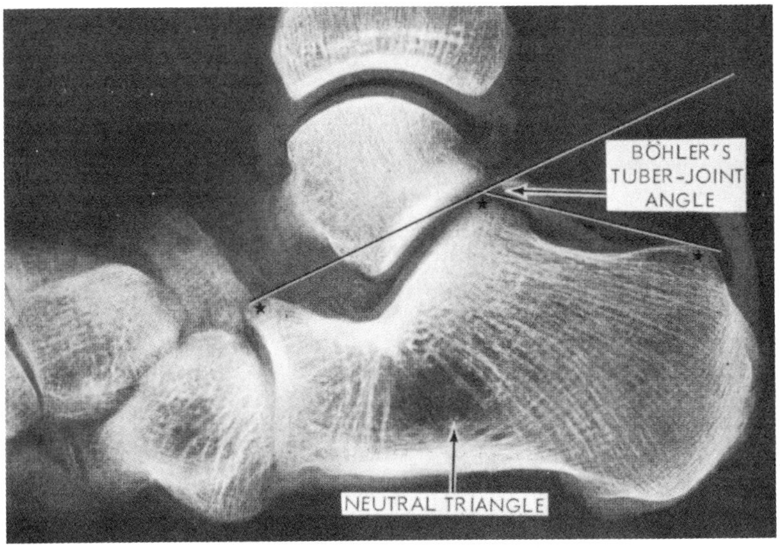

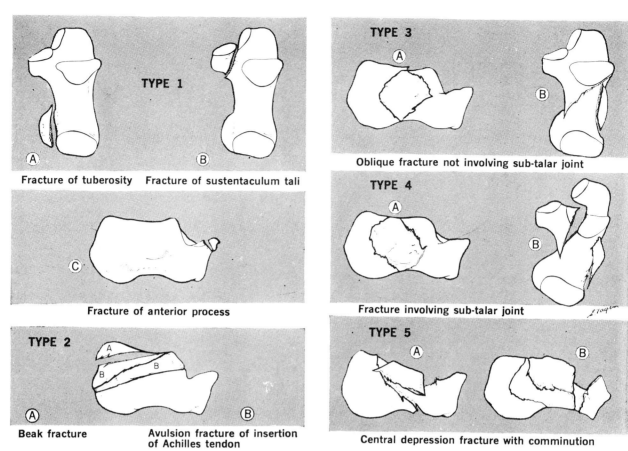

Figure 8–103. The Rowe classification of intra- and extra-articular fractures of the calcaneus. (From Rowe, C. R., Sakellarides, H. T., Freeman, P. A., et al.: Fractures of the os calcis. A long-term follow-up study of 146 patients. JAMA *184*:920, 1963. © 1963 American Medical Association.)

served involvement of the subtalar joint in about 25 percent of 180 fractures. Depressions of the articular surface in this classification are termed "central depression" fractures. In some cases, marked comminution precludes accurate diagnosis.

Radiographic Evaluation

The critical role of restoring the integrity of the subtalar joint, as often represented clinically by restoration of Böhler's angle, justifies careful roentgenographic study to determine the extent of the injury and the quality of reduction. Routine hindfoot and oblique views are mandatory. Occasionally tomography is helpful in fulfilling this requirement.

Mechanism of Injury and Associated Injuries

Indirect force, as from a twisting injury or a muscle pull, accounts for the majority of avulsion injuries. Direct violence, almost always described as falling from a height and landing on the heel, explains the majority of the severe fractures of the body of the calcaneus.

In this context it is important to recognize the associated musculoskeletal injuries that can also occur. These should be assessed both clinically and

radiographically. Associated injury has been reported in about 10 percent of the cases.[170, 189] Up to 12 percent have had an accompanying fracture of the spine,[192] and Schmidt[190] noted a 2.3 percent incidence of concurrent lower extremity fracture. This latter figure is lower than our experience would suggest.

Treatment: Extra-articular Fractures

These fractures are treated symptomatically[163, 188, 189] and rarely cause long-term problems.

Fracture of the Tuberosity (Type IA). This is an uncommon fracture usually caused by adduction or abduction of the hindfoot. On examination there is local tenderness. The fracture is readily diagnosed on an axial or PA radiograph. This fracture is almost always treated by a compressive dressing, elevation, and protective casting. Occasionally, open reduction may be required, as reported by Rowe.

Fracture of the Sustentaculum Tali (Type IB). This appears to be an uncommon injury[176] and is caused by an axial compression to an inverted hindfoot. An axial roentgenogram is necessary to demonstrate this lesion. Computed or conventional tomography may be required for an accurate

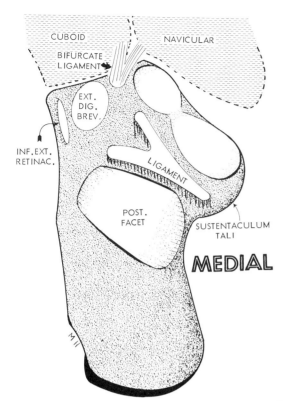

Figure 8–101. Anatomic relationship of the components of the subtalar joint. (From Harty, M.: Anatomic considerations in injuries of the calcaneus. Orthop. Clin. North Am. *4*:179, 1973.)

TABLE 8–3. Essex-Lopresti Classification of Calcaneal Fractures

I. Not involving subtalar joint
   A. Tuberosity fracture
      1. Beak type
      2. Avulsion medial border
      3. Vertical
      4. Horizontal
   B. Involving calcaneocuboid joint
      1. Parrot-nose type
      2. Vertical
II. Involving subtalar joint
   A. Without displacement
   B. With displacement
      1. Tongue type
      2. Central depression of joint
      3. Sustentaculum tali alone
   C. With gross comminution
      1. Severe tongue and joint depression
      2. Dislocation of subtalar joint

to a twisting injury; the Type II injury, the so-called beak fracture, represents an avulsion of the posterior calcaneus by the Achilles tendon. The significance of Type I and II fractures varies considerably. The anterior process avulsion may involve the calcaneocuboid joint and thus may represent a rather significant injury. Large displacements with the beak fracture may also require special attention and even, in some instances, surgical reduction.

Clearly, the most important clinical problem is the adequate recognition of the extent and treatment of fractures involving the midportion or articular aspects of this bone.

The Rowe classification is less popular than that proposed by Essex-Lopresti to describe intra-articular fractures or fractures that involve the body of this bone. The scheme proposed by Essex-Lopresti (Table 8–3) divides the fractures into two large categories: those that involve the subtalar joint and those that do not, with prognostic significance attributed to the various types.[164] Essex-Lopresti ob-

"blow-out" fracture. A general classification of the various fractures of the calcaneus was proposed by Cotton and Wilson in 1908.[160] The most revered of all general classifications of calcaneal fractures is probably that proposed by Rowe in 1963 (Fig. 8–103).[189] This classification is actually a synthesis of earlier attempts by Böhler (1931),[155] Warrick and Bremmer (1953),[196] and Watson-Jones (1955).[197]

The avulsion fractures comprise the Rowe Type I and II fractures. The Type I fracture is usually due

Figure 8–102. Böhler's tuber angle averages about 30° and is an important landmark to assess the adequacy of reduction of calcaneal fractures. (From Harty, M.: Anatomic considerations in injuries of the calcaneus. Orthop. Clin. North Am. *4*:180, 1973.)

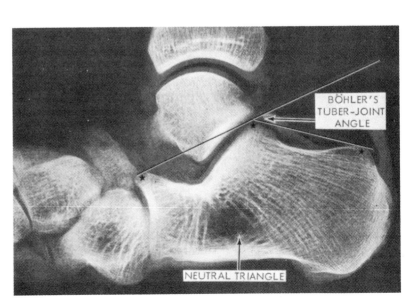

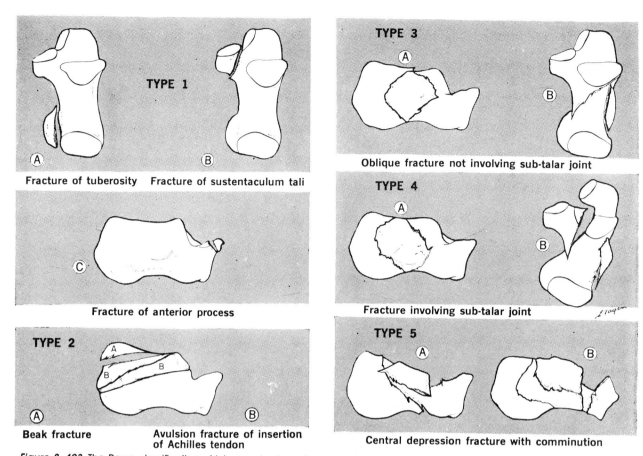

Figure 8–103. The Rowe classification of intra- and extra-articular fractures of the calcaneus. (From Rowe, C. R., Sakellarides, H. T., Freeman, P. A., et al.: Fractures of the os calcis. A long-term follow-up study of 146 patients. JAMA *184*:920, 1963. © 1963 American Medical Association.)

served involvement of the subtalar joint in about 25 percent of 180 fractures. Depressions of the articular surface in this classification are termed "central depression" fractures. In some cases, marked comminution precludes accurate diagnosis.

Radiographic Evaluation

The critical role of restoring the integrity of the subtalar joint, as often represented clinically by restoration of Böhler's angle, justifies careful roentgenographic study to determine the extent of the injury and the quality of reduction. Routine hindfoot and oblique views are mandatory. Occasionally tomography is helpful in fulfilling this requirement.

Mechanism of Injury and Associated Injuries

Indirect force, as from a twisting injury or a muscle pull, accounts for the majority of avulsion injuries. Direct violence, almost always described as falling from a height and landing on the heel, explains the majority of the severe fractures of the body of the calcaneus.

In this context it is important to recognize the associated musculoskeletal injuries that can also occur. These should be assessed both clinically and

radiographically. Associated injury has been reported in about 10 percent of the cases.[170, 189] Up to 12 percent have had an accompanying fracture of the spine,[192] and Schmidt[190] noted a 2.3 percent incidence of concurrent lower extremity fracture. This latter figure is lower than our experience would suggest.

Treatment: Extra-articular Fractures

These fractures are treated symptomatically[163, 188, 189] and rarely cause long-term problems.

Fracture of the Tuberosity (Type IA). This is an uncommon fracture usually caused by adduction or abduction of the hindfoot. On examination there is local tenderness. The fracture is readily diagnosed on an axial or PA radiograph. This fracture is almost always treated by a compressive dressing, elevation, and protective casting. Occasionally, open reduction may be required, as reported by Rowe.

Fracture of the Sustentaculum Tali (Type IB). This appears to be an uncommon injury[176] and is caused by an axial compression to an inverted hindfoot. An axial roentgenogram is necessary to demonstrate this lesion. Computered or conventional tomography may be required for an accurate

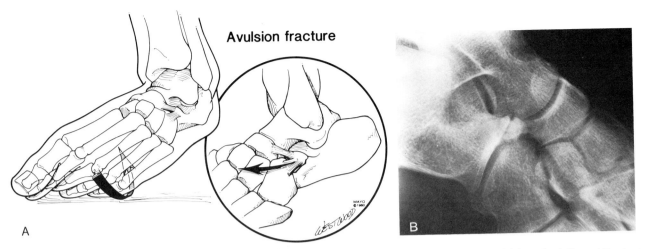

Avulsion fracture

A

B

Figure 8–104. The most common mechanism of the anterior process fracture is one of inversion and internal rotation of the foot, causing the process to be pulled off in tension *(A)*. Such a fracture is shown on the routine lateral x-ray *(B)*.

determination of the displacement. If the fracture is undisplaced, symptomatic treatment with cast immobilization for 6 to 8 weeks is all that is required. A small, displaced fragment may be excised. If a large portion of the articulation has been fractured, which is very unusual without an accompanying fracture of the body of the calcaneus, open reduction and internal fixation should be considered.

Fracture of the Anterior Process (Type IC). Fracture of the anterior process has been discussed to some extent in the recent literature.[161, 173] Termed the "fracture sprain" by Bradford,[156] this fracture is misdiagnosed initially in over 50 percent of cases. Usually it is misinterpreted as a simple sprain.[161] The mechanism of injury is typically that involved in the majority of sprains, that is, inversion and internal rotation (Fig. 8–104). This stress avulses the anterior process by virtue of the attachment of the bifurcate ligament. A dorsiflexion and eversion crush injury has also been reported as a variant of

the so-called "nutcracker fracture" of the cuboid[171] (Fig. 8–105).

Accurate diagnosis of fractures of the anterior calcaneal process is important and unfortunately may be difficult.[151] The AP and lateral roentgenograms are almost always worthless unless a large fragment with displacement is present. In the more typical case, even the routine oblique views may miss the fracture owing to the confluence of the shadows of the fracture line with the talonavicular joint. In this instance, the orientation of the x-ray should be about 10° to 15° cephalad and 10° to 15° posterior.[161, 166] This throws the anterior process into the neck of the talus, thereby demonstrating the fracture line (Fig. 8–106). If any doubt exists, a lateral tomogram readily resolves the issue (Fig. 8–107).

Treatment of the fracture is usually by immobilization for 3 to 6 weeks, depending upon the degree of symptoms. If a large fracture fragment is present, immobilization for 12 weeks or longer may be re-

Figure 8–105. A less common mechanism of the anterior process fracture is the so-called "nutcracker" injury in which the foot is dorsiflexed with a varus stress, causing a compression fracture.

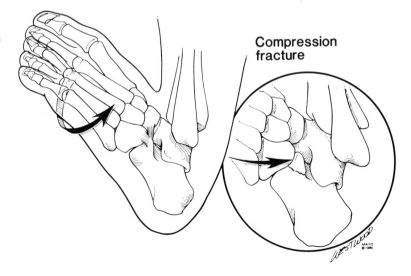

Compression fracture

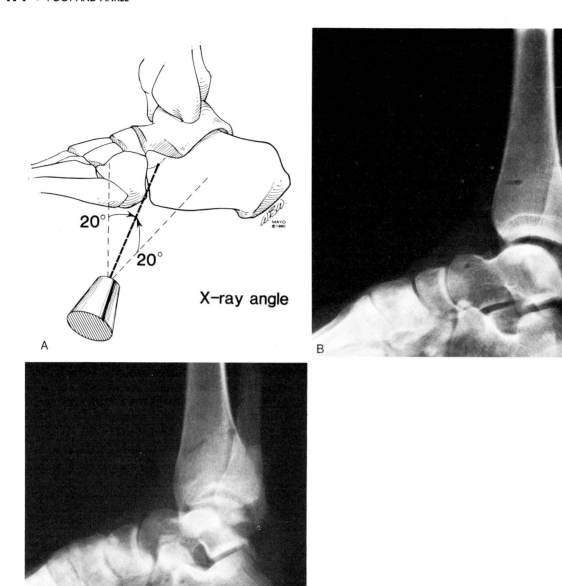

Figure 8–106. *A*, A radiograph angled 20° cephalad and 20° posterior tends to set the anterior process in relief behind the neck of the talus. *B*, Anterior process fracture is poorly seen in a cadaver specimen with routine lateral x-ray of the ankle. *C*, The fracture is better seen in this view when the radiograph is taken in the manner described in *A*.

quired. Symptoms may persist for several months. Although excision has occasionally been employed with success,[161] it should not be performed earlier than 9 to 12 months after the injury, since continued improvement is noted over this period of time in some instances.[161]

Beak Fracture of the Calcaneus (Type II). This fracture has been extensively reviewed by Korn,[175] who attributes its etiology to direct violence in combination with contracture of the Achilles tendon when the ankle is in a fixed position. This uncommon injury accounted for less than 4 percent of the cases reported by Rowe[189] and was termed a "beak fracture" by Watson-Jones[197] (Fig. 8–108). The diagnosis is readily made with routine lateral radiographs. Symptomatic treatment is usually all that is

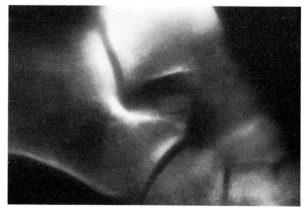

Figure 8–107. As with many of the avulsion fractures of the calcaneus, a tomogram of the lateral aspect of the calcaneus readily demonstrates the anterior process fracture.

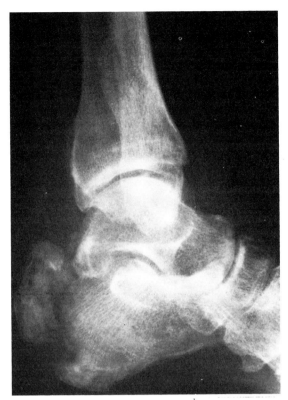

Figure 8–108. A spontaneous fracture of the posterior aspect of the calcaneus, the so-called "beak fracture." In this particular incident, the patient was a diabetic. Thus, this is a pathologic fracture.

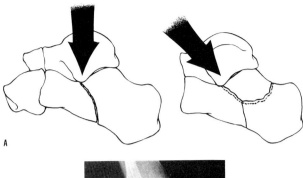

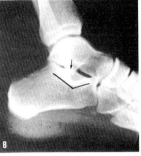

Figure 8–110. Most classifications of calcaneal fractures include the so-called "tongue type," which consists of the transverse fracture involving the posterior superior aspect of the calcaneus and includes the posterior facet. When this is badly comminuted, the posterior facet may, in fact, be depressed. The so-called "central depression" fracture is one in which the posterior facet is fractured as a free fragment and is driven plantarly into the substance of the calcaneus. (From Giannestras, N. J.: Foot Disorders. 2nd Ed. Philadelphia, Lea and Febiger, 1973.)

required. If significant displacement has occurred, then open reduction with internal fixation may be necessary.

Articular Fractures of the Calcaneus

Classification of Articular Fractures of the Calcaneus

Fractures of the calcaneus that involve the subtalar joint are a source of controversy with respect to classification and treatment. Rowe simply divides these types of fractures into those involving the subtalar joint and a so-called central depression fracture involving the articular facets.[189] Essex-Lopresti noted two patterns of fracture based on the so-called critical angle (Fig. 8–109).[164] The lateral process of the talus is situated immediately superior to the critical angle of the calcaneus and serves as

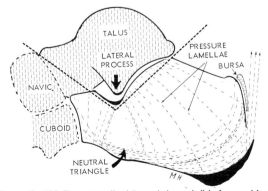

Figure 8–109. The so-called "crucial angle" is formed by the posterior and middle facets of the calcaneus. Immediately above these facets is the process of the talus, which is so situated as to result in a wedge-type effect, causing many of the calcaneal fractures. (From Harty, M.: Anatomic considerations in injuries to the calcaneus. Orthop. Clin. North Am. *4:*79, 1973.)

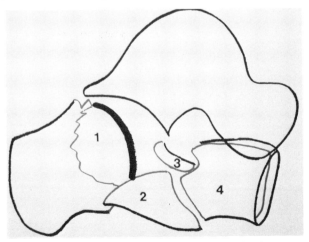

Figure 8–111. The classification of calcaneal fractures recommended by Soeur is based on the fragments that are usually present at the time of fracture and emphasizes the thalamic fragment (1). This fragment is comparable to the posterior articular facet, which has been considered an essential feature of this fracture by Essex-Lopresti and others. (From Soeur, R., and Remy, R.: Fractures of the calcaneus with displacement of the thalamic portion. J. Bone Joint Surg. *57B:*415, 1975.)

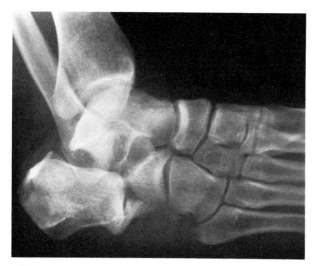

Figure 8–112. A joint-depression type fracture of the calcaneus. Notice the loss of Böhler's angle and pattern similar to that described in Figure 8–111.

a driving wedge into the body of the calcaneus with axial load.[169] The fracture that results is usually the so-called tongue-type or joint-depression type, depending upon the nature of the distributed force (Fig. 8–110). The common feature of both evaluation schemes is the focus on the posterior talofibular joint. Thus, Soeur and colleagues[192] assessed the fracture primarily in terms of the displacement of this posterior articular facet, the so-called thalamic portion (Fig. 8–111). It is of interest that all of these classifications are based primarily on the lateral roentgenogram. The axillary view demonstrates the widening and adds some further information, but in general the classification is based on a joint-depression type or is descriptive with respect to the articular surfaces involved and the maintenance of Böhler's angle.

In summary, the intra-articular fracture should be described according to the degree of involvement

TABLE 8–4. Depressed Calcaneal Fractures: Treatment Alternatives

Closed reduction
Subtalar arthrodesis
Triple arthrodesis
Resection
Open reduction
Early motion without reduction

of the subtalar joint, which is best indicated by the degree of comminution and displacement of the posterior facet as well as by the loss of Böhler's angle. These can be demonstrated with the lateral x-ray (Fig. 8–112).

Accordingly, special attention should be paid to the roentgenographic assessment of this fracture. In addition to the anatomic landmarks mentioned earlier, special features to be considered are the widening of the calcaneus and the value of the axillary view (Fig. 8–113).[149, 155, 157, 159] Involvement of the medial facet has also been implicated in late heel valgus.[179] Thus the oblique projection of the subtalar joint is often necessary to assess the sustentaculum tali fully.[150]

Treatment of Articular Fractures

Depending upon the exact nature of the fracture and the bias of the surgeon, six different treatment plans have been proposed for the more severe fractures (Table 8–4). In general, if the articular surfaces have not been comminuted but are displaced, a form of reduction is recommended. If the fragments are badly comminuted with displacement, immediate definitive reconstruction procedures or immediate initiation of functional rehabilitation is generally recommended.

Closed Reduction and Immobilization. The early literature commonly recommended closed reduction. Cotton and Wilson in 1908 reported 22 patients

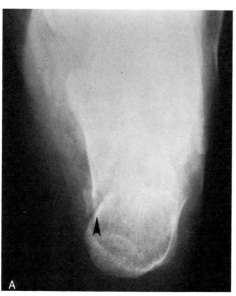 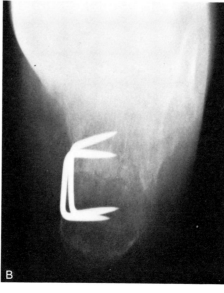

Figure 8–113. A, Widening of the calcaneus *(arrow)* is largely responsible for the sequelae of this fracture. B, Careful reduction can sometimes minimize this complication.

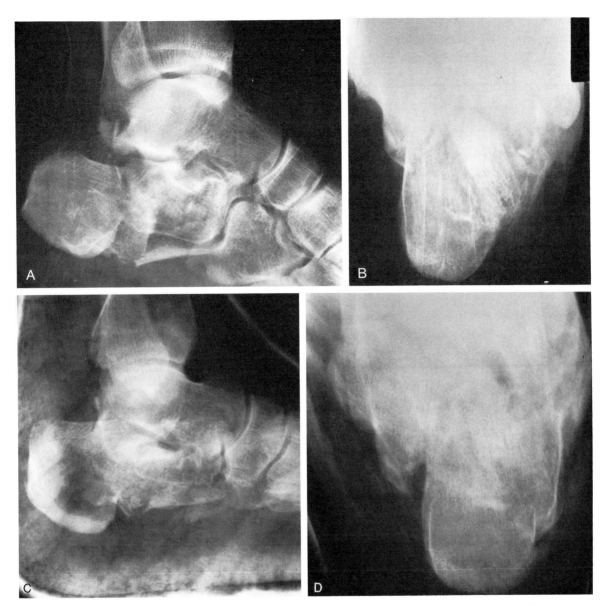

Figure 8–114. This severely comminuted fracture demonstrated comminution of the articular facets *(A* and *B)*. Since Chopart's joint was spared, a subtalar arthrodesis was performed *(C)*. The patient had a satisfactory result, but widening of the calcaneus persists *(D)*.

so treated.[160] Over 200 cases were reported in the 1930's.[155, 170, 191] Since that time, a more aggressive surgical and rehabilitative philosophy has been adopted with improved results. Reduction and prolonged immobilization is therefore not considered a viable treatment option at this time.

Subtalar Arthrodesis (Fig. 8–114). For severely comminuted fractures, immediate subtalar arthrodesis was a popular option during the Second World War. This approach allowed for relatively rapid return to military duty and was predictable in its results.* This technique has met with some popularity since it was recommended by Wilson[198] in 1927 and has been intermittently popular even to the present time. Rather encouraging results were reported by Dick (1953),[162] Hall and Pennal (1960),[167] Harris (1963),[168] Pennal and Yadow

(1973),[185] Noble (1979),[182] and as recently as 1982 by Johansson.[174]

Triple Arthrodesis (Fig. 8–115). Because of the significant disability that is associated with triple arthrodesis and because it is generally accepted that the arthrodesis is effective in selective cases, there is little present enthusiasm for this treatment modality. Although 83 cases were so treated by Conn (1935),[158] and although Thompson and Friesen reported good results in a significant number of patients (1959),[194] there is little support for this treatment of the initial fracture.

Resection of the Calcaneus. This is a theoretical option and has been suggested by Pridie (1946)[186] as one offering a high success rate. This clearly is not a viable option by today's standards.

Open Reduction and Fixation. If not the most popular, this has certainly received the most attention in the orthopedic literature, most of which has

*Personal communication, J. Janes, 1980.

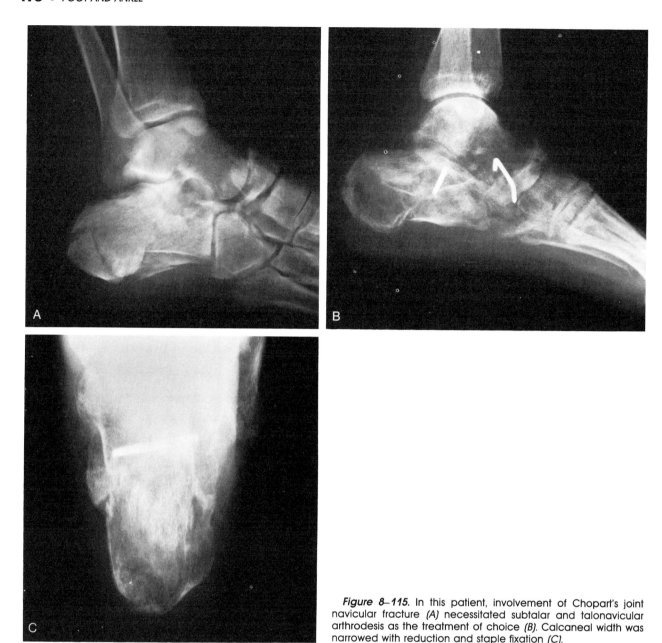

Figure 8–115. In this patient, involvement of Chopart's joint navicular fracture *(A)* necessitated subtalar and talonavicular arthrodesis as the treatment of choice *(B)*. Calcaneal width was narrowed with reduction and staple fixation *(C)*.

appeared since the Second World War.[164, 178, 184] Closed reduction with a Steinmann pin was a popular technique in the 1950's and 1960's. In the mid-1960's, however, enthusiasm waned. Interest was rekindled in the 1970's (Fig. 8–116), largely because of the excellent results of open reduction reported by McReynolds (1976)[180] (Fig. 8–117). Others subsequently have recommended various surgical techniques for the treatment of this fracture.[193, 195] The multiple techniques recommended include medial and lateral surgical approaches; fixation with sta-

ples, wires, K-wires, Steinmann pins, and screws; and supplemental bone grafting.

Variable Reduction and Immediate Motion. In the mid-1960's the attitude toward articular fractures became somewhat fatalistic, and this treatment was recommended by Rowe[189] and Lance.[176] These authors reported on over 300 patients treated with closed reduction and immediate motion. Today, most would specifically attempt reduction of the mediolateral displacement of the severely comminuted fracture in order to narrow the hindfoot.

Figure 8–117. Böhler's angle is 0° but little communication is present *(A* and *B)*. The medial approach recommended by McReynolds has been effective in restoring Böhler's angle *(C)*. This technique emphasizes the levering of this thick cortical bone into an anatomic position, which restores the critical angle *(D)* and reduces the hindfoot comminution *(E)*.

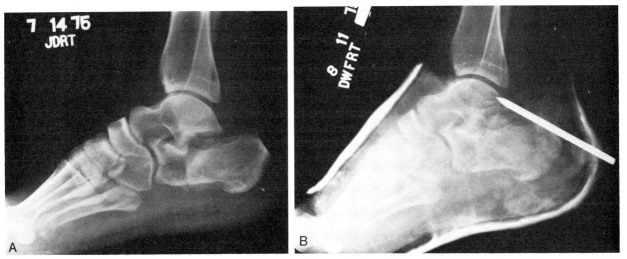

Figure 8–116. The Gasslen spike popularized by Essex-Lopresti may be used to reduce some fractures if they are not badly comminuted.

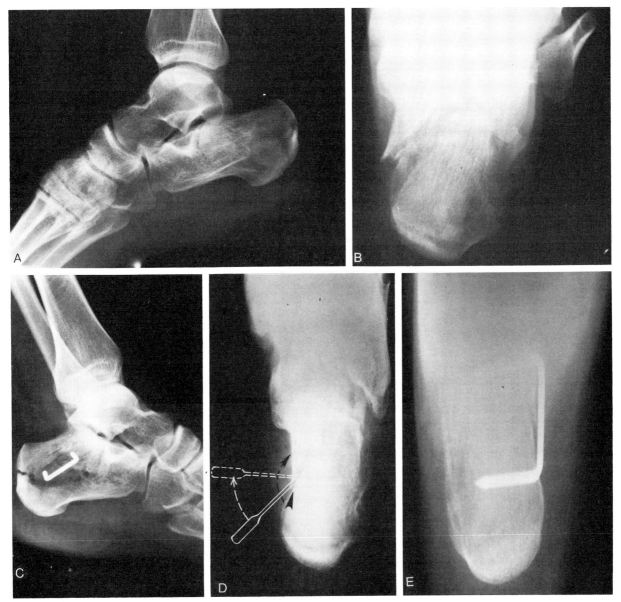

Figure 8–117. See legend on opposite page

Then, if comminution was too severe to allow fixation, early motion would be instituted.

Results

The results of these treatments of calcaneal fractures probably depended more upon the nature of the fracture than upon the specific treatment rendered.[157] Closed reduction with prolonged immobilization was demonstrated to show only 50 percent good results by some (Cotton and Wilson[160]), encouraging results by others (Bernard[153, 154]), and "all good" results by still others (Böhler[155]). In fact, on close scrutiny significant functional impairment and pain were frequently present. Thus, as mentioned earlier, this treatment is no longer considered a rational approach to the problem.

Careful analysis of the series dealing with reduction and early mobilization[153, 176, 177, 189] demonstrates that this treatment modality offers results comparable to open reduction and internal fixation and that it avoids the complications of this latter treatment option.

Somewhat surprisingly, subtalar arthrodesis demonstrates a high percentage of satisfactory results, as represented by the reports of Dick,[162] Pennal,[185] Noble,[182] and Harris.[168] Probably the most characteristic feature of this surgical approach is that patients are able to return to work at an earlier date than in the case of most other treatment options. In fact, Hall and Pennal (1960)[167] reported that 90 percent returned to work in 7 months, and Wilson (1927)[198] related that 18 of 20 returned to work in 7.2 months. This is consistent with the most recent report by Johansson (1982),[174] in which 21 patients followed for a period of 2 to 9 years showed a 90 percent satisfactory result, and most returned to work within 6 months. In spite of our inherent objection to immediate definitive treatment for intra-articular fractures, the data reported for this particular procedure are rather impressive.

As mentioned earlier, triple arthrodesis may not be considered a viable option at this time owing to the encouraging results seen after subtalar arthrodesis alone. With significant involvement of Chopart's joint, a triple arthrodesis may be considered; but we would still allow this condition to declare itself and not perform the procedure primarily. Yet, in the older literature[158] satisfactory results of up to 96 percent[194] are recorded. Such results must be interpreted with the understanding that a significant restriction of function is also associated with this treatment.

The results of open reduction and internal fixation are difficult to summarize concisely and accurately. The satisfactory results reported in the literature range from 68 percent, reported by Maxfield,[178] to 100 percent in selected cases, reported by McReynolds.[180] In general, approximately 80 to 85 percent of patients are graded as satisfactory following open reduction and internal fixation. The precise technique, including medial or lateral approaches, depends on the surgeon's preference (or bias). In certain types of fractures, for example, large fragments of the sustentaculum tali may be particularly amenable to a medial approach.[180] Additional variables of prognostic value include the patient's age as well as the effects of prolonged immobilization. Both of these variables more than double the unsatisfactory results.[164]

Immediate motion without specific reduction is no longer currently recommended. The reports in the 1960's by Rowe[189] and by Lance[176] demonstrated only 50 percent satisfactory results with this treatment modality. Most orthopedists would at least try to narrow the hindfoot with compression and to make some attempt to restore Böhler's angle prior to immediate or early motion.

Complications

The major complication of this fracture is, of course, long-term disability. In the early stages, persistent pain may be related to the altered mechanics of the hindfoot, with associated stiffness and painful periarticular joints (Fig. 8–118). Late pain may result from post-traumatic subtalar arthritis, which is inevitable in severe depression-type fractures. Widening of the calcaneus and hindfoot valgus are common[181] and are probably related to

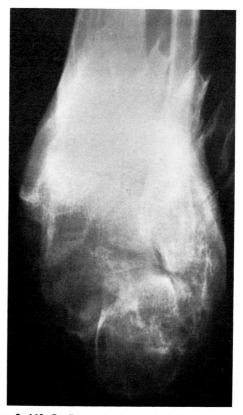

Figure 8–118. Radiograph demonstrates marked hindfoot valgus associated with a severely comminuted fracture, in which the sustentaculum tali has been comminuted.

inadequate support of the talus by a fractured sustentaculum tali.[179] Peroneal tendinitis is also a well recognized and not an uncommon source of late or continued pain. It usually is found along the lateral aspect of the heel.[149, 163, 188] Abutment of the fibula on the widened calcaneus has also been recognized as a sequela to the unreduced calcaneus fracture,[172] and medial encroachment may be a cause of tarsal tunnel syndrome.[165]

Loss of reduction is not an uncommon occurrence with this fracture, regardless of the modality and treatment. This may be lessened by a Steinmann pin inserted across the fracture.[183] Yet there has been no clear correlation of results as a function of the restoration of Böhler's angle.

With any open reduction, routine surgical complications are anticipated, including infection and wound necrosis. The medial approach to the calcaneus carries the additional potential complication of injury to the medial calcaneal branch of the posterior tibial nerve. Symptomatic paresthesias about the skin incision are likewise a problem in 5 to 10 percent of patients in our experience.

As for the severe intra-articular comminuted fractures of this bone, Bankart's pessimistic claim that "the results of treatment of the os calcis are rotten"[152] may no longer be true of today's treatment. However, in general, there has not been a dramatic improvement in our treatment of this serious injury.

INJURIES OF THE FOREFOOT REGION AND TOES

KENNETH A. JOHNSON

The forefoot is composed of those tarsal bones distal to the talus and calcaneus, i.e., the navicular, cuboid, and three cuneiforms. Also included are the five metatarsals as well as the phalanges of the toes. The tarsal bones of the forefoot, with the exception of the navicular bone, are only infrequently involved in an isolated fracture. Occasionally small chip-type fractures occur, but the most frequent tarsal injuries are associated with distal disruption of the tarsometatarsal joints.[203, 211]

Tarsometatarsal (Lisfranc) Fractures

The tarsometatarsal joints are termed the "joints of Lisfranc" after the French surgeon Jacques Lisfranc, who was an officer in the armies of Napoleon.[199, 200]

The stability of the tarsometatarsal (Lisfranc) joints depends upon both the osseous and ligamentous configurations.[209] The base of the 2nd metatarsal is distinct from the other four in that it is seated

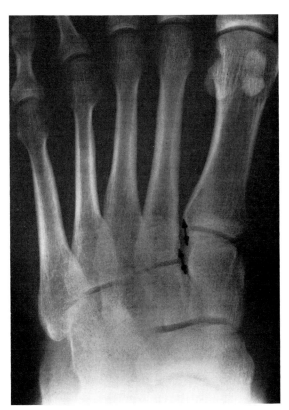

Figure 8–119. Note the "in-line" arrangement of the lateral margin of the 1st metatarsal-cuneiform and medial margin of the 2nd metatarsal-cuneiform articulations *(arrows)*. Displacements of the tarsometatarsal joints are almost invariably evident if the "in-line" configuration is assessed. The usual AP view of the foot is taken with the foot flat and the line of the x-ray beam tilted inferiorly 20°.

in a mortise between the medial and lateral cuneiforms. The proper relationship is seen on a normal AP radiograph of the foot (Fig. 8–119). The base of the 2nd metatarsal articulates directly with the distal surface of the middle cuneiform. By viewing the in-line arrangement of the medial aspect of the middle cuneiform and the medial aspect of the base of the 2nd metatarsal, it is easy to assess the proper position of the joint. Likewise, viewing the entire relationship of the lateral aspect of the medial cuneiform and the lateral aspect of the base of the 1st metatarsal is a useful way to evaluate the congruity of this joint. The bases of the lateral three metatarsals articulate with the lateral cuneiform and cuboid regions. These articulations are not easily seen on the usual AP views because of overlap of the multiple surfaces. Rotation of the x-ray beam laterally may place these joints in profile,[210] with an increase in rotation showing the more lateral joints (Fig. 8–120). Ligamentous attachments of the base of the metatarsals are also important in determining patterns of injury. The lateral four metatarsals are tightly bound to each other by transverse, dorsal, and plantar ligaments. A gap exists between the 1st and 2nd metatarsals, however; therefore, the lateral four metatarsals will usually displace as a unit away

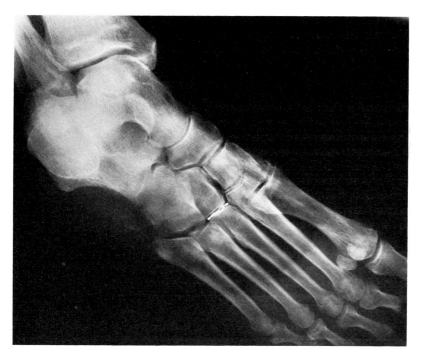

Figure 8–120. Using this same position but rotating the beam laterally places the 3rd and 4th tarsometatarsal articulations in profile (see marker in 3rd tarsometatarsal joint). Fractures and degenerative changes of these lateral joints can then be visualized.

from the 1st metatarsal. Or the 1st metatarsal will be displaced separately from the lateral four metatarsals. Recognition of these bony and ligamentous anatomic arrangements allows a better understanding of the patterns of tarsometatarsal injury.

The mechanism of injury for Lisfranc joint disruptions is not clearly defined.[200, 209, 212, 213] The most commonly cited cause is a plantarward bending of the metatarsals associated with a rotational stress. Three patterns of injury are most frequently seen and are well described (Fig. 8–121).[207] In the first pattern, all five metatarsals will displace in either a medial or lateral direction at the Lisfranc joint. This displacement is termed total incongruity. The alignment of both the 1st and 2nd metatarsal bases with the medial and middle cuneiforms is displaced. Because of the mortise arrangement of the 2nd metatarsal base, a fracture of this bone is often associated with this displacement. In the second pattern, the 1st metatarsal alone displaces medially, or the 2nd metatarsal and one or more of the successive adjacent lateral metatarsals displace laterally. This pattern is termed partial incongruity. Lateral translocation of the base of the 2nd metatarsal, usually with a fracture of the metatarsal base,[200] along with displacement of the adjacent 3rd through 5th metatarsals is probably the most common pattern of injury in this area. Directing attention to the 2nd cuneiform metatarsal alignment, however, makes the radiologic detection certain on the AP radiograph. Thirdly, a divergent pattern may be seen when the 1st metatarsal base displaces medially while the 2nd metatarsal base displaces laterally with one or more of the lateral metatarsals. This divergent pattern is unusual but is important in

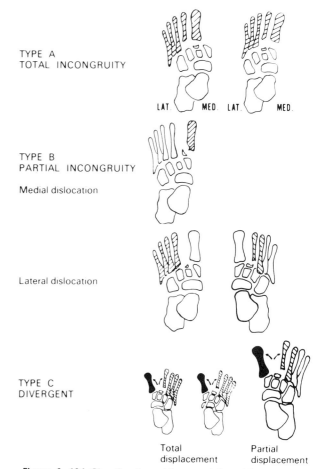

TYPE A
TOTAL INCONGRUITY

LAT. MED. LAT. MED.

TYPE B
PARTIAL INCONGRUITY

Medial dislocation

Lateral dislocation

TYPE C
DIVERGENT

Total displacement   Partial displacement

Figure 8–121. Classification of tarsometatarsal fracture-dislocations. (From Hardcastle, P. H. et al.: Injuries to the tarsometatarsal joint: Incidence, classification, and treatment. J. Bone Joint Surg. *64B*:349, 1982.)

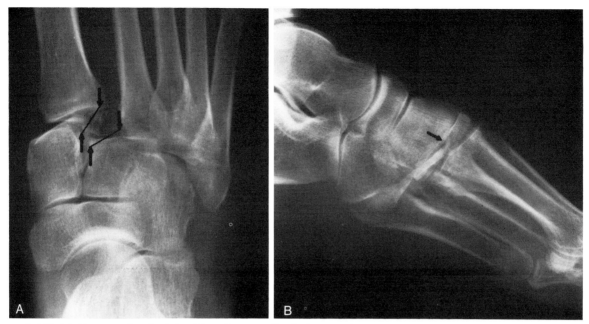

Figure 8–122. Total incongruity of a lateral type is seen with displacement *(arrows)* of all metatarsal bases. AP *(A)* and lateral *(B)* views.

that more proximal fractures and dislocations involving the cuneiforms and even the navicular bone are more commonly associated with it and should be suspected.

The example given in Figure 8–122 shows a total incongruity with lateral displacement of all the metatarsal bases. Focusing on the disruption of the

metatarsal-cuneiform alignment makes the classification easy. A lateral view is difficult to interpret because of the overlap of the involved area.

Treatment of the Lisfranc fracture-dislocation requires an accurate reduction of the disrupted joints.[200, 206, 209] Closed manipulation with adequate anesthesia may be successful. However, bone frag-

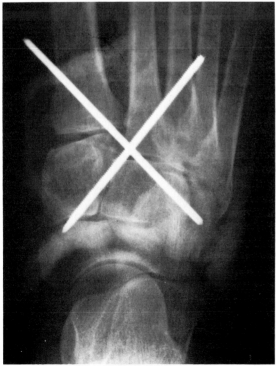

Figure 8–123. Crossed fixation wires have been used to secure the open reduction of a Lisfranc fracture-dislocation.

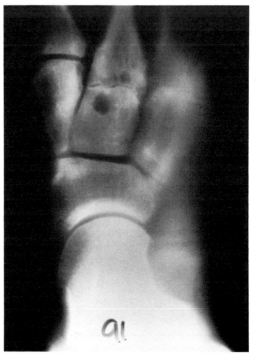

Figure 8–124. Tomogram clearly shows the late degenerative changes of the 2nd tarsometatarsal joint occurring after an undetected Lisfranc fracture-dislocation.

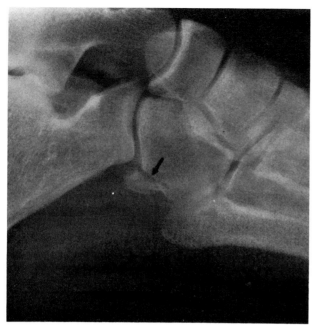

Figure 8–125. Fracture of the inferior portion of the cuboid *(arrow)*, lateral view.

ments at the 2nd metatarsal base,[200] the tibialis anterior tendon,[201, 202, 210] the peroneus longus tendon,[202] and soft tissue may all block such attempts at reduction. If the closed treatment is not perfect and stable, then open reduction through longitudinal incisions will be required.[210] This allows direct visualization of the area between the medial and middle cuneiform and the respective 1st and 2nd metatarsal bases. Any block to reduction can then be eliminated and an accurate reduction obtained. Operative AP radiographs should particularly focus on the 2nd cuneiform-metatarsal region. Kirschner-wire fixation is most commonly used to hold the

operative reduction (Fig. 8–123).[204, 211] The long-term success of treatment seems to be directly related to the accuracy of reduction. If the fracture-dislocation goes undetected or is not adequately treated, degenerative arthritis of these joints will supervene (Fig. 8–124). It is helpful to obtain AP tomograms of the tarsometatarsal articulations in these late situations to detect the specific joints and degree of arthritic involvement. Arthrodesis of the affected joints for symptoms of pain is the most common late operative treatment.[206]

Cuneiform and Cuboid Fractures

Fractures involving these midtarsal bones alone are unusual. If they occur, it is usually a result of direct trauma, such as a garage door coming down on the dorsum of the foot. When the fractures are of the chip type (Fig. 8–125), they are essentially undisplaced inasmuch as the capsule and ligament soft tissues tend to hold them in position.

The unusual compression fracture of the cuboid,[207] described as the "nutcracker" fracture, is probably caused by abduction and compression of the forefoot. A similar report[203] demonstrated an avulsion fracture of the navicular tuberosity along with compression at the calcaneal-cuboid articulation. An alternative cuboid abnormality may occur with the same abduction and compression mechanism, that is, a dislocation of the cuboid (Fig. 8–126).

Treatment of the chip-type fracture involves a short-leg walking cast for a few weeks to allow soft tissue healing. If the fracture involves a joint surface, surgical reduction and fixation are frequently necessary. In the event of later degenerative arthritis of the joint, an isolated arthrodesis may be done.

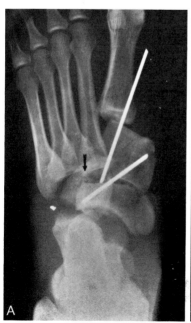
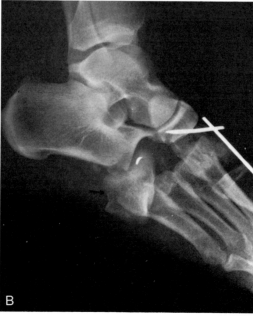

Figure 8–126. Inferior dislocation of the cuboid *(arrows)* associated with a total incongruity type of lateral tarsometatarsal fracture-dislocation. AP *(A)* and lateral *(B)* views.

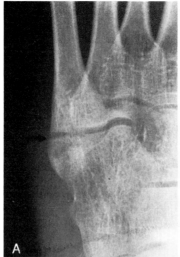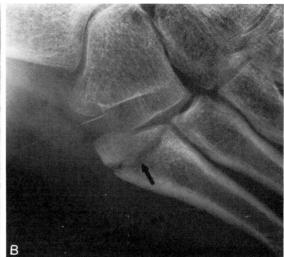

Figure 8–127. AP *(A)* and oblique *(B)* views of a 5th metatarsal base avulsion fracture *(arrows).*

Metatarsal Fractures

Fractures involving the base of the 5th metatarsal region are of two types. Both of these are most easily seen on the oblique view of the foot, which shows the base of the 5th proximal metatarsal in profile. The first is a fracture of the tuberosity (Fig. 8–127). This fracture is probably an avulsion fracture caused by a pull of the peroneus brevis, which inserts on this tuberosity. Fortunately, there are many strong ligament-capsular structures that firmly unite this tuberosity to the adjacent base of the 4th metatarsal. For this reason significant displacement of the fracture is unusual. Also, since the fracture occurs through a broad cancellous bone surface, it tends to heal well with immobilization only as necessary to provide comfort. It is important to differentiate this fracture from apophyseal growth centers and also from the sesamoid bones, the os peroneum[208] (Fig. 8–128), and os vesa-

lianum.[201, 205] The sesamoid can be distinguished from the fracture by the smooth edges of the fragments and by its usual presence on the roentgenogram of the opposite foot. The second type of 5th metatarsal base fracture occurs through the proximal metaphysis (Fig. 8–129). This is a transverse fracture, which is frequently of a stress-reaction type,[213] and is caused by jogging, hiking, jumping, or some such repetitive activity. In contrast to the tuberosity fracture, the metaphyseal fracture has a strong tendency to delayed healing. It has been suggested that internal fixation may be helpful to promote union; that is particularly indicated in the case of the professional athlete.[199, 213] Table 8–5 compares the characteristics of these two fractures of the base of the 5th metatarsal.

The term "Jones" fracture has been used loosely to refer to both fracture of the tuberosity[201] and metaphyseal fracture.[199] In fact, Sir Robert Jones, a prominent early British orthopedic surgeon, did incur a fracture of the 5th metatarsal base in 1896 while dancing. At that time the use of the roentgenograph was just emerging. He had such an

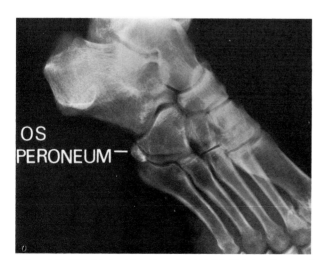

Figure 8–128. An os peroneum located in the substance of the peroneus longus tendon can be mistaken for a 5th metatarsal base avulsion fracture.

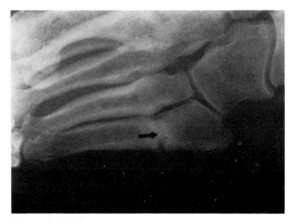

Figure 8–129. The metaphyseal fracture of proximal 5th metatarsal *(arrow)* has a tendency to delayed healing or nonunion.

image taken and described the fracture as being "about three fourths of an inch from its base."[207] Unfortunately, the published reproduction of the x-ray image was so poor that the fracture could not be seen.[202] We can only speculate that the true Jones fracture is of the tuberosity type, since it was acute in onset, healed well without operative treatment, and was common in that within weeks Jones reported that he had encountered five other patients with the same lesion.[207]*

Fracture through the neck region of the metatarsals is a result of either a direct blow or a twisting injury.[203] If direct trauma is the mechanism, a soft tissue injury may be a significant associated problem. Also, the fracture will probably be transverse and comminuted (Fig. 8–130). With a twisting injury, the fracture will be of a spiral configuration (Fig. 8–131). Again, the oblique and AP views of

---

*In this publication, which correlates radiology and orthopedic surgery, it is instructive to consider the comments of Sir Robert Jones on the relationship of these two specialties of medicine: "Radiography here, as in all branches of medicine, is an essential aid to diagnosis. No matter how experienced we may be, we cannot afford to dispense with it, even in the apparently simple and obvious case. Not only should we insist on procuring a film, but it is equally important that we should welcome the radiologist's reading of it. Some surgeons resent this and say, 'Give me the film so that I can read it myself,' but this is an arrogant and stupid attitude, and not to the patient's advantage. In Liverpool, I constantly, and with profit, confer with my friend Thurston Holland."[203]

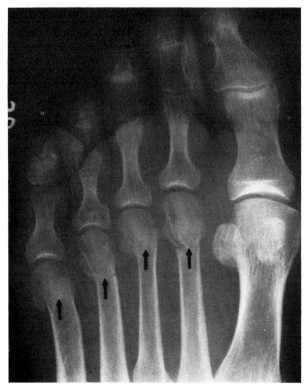

Figure 8–130. Transverse fractures of the lateral metatarsal necks were caused by direct trauma. The metatarsal heads were angulated dorsally, indicating a blow from above. AP view.

TABLE 8–5. Characteristics of Tuberosity and Metaphyseal Types of 5th Metatarsal Bone Fractures

Characteristic	Tuberosity	Metaphyseal
Onset	Acute	Acute or chronic
Mechanism	Avulsion	Fatigue (stress)
Frequency	Common	Unusual
Location	Proximal tuberosity	Metaphysis
Healing potential	Good	Poor
Need for operative fixation	Infrequent	Frequent

the foot will probably be the most useful, since they show the metatarsals in profile.

An undisplaced fracture is best treated by a walking cast. A malposition, however, should be corrected surgically if necessary to prevent the later problem of uneven weight-bearing under the metatarsal head region.[199] Kirschner-wire fixation, either obliquely if the fracture area is spiral or longitudinally with a transverse fracture, is commonly used.

Occasionally a metatarsal head will shatter as a result of direct trauma (Fig. 8–132).[202] In this situation internal fixation will not be possible, but longitudinal traction may be helpful. If the metatarsal head fracture is displaced and separated at the intra-articular surface (Fig. 8–133), open reduction and fixation may be indicated. The purpose would be to prevent late degenerative arthritis and pain.

Stress fractures can occur in the shaft of the metatarsal and most commonly involve the 2nd or 3rd rays.[213] No relationship between metatarsal length and the incidence of stress fractures has been determined.[199] This fracture (Fig. 8–134) is easily missed if the roentgenogram is taken within the first few weeks after the onset of symptoms. After a few weeks the fracture becomes evident, along with a fusiform callus (Fig. 8–135). If it is necessary to make this diagnosis early, a Tc-99m scan[202] will show the bone reaction prior to its appearance on routine x-ray views. Treatment involves decreasing the repetitive stresses that precipitated the bone reaction. Unless pain is significant, cast immobilization is not necessary.

Phalangeal Fractures

Phalangeal fractures are frequently considered insignificant. Indeed, such problems as the "night walker's" fracture of the proximal phalanx of the 5th toe do not involve an articular surface and are not angulated or displaced (Fig. 8–136). Support by taping to the adjacent toes and avoidance of direct pressure are all that is necessary.[207] However, a phalangeal fracture involving a joint surface (Fig. 8–137) should not be interpreted with such a cavalier attitude.[201] If the joint fracture is not treated adequately, late changes of stiffness and degeneration will supervene.[202]

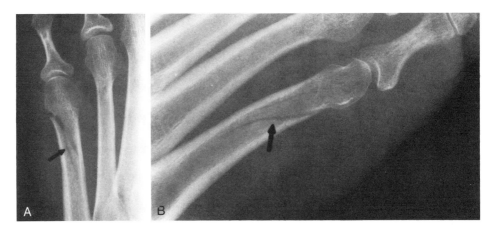

Figure 8–131. A twisting injury caused this spiral fracture of the 5th metatarsal. AP *(A)* and oblique *(B)* views.

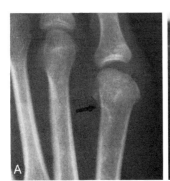
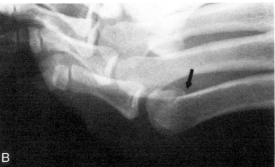

Figure 8–132. This comminuted metatarsal head fracture would not be suitable for open surgical treatment. AP *(A)* and oblique *(B)* views.

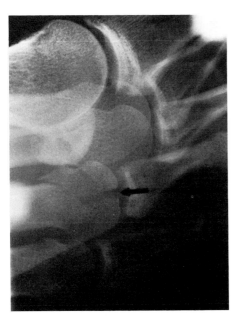

Figure 8–133

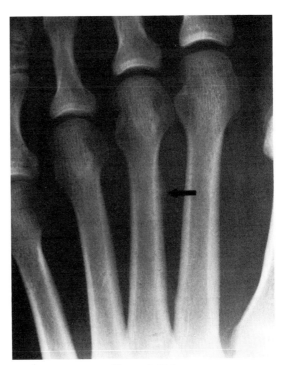

Figure 8–134

Figure 8–133. An intra-articular 4th metatarsal head fracture that may be helped by open reduction and fixation.

Figure 8–134. Third metatarsal stress fracture is seen *(arrow).* The minimal periosteal reaction may be the only early change seen on the plain radiograph.

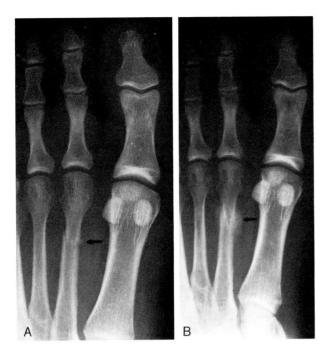

Figure 8–135. This 2nd metatarsal stress fracture was complete when initially evaluated for pain in the forefoot region with ambulation *(A)*. Three weeks later, abundant healing callus formation is present *(B)*.

Figure 8–136. AP *(A)* and oblique *(B)* views of "night walker's" fracture of the 5th proximal phalanx base.

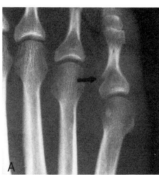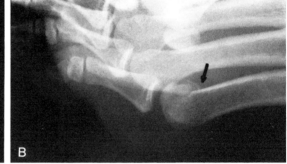

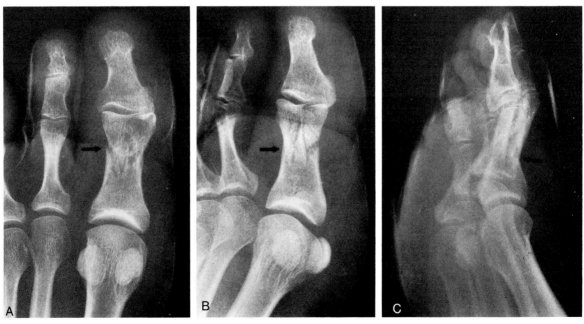

Figure 8–137. AP *(A)*, oblique *(B)*, and lateral *(C)* views show the intra-articular extension of this great toe proximal phalanx fracture.

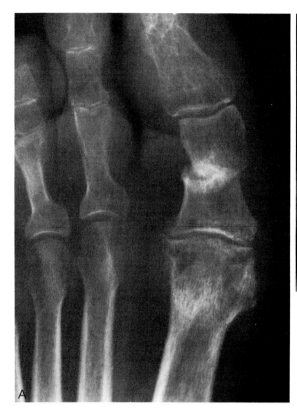

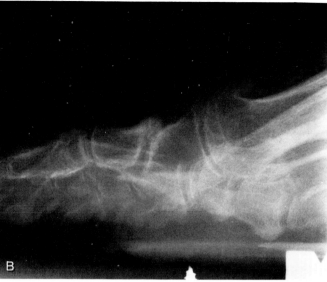

Figure 8–138. AP *(A)* and lateral *(B)* views demonstrate non-union of a great toe proximal phalanx fracture.

It is possible that a phalangeal fracture will not progress to union (Fig. 8–138). In one case of non-union the patient's pain was relieved by excision of the distal portion of the proximal phalanx through the non-united fracture site.

The other common phalangeal fracture, which may be easily overlooked, is the avulsion fracture of a portion of the phalangeal condyle by the collateral ligaments (Fig. 8–139). If suspected as a result of clinical evaluation, the fracture may be demonstrated with oblique views of the phalanx. These views show the small fragment in relief from the adjacent bone surface. The small fragment may become a chronic source of pain and thus require excision. Instability of the phalanx is not a prominent long-term problem, since footwear and the adjacent toes also provide support.

Sesamoid Fractures

A fracture of the sesamoid is infrequent but certainly can occur (Fig. 8–140). The medial tibial-oriented sesamoid beneath the 1st metatarsal head is the most common site of involvement (Fig. 8–140A). Since this sesamoid lies invested in the flexor hallucis brevis tendon, pain symptoms are increased by dorsiflexion in the proximal phalanx, which is the site of insertion of the tendon. Confusion of the sesamoid fracture with a bipartite sesamoid may occur. The bipartite sesamoid, however, is usually bilateral[207] (Fig. 8–140B), and its lines are smooth and well delineated in comparison with the jagged fracture line. A tangential view

(Fig. 8–140C) is also very helpful in showing the dorsal articular surface irregularities that may occur.

Sometimes the patient's pain symptoms will gradually increase over a few months (Fig. 8–141A and B), with no abrupt inciting onset. This change in

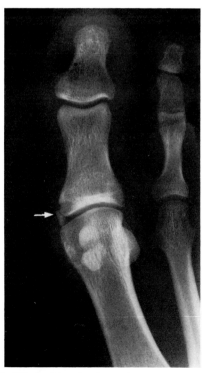

Figure 8–139. Avulsion fracture of the great toe proximal phalanx base caused by stress on the joint's tibial-oriented collateral ligament.

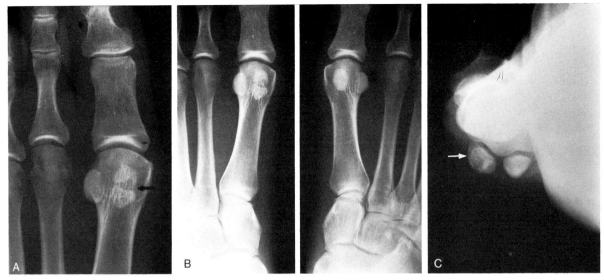

Figure 8–140. A, During a stressful athletic event this man developed acute pain beneath the 1st metatarsal head. The transverse and irregular fracture through the tibial-oriented sesamoid is seen *(arrow). B,* A view showing the affected left tibial-oriented sesamoid and asymptomatic right foot demonstrates the sesamoid fracture. A bipartite sesamoid is usually bilateral. The unilateral changes seen here support the diagnosis of the sesamoid fracture. *C,* Tangential sesamoid view gives a "double" appearance *(arrow)* indicating fracture but fortunately not much superior articular surface irregularity.

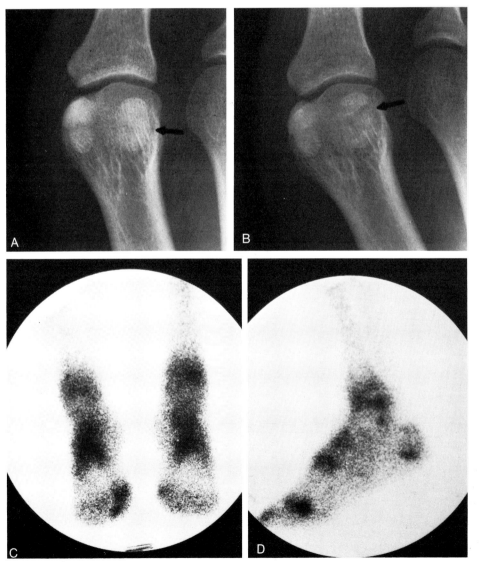

Figure 8–141. This person had the insidious onset of fibular-oriented sesamoid pain. An initial view *(A)* did not show much change. Two months later, fragmentation of that sesamoid *(arrow)* is present *(B).* Increased isotope uptake is noted in the great toe sesamoid area *(C and D),* which correlates well with the gradual changes of the sesamoid noted above.

the sesamoid suggests it might be more properly termed a stress-type fracture. As with all stress reactions of bone, a Tc-99m scan (Fig. 8–141C and D) will show increased uptake in that area.

TOTAL ANKLE ARTHROPLASTY

KENNETH A. JOHNSON

Types

Several types of ankle joint implant have become available since the satisfactory results achieved in other joint replacements have become evident.[235, 237, 241] These implants can be divided according to their design philosophy.[238] One group of implants essentially restricts motion only to the flexion-extension plane (constrained), while the other group allows for motion in multiple directions (nonconstrained). Materials utilized in each have largely been of the metal-polyethylene combination type.

The Mayo replacement for the ankle was designed by Dr. R. N. Stauffer and is of the constrained type (Fig. 8–142). It is probably fair to report that none of the prostheses available for the ankle has been shown overall to be superior to one another. The experience at the Mayo Clinic reflects the general experience of others with the ankle replacement procedure.

Results

In a report from the Mayo Clinic of 102 arthroplasties of the ankle, the "best results were obtained

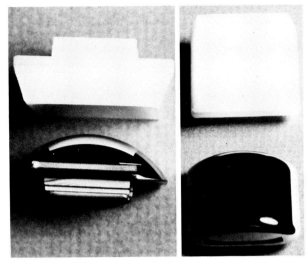

Figure 8–142. Lateral and articular surface views of the Mayo ankle arthroplasty components are shown.

in patients with rheumatoid arthritis and those with post-traumatic osteoarthritis who were older than 60 years of age."[241] More recently, expanding the evaluation to 187 arthroplasties confirmed the wisdom of this limited use of the ankle replacement arthroplasty.[236] Overall, those patients with rheumatoid arthritis had a satisfactory result in 83 percent of the ankle arthroplasties at an average follow-up of 40 months. This is in contrast to a satisfaction rate of 63 percent for the patients with traumatic primary arthritis at an average follow-up of 48 months. Also, there was a distinct tendency for the traumatic-primary group of arthroplasties to develop pain with a longer length of follow-up. Fortunately, if the underlying disease was rheumatoid arthritis, increasing pain with time was not promi-

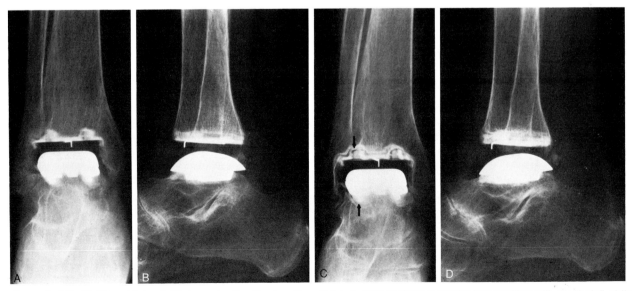

Figure 8–143. AP *(A)* and lateral *(B)* views shortly after insertion of the prosthesis show a satisfactory position with no "halo" at the interface between the methyl methacrylate and surrounding bone. AP *(C)* and lateral *(D)* views 3 years later. Resorption of bone due to infection at the junction between inserted materials and bone is evident. This is present on both the tibial and talar components *(arrows)* and is most evident on the AP view.

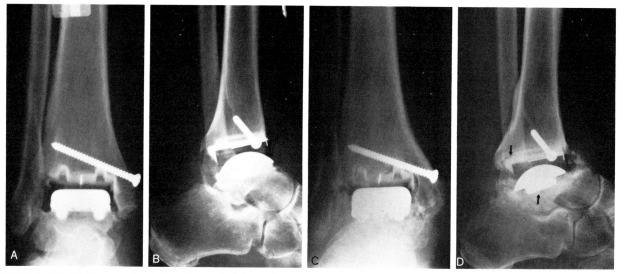

Figure 8–144. AP *(A)* and lateral *(B)* radiographs taken after insertion of an ankle prosthesis. The medial malleolar screw was used prophylactically to prevent malleolar fracture. Follow-up AP *(C)* and lateral *(D)* radiographs show loosening, which is seen primarily with the talar component. It has eroded its way into the subtalar joint *(D, lower arrow)*. Also, the tibial component shows increased tilting and a "halo" *(upper arrow)* at the bone-methacrylate interface. There was no associated infection.

nent. In fact, with rheumatoid arthritis a better result occurred when the patient was of a younger age group.

The use of an ankle arthroplasty in other diagnostic categories of ankle disease has not been successful. A previous arthrodesis, failed arthroplasty, and avascular necrosis of the talus are examples of the contraindicated diagnostic categories.

Complications

Deep infection is the major complication of all joint replacement procedures. For ankle replacement, the rate at our institution was 2.7 percent.[237] This shows itself most commonly as an increasing resorption halo of the methacrylate-bone interface (Fig. 8–143). A disproportionate number of patients with an underlying diagnosis of rheumatoid arthritis developed infection. This may represent an altered immune response, poor tissue healing, vascularity, the effect of steroids, or some other systemic abnormality associated with this disease.

Persistent pain necessitating removal of the prosthesis and an arthrodesis occurred in a further 8.0 percent of our patients. This group included cases of loosening of the prosthesis because of inadequate bone support, usually involving the talar component (Fig. 8–144). The pain that developed was not associated with infection. Impingement of the talar components beneath the fibula is also a possible cause of pain (Fig. 8–145). This occurs as a result of excessive resection of the tibia or inadequate talar resection in preparation for insertion of the prosthesis. In some instances, pain of a poorly localized nature develops, and no satisfactory explanation is present.

An arthrodesis is the salvage procedure for the total ankle arthroplasty (Fig. 8–146).[238] Union of the arthrodesis site was known to occur in 17 of 18 attempts, which demonstrates that it is a reasonable salvage possibility.

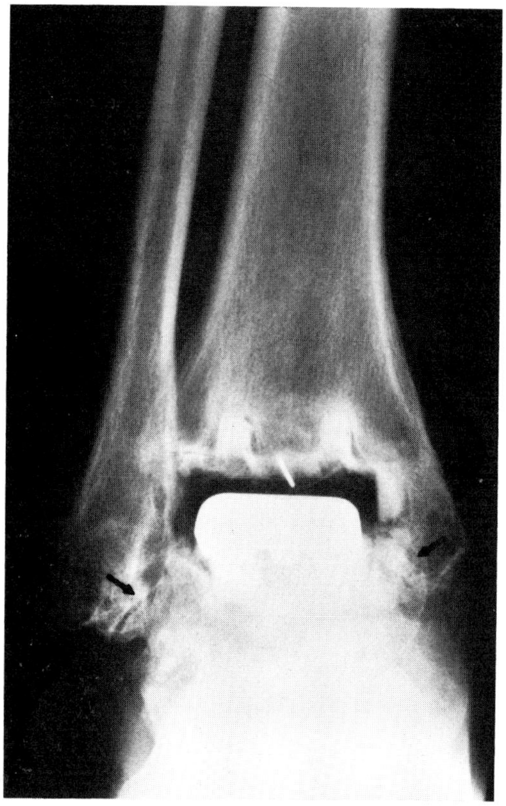

Figure 8–145. AP view shows the site of abutment of the lateral and medial malleolus on the side of the talus *(arrows)*. Resection of these areas gave relief from pain.

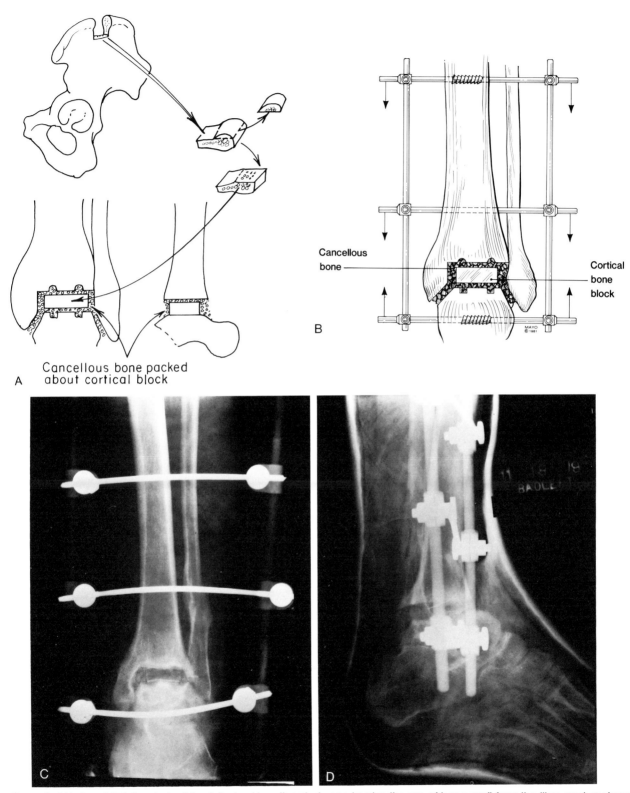

Figure 8–146. *A* and *B*, Arthrodesis of the failed ankle arthroplasty can involve the use of bone graft from the iliac crest as shown. *C* and *D*, An external fixator provides stability while the bone graft becomes incorporated. An arthrodesis of an ankle following arthroplasty has been performed.

Indications

Based on our experience with an initial 187 arthroplasties, it is evident that the number of arthroplasties inserted each year has declined after an initial "spurt" of enthusiasm. Rheumatoid arthritis remained a frequent indication for arthroplasty, while other diagnostic categories decreased with experience. The arthroplastic procedure continued to be used in the "younger" rheumatoid patient but was discontinued in the "younger" traumatic ankle patient.

Satisfactory results of arthroplasty for rheumatoid arthritis did not decline with length of evaluation but were less common with the diagnosis of traumatic primary arthritis.

The use of total ankle arthroplasty has evolved and is now indicated for painful rheumatoid arthritis in all age groups. Less often it is utilized in traumatic degenerative arthritis in older age groups.

REFERENCES

Gross Anatomy

1. Barnett, C. H., and Napier, J. R.: The axis of rotation of the ankle joint in man. J. Anat. 86:1, 1952.
2. Grant, J. C. B.: Grant's Atlas. 5th Ed. Baltimore, Williams and Wilkins, 1962.
3. Hollinshead, W. H.: Anatomy for Surgeons. Vol. 3: The Back and Limbs. 3rd Ed. New York, Harper & Row, 1982.
4. Inman, V. T.: The Joints of the Ankle. Baltimore, Williams and Wilkins, 1976.
5. Simons, G. W.: Analytical radiology of club feet. J. Bone Joint Surg. 59B:485, 1977.
6. Steel, M., Johnson, K. A., Dewitz, M. A., et al.: Radiographic measurements of the normal adult foot. Foot Ankle 1:151, 1980.

Routine Radiographic Techniques

7. Arimoto, H. K., and Forrester, D. M.: Classification of ankle fractures: An algorithm. A. J. R. 135:1057, 1980.
8. Ballinger, W. P.: Merrill's Atlas of Roentgenographic Positions and Standard Radiologic Procedures. 5th Ed. St. Louis, C. V. Mosby Co., 1982.
9. Bernau, A., and Berquist, T. H.: Orthopedic Positioning in Diagnostic Radiology. Baltimore, Urban and Schwarzenberg, 1983.
10. Brantigan, J. W., Pedegana, L. R., and Lippert, F. G.: Instability of the subtalar joint. J. Bone Joint Surg. 59A:321, 1977.
11. Brodin, B.: Roentgen examination of the subtalar joint in fractures of the calcaneus. Acta Radiol. 31:85, 1949.
12. Brostrom, L.: Sprained ankles. III. Clinical observations in recent ligament ruptures. Acta Chir. Scand. 130:560, 1965.
13. Causton, J.: Projection of sesamoid bones in the region of the first metatarsophalangeal joint. Radiology 9:39, 1943.
14. Edeiken, J., and Colter, J. M.: Ankle injury: The need for stress views. JAMA 240:1182, 1978.
15. Evans, G. A., and Frenyo, S. D.: The stress-tenogram in diagnosis of ruptures of the lateral ligament of the ankle. J. Bone Joint Surg. 61B:347, 1979.
16. Feist, J. H., and Mankin, H. J.: The tarsus: Basic relationships and motion in the adult and definition of optimal recumbent oblique projection. Radiology 79:250, 1962.
17. Foster, S. C., and Foster, R. R.: Lisfranc's tarso-metatarsal fracture-dislocation. Radiology 120:79, 1976.
18. Frolich, H., Gotzen, L., and Adam, D.: Evaluation of stress roentgenograms of the upper ankle joint. Unfallheilkunde 83:457, 1980.
19. Georgen, T. G., Danzig, L. A., Resnick, D., et al.: Roentgenographic evaluation of the tibiotalar joint. J. Bone Joint Surg. 59A:874, 1977.
20. Isherwood, I.: A radiological approach to the subtalar joint. J. Bone Joint Surg. 43B:566, 1961.
21. Johannsen, A.: Radiologic diagnosis of lateral ligament lesion of the ankle. A comparison between talar tilt and anterior drawer sign. Acta Orthop. Scand. 49:295, 1978.
22. Lewis, R. W.: Non-routine views in roentgen examination of the extremities. Surg. Gynecol. Obstet. 69:38, 1938.
23. Newmark, H. III, Olken, S. M., Melton, W. S., et al.: A new finding in the radiographic diagnosis of achilles tendon rupture. Skeletal Radiol. 8:223, 1982.
24. Norfray, J. F., Geline, R. A., Steinberg, R. I., et al. Subtleties of Lisfranc fracture-dislocations. A. J. R. 137:1151, 1981.
25. Olson, R. W.: Ankle arthrography. Radiol. Clin. North Am. 19:255, 1981.
26. Rogers, L. F., and Campbell, R. E.: Fractures and dislocations of the foot. Semin. Roentgenol. 13:157, 1978.
27. Rubin, G., and Wittin, M.: The talar tilt angle and the fibular collateral ligaments: A method for the determination of talar tilt. J. Bone Joint Surg. 42A:311, 1960.
28. Sauser, D. D., Nelson, R. C., Lavine, M. H., et al.: Acute injuries of the lateral ankle ligaments: Comparison of stress radiography and arthrography. Radiology 148:653, 1983.
29. Schultz, R. J.: The Language of Fractures. Baltimore, Williams & Wilkins, 1972.
30. Towbin, R., Dunbar, J. S., Towbin, J., et al.: Teardrop sign: Plain film recognition of ankle effusion. A. J. R. 134:985, 1980.

Arthrography and Tenography of the Foot and Ankle

31. Black, H. M., Brand, R. L., and Eicheberger, M. R.: An improved technique for evaluation of ligamentous injury in severe ankle sprains. Am. J. Sports Med. 6:276, 1978.
32. Brand, R. L., Black, H. M., and Cox, J. S.: The natural history of inadequately treated ankle sprain. Am. J. Sports Med. 5:248, 1977.
33. Brostrom, L.: Sprained ankles vs. treatment and prognosis in recent ligament ruptures. Acta Chir. Scand. 132:537, 1966.
34. Church, C. C.: Radiographic diagnosis of acute peroneal tendon dislocation. A. J. R. 129:1065, 1977.
35. Dihlman, W.: Computed tomography of the ankle joint. Chirurg 53:123, 1982.
36. Evans, G. A., and Frenyo, S. D.: The stress tenogram in the diagnosis of ruptures of the lateral ligament of the ankle. J. Bone Joint Surg. 61B:347, 1979.
37. Fitzgerald, R. H., and Coventry, M. B.: Post-traumatic peroneal tendinitis. Presented at American Society for Foot Surgery, Dallas, February 20, 1978.
38. Fitzgerald, R. H., Gross, M. R., and Johnson, K. A.: Traumatic peroneal tendinitis. A complication of calcaneal fractures. Minn. Med 58:787, 1975.
39. Freiberger, R. H., and Kaye, J. J.: Arthrography. New York, Appleton-Century-Crofts, 1979.
40. Goergen, T. G., and Resnick, D.: Arthrography of the ankle and hindfoot. In Dalinka, M. K.: Arthrography. New York, Springer-Verlag, 1980.
41. Grant, J. C. B.: Grant's Atlas of Anatomy. 5th Ed. Baltimore, Williams & Wilkins, 1962.
42. Harrington, K. D.: Degenerative arthritis of the ankle secondary to long-standing lateral ligament instability. J. Bone Joint Surg. 61A:354, 1979.
43. Kaye, J. J., and Bohne, W. H. O.: A radiographic study of the ligamentous anatomy of the ankle. Radiology 125:659, 1977.
44. Lindhilmer, E., Foge, N., and Jensen, J.: Arthrography of the ankle. Value in diagnosis of rupture of the lateral ligaments. Acta Radiol. (Diagn.) 19:585, 1978.
45. Marti, R.: Dislocation of the peroneal tendons. Am. J. Sports Med. 5:19, 1977.
46. Olson, R. W.: Ankle arthrography. Radiol. Clin. North Am. 19:255, 1981.
47. Olson, R. W.: Arthrography of the ankle: Its use in evaluation of ankle sprains. Radiology 92:1439, 1969.

48. Percy, E. C., Hill, R. O., and Callaghan, J. E.: The "sprained" ankle. J. Trauma 9:972, 1969.
49. Sauser, D. D., Nelson, R. C., Lavine, M. H., et al.: Acute injuries of the lateral ligaments of the ankle. Comparison of stress radiography and arthrography. Radiology 148:653, 1983.
50. Schweigen, J. R., Knicherbacker, W. J., and Cooperberg, P.: A study of ankle instability utilizing ankle arthrography. J. Trauma 17:878, 1977.
51. Spiegel, P. K., and Staples, O. S.: Arthrography of the ankle joint: Problems in diagnosis of acute lateral ligament injuries. Radiology 114:587, 1975.
52. Stover, C. N., and Bryan, D. R.: Traumatic dislocation of the peroneal tendons. Am. J. Surg. 103:180, 1962.
53. Termansen, N. B., Hansen, H., and Damholt, V.: Radiological and muscular status following injury to the lateral ligaments of the ankle. Acta Orthop. Scand. 50:705, 1979.
54. Vuust, M.: Arthrographic diagnosis of ruptured calcaneofibular ligament. A new projection tested on experimental injury post-mortem. Acta Radiol. (Diagn.) 21:123, 1980.

Fractures of the Ankle

55. Arimoto, H. K., and Forrester, D. M.: Classification of ankle fractures: An algorithm. A. J. R. 135:1057, 1980.
56. Ashhurst, A. P. C., and Bromer, R. S.: Classification and mechanism of fractures of the leg bones involving the ankle. Arch. Surg. 4:51, 1922.
57. Boyd, H. B.: The treatment of malunited fractures of the ankle. Instr. Course Lect. 2:60, 1944.
58. Burstein, A. H., Reilly, D. T., and Frankel, V. H.: Failure characteristics of bone and bone tissue. In Kenedi, R. M. (ed.): Perspectives in Biomedial Engineering. Baltimore, University Park Press, 1973.
59. Burwell, H. N., and Charnley, A. D.: The treatment of displaced fractures at the ankle by rigid internal fixation and early joint movement. J. Bone Joint Surg. 47B:634, 1965.
60. Cedell, C. A.: Supination-outward rotation injuries of the ankle. A clinical and roentgenological study with special reference to the operative treatment. Acta Scand. (Suppl.) 110:3, 1967.
61. Charnley, J.: The Closed Treatment of Common Fractures. Baltimore, Williams & Wilkins, 1963.
62. Fogel, G., and Morrey, B. F.: Delayed surgery for displaced ankle fractures: A long-term follow-up study. Submitted for publication, 1984.
63. Hall, H.: A simplified workable classification of ankle fractures. AAOS Symposium, 1978.
64. Joy, G., Patzakis, M. J., and Harvey, J. P. Jr.: Precise evaluation of the reduction of severe ankle fractures. J. Bone Joint Surg. 56A:979, 1974.
65. Lauge-Hansen, N.: Fractures of the ankle: Analytic survey as the basis of new experimental, roentgenographic, and clinical investigations. Arch. Surg. 56:259, 1948.
66. Lauge-Hansen, N.: Fractures of the ankle. II: Combined experimental-surgical and experimental-roentgenologic investigations. Arch. Surg. 60:947, 1950.
67. Lauge-Hansen, N.: Fractures of the ankle. III: Genetic roentgenologic diagnosis of fractures of the ankle. A. J. R. 71:456, 1954.
68. Lauge-Hansen, N.: Fractures of the ankle. IV: Clinical use of genetic roentgen diagnoses and genetic reduction. Arch. Surg. 64:488, 1952.
69. Leeds, H. C., and Ehrlich, M. G.: Instability of the distal tibiofibular syndesmosis after bimalleolar and trimalleolar ankle fractures. J. Bone Joint Surg. 66A:490, 1984.
70. Lindsjo, U.: Operative treatment of ankle fractures. Acta Orthop. Scand. (Suppl.) 189:1, 1981.
71. Mitchell, W. G., Shaftan, G. W., and Sclafani, S. J. A.: Mandatory open reduction: Its role in displaced ankle fractures. J. Trauma 19:602, 1979.
72. Pankovich, A. M.: Fractures of the fibula proximal to the distal tibiofibular syndesmosis. J. Bone Joint Surg. 60A:221, 1978.
73. Pettrone, F. H., Gail, M., Pee, D., et al.: Quantitative criteria for prediction of the results of displaced fracture of the ankle. J. Bone Joint Surg. 65A:667, 1983.

74. Ramsey, P. L., and Hamilton, W.: Changes in tibiotalar area of contact caused by lateral talar shift. J. Bone Joint Surg. 58A:356, 1976.
75. Ruedi, T.: Fractures of the lower end of the tibia into the ankle joint: Results 9 years after open reduction and internal fixation. Injury 5:130, 1973.
76. Scranton, P. E., McMaster, J. H., and Kelly, E.: Dynamic fibular function: A new concept. Clin. Orthop. 118:76, 1976.
77. Vasli, S.: Operative treatment of ankle fractures. Acta Chir. Scand. (Suppl.) 226:1, 1957.
78. Weber: As Cited by Muller, M. E., Allgower, M., and Willenegger, H.: Manual of Internal Fixation. New York, Springer-Verlag, 1970.
79. Wilson, F. C., and Skilbred, L. A.: Long-term results in the treatment of displaced bimalleolar fractures. J. Bone Joint Surg. 48A:1065, 1966.
80. Yablon, I. G., Heller, F. G., and Shause, L.: The key role of the lateral malleolus in displaced fractures of the ankle. J. Bone Joint Surg. 59A:169, 1977.

Ligamentous Injuries

81. Anderson, K. J., and LeCocq, J. F.: Operative treatment of injury to the fibular collateral ligament of the ankle. J. Bone Joint Surg. 36A:825, 1954.
82. Brantigan, J. W., Pedegana, L. R., and Lippert, F. G.: Instability of the subtalar joint. J. Bone Joint Surg. 59A:321, 1977.
83. Brostrom, L.: Sprained ankles. V. Treatment and prognosis in recent ligament ruptures. Acta Chir. Scand. 132:537, 1966.
84. Brostrom, L.: Sprained ankles. VI. Surgical treatment of "chronic" ligament ruptures. Acta Chir. Scand. 132:551, 1966.
85. Cass, J. R., Morrey, B. F., and Chao, E. Y.: Three-dimensional kinematics of ankle instability following serial sectioning of lateral collateral ligaments. Foot and Ankle 5:142, 1984.
86. Cass, J. R., Morrey, B. F., Katoh, Y., et al.: Ankle instability: Comparison of primary repair and delayed reconstruction after long-term follow-up. Submitted for publication, 1984.
87. Chrisman, O. D., and Snook, G. A.: A reconstruction of lateral ligament tears of the ankle. An experimental study and clinical evaluation of seven patients treated by a new modification of the Elmslie procedure. J. Bone Joint Surg. 51A:904, 1969.
88. Clark, B. L., Derby, A. C., and Power, G. R. I.: Injuries of the lateral ligament of the ankle: Conservative vs. operative repair. Can. J. Surg. 8:358, 1965.
89. Cox, J. S., and Hewes, T. F.: "Normal" talar tilt angle. Clin. Orthop. 140:37, 1979.
90. Dias, L. S.: The lateral ankle sprain: An experimental study. J. Trauma 19:266, 1979.
91. Drez, D. Jr., Young, J. C., Waldman, D., et al.: Nonoperative treatment of double lateral ligament tears of the ankle. Am. J. Sports Med. 10:197, 1982.
92. Elmslie, R. C.: Recurrent subluxation of the ankle-joint. Ann. Surg. 100:364, 1934.
93. Freeman, M. A. R.: Treatment of ruptures of the lateral ligament of the ankle. J. Bone Joint Surg. 47B:661, 1965.
94. Good, C. J., Jones, M. A., and Livingstone, B. N.: Reconstruction of the lateral ligament of the ankle. Injury 7:63, 1975.
95. Harrington, K. D.: Degenerative arthritis of the ankle secondary to long-standing lateral ligament instability. J. Bone Joint Surg. 61A:354, 1979.
96. Hedeboe, J., and Johannsen, A.: Recurrent instability of the ankle joint: Surgical repair by the Watson-Jones method. Acta Orthop. Scand. 50:337, 1979.
97. Jackson, D. W., Ashley, R. L., and Powell, J. W.: Ankle sprains in young athletes. Clin. Orthop. 101:201, 1974.
98. Johannson, A.: Radiological diagnosis of lateral ligament lesion of the ankle. Acta Orthop. Scand. 49:295, 1978.
99. Laughman, R. K., Carr, T. A., Chao, E. Y., et al.: Three-dimensional kinematics of the taped ankle before and after exercise. Am. J. Sports Med. 8:425, 1980.
100. Laurin, C., and Mathieu, J.: Sagittal mobility of the normal ankle. Clin. Orthop., 108:99, 1975.

101. Leonard, M. H.: Injuries of the lateral ligaments of the ankle: A clinical and experimental study. J. Bone Joint Surg. *31A*:373, 1949.
102. Meals, R. A.: Peroneal-nerve palsy complicating ankle sprain. J. Bone Joint Surg. *59A*:966, 1977.
103. O'Donoghue, D. H.: Impingement exostoses of the talus and tibia. J. Bone Joint Surg. *39A*:835, 1957.
104. O'Donoghue, D. H.: The Treatment of Injuries to Athletes. 3rd Ed. Philadelphia, W. B. Saunders, 1976.
105. Pennal, G. F.: Subluxation of the ankle. Can. Med. Assoc. J. *49*:92, 1943.
106. Prins, J. G.: Diagnosis and treatment of injury to the lateral ligament of the ankle: A comparative clinical study. Acta Chir. Scand. (Suppl.) *486*:3, 1978.
107. Rasmussen, O., and Tovborg-Jensen, I.: Anterolateral rotational instability in the ankle joint: An experimental study of anterolateral rotational instability, talar tilt, and anterior drawer sign in relation to injuries to the lateral ligaments. Acta Orthop. Scand. *52*:99, 1981.
108. Ruth, C. J.: The surgical treatment of injuries of the fibular collateral ligaments of the ankle. J. Bone Joint Surg. *43A*:229, 1961.
109. Sedlin, E. D.: A device for stress inversion or eversion roentgenograms of the ankle. J. Bone Joint Surg. *42A*:1184, 1960.
110. Staples, O. S.: Ruptures of the fibular collateral ligaments of the ankle. Result study of immediate surgical treatment. J. Bone Joint Surg. *57A*:101, 1975.
111. Staples, O. S.: Result study of ruptures of lateral ligaments of the ankle. Clin. Orthop. *85*:50, 1972.

The Talus

112. Alexander, A. H., and Lichtman, D. M.: Surgical treatment of transchondral talar-dome fractures (osteochondritis dissecans). Long-term follow-up. J. Bone Joint Surg. *62A*:646, 1980.
113. Anderson, H. G.: Medical and Surgical Aspects of Aviation. London, Oxford Medical Publications, 1919.
114. Berndt, A., and Harty, M.: Transchondral fractures (osteochondritis dissecans) of the talus. J. Bone Joint Surg. *41A*:988, 1959.
115. Campbell, C., and Ranawat, C.: Osteochondritis dissecans: The question of etiology. J. Trauma *6*:201, 1966.
116. Canale, S. T., and Kelly, F. B. Jr.: Fractures of the neck of the talus. J. Bone Joint Surg. *60A*:143, 1978.
117. Canale, S. T., and Belding, R. H.: Osteochondral lesions of the talus. J. Bone Joint Surg. *62A*:97, 1980.
118. Christensen, S. B., Lorentzen, J. E., Krogsoe, O., et al.: Subtalar dislocation. Acta Orthop. Scand. *48*:707, 1977.
119. Collins, M. C., and Collins, J. L.: Complete external dislocation of the astragalus bone. Calif. and West. Med. *51*:39, 1939.
120. Coltart, W. D.: Aviator's astragalus. J. Bone Joint Surg. *34B*:545, 1952.
121. Convery, R., Akeson, W. H., and Keown, G. H.: The repair of large osteochondral defects. Clin. Orthop. *82*:253, 1972.
122. Davidson, A. M., Steele, H. D., MacKenzie, D. A., et al.: A review of 21 cases of transchondral fracture of the talus. J. Trauma *7*:378, 1967.
123. Detenbeck, L. C., and Kelly, P. J.: Total dislocation of the talus. J. Bone Joint Surg. *52A*:283, 1969.
124. Haliburton, R. A., Sullivan, C. R., Kelly, P. J., et al.: The extraosseous and intraosseous blood supply to the talus. J. Bone Joint Surg. *40A*:1115, 1958.
125. Hawkins, L. G.: Fractures of the neck of the talus. J. Bone Joint Surg. *52A*:991, 1970.
126. Heppenstall, R. B., Farahvar, H., Balderston, R., et al.: Evaluation and management of subtalar dislocations. J. Trauma *20*:494, 1980.
127. Kappis, M.: Weitere Beiträge zur traumatisch-mechanischen Entstehung der "spontanen" Knorpelablosungen (sogen. osteochondritis dissecans). Dtsch. Z. Chir. *171*:13, 1922.
128. König, F.: Über freie Körper in den Gelenken. Dtsch. Z. Chir. *27*:90, 1888.

129. Lorentzen, J. E., Christensen, S. B., Krogsoe, O., et al.: Fractures of the neck of the talus. Acta Orthop. Scand. *48*:115, 1977.
130. McCullough, C. J., and Venugopal, V.: Osteochondritis dissecans of the talus: The natural history. Clin. Orthop. *144*:264, 1979.
131. Monson, S. T., and Ryan, J. R.: Subtalar dislocation. J. Bone Joint Surg. *63A*:1156, 1981.
132. Mukherjee, S. K., and Young, A. B.: Dome fracture of the talus. A report of 10 cases. J. Bone Joint Surg. *55B*:319, 1973.
133. Mulfinger, G. L., and Trueta, J.: The blood supply of the talus. J. Bone Joint Surg. *52B*:160, 1970.
134. Naumetz, V. A., and Schweigel, J. F.: Osteocartilaginous lesions of the talar dome. J. Trauma *20*:924, 1981.
135. Penny, N., and Davis, L. A.: Fractures and fracture-dislocations of the neck of the talus. J. Trauma *20*:1029, 1980.
136. Peterson, L., Goldie, R. F., and Irstam, L.: Fractures of the neck of the talus. Acta Orthop. Scand. *48*:696, 1977.
137. Pettine, K., and Morrey, B. F.: Long-term result of transchondral fracture of the talus. In Preparation, J. Bone Joint Surg.
138. Rendu, A.: Fracture intra-articulaire parcellaire de la poulie astraglienne. Lyon Med. *150*:220, 1932.
139. Resnick, D.: Radiology of the talocalcaneal articulations. Radiology *111*:581, 1974.
140. Roden, S., et al.: Osteochondritis dissecans and similar lesions of the talus. Acta Orthop. Scand. *23*:51, 1953.
141. Schorling, M.: Osteochondritis dissecans of the talus. Acta Orthop Scand *49*:89, 1979.
142. Sneppen, O., Christensen, S. B., Krogsoe, O., et al. Fractures of the body of the talus. Acta Orthop. Scand. *48*:317, 1977.
143. Yuan, H. A., Cady, R. B., and DeRosa, C.: Osteochondritis dissecans of the talus associated with subchondral cysts. J. Bone Joint Surg. *61A*:1249, 1979.
144. Yvars, M.: Osteochondral fractures of the dome of the talus. Clin. Orthop. *114*:185, 1976.

Navicular Fractures

145. Eichenholtz, S. N., and Levine, D. B.: Fractures of the tarsonavicular bone. Clin. Orthop. *34*:142, 1964.
146. Goergen, T. G., Watson, E. A., Rossman, D. J., et al.: Tarsonavicular stress fractures in runners. A. J. R. *136*:201, 1981.
147. Main, B. J., and Jowett, R. L.: Injuries of the midtarsal joint. J. Bone Joint Surg. *57B*:89, 1975.
148. Torg, J. S., Pavlov, H., Cooley, L. H., et al.: Stress fractures of the tarsonavicular. J. Bone Joint Surg. *64A*:700, 1982.

The Calcaneus

149. Anthonsen, W.: An oblique projection for roentgen examination of the talo-calcaneal joint of the calcaneus. Acta Radiol. *24*:306, 1943.
150. Artken, A. P.: Fractures of the os calcis—treatment by closed reduction. Clin. Orthop. *30*:67, 1963.
151. Bachman, S., and Johnson, S. R.: Torsion of the foot causing fracture of the anterior calcaneal process. Acta Chir. Scand. *105*:460, 1953.
152. Bankart, A. S.: Fracture of the os calcis. Lancet *2*:175, 1942.
153. Barnard, L.: Non-operative treatment of fractures of the calcaneus. J. Bone Joint Surg. *45A*:865, 1963.
154. Barnard, L., and Odegard, J. K.: Conservative approach in the treatment of fractures of the calcaneus. J. Bone Joint Surg. *33A*:1231, 1955.
155. Böhler, L.: Diagnosis, pathology, and treatment of fractures of the os calcis. J. Bone Joint Surg. *13*:75, 1931.
156. Bradford, C. H., and Larsen, J.: Sprain-fractures of the anterior lip of the os calcis. N. Engl. J. Med. *244*:970, 1951.
157. Cave, E.: Fracture of the os calcis—the problem in general. Clin. Orthop. *30*:64, 1963.
158. Conn, H. R.: The treatment of fractures of the os calcis. J. Bone Joint Surg. *33*:392, 1935.
159. Conwell, H. E., and Reynolds, F. C.: Key and Conwell's

Management of Fractures, Dislocations, and Sprains. 7th Ed. St. Louis, C. V. Mosby Co., 1961.

160. Cotton, F. G., and Wilson, L. T.: Fractures of the os calcis. Boston Med. Surg. J. *159*:559, 1908.
161. Degan, T. J., Morrey, B. F., and Braun, D. P.: Surgical excision for anterior-posterior fractures of the calcaneus. J. Bone Joint Surg. *64A*:519, 1982.
162. Dick, I. L.: Primary fusion of the posterior subtalar joint in the treatment of fractures of the calcaneum. J. Bone Joint Surg. *35B*:375, 1953.
163. DuVries, H. L.: Surgery of the Foot. 4th Ed. St. Louis, C. V. Mosby Co., 1978.
164. Essex-Lopresti, P.: The mechanism, reduction technique, and results in fractures of the os calcis. Br. J. Surg. *39*:395, 1952.
165. Garcia, P. G., Garcia-Rubio, M., Lopez, V. C., et al.: Tarsal tunnel syndrome: A report of fifty-six cases. J. Bone Joint Surg. *61B*:123, 1979.
166. Gellman, M.: Fracture of the anterior process of the calcaneus. J. Bone Joint Surg. *13*:877, 1931.
167. Hall, M. C., and Pennal, G. F.: Primary subtalar arthrodesis in the treatment of severe fractures of the calcaneum. J. Bone Joint Surg. *42B*:336, 1960.
168. Harris, R. I.: Fractures of the os calcis: Treatment by early subtalar arthrodesis. Clin. Orthop. *30*:100, 1963.
169. Harty, M.: Anatomic considerations in injuries to the calcaneus. Orthop. Clin. North Am. *4*:180, 1973.
170. Hermann, O. J.: Conservative therapy for the fracture of the os calcis. J. Bone Joint Surg. *19*:709, 1937.
171. Hunt, D. D.: Compression fracture of the anterior articular surface of the calcaneus. J. Bone Joint Surg. *56B*:274, 1974.
172. Isbister, J. F.: Calcaneo-fibular abutment following crush fracture of the calcaneus. J. Bone Joint Surg. *56B*:274, 1974.
173. Jahss, M. H., and Kay, B. S.: An anatomic study of the anterior superior process of the os calcis and its clinical application. Foot Ankle *3*:268, 1983.
174. Johansson, J. E., Harrison, J., and Greenwood, F. A. H.: Subtalar arthrodesis for adult trauma arthritis. Foot Ankle *2*:294, 1982.
175. Korn, R.: Der Bruch durch das hintere obere Drittel des Fersenbeines. Arch. Orthop. Unfallchir. *47*:789, 1942.
176. Lance, E. M., Carey, E. J., and Wade, P. A.: Fractures of the os calcis—treatment by early mobilization. Clin. Orthop. *30*:76, 1963.
177. Lindsay, W. R. N., and Dewar, F. P.: Fractures of the os calcis. Am. J. Surg. *95*:555, 1958.
178. Maxfield, J. E.: Os calcis fractures. Treatment by open reduction. Clin. Orthop. *30*:91, 1963.
179. McLaughlin, H. L.: Treatment of late complications after os calcis fractures. Clin. Orthop. *30*:111, 1963.
180. McReynolds, I. S.: Open reduction and internal fixation of calcaneal fractures. J. Bone Joint Surg. *54B*:176, 1972.
181. Miller, W. E.: Pain and impairment considerations following treatment of disruptive os calcis fractures. Clin. Orthop. *177*:82, 1983.
182. Noble, J., and McQuillan, W. M.: Early posterior subtalar fusion in the treatment of fractures of the os calcis. J. Bone Joint Surg. *61B*:90, 1979.
183. O'Connell, F., Mital, M. A., and Rowe, C. R.: Evaluation of modern management of fractures of the os calcis. Clin. Orthop. *83*:214, 1972.
184. Palmer, I.: The mechanism and treatment of fractures of the calcaneus. Open reduction with the use of cancellous grafts. J. Bone Joint Surg. *30A*:2, 1948.
185. Pennal, G. F., and Yadow, M. P.: Operative treatment of comminuted fractures of the os calcis. Orthop. Clin. North Am. *4*:197, 1973.
186. Pridie, K. H.: A new method of treatment for severe fractures of the os calcis. A preliminary report. Surg. Gynecol. Obstet. *82*:671, 1946.
187. Resnick, D.: Radiology of the talocalcaneal articulations. Radiology *111*:581, 1974.
188. Rockwood, C. A., and Green, D. P.: Fractures. Vol. 2. Philadelphia, J. B. Lippincott, 1975.
189. Rowe, C. R., Sakellarides, H. T., Freeman, P. A., et al.: Fractures of the os calcis. A long-term follow-up study of 146 patients. JAMA *184*:920, 1963.
190. Schmidt, T. L., and Weiner, D. S.: Calcaneal fractures in children. An evaluation of the nature of the injury in 56 children. Clin. Orthop. *171*:150, 1982.
191. Shoefield, R. O.: Fractures of the os calcis. J. Bone Joint Surg. *18*:560, 1936.
192. Soeur, R., and Remy, R.: Fracture of the calcaneus with displacement of the thalamic portion. J. Bone Joint Surg. *57B*:413, 1975.
193. Stephenson, J. R.: Displaced fractures of the os calcis involving the subtalar joint: The key role of the superomedial fragment. Foot Ankle *4*:91, 1983.
194. Thompson, K. R., and Friesen, C. M.: Treatment of comminuted fractures of the calcaneus by primary triple arthrodesis. J. Bone Joint Surg. *41A*:1423, 1959.
195. Urowitz, E., and Hall, H.: The medial approach to fracture of the os calcis. J. Bone Joint Surg. *62B*:131, 1980.
196. Warrick, C. K., and Bremner, A. E.: Fractures of the calcaneum: With an atlas illustrating the various types of fracture. J. Bone Joint Surg. *35B*:33, 1953.
197. Watson-Jones, R.: Fractures and Joint Injuries. Vol. 2. 4th Ed. Baltimore, Williams & Wilkins Co., 1955.
198. Wilson, P. D.: Treatment of fractures of the os calcis by arthrodesis of the subastragalar joint. JAMA *89*:1676, 1927.

Tarsometatarsal (Lisfranc) Fractures

199. Brown, D. C., and McFarland, G. B.: Dislocation of the medial cuneiform bone in tarsometatarsal fracture-dislocation. J. Bone Joint Surg. *57A*:858, 1975.
200. Cassebaum, W. H.: Lisfranc fracture-dislocations. Clin. Orthop. *4*:116, 1963.
201. DeBendette, M. J., Evanski, P. M., and Waugh, T. R.: The unreducible Lisfranc fracture. Clin. Orthop. *136*:238, 1978.
202. Denton, J. R.: A complex Lisfranc fracture-dislocation. J. Trauma *20*:526, 1980.
203. Engber, W. D., and Roberts, J. M.: Unreducible tarsometatarsal fracture-dislocation. Clin. Orthop. *168*:102, 1982.
204. Geckeler, E. D.: Dislocations and fracture-dislocations of the foot. Surgery *25*:730, 1949.
205. Gissane, W.: A dangerous type of fracture of the foot. J. Bone Joint Surg. *33B*:535, 1951.
206. Granberry, W. M., and Lipscomb, P. R.: Dislocation of the tarsometatarsal joints. Surg. Gynecol. Obstet. *114*:467, 1962.
207. Hardcastle, P. H., Reachauer, R., Kutscha-Lissberg, E., et al.: Injuries to the tarsometatarsal joint. J. Bone Joint Surg. *64B*:349, 1982.
208. Holstein, A., and Joldersma, R. D.: Dislocation of first cuneiform in tarsometatarsal fracture-dislocations. J. Bone Joint Surg. *32A*:419, 1950.
209. Jeffreys, T. E.: Lisfranc's fracture-dislocation. J. Bone Joint Surg. *45B*:546, 1963.
210. Parlasca, R.: Personal Communication.
211. del Sel, J. M.: The surgical treatment of tarsometatarsal fracture-dislocations. J. Bone Joint Surg. *37B*:203, 1955.
212. Wiley, J. J.: The mechanism of tarsometatarsal joint injuries. J. Bone Joint Surg. *53B*:474, 1971.
213. Wilson, D. W.: Injuries of the tarsometatarsal joints. J. Bone Joint Surg. *54B*:677, 1972.

Cuneiform and Cuboid Fractures

214. Dewar, F. P., and Evans, D. C.: Occult fracture-subluxation of the midtarsal joint. J. Bone Joint Surg. *50B*:386, 1968.
215. Hermel, M. B., and Gershan-Cohen, J.: The nutcracker fracture of the cuboid by indirect violence. Radiology *60*:850, 1953.

Metatarsal Fractures

216. Blodgett, W. H.: Disorders of the Foot and Ankle. Philadelphia, W. B. Saunders, 1982.
217. Dameron, T. B.: Fractures and anatomical variations of the proximal portion of the fifth metatarsal. J. Bone Joint Surg. *57A*:788, 1975.
218. DeLee, J. C., Evans, J. P., and Julian, J.: Stress fracture of the fifth metatarsal. Am. J. Sports Med. *11*:349, 1983.

219. Drez, D., Young, J. G., Johnston, R. D., et al.: Metatarsal stress fractures. Am. J. Sports Med. *8*:123, 1980.
220. Garcia, A., and Parks, J. C.: Foot Disorders. 2nd Ed. Philadelphia, Lea and Febiger, 1973.
221. Harrison, M.: Fracture of the metatarsal head. Can. J. Surg. *11*:511, 1968.
222. Jones, R.: Fracture of the fifth metatarsal bone. Liverpool Med. Chir. J. *22*:103, 1902.
223. Jones, R.: Manipulation as a therapeutic measure. Proc. Roy. Soc. Med. *25*:1405, 1931–1932.
224. Kavanaugh, J. H., Brower, T. D., and Mann, R. V.: The Jones fracture revisited. J. Bone Joint Surg. *60A*:776, 1978.
225. Levy, J.: Stress fractures of the first metatarsal. A. J. R. *130*:679, 1978.
226. Peltiey, L. F.: Eponymic fractures: Robert Jones and Jones's fracture. Surgery *71*:522, 1972.
227. Prather, J. L., Nusynowitz, M. L., Snowdy, H. A., et al.: Scintigraphic findings in stress fractures. J. Bone Joint Surg. *59A*:869, 1977.
228. Smith, A. D., Carter, J. R., and Marcus, R. E.: The os vesalianum: An unusual cause of lateral foot pain. Orthopedics *7*:86, 1984.
229. Stormont, D. M.: Stabilizers of the Ankle. M. S. Thesis, Mayo Clinic, University of Minnesota, 1984.

Phalangeal Fractures

230. Anderson, L. D.: Injuries of the forefoot. Clin. Orthop. *122*:18, 1977.

231. Cobey, J. C.: Treatment of undisplaced toe fractures with a metatarsal bar mode from tongue blades. Clin. Orthop. *103*:56, 1974.
232. Connolly, J. F. (ed.): DePalma's Management of Fractures and Dislocations. 3rd Ed. Philadelphia, W. B. Saunders, 1981.
233. Giannestras, N. J., and Sammarco, G. J.: Fractures. Philadelphia, J. B. Lippincott Co., 1975.

Sesamoid Fractures

234. Jahss, M. A.: The sesamoids of the hallux. Clin. Orthop. *157*:88, 1981.

Total Ankle Arthroplasty

235. Evanski, P. M., and Waugh, T. R.: Management of arthritis of the ankle. Clin. Orthop. *122*:110, 1977.
236. Johnson, K. A.: Umpublished Data.
237. Newton, S. E.: Total ankle arthroplasty. J. Bone Joint Surg. *64A*:104, 1982.
238. Pappas, M., Buechel, F., and De Palma, A. F.: Cylindrical total ankle joint replacement. Clin. Orthop. *118*:82, 1976.
239. Scholz, K. C.: Total ankle replacement arthroplasty. *In* Bateman, J. E. (ed.): Foot Science. Philadelphia, W. B. Saunders Co., 1976.
240. Stauffer, R. N.: Salvage of painful total ankle arthroplasty. Clin. Orthop. *170*:184, 1982.
241. Stauffer, R. N., and Segal, N. M.: Total arthroplasty: Four years' experience. Clin. Orthop *160*:217, 1981.

9

THE SHOULDER

ROBERT H. COFIELD • THOMAS H. BERQUIST

ANATOMY

The shoulder is anatomically complex, and a review of certain anatomic features is helpful in understanding how to perform imaging procedures and interpret radiographic findings properly.

Osteology

Clavicle

The clavicle is a slightly curved (S-shaped) bone that lies ventral to the shoulder girdle (Fig. 9–1). It is one of the first bones to ossify.[3] The medial epiphysis does not unite until the end of the second decade. This should not be mistaken for a fracture. There are no secondary ossification centers distally. The clavicle articulates with the acromion distally and rarely with the coracoid.[2, 8] Medially the pestle-shaped portion of the clavicle articulates with the sternum and first rib. The midportion of the clavicle is tubular, and the distal portion is relatively flat.[6, 7] The dorsal surface of the clavicle is roughened proximally and distally. The trapezius and deltoid muscles insert distally, and the sternocleidomastoid

Figure 9–1. Radiographs of the clavicle with location of major muscle attachments. *A,* Superior surface. *B,* Inferior surface.

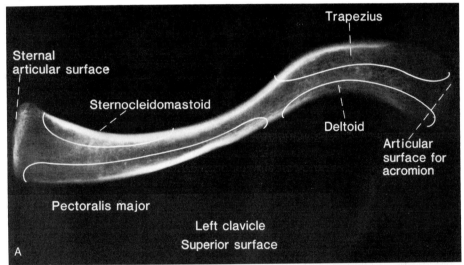

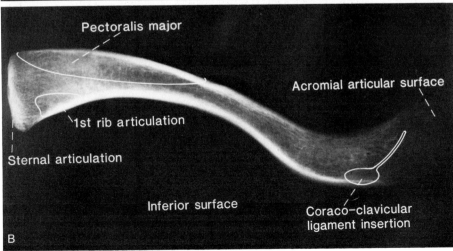

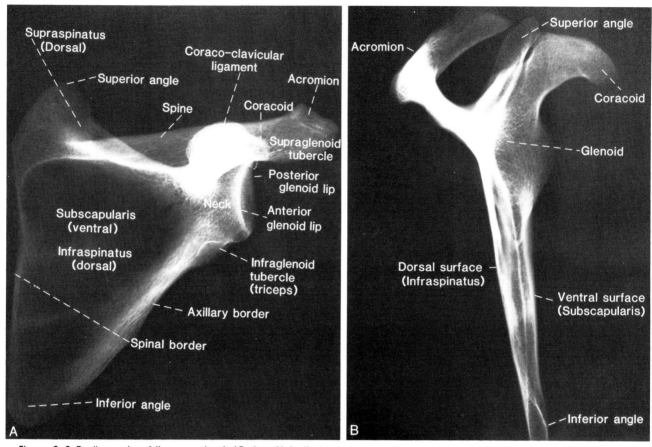

Figure 9-2. Radiographs of the scapula. A, AP view. Note that the anterior glenoid lip is medial to the posterior glenoid lip. B, Lateral scapula.

and pectoralis major insert proximally (Fig. 9-1). Inferiorly the conoid and trapezoid bands of the coracoclavicular ligament attach as the clavicle bows dorsally. They insert in the conoid tubercle and trapezoid ridge, respectively.

Scapula

The scapula is dorsal to the chest wall. The wing (body) of the scapula is a large, flat triangular bone that is almost entirely covered with muscles dorsally

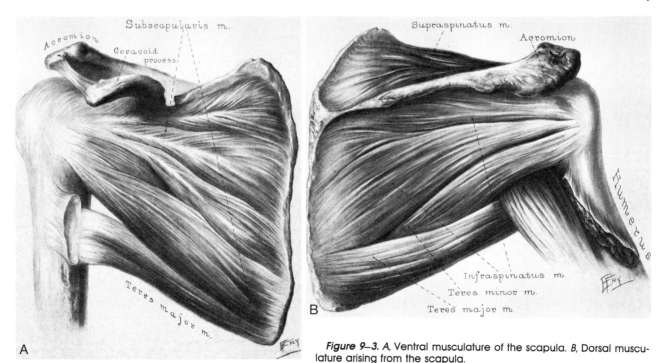

Figure 9-3. A, Ventral musculature of the scapula. B, Dorsal musculature arising from the scapula.

and ventrally (Fig. 9–2). The subscapularis covers the ventral surface. Dorsally the supraspinatus takes its origin above the spine of the scapula and the infraspinatus below (Fig. 9–3). The teres major and minor arise from the inferior scapula. The triceps originates from a tubercle just below the glenoid (Fig. 9–2). This tubercle is usually easily visible radiographically. The supraglenoid tubercle is located just superior to the glenoid and serves as the origin of the long head of the biceps brachii. When seen *en face*, the glenoid lies at the junction of the scapular body, the scapular spine posteriorly, and coracoid anteriorly (Fig. 9–2). This forms a "Y" with the glenoid at the junction of the limbs.

With the patient positioned for the AP view the scapula appears oblique. Therefore, the anterior lip of the glenoid is projected medially to the posterior lip (Fig. 9–2). Approximately 40° of posterior rotation is required to obtain a true tangential view of the glenoid (Fig. 9–2). The broad dorsal convex surface of the coracoid serves as the origin of the coracoclavicular ligaments.

There are several secondary ossification centers that should not be confused with fractures. These include the superior glenoid, inferior glenoid, acromial, coracoid, and infrascapular. These ossification centers usually fuse in the second decade.[10] The glenoid ossification centers may be a source of confusion in patients with shoulder instability.

Proximal Humerus

The humeral head is nearly hemispheric and has four times the surface area of the glenoid.[14] The anatomic neck is located at the margin of the articular surface and lies in an oblique plane running superiorly from medial to lateral zones (Fig. 9–4). The surgical neck lies more inferiorly below the tuberosities.

The greater tuberosity is located laterally below the anatomic neck. This structure is seen in profile with the shoulder externally rotated (Fig. 9–4A). There are three facets on the greater tuberosity for insertion of three of the muscles of the rotator cuff.[9]

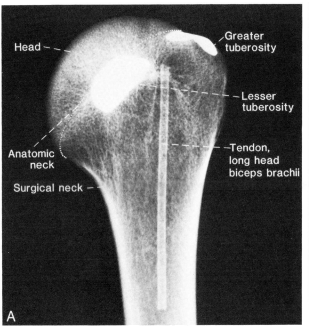

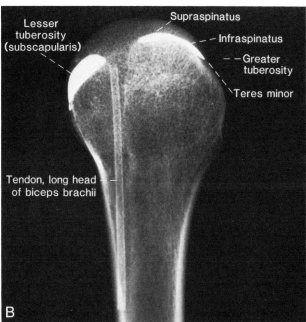

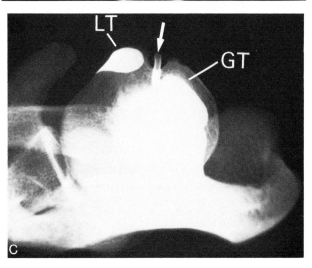

Figure 9–4. Radiographs of the proximal humerus. (Metal markers on the tuberosities.) A, AP view, external rotation. B, AP view, internal rotation. C, Tangential view of bicipital groove (arrow).

The insertion for the supraspinatus is most anterior, lying near the intertubercular sulcus. The infraspinatus and teres minor insert just posteriorly to the supraspinatus (Fig. 9–4). The intertubercular sulcus lies between the greater and lesser tuberosities. Radiographically this groove normally measures about 11 mm in width and 4.6 mm in depth.[3] The tendon of the long head of the biceps brachii runs through this groove.[3, 8, 12] The lesser tuberosity lies medially to the intertubercular sulcus and serves as the insertion for the subscapularis (Fig. 9–4C).

The osteology for the remainder of the humerus is discussed in Chapter 10, The Humeral Shaft.

Articular Anatomy

Glenohumeral Joint

The glenohumeral joint is a ball and socket (spheroidea) joint.[4, 6, 7] The normally shallow glenoid cavity is much smaller than the humeral head.[7, 13, 14] The cavity is deepened by a fibrocartilaginous labrum which extends around the entire peripheral margin of the glenoid cavity (Fig. 9–5).

The synovial lined capsule attaches proximally to the glenoid labrum and extends peripherally to the anatomic neck of the humerus.[4, 7, 8] The total capsular volume is nearly twice that of the humeral head.[13] The capsule is stronger anteriorly and inferiorly and is reinforced by surrounding muscles, tendons, and ligaments. Superiorly reinforcement is achieved by the rotator cuff muscles, specifically by the supraspinatus (Fig. 9–6). Inferiorly there is support of the glenoid attachment by the triceps

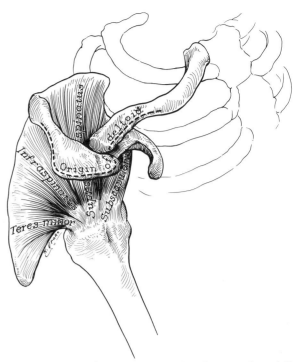

Figure 9–6. Illustration demonstrating the muscles of the rotator cuff. (Courtesy of Mark B. Coventry, Mayo Clinic, Rochester, Minnesota.)

brachii, which originates from the infraglenoid tubercle. Anterior reinforcement is provided by the subscapularis tendon. Posteriorly the teres minor and infraspinatus are adjacent to the capsule[7, 8] (Fig. 9–5). Superiorly the tendon of the long head of the biceps brachii arises from the supraglenoid tubercle

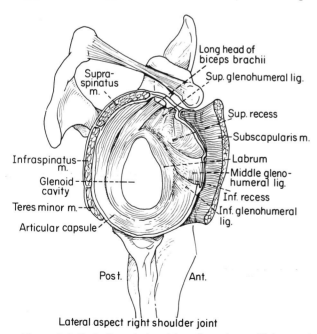

Figure 9–5. Illustration of glenoid cavity en face with humeral head removed. (From Morrey, B. F., and Chao, E. Y.: Recurrent anterior dislocation of the shoulder. *In* Black, J., and Dumpleton, J. H. (eds.): Clinical Biomechanics: A Case History Approach. New York, Churchill Livingstone, 1981.)

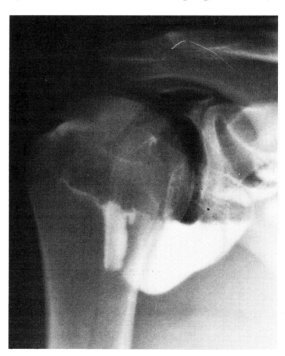

Figure 9–7. AP view of double-contrast arthrogram demonstrating the course of the tendon of the long head of the biceps brachii and its sheath.

and labrum.[14] The tendon crosses the superior joint and exits through the intertubercular sulcus.[3] (Fig. 9–7). This sulcus is formed by the greater and lesser tuberosities. The roof of the groove is covered by the transverse humeral ligament. The biceps tendon is covered by a synovial sheath that extends several cm beyond the normal capsule to about the level of the surgical neck.[6–8, 14]

Additional support is provided by four ligament complexes: (1) the coracohumeral ligament, which arises from the coracoid to insert in the greater and lesser tuberosities; (2) the superior glenohumeral ligament, which originates just below the coracohumeral ligament and blends with the capsule as it inserts in the lesser tuberosity; (3) the middle glenohumeral ligament, which arises from the anterior glenoid and crosses inferiorly to the superior glenohumeral ligament to insert in the lower portion of the lesser tuberosity; and (4) the inferior glenohumeral ligament, which arises from the anterior glenoid and inserts in the region of the surgical neck below the middle glenohumeral ligament.[2, 7, 8, 14, 17] Stability supplied by the capsule and ligaments is augmented considerably by the rotator cuff.[14]

There may be numerous bursae about the shoulder, but most do not communicate with the joint, and they are not always constant (Table 9–1). The most important are the subscapularis, subdeltoid, subcoracoid, and subacromial. The subscapularis bursa is situated anteriorly beneath the coracoid process and lies dorsal to the subscapularis tendon. The infraspinatus bursa communicates with the posterior joint and lies between the capsule and the infraspinatus tendon. This is not always present.[7, 8] Communication with the tendon sheath of the long head of the biceps is almost always present in the normal shoulder.[7, 8, 14] A large bursa lies between the rotator cuff and acromion. It is composed of subdeltoid, subacromial and subcoracoid portions.[6] This does not communicate with the capsule if the rotator cuff is intact.[7, 8, 13, 15, 16]

Acromioclavicular Joint

The acromioclavicular joint is a synovial joint that joins the distal clavicle and medial portion of the acromion. An intra-articular disk is occasionally present.[7] Both gliding and rotary motion (scapula) are possible.[7, 11, 13] The capsule of the joint is supported by the superior and inferior acromioclavicular ligaments; however, major support is derived from the coracoclavicular ligament (trapezoid and coracoid ligaments). Rarely, a joint is present between the coracoid and clavicle.[2, 8]

Sternoclavicular Joint

The medial articular portion of the clavicle forms a gliding synovial joint with the manubrium and cartilaginous portion of the first rib. The clavicular surface is larger than the articular surface of either the manubrium or the first rib.[7, 14] Ligamentous support includes the interclavicular ligament superiorly, the costoclavicular ligament inferiorly, and the anterior and posterior sternoclavicular ligaments. An articular disk extends from the upper clavicle to the cartilage of the first rib, dividing the joint into medial and lateral compartments.

Neurovascular Anatomy

The relationships of the neurovascular structures to the clavicle and sternoclavicular joint deserve mention.

The subclavian artery and vein pass posteriorly to the sternoclavicular joint. The second portion of the artery passes posteriorly to the scalenus anterior, which inserts into the upper portion of the first rib (Fig. 9–8). The brachial plexus (C5–T1 ventral roots) descends to join the vessels at this point. The axillary artery, a continuation of the subclavian artery, begins at the lateral margin of the first rib and extends to the distal border of the teres major. The neurovascular structures pass between the midclavicle and first rib through the axilla and along the medial aspect of the upper humerus. The major blood supply to the humerus and surrounding musculature is derived from branches of the axillary artery. These include the anterior and posterior humeral circumflex, clavicular, acromial, and deltoid branches from the thoracoacromial axis.[7]

Fracture-dislocations of the sternoclavicular joint and glenohumeral joint may result in neurovascular

TABLE 9–1. Shoulder Bursae

Bursa	Location	Normal Joint Communication
Subscapular	Between subscapulosus tendon and capsule	Yes
Infraspinatus	Between capsule and infraspinatus tendon	Inconstant
Subdeltoid	Between deltoid and rotator cuff	No
Subacromial	Between acromion and rotator cuff (usually contiguous with subdeltoid)	No
Subcoracoid	Between coracoid and subscapularis (may be contiguous with subacromial)	No
Coracobrachialis	Between coracobrachialis and subscapularis	No
Latissimus dorsi	Between latissimus and teres major	No
Teres major	Between teres and humeral insertion	No
Pectoralis major	Between pectoralis and humeral insertion	No

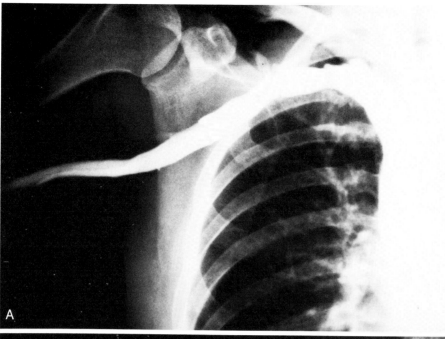

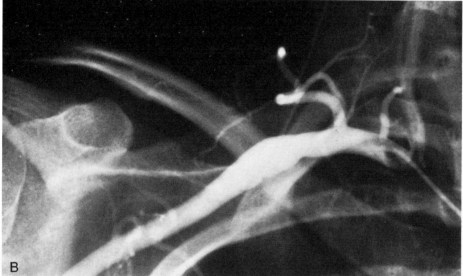

Figure 9–8. A, Venogram with humerus abducted. Note relationship of the vessels to the sternoclavicular joint, first rib and clavicle, and glenohumeral joint. *B,* Arteriogram demonstrating subclavian branches and relationship to clavicle and first rib.

complications. These will be discussed in more detail later in this chapter.

Biomechanics

The glenohumeral configuration and supporting structures of the shoulder allow uniquely complex motion.[2, 9, 11, 15, 16] The muscles involved in glenohumeral motion are the rotator cuff, deltoid, pectoralis major, latissimus dorsi, and teres major.[16] Motion occurs primarily at the glenohumeral joint. However, motion also occurs in the acromioclavicular and sternoclavicular joints.[13] Glenohumeral motion is responsible for 120° of the 180° abduction arc. More than 120° of abduction requires scapular and clavicular motion. If the humerus cannot externally rotate, motion is restricted owing to impingement of the greater tuberosity on the acromion.

With full abduction (180°) the scapula is capable of rotating 60°. The major muscles producing full abduction are the deltoid, supraspinatus, trapezius, and serratus anterior.[1, 7, 11]

The biomechanics of abduction have been stressed owing to common clinical problems involving the rotator cuff (tears and impingement).[2, 11, 12] This movement can be studied fluoroscopically as a part of shoulder arthrography. The shoulder is also capable of flexion, extension, adduction, and rotation.[7] The main flexors are the pectoralis major and anterior deltoid fibers, with some contribution from the biceps brachii.[1, 7] Extension is accomplished with fibers from the posterior deltoid, teres major, and latissimus dorsi. Adduction is achieved by contraction of the subscapularis, infraspinatus, teres minor, pectoralis major, latissimus dorsi, and teres major.[7] External rotation is powered by the

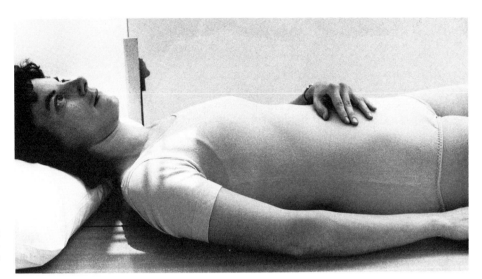

Figure 9-9. Patient positioned for standard AP views of the shoulder, internal rotation view. The hand is palm down.

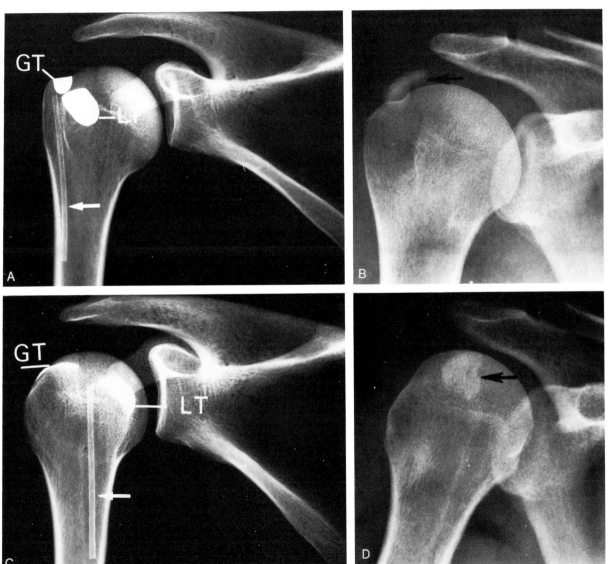

Figure 9-10. A, Dried skeletal specimen demonstrating the position of the tuberosities and bicipital groove with external rotation. (GT, greater tuberosity; LT, lesser tuberosity; arrow indicates position of tendon of long head of the biceps.) *B,* External rotation view in a patient with calcific tendinitis *(arrow).* Note the overlap of the humeral head and glenoid. *C,* Dried skeletal specimen. The lesser tuberosity is rotated medially, demonstrating the relationship of the tendon *(arrow)* to the tuberosities. *D,* Internal rotation view in the same patient as shown in *B.* The calcific deposit is indicated by the arrow.

infraspinatus and teres minor; and internal rotation is powered by the pectoralis major, latissimus dorsi, teres major, and subscapularis.

ROUTINE RADIOGRAPHY

Radiographic analysis of the shoulder has proved to be more difficult and less fruitful than x-rays of other anatomic regions of the musculoskeletal system. Golding has most succinctly stated this problem and has offered one—and a major— solution: "The commissioner who sends a patient to the x-ray department for an examination of his shoulder is frequently disappointed in the disparity between the lack of radiologic evidence and the marked clinical signs which are present. . . . A fundamental principle established in the early days of radiography was to obtain an anterior-posterior and a lateral film of every bone or joint. It is not a fact, therefore,

that an axial film of the shoulder joint is a routine procedure in every x-ray department."[34] This failure to include a "lateral" view of the shoulder has been one major problem. Another has been a lack of analysis of the various views and lack of uniformity in the radiographic techniques that apply to the investigation of an individual with shoulder injury or disease.

This section presents the plain film alternatives for evaluation of shoulder problems and suggests groupings of these films. Special techniques are then discussed as an augmentation of the basic x-ray examination. These include tomography, nuclear scanning, the contrast studies of bursography and arthrography, computed tomography, and ultrasound. The evaluation of trauma and reconstructive conditions will also be presented. Magnetic resonance imaging, as it applies to shoulder evaluation, has not achieved the level of clarity that would warrant its inclusion here. As it supplements

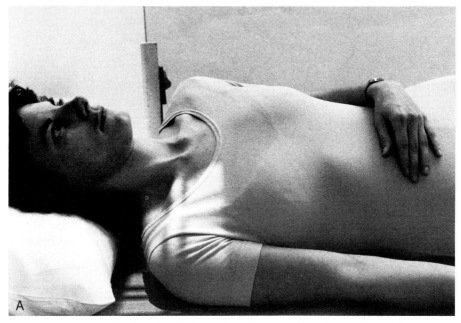

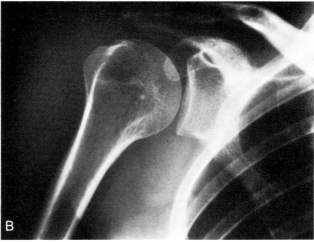

Figure 9–11. *A,* Patient positioned for 40° posterior oblique view with wedge for support under opposite shoulder. *B,* Radiograph clearly demonstrates the glenohumeral joint. The coracoid is projected over the upper joint space.

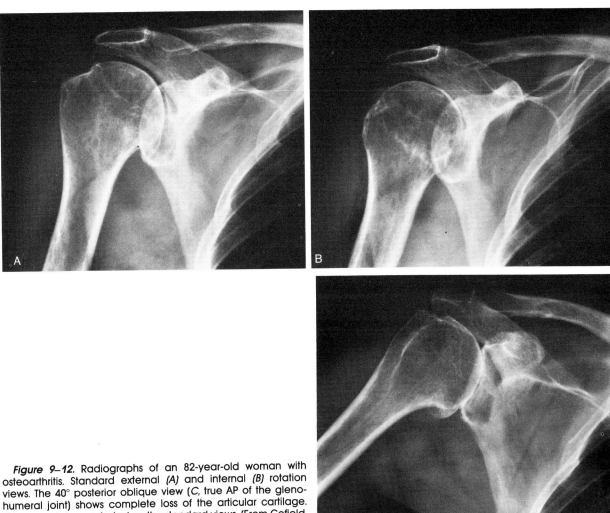

Figure 9–12. Radiographs of an 82-year-old woman with osteoarthritis. Standard external *(A)* and internal *(B)* rotation views. The 40° posterior oblique view (*C,* true AP of the gleno-humeral joint) shows complete loss of the articular cartilage. This was not demonstrated on the standard views. (From Cofield, R. H.: Unconstrained total shoulder prostheses. Clin. Orthop. *173*:97, 1983.)

diagnosis, arthroscopy will be presented; but it is certainly less useful in the shoulder than in the knee.

AP Views

Standard Shoulder Projections. The standard shoulder projections have been AP views of the humerus in external and internal rotation. These views should be obtained in the upright position when possible. However, following trauma the supine position is most often used. The external rotation view is obtained with the arm rotated externally so that the hand is palm up. The central beam is centered on the coracoid and is perpendicular to the 8 × 10 inch cassette. The internal rotation view requires the arm to be internally rotated. This can be best accomplished with the elbow flexed and the hand on the abdomen or side[19, 20] (Fig. 9–9).

These films have advantages and limitations. Their major advantage is familiarity. They offer a useful survey for the presence or absence of severe or advanced shoulder diseases: metastatic or pri-

mary cancer, arthritis, calcific tendinitis (Fig. 9–10), chronic rotator cuff tears, or old trauma. However, these views alone are usually not satisfactory, as implied by Golding, for a careful analysis of acute trauma or for an evaluation of musculoskeletal pathology in the shoulder being considered for reconstructive surgery. The standard shoulder projections essentially represent AP views of the chest centered over the shoulder girdle. They are oblique to the glenohumeral joint because of the position of the scapula on the chest wall and do not depict the joint line free of bony overlap.

Posterior Oblique View

The basic shoulder projections, being oblique to the glenohumeral joint, may not clearly show joint space narrowing. A 40° posterior oblique view will visualize the joint space and offers the advantage of an angle nearly 90° to the anterior oblique view. The patient is rotated 40° to the affected side. In the supine position a wedge should be used for support (Figs. 9–11*A* and 9–12). The central beam is centered on the shoulder joint and is perpendicular to the cassette.

Scapular Y-View

The scapular Y-view,[48] the 60° anterior oblique view, or the lateral scapular view represents an alternative for obtaining a lateral x-ray of the shoulder. In the upright position the patient is rotated 60° toward the wall-mounted cassette. Following trauma it is often necessary to elevate the involved shoulder 60° and to support the patient with a foam wedge (Fig. 9–13A). In the latter situation, the central beam is centered on the medial edge of the shoulder and is perpendicular to the cassette.[19] The "Y" (Figs. 9–13B and 9–4) is formed by the junction of the coracoid process, the body of the scapula, and the spine of the scapula. These limbs meet at the glenoid, and in this projection the humeral head should be centered over the glenoid. The x-ray technique is simple, and the bony anatomy is clearly delineated. In one study evaluating 19 shoulder fractures, 4 fractures were not seen on any other views of the shoulder.[27]

Transthoracic Lateral View. A number of additional or alternative views have been described and suggested. Their goal is to visualize the glenohumeral joint at or near 90° to the standard projection. The transthoracic lateral view is a projection at 90° to the standard views, but the superimposed chest structures render interpretation difficult at best and typically uncertain. As in the case of the standard projections, another disadvantage of this view is that it is oblique to the glenohumeral joint surface. This technique will be the auxiliary view discussed in Chapter 10.

Axillary View

The axillary shoulder projection has largely replaced the transthoracic lateral view. The patient is supine with the arm abducted 90°, and the cassette on the table top is cranial to the shoulder (Fig. 9–14A). The central beam is centered on the axilla and is perpendicular to the cassette. Alternate positions have also been described by Bernau[20] and Ballinger.[19] In the absence of acute trauma the arm is widely abducted, and excellent visualization of the bony architecture is easily accomplished. In the presence of an acute injury, the x-ray can still be obtained without the use of special equipment by abducting the arm only the width of the x-ray tube (Fig. 9–14B). An alternative method has been described by Wallace and Hellier.[52] Several authors have proclaimed the value of this view (Fig. 9–14C). In a series of patients without acute trauma, 15 abnormalities[23, 29, 34] in 130 abnormal x-rays would not have been identified without using this view.[26]

It is apparent that several options are available to depict the shoulder joint radiographically. An incomplete examination need no longer be accepted. In the absence of acute trauma, the largest amount of information is obtained from a combination of several views. These include a 40° posterior oblique x-ray in internal and external rotation and an axillary view. With further experience, it may prove

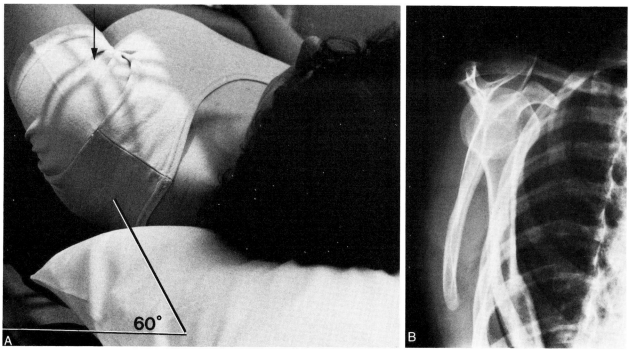

Figure 9–13. A, Patient positioned for Y-view of the shoulder. (Arrow-tube angle, patient shoulder elevated 60°.) *B,* Radiograph clearly demonstrates the relationship of the humeral head to the glenoid and coracoacromial arch. The acromion and coracoid are well seen.

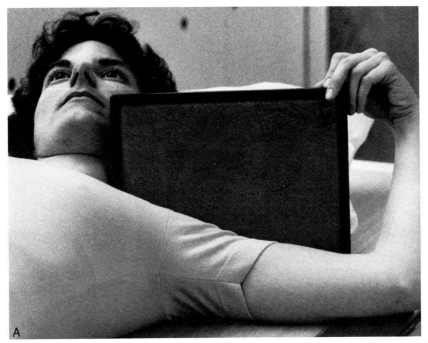

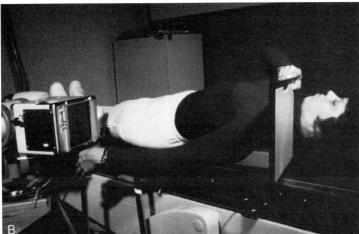

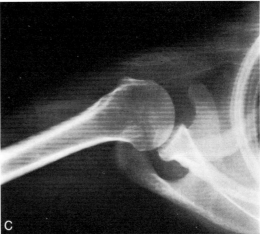

Figure 9–14. A, Patient positioned for routine axillary view of the shoulder. *B,* Patient positioned for "emergency" axillary view of the shoulder. *C,* Radiograph demonstrating axillary view.

possible to eliminate the internal rotation view. This grouping of three x-rays might be called an elective shoulder series. When acute trauma is being evaluated, arm rotation is often not desirable, and arm movement is kept to a minimum. In this situation, a shoulder trauma series is more effective, including a 40° posterior oblique, a 60° anterior oblique, and an emergency axillary view.[32, 43]

Scapula

AP View

The AP view of the scapula can be obtained with the patient supine or upright. The arm should be fully abducted, if possible[19] (Fig. 9–15A). The hand may be placed on the hip with the elbow slightly flexed, if abduction is limited. The beam is centered

on the midscapula and is perpendicular to the cassette. Breathing during the procedure will diminish the shadows caused by the overlying ribs.[19]

The radiograph demonstrates the lateral portions of the scapula, but the medial scapula is partially obscured by thoracic structures (Fig. 9–B).

Lateral View

The lateral view of the scapula may be difficult to obtain in the acutely injured patient. The patient can be rotated from the supine position to an almost lateral position, with the affected shoulder adjacent to the table. The elbow should be flexed, with the forearm anterior to the chest.[41] This will prevent the humerus from overlapping the scapula (Fig. 9–16B). The central beam is centered parallel to the scapular border (palpable) and is perpendicular to

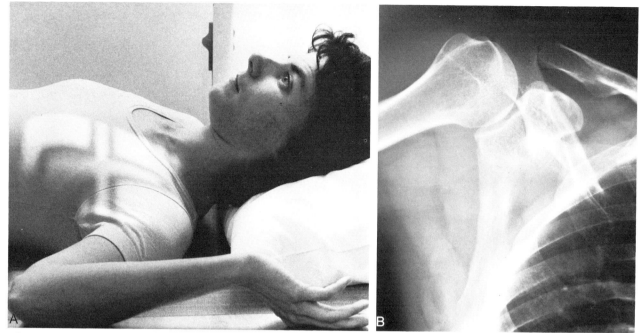

Figure 9–15. A, Patient positioned for AP scapular view. The beam is centered on the midscapula and is perpendicular to the table. *B,* AP view of scapula. The medial margin is partially obscured by ribs.

the cassette (Fig. 9–16A). When possible, this view should be obtained in the upright position.

The radiograph (Fig. 9–16B) demonstrates the scapular body and spine, the coracoid, and the acromion. Excellent rib detail is also obtained in the area adjacent to the clavicle.

Acromioclavicular Joint

X-rays of the clavicle and its articulations can be difficult to obtain and may require special projections. The acromioclavicular joint is seen on AP or posterior oblique views of the shoulder and on the

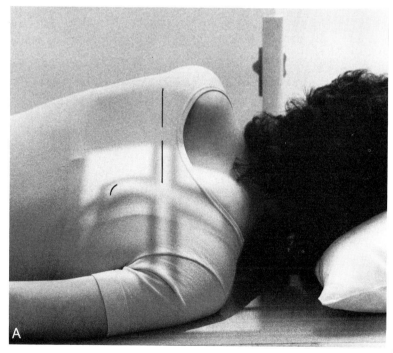

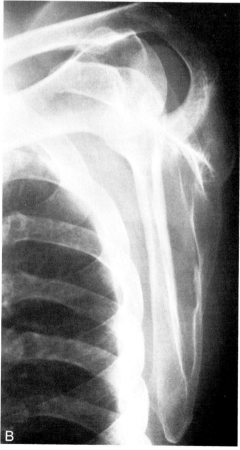

Figure 9–16. A, Patient positioned for lateral view of the scapula; demonstrating inferior scapular angle *(curved line)* and central beam *(broken line).* *B,* Lateral view of the scapula. Note that the humerus is not overlying the scapula.

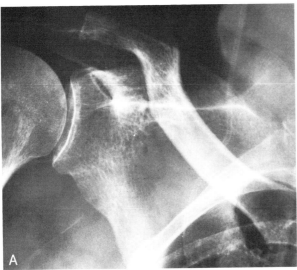
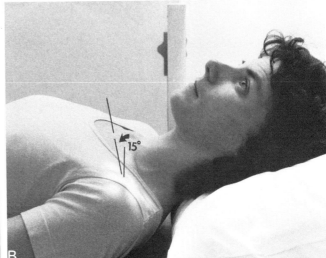
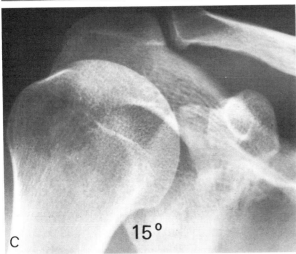

Figure 9–17. *A*, AP view of the clavicle. The acromioclavicular joint is overpenetrated and not well demonstrated. *B*, Patient positioned for AP view of the acromioclavicular joint. The tube is angled 15°, and the beam is coned down over the joint. *C*, Radiograph of acromioclavicular joint.

axillary view. The typical x-ray exposure for the shoulder joint may, however, be too great, overpenetrating the acromioclavicular joint and rendering this portion of the film too dark for interpretation (Fig. 9–17A). The technician may have to decrease the intensity of the beam to obtain better detail. Best results are obtained with localized views.

The injured patient is most easily examined in a supine position. The beam is coned down over the acromioclavicular joint and angled 15° to the head (Fig. 9–17B).[19, 20] The resulting image provides better detail and projects the joint free of overlying structures (Fig. 9–17C).

With injuries of the acromioclavicular joint, stress x-rays may be helpful to diagnose the degree of ligamentous damage. This is done by hanging 8 to 10 lb of weight from both wrists, using a device such as the one illustrated in Figure 9–18. If the patient is asked to hold the weights, contraction of the extremity muscles may create false negative results. Figure 9–19 illustrates an acromioclavicular dislocation as demonstrated on stress views. On this x-ray the distance between the undersurface of the clavicle and the upper surface of the coracoid is almost twice as great on the left as on the right. If

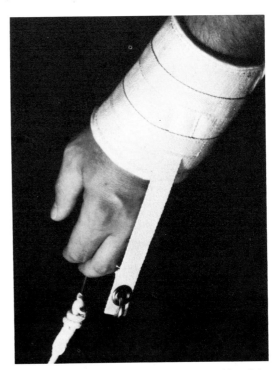

Figure 9–18. Ankle traction cuff used as a wrist cuff for stress views of the acromioclavicular joint.

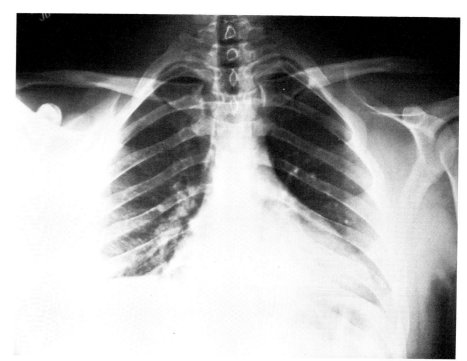

Figure 9–19. Stress views of the acromioclavicular joint. Note the marked increase in coracoclavicular distance on the left compared with the distance on the right.

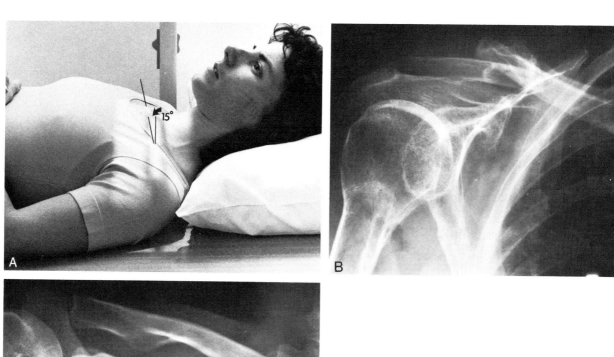

Figure 9–20. A, Patient positioned for AP view of the clavicle. The tube is angled 15° to the head. (Note cone-light size compared with acromioclavicular joint view in Fig. 9–17B). *B,* AP view of the clavicle with no angulation. There is overlap of the distal clavicle, acromion, and scapula. Note the displaced midshaft fracture. *C,* Angled (15°) view of the clavicle more clearly demonstrates the distal clavicle, as it is projected above the spine of the scapula.

the difference on the injured side is more than 5 mm greater than the noninjured side, a complete coracoclavicular ligament disruption is likely to have occurred.[46] The coracoclavicular distance normally measures about 1.3 cm.[21]

Clavicle

AP Views

The PA view of the clavicle (AP may also be used) places the clavicle against the cassette; this increases image quality. In severely injured patients the AP view (supine) is most often used (Fig. 9–20A). With the AP projection the acromioclavicular joint is superimposed on the posterior acromion and spine of the scapula. Angling the central beam 15° cephalad will eliminate this difficulty.[18, 55]

Oblique View

The oblique view (tangential view) provides better visualization of the midclavicle. The patient's affected side is elevated, and the cassette (angled 45° to the table) is placed above the shoulder (Fig. 9–21A). The central beam is also angled 45° to be perpendicular to the cassette. The resulting radiograph projects the clavicle above the ribs (Fig. 9–21B). This allows better evaluation of the midclavicle.[19] The alternate method (Fig. 9–21C) is performed with the patient supine. With this technique the acromioclavicular joint is more often obscured.

Sternoclavicular Joints

With lesions in the middle third of the clavicle or involving the sternoclavicular joint, views other than an AP or slightly oblique projection will be difficult to obtain. Bernau and Berquist[20] describe a prone technique with the cassette angled 15° to place it next to the sternoclavicular joints. The tube is centered on T2 and angled perpendicularly to the cassette (15° to the head) (Fig. 9–22A). This view is useful in most situations. Quesada has suggested placing the patient prone and obtaining two views, one with the central ray angled cephalad 45° and

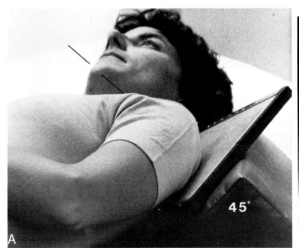
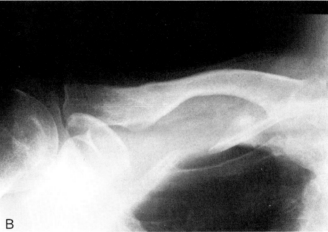
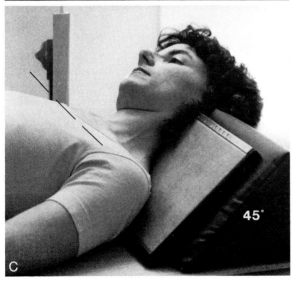

Figure 9–21. A, Patient positioned for the oblique tangential view. The cassette is angled at about 45°. The central beam is perpendicular to the cassette. B, Radiograph demonstrates the midclavicle and acromioclavicular joint. Fractures will be projected free from overlying bone shadows. C, Patient positioned for supine tangential view.

Text continues on page 516

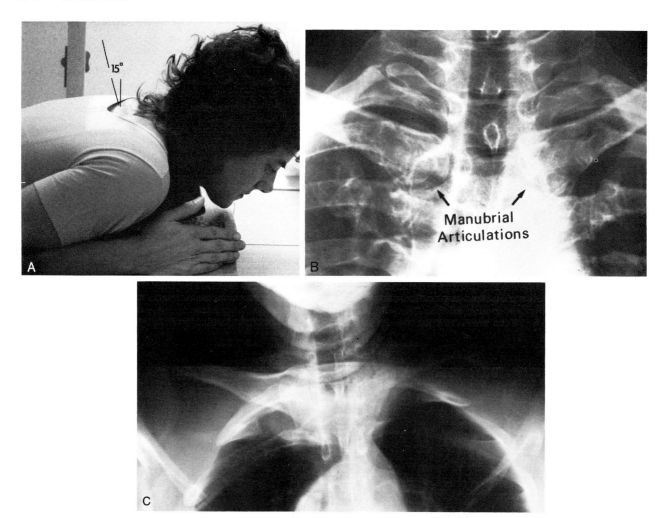

Figure 9–22. *A*, Patient positioned for routine PA view of the sternoclavicular joint. Normally the tube is angled at 15°. *B*, Normal sternoclavicular joints. Even with excellent technique this view is difficult to interpret owing to overlying structures. *C*, 40° view showing asymmetrical clavicles due to posterior dislocation on the right.

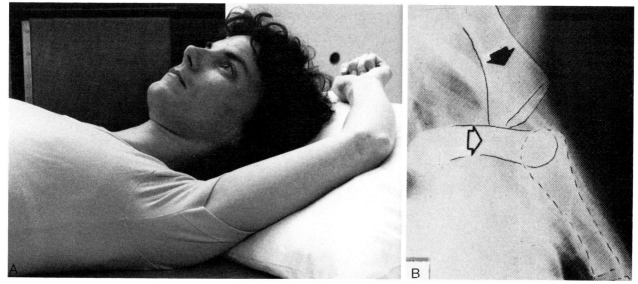

Figure 9–23. *A*, Patient positioned for Heinig view.[36, 40] The arm closest to the tube is elevated, with the tube angled through the joint at about 45°. The cassette is above the opposite shoulder and perpendicular to the beam. *B*, Retouched radiograph of Heinig projection. (*B*, From Lee, F. A., and Gwinn, J. L.: Retrosternal dislocation of the clavicle. Radiology *110*:631, 1974.)

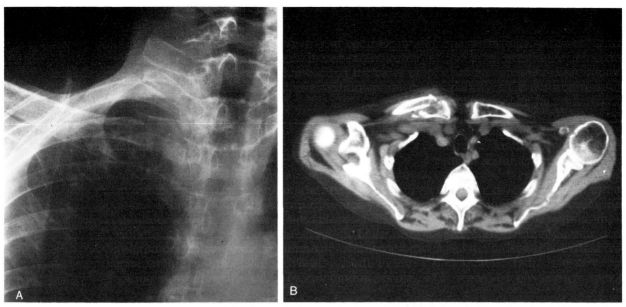

Figure 9-24. Trauma to the medial clavicle. *A,* Radiograph shows a fracture of the medial end of the clavicle. *B,* CT scan clearly demonstrates this overriding fracture of the proximal clavicle.

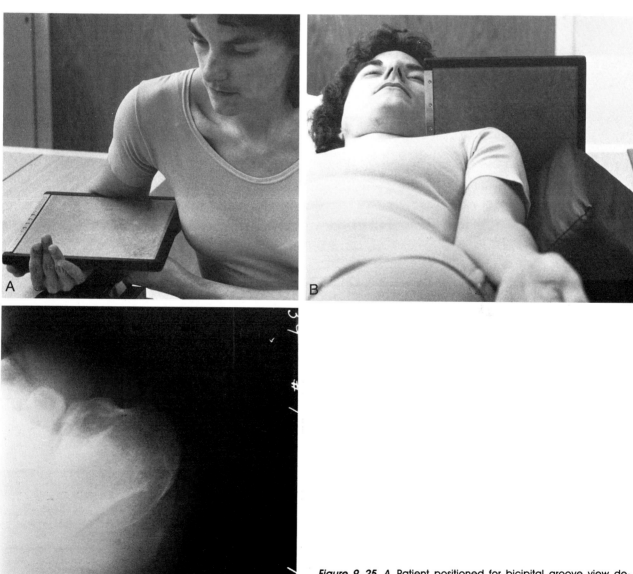

Figure 9-25. *A,* Patient positioned for bicipital groove view described by Fisk.[31] *B,* Alternate method for bicipital groove view. *C,* AP radiograph demonstrating the bicipital groove.

one with the central ray angled caudad 45°.[44] A 40° cephalic tilt view (serendipity technique)[46] with the patient supine has proved to be more practical. The patient is positioned as for the AP clavicle view, but the tube is angled 40° to the head and centered on the manubrium. With this technique an anteriorly displaced structure will appear to be upwardly displaced, and a posteriorly displaced structure will appear inferior to its normal position (Fig. 9–22C). Heinig has suggested a technique for obtaining a lateral view of the medial end of the clavicle and the sternoclavicular joint (Fig. 9–23). This may prove helpful in difficult situations, but interpretation is still difficult because of the superimposition of chest structures.[36] Computed tomography may provide the best evaluation of the sternoclavicular joint (Fig. 9–24).

Special Views

The views already discussed represent the general x-ray alternatives for investigation of the shoulder girdle. There are additional views that can be obtained to visualize specific structures or search for discrete pathologic changes.

On occasion it may be desirable to obtain x-rays of the bicipital groove. With the extremity in the anatomic position, the groove is positioned approximately 15° lateral to the midportion of the anterior aspect of the humeral head. Fisk[31] suggested one method of visualizing this groove (Fig. 9–25A). We have as an alternative positioned the patient as illustrated in Figure 9–25B.[20] The involved side is elevated slightly with cushion support. The cassette

is positioned above the shoulder, with the hand in an anatomic position. The central beam is centered on the upper aspect of the humeral head.[20] This view offers a projection of the length of the groove. The upper angle of the groove is better shown in the Fisk projection (Fig. 9–25C).

A number of views have been developed to augment the evaluation of the unstable or recurrently dislocating shoulder. These views are designed to visualize a bony or calcific reaction, a fracture of the anterior glenoid rim, or a compression fracture of the posterior aspect of the humeral head—the Hill-Sachs lesion.[38] In the acute anterior dislocation the Hill-Sachs deformity is seen on an AP view and is usually characteristic (Fig. 9–26). On occasion the humeral head can be seen to be indented posteriorly and impacted on the anterior glenoid rim—the genesis of the humeral head defect. The anterior nature of this dislocation can be confirmed with an emergency axillary or anterior oblique shoulder x-ray (Fig. 9–26B).

In the nonacute setting, the diagnosis of continuing shoulder instability may be difficult and x-ray confirmation of the presence of lesions associated with shoulder instability is sought. Hill and Sachs suggested using an AP x-ray with the arm in marked internal rotation to visualize the humeral impaction-fracture. Rokous and colleagues[47] suggested a modified axillary view (the West Point axillary) to accomplish these ends (Fig. 9–27A-C). The patient is prone, and the shoulder is elevated 3 inches from the tabletop. The arm is abducted 90° and rotated so that the forearm hangs off the x-ray table and is pointed directly at the floor. The x-ray tube is positioned with the central ray projecting

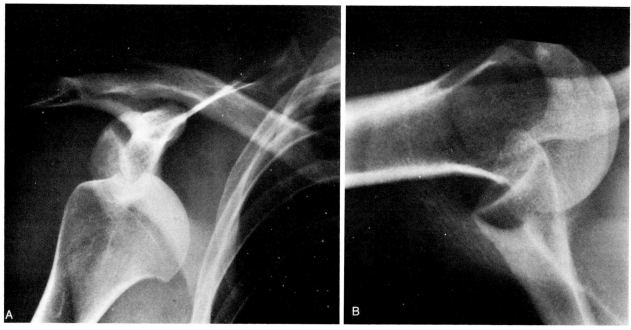

Figure 9–26. A, Anterior dislocation with typical Hill-Sachs impression fracture. The head rests on the glenoid rim. B, Axillary view of the anteriorly dislocated shoulder.

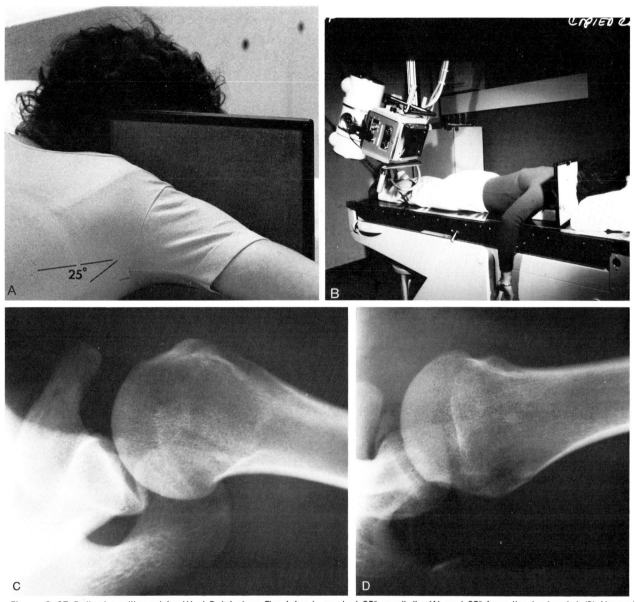

Figure 9–27. Patient positioned for West Point view. The tube is angled 25° medially (A) and 25° from the horizontal (B). Normal axillary view (C). West Point view in a patient with a small Hill-Sachs fracture and reactive bone along the anterior inferior glenoid rim (D).

25° from the horizontal and 25° medially. This projects the anterior inferior glenoid rim better than the standard axillary x-ray, which projects the anterior glenoid rim. The fixed arm position and rotation usually demonstrates the Hill-Sachs lesion when it is present. In their 63 patients with chronic subluxation of the shoulder, 53 (84 percent) demonstrated abnormalities of the glenoid rim. No cases of acute anterior dislocation demonstrated this abnormality, but 6 of 19 cases (32 percent) with recurrent anterior dislocation did have this lesion.

Hall and colleagues described a view developed by William S. Stryker, the Stryker notch view[35] (Fig. 9–28A and B). The patient is supine, with the hand adjacent to or on top of the head and the elbow directed vertically. The central beam is angled 10° cephalad and centered on the coracoid (palpable). In patients with recurrent anterior dislocation, Hall and colleagues could identify the humeral head lesion in 18 of 20 shoulders (90 percent). Additional x-ray views also designed to depict the humeral head lesion and recurrent anterior instability are modifications of the Hermodsson[37] or the Didiee[28] views.

In patients who are being evaluated for recurrent anterior shoulder instability, multiple views are necessary to outline all of the bone pathology, as one single view does not always depict these two lesions. In these situations, the basic AP views in internal and external rotation are supplemented by

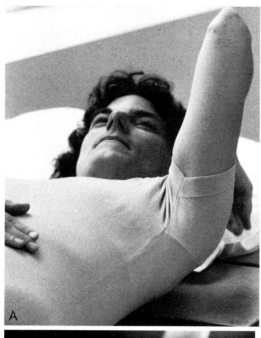
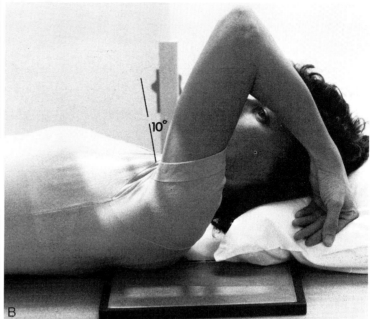
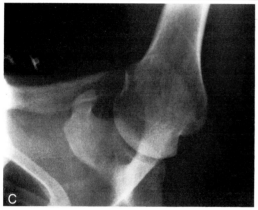

Figure 9–28. A and *B*, Patient positioned for the Stryker notch view.[35] *C*, Radiograph demonstrating a large Hill-Sachs defect.

a West Point axillary and a Stryker notch view. With these two additional x-rays, it is unlikely that important findings will be missed (Fig. 9–29).

Soft Tissue Radiography

Various technical adjustments have been made to improve contrast between soft tissues, including the edge-contrast enhancement that occurs with xeroradiography[45] (see Xeroradiography in Chapter 1). The value of these techniques rests on the assumption that inflammatory processes will cause tissues to become edematous and thus will reduce the difference in attenuation between muscle, tendon or fascia, and fat. Even on standard shoulder x-rays a subdeltoid fat layer is often seen. When there is subdeltoid bursal enlargement, this fatty layer will be pushed outward and appear elliptical rather than almost straight.[53] In the presence of bursal inflammation, as occurs with infection or in the advanced bursitis associated with degenerative tendon changes, this layer may not be visible. In one series using special soft tissue techniques, there were discrepancies in x-ray interpretation in only 5 of 108 shoulders examined to analyze this subdeltoid fatty layer.[25] Thus, a potential for a high degree of accuracy exists. From the clinical standpoint, this information is seldom critical, but it is one more bit of data used in evaluating a patient's problem. This is especially true when there is a possibility of sepsis.

Tomography

In the shoulder tomography is seldom necessary. However, it may be a useful adjunct to routine x-ray evaluation or coned-down views. This is especially true of the medial third of the clavicle and the sternoclavicular joint, as thoracic contents may obscure alterations in bone structure or joint relationships. Shoulder pain is often traumatic or degenerative in origin, but small neoplasms such as an osteoid osteoma may cause difficulty in diagnosis. Plain x-rays may not localize the problem. A radioisotope scan can localize the lesion, allowing selection of a tomographic projection to define the lesion (Fig. 9–30).

Recently several authors have combined arthrography and tomography to yield a better definition

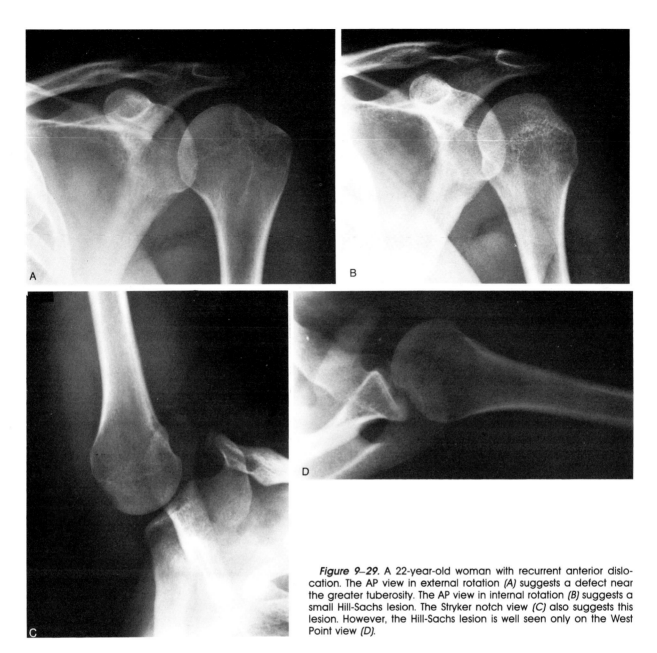

Figure 9–29. A 22-year-old woman with recurrent anterior dislocation. The AP view in external rotation *(A)* suggests a defect near the greater tuberosity. The AP view in internal rotation *(B)* suggests a small Hill-Sachs lesion. The Stryker notch view *(C)* also suggests this lesion. However, the Hill-Sachs lesion is well seen only on the West Point view *(D)*.

Figure 9–30. A 24-year-old man with pain in the shoulder. The pain was said to be worse at night and relieved by aspirin. *A*, Tc = 99m scan demonstrates increased uptake in the left glenoid. *B*, A Stryker Notch view demonstrates a lucent area in the glenoid *(arrow)*. *C*, Tomograms further define the osteoid osteoma.

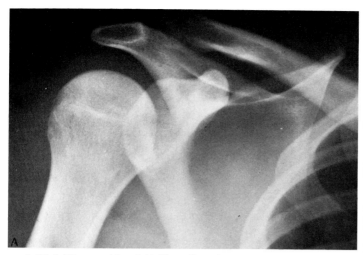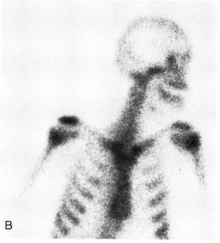

Figure 9–31. A 20-year-old weight lifter with pain on the top of the shoulder. *A,* Routine radiograph shows slight resorption of the distal clavicle. *B,* Tc-99m scan demonstrates increased uptake at the acromioclavicular joint.

of structures outlined by the contrast material.[39] Arthrotomography will be discussed later in this chapter along with arthrography.

Ultrasonography

The value of ultrasonography is uncertain and currently experimental. As resolution improves, it may well have a role. Farrar and colleagues[30] reported on dynamic sonographic studies of the rotator cuff. Forty-eight patients were evaluated. Features consistently associated with tendon tears included abnormal motion patterns of the supraspinatus with arm rotation and persistently disrupted echoes within the tendon substance. Very large tears were imaged as regions of diminished echo density. Arthrography was also performed on these patients. Sonography was falsely positive in 6 and falsely negative in 2. Farrar and colleagues pointed out the need for operator experience. They maintained that ultrasound may be a useful screening tool and that it yields information not only about tearing but also about tissue quality.

A review of this material shows that ultrasonography may have a role as a screening procedure to identify medium-sized rotator cuff tears. For smaller tears when ultrasonographic diagnosis is in question or questionable, arthrography is probably still a more effective technique. Ultrasound may have a role in the evaluation of shoulder pain when the arthrogram is negative. Abnormal tendon echoes may suggest internal tendon damage as a source of the pain. This is a promising area, as the technique is almost to the point of clinical usefulness.

Radionuclide Scanning

Nuclear scanning using Tc-99m–labeled phosphate compounds is very sensitive to increased vascularity or increased metabolic activity in bone. On the other hand, it is not very specific. Certainly the shoulders are most commonly scanned as part of a whole body scan to screen for metastatic disease. Radionuclide scanning can also be used to evaluate a number of other shoulder conditions and has particular importance in a few. Overinterpretation of increased uptake may be a problem, however, as there can be increased uptake in the glenohumeral, acromioclavicular, or sternoclavicular joint areas when no symptoms or routine x-ray findings are present.[33] There may also be increased activity seen around the glenohumeral or acromioclavicular joints of the dominant extremity. In the study of Sebes and colleagues, scans of 100 right-handed people showed that 30 had increased radioactivity on the right, and only 5 showed this increase on the left.[49] In 8 left-handed people, 3 had increased activity on the left and none had this increase on the right.

The scan can be used to screen for certain benign neoplasms (e.g., osteoid osteoma) as mentioned earlier. It can also be used to assess soft tissue pathology about the shoulder, such as rotator cuff disease or periarthritis.[51, 54] This is probably related to the inflammation that accompanies these disorders. In studying these patients the history, physical examination, routine shoulder x-rays, and possibly an arthrogram will usually establish the diagnosis, thus making scanning unnecessary. However, some of these patients, especially those with incomplete-thickness rotator cuff tears and bursal inflammation, remain so symptomatic for so long that some visual means of confirming their diagnosis seems worthwhile. The bone scan, being a sensitive test, may well do so.

It has been noted that weight lifters and some other athletes develop osteolysis of the distal clavicle.[22] X-ray findings include osteoporosis of the distal clavicle, loss of subchondral bone detail, cystic changes, or bone resorption. However, the x-ray findings may be subtle. The nuclear scan shows intense uptake related to the inflammation and traumatic arthritis, thus pinpointing the location of the pathology (Fig. 9–31).

Infectious arthritis or rheumatoid diseases in the shoulder are more specifically evaluated by arthrography rather than by scanning. Following the progress of these patients by scanning has not proved to be practical. The evaluation of the painful total shoulder arthroplasty by nuclear scanning is occasionally helpful but in general has been disappointing (Fig. 9–32). This is probably due to a number of factors: the normal variability in shoulder uptake, the expected increase in uptake with soft tissue inflammation in the shoulder, the small area of glenoid-component bone fixation, and the limited amount of bone reaction adjacent to the implant when loosening occurs. The painful total shoulder arthroplasty often shows a slightly increased general uptake in the joint area, similar to nonpainful total shoulder arthroplasties, and all too often this is not well localized in the glenoid region. Thus, in these situations, if the uptake is concentrated in the glenoid region in deference to other areas, it can be considered as an indication of loosening (if the study is done more than 6 months postoperatively). However, if the uptake is slightly increased in general, not much useful information is obtained.

Computed Tomography

Some of the difficulties involved in obtaining an alternative to the AP views for sternoclavicular and medial clavicular lesions have been mentioned earlier. Computed tomographic scanning is very useful for overcoming these difficulties Fig. 9–24B). Scapular spine or body lesions may also be further defined using this technique. Using computed to-

mography the scapulothoracic junction is well outlined, and the osteochondromas or chest wall lesions in this region can be well visualized. However, recent experience has demonstrated that magnetic resonance imaging is superior to CT in the evaluation of chest wall lesions.

Computed tomography has proved to be especially useful for better definition of glenoid fractures and more complex fractures, as often the shoulder views are not adequate to make a decision about the need for surgery (Fig. 9–33). As an extension of the application of computed tomographic scanning, Danzig and colleagues have suggested its use for identification of glenoid-Bankart type lesions and humeral head, Hill-Sachs lesions in the evaluation of unstable shoulders.[24]

Experience with magnetic resonance imaging is limited. Soft tissue contrast and resolution may make this technique useful in evaluation of cuff tears and bicipital tendon injury.

SPECIAL DIAGNOSTIC TECHNIQUES

Multiple radiographic techniques are available to assist the orthopedic surgeon or clinician in evaluating shoulder problems that may not be detectable or fully defined with the previously discussed imaging techniques. This section will discuss the utilization of arthrography, bursography, and aspiration and injection techniques as well as arthroscopy in the evaluation of patients with pain and other symptoms pertaining to the shoulder.

One cannot overemphasize the importance of a systematic approach to the diagnosis of shoulder disorders. The first and most important step is good

Figure 9–32. Tc-99m scan in a patient with painful shoulder arthroplasties shows increased uptake bilaterally. This is particularly prominent on the posterior scans shown in the lower half of the figure. Loose glenoid components were present.

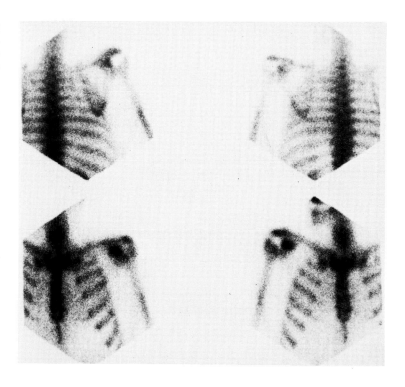

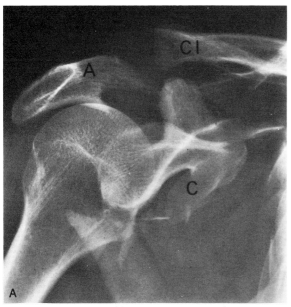

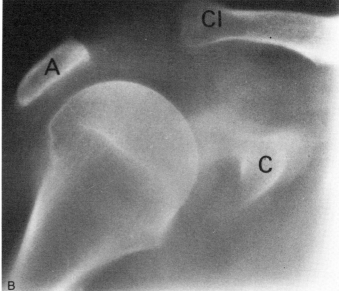

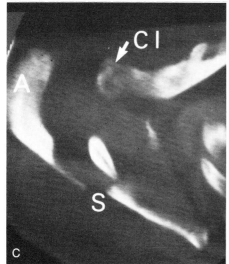

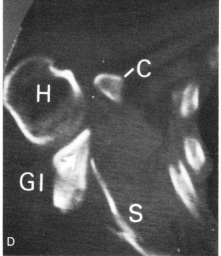

Figure 9–33. Complex scapular fracture. *A,* AP view demonstrates multiple fragments. *B,* Tomography is not of great value in demonstrating the position of the fragments. *C,* CT scan at the acromial level shows comminution of the spine of the scapula and acromioclavicular separation. The midclavicle is fractured. *D,* Image taken just below this level shows an intact glenoid articular surface and the anterior-most portion of the coracoid. (Gl, glenoid; A, acromion; Cl, clavicle; C, coracoid; S, scapula.)

TABLE 9–2. Indications and Techniques for Shoulder Arthrography in 552 Arthrograms

Suspected Clinical Problem	% Cases	Technique
Rotator cuff tear (partial and/or complete)	57%	Double-contrast
Adhesive capsulitis, diagnosis and treatment	15%	Single-contrast ± dilatation
Impingement syndrome	8%	Double-contrast ± bursogram
Evaluation of the PO shoulder	6%	
1. Previous cuff tears		Double-contrast
2. TSA		Subtraction technique
Instability or chronic subluxation	5%	Double-contrast with tomography or CT
Biceps tendon tear	4%	Double-contrast
Post-traumatic deformities	3%	Double-contrast ± tomography or CT
Tendinitis	2%	Double-contrast

TABLE 9–3. Plain Film Findings in Rotator Cuff Tears

	Humeroacromial Distance (Superior Subluxation)			Location of Abnormal Findings			
	>1 cm	<1 cm	<0.7 cm	Greater tuberosity	Acromio-clavicular joint	Inferior glenoid spurring	Humeral spurring
145 complete thickness cuff tears	5%	30%	65%	90%	75%	25%	25%
38 partial thickness cuff tears	44%	40%	16%	11%	0%	0%	10%

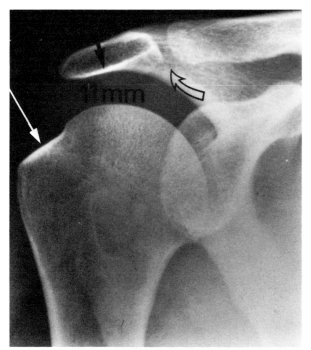

Figure 9–34. Normal humeroacromial distance with convex acromion *(upper black arrow)* and a well-defined smooth greater tuberosity *(lower black arrow)*. Normal acromioclavicular joint *(open arrow)*.

communication between the referring physician and the radiologist. Such communication combined with a thorough evaluation of the routine radiographs will allow the radiologist to determine the proper procedure and film sequence for the best evaluation of the patient's clinical problems.

Shoulder Arthrography

Proper choice of arthrographic technique requires an awareness of the patient's clinical problem, such as a rotator cuff tear or impingement syndrome, as well as an understanding of the plain-film findings. Shoulder arthrography is most often utilized in the evaluation of the rotator cuff.[65–67, 85, 94, 95, 100, 103, 106] However, more subtle changes in the shoulder may also be detected, especially with double-contrast techniques.

In our series of 552 shoulder arthrograms, 38 percent of patients were referred with pain and diminished range of motion. The majority of these patients were suspected to have rotator cuff lesions. An additional 19 percent were referred with definite clinical evidence of cuff tears. Thus, 57 percent of the arthrograms were performed with cuff disease specifically in mind. Table 9–2 summarizes the other common indications in our practice. The techniques most often used are also included in Table 9–2. Arthrography is less commonly performed to exclude synovitis, loose bodies, and arthritis.[66, 72]

Knowledge of the patient's suspected problem and careful evaluation of routine radiographs can assist one in proper performance of the arthrogram and choice of filming sequence to best define the patient's problem.

Review of plain-film findings on 552 patients undergoing shoulder arthrography has provided extensive data regarding these findings. Previous reports of plain-film findings in patients with rotator cuff tears describe superior subluxation of the humeral head (distance from humeral head to acromion ≤ 7 mm), reversal of the normal acromial convexity, sclerosis or cystic changes in the greater tuberosity, and bony eburnation of the glenoid or humeral head inferomedially.[63, 75, 81, 111] The latter finding (hypertrophic spurring involving the humeral head inferomedially) is not a reliable indicator of rotator cuff tearing and can be seen with many chronic shoulder problems.[81, 111] DeSmet reported plain-film abnormalities in 90.4 percent of 42 pa-

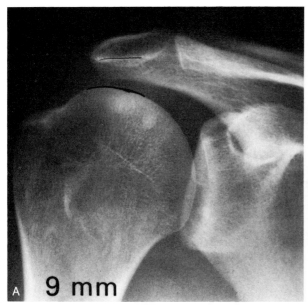
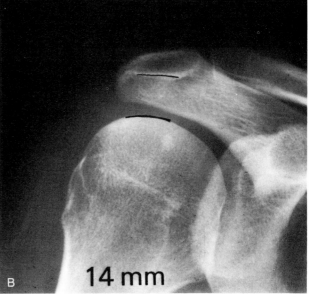

Figure 9–35. The acromiohumeral distance in external rotation *(A)* measures 9 mm. In internal rotation *(B)* the measurement is 14 mm, a difference of 5 mm with change of position.

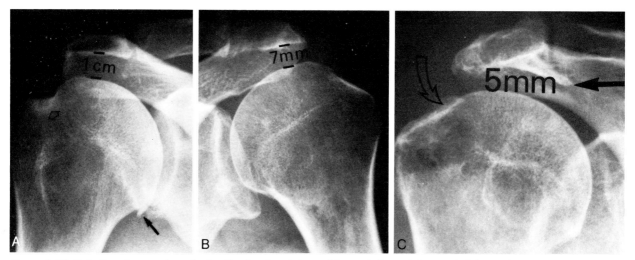

Figure 9–36. Plain film changes in patients with chronic rotator cuff tears. *A,* Acromiohumeral distance 1 cm. Note cystic changes in the greater tuberosity *(open arrow)* and spurring of the head and glenoid *(black arrow)*. *B,* Superior subluxation with acromiohumeral distance of 7 mm. Relatively normal glenoid and greater tuberosity. *C,* Superior subluxation with acromiohumeral distance of 5 mm. Note large acromial spur *(black arrow)* impinging on the cuff and bursa. There is new bone formation at the cuff insertion into the greater tuberosity *(open arrow)*.

tients with rotator cuff tears.[63] Our review of 552 arthrograms revealed 145 complete and 38 partial tears of the rotator cuff. As would be expected, changes on plain radiographs were much more common with complete chronic cuff tears (Table 9–3). Patients with acute cuff tears (no associated fractures) less frequently demonstrate bony abnormalities on plain films.

Superior subluxation of the humeral head causes a reduction of the distance between the acromion, which is normally convex inferiorly, and the humeral head. Consistency in measurement is essential if one is to utilize this measurement properly. We measure all cases in external rotation. This

measurement is virtually always greater than 1 cm in normal individuals (Fig. 9–34).

Measurements on the same shoulder may vary up to 5 mm between external and internal rotations (Fig. 9–35). Also, one must consider target-film distance and tube centering. We measured the acromiohumeral distance in external rotation with a 48-inch target-film distance. The patient was placed in a straight AP position and then positioned obliquely for a true AP view of the glenohumeral joint. We also centered the tube over the coracoid and directly over the acromiohumeral joint. There was less than 1 mm difference in the measurements. Thus, consistency in obtaining the measurements

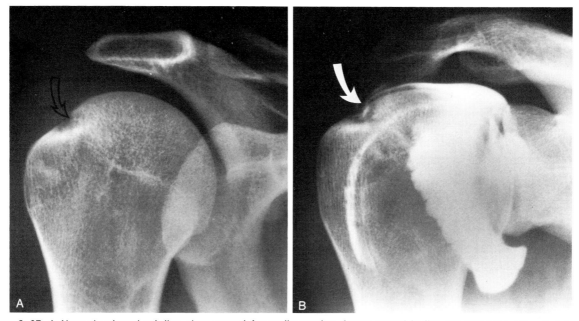

Figure 9–37. A, Normal external rotation view except for cystic erosion *(open arrow)* in the greater tuberosity. *B,* Arthrogram demonstrates a corresponding incomplete thickness tear in the rotator cuff *(arrow)*.

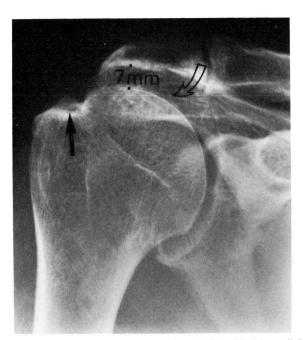

Figure 9–38. Chronic rotator cuff tear with "double tuberosity" *(black arrow)*. Also radiograph shows subluxation with acromiohumeral measurement of 7 mm and cartilaginous calcification *(open arrow)*.

is all that is necessary for constitutional accuracy. In patients with rotator cuff tears, the acromiohumeral distance was less than 1 cm in 95 percent of cases, with 65 percent measuring less than 0.7 cm (Fig. 9–36). The small percentage of patients with 1 cm in distance and rotator cuff tears were younger patients with small cuff tears. In less than 5 percent of cases, measurements of less than 0.7 cm were noted, and no cuff tears were detected arthrographically. We must strongly question whether proper arthrographic technique and exercise were accomplished during the procedures in this group of patients.

Changes in the greater tuberosity were evident in 90 percent of patients with complete cuff tears. These findings included cystic changes (Fig. 9–37), sclerosis, small erosions, and in 6 patients a "double tuberosity" (Fig. 9–38). This latter finding is of interest in that 2 cuff tears were missed arthrographically. These patients also demonstrated some degree of superior subluxation. At surgery large cuff tears were found as well as extensive capsular scarring. We suspect that the area of ossification adjacent to the tuberosity may represent an ossified or calcified supraspinatus remnant. This finding

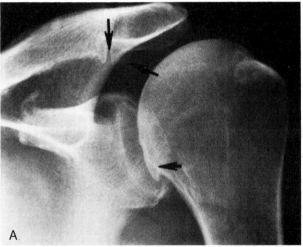

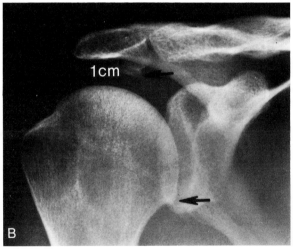

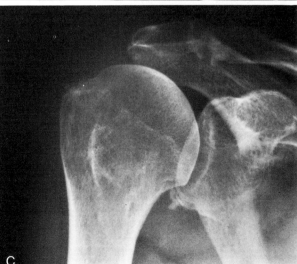

Figure 9–39. A, Spurring of the inferior margins of the acromioclavicular joint *(upper black arrows)* in a patient with symptoms of impingement and a proven rotator cuff tear. Inferior humeral head spurring *(lower black arrow)*. B, Normal acromiohumeral distance. Large acromial spur *(upper black arrow)*. Small spur on lower humeral head *(lower black arrow)*. C, Almost all secondary changes described with chronic cuff tears are present, i.e., superior subluxation of the humeral head, eburnation on the greater tuberosity, spurring of the acromioclavicular joint margin, and osteolytic changes of the acromion.

should alert one to look harder for a cuff tear if the initial films are normal.

Subtle changes on the inferior surface of the acromion or distal clavicle were present in 75 percent of patients with complete cuff tears (Fig. 9–39). These findings were also noted in a high percentage of patients with impingement syndrome. Therefore, such changes are less specific for a rotator cuff tear than changes in the greater tuberosity or superior subluxation of the humeral head.

Eburnation along the glenoid rim and spurring of the inferior medial aspect of the humeral head were present in 25 percent of patients (Fig. 9–39A and B), but this finding can also be seen with degenerative arthritis and in adhesive capsulitis. Other routine radiographic findings not usually associated with cuff tears included chondrocalcinosis, soft tissue calcification (Fig. 9–40), loose bodies and calcified phleboliths (from hemangioma or arteriovenous malformation). These changes suggest other etiologies as the cause of the patient's pain.

Other views should also be reviewed for findings suggesting instability or previous dislocation (Hill-Sachs lesions, Bankart deformity). Older films may indicate subtle loss of articular cartilage in patients with arthritis or joint space infection (see Radiographic Technique section). Once one has conferred with the clinician and examined the routine radiographs, the proper approach for the arthrogram will become evident.

Technique

Shoulder arthrography is performed on a fluoroscopic table with an overhead tube and small (≤ 6 mm) focal spot. This has the advantage of better geometry than conventional fluoroscopic equipment, resulting in better film quality. It also allows greater patient access for the physician performing the examination (see Introduction to Arthrography in Chapter 1).

With the patient in the supine position, the arm to be examined is externally rotated. A scout film is obtained to be certain the radiographic technique is optimum. The technical quality of the films taken following injection is critical, and pre-injection scout films minimize the problem of inadequate technique and repeat injections. Scout films are especially important if the radiographic technician does not perform arthrography on a regular basis.

Following establishment of optimum radiographic technique, the patient is prepared for the procedure with a 5-minute surgical scrub followed by application of povidone-iodine (Betadine) to the skin in the area to be injected. A 5-ml syringe with 1 percent lidocaine (Xylocaine) and a 25-gauge needle is used to mark the site of injection. The site is chosen over the glenohumeral joint below the coracoid and approximately at the junction of the mid- and distal thirds of the glenoid articular surface (Fig. 9–41). A wheal is made in the skin over the joint-entrance point. The soft tissues are also infiltrated with lidocaine. We err toward the medial margin of the humeral head. This insures an intra-articular positioning of the needle. The needle enters the joint or strikes the humeral head. With this technique the glenoid labrum is avoided.

The injection is made after fluoroscopic control to be certain that the needle is properly positioned. If the needle is not in the joint, a small collection of contrast material will accumulate at the needle tip with the initial injection. If properly positioned, the contrast material flows away from the needle around the humeral head (Fig. 9–42). An extensive literature is available concerning variations in this technique.[66, 85, 103, 107]

If single-contrast technique is utilized, 6 to 10 ml

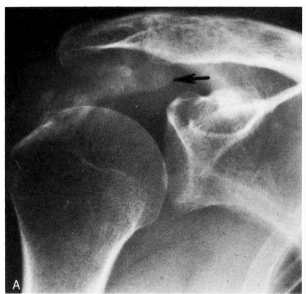
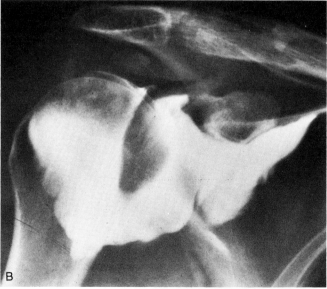

Figure 9–40. A, Extensive calcification in the rotator cuff. Note increased acromiohumeral space due to inflamed fluid-filled bursa *(arrow).* B, Arthrogram demonstrates an intact rotator cuff.

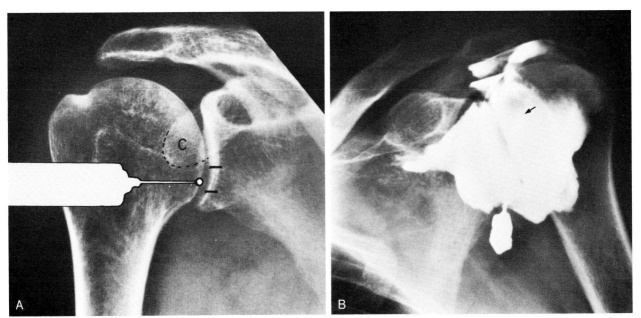

Figure 9–41. A, Needle tip marking entry site. B, Improper needle placement. The tip of the needle *(arrow)* is too far lateral and superior. This resulted in filling of both the joint and subdeltoid subacromial bursa. No cuff tear was identified at surgery.

of diatrizoate meglumine (Hypaque-M-60) is injected. Too much contrast material obscures detail, and the arthrogram is less informative (Fig. 9–43). With experience one can judge capsular volume early and avoid excessive amounts of contrast material. In double-contrast examinations, 4 ml of contrast material is injected followed by 10 to 15 ml of air, depending upon the capsule size. Again, too much contrast material defeats the purpose of a double-contrast examination. The injection must be observed fluoroscopically. If contrast is seen to leak into the subacromial bursa during the injection, the exact site of a rotator cuff tear can be visualized.

Following the injection the patient is exercised under fluoroscopic control, and any symptoms and radiographic changes are carefully noted. The relationship of the head and tuberosities to the acromion and coracoid can be examined, if impingement is suspected clinically. The patient is then fluoroscopically positioned for tangential AP views of the glenohumeral joint. Films are taken in external and internal rotation. The tangential projection allows better evaluation of the articular cartilage (Fig. 9–44). Goldman and colleagues recommend over-

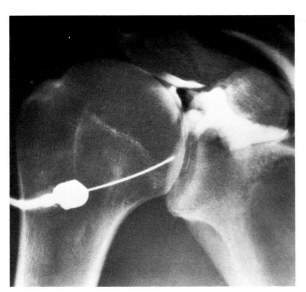

Figure 9–42. With needle properly positioned, contrast material flows around the humeral head. Note the contrast above the origin of the biceps tendon. This should not be confused with a tear.

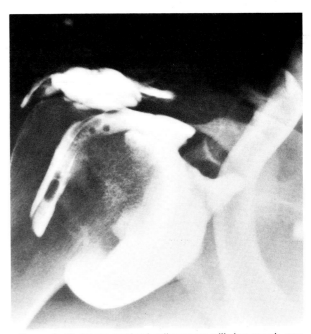

Figure 9–43. Single-contrast arthrogram with too much contrast material. A complete rotator cuff tear is noted. Other detail is obscured by the contrast material.

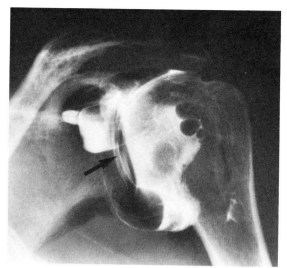

Figure 9–44. Normal double-contrast arthrogram. External rotation view with patient positioned for tangential view of the articular surface *(arrow).*

penetrated views for evaluation of the articular cartilage and underpenetrated views for evaluation of soft tissue anatomy.[72]

The patient is then moved to a different radiographic suite, and the remainder of the films are performed. With a routine single-contrast examination, axillary, upright weight-bearing[68] and scapular lateral Y-views are obtained in addition to the internal and external rotation views. Bicipital groove views are obtained if symptoms dictate. If routine film findings lead one to suspect a rotator cuff tear but none is found on the initial arthrograms, further

exercise and occasionally reinjection are performed to prevent false negative studies.

If a double-contrast examination is performed, the same views are obtained. However, axillary views are taken in the prone and supine position to demonstrate the glenoid labrum to better advantage. Conventional or computed tomography is occasionally necessary to evaluate the labrum and other subtle changes, especially in patients with previous dislocations or chronic shoulder instability.[64, 84, 108]

When conventional or computed tomography is anticipated, we often inject 0.3 ml of 1:1000 epinephrine with the contrast material. This allows more time to obtain the adequate films, as dilution and absorption of the contrast material are decreased.

Normal Arthrogram

Review of the normal film series utilized with single- and double-contrast arthrography will emphasize the usefulness of each exam (Figs. 9–45 and 9–46). It is obvious that the double-contrast examination provides better detail of certain structures. The synovium and articular cartilages are seen to better advantage, as is the undersurface of the cuff, which is coated with contrast material and outlined by air (Figs. 9–47 and 9–48). The intercapsular portion of the biceps tendon is also more clearly demonstrated, especially with the upright weight-bearing view. Advantages in the visualization of various pathologic conditions will be discussed later in this section.

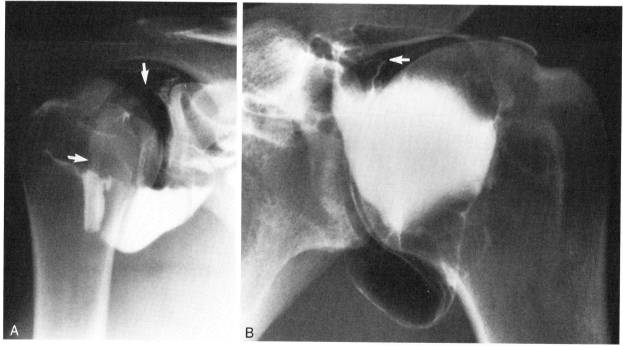

Figure 9–45. A, External rotation with upright weight bearing using double-contrast technique. Note that the biceps tendon can be seen from its origin to the point where it leaves the tendon sheath *(small arrows).* The undersurface of the cuff is well demonstrated. The subscapularis recess is small and compressed by the subscapularis during external rotation. *B,* View without weight bearing. Note superior glenoid labrum *(arrow).*

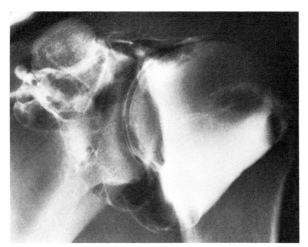

Figure 9–46. Internal rotation view. The subscapularis bursa is larger than that seen on the external view. The biceps tendon is obscured by contrast material and the medial humeral cortex.

Single-contrast examinations are effective for demonstrating cuff tears and are perhaps the study of choice for adhesive capsulitis. However, the synovium, articular cartilages, and labrum are often obscured using single-contrast technique. The biceps tendon is also more difficult to evaluate. Extravasation may be noted from the biceps tendon sheath and subscapularis bursa in normal individuals (Fig. 9–49).

Abnormal Arthrograms

Rotator Cuff Tears. The most common indication for shoulder arthrography is evaluation of patients with suspected tears in the rotator cuff. Many

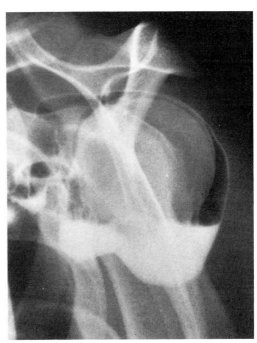

Figure 9–48. The scapular lateral view allows one to assess the capsular volume and entire circumferential synovial surface. Note also the normal relationship of the humeral head to the acromion.

patients with rotator cuff tear have a history of trauma. The incidence is higher in patients over 50 years of age.[94, 95, 100, 114] In our experience (552 cases), 91 percent were over 40 years of age.

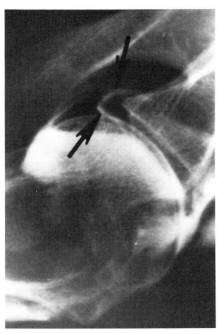

Figure 9–47. Prone axillary view with double-contrast technique. Note the glenoid labrum *(arrows)* and articular cartilage. Contrast medium pools in the anterior capsule.

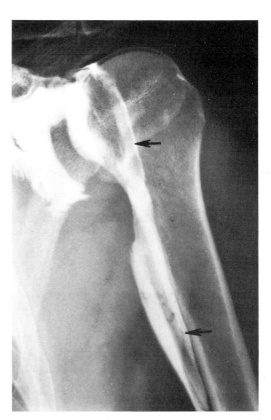

Figure 9–49. Contrast medium may leak from the biceps tendon sheath *(arrows)* in normal individuals.

The patient presentation as described by Neviaser[94] may include any of the following:

1. Trauma without fracture dislocation
2. Anterior dislocation
3. Dislocation with avulsion of the greater tuberosity
4. Chronic pain without history of trauma
5. Avulsion of the greater tuberosity.

In our study, all but 9 percent were chronic tears, with a history of trauma within 2 years in over 60 percent of patients. Of the 552 arthrograms reviewed, 145 patients were found to have complete tears of the cuff, as demonstrated by communication of the glenohumeral joint with the subacromial bursa (Fig. 9–50).

The most important views are the AP views with internal and external rotation. Almost all rotator cuff tears start in or are confined to the supraspinatus tendon. With external rotation of the shoulder, this tendon is the most lateral when compared with the other tendons of the rotator cuff. In rotator cuff tears, upward subluxation is most severe in this view, as the amount of tendon between the humeral head and the acromion is least. In the external rotation view, the distance from the edge of the humeral head cartilage to the tendon edge as defined by the dye is significant. This will depict the medial to lateral length of the tear. The extent of the tear in a posterior direction or the width of the tear, on the other hand, is assessed on the internal rotation view. When the shoulder is internally rotated, the infraspinatus beomes more lateral and lies under the acromion, as seen on the AP view. If the upper surface and undersurface of the tendon are well outlined and complete to the tendon insertion, the tear has not extended to any degree into the infraspinatus, and it is a small or medium-sized tear. If the tendon is

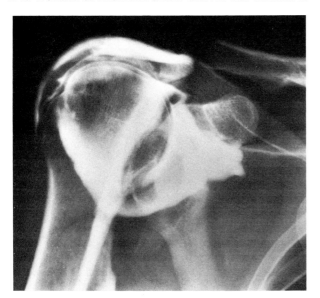

Figure 9–50. Single-contrast arthrogram demonstrating a complete rotator cuff tear. Contrast medium fills the subacromial and subdeltoid bursa. The articular cartilage and nature of the tear are difficult to evaluate.

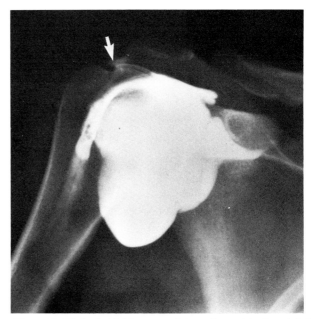

Figure 9–51. Partial-thickness cuff tear (arrow) in the distal supraspinatous portion of the cuff seen on external rotation.

not well outlined on both surfaces but another tendon gap is seen, the tear has extended into the infraspinatus and is at least large in size. If the axillary view shows a normal posterior capsule pouch, the tear is large; but if the posterior pouch is also obliterated, as mentioned previously, the tear likely extends to include the posterior aspect of the infraspinatus also and is global or massive in size. Finally, an anterior oblique view should be obtained to confirm observations of the extent of the tendon tearing.

In our series 38 patients had partial tears in which the arthrogram revealed extravasation of contrast material into the partial thickness of the rotator cuff (Figs. 9–51; also see Figs. 9–15 and 9–37B). Partial thickness tearing of the rotator cuff usually occurs in the supraspinatus. This can be seen as an extension of dye into the tendon substance but not into the bursa. If the contrast material extends past the end of the cartilage surface laterally, a portion of the tendon attachment is torn or has degenerated. These findings may be clarified by using a traction view in the upright position. Such findings also suggest that a careful evaluation is necessary, as a component of the impingement syndrome[41] related to anterior acromial osteophyte formation may well be present. Figure 9–52 points out the importance of multiple views in assessing the rotator cuff. The AP views were normal in this case.

Surgery or arthroscopy was performed in 140 of 183 patients and confirmed the arthrographic findings in 99 percent of the cases. False negative arthrograms are due to improper technique. Technical failures included improper injections, failure to exercise the patient sufficiently (Fig. 9–53), and a lack of awareness of the radiographic appearance of partial cuff tears. There were no false positives.

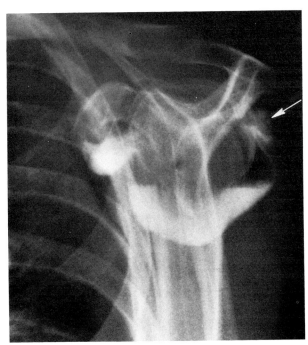

Figure 9–52. Partial-thickness cuff tear posteriorly *(arrow)*, which could only be identified on the scapular lateral view.

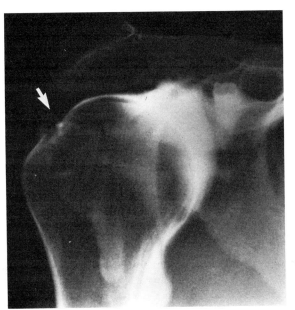

Figure 9–53. External rotation view with no evidence of a cuff tear. Note the bony projection from the greater tuberosity *(arrow)*. At surgery a large tear was present with fibrous scarring.

Eighty-five percent of complete tears involved the supraspinatus near its insertion into the greater tuberosity; the adjacent infraspinatus was also involved in 39 percent of the cases. Tears in the subscapularis and teres minor were much less common, occurring in only 12 percent of the patients.

The accuracy rate did not differ significantly when comparing single- versus double-contrast techniques. However, partial tears were more readily detected by utilizing double-contrast techniques. This technique allows one to evaluate the size of the tear and the appearance of the tendon ends

(Fig. 9–54). These findings may aid the surgeon in determining the best treatment.[69, 79, 102] We find that in tears of 1 to 2 cm in length evaluation of tendon ends is of value, but in larger chronic tears with extensive plain-film findings the tendon ends are more difficult to visualize owing to scarring (Fig. 9–54). In patients with superior subluxation and an acromiohumeral distance of 5 mm or less, we have found double-contrast technique to add little to the diagnosis. Also, in this setting, unless surgery is contemplated, we see little need to perform the arthrogram in the first place. Double-contrast arthrography is not utilized prior to arthroscopy, as the air hinders the arthroscopist.

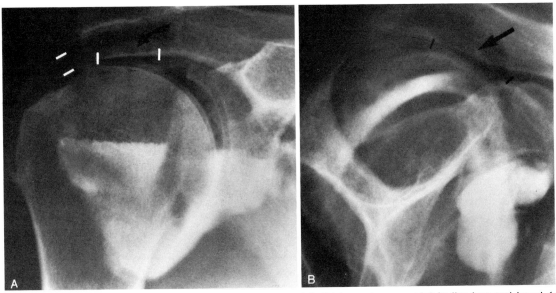

Figure 9–54. A, Double-contrast technique demonstrating a complete-thickness tear superior to the humeral head *(arrow)* on external rotation. Tendon thickness is easily assessed. *B,* The scapular lateral view demonstrates the AP dimensions of the tear.

TABLE 9–4. Arthrographic Findings in Adhesive Capsulitis

Diminished capsular volume (usually less than 10 ml)
Small axillary recess and subcapsularis bursa
Lymphatic filling
Irregularity at the capsular insertions

Adhesive Capsulitis. The term adhesive capsulitis was coined by Neviaser in 1953.[92, 93] Patients present with pain and varying degrees of reduction in the range of motion of the involved shoulder. The etiology is unclear, but it has been stated that the condition may be due to capsular thickening or adhesions involving the capsule, biceps, and subacromial bursa.[103] Simmonds and DePalma postulated that inflammation may be secondary to degeneration of the supraspinatus tendon and biceps tendon, respectively.[62, 109] To add to the confusion, a recent report in which arthroscopy was performed on patients with adhesive capsulitis noted no adhesions or intra-articular abnormalities. It stated that the etiology was more than likely extra-articular.[76] The final common result is cuff and capsular stiffness secondary to scarring.[115] Regardless of the etiology, however, arthrography is an effective diagnostic tool.

Suspected adhesive capsulitis was the third most common indication for arthrography in our series. Fifty-eight of 82 patients with decreased capsular volume had associated rotator cuff tears. Only 25 percent of patients with adhesive capsulitis alone demonstrated changes on the routine radiographs, and when present these were nonspecific, such as spurring of the glenoid or humeral head.

Arthrograms revealed a group of characteristic findings, which are presented in Table 9–4 (Fig. 9–55). The most common feature is decreased capsular volume, with reduced size of the axillary recess and subscapular bursa (Fig. 9–55). Patients may complain of shoulder discomfort after only several ml of contrast material has been injected.[66, 93, 94, 102] If double-contrast technique is used, the air will not be retained in the small capsule, and the joint will often decompress via the needle. After injecting 2 to 4 ml of contrast material it may become apparent that the capsule volume is only minimally reduced. Double-contrast technique adds little to the diagnosis.

In our series the biceps tendon sheath was not filled or only incompletely filled in 20 percent of patients with adhesive capsulitis. The significance of this finding is uncertain, but biceps adhesions have been described by several authors.[30–32, 69, 97, 100, 106]

Once the diagnosis is established, the arthrogram may then become a therapeutic tool to distend the contracted capsule and relieve, at least temporarily, the patient's symptoms.[69, 97] This can be accomplished by gradually distending the capsule with a mixture of contrast material and 1 percent lidocaine (Xylocaine).[56, 66, 70, 92, 100, 103] The injection volume is gradually increased until the capsule ruptures, and at this point further injection is unnecessary. The extravasation usually occurs along the subscapularis. This is followed by a set of assisted exercises with a gradually increasing range of motion (Fig. 9–56). To use this technique other precipitating or continuing sources of pain must be excluded. Unless a formal manipulation accompanies the procedure, the amount of success one will have in gaining more movement is uncertain. Our experience has

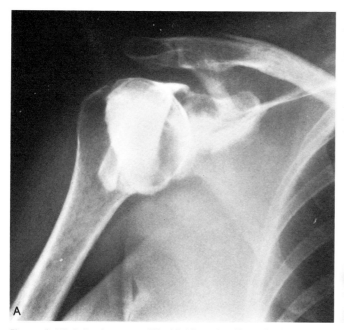
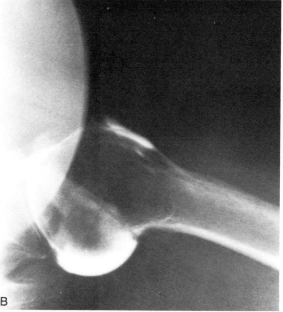

Figure 9–55. Adhesive capsulitis. AP *(A)* and axillary *(B)* views showing small axillary and subscapularis recesses. Biceps tendon is normal.

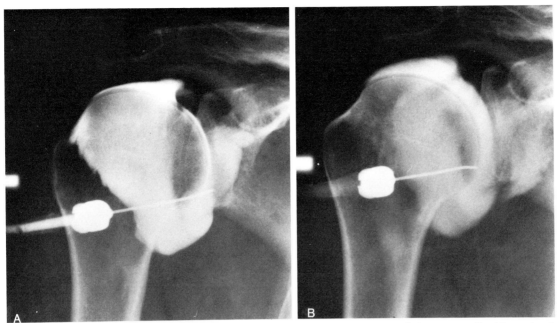

Figure 9–56. *A*, Adhesive capsulitis with reduced volume and small axillary and subscapularis recesses. The biceps tendon sheath is not filled. *B*, Following dilatation with contrast material and Xylocaine the volume is significantly increased. The tendon and sheath are now identified.

shown moderate success at best. Most patients do not seem to benefit particularly, but a few do. In patients with a rotator cuff tear dilatation is of little value, as the capsule will decompress into the subacromial bursa.

Biceps Tendon Abnormalities. Arthrography, if properly utilized, may aid in diagnosis of biceps tendon abnormalities. Again, plain film evaluation is important. A bicipital groove view should be obtained in cases of clinically suspected biceps tendon lesions. The bony appearance of the groove may provide some clue to the diagnosis. Cone and colleagues noted an average medial wall angle of 48°.[60] The average width was 11 mm and the depth 4.6 mm. Medial wall bone spurs and spurs in the groove were noted in 33 percent and 8 percent, respectively (Fig. 9–57). If the angle approaches 90°, constriction and tenosynovitis is said to be a diagnostic consideration. Angles less than 30° may be associated with subluxation of the biceps tendon.[60, 97]

The main difficulty in detecting biceps tendon abnormalities arthrographically is the lack of consistent filling of this tendon sheath. Preston[100] and Nelson[91] have reported nonfilling as abnormal; however, other authors,[66, 71, 103] including our group, cannot concur with this statement. Killoran reports that 11 percent of tendon sheaths failed to fill in otherwise normal arthrograms.[80] Normal tendon sheaths with nonfilling of the sheath were noted surgically in a significant number of patients during the preoperative arthrograms. Only when the tendon sheath is filled can evaluation of the tendon be accomplished. This is most accurate with double-contrast technique and bicipital groove views combined with weight-bearing internal and external

rotation views.[68, 69, 72] The number of tendon sheaths filled does not differ significantly with single- or double-contrast technique, but the detail, especially in the intracapsular portion, is much improved with the double-contrast technique (Fig. 9–45A). Goldman[73] described 9 biceps tendon abnormalities in 158 patients with double-contrast technique. Single-contrast exams in 198 patients failed to detect any abnormalities and missed 2 complete tears.[73] In our experience, biceps tendon involvement (nonfilling or synovitis of the sheath on the arthrogram) occurred in 20 percent of patients with complete rotator cuff tears and in 20 percent of patients with adhesive capsulitis. However, nonfilling and extrav-

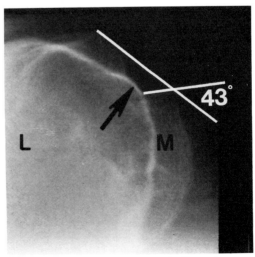

Figure 9–57. Bicipital groove *(arrow)* with angle of 43° measured by a line across the top of the tuberosities and a line along the medial wall.

TABLE 9–5. Arthrographic Biceps Tendon Abnormalities

> Tears—complete or partial
> Subluxation
> Tendinitis and entrapment
> Loose bodies

asation of the tendon sheaths are not necessarily significant findings.[66, 73, 103] Positive findings (Table 9–5) include complete or partial tears noted by absence of the tendon in the sheath, irregularity of the tendon, or distortion of the sheath (Fig. 9–58). Subluxation of the tendon is best seen on the bicipital groove view, but it can also be detected by failure of the tendon to change position properly on internal and external rotation views (Fig. 9–59).[66, 73, 103] Additional findings in our series included synovitis, loose bodies in the tendon sheath (Fig. 9–60), and surgically absent or transplanted tendons. In the total series of 552 arthrograms, excluding associated cuff tears, only 16 biceps abnormalities were detected (3 percent).

Articular Cartilage and Other Abnormalities. Arthrography is also valuable in evaluating the articular cartilage, glenoid labrum, and synovium. Cartilaginous lesions can be detected before they are obvious on plain films in rheumatoid arthritis, ankylosing spondylitis, and infection. More commonly, the arthrogram is utilized in patients with shoulder instability. Evaluation of the glenoid labrum for Bankart lesions and the humeral head for Hill-Sachs deformities may indicate dislocations.[8, 35, 36, 67, 73, 82, 91, 96] The capsule may be generous as well, indicating an additional factor contributing to the instability.

In evaluating the glenoid labrum and articular cartilage, double-contrast arthrography provides much greater detail. Care must be taken not to utilize more than 4 ml of positive contrast or large

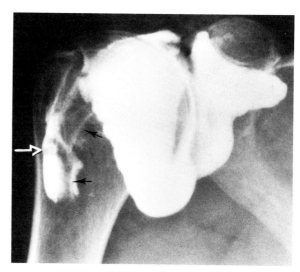

Figure 9–59. External rotation view. Note medial subluxation and irregularity of the biceps tendon *(black arrows)*. There is a partial tear and synovitis with a small loose body lateral to the tendon *(open arrow)*.

portions of the articular cartilage may be obscured. This is true in single-contrast arthrography as well (Fig. 9–61).

We prefer both supine and prone axillary views as well as fluoroscopically positioned internal and external rotation views for the best evaluation of the labrum and articular cartilage. In patients with shoulder instability better detail is offered by arthrotomography or double-contrast computed tomography[64, 84, 108] (Fig. 9–62). A Stryker notch view should be obtained to exclude a subtle Hill-Sachs deformity.

Double-contrast examination with a scapular lat-

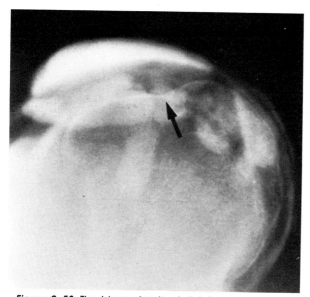

Figure 9–58. The biceps tendon is totally absent *(arrow)*. It was detached from its point of origin.

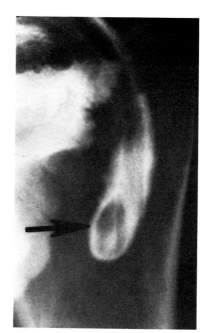

Figure 9–60. Localized view of biceps tendon with loose body *(arrow)*. Note also the irregular synovial pattern in the upper capsule and sheath.

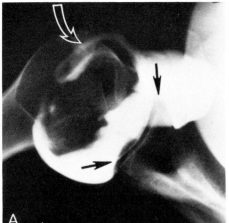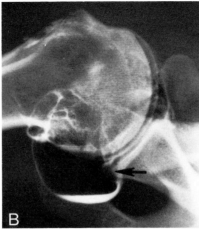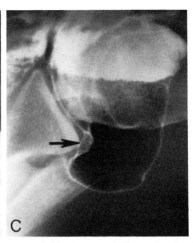

Figure 9–61. A, Single-contrast arthrogram, axillary view. The glenoid labrum is partially obscured *(black arrows).* Biceps tendon is well seen *(open arrow).* B, Double-contrast arthrogram in prone axillary view revealing normal rounded appearance of the posterior labrum *(arrow).* Articular cartilage is well demonstrated. Posterior capsule is normal. *C,* Previous posterior dislocation with slightly irregular posterior labrum *(arrow)* and generous capsule posteriorly. Compare capsule with Figure 9–61A.

eral view is also critical to evaluate capsule size and to detect any changes in the configuration of the anterior, posterior, and inferior recesses of the capsule (Fig. 9–63). With anterior dislocations the capsule may be stripped from the glenoid, resulting in a generous anterior capsule and loss of the separation between the axillary recess and subscapularis bursa.[67] To attach any significance to this, the arm must be in external rotation, as it is common for this confluence to occur without instability when the arm is internally rotated. Partial or complete rotator cuff tears may also be detected in association with chronic instability. Evaluation of patients with previous trauma or surgery may be aided by an upright weight-bearing view, which assists in determining the degree of laxity (Fig. 9–64).

Loose bodies may be sufficiently ossified to be detected on routine radiographs. However, arthrography can be helpful, especially when the loose bodies are in such unusual locations as the biceps tendon sheath (Fig. 9–60). Care must be taken not

to mistake air bubbles for loose bodies. If the arthrogram is specifically requested for the detection of osteocartilaginous fragments, single-contrast examinations, with or without tomography, may be more useful.

Synovitis, though nonspecific, indicates inflammation and along with other findings may aid in determining the patient's clinical problem. We detected synovial changes in 56 patients (10 percent) of 552 cases (Figure 9–65). Most patients with synovitis also had advanced degenerative arthritis and chronic rotator cuff tears. Dissecting synovitis was noted in 4 patients. The etiology of this condition is not clear, but synovitis has been associated with chronic cuff tears and rheumatoid arthritis, and it is also noted following local steroid injections.[89] We have also demonstrated this condition with adhesive capsulitis (Fig. 9–66). Steroids may result in connective tissue weakness, leading to synovial dissection. Subtle synovial changes are best detected with double-contrast technique, though gross

Figure 9–62. A, Axillary view demonstrating a torn anterior labrum. B, Double-contrast CT scan showing an intact anterior labrum *(arrow).* Note air in the sheath around the bicipital tendon *(arrow).*

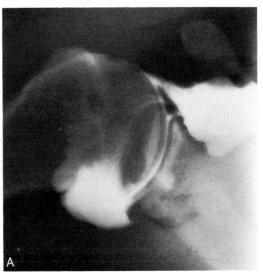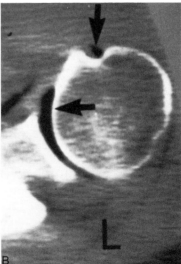

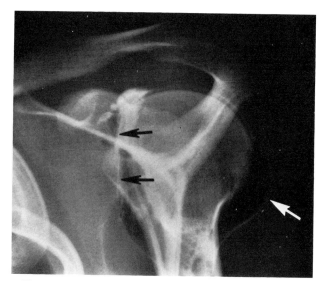

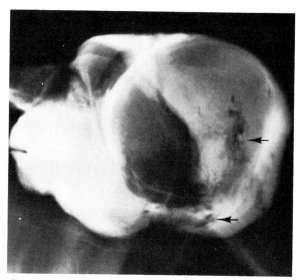

Figure 9–63. Previous anterior repair with straightening and reduction of the anterior recess *(double arrows)*. The posterior capsule is generous *(single arrow)*.

Figure 9–65. Irregular synovial filling defects *(arrows)* due to synovitis in a patient with degenerative arthritis. No evidence of a rotator cuff tear.

changes are usually obvious with single-contrast technique.

Chondromalacia is best detected arthroscopically, but it can also be seen with double-contrast arthrography. Findings include irregular thinning and subchondral sclerosis (Fig. 9–67).

Subtraction Arthrography of the Shoulder

With the increasing utilization of joint replacement, an arthrographic technique for postoperative evaluation has become necessary. Subtraction arthrography serves this need.

This technique differs only slightly from conventional arthrography of the shoulder. The patient is positioned as he or she would be for the usual shoulder arthrogram. Sandbags or some stabilizing device can be used to minimize any possible change in position of the arm and shoulder. Again, slight external rotation is best if possible. Following the usual sterile preparation, the skin is anesthetized over the medial margin of the head of the humeral component. A 22-gauge spinal needle is directed vertically, and when properly positioned, the metal head can be felt at the needle tip. The joint is aspirated and any contents sent for culture and

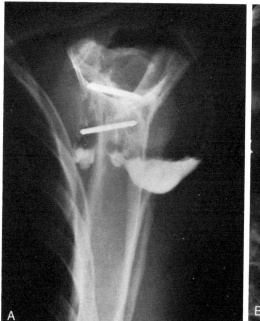

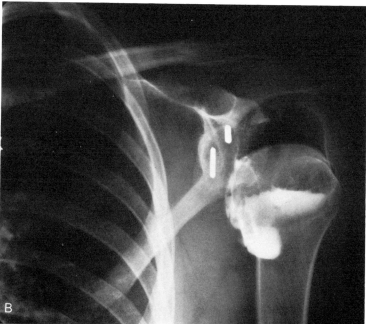

Figure 9–64. *A,* Scapular lateral view in patient with previous anterior repair and continued instability. Absent biceps tendon with inferior subluxation and slight reduction in capsular volume. (Compare with Fig. 9–63.) *B,* Upright weight-bearing view demonstrates marked inferior instability.

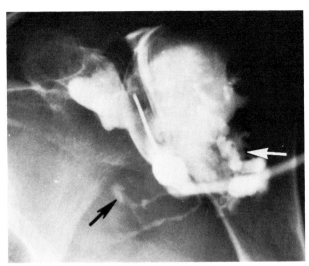

Figure 9–66. Reduced capsular volume with small axillary and subscapularis recesses. Note dissecting synovial cysts and lymphatic filling in the axillary region *(arrows).*

sensitivity. If no fluid is obtained, the joint is irrigated with sterile nonbacteriostatic saline, and the aspirate is then sent for culture. A film is taken to serve as the mask (see the discussion on subtraction in Chapter 1 for technical details). Hypaque-M-60 is injected until the capsule is distended. This must be accomplished for the accurate assessment of loosening. The end point for the injection occurs when (1) the patient experiences discomfort, (2) there is lymphatic filling, or (3) the contrast flows back into the syringe when pressure is released from the barrel. Following the injection, a film is taken for subtraction purposes and the needle is removed.

The patient is positioned for tangential internal and external rotation views, which are taken fluoroscopically. The shoulder is exercised under fluoroscopic monitoring, and push-pull maneuvering is performed. Axillary, scapular lateral, and upright weight-bearing views are also obtained.

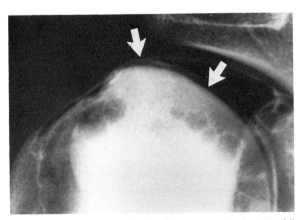

Figure 9–67. Double-contrast arthrogram with sclerosis of the humeral head, thinning of the articular cartilage *(arrows),* and increased density of the subchondral bone.

In evaluating these views one must examine the capsule size and synovium and also check for extravasation of contrast material at the bone-methacrylate interface. The latter indicates loosening (Fig. 9–68). If findings are equivocal, we have found it helpful to inject bupivacaine (Marcaine). Relief of the patient's symptoms suggests intra-articular pathology.

Subtraction arthrography offers three diagnostic tools: (1) culture or fluid study, (2) anatomic detail, and (3) diagnostic anesthetic for confirmation of the location of the patient's symptoms.

Pitfalls in Shoulder Arthrography

Inaccuracy in shoulder arthrography should not occur if proper attention is given to clinical data, plain film findings, and choice of technique. Proper needle position is essential. Improper position can result in extravasation, which if not detected fluoroscopically results in an indeterminate examination. Also, if the needle is inadvertently placed in the subacromial bursa (see Fig. 9–41*B*), a false diagnosis of rotator cuff tear may result. A most important and often overlooked factor is the necessity of quality films, in which proper projections are obtained by an experienced arthrographic technician. If such a person is not available, preliminary films in the prechosen postinjection positions should be obtained to avoid poor-quality films and repeat injections.

One must also take care not to utilize too much contrast material, which may obscure subtle changes. Injection of 20 ml of positive contrast material to exclude a complete cuff tear will totally obliterate any additional findings. This, then, dictates individualization of cases depending on the size of the capsule, which can be observed during the initial portion of the injection. Marked adhesive capsulitis will be obvious. In a normal capsule no more than 4 ml of contrast material and 10 to 15 ml of air is necessary for high-quality double-contrast examinations.

Proper evaluation of routine films can also aid in proper technique and diagnosis. A good example is the "double tuberosity" sign that was noted in 6 patients—all with complete rotator cuff tears. Because of the chronic nature of their clinical status, a bursal membrane or scarring partially seals the tear and makes arthrographic evaluation difficult. When this situation arises, further exercise or in some cases reinjection will identify the surprisingly large tears. Assuming proper technique has been employed, there are certain findings which may be confused with rotator cuff tears. Freiberger and Kaye report that contrast medium in the biceps tendon sheath may project laterally to the humeral head on the external rotation view and mimic a complete cuff tear.[66] Also, occasionally a small streak of contrast may be present above the origin of the biceps tendon near the superior glenoid labrum. This should not be confused with a rotator cuff tear (see Fig. 9–42).

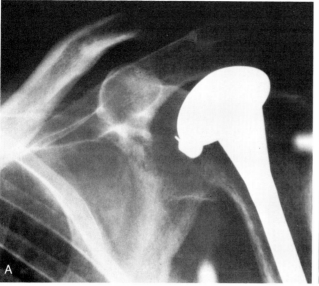

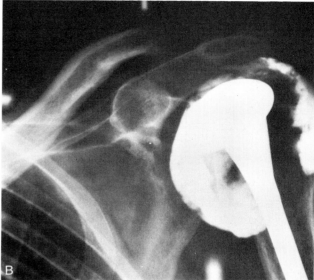

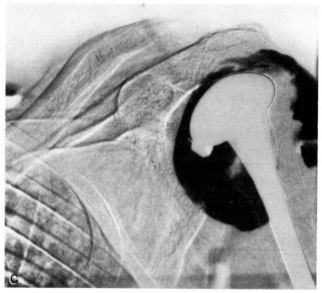

Figure 9–68. A, Neer prosthesis with needle tip positioned just medial to the head of the metal component. *B,* Conventional radiograph following injection of contrast material. Note extensive capsular irregularity due to synovitis. There is no evidence of loosening. *C,* Subtraction view confirms the findings in *B.* There is slight extravasation of contrast medium along the upper lateral humeral component. This was not evident on the routine arthrogram. Aspirated joint fluid did not demonstrate infection.

Healed partial or complete tears with fibrous nodules, deep central tears, and incomplete tears on the bursal side of the cuff may go undetected arthrographically.[100]

Complications in Shoulder Arthrography

Shoulder arthrography is a simple, relatively benign procedure with few potential complications.

No infections occurred in our 552 cases. Freiberger reports an incidence of infection of 1 in 25,000 cases.[66]

However, allergic reactions to contrast medium may occur and proper emergency medications (see Introduction to Arthrography in Chapter 1) should be available. Urticaria has been reported.[66, 67] Four percent of our patients developed urticaria following the procedure. In only one instance (1 of 552) were symptoms sufficient to warrant treatment with antihistamines.

Pain may occur following the arthrogram. Hall[77] and Pastershank[99] report increased pain in 74 percent of patients 24 to 48 hrs following arthrography. Mixtures of contrast material with small amounts of lidocaine may result in less discomfort, but especially with double-contrast technique this causes significant dilution of the contrast material and thus poor-quality films. Increased pain typically occurs 4 to 6 hr following the procedure in Hall's experience, and the pain may persist for up to 2 days.[77] This pain does not correlate with the arthrographic findings. Double-contrast technique results in less postprocedural pain than single-contrast examinations, perhaps owing to smaller volumes of contrast material.[77]

Goldberg reported increased pain with CO_2 as compared to room air in double-contrast examination of the knee. Reaspiration of the contrast material following the examination had no noticeable effect.[71]

Sterile effusions, perhaps owing to contrast medium irritation of the synovium, have been reported in the knee and aspiration is indicated for relief of pain. To date we have not experienced this problem with shoulder arthrography.

Shoulder Arthroscopy

Arthroscopy has become a valuable tool for the investigation and treatment of knee pathology. Burman, a pioneer in arthroscopy, recognized that shoulder arthroscopy was possible and not too difficult.[58] More recently, suggestions have been offered concerning the usefulness of arthroscopy in evaluating shoulder lesions. These include investigation of rotator cuff tears, biceps tendon lesions, periarthritis, shoulder instability, glenoid labral tears, degenerative joint disease, rheumatoid arthritis, congenital abnormalities, and postoperative pain.[57, 78] Certainly arthroscopy has a role in the evaluation or treatment of shoulder diseases (Fig. 9–69), but it is probably not as extensive as has been suggested.

The authors reviewed their recent experience with shoulder arthroscopy, and a number of points emerged.[59] For rotator cuff tears, arthrography is a highly diagnostic tool, and arthroscopy offers little or nothing in addition to this test. Bicipital tendon problems occur within the groove on the upper humerus and only rarely occur within the shoulder joint. Periarthritis is diagnosed by physical examination and, if necessary, arthrography. It is best treated by physiotherapy with or without manipu-

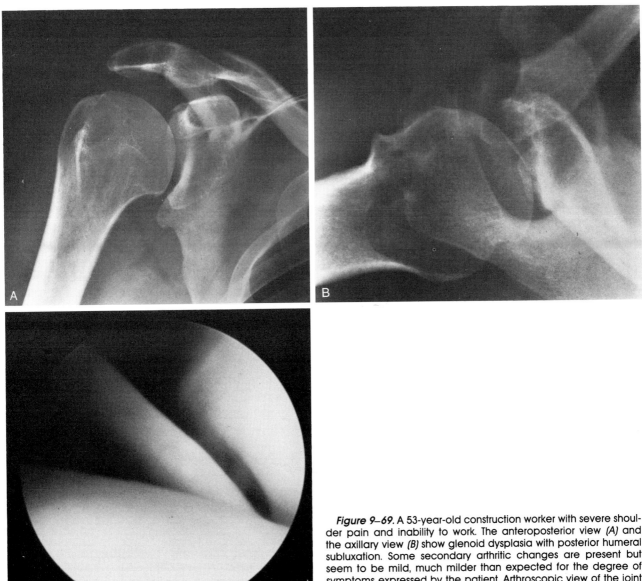

Figure 9–69. A 53-year-old construction worker with severe shoulder pain and inability to work. The anteroposterior view *(A)* and the axillary view *(B)* show glenoid dysplasia with posterior humeral subluxation. Some secondary arthritic changes are present but seem to be mild, much milder than expected for the degree of symptoms expressed by the patient. Arthroscopic view of the joint *(C)* shows normal cartilage of the humeral head. The biceps tendon is without inflammation or fraying, and the anterior aspect of the supraspinatous tendon is normal.

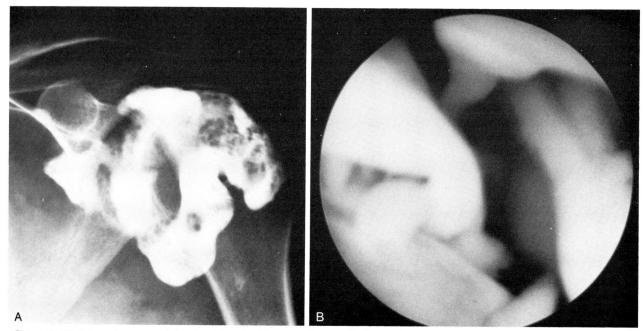

Figure 9–70. A, An arthrogram of the shoulder of a 22-year-old man with rheumatoid arthritis. The joint abnormalities in this patient were limited to the shoulder; before arthrography and arthroscopy with synovial biopsy, the diagnosis was uncertain. B, The arthroscopic view shows the drumstick-shape of the hypertrophic synovial fronds often seen in rheumatoid arthritis.

lation. In difficult cases with shoulder instability, arthroscopy was occasionally of value, but examination under anesthesia was more often helpful.

On the other hand, when x-rays are not compatible with the degree of joint related symptomatology, arthroscopy can stage arthritic diseases. It can also diagnose the disease with certainty when an atypical clinical picture is present (Fig. 9–70). Arthroscopy is valuable in the diagnosis and treatment of acute septic arthritis, though in chronic sepsis operative treatment is probably better. Computed tomographic scanning will now define glenoid fractures quite well, eliminating the need for arthroscopic evaluation. As one can see, the potential for arthroscopy, as for many other powerful diagnostic tools, is evolving and is not fully established.

Bursography

Contrast studies of the subacromial bursa (Fig. 9–71) are rarely performed but have been suggested as a means of evaluating partial tears in the superior surface of the rotator cuff, adhesive capsulitis,[102] and impingement syndrome.[61, 83, 110] The bursa may also be enlarged and inflamed in rheumatoid arthritis or any chronic inflammatory process.[103, 109, 111] Subacromial bursography, rather than arthrography, has been used in Japan to diagnose rotator cuff tears.[86]

We have utilized bursography infrequently, and to date the indications are still somewhat unclear. However, this technique may become more efficacious in the future, and certainly radiologists or orthopedists should be familiar with injection or aspiration of this bursa.

The subacromial bursa is a caplike structure between the rotator cuff and acromion with subdeltoid, subacromial, and subcoracoid portions. The normal bursa may be difficult to inject accurately.[82, 109]

Technique

The patient is placed on the fluoroscopic table in the supine position. The anterior shoulder is prepared with povidone-iodine (Betadine) solution as

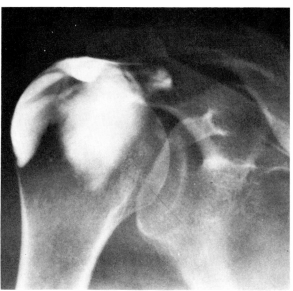

Figure 9–71. Normal single-contrast bursogram.

in arthrographic technique. The bursography set is the same as the tray used for arthrography. A 5-ml syringe with a 25-gauge needle is used to mark the subacromial region, and a wheal is made in the skin with 1 percent lidocaine (Xylocaine). The soft tissues are also anesthetized. Following injection of the local anesthetic, a 1 1/2-inch 22-gauge needle is advanced vertically and slightly superiorly under the acromion. When the undersurface of the acromion is reached, the needle can be withdrawn 1 to 2 mm, and the tip should be in the subacromial bursa. Any fluid should be aspirated at this time and sent for the appropriate laboratory studies. Three ml of Hypaque-M-60 and 5 or more ml of room air are used to distend the bursa. This promotes better elevation of the synovium and upper surface of the cuff, allowing these as well as any extrinsic ligamentous or bony deformity of the bursa to be evaluated. Radiographs are obtained in internal and external rotation, axillary, and scapular positions. The scapular lateral view allows the most advantageous study of the acromial and coracoid relationships to the bursa.

Following the radiographic study, diagnostic or therapeutic injection with bupivacaine or lidocaine and betamethasone (Celestone) may be performed, thus adding to the versatility of the study.

Acromioclavicular Arthrography

Radiographic approach to the acromioclavicular joint, though not commonly employed compared with glenohumeral arthrography, may be of diagnostic and therapeutic value.

Arthrography has been reported to be useful in determining the extent of ligamentous injury following acromioclavicular separations.[116] Resnick[102]

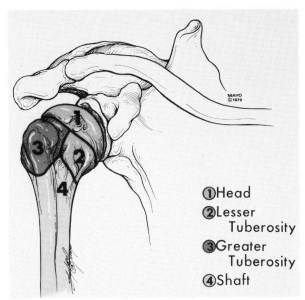

Figure 9–72. The four major anatomic fragments used to describe proximal humeral fractures in the displacement system of Neer.[8]

① Head
② Lesser Tuberosity
③ Greater Tuberosity
④ Shaft

describes potential utilization of this technique in rheumatoid arthritis to diagnose cystic formation and synovitis, but it is likely that acromioclavicular arthrography will be restricted to therapeutic injections or diagnostic aspirations and will remain an infrequently performed procedure.

The anatomy of the acromioclavicular joint results in an "L"-shaped cavity, with the leg of the "L" projecting under the distal clavicle.[112] The capsule is lined with synovium and is reinforced by the superior and inferior acromioclavicular ligaments. The normal joint capacity is 1 to 2 ml.[102, 112]

Patients to be studied are prepared in the usual

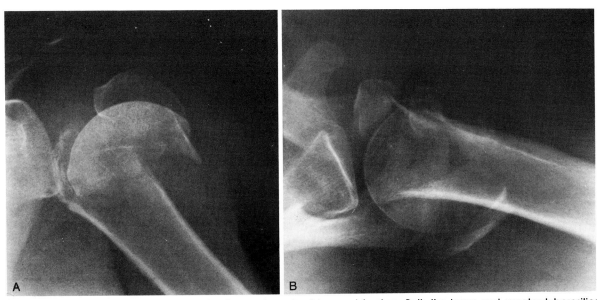

Figure 9–73. AP *(A)* and axillary *(B)* views of a four-part proximal humeral fracture. Both the lesser and greater tuberosities are fractured from the humeral head and displaced from their normal positions in relation to the humeral head. The humeral head is also displaced relative to the humeral shaft and is angled upward and posteriorly.

TABLE 9–6. Proximal Humerus Fractures: Classification and Incidence*

Type	Incidence (%)
Two-part (one segment displaced in relation to other three)	13
Three-part (two segments displaced in relation to other two)	3
Four-part (all segments displaced)	4

*After Greenway and colleagues[133] and Neer and Rockwood.[154]

manner with sterile technique. The needle is advanced from a position superior to the joint following injection of local anesthetic. Fluoroscopic guidance assures proper positioning. One to 2 ml of Hypaque-M-60 can be injected. This normally should not extend beyond the capsule. Extension of contrast material medially toward the coracoid indicates coracoclavicular ligament injury.[99]

Other Procedures

Diagnostic injections of local anesthetic may be useful. Also, areas of tendon calcification may be helped through irrigation of the calcium with sterile saline via injection. This results in a breakup of the calcium, and some fragments may actually be aspirated. The procedure is followed by injection of the involved area with a 1:1 mixture of bupivacaine (0.5 percent) and betamethasone. This procedure may result in significant symptomatic relief of calcific tendonitis.

TRAUMA

Fractures of the Proximal Humerus

Fractures of the proximal humerus usually occur in older patients. If one considers all fractures, about 5 percent involve the proximal humerus.[129, 133, 154] In older patients, the fracture most often occurs after minor trauma, such as a fall. In younger individuals, the skeletal strength is greater than provided by ligaments, so that dislocations usually occur instead of fractures.[138, 154] When fractures occur in this age group, they usually result from significant trauma (motor vehicle or motorcycle accidents).

Codman[128] demonstrated that fractures of the proximal humerus tend to follow the physeal lines that divide the humerus into four parts, the humeral head, lesser tuberosity, greater tuberosity, and shaft (Fig. 9–72). Neer[150] proposed the most widely accepted classification of fractures of the proximal humerus. This classification is based on the number of fragments and the degree of displacement or angular deformity. If there is 1 cm of displacement between the fragments or greater than 45° of angular malposition, the fragment is considered to be displaced (Figure 9–73).

The majority of proximal humeral fractures (80 to 85 percent) are undisplaced. Fractures most commonly involve the surgical neck.[136, 165] The rotator cuff, capsule, and periosteum assist in maintaining position of the fragments[133, 154] (Table 9–6). A two-part fracture indicates that one fragment is displaced more than 1 cm or angulated more than 45°.

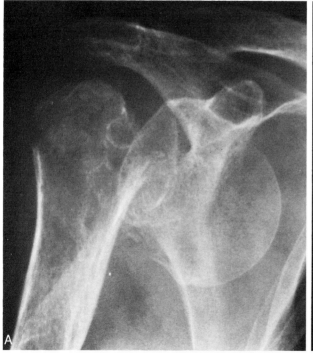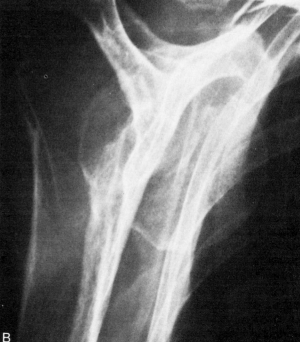

Figure 9–74. Three-part anterior fracture-dislocation. AP view *(A)* and scapular Y-view *(B)* demonstrate anterior dislocation of the humeral head with superior positioning of the shaft. The greater tuberosity remains in the joint space.

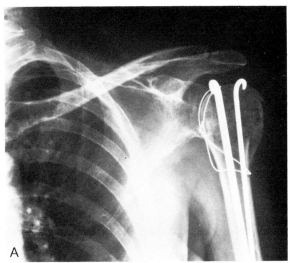
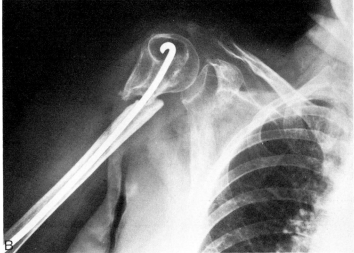

Figure 9–75. A, Internal fixation of a three-part fracture with two Rush rods and wire. There is good anatomic reduction. B, Non-united fracture with loose Rush rod. Note the sclerotic fracture ends and lucency around the rod due to motion.

Three-part fractures have two displaced or angulated fragments (Fig. 9–74). With four-part fractures (Fig. 9–73), all fragments are displaced. Isolated fractures of the tuberosities are rare unless there is an associated dislocation.

As a general rule, with two-part displacement closed manipulation restores acceptable position. Immobilization with a sling or Velpeau immobilizer is followed with early exercise to avoid adhesive capsulitis.[154] Open reduction is occasionally attempted to restore position. The pectoral muscles may cause medial displacement of the shaft (Fig. 9–75). Open reduction is generally required with three-part fractures. When all four fragments are

displaced, a proximal humeral prosthesis is considered because of the relatively high frequency of late avascular necrosis of the separated head fragment. If there is an associated shoulder dislocation, the displacement classification is still useful to classify the injury and to predict the type of treatment that will be needed (Figs. 9–74 and 9–76).

Other classifications of surgical or anatomic neck fractures do not adequately describe the variety of injuries seen. The classification of humeral fractures as abduction or adduction fractures is usually spurious, as the direction of arm rotation will affect the x-ray appearance. In most of these fractures, the apex of the head-shaft angulation is actually anterior

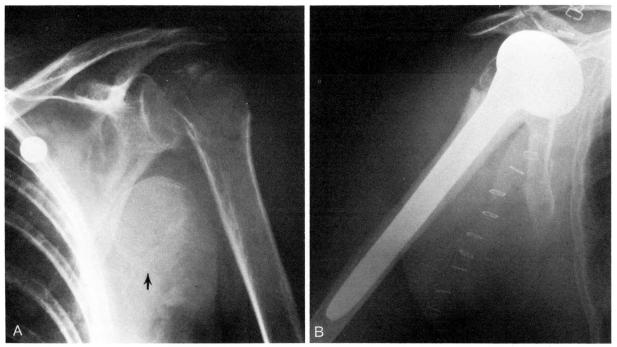

Figure 9–76. A, Fracture-dislocation with humeral head *(arrow)* in the axillary region. B, Treated with a Neer prosthesis and fixation of tuberosities.

(Fig. 9–75). Accurate radiographic evaluation can be obtained with the shoulder trauma series (40° posterior oblique in external rotation, axillary view, scapular view). In certain situations, tomography may be indicated.

Significant complications in undisplaced proximal humeral fractures are uncommon.[141] Adhesions may cause a reduced range of motion and pain. This can be reduced by including early mobilization as a part of the treatment plan.[154, 165]

Injury to the axillary artery and vein or brachial plexus may occur with significant displacement of the surgical neck. These structures lie just anterior and inferior to the capsule.[154, 165]

Non-union or malunion may occasionally occur (Fig. 9–75B). Neer reported non-union more commonly in patients treated with hanging casts.[151]

Malunion due to fracture of the greater tuberosity or significant angulation of neck fractures can result in decreased range of motion. Joint reconstruction may be necessary in the most severe cases (Fig. 9–76).

Avascular necrosis is common following four-part fractures or displaced fractures of the anatomic neck. The blood supply to the head is disrupted in these cases.[154]

Glenohumeral Dislocations

Dislocations of the glenohumeral joint occur more frequently than dislocations at any other articulation. They account for 50 percent of all dislocations.[154, 165] Most dislocations are anterior (97 per-

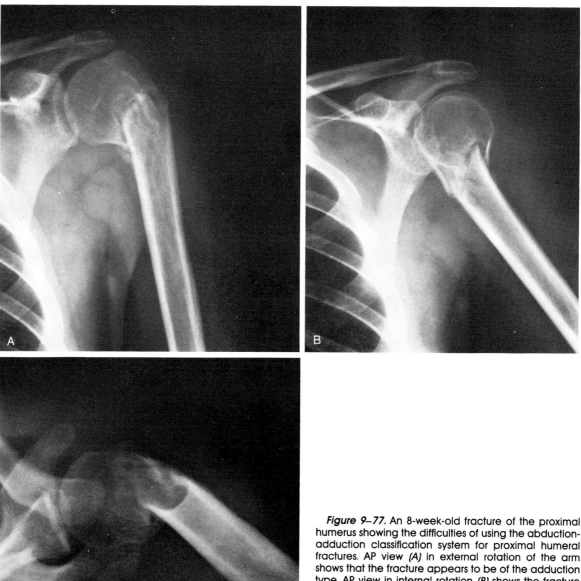

Figure 9–77. An 8-week-old fracture of the proximal humerus showing the difficulties of using the abduction-adduction classification system for proximal humeral fractures. AP view *(A)* in external rotation of the arm shows that the fracture appears to be of the adduction type. AP view in internal rotation *(B)* shows the fracture to be of the abduction type. The axillary view *(C)* shows that the actual angulation is anterior. This is the usual direction of displacement seen with this type of fracture.

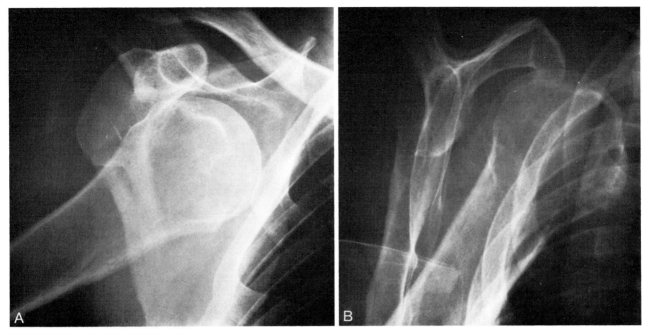

Figure 9–78. Subcoracoid anterior dislocation, AP view *(A)* and scapular Y-view *(B)*. The Y-view most clearly demonstrates the humeral head relationship to the glenoid.

cent). Posterior dislocations occur in 2 to 4.3 percent of patients, and superior and inferior dislocations are rare.[131, 154, 159, 164, 165]

Anterior Dislocations. Most anterior dislocations (96 percent) are due to trauma, though certain individuals can voluntarily dislocate their shoulders.[168] Traumatic dislocations usually result from a fall with the arm in abduction and external rotation. Rarely, the dislocation is due to direct posterolateral trauma. In adolescence, dislocations in males outnumber those in females 5:1.[154, 161] As the humeral head dislocates, it is forced anteriorly and inferiorly against the capsule, glenohumeral ligaments, and subscapularis (Fig. 9–77). These structures provide the majority of the shoulder's anterior stability.[130, 176] The posterolateral aspect of the humeral head comes in contact with the glenoid rim, which may result in an associated impaction fracture. This was described by Hill and Sachs and bears their name, the Hill-Sachs deformity.[137] This lesion occurs in 67 to 76 percent of cases.[159, 171] Associated lesions of the anterior inferior glenoid rim reportedly occur less frequently, appearing in approximately 50 percent.[154, 161, 165] However, Rowe determined that the Bankart lesion was the most common finding in patients with recurrent dislocations.[171]

Most anterior dislocations are obvious on the conventional AP radiograph. However, a routine trauma series is most accurate (40° posterior oblique, axillary, "Y"-view) for complete assessment of the dislocation and associated fractures. Dislocations are described according to their location. In order of decreasing frequency, dislocation may be subcoracoid (Fig. 9–78), subglenoid, subclavicular, or intrathoracic. Intrathoracic dislocations are rare but

are associated with more significant complications.[154]

Following closed reduction, the radiographic trauma series, except for the axillary view, should be repeated. The radiographs must be carefully studied to assure adequate reduction and to exclude associated fractures (greater tuberosity, Hill-Sachs, or glenoid rim). For example, if the anterior dislocation results in the humeral head lying medial to the coracoid, reduction may be more difficult. Interposition of the tendon of the long head of the biceps may occur with this type of dislocation, making reduction difficult or impossible. Displacement of the biceps tendon should also be considered in dislocations with large greater tuberosity fractures, for the bicipital groove may be involved.[139] Fractures of the greater tuberosity occur in up to 15 percent of anterior dislocations.

Additional views (described in the earlier section on radiographic techniques) are useful in detecting subtle Hill-Sachs deformities and glenoid rim fractures. The Stryker notch view is easy to duplicate and for Hill-Sacks deformities in 90 percent of patients with recurrent dislocation.[134] AP internal rotation views will detect Hill-Sachs deformity in 50 percent of patients with recurrent dislocation.[150] Glenoid rim fractures may be obvious on the routine axillary or West Point views.[121, 166] However, labral injuries may be present with no obvious bony changes. Therefore, double-contrast arthrography, with or without CT, or arthrotomography may be indicated in patients with recurrent dislocations.

Treatment of anterior dislocation can usually be accomplished with closed reduction (Fig. 9–79). Exceptions include patients with soft tissue inter-

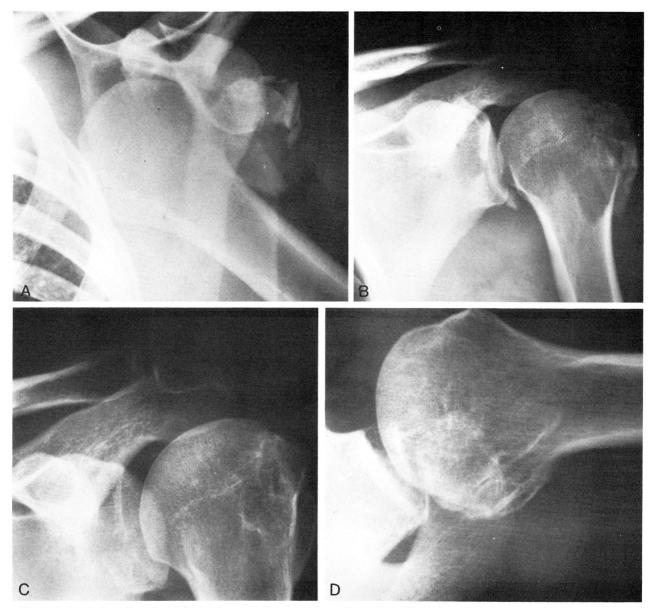

Figure 9-79. AP view *(A)* of the shoulder demonstrating an anterior dislocation with fracture of the greater tuberosity and glenoid. Following closed reduction, the greater tuberosity is close to normal anatomic position *(B)*. There is a fragment below the glenoid. This could have been localized with axillary views or CT. AP *(C)* and axillary *(D)* views after healing.

position, subacromial greater tuberosity displacements, and large (> 5 mm) glenoid rim fractures.[5] Glenoid fractures can lead to recurrent dislocation or traumatic arthritis.[120, 140, 154, 177] Internal fixation is considered in these patients.

Posterior Dislocations. Only about 2 to 4.3 percent of shoulder dislocations are posterior.[128, 144, 154, 157, 159, 165, 178] The injury may follow electric shock therapy, seizures, or falls with the arm adducted and internally rotated. Direct trauma to the anterior shoulder may also cause dislocation, but this is not common.[161, 178]

Clinically, the patient's arm may be held in slight abduction and internal rotation. External rotation is blocked. Unfortunately, the diagnosis is missed clinically in many patients.[154, 165]

The injury may be easily overlooked on the conventional AP view. There are, however, several signs present:

1. The humeral head is fixed in internal rotation (100 percent).

2. The joint may appear abnormally widened or narrowed.

3. The usual "half moon" overlap of the humeral head and glenoid may be absent or distorted (55 percent).

4. A "trough line" may appear in the humeral head, representing a compression-fracture of the anterior aspect of the humeral head (75 percent).

5. There may be an associated fracture of the lesser tuberosity (25 percent).[127]

Routine use of the 40° posterior oblique AP,

scapular Y-view, and axillary view (trauma series) should prevent missed diagnoses of posterior dislocation. The Y-view is particularly useful, as the relationship of the humeral head to the glenoid is easy to access. Also, the view can be obtained without moving the arm (Fig. 9–80). Rather than memorize the various signs on the conventional AP view, we suggest use of these alternative views for more accurate diagnoses.

Normally, the distance from the medial margin of the humeral head to the anterior glenoid rim is no more than 6 mm.[118] Posterior dislocation results in an increase in this distance, the rim sign.[118, 165] The normal overlap between the head and posterior rim of glenoid will be absent.

Posterior dislocations are also described by loca-

tion. The majority (98 percent) are subacromial, but subglenoid and subspinal (scapular spine) dislocations also occur.[157, 161] On the AP view, posterior subglenoid and subspinal dislocations may mimic an anterior dislocation.[154] The problem is easily solved with the scapular Y-view. Fractures of the lesser tuberosity and less commonly of the glenoid and posterior capsule tears with rim fractures are associated with posterior dislocations.[127, 154, 165]

Posterior dislocations can usually be treated with closed reduction. The incidence of recurrence is much lower than that with anterior dislocations.[135, 154]

Superior and Inferior Dislocations. Superior and inferior (luxatio erecta) dislocations are rare.[131, 154, 161] Superior dislocations overlie the acromion or

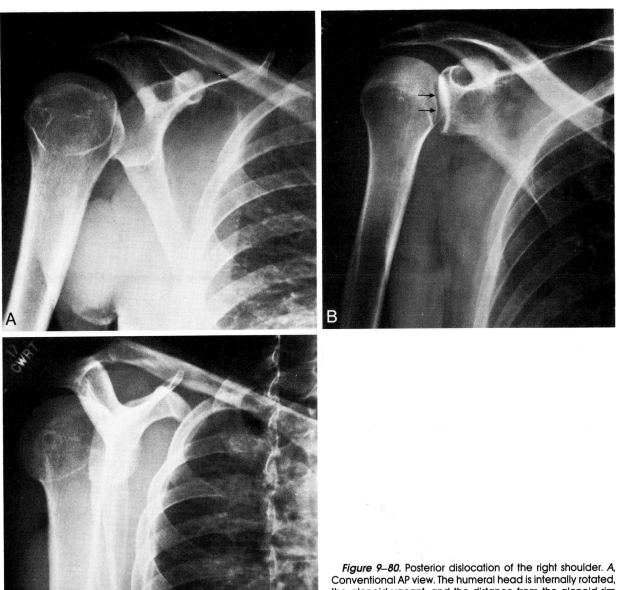

Figure 9–80. Posterior dislocation of the right shoulder. *A,* Conventional AP view. The humeral head is internally rotated, the glenoid vacant, and the distance from the glenoid rim to humeral head increased. *B,* 40° oblique AP view. There is overlap of the joint spaces (compare to normal view in Fig. 9–11*B*). Note the "trough line" due to the impacted head fracture *(arrows). C,* The scapular Y-view clearly demonstrates the posterior dislocation.

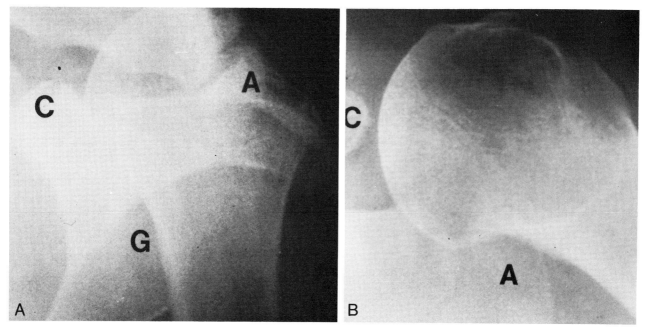

Figure 9–81. Superior dislocation of the shoulder. *A,* AP view with acromion (A), coracoid (C), and glenoid (G) labeled. The humeral head overlies the acromioclavicular joint. *B,* The axillary view shows the relationship of the humeral head to the coracoid (C) and acromion (A). (From Downey, E. F., Jr., Curtis, D. J., and Brower, A. C.: Unusual dislocations fo the shoulder. AJR *140:*1207, 1983 © 1983, Am. Roentgenic Ray Soc.)

clavicle on the AP view (Fig. 9–81). This dislocation is usually due to a severe upward force on the adducted arm.[131] With luxatio erecta, the humerus becomes parallel to the spine of the scapula, and the arm is abducted (Fig. 9–82). Downey reported

this type of dislocation in 0.5 percent of all dislocations.[131] This injury is due to force on the flexed arm (above the head). As a result the humeral head is forced downward. These types of dislocations can usually be managed initially with closed reduction, but more injuries and rotation cuff tears may be present.

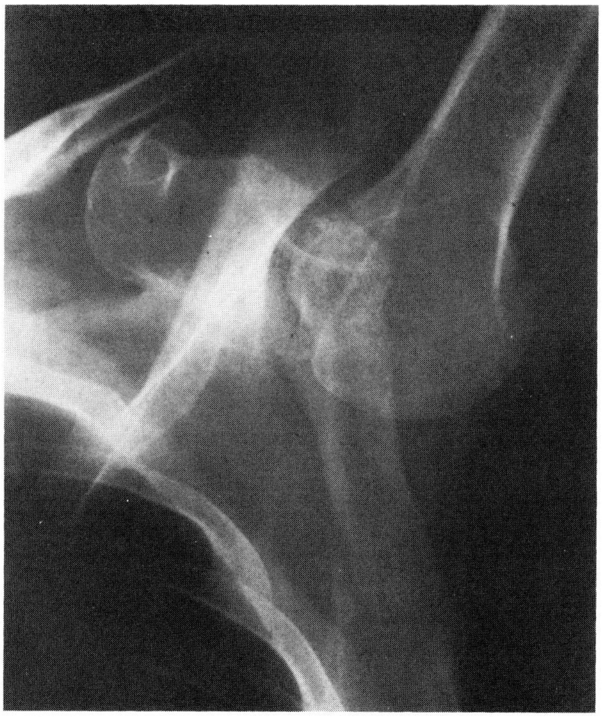

Complications of Glenohumeral Dislocations

Complications of glenohumeral dislocations and fracture-dislocations are more common than complications of proximal humeral fractures. Associated fractures and recurrent dislocations are the most common problem.[154, 165] Rowe[171] reviewed 39 patients with recurrent anterior dislocation. He noted Bankart fractures in 84 percent, Hill-Sachs deformities in 76 percent, and capsular laxity in 83 percent of operated shoulders. Radiographic assessment of these complications has been discussed earlier in this chapter. Rupture of the capsule and tears on the rotator cuff may occur either acutely or with recurrent dislocations.[144, 163] Arthrography is important in the evaluation of patients with suspected soft tissue or cartilaginous injury following dislocation (see section on Shoulder Arthrography).

Neurovascular injury may occur in the axillary region following dislocations. Vascular injuries include laceration, thrombosis, intimal laceration, and false aneurysms of the axillary artery.[136, 141, 154, 161, 179] Axillary artery injuries may be overlooked initially owing to collateral circulation. Peripheral pulses may be present even with significant axillary artery injury.[136, 141] Early diagnosis with selective angiographic techniques is essential to determine the

Figure 9–82. Erect dislocation (luxatio erecta). The humerus is parallel to the scapular spine, with the humeral head inferior to the glenoid. (From Downey, E. F., Jr., Curtis, D. J., and Bower, H. C.: Unusual dislocations of the shoulder. AJR *140:*1207, 1983 © 1983, Am. Roentgenic Ray Soc.)

TABLE 9–7. Acromioclavicular Dislocation: Classification and Prognosis*

Classification	X-ray	Prognosis
Type I. Ligament sprain, a few ligament fibers torn	Normal	No instability; excellent
Type II. Rupture of the capsule and acromioclavicular ligaments	Joint wide, clavicle may be slightly elevated	May require arthroplasty if symptoms persist; 90% recover, 10% may require surgery
Type III. Rupture of capsule, acromioclavicular ligaments, and coracoclavicular ligaments	Elevated clavicle, increased coracoclavicular distance	Internal fixation; 80% good, 20% reoperation

*After Neer and Rockwood.[154]

extent of injury. Amputation rates following axillary artery occlusion have been reported to be as high as 43 percent.[136]

The axillary nerve crosses the subscapularis anteriorly.[154] Stretching or compression can occur, especially with anterior dislocations. Fortunately, complete disruption is uncommon, and loss of function is rare.[154, 175] Simeone recommends exploration only if neural deficit persists beyond 3 months after reduction.[175]

Acromioclavicular Dislocations

Dislocations of the acromioclavicular joint (12 percent) occur less commonly than glenohumeral dislocations (85 percent). Rowe and Marble reported only 52 cases in 1,603 patients with shoulder trauma.[169] The mechanism of injury is usually a fall in which force is directed to the point of the shoulder. Dislocations due to indirect forces directed superiorly through the humeral head have also been reported.[154, 161] Nielsen found that the majority of injuries were due to direct trauma and that only 5 percent were due to falls on the outstretched hand.[156]

Allman[117] classified acromioclavicular joint injuries based on the degree of ligament injury. Table 9–7 describes the categories of injury, the radiographic findings, and the prognosis used in Allman's classification. Radiographic changes in Type I and Type II injuries may be subtle. The radiographs are normal in Type I (Fig. 9–83). Generally, radiographs of the shoulder will overpenetrate the acromioclavicular joint. Therefore, it is best to obtain well coned views centered on the joint, with the tube angled 15° to the head. This will reduce the amount of bony overlap. Weight-bearing views are essential to diagnose Type II lesions and to differentiate Type II from Type III injuries[122, 154, 161] (Fig. 9–84). In Type III injuries, the coracoclavicular ligaments are torn if the distance between the upper aspect of the coracoid and the undersurface of the clavicle is greater than 50 percent or increased > 5 mm compared with the normal shoulder.[122, 154]

Treatment of most Type I and II injuries is successful with closed methods. Occasionally, closed reduction fails with Type II lesions and late distal clavicle excision is necessary. Internal fixation is more often necessary with Type III injuries.[154, 161]

Adjacent fractures can accompany acromioclavicular dislocation (Fig. 9–85). In our experience the coracoid and clavicle are fractured most frequently. Intra-articular acromial fractures may also occur.

Heterotopic ossification in the coracoclavicular and acromioclavicular region has been reported (Fig. 9–86).[119, 154] The incidence reported varies from 57 to 82 percent.

Migration of pins has also been reported following internal fixation.[812]

Sternoclavicular Dislocations

Dislocations of the sternoclavicular joint are uncommon. Rowe reported that this injury occurred in 3 percent of all shoulder dislocations.[169] Dislocation usually results from indirect trauma to the shoulder. Posterolateral forces transmitted medially cause anterior dislocation, and anterolateral forces result in posterior dislocation. Direct anterior trauma can occur in sports such as football. This causes posterior dislocation.[154, 160, 161, 169] Anterior dislocations occur much more frequently than pos-

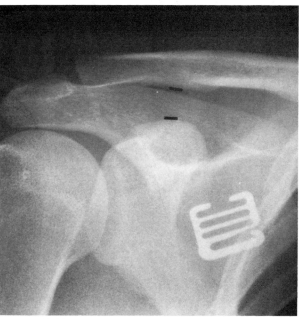

Figure 9–83. Mild sprain of the acromioclavicular ligaments. The joint space and coracoclavicular distance *(lines)* are normal even with weight bearing.

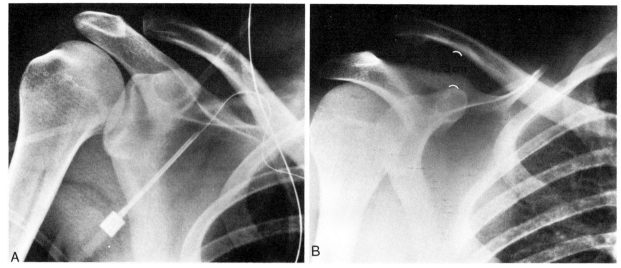

Figure 9–84. *A,* Widening of the right acromioclavicular joint with apparently normal coracoclavicular distance. View without weight bearing (Type II versus Type III). *B,* Weight-bearing views clearly demonstrates the complete dislocation and coracoclavicular ligament disruption (Type III).

terior dislocations.[150, 155] Nettles and Linscheid reported that 3 of 60 sternoclavicular dislocations were posterior.[155]

Anterior dislocations may be easily palpable. Posterior dislocations can be more difficult to diagnose clinically owing to swelling. Unfortunately, early diagnosis is necessary, as reduction after 48 hours is difficult.[174] In addition, posterior dislocations may be potentially fatal injuries owing to involvement of the trachea and great vessels.

Allman[117] classified sternoclavicular dislocations in the same manner as acromioclavicular dislocations. Type I injuries cause only slight tearing of

the sternoclavicular ligament. In Type II lesions the sternoclavicular ligament is torn, and Type III injury results in tears of both the sternoclavicular and costoclavicular ligaments. In the latter situation, either anterior or posterior dislocation occurs.

Radiographic evaluation of this injury is difficult. Overlying structures often cause confusion. Since the lesion is uncommon, radiographic technicians are often unfamiliar with appropriate techniques. However, a simple technique described by Hobbs is usually sufficient for complete dislocations (see section on Radiography). Angling the tube 40° to the head projects the sternoclavicular joints supe-

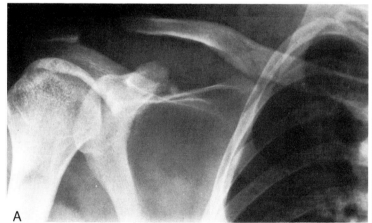

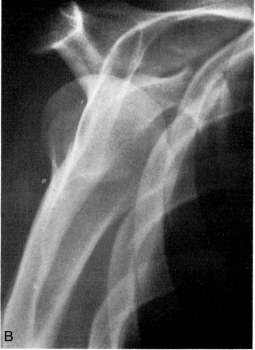

Figure 9–85. *A,* Acromioclavicular separation and undisplaced clavicle fracture seen on the AP view. *B,* The scapular Y-view more clearly demonstrates the coracoid fracture.

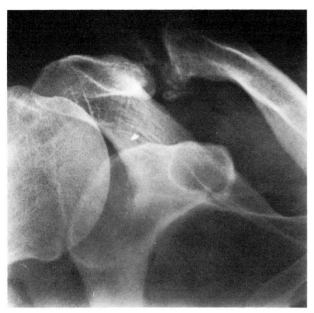

Figure 9–86. Ossification following unsuccessful closed reduction of the acromioclavicular joint.

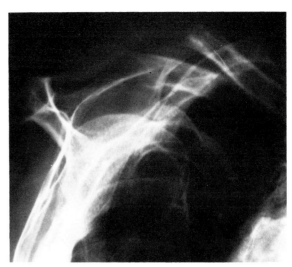

Figure 9–87. Scapular Y-view demonstrating overriding of a midclavicle fracture.

riorly. If the anterior dislocation is present, the involved clavicle will be higher than the normal side. With posterior dislocations, the involved clavicle is lower (see Fig. 9–22C). Conventional and computed tomography may be helpful in more difficult cases.[142, 174] Actually, CT provides sufficient images for accurately evaluating subluxations as well as complete dislocations (see Fig. 9–91C). Subtle changes in the joint are much more obvious with CT than with routine films or tomography. The direction of displacement is also more obvious. An additional advantage of CT is the ability to assess the trachea, great vessels, and adjacent soft tissues. Magnetic resonance imaging may prove to be equally effective in this regard.

Treatment of sternoclavicular dislocation is usually successful with closed techniques.[126, 154, 158, 161] Problems can occur with internal fixation. Migration or fracture of pins and screws may result in injury to the retrosternal vessels or airway.[154, 182]

Most significant complications are associated with posterior dislocation. Fortunately, this injury is not common. Injuries to the arch vessels, trachea, and esophagus have been reported.[154, 161, 172, 181] Nerve injury may also occur. Injuries to the great vessels and trachea may be life threatening, indicating the urgency of early diagnosis of posterior dislocation.[167] The incidence of complications is 25 percent.[154, 172, 181]

Surgical complications may occur as well, and closed reduction is attempted in most cases.[126] A major problem is migration of Steinmann pins or Kirschner wires into the anterior superior mediastinum. Omer[158] reported operative complications in 5 patients who had metal fixation of a sternoclavicular dislocation. Complications included infection, pin fracture, and pin migration.

Clavicle Fractures

Clavicle fractures are common, especially in children.[154, 161, 165] The injury usually is caused by a fall on the outstretched hand. The lateral force directed through the shoulder results in fracture of the midclavicle (Fig. 9–87). Less frequently direct trauma to the clavicle or shoulder results in fracture.

Fractures of the middle third of the clavicle are most common (80 percent).[117, 153, 165] Allman[117] classified clavicle fractures anatomically. Group I fractures involve the middle third of the clavicle. Displacement of these fractures is common (Fig. 9–88). The sternocleidomastoid elevates the proximal fragment, and the weight of the arm tends to lower the distal fragment.[1, 3, 42] This results in a superior tented radiographic appearance. Group II fractures involve the distal clavicle (lateral to the coracoclavicular

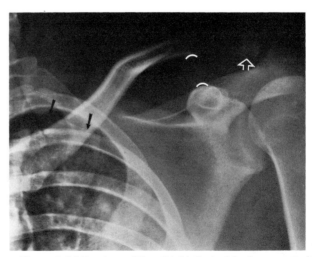

Figure 9–88. Fracture of the distal left clavicle *(open arrow)* with rupture of the coracoclavicular ligaments (Neer Group II). Note the pneumothorax *(black arrows)* and upper-lobe pulmonary contusion.

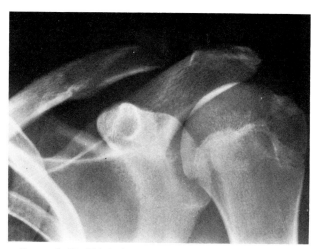

Figure 9–89. Distal clavicle fracture involving the articular surface with associated widening of the joint.

ligament). These fractures make up 15 percent of clavicle fractures.[117, 165] Group III fractures (5 percent) involve the medial clavicle.

Radiographic evaluation of the mid- and distal clavicle is not difficult. AP or oblique views of the clavicle (see section on Radiography), with the tube angled 15° to the head, will allow good visualization of the mid- and distal clavicle (Fig. 9–89). The angulation projects the clavicle above the chest. A coned-down 15° angled view is best to overcome the problem of overpenetrating the acromioclavicular joint. Subtle midclavicle fractures may be overlooked. If symptoms dictate, a 40° cephalic angle may make detection less difficult (Fig. 9–90). Evaluation of the proximal clavicle is more difficult. Forty-degree angled views and oblique views are usually adequate if the fracture is displaced. In selected cases, especially undisplaced fractures, tomograms or computed tomography may be necessary (Fig. 9–91).

Most clavicle fractures can be treated with closed reduction using shoulder support (sling, "Figure of 8," etc.).[154, 161] Group II fractures of the distal clavicle may require internal fixation. Resection of the distal clavicle may be required in patients with persistent symptoms.

Significant complications are less common with clavicle fractures than with glenohumeral fracture-dislocations. Malunion of midclavicle fractures or excessive callus formation does occur. This may result in compression of the adjacent neurovascular structures between the clavicle and first rib.[146, 161]

Non-union occurs in only 1 to 2 percent of cases.[180] Osteoarthritis may occur following intra-articular fracture. This is more common at the acromioclavicular joint. Post-traumatic osteolysis may be seen in the distal clavicle following trauma. This is usually not associated with fractures of the distal clavicle. Patients present with continued pain and weakness after trauma. Erosive changes develop on the distal clavicle, which are visible on the radiograph (Fig. 9–92). Involvement may progress to the level of the coracoclavicular ligaments.[162] Changes may be due to synovial hyperplasia, but this is uncertain. Following treatment with immobilization some degree of bone healing occurs, though the joint often remains widened.[162]

Scapular Fractures

Fractures of the scapula are uncommon (1 percent of all fractures).[161] Injury to the body of the scapula is caused by direct force. The scapula is well protected by an envelope of muscles. Therefore, considerable force is required to cause the fracture, and displacement of body fractures is usually not significant. Associated fractures of the ribs, clavicle, and spine, however, are not unusual. Injury to the lungs and bronchi may also occur. Evaluation of

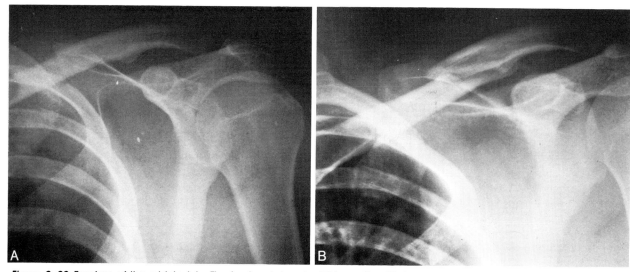

Figure 9–90. Fracture of the midclavicle. The fracture is barely visible on the AP view *(A)*. The 15° cephalic angle view *(B)* makes the diagnosis obvious.

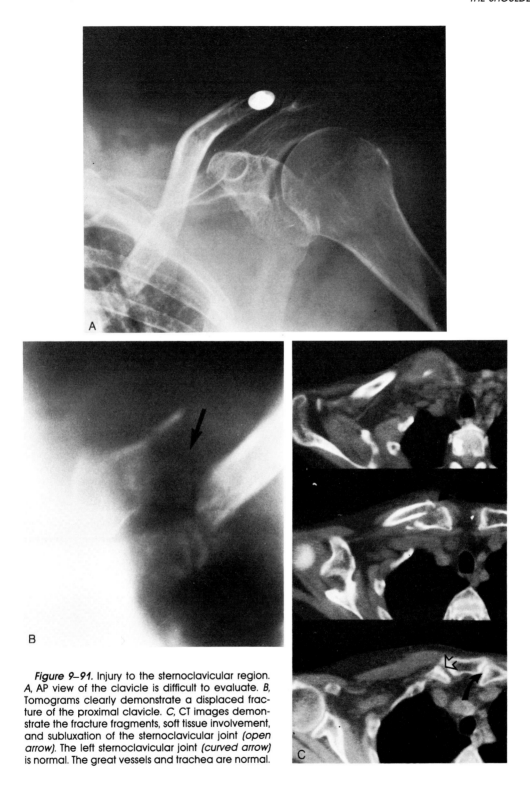

Figure 9–91. Injury to the sternoclavicular region. *A*, AP view of the clavicle is difficult to evaluate. *B*, Tomograms clearly demonstrate a displaced fracture of the proximal clavicle. *C*, CT images demonstrate the fracture fragments, soft tissue involvement, and subluxation of the sternoclavicular joint *(open arrow)*. The left sternoclavicular joint *(curved arrow)* is normal. The great vessels and trachea are normal.

the body of the scapula is usually successful with AP and lateral views.

Fractures of the body may extend to the glenoid articular surface (Fig. 9–93). Most commonly, glenoid fractures are associated with dislocations. However, Varriale and Adler[177] have described glenoid fractures that are not associated with dislocation. Fractures may be undisplaced, displaced, or bursting. Detection of glenoid fractures is critical

because, if displaced, they lead to traumatic arthritis. Scapular Y, West Point, and axillary views are most useful in demonstrating these fractures[120, 177] (Fig. 9–94). Occasionally CT images are needed, especially if open reduction is considered. Avulsion fractures of the infraglenoid tubercle are due to forceful triceps contraction.[124] This fracture may also lead to recurrent dislocation, especially if a portion of the rim is involved.[124, 154] Subtle avulsions of the

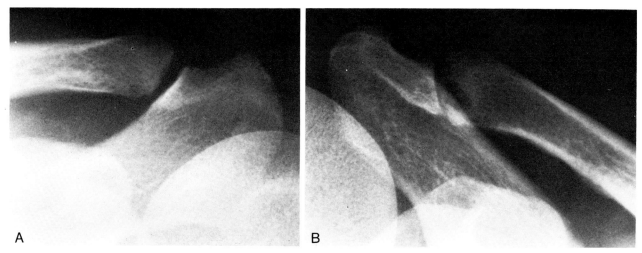

Figure 9–92. Post-traumatic osteolysis. *A,* Normal clavicle. *B,* Erosions in the involved clavicle.

infraglenoid tubercle may require a Bennett view for detection. This view is taken with the arm abducted 90° and the elbow flexed. The tube is angled 5° to the head and centered on the shoulder.[124]

Fractures of the acromion are due to a direct blow from above. Radiographic diagnosis is not difficult in most cases. The axillary and Y-view are particularly useful in the diagnosis of subtle acromial fractures (Fig. 9–95).

Fractures of the coracoid process may be due to direct trauma or avulsion. Most fractures occur at the base. Displacement is usually prevented by ligament attachment.

Muscular origins of the scapula include the coracobrachialis, short head of the biceps, and pectoralis minor.[167] Repeated trauma in trapshooters may result in a coracoid stress fracture.[125, 173] Radiographic evaluation of coracoid fractures should include the scapular Y-view and axillary views[173] (Fig. 9–96). In addition, weight-bearing views should be consid-

ered. Fractures of the coracoid are associated with acromioclavicular dislocation.[143] Subtle injury may also be identified with the oblique angled view described by Goldberg and Vicks.[132] The patient is rotated 20° posteriorly, and the tube is angled 20° toward the head. This view projects the coracoid above the adjacent skeletal structures.

Most scapular fractures are managed conservatively. Internal fixation may be necessary if significant displacement has occurred (Fig. 9–33).

RECONSTRUCTIVE SURGERY

The use of x-rays in the analysis of shoulder subluxations or dislocations has been described. The two other major areas of reconstructive shoulder surgery are rotator cuff disease and arthritis.

The many nonspecific changes seen in rotator cuff disease on the greater humeral tuberosity or the acromion have been mentioned in many studies and have been emphasized by Golding.[189] His claim that there are changes on the routine x-ray of a shoulder with rotator cuff disease is, of course, in contrast with Codman's classic description of normal x-rays in those with supraspinatus tendon tearing.[183] The humerus may show cystic changes near the tuberosity, sclerosis, or, in advanced cases, resorption or erosion. The acromion may also show sclerosis or osteophytes in people with rotator cuff disease.[192] This has recently been re-emphasized, as have the frequently accompanying osteophytic changes at the acromioclavicular joint.[195] In more advanced rotator cuff disease with tendon tearing, the inferiorly convex appearance of the acromion will become inferiorly concave.

Much attention has been directed to the superior subluxation of the humeral head in which there is a decrease in the distance between the top of the humeral head and the undersurface of the acromion.[187, 190] According to Golding, the acromiohu-

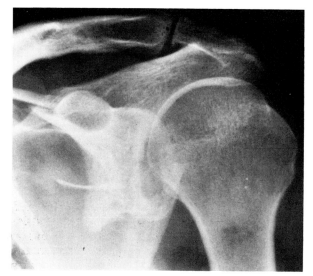

Figure 9–93. Fracture of the body and neck of the scapula.

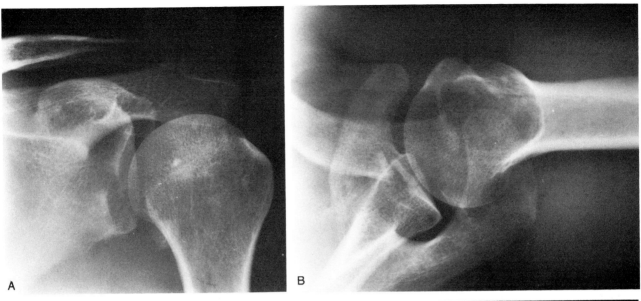

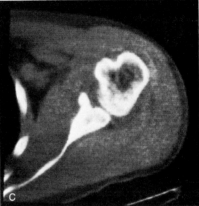

Figure 9–94. Glenoid fracture demonstrated on AP view *(A).* The axillary view *(B)* shows the fracture anteriorly. CT scan *(C)* demonstrates the position of the fragment most accurately.

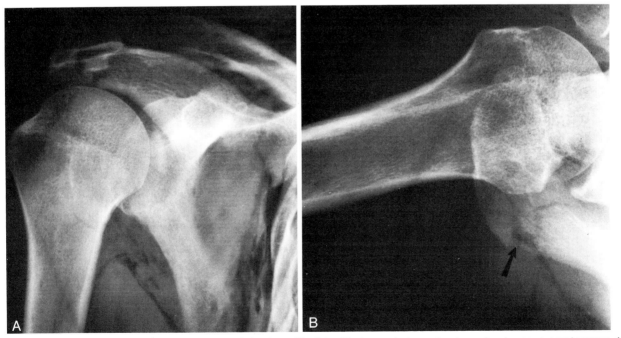

Figure 9–95. Undisplaced comminuted acromial fracture. AP view *(A)* demonstrates extensive subcutaneous emphysema. Air overlying the bone makes detection of fracture difficult. Axillary view *(B)* demonstrates the acromial fracture *(arrow).*

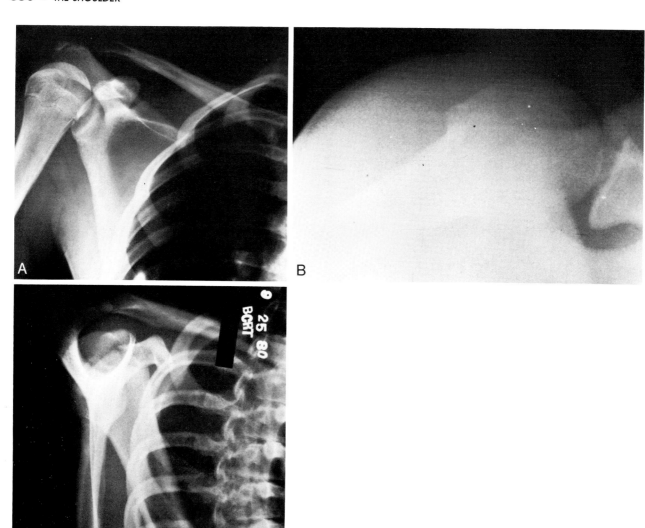

Figure 9–96. Shoulder pain after anterior trauma. AP *(A)* and axillary *(B)* views are negative. Scapular Y-view *(C)* clearly demonstrates the coracoid fracture.

meral interval was found to vary between 7 and 13 mm in 150 normal shoulders. In a series by Cotton and Rideout[186] a range from 6 to 14 mm was considered normal. Weiner and MacNab[196] reviewed 60 patients with normal shoulders; the normal acromiohumeral space seemed to be 7 to 14 mm. Our data indicate that 95 percent of patients with an acromiohumeral measurement ≤ 7 mm had rotator cuff tears. Subluxation of the humeral head superiorly is not an early change, and in small rotator cuff tears there may be no subluxation. However, in the Weiner and MacNab data, of those with rotator cuff tears only 24 percent had an interval of 9 mm or more. Eighty percent of normal shoulders had an interval of 9 mm or more. They felt that an interval of 5 mm or less should be considered an indication of a significant rotator cuff tear. The acromiohumeral interval in rotator cuff tears is usually smaller with external rotation of the humerus.

This is most often true in medium-sized rotator cuff tears. With external rotation the supraspinatus is positioned laterally under the acromion, and when it is torn the humerus can subluxate upward, which represents a minor joint contracture from the unbalanced muscle activity in the deltoid. When subluxation upward is pronounced in both internal and external rotation views, a larger tear including the infraspinatus is present. In diseases with a chronic synovitis (most notably rheumatoid arthritis), the tendon thickness can be rather uniformly diminished with secondary upward humeral subluxation and no rotator cuff tearing; thus, in rheumatoid disease the decreased acromiohumeral interval is indicative of rotator cuff disease, but the tendons may not have full-thickness tearing. Rotator cuff disease in rheumatoid arthritis has been studied with arthrography,[188] and the surgical pathology in rheumatoid arthritis has been determined in those

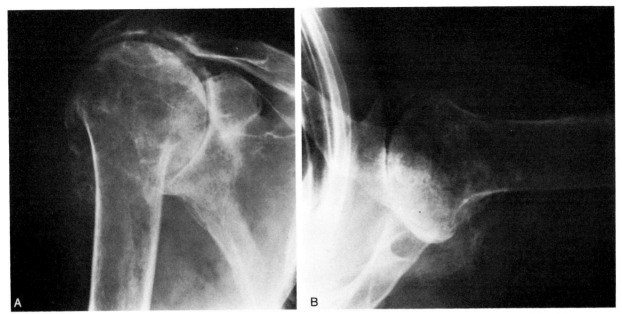

Figure 9–97. Radiographs of a 68-year-old man with a long-standing history of shoulder tendinitis, weakness of shoulder movement, and now stiffness with pain. The x-rays *(A and B)* show a severe upward subluxation of the humeral head with abutment against the acromion and loss of the articular cartilage. This has been termed cuff tear arthritis.

individuals requiring prosthetic arthroplasty.[185, 194] Rotator cuff tearing in rheumatoid arthritics with significantly symptomatic shoulder disease is present in only 25 to 40 percent of shoulders.

Recently, an entity called cuff tear arthritis has been described (Fig. 9–97).[194] It seems as if severe long-standing rotator cuff disease may, in some cases, cause enough instability, joint destruction by rubbing of the humeral head cartilage against the acromion, or alteration of the cartilage nutrition to create this picture. The "Milwaukee shoulder"[191]—rotator cuff defects often associated with some cartilage loss—may have a similar x-ray appearance.

In patients with this syndrome, microspheroids containing hydroxyapatite crystals, active collagenase, and protease activity are present in the synovial fluids. These findings have led to speculation on a scheme for causation of this problem.

Until the last decade little attention was directed to the clinical or x-ray evaluation of shoulder arthritis. Probably this neglect can be attributed to how little was available for effective treatment or confirmation of the pathology. Neer[193] did describe the pathology seen in osteoarthritis of the shoulders (Fig. 9–98). The humeral head is well seated in the glenoid, with flattening of the central aspect of the

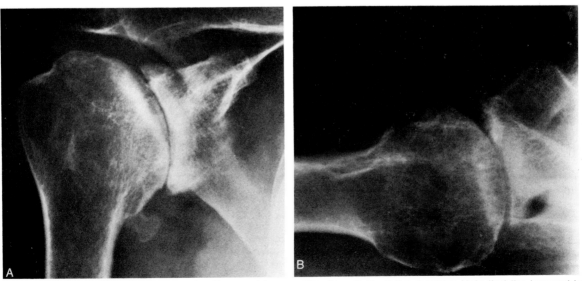

Figure 9–98. AP *(A)* and axillary *(B)* views of a 68-year-old man with osteoarthritis of the shoulder. Note that the humeral head is well centered on the glenoid in the AP view. There is flattening of the central portion of the humeral head, cartilage loss, subchondral bony sclerosis, and osteophyte formation along the humeral neck region. The axillary view shows the posterior humeral subluxation and the asymmetrical glenoid erosion with more glenoid erosion posteriorly than anteriorly.

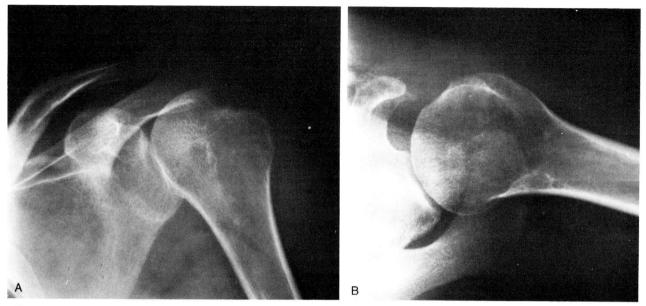

Figure 9–99. A 24-year-old man with rheumatoid arthritis of the shoulder. *A,* AP view shows erosion at the junction of the articular surface of the humerus with the greater tuberosity. This often simulates a Hill-Sachs type of lesion. *B,* Axillary view shows narrowing of the cartilage joint space.

humeral head, and often there is osteophyte formation along the humeral neck. It is also important to recognize the asymmetrical glenoid erosion that occurs, which may be associated with posterior humeral subluxation. This radiographic picture should not be confused with cuff tear arthritis, as reconstructive surgical planning and expectations for results are vastly different in the two cases.

X-ray appearance in rheumatoid arthritis varies greatly. There may simply be osteoporosis. Early signs of synovitis and joint space narrowing (best seen on the axillary view) may be apparent. The synovitis can cause juxta-articular erosion on the humeral head mimicking a Hill-Sachs lesion (Fig. 9–99). Cartilage loss, osteoporosis, and slight upward humeral subluxation is a most typical appearance of a significantly symptomatic rheumatoid shoulder (Fig. 9–100). Variations in bone erosion may be seen with loss of the humeral head (Fig. 9–101), central erosion of the glenoid (arthrokatad-

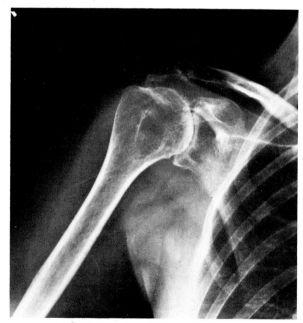

Figure 9–100. The most typical x-ray appearance of rheumatoid arthritis in the shoulder. AP view shows osteoporosis, loss of the cartilaginous joint space, and slight upward subluxation of the humeral head.

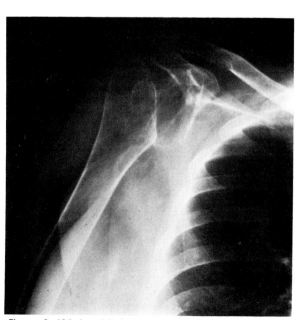

Figure 9–101. An elderly woman with long-standing severe rheumatoid arthritis. X-ray shows osteoporosis and loss of substance of the humeral head.

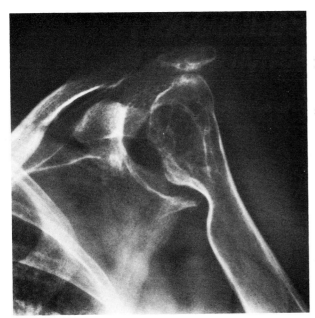

Figure 9–102. An elderly woman with long-standing rheumatoid arthritis severely involving both shoulders. The radiograph shows upward subluxation of the humeral head and loss of bone substance both on the humeral head and the glenoid. The resorption of bone is most striking in the glenoid, with central erosion present. This condition has been termed arthrokatadysis of the scapula.

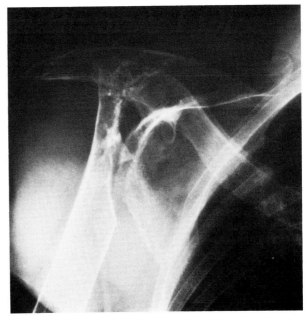

Figure 9–103. Advanced rheumatoid arthritis showing the severe resorption of both the humeral head and the glenoid.

ysis of the scapula) (Fig. 9–102), or loss of both the humeral head and the glenoid (Fig. 9–103). Rotator cuff disease and upward subluxation in rheumatoid arthritis have been mentioned earlier. Loss of the subscapularis may cause anterior subluxation, and some rheumatoid arthritic shoulders actually pres-

ent with anterior dislocations in the absence of trauma (Fig. 9–104).

In arthritis secondary to old fractures or fracture-dislocations, the various components of the shoulder must be analyzed with an eye toward reconstructive planning. The glenohumeral cartilage is assessed on 40° posterior oblique and axillary views. Humeral head positioning on the glenoid and on the humeral shaft are analyzed on these views and

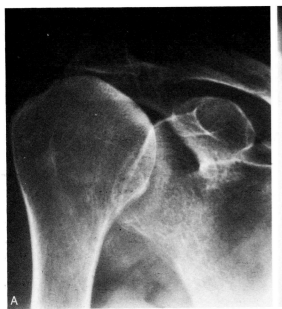
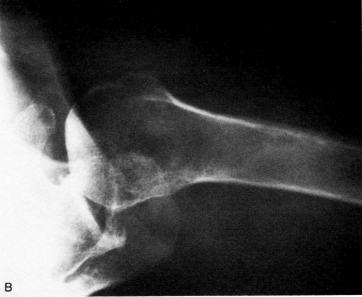

Figure 9–104. A middle-aged patient with long-standing rheumatoid arthritis. AP view *(A)* shows some cartilage loss and upward subluxation of the humeral head on the glenoid. Axillary view *(B)* shows anterior subluxation of the humeral head on the glenoid in addition to the cartilage loss. This indicates damage to the rotator cuff and capsule, particularly in the anterior and superior aspects of these structures.

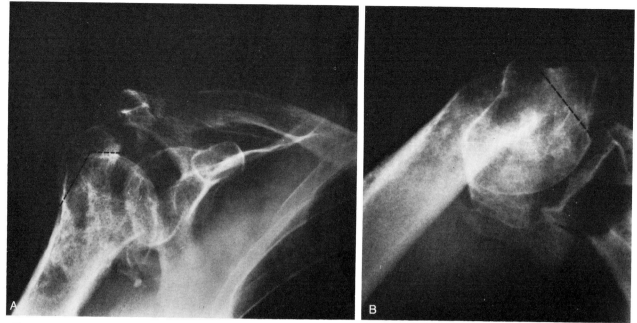

Figure 9–105. A 66-year-old man with glenohumeral arthritis secondary to an old four-part proximal humeral fracture. Multiple x-ray views are necessary for surgical planning. AP view *(A)* indicates the lines of osteotomy necessary to restore greater tuberosity position. Axillary view *(B)* indicates the line of lesser tuberosity osteotomy necessary for reconstruction of this tuberosity behind a prosthesis. (From Tanner, M. W., and Cofield, R. H.: Prosthetic arthroplasty for fractures and fractures-dislocations of the proximal humerus. Clin. Orthop. *179:*116, 1983.)

the anterior oblique view. Tuberosity position is assessed on all three views. With this information osteotomies can be planned (Fig. 9–105).

There are other more rare causes of arthritis requiring the need for reconstructive surgery. Septic arthritis of the shoulder does not differ in appearance from that seen in other joints. Idiopathic avascular necrosis is similar in appearance to that seen in the hip. The "crescent sign" is less frequently seen, but when seen it is best appreciated on the axillary view. Radiation necrosis of the shoulder, subchondral humeral bone collapse, and cartilage loss can occur one or more decades following radiation therapy treatment for carcinoma of the breast (Fig. 9–106). This is amenable to reconstruction, but added difficulties are expected, notably wound healing problems and joint stiffness owing to the extensive tissue destruction and reactive scarring.

Postoperative analysis of prosthetic shoulder arthroplasties is quite difficult. After proximal humeral prosthetic replacement, the x-ray may look quite good, though pain is present, or the converse may obtain. This is not surprising, as the same situation appears in replacement surgery of the proximal femur, using a Moore or Thompson replacement. Loosening of the prosthetic stem in the bone may be present without an abnormality present on the x-ray. If the prosthesis is articulating against a glenoid surface without cartilage, the symptoms are probably related to this absence of cartilage. The rotator cuff is difficult to evaluate after prosthetic surgery with either a proximal hu-

meral component alone or a total shoulder replacement. The healing response to surgery and a foreign implant is to deposit fibrous tissue. X-ray dye injected into the joint usually outlines the joint and prosthesis but rarely depicts a subacromial or sub-

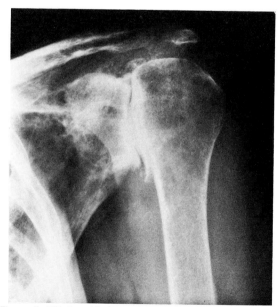

Figure 9–106. An elderly woman who had a mastectomy for carcinoma of the breast and radiation therapy 20 years prior to obtaining this AP shoulder x-ray. The x-ray shows changes in the bone pattern secondary to radiation necrosis, loss of the glenohumeral cartilage, and collapse of a portion of the humeral head.

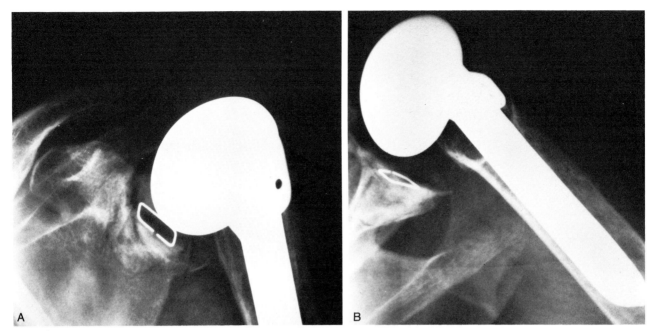

Figure 9–107. An elderly woman with long-standing rheumatoid arthritis 4 months after a total shoulder arthroplasty. AP *(A)* and axillary *(B)* views show difficulties in positioning to obtain the optimum view of the glenoid bone-cement junction and the rather innocuous appearance of the glenoid bone-cement lucent lines. In surgery this glenoid was found to be grossly loosened.

deltoid bursa in the presence of a rotator cuff tear. The reactive scarring obscures this appearance.

In total shoulder replacement, few problems have been noted with loosening of the proximal humeral component, but glenoid loosening occurs with at least the frequency of acetabular loosening.[184] Radiographic evidence of loosening is difficult to obtain. Often a lucent line appears at the glenoid bone-cement junction. Seldom, however, is it greater than 1 to 1.5 mm in width (Fig. 9–107). It is also difficult to see the entire interface because of the irregular shape of the fixation. When the components include a metal backing, a very slight obliquity will prevent visualization of the glenoid

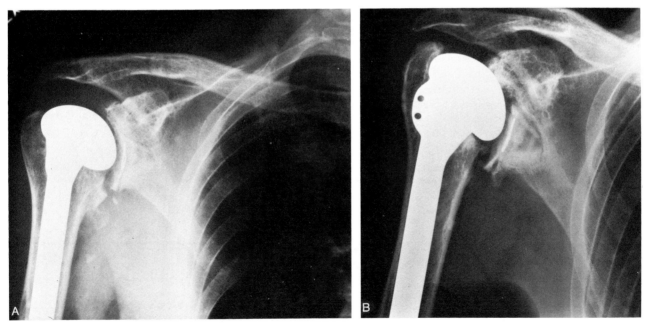

Figure 9–108. A, AP x-ray taken 2 months following total shoulder arthroplasty. A small lucent line is apparent at the glenoid bone-cement junction. *B,* An x-ray of the same shoulder taken 6 years later showing medial migration of the glenoid component due to loosening. The humeral head has also become impacted slightly further in the humeral shaft.

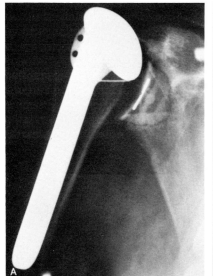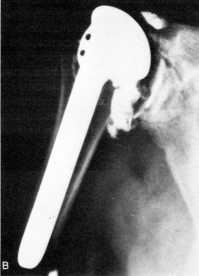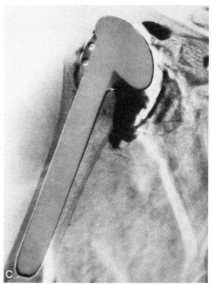

Figure 9–109. A, The plain x-ray of a 62-year-old man with a painful total shoulder arthroplasty. The x-ray shows upward subluxation of the humerus on the glenoid and suggests loosening of the glenoid with medial migration and upward tilting of the glenoid component. There is a small surrounding radiolucent line at the glenoid bone-cement junction. B, The shoulder arthrogram illustrates the difficulties of arthrography in this situation. The capsule is very contracted and the dye does not flow freely through the joint. C, A subtraction view of the arthrogram is slightly clearer, showing some extravasation of the dye around both the upper humeral component and the glenoid component.

bone-cement interface and the radiolucent line. Later, in the presence of glenoid component loosening, there will be a medial migration of the component with its cement. This is usually accom-

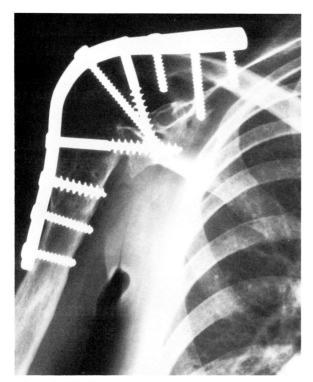

Figure 9–110. X-ray done immediately following a shoulder arthrodesis procedure. Because of the cancellous bone at the junction of the arthrodesis site, it is very difficult to assess the degree of bone healing. This x-ray, taken immediately following surgery, appears to show fused bone when, of course, bony healing has not yet occurred.

panied with slight upward tilting of the articular surface of the glenoid component (Fig. 9–108).

Technetium-labeled diphosphonate scans may show increased uptake in the region of the glenoid when there is loosening, but uptake in this area is somewhat variable, making the test less valuable than might be hoped for. Usually the test is not diagnostic (Fig. 9–32). Arthrograms of total shoulders not only do not help much in analyzing the rotator cuff, but in the presence of normal or near normal postoperative x-rays, arthrograms are almost without exception not diagnostic in the evaluation of glenoid loosening (Fig. 9–109). One is then left with a clinical picture combined with analysis of sequential x-rays; but perhaps temporizing in confirmation of the diagnosis in this situation is better, as some patients who have glenoid loosening have resolution of their pain with time, and others who subsequently require operation find that revision is not uniformly successful for them.

Prosthetic replacement is currently the most useful form of reconstructive surgery for a destroyed glenohumeral joint; however, in the presence of sepsis with cartilage loss or deltoid and rotator cuff paralysis, a shoulder fusion is still indicated. It is very difficult to be certain of bone union following an arthrodesing procedure. The bone is largely cancellous, and with accurate fitting the bone may actually look fused immediately after surgery (Fig. 9–110). In follow-up films, the x-ray beam must be oriented parallel to the newly sculptured junction between the two bones (Fig. 9–111). Fluoroscopy may be necessary for the alignment of the beam, as slight obliquity will prevent visualization of the line of bony healing between the humeral head and glenoid.

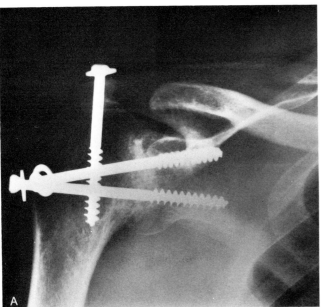
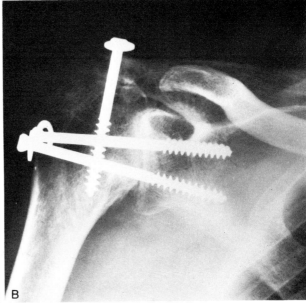

Figure 9–111. X-rays taken 4 years after the shoulder arthrodesis procedure. The patient is asymptomatic relative to the shoulder except for typical limitation of shoulder movement. The slightly oblique view to the joint line *(A)* will not allow accurate assessment of bone healing. View taken more nearly perpendicular to the joint line *(B)* suggests that a fibrous ankylosis rather than bony union may be present.

REFERENCES

Anatomy

1. Basmajian, J. V.: The surgical anatomy and function of the arm-trunk-mechanism. Surg. Clin. North Am. *43*:1471, 1963.
2. Cockshott, P.: The coracoclavicular joint. Radiology *131*:313, 1979.
3. Cone, R. O., Danzig, L., Resnick, D., et al.: The bicipital groove: Radiographic, anatomic, and pathologic study. A. J. R. *141*:781, 1983.
4. DePalma, A. F.: Surgery of the Shoulder. Philadelphia, J. B. Lippincott, 1973.
5. Gardner, E.: The prenatal development of the human shoulder joint. Surg. Clin. North Am. *43*:1465, 1963.
6. Grant, J. C. B.: Grant's Atlas of Anatomy. 5th Ed. Baltimore, Williams and Wilkins, 1962.
7. Gray, H.: Anatomy of the Human Body. 28th Ed. Goss, C. M. (ed.). Philadelphia, Lea and Febiger, 1966.
8. Greenway, G. D., Danzig, L., Resnick, D., et al.: The painful shoulder. Med. Radiogr. Photogr. *58*:21, 1982.
9. Hitchcock, H. H., and Bechtol, C. O.: Painful shoulder. J. Bone Joint Surg. *30A*:262, 1948.
10. Keats, T. E.: Atlas of Normal Roentgen Variants Which May Simulate Disease. 2nd Ed. Chicago, Year Book Medical Publishers, 1973.
11. Lucas, D. B.: Biomechanics of the shoulder joint. Arch. Surg. *107*:425, 1973.
12. Meyer, A. W.: Spontaneous dislocation and disruption of the tendon of the long head of the biceps brachii: 59 instances. Arch. Surg. *17*:493, 1928.
13. Neer, C. S., and Rockwood, C. A.: Fractures and dislocations of the shoulder. *In* Rockwood, C. A. Jr., and Green, D. P. (eds.): Fractures. Philadelphia, J. B. Lippincott, 1975.
14. Post, M.: The Shoulder: Surgical and Nonsurgical Management. Philadelphia, Lea and Febiger, 1978.
15. Saha, A. K.: Dynamic stability of the glenohumeral joint. Acta Orthop. Scand. *44*:668, 1973.
16. Saha, A. K.: Theory of Shoulder Mechanism. Springfield, Ill., Charles C Thomas, 1961.
17. Turkel, S. J., Pono, M. W., Marshall, J. L., et al.: Stabilizing mechanisms preventing anterior dislocation of the glenohumeral joint. J. Bone Joint Surg. *63A*:1208, 1981.

Routine Radiography

18. Alexander, O. M.: Radiography of the acromioclavicular articulation. Med. Radiogr. Photogr. *30*:34, 1954.
19. Ballinger, P. W.: Merrill's Atlas of Roentgenographic Positions and Standard Radiologic Procedures. 5th Ed. St. Louis, C. V. Mosby, 1982.
20. Bernau, A., and Berquist, T. H.: Orthopedic Positioning in Diagnostic Radiology. Baltimore, Urban and Schwarzenberg, 1983.
21. Bosworth, B. M.: Complete acromioclavicular dislocation. N. Engl. J. Med. *241*:221, 1949.
22. Cahill, B. R.: Osteolysis of the distal part of the clavicle in male athletes. J. Bone Joint Surg. *64A*:1053, 1982.
23. Clements, R. W.: Adaptation of the technique for radiography of the glenohumeral joint in the lateral position. Radiol. Technol. *51*:305, 1979.
24. Danzig, L., Resnick, D., and Greenway, G.: Evaluation of unstable shoulders by computed tomography. Am. J. Sports Med. *10*:138, 1982.
25. Deichgraber, E., and Olsson, B.: Soft tissue radiography in painful shoulder. Acta Radiol. (Diagn.) *16*:393, 1975.
26. DeSmet, A. A.: Axillary projection in radiography of the nontraumatized shoulder. A. J. R. *143*:511, 1980.
27. DeSmet, A. A.: Anterior oblique projection in radiography of the traumatized shoulder. A. J. R. *134*:515, 1980.
28. Didiee, J.: Le radiodiagnostic dans la luxation recidivante de l'épaule. J. Radiol. Electrol. *14*:209, 1930.
29. Fagerland, M., and Ahlgren, O.: Axial projection of the humeroscapular joint. Acta Radiol. (Diagn.) *22*:203, 1981.
30. Farrar, E., Matsen, F., Rogers, J., et al.: Dynamic sonographic study of lesions of the rotator cuff. Presented at the Annual Meeting of the AAOS, Anaheim, CA, 1983.
31. Fisk, C.: Adaptation of the technique for radiography of the bicipital groove. Radiol. Technol. *37*:47, 1965.
32. Flinn, R. M., MacMillan, C. L., Campbell, D. R., et al.: Optimal radiography of the acutely injured shoulder. J. Can. Assoc. Radiol. *34*:128, 1983.
33. Genoe, G. A., and Moeller, J. A.: Normal shoulder variations in the technetium-99m polyphosphate bone scan. South. Med. J. *67*:659, 1974.
34. Golding, F. C.: The shoulder: The forgotten joint. Br. J. Radiol. *35*:149, 1962.
35. Hall, R. H., Isaac, F., and Booth, C. R.: Dislocation of the

shoulder with special reference to accompanying small fractures. J. Bone Joint Surg. *41A*:489, 1959.

36. Heinig, C. F.: Retrosternal dislocation of the clavicle: Early recognition, x-ray diagnosis, and management. J. Bone Joint Surg. *50A*:830, 1968.

37. Hermodsson, I.: Roentgenologische Studien über die traumatischen und habituellen Schultergelenkverrenkungen nach vorn und nach unten. Acta Radiol. (Suppl.) *20*:1, 1934.

38. Hill, N. H., and Sachs M. D.: The grooved defect of the humeral head. A frequently unrecognized complication of dislocations of the shoulder joint. Radiology *35*:690, 1940.

39. Kilcoyne, R. F., and Matsen, E. A. III: Rotator cuff tear measurement by arthropneumotomography. A. J. R. *140*:315, 1983.

40. Lee, F. A., and Gwinn, J. L.: Retrosternal dislocation of the clavicle. Radiology *110*:631, 1974.

41. Mazujian, M.: Lateral profile view of the scapula. X-Ray Tech. *25*:24, 1953.

42. McGlynn, F. J., El-Khoury, G., and Albright, J. P.: Arthrotomography of the glenoid labrum in shoulder instability. J. Bone Joint Surg. *64A*:506, 1982.

43. Neer, C. S. II: Displaced proximal humeral fractures. Part I. Classification and evaluation. J. Bone Joint Surg. *52A*:1007, 1970.

44. Quesada, F.: Technique for the roentgen diagnosis of fractures of the clavicle. Surg. Gynecol. Obstet. *42*:424, 1926.

45. Reichman, S., Astrand, K., Deichgraber, E., et al.: Soft tissue xeroradiography of the shoulder joint. Acta Radiol. *16*:572, 1975.

46. Rockwood, C. A. Jr.: Part II: Dislocations about the shoulder. *In*: Rockwood, C. A. Jr., and Green, D. P. (eds.): Fractures. Philadelphia, J. B. Lippincott, 1975.

47. Rokous, J. R., Feagin, J. A., and Abbott, H. G.: Modified axillary roentgenogram. A useful adjunct in the diagnosis of recurrent instability of the shoulder. Clin. Orthop. *82*:84, 1972.

48. Rubin, S. A., Gray, R. L., and Green, W. R.: The scapular "Y": A diagnostic aid in shoulder trauma. Radiology *110*:725, 1974.

49. Sebes, J. I., Vasinrapee, P., and Friedman, B. I.: The relationship between radiographic findings and asymmetrical radioactivity in the shoulder. Radiology *120*:139, 1976.

50. Slivka, J., and Resnick, D.: An improved radiographic view of the gleno-humeral joint. J. Can. Assoc. Radiol. *30*:83, 1979.

51. Stodell, M. A., Nicholson, R., Scott, J., et al.: Radioisotope scanning in the painful shoulder. Rheum. Rehab. *19*:163, 1980.

52. Wallace, W. A., and Hellier, M.: Improving radiographics of the injured shoulder. Radiography *49*:229, 1983.

53. Weston, W. J.: Subdeltoid bursa. Australas. Radiol. *17*:214, 1973.

54. Wright, M. G., Richards, A. J., and Clarke, M. B.: Letter: 99mTc-pertechnetate scanning in capsulitis. Lancet *2*:1265, 1975.

55. Zanca P.: Shoulder pain: Involvement of the acromioclavicular joint. Analysis of 1000 cases. Am. J. Roentgenol. *112*:493, 1971.

Special Diagnostic Techniques

56. Andrew, L., and Lundberg, B. J.: Treatment of rigid shoulders by joint distension arthrography. Acta Orthop. Scand. *36*:45, 1965.

57. Bateman, J. E.: The Shoulder and Neck. 2nd Ed. Philadelphia, W. B. Saunders Co., 1978.

58. Burman, M. S.: Arthroscopy of the direct visualization of joints: An experimental cadaver study. J. Bone Joint Surg. *13*:669, 1931.

59. Cofield, R. H.: Arthroscopy of the shoulder. Mayo Clin. Proc. *58*:501, 1983.

60. Cone, R. O., Danzig, L., Resnick, D., et al.: The bicipital groove. Radiographic, anatomic, and pathologic study. A. J. R. *141*:781, 1983.

61. Cone, R. O., Resnick, D., and Danzig, L.: Shoulder impingement syndrome: Radiographic evaluation. Radiology *150*:29, 1984.

62. DePalma, A. F.: Loss of scapulohumeral motion. Ann. Surg. *135*:193, 1952.

63. DeSmet, A. A., and Ting, Y. M.: Diagnosis of rotator cuff tear on routine radiographs. J. Can. Assoc. Radiol. *28*:54, 1977.

64. El-Koury, G. Y., Albright, J. B., Yousef, M. A., et al.: Arthrotomography of the glenoid labrum. Radiology *131*:333, 1979.

65. Ellis, V. H.: The diagnosis of shoulder lesions due to injuries to the rotator cuff. J. Bone Joint Surg. *35B*:72, 1953.

66. Freiberger, R. H., and Kaye, J. J.: Arthrography. New York, Appleton-Century-Crofts, 1979.

67. Garcia, J. F.: Arthrography. Curr. Probl. Diagn. Radiol. *9*:1, 1980.

68. Garcia, J. F.: Arthrographic visualization of rotator cuff tears. Optimal application of stress to the shoulder. Radiology *150*:595, 1984.

69. Ghelman, B., and Goldman, A. B.: Double-contrast shoulder arthrogram: Evaluation of rotator cuff tears. Radiology *124*:251, 1977.

70. Gilula, L. A., Schoenecker, P. L., and Murphy, W. A.: Shoulder arthrography as a treatment modality. A. J. R. *131*:1047, 1978.

71. Goldberg, R. P., Hale, F. M., and Wyshak, E.: Pain in knee arthrography. Air vs. CO_2 and aspiration vs. no reaspiration. A. J. R. *136*:377, 1981.

72. Goldman, A. B., Dines, D. M., and Warren, R. F.: Shoulder Arthrography: Technique, Diagnosis, and Clinical Correlation. Boston, Little, Brown and Co., 1982.

73. Goldman, A. B., and Ghelman, B.: The double-contrast shoulder arthrogram. A review of 158 studies. Radiology *127*:655, 1978.

74. Goldman, A. B., Katz, M. C., and Freiberger, R. H.: Posttraumatic adhesive capsulitis of the ankle: Arthrographic analysis. A. J. R. *127*:585, 1976.

75. Ha'eri, G. B.: Ruptures of the rotator cuff. Can. Med. Assoc. J. *123*:620, 1980.

76. Ha'eri, G. B., and Maitland, A.: Arthroscopic findings in the frozen shoulder. J. Rheumatol. *8*:149, 1981.

77. Hall, F. M.: Morbidity from shoulder arthrography. Etiology, evidence, and prevention. A. J. R. *136*:59, 1981.

78. Johnson, L. L.: Diagnostic and Surgical Arthroscopy: The Knee and Other Joints. 2nd Ed. St. Louis, C. V. Mosby Co., 1981.

79. Kilcoyne, R. F., and Matsen, F. A. II: Rotator cuff tear measurement by arthropneumotomography. A. J. R. *140*:315, 1983.

80. Killoran, P. J., Marcove, R. C., and Freiberger, R. H.: Shoulder arthrography, A. J. R. *103*:658, 1968.

81. Kotzen, L. M.: Roentgen diagnosis of rotator cuff tears. A. J. R. *112*:507, 1971.

82. Kunnel, B. M.: Arthrography in anterior capsular derangements of the shoulder. Clin. Orthop. *83*:170, 1972.

83. Lie, S., and Mast, W. A.: Subacromial bursography. Radiology *144*:626, 1982.

84. McGlynn, F. J.: Arthrotomography of the glenoid labrum in shoulder instability. J. Bone Joint Surg. *64A*:506, 1982.

85. McLaughlin, H. L.: Rupture of the rotator cuff. J. Bone Joint Surg. *44A*:979, 1963.

86. Mikasa, M.: Subacromial bursography. J. Jap. Orthop. Assoc. *53*:225, 1979.

87. Mink, J. H., Richardson, H., and Grant, T. T.: Evaluation of the glenoid labrum by double-contrast arthrography. A. J. R. *133*:883, 1979.

88. Mosely, H. F., and Goldie, I.: Arterial pattern of the rotator cuff. J. Bone Joint Surg. *48B*:780, 1963.

89. Nance, P. F., Jones, T. R., and Kaye, J. J.: Dissecting synovial cysts of the shoulder. A complication of chronic rotator cuff tears. A. J. R. *138*:739, 1982.

90. Neer, C. S. II: Anterior acromioplasty for the chronic impingement syndrome in the shoulder. J. Bone Joint Surg. *54A*:41, 1972.

91. Nelson, C. L., and Burton, R. I.: Upper extremity arthrography. Clin. Orthop. *107*:72, 1975.

92. Neviaser, J. S.: Adhesive capsulitis of the shoulder. J. Bone Joint Surg. *27*:211, 1953.

93. Neviaser, J. S.: Arthrography of the shoulder joint. Study of the findings in adhesive capsulitis. J. Bone Joint Surg. *44A*:1321, 1962.
94. Neviaser, R. J.: Tears of the rotator cuff. Orthop. Clin. North Am. *11*:295, 1980.
95. Nixon, J. E., and DiStefano, V. S.: Rupture of the rotator cuff. Orthop. Clin. North Am. *6*:423, 1975.
96. Nixon, J. R., and Young, W. S.: Arthrography of the shoulder in anterior dislocations: A study of African and Asian patients. Injury *9*:287, 1978.
97. O'Donoghue, D. H.: Subluxing biceps tendon in the athlete. J. Sports Med. *1*:20, 1973.
98. Older, M. W. J., McIntyre, J. L., and Lloyd, G. J.: Distension arthrography of the shoulder joint. Can. J. Surg. *19*:203, 1976.
99. Pastershank, S. P.: The effect of water-soluble contrast medium on the synovial membrane. Radiology *143*:331, 1982.
100. Preston, B. J., and Jackson, J. P.: Investigation of shoulder disability by arthrography. Clin. Radiol. *28*:259, 1977.
101. Reeves, B.: The natural history of frozen shoulder syndrome. Scand. J. Rheum. *4*:193, 1975.
102. Resnick, D.: Arthrography, tenography, and bursography. *In* Resnick, D., and Niwayama, G. (eds.): Diagnosis of Bone and Joint Disorders. Philadelphia, W. B. Saunders, 1981.
103. Resnick, D.: Shoulder arthrography. Radiol. Clin. North Am. *19*:243, 1981.
104. Rothburn, J. B., McNab, I.: Microvascular pattern of the rotator cuff. J. Bone Joint Surg. *52B*:540, 1970.
105. Rothman, R. H., and Park, W. W.: Vascular anatomy of the rotator cuff. Clin. Orthop. *41*:176, 1965.
106. Samolson, R. C., and Binder, W. F.: Symptomatic full thickness tears of the rotator cuff. Orthop. Clin. North Am. *6*:449, 1975.
107. Schneider, R., Ghelman, B., and Kaye, J. J.: A simplified technique for shoulder arthrography. Radiology *114*:738, 1975.
108. Shuman, W. B., Kilcoyne, R. F., Matsen, F. A., et al.: Double-contrast computed tomography of the glenoid labrum. A. J. R. *141*:581, 1983.
109. Simmonds, F. A.: Shoulder pain with particular reference of "frozen" shoulder. J. Bone Joint Surg. *31B*:426, 1949.
110. Strizak, A. M., Danzig, L., Jackson, W., et al.: Subacromial bursography. An anatomical and clinical study. J. Bone Joint Surg. *64A*:196, 1982.
111. Weiner, D. S., and MacNab, I.: Superior migration of the humeral head: A radiographic aid to diagnosis of rotator cuff tear. J. Bone Joint Surg. *52B*:524, 1970.
112. Weston, W. J.: Arthrography of the acromioclavicular joint. Australas. Radiol. *18*:213, 1974.
113. Weston, W. J.: The subdeltoid bursa. Australas. Radiol. *17*:214, 1973.
114. Wolfgang, G. L.: Rupture of the musculotendinous cuff of the shoulder. Clin. Orthop. *134*:230, 1978.
115. Wright, V., and Haj, A. M.: Periarthritis of the shoulder. Assoc. Rheum. Dis. *35*:220, 1976.
116. Zachrisson, B. E., and Ejeskar, A.: Arthrography in dislocation of the acromioclavicular joint. Acta Radiol. (Diagn.) *20*:81, 1979.

Trauma

117. Allman, F. L.: Fractures and ligamentous injuries of the clavicle and its articulations. J. Bone Joint Surg. *49A*:774, 1967.
118. Arndt, J. H., and Sears, A. D.: Posterior dislocation of the shoulder. A. J. R. *94*:639, 1965.
119. Arner, O., Sandahl, U., and Orhleng, H.: Dislocation of the acromioclavicular joint: A review of the literature and report of 56 cases. Acta Chir. Scand. *113*:140, 1957.
120. Aston, J. W. Jr., and Gregory, C. F.: Dislocation of the shoulder with significant fracture of the glenoid. J. Bone Joint Surg. *55A*:1531, 1973.
121. Bankart, A. S. B.: Recurrent or habitual dislocation of the shoulder joint. Br. Med. J. *2*:1132, 1923.
122. Bearden, J. M., Hughston, J. C., and Whatley, G. S.: Acromioclavicular dislocation: Method of treatment. J. Sports Med. *1*:5, 1973.
123. Bosworth, B. M.: Complete acromioclavicular dislocation. N. Engl. J. Med. *241*:221, 1949.
124. Bowerman, J. W., and McDonnell, E. J.: Radiology of athletic injuries: Baseball. Radiology *116*:611, 1975.
125. Boyer, D. W. Jr.: Trapshooter's shoulder: stress fracture of the coracoid process. J. Bone Joint Surg. *57A*:862, 1975.
126. Buckerfield, C. T., and Castle, M. E.: Acute traumatic retrosternal dislocation of the clavicle. J. Bone Joint Surg. *66A*:379, 1984.
127. Cisternino, S. J., Rogers, L. F., Stuffleban, B. C., et al.: The trough line: A radiographic sign of posterior dislocation. A. J. R. *130*:951, 1978.
128. Codman, E. A.: The Shoulder: Rupture of the Supraspinatus Tendon and Other Lesions in or about the Subacromial Bursa. Boston, Thomas Todd, 1934.
129. DePalma, A. F., and Cantilli, R. A.: Fractures of the upper end of the humerus. Clin. Orthop. *20*:73, 1961.
130. DePalma, A. F., Groke, A. J., and Probhakasm, M.: The role of the subscapularis in recurrent anterior dislocation of the shoulder. Clin. Orthop. *54*:35, 1967.
131. Downey, E. F. Jr., Cartes, D. J., and Bower, A. C.: Unusual dislocations of the shoulder. A. J. R. *140*:1207, 1983.
132. Goldberg, R. P., and Vicks, B.: Oblique angled view for coracoid fractures. Skeletal Radiol. *9*:195, 1983.
133. Greenway, D. G., Danzig, L., Resnick, D., et al.: The painful shoulder. Med. Radiogr. and Photogr. *58*:21, 1982.
134. Hall, R. H., Isaac, E., and Booth, C. R.: Dislocation of the shoulder with special reference to accompanying small fractures. J. Bone Joint Surg. *41A*:489, 1959.
135. Hawkins, R. J., Koppert, G., and Johnston, G.: Recurrent posterior instability (subluxation) of the shoulder. J. Bone Joint Surg. *66A*:169, 1984.
136. Hayes, J. M., and Van Winkle, G. N.: Axillary artery injury with minimally displaced fracture of the neck of the humerus. J. Trauma *23*:431, 1983.
137. Hill, A. A., and Sachs, M. D.: The grooved defect of the humeral head—a frequently unrecognized complication of dislocations of the shoulder joint. Radiology *35*:690, 1940.
138. Horak, J., Nilsson, B. E.: Epidemiology of fractures of the upper end of the humerus. Clin. Orthop. *112*:250, 1975.
139. Janecki, C. J., and Barnett, D. C.: Fracture-dislocation of the shoulder with biceps tendon interposition. J. Bone Joint Surg. *61A*:142, 1979.
140. Kummel, B. M.: Fracture of the glenoid causing chronic dislocation of the shoulder. Clin. Orthop. *69*:189, 1970.
141. Linson, M. A.: Axillary artery thrombosis after fracture of the humerus. J. Bone Joint Surg. *62A*:1214, 1980.
142. Lourie, J. A.: Tomography in diagnosis of posterior dislocation of the sterno-clavicular joint. Acta Orthop. Scand. *51*:579, 1980.
143. Mariani, P. P.: Isolated fracture of the coracoid process in an athlete. Am. J. Sports Med. *8*:129, 1980.
144. McLaughlin, H. L.: Posterior dislocations of the shoulder. J. Bone Joint Surg. *34A*:584, 1952.
145. McLaughlin, H. L., and MacLellan, D. I.: Recurrent anterior dislocation of the shoulder. II. A comparative study. J. Trauma *7*:191, 1967.
146. Miller, D. S., and Boswick, J. A.: Lesions of the brachial plexus associated with fractures of the clavicle. Clin. Orthop. *64*:144, 1969.
147. Moseley, H. F.: The basic lesions of recurrent anterior dislocation. Surg. Clin. North Am. *43*:1631, 1963.
148. Natter, P. D.: Coracoclavicular articulation. J. Bone Joint Surg. *23*:177, 1941.
149. Nedecker, A., and Cooke, G. M.: Hill-Sachs deformity with an unusually large defect. J. Can. Assoc. Radiol. *30*:116, 1979.
150. Neer, C. S. II: Anterior acromioplasty for the chronic impingement syndrome in the shoulder: A preliminary report. J. Bone Joint Surg. *54A*:41, 1972.
151. Neer, C. S. II: Displaced proximal humeral fractures. Part I. Classification and evaluation. J. Bone Joint Surg. *52A*:1077, 1970.
152. Neer, C. S. II: Fractures of the distal clavicle with detachment of the coracoclavicular ligament in adults. J. Trauma *3*:99, 1963.

153. Neer, C. S. II: Fractures of the distal third of the clavicle. Clin. Orthop. *58*:43, 1968.
154. Neer, C. S. II, and Rockwood, C. A.: Fractures and dislocations of the shoulder. *In*: Rockwood, C. A., and Green, D. P. (eds.): Fractures. Philadelphia, J. B. Lippincott, 1975.
155. Nettles, J. L., and Linscheid, R.: Sternoclavicular dislocations. J. Trauma *8*:158, 1968.
156. Nielsen, W. B.: Injury to the acromioclavicular joint. J. Bone Joint Surg. *45B*:207, 1963.
157. Nobel, W.: Posterior traumatic dislocation of the shoulder. J. Bone Joint Surg. *44A*:523, 1962.
158. Omer, G. E.: Osteotomy of the clavicle in surgical reduction of anterior sternoclavicular dislocation. J. Trauma *7*:584, 1967.
159. Pavlov, H., and Freiberger, R. H.: Fractures and dislocations about the shoulder. Semin. Roentgenol. *13*:85, 1978.
160. Peterson, D. C.: Retrosternal dislocation of the clavicle. J. Bone Joint Surg. *43B*:90, 1961.
161. Post, M.: The Shoulder: Surgical and Non-Surgical Management. Philadelphia, Lea and Febiger, 1978.
162. Quinn, S. F., and Glass, T. A.: Post-traumatic osteolysis of the clavicle. South. Med. J. *76*:307, 1983.
163. Reeves, B.: Arthrography of the shoulder. J. Bone Joint Surg. *48B*:424, 1966.
164. Resnick, D.: Shoulder pain. Orthop. Clin. North Am. *14*:81, 1983.
165. Rogers, L. F.: Radiology of Skeletal Trauma. New York, Churchill Livingstone, 1982.
166. Rokous, J. R., Feegin, J. A., and Abbott, H. G.: Modified axillary roentgenogram. A useful adjunct in diagnosis of recurrent instability of the shoulder. Clin. Orthop. *82*:84, 1972.
167. Rowe, C. R.: Fractures of the scapula. Surg. Clin. North Am. *43*:1565, 1963.
168. Rowe, C. R.: Prognosis in dislocation of the shoulder. J. Bone Joint Surg. *38A*:957, 1956.
169. Rowe, C. R.: Shoulder girdle injuries. *In*: Cave, E. F.: Trauma Management. Chicago, Year Book Publishers, 1974.
170. Rowe, C. R., and Sakellarides, H. T.: Factors related to recurrence of anterior dislocation of the shoulder. Clin. Orthop. *20*:40, 1961.
171. Rowe, C. R., Zarins, B., and Ciullo, J. V.: Recurrent anterior dislocation of the shoulder after surgical repair. Apparent causes of treatment failure. J. Bone Joint Surg. *66A*:159, 1984.
172. Salvatore, J.: Sternoclavicular joint dislocation. Clin. Orthop. *58*:51, 1968.
173. Sandrock, A. R.: Another sports fatigue fracture: Stress fracture of the coracoid process of the scapula. Radiology *117*:274, 1975.
174. Selesnick, F. H., Jablow, M., Frank, C., et al.: Retrosternal dislocation of the clavicle. Report of 4 cases. J. Bone Joint Surg. *66A*:287, 1984.
175. Simeone, F. A.: Neurological complications of closed shoulder injuries. Orthop. Clin. North Am. *6*:499, 1975.
176. Turkel, S. J., Pinto, M. W., Marshall, J. L., et al.: Stabilizing mechanisms preventing anterior dislocation of the gleno-humeral joint. J. Bone Joint Surg. *63A*:1208, 1981.
177. Varriale, P. L., and Adler, M. L.: Occult fracture of the glenoid without dislocation. J. Bone Joint Surg. *65A*:688, 1983.
178. Vastamaki, M., and Solonen, K. A.: Posterior dislocations and fracture-dislocations of the shoulder. Acta Orthop. Scand. *51*:479, 1980.
179. White, E. M., Kattapuram, S. V., and Jupiter, J. B.: Case report 241. Post-traumatic pseudoaneurysm. Skeletal Radiol. *10*:178, 1983.
180. Wilkins, R. M., and Johnson, R. M.: Ununited fractures of the clavicle. J. Bone Joint Surg. *65A*:773, 1983.
181. Worman, L. W., Leagus, C.: Intrathoracic injury following retrosternal dislocation of the clavicle. J. Trauma *7*:416, 1967.
182. Zuckerman, J. D., and Matsen, F. A.: Complications about the gleno-humeral joint related to the use of screws and staples. J. Bone Joint Surg. *66A*:175, 1984.

Reconstructive Surgery

183. Codman, E. A.: The Shoulder: Rupture of the Supraspinatus Tendon and Other Lesions in or about the Subacromial Bursa. Boston, Thomas Todd Co., 1934.
184. Cofield, R. H.: Total shoulder arthroplasty with the Neer prosthesis. J. Bone Joint Surg. In publication.
185. Cofield, R. H.: Unconstrained total shoulder prosthesis. Clin. Orthop. *173*:97, 1983.
186. Cotton, R. E., and Rideout, D. F.: Tears of the humeral rotator cuff. J. Bone Joint Surg. *46B*:314, 1964.
187. DeSmet, A. A., and Ting, Y. M.: Diagnosis of rotator cuff tear on routine radiographs. J. Can. Assoc. Radiol. *28*:54, 1977.
188. Ennevarra, K.: Painful shoulder joint in rheumatoid arthritis. Acta Rheum. Scand. (Suppl.) *2*:1, 1967.
189. Golding, F. C.: The shoulder: The forgotten joint. Brit J. Radiol *35*:149, 1962.
190. Kotzen, E.: Roentgen diagnosis of rotator cuff tear: Report of 48 surgically proven cases. A. J. R. *112*:507, 1971.
191. McCarty, D. J., Halverson, P. B., Carrerra, G. F., et al.: "Milwaukee shoulder"—association of microspheroids containing hydroxyapatite crystals, active collagenase, and neutral protease with rotator cuff defects. I. Clinical aspects. Arthritis Rheum. *24*:464, 1981.
192. Neer, C. S. II: Anterior acromioplasty for chronic impingement syndrome of the shoulder. J. Bone Joint Surg. *54A*:41, 1972.
193. Neer, C. S. II: Replacement arthroplasty for gleno-humeral osteoarthritis. J. Bone Joint Surg. *56A*:1, 1974.
194. Neer, C. S. II, Watson, K. C., and Stanton, F. J.: Recent experience in total shoulder replacement. J. Bone Joint Surg. *64A*:319, 1982.
195. Petersson, C. H., and Gentz, C. F.: Rupture of the supraspinatus tendon. The significance of distally pointing acromioclavicular osteophytes. Clin. Orthop. *174*:143, 1983.
196. Weiner, D. S., and MacNab, I.: Superior migration of the humeral head. A radiological aid in the diagnosis of rotator cuff tears. J. Bone Joint Surg. *52B*:524, 1970.

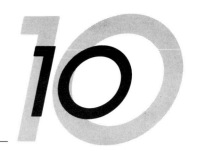

FRACTURES OF THE SHAFT OF THE HUMERUS

CLAIRE E. BENDER • DONALD C. CAMPBELL II

Humeral shaft fractures compose 1 percent of all fractures.[10] Most of these fractures heal with closed reduction. Radial nerve and vascular complications occur occasionally.

ANATOMY

The key to proper treatment of fractures of the humeral shaft is a good understanding of the anatomy of the humerus. The shaft extends proximally from the upper border of the insertion of the pectoralis major muscle on the greater tubercle to the supracondylar ridges distally[2] (Figs. 10–1A, 10–2A). On a cross-sectional view the proximal half of the shaft is circular; the distal half flattens in the AP dimension. The humeral shaft is described as having three surfaces and three borders. The anterior border, between the anterolateral and anteromedial surfaces, begins with the crest of the greater tubercle, includes the medial edge of the deltoid tuberosity, becomes indistinct on the more flattened lower part of the body, and ends at the sharp lateral edge of the coronoid fossa. The medial border begins with the crest of the lesser tubercle, which often fades out in the midshaft, and ends as the medial supracondylar ridge. The lateral border, although poorly defined superiorly, ends as the lateral supracondylar ridge (Figs. 10–1 and 10–2).

The anterolateral surface contains the deltoid tu-

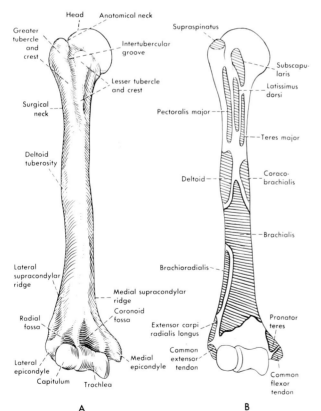

Figure 10–1. Illustrations of anterior humerus and muscle insertions. *A,* Bony landmarks of the humerus. *B,* Muscle insertions. (From Hollinshead, W. H.: Anatomy for Surgeons, Vol. 3: The Back and Limbs. 3rd Ed. New York, Harper and Row, 1982.)

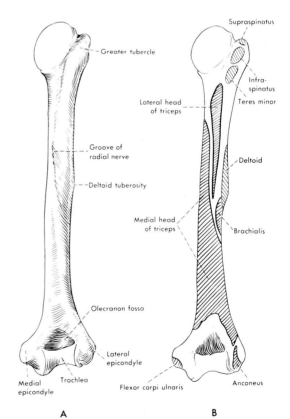

Figure 10–2. Illustrations of posterior humerus and muscle insertions. *A,* Bony landmarks. *B,* Muscle insertions. (From Hollinshead, W. H.: Anatomy for Surgeons, Vol. 3: The Back and Limbs. 3rd Ed. New York, Harper and Row, 1982.)

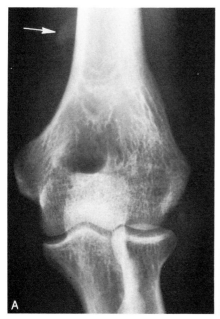
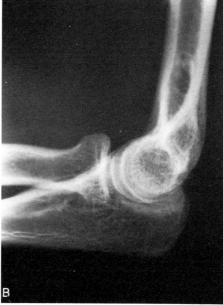

Figure 10–3. Supracondylar process seen on AP *(A)* and lateral *(B)* views.

berosity above; below, where the anterior border becomes poorly defined, the anterolateral and anteromedial surfaces tend to blend, as they both give rise to the brachialis muscle. There are no distinguishing landmarks on the anteromedial surface. The posterior surface is crossed obliquely by a shallow groove, the radial or spiral groove (Fig. 10–2A). The radial nerve courses in this groove, which runs downward and laterally from behind the deltoid tuberosity.[6]

Anterior and posterior compartments are formed by medial and lateral intermuscular septa. The biceps brachii, brachialis, and coracobrachialis are muscles included in the anterior compartment; the posterior compartment includes the triceps.

A relatively common variation in the distal humerus is the supracondylar process (Fig. 10–3). It represents an anomalous beaklike projection of variable size along the anteromedial surface of the humerus about 5 cm above the medial epicondyle. A well developed supracondylar process is often connected to the medial epicondyle by a fibrous band, the ligament of Struthers. Fracture of the supracondylar process is clinically important, as it may result in damage to the median nerve and brachial artery, which pass beneath it.[6]

The muscles of the arm are the biceps brachii, coracobrachialis, and brachialis muscles anteriorly and the triceps and anconeus posteriorly. Of these muscles the brachialis and medial and lateral heads of triceps arise from the humeral shaft. Only the coracobrachialis inserts on the shaft of the humerus (see Figs. 10–1B and 10–2B).

The musculocutaneous nerve supplies the anterior compartment arm muscles. Posteriorly the radial nerve supplies the triceps.

In the upper arm the radial nerve lies behind the axillary artery and on the front of the long head of the triceps. It then passes laterally and posteriorly with the profunda brachii artery, deep to the long head of the triceps. As it passes along the posterior aspect of the humerus, it moves between the lateral

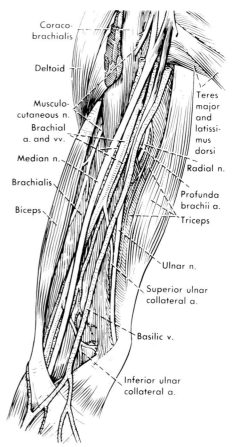

Figure 10–4. Illustration of the major vessels and nerves of the arm. (From Hollinshead, W. H.: Anatomy for Surgeons, Vol. 3: The Back and Limbs. 3rd Ed. New York, Harper and Row, 1982.)

and medial heads of the triceps. The radial nerve is positioned close to, but not actually in, the spiral groove. The nerve then pierces the lateral intermuscular septum (along with the radial collateral branch of the brachial artery) to pass forward and distally in close association with the brachialis.[6]

Usually the median and ulnar nerves do not supply any muscles of the arm. The median nerve is formed anterior or anterolateral to the brachial artery. It then descends lateral or anterolateral to the artery to the midshaft level. Thereafter, it usually crosses in front of the artery to lie on the medial side and passes down to the cubital fossa. The ulnar nerve lies medial or posterior to the brachial artery in the upper arm. At the midarm level it pierces the medial intermuscular septum to lie in front of the medial head of the triceps. It courses inferiorly with the superior ulnar collateral artery[6] (Fig. 10–4).

The brachial artery roughly parallels the shaft of the humerus. At the lower border of the teres major, the axillary artery becomes the brachial artery. Proximally the artery lies first on the medial side of the arm in front of the long head of the triceps and then on the medial head of the triceps (Fig. 10–5). As it continues distally, it slopes forward along the medial border of the biceps to lie on the anterior surface of the brachialis muscle. It then passes into the cubital fossa, where it divides into the radial

and ulnar arteries. The brachial artery is usually accompanied by two brachial veins, one lying medial and one lateral to it, but with numerous anastomoses between them.

Branches of the brachial artery in the arm include the profunda brachii, the nutrient artery of the humerus, and the superior and ulnar collateral arteries (Fig. 10–5).

Blood is supplied to the humerus from branches of the brachial artery, including one or more nutrient arteries, and from the vessels intimately associated with the ends of the bone. The chief nutrient artery of the humerus is a slender branch that arises from the brachial artery (or sometimes from the superior ulnar collateral) about the middle of the arm, which enters the anteromedial surface of the humerus. The nutrient artery foramen travels inferiorly and obliquely. Its external end is usually located in the middle third of the bone, but it may vary considerably, appearing anywhere from a position at the inferior level of deltoid tuberosity to the junction of the mid- and lower third of the humerus.

The profunda brachii artery is the largest branch vessel in the arm. Usually it originates on the posteromedial side of the brachial artery in the upper arm and runs downward and laterally behind the brachial artery to parallel the radial nerve in a spiral around the humerus. It passes deep to the long head of the triceps, then deep to the lateral head, and then between it and the medial head of the triceps. At the level of the lateral intermuscular septum, the profunda divides into the radial and middle collateral arteries. The profunda brachii artery usually gives off a nutrient branch to the body of the humerus as it starts its course around the bone. Usually this nutrient branch enters the bone above and medial to the radial groove. It may be the largest nutrient artery of the humerus.[6]

MECHANISM OF INJURY AND CLASSIFICATION

There are several unique features of the humerus that present special problems in fracture treatment. First, the humerus is the most freely movable long bone. Scapulohumeral motion can amplify its motions. Second, the humerus functions as a lever; therefore, nearly all stress to the bone is in tension form or is at an angle to the long axis of the bone. Thus, weight-bearing or compression forces are not problems in fracture management. Finally, when the person is upright, the bone hangs vertically and thus is influenced by gravity alone, allowing realignment of fracture fragments.[1, 7]

The location of the fracture and its relationship to muscle attachments will affect the direction of displacement of bone fragments. Fractures of the proximal third (between the pectoralis major and deltoid insertions) result in medial displacement of the proximal fragment owing to the pull of the

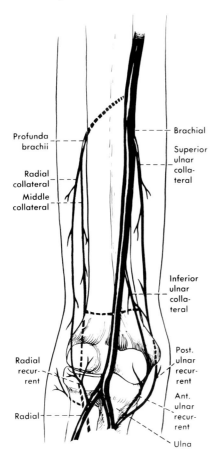

Figure 10–5. Brachial artery and its branches. (From Hollinshead, W. H.: Anatomy for Surgeons, Vol. 3: The Back and Limbs. 3rd Ed. New York, Harper and Row, 1982.)

pectoralis major muscle. Fractures distal to the deltoid tuberosity result in abduction of the proximal fragment from pull by the deltoid and proximal displacement of the distal fragment from pull by the brachialis and biceps.

Direct force, from either blunt or penetrating injury, is the most frequent cause of fracture of the humeral shaft. A transverse fracture is the result of a bending force; a spiral fracture results from a combination of bending and torsion forces.[3]

Compression forces acting on the humerus tend to affect either end but not the shaft.[3] Indirect forces, such as falling directly on the elbow or on an outstretched hand, vigorous throwing of objects, or even violent muscle contraction can also result in fracture of the humeral shaft.

Depending on the age of the patient and the type of injury, the fracture can be open or closed, complete or incomplete, simple or comminuted.

The level of the fracture is described as being in

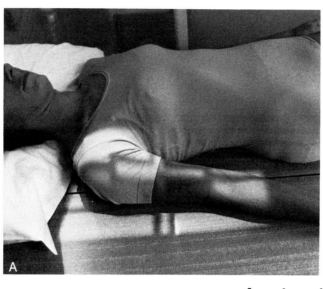

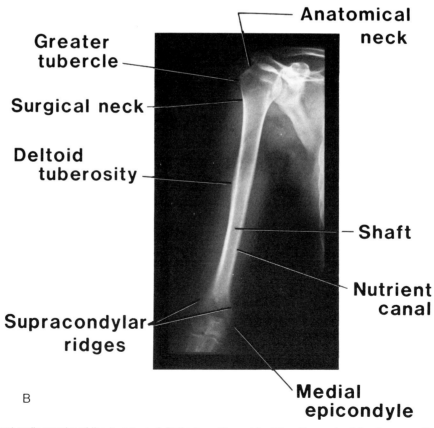

Figure 10–6. Standard radiographs of the humerus. A, Patient positioned for AP radiograph of the humerus. The film is centered on the midshaft with both the elbow and shoulder included on the film. B, AP radiograph of the humerus.

Illustration continued on opposite page

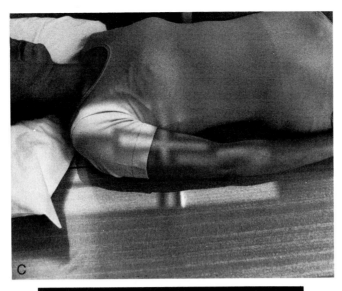

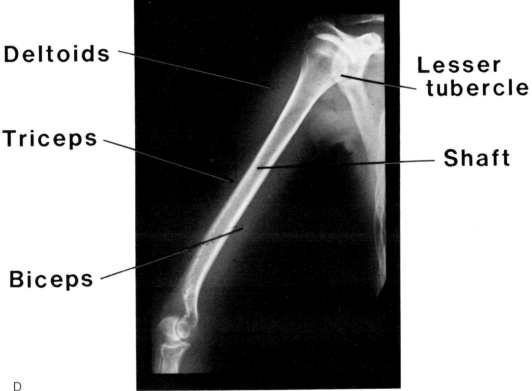

Deltoids

Triceps

Biceps

Lesser tubercle

Shaft

D

Figure 10–6 Continued. *C,* Patient positioned for lateral view of the humerus. The forearm is pronated. *D,* Lateral radiograph of the humerus.

the upper, middle, or lower third of the shaft. In Mast's series of 240 patients, 69 percent of the fractures occurred at midshaft level.[11] Of the total fractures, 61 percent were transverse, 18 percent oblique, 17 percent spiral, and 4 percent segmental. Severe comminution occurred in 12 percent.

Fractures at the junction of the middle and distal third of the humeral shaft may be particularly troublesome. Injury to the main nutrient artery may contribute to delayed union or non-union. Holstein and Lewis have emphasized that the radial nerve is at great risk of entrapment in the fracture because it passes close to the bone near the lateral supra-

condylar ridge.[8] The mobility of the nerve is reduced as it passes through the lateral intermuscular septum. Closed reduction may damage the nerve. For this reason open reduction and internal fixation of these fractures is recommended, especially if there is any evidence of radial nerve paresis.

RADIOLOGIC EVALUATION

Standard recumbent views include the AP and lateral projections (Fig. 10–6). The selected film must be long enough to include both the shoulder and elbow joints. This is necessary in order to exclude associated injuries as well as to assist in determining the position in which the film was obtained. All films are obtained using the Potter-Bucky technique. For the AP projection the arm is placed at the patient's side with the elbow extended and hand supinated (Fig. 10–6A). This places the epicondyles parallel to the plane of the film.

The lateral projection is obtained with the elbow extended and hand pronated (Fig. 10–6C). If the patient is in a hanging case or splint, the arm is abducted slightly and internally rotated. The hand will then be over the abdomen.

The central ray of the x-ray beam is directed perpendicular to the midshaft of the humerus in the standard projections.

The transthoracic lateral projection should be obtained when additional injuries or immobilization precludes the standard lateral view. With the patient in the recumbent position, the affected extremity is placed next to the cassette. The uninjured arm is raised, resting the forearm on the head (Fig. 10–7A). This elevates the normal shoulder and depresses the injured extremity. Superimposition of the shoulders is therefore minimized. The cassette is centered at the area of interest of the humerus.

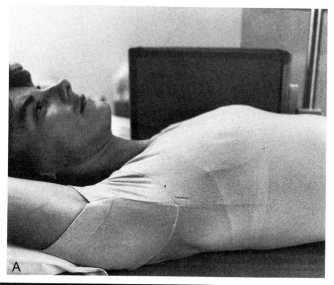

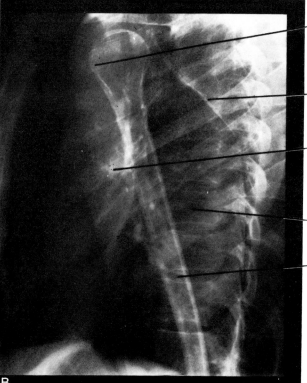

Lesser tubercle

Lateral margin of scapula

Pulmonary hilus

Thoracic vertebra

Shaft

Figure 10–7. A, Patient positioned for transthoracic view. The unaffected arm is elevated. *B,* Radiograph taken with transthoracic technique.

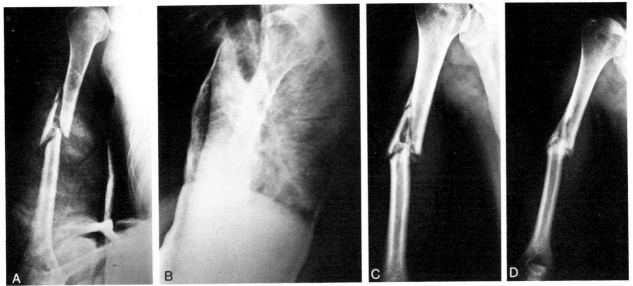

Figure 10–8. A, AP view of comminuted fracture of the midshaft of the humerus in hanging cast. *B,* Transthoracic view reveals slight anterior angulation. *C,* Follow-up film 5 weeks later demonstrates healing with callus formation. *D,* Film taken 4 months after injury with healed fracture.

The unaffected shoulder should be turned slightly posterior to visualize the injured humerus properly. The central ray is directed perpendicularly to the midpoint of the film. Film exposure is made at full inspiration in order to improve the anatomic contrast as well as to minimize the exposure factors (Fig. 10–7B).

A lead apron is used for gonadal shielding.

With severe trauma, additional injury to the radius and ulna may occur. Pierce described 21 cases of combined injury, with 6 cases in which the fractures were of the midshafts of all three bones.[12] He also noted that 11 of 21 patients had acute neural injuries.

MANAGEMENT OF HUMERAL FRACTURES

Initial Management

Humeral shaft fractures usually heal without problems. Nevertheless, treatment must be individualized because of several factors. Treatment depends upon (1) the patient's age, (2) the type and level of fracture, (3) the degree of fracture displacement, (4) muscular development, and (5) associated injuries.[7] Closed primary treatment may include (1) dependency traction (e.g., long-arm hanging cast) and (2) thoracobrachial immobilization (e.g., open Velpeau-type cast).[7] Abduction

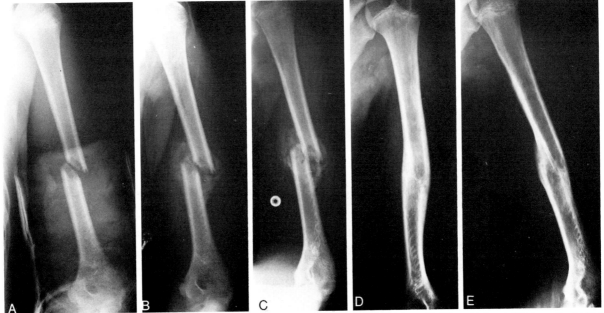

Figure 10–9. Simple fracture of the midshaft of the humerus. AP view *(A)* at time of injury. AP *(B)* and lateral *(C)* views 3 weeks after injury show abundant callus. Healing is evident on AP *(D)* and lateral *(E)* views 3 months after the fracture.

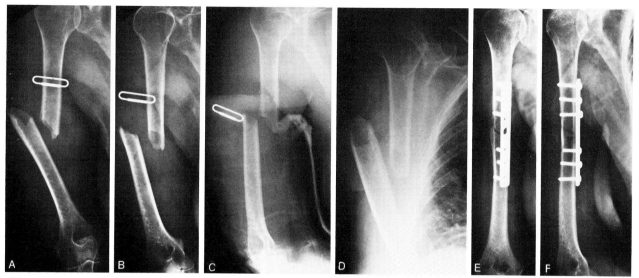

Figure 10–10. AP *(A)* and lateral *(B)* radiographs demonstrating a short, oblique fracture of the midhumerus with significant displacement. Immediate post-reduction view *(C)* in hanging cast. Three week follow-up film *(D)* shows progressive displacement and overriding of the fragments. AP *(E)* and lateral *(F)* views show good reduction with plate and screw fixation.

splints or casts and various forms of functional bracing may also be used in closed primary treatment.

Perfect alignment and apposition of fracture components are not essential. Anterior angulation of up to 20° and varus angulation of up to 30° can usually be accepted without compromising function or appearance.[9] However, the closer the fracture is to the elbow joint, the more important alignment becomes.

Immediately after initial closed reduction and immobilization, repeat radiographs are obtained in the AP and lateral (or transthoracic) views (Figs.

10–8 and 10–9). Follow-up radiographs are obtained periodically until evidence of healing is seen.

Indications for primary operative treatment include (1) displaced transverse fractures and short oblique fractures, (2) long spiral fractures with displacement suggestive of soft tissue interposition,[9] and (3) compound wounds and vascular complications. Mast reports vascular injury at a frequency of 3 percent.[11]

Radial nerve paralysis secondary to injury from humeral shaft fractures does not imply the need for early operative management. Although the frequency of radial nerve injury varies from 3 to 16

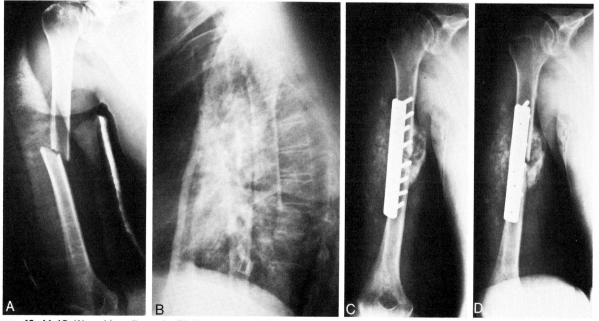

Figure 10–11. AP *(A)* and transthoracic *(B)* views demonstrate a fracture of the midhumerus with anterior displacement of the distal fragment. The fracture was treated with bone graft and plate and screw fixation *(C and D).*

percent,[10] most cases of radial nerve injury resolve spontaneously.[4] Exploration of the fracture and nerve may itself result in nerve injury. Since the results of late nerve repair are equal to those following early repair, it is wise to wait at least 2 weeks to evaluate nerve status further. Electromyography may become useful at this point. The incidence of median and ulnar nerve palsy is less than 3 percent.

Methods of internal fixation include plating with the option of bone grafting, which is the most common technique (Figs. 10–10 and 10–11), and use of intramedullary rods and nails. The latter help to preserve alignment and maintain length. The level of the fracture may influence the choice of internal

fixation. Midshaft fractures may be treated with plates and screws or intramedullary rods. Fractures at the ends of the humeral shaft must be carefully evaluated in order to choose the best method of fixation.[3]

Delayed Management

Delayed union (defined as clinical absence of union at 8 weeks) or non-union may be associated with (1) poor apposition or distraction of fracture fragments, (2) initial internal fixation, (3) interference of blood supply to the humeral shaft, (4) open

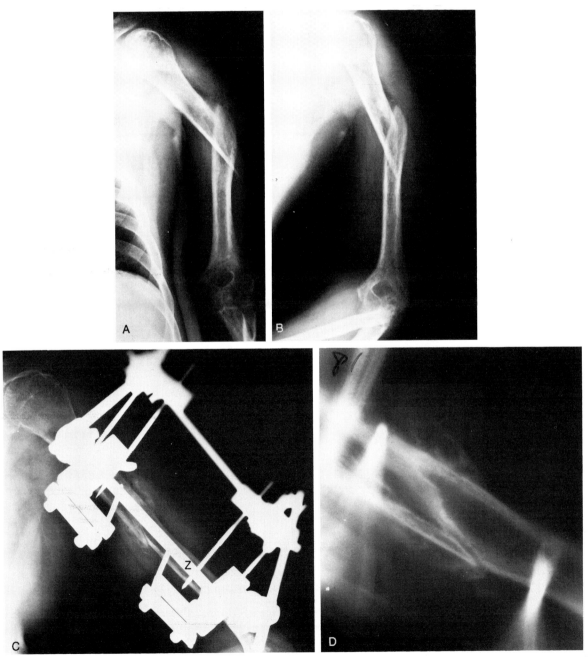

Figure 10–12. AP *(A)* and lateral *(B)* views of an overriding non-united humeral fracture. Reduction was maintained with a Hoffman apparatus *(C)*. Tomogram *(D)* demonstrates healing with early callus formation.

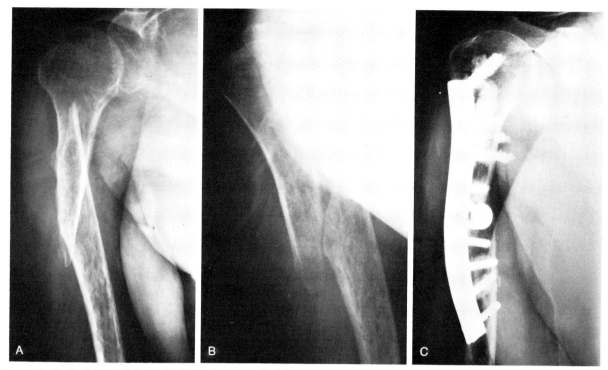

Figure 10–13. AP *(A)* and oblique *(B)* views of a non-united fracture of the humeral shaft and osteoporosis. Stabilization achieved through application of plate and screws, with methyl methacrylate used to improve fixation of screws *(C)*.

injury and infection, and (5) soft tissue interposition.[5] Treatment of delayed union consists of further conservative measures or internal fixation. Nonunion of the humerus may be treated with plating, nailing, intramedullary rod fixation, or, more rarely, external fixation devices[13] (Fig. 10–12). Delayed unions and non-unions may be complicated by osteoporosis. In such cases it may be useful to utilize methyl methacrylate to enhance fixation of the screws and plate (Fig. 10–13).

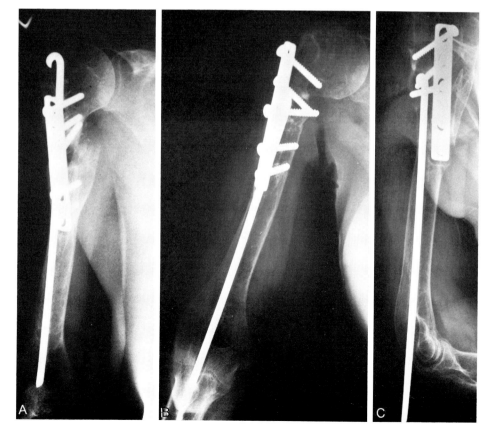

Figure 10–14. Osteoporotic humerus with Rush rod and plate and screw fixation of a proximal humeral fracture *(A)*. Follow-up AP *(B)* and lateral *(C)* views demonstrate migration of the rod through the distal humerus and loosening of the plate and screws. The fracture is not united.

Unstable fractures in osteoporotic bone can defeat efforts at stabilization by internal fixation as a result of loosening and migration of fixation devices[8] (Fig. 10–14).

Body-section tomography is performed for evaluation of delayed fracture healing (Fig. 10–12D). Linear or complex motion tomography is used, depending upon the presence of metallic fixation devices (see Chapter 1, Conventional Tomography). AP and lateral views are obtained at 0.5-cm slices, depending on the thickness of the body part. A persistent fracture line is usually readily identified by this technique. Gupta and colleagues have performed osteomedullograms in cases of delayed union and non-union of diaphyseal fractures.[5] While visualizing the proliferating venous endothelium across the fracture site, conservative treatment was continued, which led to complete healing in all 12 cases.

REFERENCES

1. Caldwell, J. A.: Treatment of fractures of the shaft by hanging cast. Surg. Gynecol. Obstet. *70*:421, 1940.
2. Christensen, N. O.: Küntscher intramedullary reaming and nail fixation for nonunion of the humerus. Clin. Orthop. *116*:222, 1976.
3. Epps, C. H. Jr.: Fractures of the shaft of the humerus. *In*: Rockwood, C. A., and Green, D. P. (eds.): Fractures. Philadelphia, J. B. Lippincott, 1975.
4. Fenjo, G.: On fractures of the shaft of the humerus. Acta Chir. Scand. *137*:221, 1971.
5. Gupta, R. C., Kumar, S., and Gupta, K. K.: A clinical evaluation of osteomedullography in diaphyseal fractures. J. Trauma *20*:507, 1980.
6. Hollinshead, W. H.: Anatomy for Surgeons. Vol. 3: The Back and Limbs. 3rd Ed. New York, Harper and Row, 1982.
7. Holm, C. L.: Management of humeral shaft fractures. Clin. Orthop. *71*:132, 1970.
8. Holstein, A., and Lewis, G. B.: Fractures of the humerus with radial-nerve paralysis. J. Bone Joint Surg. *45A*:1382, 1963.
9. Klemerman, L.: Fractures of the shaft of the humerus. J. Bone Joint Surg. *48B*:105, 1966.
10. Mann, R. J., and Neal, F. G.: Fractures of the shaft of the humerus in adults. South. Med. J. *58*:264, 1964.
11. Mast, J. W., Spiegel, P. G., Harvey, J. P. J., et al.: Fractures of the humeral shaft. Clin. Orthop. *112*:254, 1975.
12. Pierce, R. O., and Hodurski, F.: Fractures of the humerus, radius and ulna in the same extremity. J. Trauma *19*:182, 1979.
13. Shaw, J. L., and Sakellarides, H.: Radial nerve paralysis associated with fractures of the humerus. J. Bone Joint Surg. *49A*:889, 1967.

THE ELBOW

BERNARD F. MORREY • *THOMAS H. BERQUIST*

ANATOMY

Understanding the basic anatomy of the elbow is essential for the proper interpretation of the various manifestations of trauma that can affect this joint.

The distal humerus flares just above its articulation to form the medial and lateral supracondylar bony columns. These stabilize the articular surface, which is composed of the capitellum and trochlea (Fig. 11–1). The distal half of the elbow is composed of the proximal radius and ulna. These in turn articulate with the capitellum and trochlea in a very tightly constrained configuration. The lateral aspect of the distal humerus demonstrates a normal anterior articulatory rotation of approximately 30° with respect to the long axes of the humeral shaft (Fig. 11–2). The proximal radius is composed of a disk-shaped radial head with an indentation in the center that articulates with the capitellum. The neck of the radius makes a 15° angle with the shaft (Fig. 11–3).[5] The proximal ulna consists of the sigmoid notch with an arc of approximately 180°. This notch is rotated posteriorly to articulate with the trochlea (Fig. 11–4). On the AP view the distal humerus makes a valgus angle of approximately 6°. The proximal humerus makes a 4° valgus angle, thus explaining the normal 10° to 13° carrying angle (Fig. 11–5).[2, 3] The carrying angle changes with flexion.[11] Thus, flexion-contractures make radiographic estimates of carrying angle meaningless.

The elbow articulation is one of the most congruent in the body.[11] As such, the cartilage thickness varies inversely with the congruence.[4, 12] Thus, the anticipated radiographic appearance of the joint space would be less at the elbow than at other joints. The distribution of the articular cartilage about the greater sigmoid notch is also of interest, since in most individuals the hyaline cartilage is not continuous (Fig. 11–6).[14] This finding is significant in that comminuted intra-articular fractures of the olecranon usually occur through this area, just as

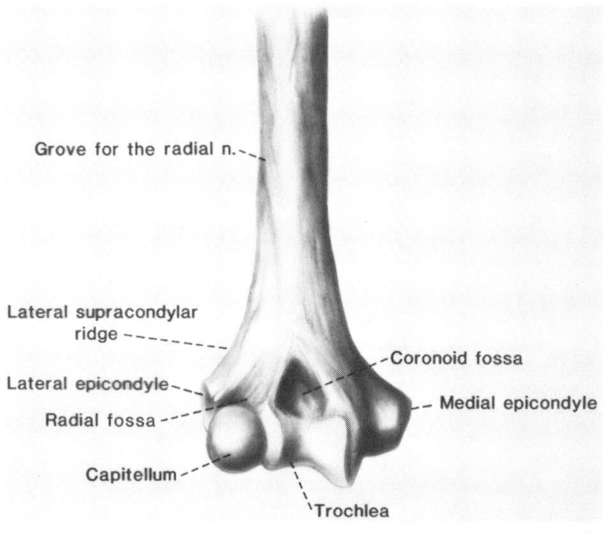

Figure 11–1. Osseous anatomy of the distal humerus. Note the supracondylar bone that supports the articular trochlea and capitellum. The bone laterally is more substantial than that medially. (From Morrey, B. F. (ed.): The Elbow and Its Disorders. Philadelphia, W. B. Saunders Co., 1985.)

Grove for the radial n.

Lateral supracondylar ridge

Lateral epicondyle

Radial fossa

Capitellum

Coronoid fossa

Medial epicondyle

Trochlea

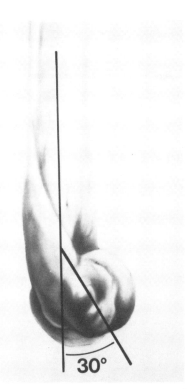

Figure 11–2. Lateral projection of the humerus demonstrates the anterior angulation of the distal condyles. This angulation is important in assessing the adequacy of reduction. (From Morrey, B. F. (ed.): The Elbow and Its Disorders. Philadelphia, W. B. Saunders Co., 1985.)

30°

579

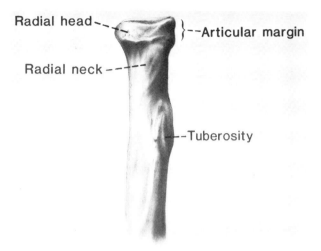

Figure 11–3. Proximal radius reveals approximately 15° angulation of the neck with respect to the shaft. (From Morrey, B. F. (ed.): The Elbow and Its Disorders. Philadelphia, W. B. Saunders Co., 1985.)

Figure 11–4. The lateral aspect of the proximal ulna reveals the greater sigmoid notch with an arc of approximately 180°. This articulation helps account for the stability of the joint. (From Morrey, B. F. (ed.): The Elbow and Its Disorders. Philadelphia, W. B. Saunders Co., 1985.)

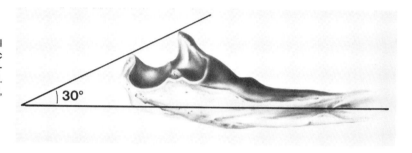

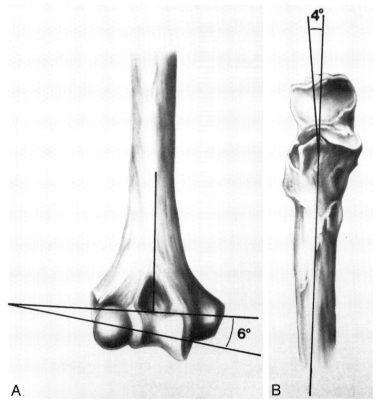

Figure 11–5. The carrying angle is formed by the valgus tilt of both the humeral (A) and ulnar (B) articulations.

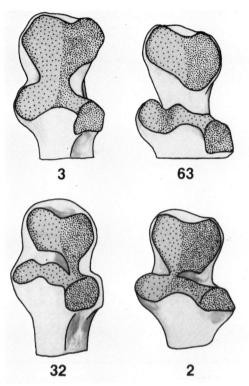

3   **63**

32   **2**

Figure 11–6. In approximately 95% of patients, virtually no articular cartilage is present at the midportion of the olecranon. (After Tillmann, B.: A Contribution to the Functional Morphology of Articular Surfaces. Bargmann, W., and Doerr, W., eds. Konorz, G., trans. Littleton, Mass., P.S.G. Pub. Co., 1978.)

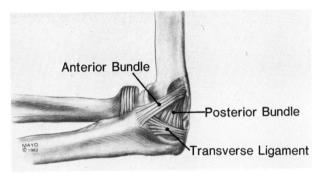

Anterior Bundle

Posterior Bundle

Transverse Ligament

Figure 11–7. Classic demonstration of the medial collateral ligaments. Notice that the anterior bundle of the medial collateral ligament inserts onto the coronoid. This accounts for the stability of the joint even when the proximal ulna has been removed. (From Morrey, B. F. (ed.): The Elbow and Its Disorders. Philadelphia, W. B. Saunders Co., 1985.)

some surgical approaches to the joint are undertaken here. The highly congruent articulation, coupled with its lateral ligaments, provides the stability of the elbow joint.

The medial aspect of the elbow and the medial collateral ligaments are dominated by the anterior ulnar collateral ligament (Fig. 11–7).[7] The posterior ulnar collateral ligament is taut only in flexion, and

a transverse component is of relatively little clinical significance. It is the medial complex that tends to render the elbow stable. On the lateral aspect, the lateral collateral ligament attaches to the annular ligament and then onto the ulnar ligament with accessory fibers (Fig. 11–8).

The supracondylar bone that supports the articulation is vulnerable to fracture and comminution. The medial bone is much thinner and less substantial than the lateral supracondylar column. Fractures of the distal humerus, then, are difficult to reduce and treat, whether by open or closed techniques.

The medial epicondyle is much more prominent than the lateral. The medial collateral ligament attaches to the undersurface of the medial epicondyle. Thus, any disruption of the epicondyle is indicative of disruption of the medial collateral ligament complex.[9] The radial collateral ligament attaches to the lateral epicondyle, which is much less prominent and thus less vulnerable to injury.

Four major muscle groups are distributed about the elbow (Fig. 11–9).[1, 8] The first, or flexor group,

Figure 11–8. Lateral collateral ligament complex. The radial collateral ligament inserts into the annular ligament, but accessory components provide additional stability to this joint. (From Morrey, B. F. (ed.): The Elbow and Its Disorders. Philadelphia, W. B. Saunders Co., 1985.)

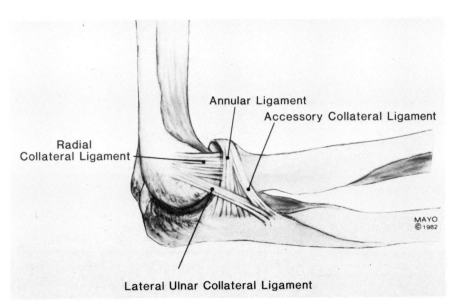

Annular Ligament

Accessory Collateral Ligament

Radial Collateral Ligament

Lateral Ulnar Collateral Ligament

muscle.[13] The extension of the elbow is provided almost exclusively by the second muscle group, the triceps mechanism. The triceps inserts onto the tip of the olecranon and is rarely involved with traumatic conditions or diseased prostheses. The insertion, however, is protected from the skin by the olecranon bursa, which is a common source of inflammation in occupational and recreational injuries. On the lateral aspect of the joint, the third muscle group, the so-called extensor-supinator group, is intimately associated with the lateral epicondyle. The undersurface of the supinator muscle is associated with the collateral ligament structures. These are rarely the source of direct trauma, and calcification is unusual. The medial aspect attaching to the region of the medial epicondyle gives rise to the origin of the fourth muscle group, the flexor-pronator group. Both of these common tendinous regions are subject to tennis elbow. In the youth these regions are vulnerable to avulsion fractures, particularly along the medial aspect.

The neurovascular structures across the elbow are well recognized (Fig. 11–10). The brachial artery closely accompanies the median nerve; both cross the medial aspect of the biceps as each structure enters the antecubital fossa.[8] In this position, these structures are vulnerable to injury after supracondylar fractures and elbow dislocation. Entrapment in the fracture or in the joint has been occasionally reported. The ulnar nerve is particularly susceptible to direct trauma to the joint. In addition, non-union of condylar fractures commonly result in a "tardy ulnar nerve palsy."[6] The radial nerve emerges from the lateral aspect of the biceps and under the brachioradialis. This nerve is particularly vulnerable to injury with midshaft humeral fractures, but it is

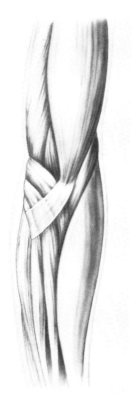

Figure 11–9. The muscular envelope of the elbow joint accounts for both the deforming forces seen in supracondylar-type fractures and the ectopic calcification seen after injury.

consists of the brachialis and biceps muscles. The brachialis crosses the joint closely applied to the capsule, thus making it vulnerable to injury during elbow dislocations and in trauma.[10] Myositis ossificans may be distributed along the course of this

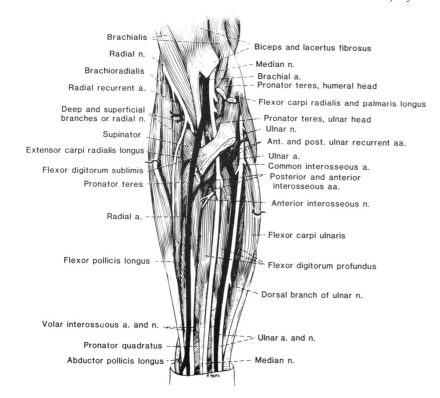

Brachialis
Radial n.
Brachioradialis
Radial recurrent a.
Deep and superficial branches or radial n.
Supinator
Extensor carpi radialis longus
Flexor digitorum sublimis
Pronator teres
Radial a.
Flexor pollicis longus
Volar interosseous a. and n.
Pronator quadratus
Abductor pollicis longus

Biceps and lacertus fibrosus
Median n.
Brachial a.
Pronator teres, humeral head
Flexor carpi radialis and palmaris longus
Pronator teres, ulnar head
Ulnar n.
Ant. and post. ulnar recurrent aa.
Ulnar a.
Common interosseous a.
Posterior and anterior interosseous aa.
Anterior interosseous n.
Flexor carpi ulnaris
Flexor digitorum profundus
Dorsal branch of ulnar n.
Ulnar a. and n.
Median n.

Figure 11–10. The neurovascular relationship with the muscles as they cross the antecubital fossa is a complex anatomic relationship that accounts for the rather frequent incidence of compromise of these structures with elbow trauma. (From Hollinshead, W. H.: Anatomy for Surgeons, Vol. 3: The Back and Limbs. 3rd Ed. New York, Harper and Row, 1982.)

not uniquely vulnerable to trauma at the elbow joint.

The supracondylar bone that supports the articulation of the joint is vulnerable to fracture-comminution. As mentioned earlier, the medial bone is much thinner and less substantial than the lateral supracondylar column, making fractures of the distal humerus difficult to reduce and treat. Finally, the fat pads of the elbow joint, present both anteriorly and posteriorly, are extrasynovial but intracapsular. Hence, any effusion or hemarthrosis tends to displace them. This displacement makes the fat pads visible on the lateral roentgenogram. The anterior fat pad may occasionally be seen in a routine radiograph. Demonstration of the posterior fat pad, on the other hand, is generally considered pathognomonic of an intra-articular effusion.

ROUTINE RADIOGRAPHIC TECHNIQUES

A minimum of two projections are necessary to evaluate the joint extremity.[37] The AP and lateral views of the elbow provide two views taken at 90° angles and fulfill this criterion. In trauma patients we also routinely obtain oblique views.

AP View

The view is obtained with the patient sitting adjacent to the x-ray table (the supine position may be used in the injured patient). The patient should be positioned so that the extended elbow is at the same level as the shoulder; thus, the extremity is in contact with the full length of the cassette.[16, 18] The extended elbow with the hand supinated is positioned with the central beam perpendicular to the joint, as shown in Figure 11–11A. The AP view is of value in studying the medial and lateral epicondyles as well as the radial capitellar articular

surface. With this view the invariant relationship of the radial head centered on the capitellum is observed (Fig. 11–11B). Assessment of the ulnotrochlear articular surface and at least a portion of the olecranon fossa is also possible. The normal carrying angle (5° to 20°, average 15°) can be measured on this view.[3]

Lateral View

The lateral view is obtained by flexing the elbow 90° and placing it directly upon the cassette. Again, the beam is perpendicular to the joint, as shown in Figure 11–12A. The hand must also be carefully placed in the lateral position.[16, 18] This view provides good detail of the distal humerus, elbow joint, and proximal forearm. The coronoid of the ulna, which cannot be readily visualized on the AP view, and the olecranon are well visualized in the lateral projection (Fig. 11–12B and C). With a true lateral projection the presence of three concentric arcs can be identified (Fig. 11–13).[29] The smaller arc is the trochlear sulcus, the intermediate arc represents the capitellum, and the larger arc is the medial aspect of the trochlea. If the arcs are interrupted, one has not obtained a true lateral projection.

Unfortunately, in patients with elbow injury the true AP and lateral views are difficult to obtain. Patients will frequently be unable to extend the elbow fully or flex the elbow to 90°. In these situations, the cassette should be placed under or adjacent to the extremity, and the tube should be angled to approximate these views as closely as possible.

Oblique Views

Oblique views are obtained by initially positioning the arm as one would for the usual AP film. For the medial oblique view (Fig. 11–14), the patient's arm is positioned with the forearm and arm

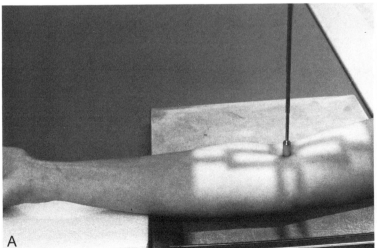
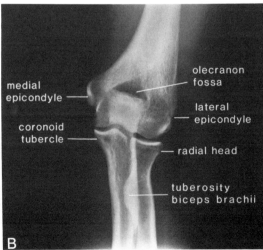

Figure 11–11. *A*, Patient positioned for AP view of elbow. Arm is level with cassette with the hand palm up. The central beam (pointer) is perpendicular to the elbow. *B*, Radiograph demonstrating bony relationships and anatomy. (From Berquist, T. H.: Imaging techniques in the elbow. *In* Morrey, B. F. (ed.): The Elbow and Its Disorders. Philadelphia, W. B. Saunders Co., 1985.)

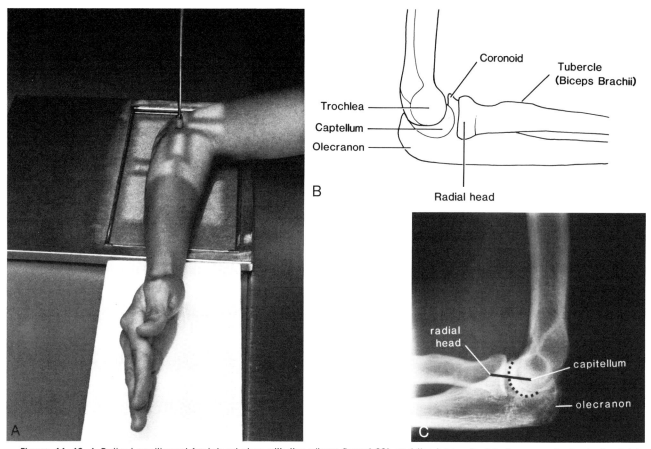

Figure 11–12. A, Patient positioned for lateral view with the elbow flexed 90° and the beam (pointer) perpendicular to the joint. The shoulder is at the same level as the cassette. This is required to obtain a true lateral view. B, and C, Illustration and radiograph demonstrating lateral view of the elbow. (From Berquist, T. H.: Imaging techniques in the elbow. In Morrey, B. F. (ed.): The Elbow and Its Disorders. Philadelphia, W. B. Saunders Co., 1985.)

internally rotated approximately 45°.[16] This view allows improved visualization of the trochlea, olecranon, and coronoid. The radial head is obscured by the proximal ulna. The lateral oblique view (Fig. 11–15) is taken with the forearm, arm, and hand externally rotated (Fig. 11–15A).[16] This projection provides excellent visualization of the radiocapitellar articulation, medial epicondyle, radioulnar articulation, and coronoid tubercle (Fig. 11–15B).

Radial Head View

Radial head fractures are a common clinical problem and are often difficult to visualize. Several other techniques may be utilized when such a lesion is suspected.[25, 26, 37, 38] The radial head view (Fig. 11–16) is easily performed by positioning the patient as one would for a routine lateral examination. The tube is then angled 45° toward the joint.[25] This view

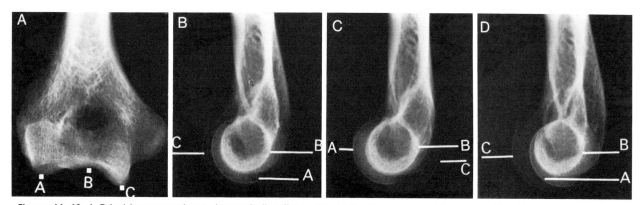

Figure 11–13. A, Dried bone specimen demonstrating the points of the three concentric arcs on the AP view: A, capitellum; B, trochlear sulcus; C, medial aspect of the trochlea. B, On true lateral view these arcs are perfectly aligned. C and D, With slight angulation (5° lateral and 5° medial), the arcs are no longer aligned, indicating that the view is not a true lateral. (From Berquist, T. H.: Imaging techniques in the elbow. In Morrey, B. F. (ed.): The Elbow and Its Disorders. Philadelphia, W. B. Saunders Co., 1985.)

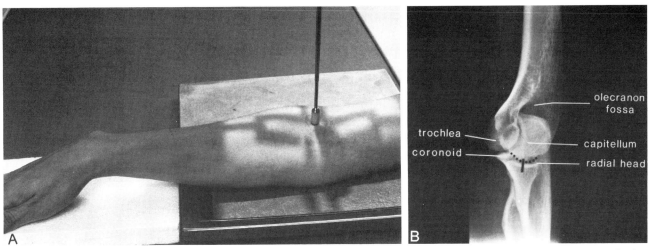

Figure 11–14. A, The patient's arm and forearm are internally rotated and the hand pronated. The central beam is perpendicular to the elbow joint (pointer). *B,* Radiograph of medial view. The radial head is obscured by the ulna. Note the constant radiocapitellar alignment (*dotted line* indicates capitellum). (From Berquist, T. H.: Imaging techniques in the elbow. *In* Morrey, B. F. (ed.): The Elbow and Its Disorders. Philadelphia, W. B. Saunders Co., 1985.)

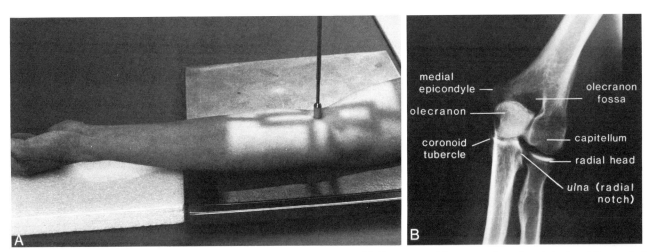

Figure 11–15. A, The patient is positioned for the lateral oblique view, with the arm and forearm externally rotated and the central beam perpendicular to the elbow joint (pointer). *B,* Radiograph of lateral oblique view. Note good visualization of radial head and capitellum, medial epicondyle, and radioulnar articulation. (From Berquist, T. H.: Imaging techniques in the elbow. *In* Morrey, B. F. (ed.): The Elbow and Its Disorders. Philadelphia, W. B. Saunders Co., 1985.)

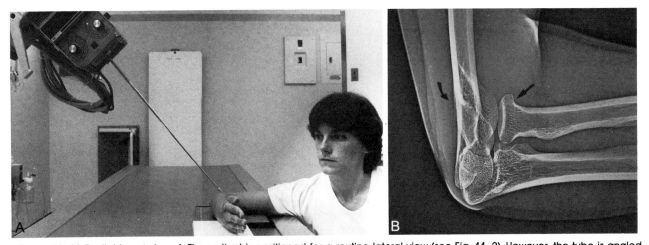

Figure 11–16. Radial head view. *A,* The patient is positioned for a routine lateral view (see Fig. 11–2). However, the tube is angled 45° toward the joint rather than perpendicularly. *B,* Radial head view with xeroradiographic technique (see xeroradiography in Chapter 1). Note excellent visualization of the radial head with an unpacked fracture *(straight arrow)*. Posterior fat pad *(curved arrow)* is definitely seen. (From Berquist, T. H.: Imaging techniques in the elbow. *In* Morrey, B. F. (ed.): The Elbow and Its Disorders. Philadelphia, W. B. Saunders Co., 1985.)

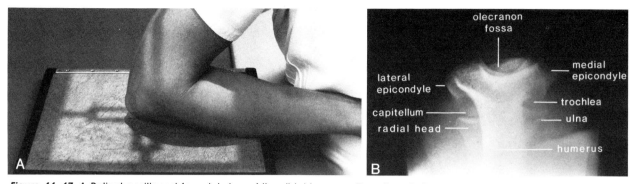

Figure 11–17. *A,* Patient positioned for axial view of the distal humerus. The elbow is flexed approximately 110°, with the forearm and elbow on the cassette. The central beam is perpendicular to the cassette and centered in the region of the olecranon fossa. *B,* Radiograph provides excellent visualization of the epicondyles, ulnar sulcus, and radiocapitellar and ulnar trochlea articulations. (From Berquist, T. H.: Imaging techniques in the elbow. *In* Morrey, B. F. (ed.): The Elbow and Its Disorders. Philadelphia, W. B. Saunders Co., 1985.)

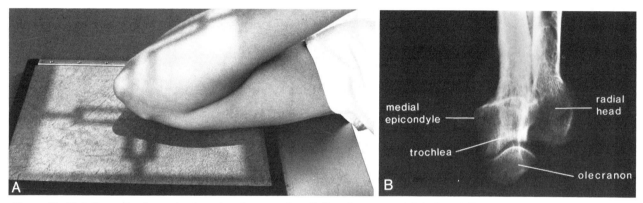

Figure 11–18. *A,* The patient's arm is placed on the cassette with the elbow completely flexed. The central beam is perpendicular to the cassette. *B,* Radiograph demonstrates the olecranon, trochlea, and medial epicondyle. (From Berquist, T. H.: Imaging techniques in th elbow. *In* Morrey, B. F. (ed.): The Elbow and Its Disorders. Philadelphia, W. B. Saunders Co., 1985.)

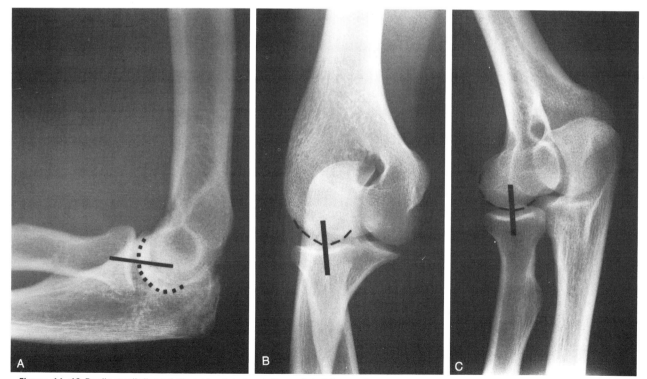

Figure 11–19. Radiocapitellar relationship. *A,* Lateral; *B,* medial oblique; *C,* lateral oblique. (From Berquist, T. H.: Imaging techniques in the elbow. *In* Morrey, B. F. (ed.): The Elbow and Its Disorders. Philadelphia, W. B. Saunders Co., 1985.)

projects the radius away from the remaining bony structures, allowing subtle changes to be more readily detected (Fig. 11–16*B*). This view may also allow the fat pads to be more easily visualized.

Axial Views

Occasionally, suspected pathology of the olecranon or epicondyles prompts further evaluation using axial projections. Figure 11–17 demonstrates the axial projection utilized to evaluate the medial and lateral epicondyles as well as the olecranon fossa and ulnar sulcus. The patient's elbow is flexed approximately 110° with the forearm on the cassette, the beam directed perpendicularly to the cassette, and the casette centered on the olecranon fossa.[16] This projection is also helpful in detecting subtle tendon calcifications in athletes with tendinitis and is often used to evaluate the reduction of unstable supracondylar fractures. The olecranon process itself is best demonstrated on the axial projection taken with the elbow completely flexed, as shown in Figure 11–18.[16]

Assessment of Standard Radiographic Views

Other views of the elbow can be performed in different clinical situations, but these studies are the most commonly utilized views. Assessment of these views should be complete and systematic. Certain features should be checked consistently and, when necessary, further views or modalities should be employed.

The relationship of the radial head to the articular surface of the capitellum is constant regardless of the view obtained (Fig. 11–19). The radius is normally bowed at the level of the tubercle. Therefore, while a line through the midpoint of the head and neck provides consistency, the line should not be extended to include this portion of the shaft.

Careful evaluation of the fat pads is essential. These structures are intracapsular but extrasynovial.[20, 28, 31, 33, 37] The anterior fat pad is normally seen on the lateral view. The posterior fat pad is obscured owing to its position in the olecranon fossa (Fig. 11–20). Displacement of the fat pads, particularly the posterior, is indicative of an intra-articular fracture with hemarthrosis.[19, 20, 32, 37] Norell[32] reported that 90 percent of children with posterior fat pad signs had elbow fractures. This finding is somewhat less common in the adult, but if it is present a fracture is likely. Cross-table lateral views may be more specific. A lipohemarthrosis may be evident, which is more specific for an intra-articular fracture.[15, 33, 41]

The supinator fat stripe lies ventral to the radial head and neck on the surface of the supinator muscle (Fig. 11–21). Fractures about the elbow will frequently displace or obliterate this structure, providing a clue to the underlying injury. Rogers and MacEwan[37] reported changes in this fat stripe in 100 percent of fractures of the radial head and neck and in 82 percent of other elbow fractures.

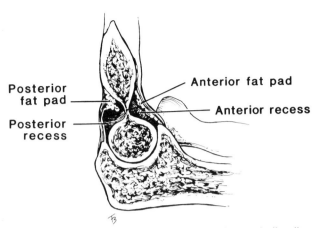

Figure 11–20. Lateral illustration of elbow demonstrating the anterior and posterior fat pads. (From Berquist, T. H.: Imaging Techniques in the elbow. *In* Morrey, B. F. (ed.): The Elbow and Its Disorders. Philadelphia, W. B. Saunders Co., 1985.)

The anterior humeral line is helpful in detecting subtle supracondylar fractures in children but it is not frequently used in adults.[36] This line, drawn along the anterior humeral cortex, should pass through the middle third of the capitellum.

SPECIAL RADIOGRAPHIC TECHNIQUES

Several special techniques are available to assess elbow pathology not clearly demonstrable on routine views.

Arthrography

Elbow arthrography, though less frequently performed than arthrography of the knee, shoulder, and hip, is a simple and valuable technique in selected patients with elbow disorders. The proce-

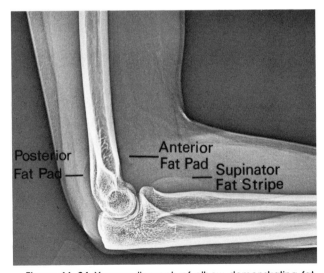

Figure 11–21. Xerogradiograph of elbow demonstrating fat pads and supinator fat stripe. (From Berquist, T. H.: Imaging techniques in the elbow. *In* Morrey, B. F. (ed.): The Elbow and Its Disorders. Philadelphia, W. B. Saunders Co., 1985.)

TABLE 11–1. Elbow Arthrography: Indications and Techniques

Indication	Procedure
Loose bodies	Double-contrast ± tomography
Osteochondromatosis	
Osteochondritis dissecans	
Fracture fragments from acute trauma	Double-contrast ± tomography
Ligament and capsule tears	Single-contrast
Synovitis	Double-contrast with tomography
Synovial cysts	Single-contrast
Articular cartilage abnormalities	Double-contrast with tomography
Capsule size	Single-contrast
Needle position prior to aspiration	Single-contrast
Postoperative	
Total joint replacement	Subtraction technique for total elbow arthroplasty
Other	Double-contrast with tomography

dure, when properly performed, can provide valuable information regarding the synovial lining, articular surfaces, and configuration of the elbow joint. Elbow arthrography is most commonly indicated for evaluation of loose bodies or subtle synovial or articular changes (Table 11–1).[23, 34, 39, 40] Such osteocartilaginous bodies may result from osteochondromatosis, osteochondritis dissecans, or osteochondral fragments from acute trauma. The articular cartilage in patients with osteochondritis dissecans and the various arthritides is also effectively studied with elbow arthrography.[22] Less commonly, arthrograms are performed to evaluate ligament tears or the articular capsule. In our experience as well as that of several other authors, patients with chronic elbow instability frequently demonstrate an enlarged, irregular capsule.[23, 30, 39]

Elbow arthrography may reveal diminished capsular volume in patients with a decreased range of motion and pain, changes similar to those described for adhesive capsulitis involving the shoulder.[30] Arthrograms are occasionally performed to evaluate patients with pain thought to be due to loosening or infection of a prosthesis following total joint replacement. Arthrograms may also be indicated in certain instances following other surgical procedures on the elbow in which unexplained chronic pain or disability persists.[30, 39]

Technique

To obtain maximum information, arthrography should be performed by an experienced physician with a thorough understanding of the patient's clinical situation. Review of routine radiographs is essential, as these films may provide clues that dictate subtle changes in film technique. The choice of contrast material and indications for tomography are also highly dependent upon the patient's clinical situation (see Table 11–1). Simply stated, arthrography should be tailored to the individual patient.

The radiographic equipment utilized in arthrography requires excellent detail and must also allow adequate work space to simplify patient positioning and needle placement. An overhead tube provides better geometry, resulting in improved film quality compared with the conventional fluoroscopic unit (see Introduction to Arthrography in Chapter 1).

The contrast agent for arthrography can be air, a positive contrast material, or a combination of the two. Several contrast media are available that can be utilized effectively in single- or double-contrast arthrography. We most commonly use Hypaque-M-60. Renografin 60 and Reno-M-60 are also commonly used. Because of increased osmolality and rapid absorption, the contrast medium rapidly be-

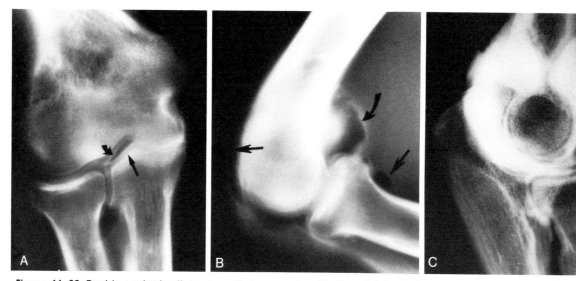

Figure 11–22. Double-contrast arthrogram with tomography. AP *(A)* and lateral *(B)* views demonstrate excellent articular and synovial detail *(arrows).* Single-contrast arthrogram *(C)* with too much contrast medium obscures anatomic detail.

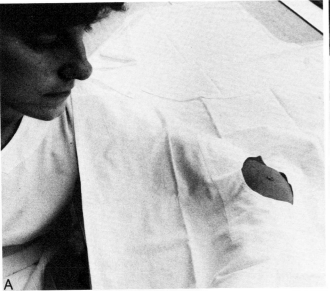

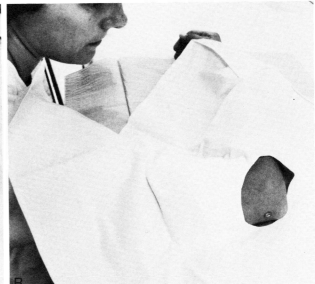

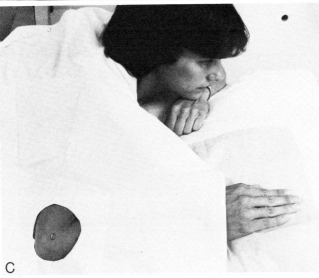

Figure 11–23. Patient positioning for elbow arthrography. *A,* Sitting with elbow flexed and marker over radiocapitellar joint for lateral approach. *B,* Sitting with elbow flexed and marker set for posterior approach. *C,* Prone with marker positioned for lateral approach. (From Berquist, T. H.: Imaging Techniques in the Elbow. *In* Morrey, B. F. (ed.): The Elbow and Its Disorders. Philadelphia, W. B. Saunders Co., 1985.)

comes diluted in the joint, resulting in loss of detail with filming. This may occur as early as 5 to 10 min following injection. If an effusion is present, dilution may occur even more rapidly. This dilution and loss of detail can be prevented to some degree by combining 0.3 ml of 1:1,000 epinephrine with the contrast material.[23] The latter step is especially indicated if tomography is used.

Multiple techniques for performing elbow arthrography have been described by other authors.[23, 30, 34, 35, 39, 40] In most cases, we utilize double-contrast technique. This provides better detail in the visualization of the articular surfaces and synovial lining of the capsule. Subtle changes can be obscured if single-contrast technique is utilized (Fig. 11–22).[23, 27] We frequently employ trispiral tomography to define the articular and intracapsular detail most effectively. Linear tomography is helpful if trispiral tomography is not available.[35]

The patient is positioned either sitting next to the table or lying prone (Fig. 11–23). In either position

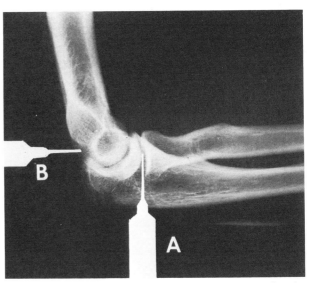

Figure 11–24. Lateral (A) and posterior (B) approaches for elbow arthrography or joint aspiration.

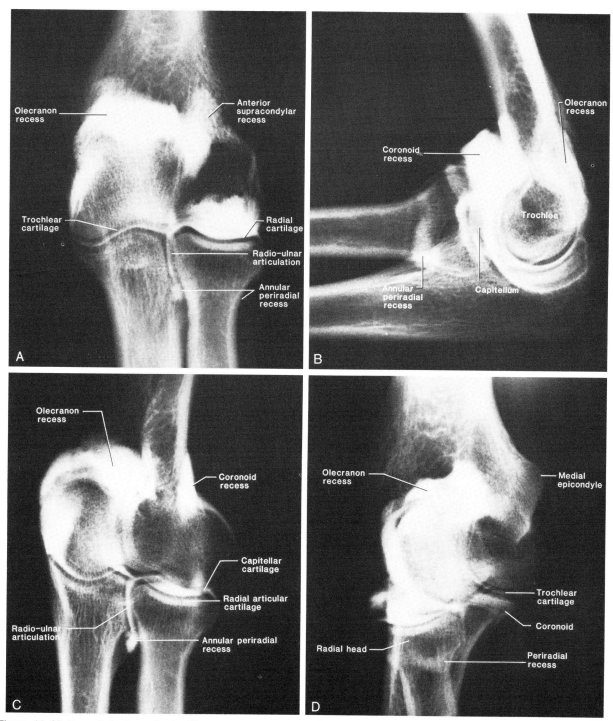

Figure 11–25. Normal single-contrast arthrograms. AP *(A)*, lateral *(B)* and oblique views (*C* and *D*). (From Berquist, T. H.: Imaging techniques in the elbow. *In* Morrey, B. F. (ed.): The Elbow and Its Disorders. Philadelphia, W. B. Saunders Co., 1985.)

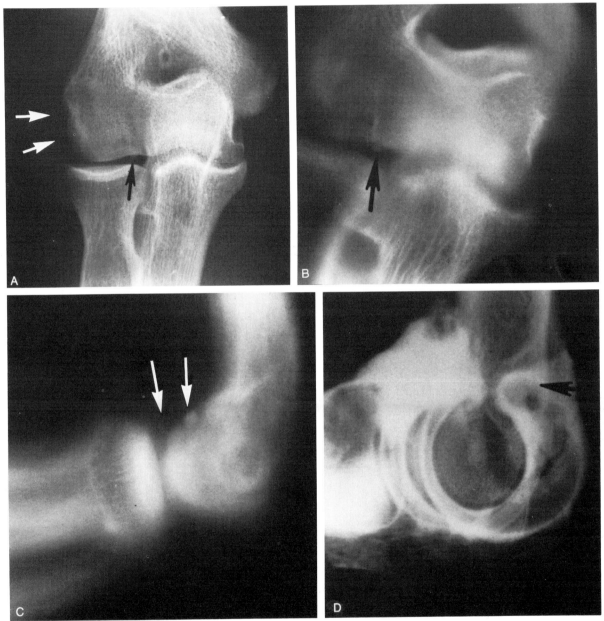

Figure 11–26. Patient with chronic elbow pain and clicking. AP view of the elbow *(A)* with irregularity or loose body near the capitellum *(single arrow)* and subtle densities laterally *(arrows).* AP *(B)* and lateral *(C)* tomograms reveal that the fragment is attached to the capitellum. The densities seen laterally should be extra-articular. Lateral arthrogram *(D)* demonstrates several lucent loose bodies *(arrow).*

the elbow is flexed 90° with the lateral aspect of the elbow toward the examiner. The determination of which position is best depends somewhat upon the equipment available and the patient's condition. Prior to the procedure, fluoroscopic evaluation of the range of motion, examination for stability, and observations for possible loose bodies should be performed.[23, 27] The elbow is then prepared using sterile technique, and one of two needle sites may be chosen for entering the joint. In most instances, a lateral approach into the radiocapitellar joint is chosen (Fig. 11–24). However, following resection of the radial head or other operative techniques, or if a lateral injury is suspected, a posterior approach may occasionally be required. With the posterior approach, the elbow is again flexed 90°, and the medial and lateral epicondyles and olecranon are palpated. The needle is then placed at an equal distance between these landmarks (Figs. 11–23B and 11–24).[27] The needle is positioned with fluoroscopic guidance in both situations.

When the needle enters the joint space, a small amount of contrast material is introduced to check needle position. If the needle is properly located within the joint space, the contrast material will flow away from the needle tip. Contrast material will collect at the needle tip if the needle is not properly positoned. Significant resistance is also noted if the needle is not within the joint space. The joint should be aspirated prior to injection of the balance of the contrast medium. If fluid is present, laboratory studies can be obtained (culture, crystals, etc.) Large amounts of fluid will result in dilution of the contrast medium and a suboptimal arthrogram.

Depending on the clinical setting, the injection may consist of three different techniques (see Table 11–1). As mentioned previously, we most fre-

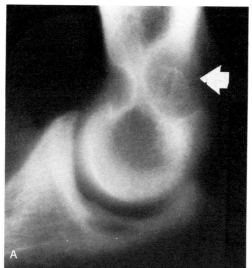

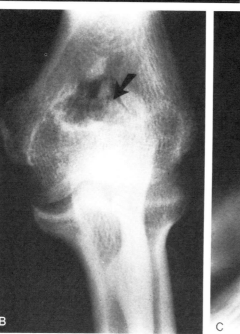

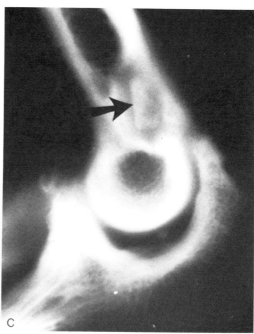

Figure 11–27. Lateral tomogram (A) of the elbow in patient with os supratrochleare dorsale. Note the thin cortical margin and lack of trabecular pattern. AP radiograph (B) and lateral tomogram (C) demonstrate marked thickening and trabeculation in a symptomatic patient.

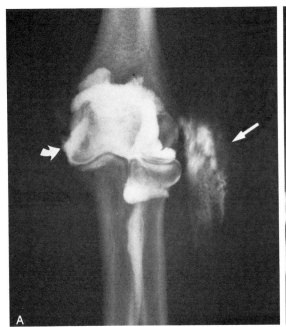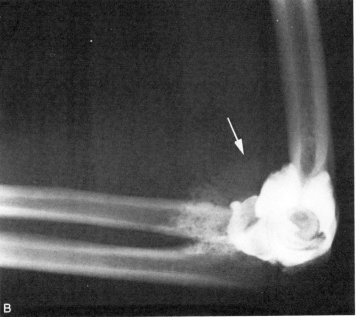

Figure 11–28. Patient with suspected lateral capsule tear. Posterior injection was used. AP *(A)* and lateral *(B)* views of a single-contrast arthrogram demonstrate lateral extravasation from a capsular tear *(arrows).* (From Berquist, T. H.: Imaging techniques in the elbow. *In* Morrey, B. F. (ed.): The Elbow and Its Disorders. Philadelphia, W. B. Saunders Co., 1985.)

quently use the double-contrast technique, which requires approximately 0.5 to 1 ml of positive contrast material and 6 to 12 ml of air. This mixture varies depending upon the size of the joint capsule and the patient being studied. If a significant allergy to contrast material is elicited in the patient's history, air alone may be utilized; however, with air alone the detail is not ideal, and even with tomography the examination may be suboptimal. Single-contrast injections of 5 to 6 ml may be adequate in certain situations (examination of capsule size and disruptions);[23, 40] however, we rarely use single-contrast technique (see Table 11–1).

Following the injection, the needle is removed, and the elbow is slowly exercised to avoid rupturing the capsule. This also avoids the formation of excessive air bubbles. While being exercised, the elbow is studied fluoroscopically. This assists in evaluating the joint's range of motion as well as the presence of loose bodies. In addition, stress can be applied to the elbow in patients with suspected elbow instability. Routine filming includes AP, lateral, and both oblique views. Medial and lateral cross-table views (with double-contrast technique) enhance the air-contrast component in the superior portion of the capsule. Routine films are followed by tomography, when indicated.

Normal Arthrogram

In the normal arthrogram (Fig. 11–25), the three articular compartments of the joint are readily identified (radiocapitellar, ulnotrochlear, radioulnar). There are three recesses: anterior (coronoid), posterior (olecranon), and annular.[24, 39, 40] The posterior

recess is particularly difficult to visualize. Tomograms taken in the lateral projection with the elbow flexed 90° are most helpful in evaluating this region.

The normal joint capacity is 10 to 12 ml. This capacity may decrease in cases of capsulitis or increase to 18 to 22 ml in patients with chronic instability or recurrent dislocations.[27]

Abnormal Arthrogram

Abnormalities encountered during arthrography are frequently related to loose bodies. These so-called "loose bodies" may actually be free or attached. If contrast material completely surrounds the object, it may properly be considered a loose body. In certain cases tomography may be useful in detection of loose bodies and in evaluation of articular defects,[22] though arthrography is often more definitive (Fig. 11–26).

Intra-articular bodies in the olecranon fossa may be due to trauma associated with enlarging osteochondral fragments. Fragments are nourished by synovial fluid.[17] An ossicle, the os supratrochleare dorsale, has also been described by Obermann (Fig. 11–27).[33] This may be symptomatic owing to repeated olecranon trauma. In patients with symptoms, the ossicles are sclerotic and irregular (Fig. 11–27B and C). This feature allows the ossicles to be radiographically differentiated from asymptomatic densities. The majority of symptomatic ossicles (87 percent) are on the right.[33]

Occasionally arthrography is performed for suspected capsular tears or ligament injury. Extravasation of contrast material indicates a tear (Fig. 11–28). Care must be taken not to mistake this

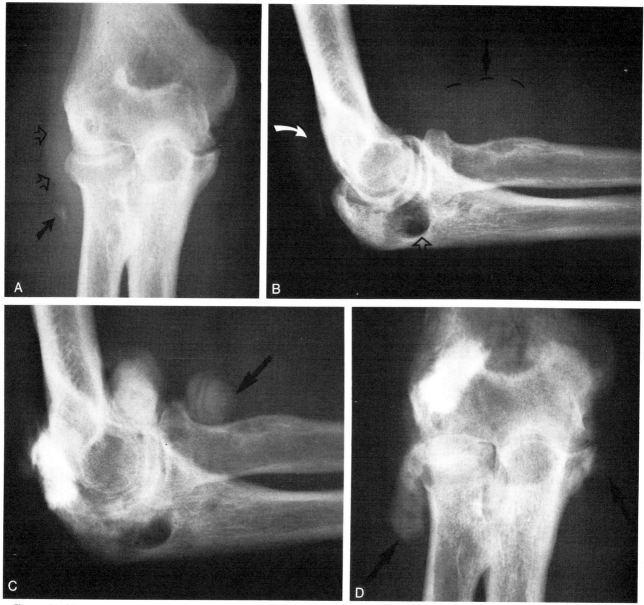

Figure 11–29. Patient with previous surgery for ligament repair and degenerative cyst in the ulna. The AP *(A)* view demonstrates lateral soft tissue swelling *(open arrows)* with a bony density *(black arrow)* in the soft tissues. The joint space is narrowed with degenerative changes. The lateral view *(B)* demonstrates the cyst with postoperative changes *(open arrow)*, and shows displacement of the posterior fat pad *(curved arrow)* and supinator fat stripe *(upper straight arrow and broken lines)*. The single-contrast arthrograms *(C* and *D)* demonstrate a walled-off leak in the annular recess *(black arrow)* and a second area laterally that contains the bony density seen in *A (arrow in D)*.

extravasation with extravasation at the needle site. This latter extravasation is frequent with capsulitis but can usually be avoided with good technique. If a lateral ligament tear is suspected, a posterior approach should be utilized. Ideally, the injection should be placed on the side opposite that of the suspected tear.

Persistent pain and limited range of motion following surgery may also require arthrographic evaluation (Fig. 11–29). The integrity of the capsule, ligaments, and articular surface can be accurately assessed.

TRAUMA

Soft Tissue Injury

Soft tissue injury about the elbow is most often secondary to hyperextension or valgus stress commonly due to a fall on the outstretched hand. An associated blow directed to the posterior aspect of the elbow coincident with the fall is occasionally reported. While the radiographs will not show an injury to bone, tearing of the anterior capsule, stretching of the medial collateral ligament, or possibly tearing of the synovium can all result in a painful hemarthrosis. The fat pad sign will be positive, physical examination may reveal a local tenderness, and the joint will not fully extend. It should be recognized that a significant injury to this joint is possible even without roentgenographic evidence of fracture. Recovery may be slow, and some loss of extension may occasionally be seen even without fracture.

Ligament Injury

The most extreme example of ligamentous disruption is posterior dislocation of the elbow (Fig. 11–30). Some have classified elbow dislocation according to the position of the displaced ulna with respect to the humerus. This criterion gives rise to the following types of dislocation: posterior, posterolateral, lateral, posteromedial, pure lateral, or anterior. The posterolateral type of dislocation is most common. Anterior dislocation is extremely rare. This classification implies little about the prognosis of such injuries, and it probably has relatively little value to the clinician. However, it does serve to describe the radiographic appearance of the displacement accurately.

While the degree of dislocation will vary, injury to the anterior portion of the medial collateral ligament is considered present in all such events.[59] Associated injuries are common, and fractures of the coronoid, epicondyles,[58] or radial head occur in approximately 28 percent of patients with the dislocation.[51] Of these fractures, involvement of the radial head (Fig. 11–31) or coronoid is most common. The mechanism of injury is a fall on the outstretched hand possibly combined with a hyperextension injury or a significant axial load.[60]

Physical examination clearly reveals an elbow that is markedly painful to examination and is usually held in a position of approximately 60° to 70° of flexion. The prominent proximal ulna is palpable posteriorly. If the injury has gone without attention for more than 3 to 4 hr, a significant amount of swelling may be present. Treatment consists of immediate reduction of the dislocation regardless of the presence of a fracture. If the dislocation is complete, this is performed under a general anesthetic or an axillary block. If the coronoid is perched on the trochlea, reduction may be performed using intravenous sedation. Following the reduction, AP, lateral, and occasionaly oblique radiographs are necessary to ensure that no fracture is present, or if one is present, that the fracture fragment will not interfere with motion. Tomography and occasionally arthrography may be required to evaluate the joint space completely. Calcification of the ligaments has been variously described in 10 to 15 percent of these individuals.[58] The calcification can occur either medially or laterally but is most common in the medial ligament complex (Fig. 11–31).

Isolated ligamentous injury is occasionally diagnosed after a fall on the outstretched hand when a valgus stress imparted to the joint results in disruption of the medial collateral ligament.[53] This is an injury that is not commonly recognized, and radiographically there are virtually no clues to its presence except a possible fat pad sign or calcification at the medial epicondyle.[51]

Additional mechanisms of ligamentous injury include the stress at the medial epicondyle that is seen with ballplayers, particularly in the case of adolescents.[43, 46] Frank avulsions of the medial epicondyle can also occur that might be considered a variant of ligamentous disruption.[61]

Confirmation of ligamentous disruption is ob-

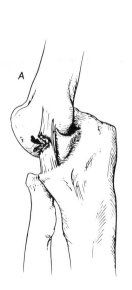 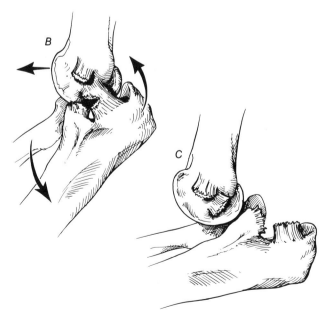

Figure 11–30. Dislocation of the elbow caused by hyperextension injury, resulting in disruption of the medial and lateral collateral ligament complex. (From Schwab, G. H., Bennett, J. B., Woods, G. W., et al.: Biomechanics of elbow instability: The role of the medial collateral ligament. Clin. Orthop. 146:42, 1980.)

©1978 Baylor College of Medicine

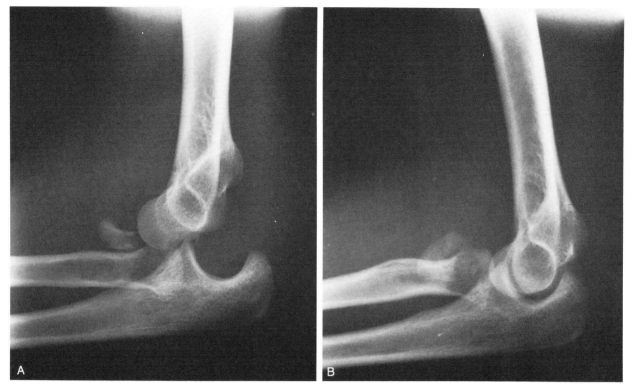

Figure 11–31. Type IV fracture-dislocation of the elbow with displacement of the radial head fragment *(A).* With reduction the radial head aligns to the capitellum, but the fragment remains displaced *(B).*

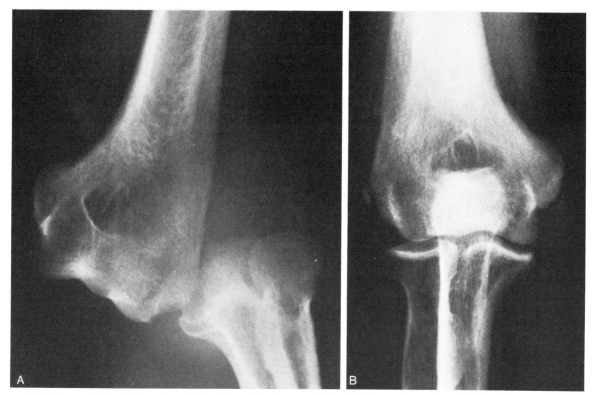

Figure 11–32. A pure lateral dislocation of the elbow *(A)* subsequently treated by reduction. Although there was no fracture, with healing ectopic ossification, or calcification, is noted in both the medial and collateral ligaments *(B).*

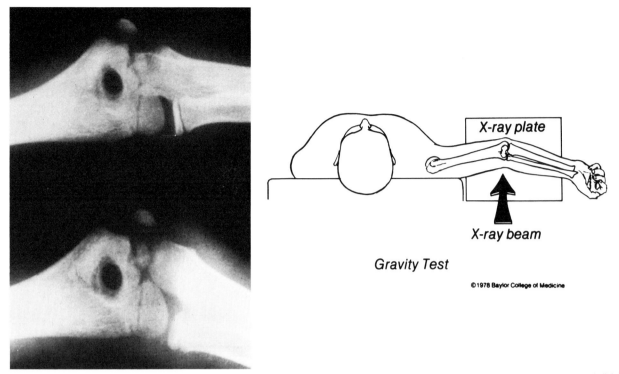

Figure 11–33. The valgus stress view of the elbow is demonstrated with the gravity test in which the arm is allowed to fall into "valgus." (From Schwab, G. H., Bennett, J. B., Woods, G. W., et al.: Biomechanics of elbow instability: The role of the medial collateral ligament. Clin. Orthop. 146:1980.)

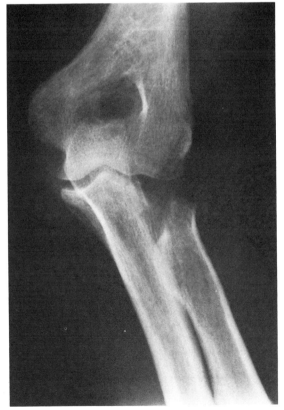

Figure 11–34. An extreme valgus deformity of the elbow with surprisingly little medial opening of the ulnohumeral joint.

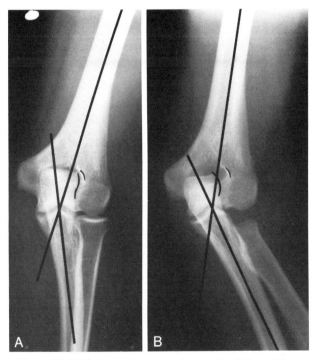

Figure 11–35. Normal valgus carrying angle of the uninjured extremity (A) with an increased valgus carrying angle after radial head has been excised. Once again, notice the surprisingly normal ulnohumeral joint, but the tip of the proximal ulna moves out of the olecranon fossa (B). (From Berquist, T. H.: Imaging techniques in the elbow. In Morrey, B. F. (ed.): The Elbow and Its Disorders. Philadelphia, W. B. Saunders Co., 1985.)

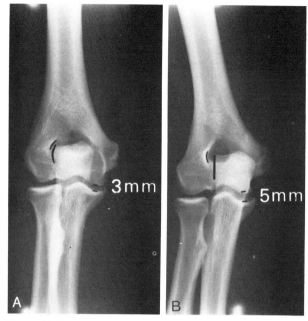

Figure 11–36. Normal AP roentgenogram of the elbow *(A)* with increased valgus stress opening 2° at the medial joint line. The tip of the olecranon moves medially *(B)*. (From Berquist, T. H.: Imaging techniques in the elbow. *In* Morrey, B. F. (ed.): The Elbow and Its Disorders. Philadelphia, W. B. Saunders Co., 1985.)

tained with a stress view. The valgus stress view as recommended by Schwab and colleagues is demonstrated in Figure 11–32.[59] This view cannot be obtained in the acute instance unless the joint has been anesthetized. Stress views of the elbow are difficult to interpret, since a significant valgus angulation can occur without a concurrent amount of widening of the ulnohumeral joint (Fig. 11–33). On the AP roentgenogram, the tip of the olecranon is not symmetrically aligned in the olecranon fossa (Figs. 11–34 and 11–35). This finding should alert the radiologist to the instability even if the joint line does not appear tilted. Ideally, stress views should be performed with fluoroscopic guidance. This allows proper positioning and facilitates detection of subtle changes during the stressing maneuver. Comparison with the normal elbow is essential. A widening of the joint space greater than 1 mm above the neutral measurement may be arbitrarily considered abnormal (Fig. 11–36). Magnetic resonance imaging may provide a new method of examining elbow ligament injury. The anatomic detail provided allows one to visualize the tendons and ligaments. This should allow detection of significant ligament tears. Arthrography may also be of value in detecting ligament disruption and in evaluating capsule size.

Complications of ligamentous disruption can include recurrent dislocations of the elbow.[54] The brachial artery may be entrapped in the joint upon reduction,[49] or the median nerve may likewise become incarcerated.[56] The most commonly recognized radiographic complication of elbow disloca-

tion is probably the entrapment of the medial epicondyle in the joint. This occurs in adolescents who have sustained avulsion of this structure at the time of the traumatic event.[61]

Treatment of most soft tissue injuries about the elbow consists simply of rest and immobilization for variable periods of time. Usually less than 2 or at most 3 weeks of immobilization is required after dislocation because late instability occurs in only about 1 or 2 percent and because a flexion-contracture can result with prolonged immobilization.[48, 54] Most clinicians recommend early motion at least through a safe or protected arc, for example, from 30° to 100°.

Tendon Injury

Traumatic tendon avulsions about the elbow are distinctly uncommon.[51] Some authors have implicated systemic disease processes, such as hyperparathyroidism[43] or osteogenesis imperfecta,[50] for these avulsions. Associated injuries may also occur with tendon injury, such as fracture of the radial head. Levy demonstrated that these fractures occur with avulsion injuries of the triceps.[47]

It is of special interest that characteristic radiographic features have been described for both the biceps[44] and triceps avulsion.[45] The most commonly recognized tendon injury about the elbow is avulsion of the biceps tendon from the radial tuberosity. Radiographically the radial tuberosity will often reveal hypertrophic changes or irregularity. This is best demonstrated on the lateral radiograph with the forearm in neutral rotation (Fig. 11–37).[44] Davis has found that this finding implicates a degenerative process as the etiology of the disruption. The diagnosis is suspected when the patient complains of a ripping or tearing pain in the antecubital space during a lifting episode. Examination reveals ten-

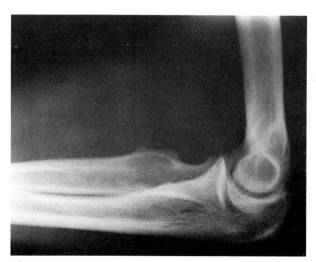

Figure 11–37. Rupture of the biceps tendon is often associated with degenerative changes of the radial tuberosity, as demonstrated here.

derness in the antecubital fossa, and flexion causes a proximal retraction of the muscle as opposed to the distal retraction that is seen in rupture of the long head of the biceps. The injury is treated with primary reattachment of the biceps tendon to the tuberosity[51] within the first several days.

Avulsion of the triceps from the tip of the olecranon is even less common. The mechanism of injury is unexpected resistance to extension of the elbow. The clinical features include local tenderness and loss of extension function. On the routine lateral roentgenogram an osseous density is regularly observed about the olecranon fossa.[45] This finding is pathognomonic for triceps avulsion. As with biceps rupture, the treatment is an immediate reattachment to the tip of the olecranon.

FRACTURES

Humeral Fractures

Supracondylar and Transcondylar Fractures of the Distal Humerus

Mechanism of Injury. Approximately 80 percent of distal humeral fractures occur in children.[51] The usual mechanism of injury for the most common type of fracture is a fall on the outstretched hand causing extension at the elbow joint (Fig. 11–38) and a shearing fracture of the distal humerus. The flexion fracture occurs from a direct blow to the

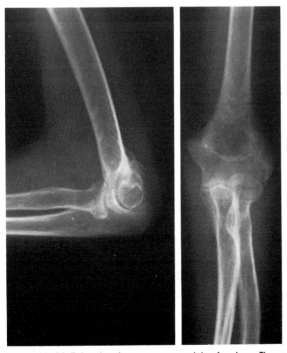

Figure 11–38. Extension-type supracondylar fracture. There is relatively little deformity on the AP projection, but the loss of the anterior angulation and displacement of the condyles is noted on the lateral view. (From Bryan, R. S.: Fractures about the elbow in adults. Instr. Course Lect. *30*:200, 1981.)

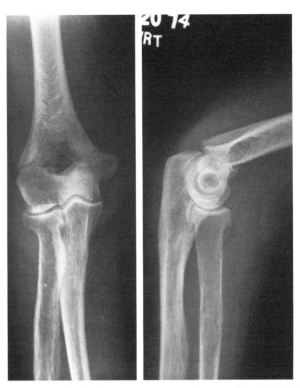

Figure 11–39. Flexion-type supracondylar fracture. Again, the AP view looks essentially normal, but the important anterior angulation of the articular surface clearly demonstrates the fracture. (From Bryan, R. S.: Fractures about the elbow in adults. Instr. Course Lect. *30*:200, 1981.)

posterior aspect of the flexed elbow and is much less common.

Classification. Fractures of the distal humerus have been classified as flexion and extension injuries. The extension injury occurs approximately ten times more often than the flexion injury. In the extension injury the fracture line is usually oblique, and displacement occurs posteriorly and proximally. The flexion injury occurs in the older age group. It entails a more transverse fracture line. Displacememt occurs anteriorly and proximally (Fig. 11–39).[51]

Physical Examination. Physical examination usually demonstrates variable amounts of swelling in the distal humeral region. The important bony landmarks retain their nominal relationships. With the elbow flexed, the medial and lateral epicondyle form the base of a triangle with the olecranon at the tip (Fig. 11–40). The deforming force from the muscle causes displacement but does not alter the relationship. A careful neurologic and vascular examination is of paramount importance in the patient with a supracondylar fracture, since the brachial artery as well as the median and ulnar nerve can be injured by the distal humeral fracture fragment (Fig. 11–41).[77] Injury to the brachial artery can result in muscle and nerve ischemia of the extremity in the severe form known as Volkmann's ischemic contracture.[79]

The lateral radiograph reveals variable amounts

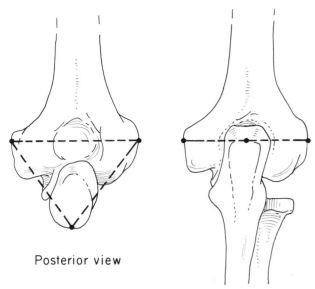

Posterior view

Figure 11–40. The posterior bony landmarks of the medial and lateral epicondyle and the tip of the olecranon form a triangle in the flexed position and a straight line in the extended position. (From Morrey, B. F. (ed.): The Elbow and Its Disorders. Philadelphia, W. B. Saunders Co., 1985.)

of displacement caused by the triceps mechanism, which pulls the condylar fragment proximally and posteriorly in the extension injury. The flexion fracture usually has less deformity, with anterior and proximal displacement as seen in the lateral radiograph. The transcondylar fracture occurs more commonly in older patients and usually shows less displacement.[62] The diagnosis is readily made by routine AP and lateral radiographs.

Treatment. Treatment of these fractures consists

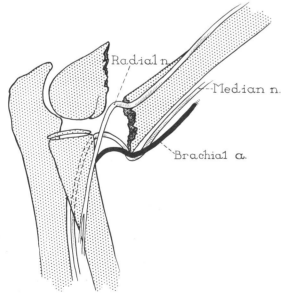

Figure 11–41. The displaced-extension supracondylar injury of the elbow can result in neurovascular compromise. (From Lipscomb, P. R., and Burleson, R. J.: Vascular and neural complications in supracondylar fractures of the humerus in children. J. Bone Joint Surg. *37A*:468, 1955.)

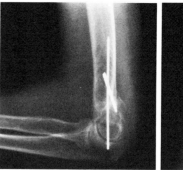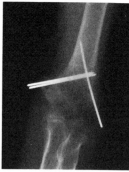

Figure 11–42. Supracondylar fracture fixed with crossed K-wires. Notice that in the lateral projection an anatomic reduction has not been obtained. (From Morrey, B. F. (ed.): The Elbow and Its Disorders. Philadelphia, W. B. Saunders Co., 1985.)

of closed reduction or reduction by skeletal traction.[68, 73, 84, 87] In either instance an AP image is important to ensure the proper varus-valgus orientation of the articulation, thus avoiding a varus or "gun stock" malunion deformity. Since the elbow is stable in flexion, routine views do not show this relationship. Hence, special flexion axial views of

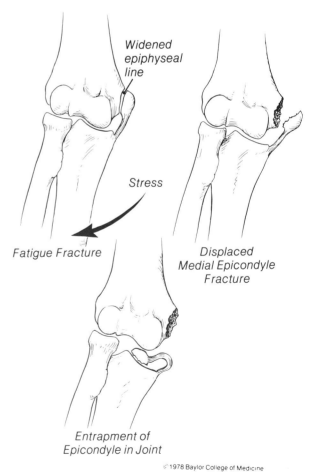

Figure 11–43. Valgus stress to the elbow can result in avulsion of the medial epicondyle, which can occasionally result in entrapment in the joint. (From Schwab, G. H., Bennett, J. B., Woods, G. W., et al.: Biomechanics of elbow instability: The role of the medial collateral ligament. Clin. Orthop. *146*:42, 1980.)

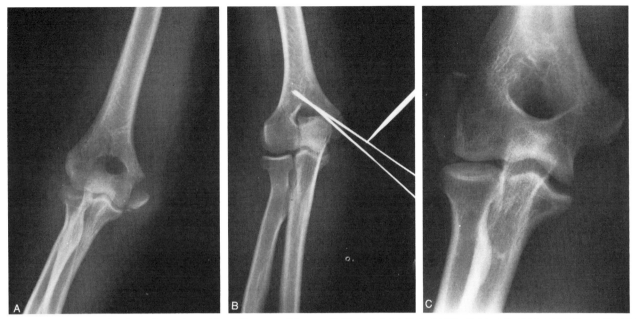

Figure 11–44. *A,* Avulsed medial epicondyle. *B,* Because this was displaced more than 3 mm, open-reduction and internal fixation were carried out. *C,* A rare avulsion injury of the lateral epicondyle. (From Morrey, B. F. (ed.): The Elbow and Its Disorders. Philadelphia, W. B. Saunders Co., 1985.)

the distal humerus are required in order to appreciate fully the quality of the reduction (Fig. 11–17). The normal anterior orientation of the articular surface (see Fig. 11–2) should be considered in assessing the reduction. This is readily accomplished with a routine lateral radiograph (Fig. 11–42).

Epicondylar Fractures

Mechanisms of Injury. Avulsion fractures of the epicondyle are distinctly unusual in the adult, since the physis has closed. Varus or valgus stresses that ordinarily cause an avulsion fracture of the epicondyle in the child result in a complex injury or fracture in the adult.[62] The mechanism of the medial epicondyle fracture is an avulsion force that is transmitted across the medial collateral ligament from a valgus stress imparted to the extended elbow (Fig. 11–43). The lateral epicondylar fracture is extremely rare (Fig. 11–43C).[51, 91] It probably occurs with a mechanism of injury similar but opposite in direction to that involved in fractures of the medial epicondyle. The lateral epicondyle may be treated in a closed fashion if the displacement is less than 2 to 3 mm.[87] An accurate reduction of the medial epicondyle, however, is more critical, since the ligamentous integrity of the joint depends upon the position of the medial epicondyle.[62] Thus, we recommend anatomic replacement of this fracture if more than 2 to 3 mm of displacement has occurred (Fig. 11–44).[51]

Complications. Occasionally, a severe displacement of the medial epicondyle associated with elbow dislocation can result in entrapment of this fracture fragment in the joint after reduction (Fig. 11–45). This entrapment is often difficult to diagnose on the lateral x-ray but is suggested by medial joint widening or visualization of the loose body on the radiograph. When this occurs, closed reductions

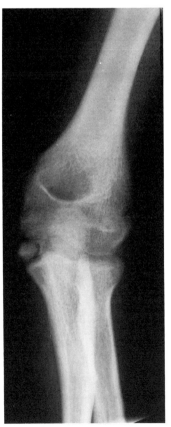

Figure 11–45. Example of a trapped medial epicondyle in the medial joint line.

are unsuccessful, and the fracture should be opened and anatomically pinned. Usually two smooth K-wires or a small compression screw is adequate for fixation. If closed treatment is used, immobilization for approximately 2 weeks is followed by gentle, progressive, active motion in an arc of 30° to 90°. Gradual increase in activity, as tolerated, is allowed after this period of time. Residual deformity, weakness, or instability following the fracture is considered very unusual.[87]

T and Y Condylar Fractures

Mechanism of Injury. These fractures occur from a direct blow to the proximal ulna usually, but not always, with the elbow in flexion. The fracture line is initiated in the central groove of the trochlea, propagates across the olecranon and coronoid fossa, and emerges across the medial and lateral supracondylar bony columns.

Classification. The most useful classification of this fracture is that proposed by Riseborough and Radin in 1969.[86] This classification aids in clarifying the mechanism and severity of the injury as well as the appropriate treatment program (Fig. 11–46). Riseborough and Radin distinguished four types of fracture. Type I fractures consist of undisplaced T or Y condylar fractures. The Type II injury is one in which the condyles are displaced but not rotated. Type III fractures are those in which the medial and lateral condylar components are rotated. This rotation is caused by the action in the flexor and extensor muscle masses and results in the so-called inverted V sign (Figure 11–47). The Type IV fracture is one with marked comminution.

Clinical and Radiographic Evaluation. In the T and Y supracondylar fracture, the epicondyles are displaced, so that the posterior triangle relationship is altered. There is usually massive swelling, and flexion-extension of the elbow is not possible. The

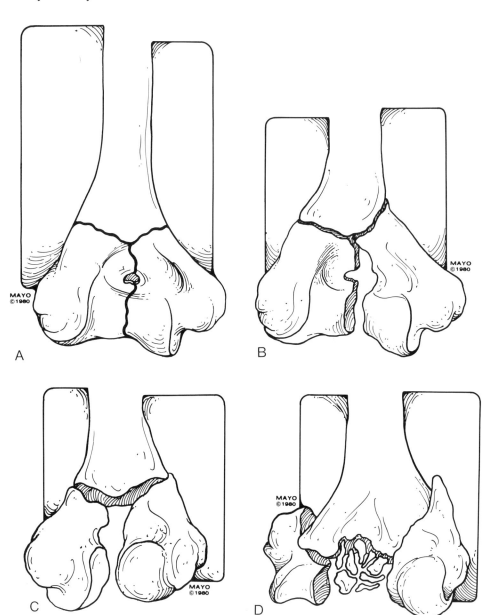

Figure 11–46. Classification of T and Y condylar fractures. *A,* Type I, undisplaced fracture; *B,* Type II, displacement without significant rotation; *C,* Type III, displacement with rotation of the condyle; *D,* Type IV, displacement and comminution. (From Bryan, R. S.: Fractures about the elbow in adults. Instr. Course Lect. *30:*200, 1981.)

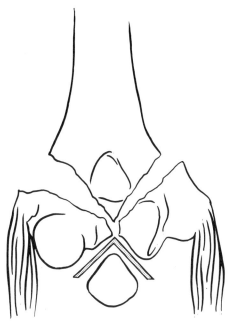

Figure 11–47. The medial and lateral musculature results in the deforming rotation of the articular condyles. The ulna serves as a wedge that initiates the fracture. (From Morrey, B. F. (ed.): The Elbow and Its Disorders. Philadelphia, W. B. Saunders Co., 1985.)

radiographs clearly demonstrate the fracture. No special techniques or views are required for the diagnosis. However, the severity and degree of comminution is often more extensive than can be appreciated on the simple AP and lateral views. Oblique views are sometimes helpful to appreciate fully the precise nature of the fracture.

Treatment. Treatment is controversial. In the Type I and Type II injuries, closed reduction is often employed and is usually adequate, particularly if there is not a great deal of displacement.[72, 76, 89] With the Type III fracture, many recommend open reduction and internal fixation (Fig. 11–48).[63, 65, 74, 90] This is the treatment of choice in our experience, but we would emphasize that significant experience and expertise with open techniques is mandatory. Skeletal traction is a safe and frequently employed technique for these fractures.[84, 89]

An accurate evaluation of the reduction during traction or after closed reduction is, in any case, of paramount importance. The quality of reduction can be readily followed with serial AP and lateral roentgenograms. The flexed axial view is frequently employed in this setting. Posterior angulation is not uncommon and must be avoided in the adult. Rigid fixation should be obtained with these fractures if an open technique is employed. Cortical cancellous lag screws, medial and lateral plates, Y-plates (Fig. 11–49), and multiple K-wires have been used for this purpose. The radiograph not only helps assess the adequacy of the reduction; it also ensures that the fixation device has not impinged on the olecranon fossa.

Complications. Complications of this fracture include improper reduction (Fig. 11–50) and the development of exuberant callus that can fill the olecranon fossa and thus limit motion. Internal fixation devices can likewise limit motion if the fossae are crossed by screws or pins (Fig. 11–51). These features of treatment can be detected radiographically with routine views, but occasionally tomography or flexion-extension views will be helpful. Non-union occurs in about 5 percent[51] and is usually associated with inadequate surgical procedure.[82]

Figure 11–48. A Type III T condylar fracture in which the fracture fragments are rotated but gross comminution has not occurred *(A)*. This is readily fixed by restoring the articular integrity with a lag screw. The supracondylar component is then initially sutured with K-wires *(B and C)*. (From Morrey, B. F. (ed.): The Elbow and Its Disorders. Philadelphia, W. B. Saunders Co., 1985.)

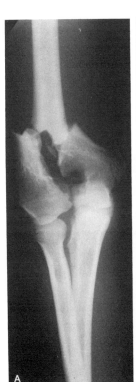
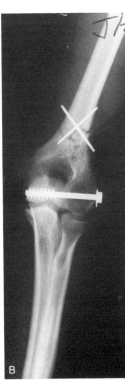
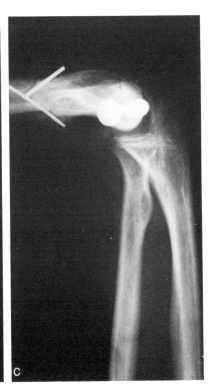

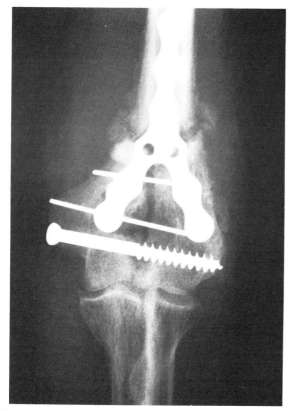

Figure 11–49. The Y plate is often used for Type III fractures.

Capitellar Fractures

This fracture is one of the most difficult to diagnose accurately by the radiograph. The mechanism of injury is either a direct blow or a fall on the outstretched hand.

Classification. Three types of capitellar fractures have been described (Fig. 11–52).[51] The Type I fracture involves the entire capitellum or a major portion of it, often with a small portion of the trochlea. This fracture is virtually never seen on the AP radiograph but is readily seen on the lateral view (Fig. 11–53). Type II injury consists of a shearing fracture. Often there is little or no cancellous bone on the cartilage; as a result, this fracture is notoriously misdiagnosed. The fat pad sign is helpful in detecting an injury, and aspiration showing fat globules and a hemarthrosis should also raise one's suspicion of the likelihood of this fracture.[67] The Type III injury is a comminuted fracture of the capitellum, often associated with fracture of the radial head.[85] The mechanism of injury is a fall on the outstretched hand, causing a compression injury.

Roentgenographic Assessment. The AP view is usually unrewarding for all three types of fractures. The lateral view is sufficient for Type I, but oblique views of the elbow joint may be needed for detection of Type II fractures. Occasionally, a lateral tomogram may be needed for Type II and III fractures. The differential diagnosis for Type II fracture includes fracture of the radial head. An important point of distinction is that the displacement of the capitellar fracture fragment is commonly superior to the capitellum (Fig. 11–53B), while the displacement of the radial head fracture fragments is not (see Fig. 11–31B). For the Type II fractures, the sheared cartilage may have little or no osseous compartment. In this instance, evidence of a lipohemarthrosis from radiography or arthrocentesis will be helpful.

Physical Examination. While the physical exam-

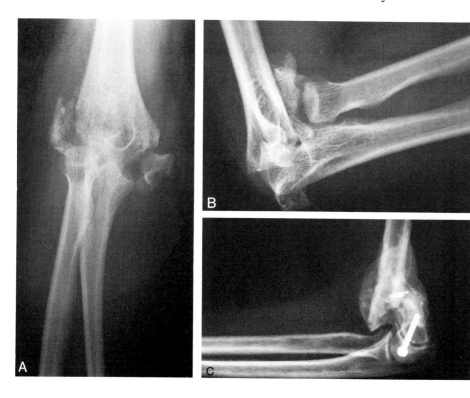

Figure 11–50. AP view of severely comminuted fracture involving primarily the condyles (A), with further extent of damage being demonstrated by the lateral view (B). These fractures are usually very difficult, and this one has healed in a malunited position, as demonstrated on the follow-up lateral view (C).

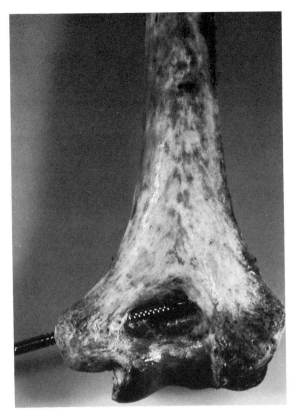

Figure 11–51. Limitation of motion can result from fixation devices being present in the olecranon fossa. (From Morrey, B. F. (ed.): The Elbow and Its Disorders. Philadelphia, W. B. Saunders Co., 1985.)

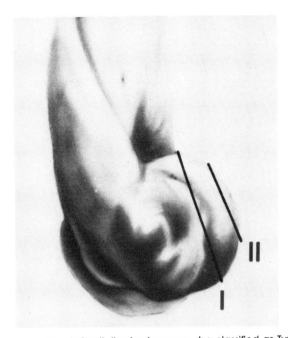

Figure 11–52. Capitellar fractures may be classified as Type I, in which a large fragment is sheared from the capitellum, or Type II, in which a very thin cartilaginous fragment is fractured. The Type III, not shown, is an impaction-type fracture that usually cannot be diagnosed by the radiograph. (From Morrey, B. F. (ed.): The Elbow and Its Disorders. Philadelphia, W. B. Saunders Co., 1985.)

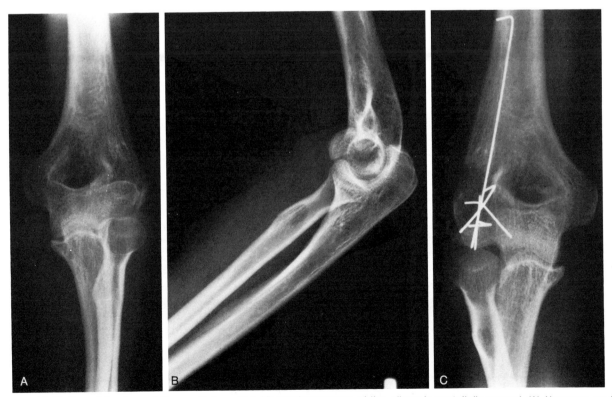

Figure 11–53. Type I fracture of the capitellum. The AP roentgenogram of the elbow is essentially normal (A). However, on the lateral view, the fractured capitellum is easily visualized (B). In this instance, the fracture was stabilized with multiple K-wires (C). (From Morrey, B. F. (ed.): The Elbow and Its Disorders. Philadelphia, W. B. Saunders Co., 1985.)

ination is not very helpful in most other fractures, it is helpful in the diagnosis of capitellar fractures. Hemarthrosis with crepitus and pain over the radiohumeral articulation, which is aggravated by pronation and supination but not by flexion-extension, are specific and characteristic physical features.

Treatment. The treatment of Type I fractures is somewhat controversial.[66, 70, 71] Closed reduction is possible, and the fracture may appear to be anatomically reduced on the lateral roentgenogram. However, limitation of motion may persist. Internal fixation may be effected by K-wires if the fracture is not too large (Fig. 11–53C). If the fragment is large, screw fixation lagged from posterior to anterior is our preferred treatment. The small Type I fragment and the Type II fragment may simply be excised.[69] Loose fragments are removed for the Type III fracture if motion is limited. If the radial head requires removal, the capitellar fracture is ignored, but loose fragments are removed.

Fracture of the Condyles

Fracture of a humeral condyle is uncommon but may be seen to involve either the medial or the lateral structure.

Mechanism of Injury. An isolated fracture of the condyle can occur from one of two mechanisms. Both essentially involve an avulsion or a shearing type of fracture. A fall on the outstretched hand with the forearm in valgus can produce an axial load which, depending upon the distribution of the forces, may result in a shearing type of lateral

condylar fracture or an avulsion type of medial condylar fracture. Conversely, a fall on the outstretched hand with axial load and a varus angular component may produce a shearing type of medial condylar fracture and an avulsion type of lateral condylar fracture. Thus, four possible mechanisms obtain: shearing or avulsion of the medial condyle and shearing or avulsion of the lateral condyle.

Classification. This fracture has been classified into two types by Milch.[80, 81] The Type I lateral fracture involves only the capitellum and lateral epicondyle; the Type I medial fracture includes the medial lip of the trochlea and the medial epicondyle. The Type I lateral fracture includes no or only a small part of the lateral trochlea (Fig. 11–54). The Type II lateral fracture involves the lateral half of the trochlea; the Type II medial fracture involves the entire trochlea. This classification is of major significance, since the Type II fracture, usually lateral, is associated with marked elbow instability. If this fracture is not appropriately treated with surgery, permanent and significant residual impairment can result.

Diagnosis. The diagnosis of an articular fracture of some type is suspected as a result of physical examination, which demonstrates that the posterior triangular relationship has been altered. In the adult, routine radiography readily demonstrates the nature of the injury. However, because the distal humerus is primarily cartilaginous in the young child, this fracture, representing a Salter-Harris Type IV, can be very difficult to diagnose correctly.

Treatment. The Type I injury is frequently an undisplaced fracture and can be treated by closed

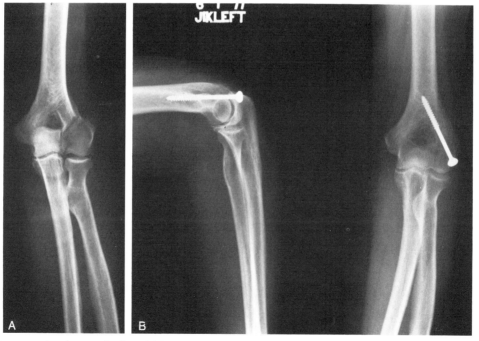

Figure 11–54. An example of an undisplaced lateral condylar fracture. Notice that this fracture involves the supracondylar and bony column *(A)*. Although undisplaced in order to allow early motion, this fracture was stabilized with a single screw *(B)*. (From Morrey, B. F. (ed.): The Elbow and Its Disorders. Philadelphia, W. B. Saunders Co., 1985.)

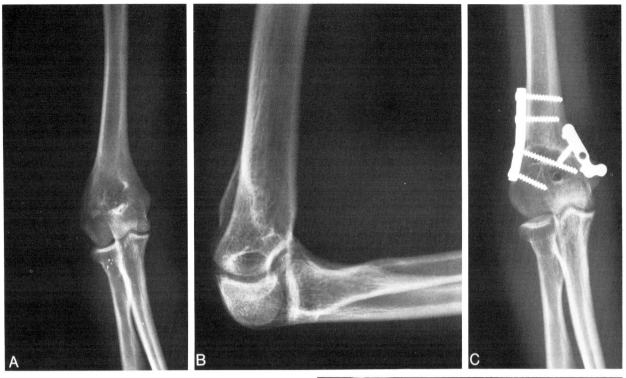

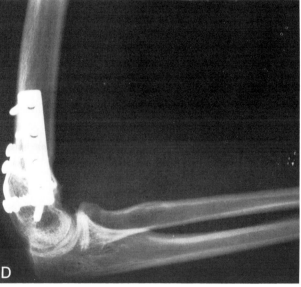

Figure 11–55. Healed fracture of the humeral condyles demonstrates approximately 5° of varus angulation *(A)* and also limitation of flexion due to the posterior displacement of the condyles *(B)*. A corrective osteotomy was performed with screw and plate fixation and is shown in both the AP *(C)* and the lateral projection *(D)*. The normal anterior rotation of the articular surface is restored. This resulted in resumption of normal motion of the joint. (From Morrey, B. F. (ed.): The Elbow and Its Disorders. Philadelphia, W. B. Saunders Co., 1985.)

reduction and immobilization for 3 to 6 weeks, depending upon the age and severity of the injury. Any displaced Type I fractures should be treated with open reduction and internal fixation (Fig. 11–54*B*). Surgical correction of all Type II fractures is recommended.[80] Usually a lateral Kocher incision or a medial triceps reflecting approach, as described by Bryan and Morrey, is used.[64] In most instances, the condyles are readily fixed with interfragmentary compression by lag screws. Early motion is begun at 1 to 2 weeks. In the child the fracture must be followed carefully for 1 to 2 years because of potential disturbance of growth.

Complications. Untoward events with this fracture include neurovascular compromise, as the proximal fragment may impinge on or impale the neurovascular bundle.[77] The development of ischemic contracture of the forearm, the so-called Volkmann's ischemic contracture, is notorious following supracondylar types of fractures.[79] The more common types of complications, however, involve inadequate reduction and the subsequent loss of proper position, motion, and stability owing to an incongruous joint. Even internal fixation can contribute to this complication if the fixation device impinges on the olecranon fossa and thereby limits motion (see Fig. 11–51). Lack of proper reduction can cause malorientation of the articular surface, which further limits motion or function (Fig. 11–55).[83] Soft tissue calcification and scarring about

Text continues on page 611

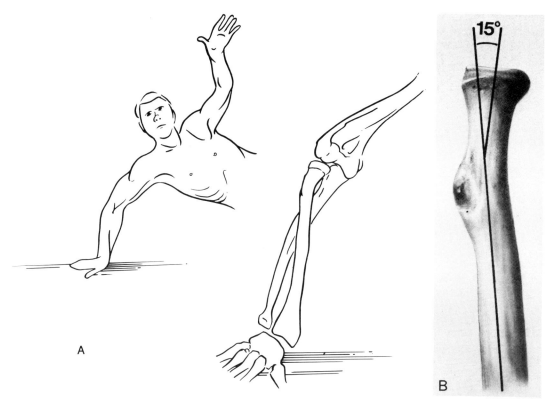

Figure 11–56. Mechanism of radial head fracture or fall on the slightly flexed pronated upper extremity *(A)*. Normal neck-shaft angle of the proximal radius *(B)*. (From Morrey, B. F. (ed.): The Elbow and Its Disorders. Philadelphia, W. B. Saunders Co., 1985.)

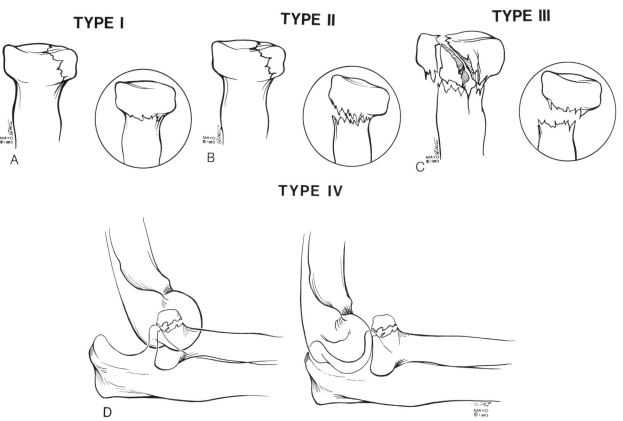

Figure 11–57. *A,* Type I radial head fracture is undisplaced. *B,* Type II demonstrates more than 2 mm displacement and less than 30% involvement and/or less than 30° angulation. *C,* Type III is a comminuted fracture of the radial head or a displaced radial neck fracture. *D,* Type IV is represented as a fracture-dislocation of the radial head and ulnohumeral joint. (From Morrey, B. F. (ed.): The Elbow and Its Disorders. Philadelphia, W. B. Saunders Co., 1985.)

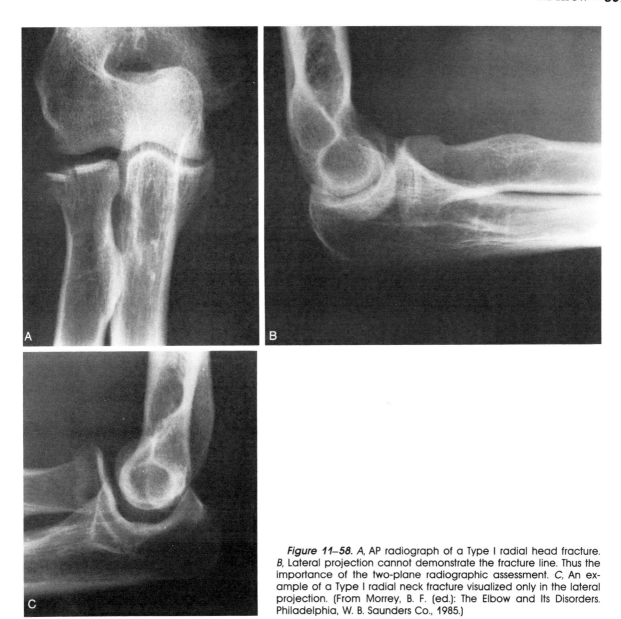

Figure 11–58. A, AP radiograph of a Type I radial head fracture. *B,* Lateral projection cannot demonstrate the fracture line. Thus the importance of the two-plane radiographic assessment. *C,* An example of a Type I radial neck fracture visualized only in the lateral projection. (From Morrey, B. F. (ed.): The Elbow and Its Disorders. Philadelphia, W. B. Saunders Co., 1985.)

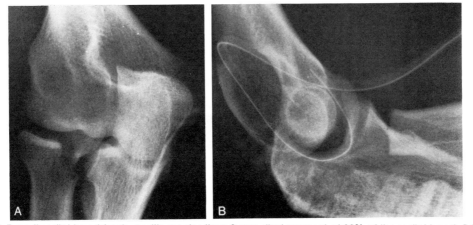

Figure 11–59. A, Type II radial head fracture with greater than 2 mm displacement of 30% of the radial head. *B,* This is treated by radial head excision. (From Morrey, B. F. (ed.): The Elbow and Its Disorders. Philadelphia, W. B. Saunders Co., 1985.)

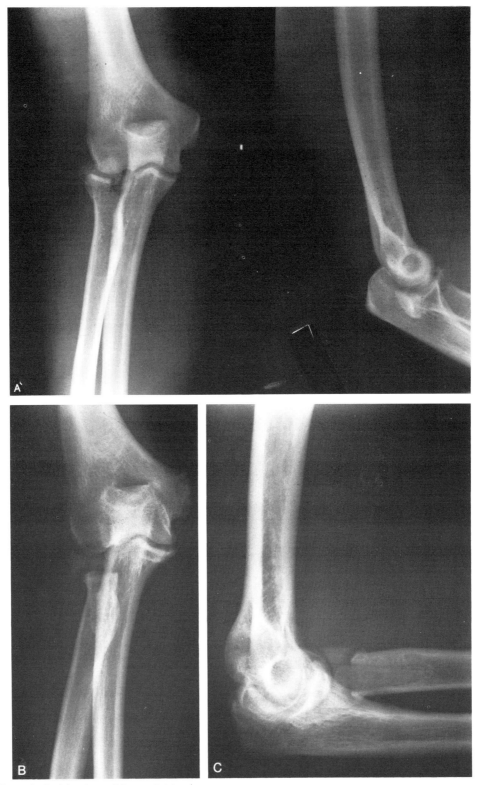

Figure 11-60. Comminuted fracture of the radial head demonstrated in both the AP and lateral projections *(A)*. This particular fracture was treated at 8 years and is shown in follow-up AP *(B)* and lateral *(C)* projections. As is often the case, this radiographic finding did not correlate with any clinical symptomatology. (From Morrey, B. F. (ed.): The Elbow and Its Disorders. Philadelphia, W. B. Saunders Co., 1985.)

this joint are common even with minimal trauma, but they are particularly significant and disastrous after the more severe intra-articular injuries. They require prompt treatment.[78] Hypertrophic callus can sometimes develop either posteriorly or anteriorly. Often the olecranon fossa will be obliterated. Once again, motion is lost.

To conclude, the current philosophy of treatment for distal humeral fractures emphasizes early motion and relies upon open reduction and internal fixation with rigid devices as the treatment of choice. If the injury has resulted in hopeless comminution, then traction and motion is recommended. With single large fragments that are not badly displaced, early motion is likewise suggested. In any event, prolonged casting is to be discouraged.

Fractures of the Proximal Radius

Fractures of the head and neck of the radius are a common injury, accounting for approximately one third of all elbow fractures and 1 to 2 percent of all fractures seen by the physician.[91, 107] The mechanism of injury has been carefully described by Thomas. These fractures occur from a fall on the outstretched hand with the elbow partially flexed and pronated (Fig. 11–56).[60] Because the neck of the radius makes an angle of about 15° with the shaft of the bone, in the pronated position the anterolateral margin comes into contact with the capitellum. Thus, the proximal radius is vulnerable to a shearing type of fracture. Increasing amounts of force with this orientation result in a more extensive injury.

Classification. We feel that the most useful classification is one modified from Mason.[110] It consists of four types (Fig. 11–57). The type I fracture is an undisplaced or minimally displaced (< 2 mm) fracture of the head or neck (Fig. 11–58). The Type II fracture involves approximately one third of the radial head, with greater than 2 mm of displacement or 20° to 30° of angulation (Fig. 11–59). The Type III fracture involves comminution of the radial head (Fig. 11–60). The Type IV fracture is any fracture of the radial head with dislocation of the ulnohumeral joint (Fig. 11–61).[106] In the pediatric age group, most of these injuries occur as fractures of the radial neck, with varying degrees of angulation and displacement. If the fracture is of the radial neck, angulation of less than 20° to 30° is considered a Type I fracture; angulation of greater than 20° to 30° is considered a Type II fracture; and angulation of greater than 60° or dislocation is considered a Type III radial neck fracture.

The diagnosis is suspected by a history of the injury. Marked local tenderness of the radiohumeral joint with extreme pain on pronation-supination is demonstrated on the physical examination.

Radiographic Findings. Routine AP and lateral radiographs are usually sufficient to demonstrate this fracture (Figs. 11–58 to 11–61). However, a single view will often not reveal the fracture line,

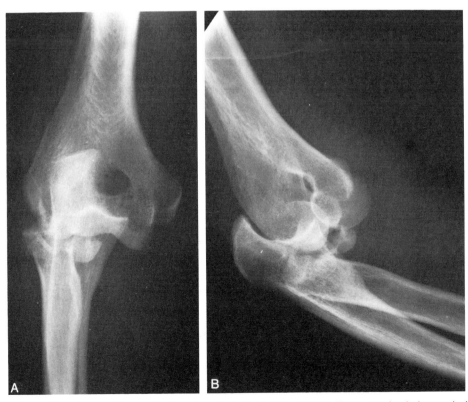

Figure 11–61. Fracture-dislocations of the radial head and ulnohumeral joint *(A).* These are best demonstrated on the lateral projection *(B).* (From Morrey, B. F. (ed.): The Elbow and Its Disorders. Philadelphia, W. B. Saunders Co., 1985.)

and oblique or radial head views are sometimes required before the true extent of the fracture is appreciated. A fat pad sign with the features of the physical examination discussed earlier may be the only indication, but these should allow diagnosis even of minimally displaced Type I fractures.[67] Distinction between a Type II capitellar and a Type I radial head fracture may be difficult.[51] Additional views should be taken when there is doubt. Occasionally a tomogram may be necessary to resolve the issue.

Treatment. The appropriate treatment of this fracture is one of the most controversial areas in orthopedic surgery. The Type I fracture is treated nonoperatively with early motion after the joint has been aspirated.[92, 109, 112] Surgical excision of Type II and III fractures has been the standard treatment.[100, 101, 110, 114, 115, 117] In our opinion, the Type II or III uncomplicated fracture should be surgically excised only if displacement limits motion in the anesthetized joint.[51, 92, 93, 95]

We begin motion on the day of the injury, if possible. If there have been associated injuries of the distal radioulnar stabilizers[104] or of the medial collateral ligament,[94, 99] a radial head prosthesis should be considered.[105, 108] A cleavage fracture of a single fragment involving approximately one third of the radial head with associated ligament injury is amenable to open reduction and internal fixation. This treatment should be considered (Fig. 11–62) in a patient under 40 to 50 years of age.[113] If elbow

ligaments have been torn, the joint can be unacceptably unstable after radial head excision.[105, 111] In this case a radial head prosthesis may also be used to improve stability and to allow early rehabilitation. Although acrylic and metal prostheses have been used in the past, the Silastic prosthesis designed by Swanson is most commonly used in this country.[103, 108, 119] This material is subject to fracture and the implant can dislocate. To assess these radiographic features properly, routine and oblique views may be necessary. Since Silastic is radiolucent, xeroradiography has been recommended to evaluate this implant.[96] While not necessary routinely, it is of value in the symptomatic joint.

Results. The results of treatment of the Type I fracture tend to be very good, although a surprisingly high number of patients will have some complaints.[115] In general, Type II and III fractures are associated with about 80 to 90 percent satisfactory results[92, 93, 95, 100, 110] with both operative and closed treatment. Patient selection remains controversial, although early motion is generally becoming accepted regardless of the nature of initial treatment.[51]

Complications. Multiple complications are seen both as associated injuries and following treatment of radial head fractures, particularly after radial head excision. Associated fractures of the ulna[116] are not uncommon and represent a variant of the Monteggia lesion described later. Ectopic ossification or overgrowth of the resected stump of the radius can be so prominent that it gives rise to a

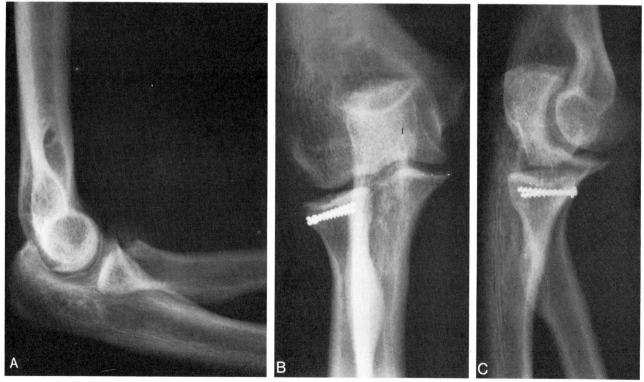

Figure 11–62. Fracture of the radial head as demonstrated on the lateral projection (A). This fracture was treated with internal fixation (B and C). Two views are helpful to ensure containment of the screws. (From Morrey, B. F. (ed.): The Elbow and Its Disorders. Philadelphia, W. B. Saunders Co., 1985.)

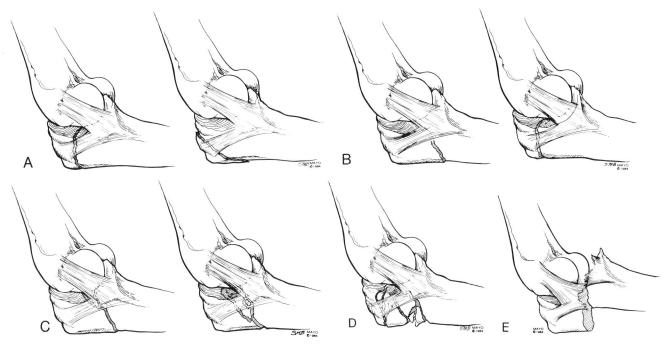

Figure 11–63. Classification of olecranon fractures. The avulsion type fracture may or may not involve the articular joint (A). The oblique or transverse fracture usually involves the midportion of the olecranon (B). An oblique fracture with comminution usually involves the nonarticular portion of the olecranon (C). The comminuted fracture involves the majority of the olecranon process (D). In fracture-dislocation the fracture occurs distally with associated injury of the medial collateral ligament, thus resulting in instability (E). (From Morrey, B. F. (ed.): The Elbow and Its Disorders. Philadelphia, W. B. Saunders Co., 1985.)

radiographic appearance of an apparent regrowth of the radial head, particularly in the younger individual.[118] Ligamentous instability is so common that it may be termed a Type IV fracture. Our experience with this injury indicates that immobilization for more than 4 weeks will result in a poor prognosis,[98] and thus a Silastic implant might be considered a source of stability in this setting.[105, 119] If radial head excision has occurred, shortening of the radius can cause some symptoms at the wrist.[103, 119] This injury can result in a decrease in forearm rotation due to shortening of the interosseous membrane.[120] For this reason, some people recommend that the radial head be left alone and excised only if it becomes symptomatic later. Interestingly very few data have been gathered to demonstrate whether this is an effective means of treatment. We have recently analyzed our experience with delayed excision of the radial head. Our review demonstrated that, in fact, improved motion and relief of pain can be rather predictably observed in about 75 percent of the patients treated this way.[97]

Fractures of the Ulna

Because of its subcutaneous position, the olecranon is particularly susceptible to trauma. Most fractures are intra-articular and thus can compromise both the stability and function of the joint. If the triceps with its fascial expansions has been disrupted, the fracture becomes even more displaced. Without this feature, the displacement is usually minimal. Persistent fascial lines, usually bilateral, have been reported and are usually differentiated from fractures.[138]

Mechanism. Fractures of the olecranon occur from a direct blow, usually from a fall on the flexed elbow or, less commonly, as a result of a hyperextension injury. The hyperextension injury is usually associated with other injury, for example, elbow dislocation or radial head fracture. Greater comminution is observed in the older and younger age groups. A clean transverse line is often observed.

Classification. The most common classification of olecranon fractures is that described by Colton[126] and consists, with minor modifications, of the following types (Fig. 11–63):

Type I. Undisplaced fracture. This fracture usually results from a direct blow, with the fragment separated less than 2 mm.

Type II. Displaced fracture involving avulsion and a transverse or oblique fracture line. This fracture probably occurs from a direct pull of the triceps during a forced elbow flexion or from a fall on the tip of the olecranon (Fig. 11–63A).

Type III. Transverse or oblique olecranon fracture (Fig. 11–63B). This fracture usually occurs by way of a more indirect mechanism of injury. The elbow is flexed against resistance and receives a direct blow, with the trochlea serving as a wedge that fractures the midportion of the olecranon. With more severe violence, comminution is again usually found in the midportion of the olecranon, which is the nonarticular part of the elbow (Fig. 11–63C).

Type IV. Comminuted fracture. A direct blow,

severe in a younger individual, less severe in the older patient, may cause significant comminution involving not only the midportion but also the proximal portion of the olecranon (Fig. 11–63D).

Type V. Fracture-dislocation. As the fracture is more distal about the area of the coronoid, associated disruption of the collateral ligament occurs, which results in a more unstable type of fracture. Often the forearm is dislocated or subluxated anteriorly (Fig. 11–63E). This may also be considered a Monteggia variant.

Radiographic Evaluation. The AP radiograph of the elbow is not particularly helpful in defining the severity of the injury unless there is either medial or lateral displacement. Even rather severe fractures may demonstrate a reasonably normal AP view (Fig. 11–64A). The lateral view, on the other hand, not only demonstrates the precise orientation, displacement, and comminution of the fracture but also is most helpful in revealing any associated fracture of the radial head or displacement of the distal fragment (Fig. 11–64B). Failure to obtain a true lateral view before treatment is probably the most common error in the initial radiographic assessment of this type of injury.

Treatment. The specific goals of treatment of this fracture include maintenance or restoration of congruity, attainment of stability, and preservation of function, particularly avoiding limitation of motion. Thus, surgical intervention is indicated in most displaced fractures unless rather significant extenuating circumstances obtain.[143]

If the fracture is undisplaced, a relatively brief period of immobilization (2 or 3 weeks) followed by

gentle controlled motion and careful recheck evaluation is indicated. Follow-up roentgenograms should be obtained 6 to 10 days after the initial injury and then on a weekly basis for approximately 1 month. Flexion at greater than 90° is usually avoided until union is complete. Union often occurs in the second and almost always by the third month.

Treatment of Displaced Fractures

Treatment of displaced fractures of the olecranon depends upon the degree of comminution and displacement and the age of the patient. As long ago as 1876, surgical fixation was reported by Shelton.[146] Various devices were used in the early 1900's, including wires, nails, bone pegs, kangaroo tendon, and fascia lata.[128] Simple wiring of the fracture was the most common method of treatment until the last decade.[121, 129, 133, 147] Because of the inadequate stability, the reduction was often lost.

The most common means of fixation now is that recommended by the AO Group, termed "tension band wiring" (Fig. 11–65A and B). This technique converts the distraction forces of the fracture into compression forces during elbow flexion (Fig. 11–65C). The two Kirschner wires directed down the shaft of the olecranon allow reduction of the fracture, which is converted to a stable configuration by the addition of the "Figure of 8" wire loop. This wire is placed through a transverse hole in the distal portion of the fracture and across the pins as they protrude from the olecranon more proximally (Fig. 11–65C).

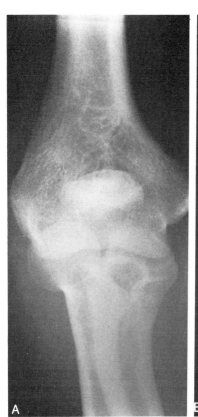
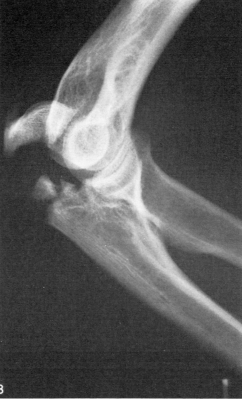

Figure 11–64. A, AP roentgenogram of an olecranon fracture demonstrating relatively little pathology. *B,* Lateral projection showing a marked comminution and displacement of the olecranon fracture. (From Morrey, B. F. (ed.): The Elbow and Its Disorders. Philadelphia, W. B. Saunders Co., 1985.)

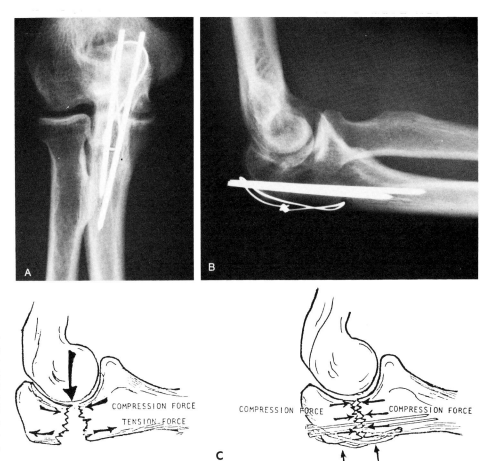

Figure 11–65. A, AP radiograph of the most common type of fixation, the AO-recommended tension band wiring. B, Lateral projection. C, The fixation should be placed so as to provide compression of the joint during flexion. (From Morrey, B. F. (ed.): The Elbow and Its Disorders. Philadelphia, W. B. Saunders Co., 1985.)

Intramedullary fixation with Rush rods and Leinbach screws or a flexible device[127] has been recommended, but, in general, these modalities are unable to stabilize the fracture adequately. Because of this inadequate stabilization, fatigue failure of such devices is not uncommon.

The use of a single screw across the oblique fracture is sometimes used, and this fixation is effective in stabilizing uncomminuted fractures owing to compression of the fracture surface (Fig. 11–66).

The use of plates is less commonly used for this

Figure 11–66. An oblique, relatively noncomminuted fracture of the proximal ulna with a fracture of the medial head *(A)*. The fracture was treated with a compression screw *(B)*.

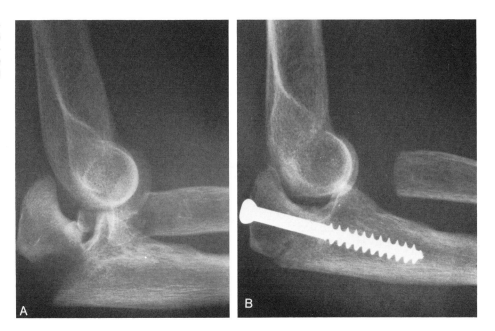

fracture because of the subcutaneous nature of the bone and the difficulty in obtaining soft tissue cover. For badly displaced fractures or in uncertain circumstances, one of the special plates may be used (Fig. 11–67), but generally in this instance one of the other modalities is preferred.

A third treatment option other than casting or splinting and open reduction with internal fixation is excision of fracture fragments. The principle for this approach has been well defined by Mac-Ausland.[134] If at least 20 percent of the olecranon is present and intact, the procedure maintains stability for badly comminuted fractures in older individuals. The major attractions of this particular procedure are its relative ease and freedom from complications (Fig. 11–68).[131]

Results. The results of prolonged splinting have been universally bad; thus, as mentioned earlier, this is not commonly performed unless the fracture is stable and relatively undisplaced, and unless reasonable early motion can be begun. Surprisingly,

relatively little information is available with respect to the long-term follow-up of many of these techniques. Weseley has reported the results of a specialized hooked plate for fixation of this fracture. He reported excellent to good results in all 25 patients so treated.[148] A careful assessment of the long-term follow-up of excision compared with one of the other modalities of fixation has been recently reported by Gartsman and colleagues.[131] They found no significant difference between these two groups and, in general, quite gratifying results in both. However, there were more complications in the group treated by reduction and fixation. These were usually related to removal of the fixation device.

Complications. In general, complications from this fracture involve loss of motion, sometimes ulnar neuropathy, post-traumatic arthritis, and rarely instability or non-union. Loss of 30° of extension is not uncommon, and some loss of motion is reported in about half of the cases.[129, 131, 142] Ulnar neuropathy has been reported in 2 percent[142] to 10

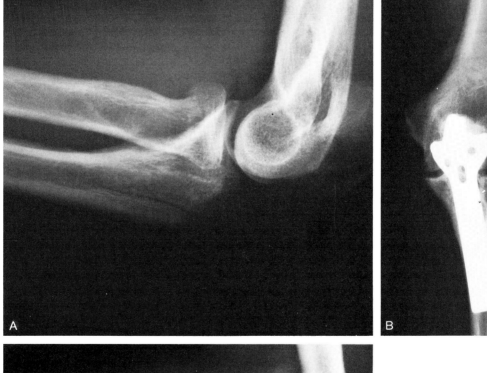

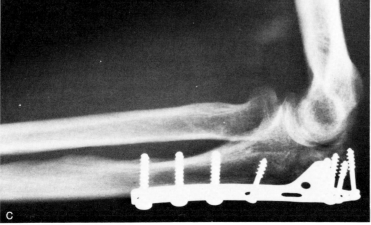

Figure 11–67. Badly displaced but minimally comminuted fracture with a linear component down the shaft of the ulna *(A)*. This was treated with a special AO-type plate, as seen on the AP *(B)* and lateral *(C)* projections. (From Morrey, B. F. (ed.): The Elbow and Its Disorders. Philadelphia, W. B. Saunders Co., 1985.)

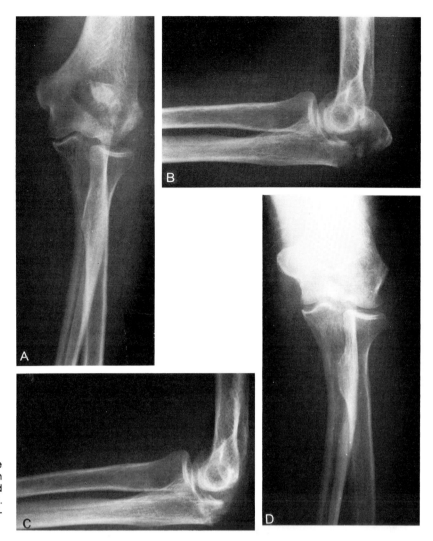

Figure 11–68. Comminuted fracture of the olecranon in an elderly patient, as shown on the AP *(A)* and lateral *(B)* projections. Treated by excision *(C)* and *D).* (From Morrey, B. F. (ed.): The Elbow and Its Disorders. Philadelphia, W. B. Saunders Co., 1985.)

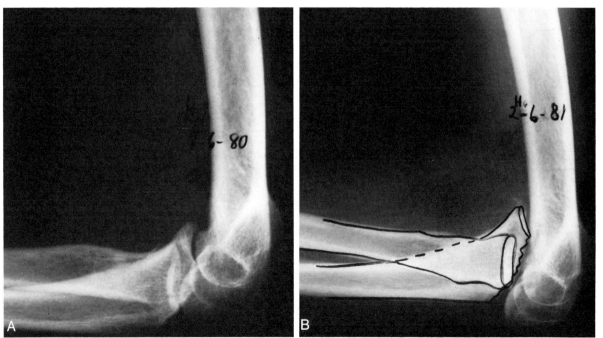

Figure 11–69. Lateral projection showing excision of greater than 80 percent of the olecranon *(A).* Resulting instability was predictable because the medial collateral ligament had been disrupted *(B).* (From Morrey, B. F. (ed.): The Elbow and Its Disorders. Philadelphia, W. B. Saunders Co., 1985.)

percent[129] of patients. Obviously, this nerve must be carefully inspected and protected during any surgical procedure. Instability of the forearm after resection of the olecranon (Fig. 11–69) is very uncommon but has been reported.

Non-union of the olecranon is uncommon. When

it occurs, it is almost always a result of inadequate surgical intervention (Fig. 11–70). Olecranon non-union less commonly occurs as a result of a trans-olecranon approach to distal humeral fractures (Fig. 11–69). This occurs in only about 5 percent of such exposures.[51]

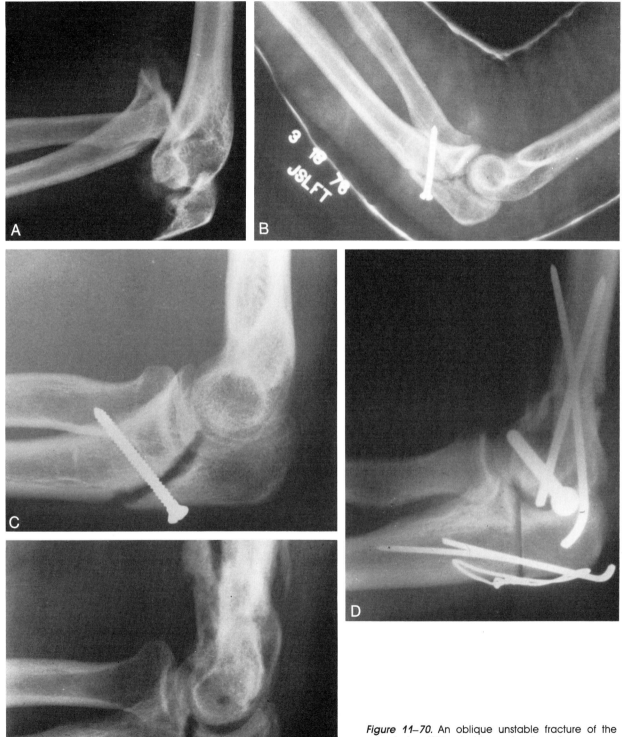

Figure 11–70. An oblique unstable fracture of the proximal ulna *(A)* treated by an inadequate compression screw *(B)*. This fracture did not unite *(C)*. Olecranon osteotomy was performed to fix the supracondylar fracture *(D)*. Union followed *(E)*. (From Morrey, B. F. (ed.): The Elbow and Its disorders. Philadelphia, W. B. Saunders Co., 1985.)

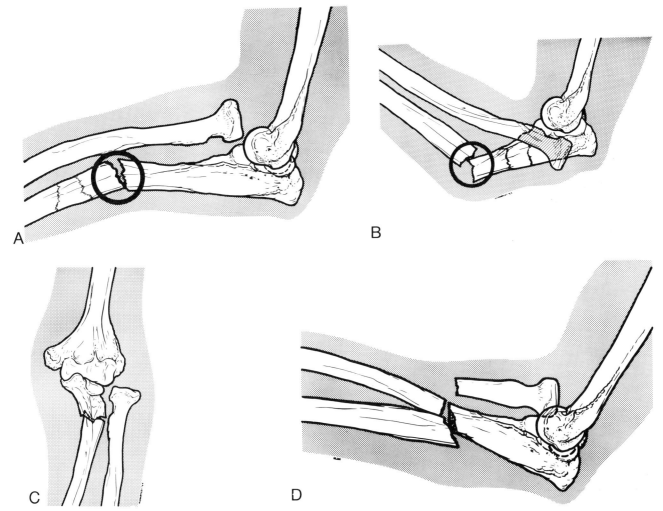

Figure 11-71. Classification of Monteggia fractures. *A,* Type I: the radial head is displaced anteriorly; *B,* Type II: the radial head displacement is posterior or posterolateral; *C,* Type III: lateral or anterolateral dislocation of the radial head associated with fracture of the ulnar metaphysis; *D,* Type IV: unusual anterior dislocation of the radial head with fracture of the proximal third of the radius and ulna at the same level. (*A, B,* and *C* from Reckling, F. W. and Cordell, L. D.: Unstable fracture-dislocation of the forearm. The Monteggia and Galeazzi lesions. Arch. Surg. *96:*999, 1968; and *D* from Reckling, F. W.: Unstable fracture-dislocations of the forearm [Monteggia and Galeazzi lesions]. J. Bone Joint Surg. *64A:*857, 1982.)

The Monteggia Lesion

A very specialized type of fracture that occurs about the elbow involves fracture of the proximal ulna with dislocation of the radial head. Described in 1814 by Monteggia of Milan,[136] this fracture has been termed the Monteggia lesion by Bado.[122] These fractures are not common and compose about 7 percent of all ulnar fractures and thus about 0.7 percent of elbow injuries.[123]

Classification. The relatively simple classification of this fracture has been proposed by Bado[122] and consists of the following types:

Type I. Fracture of the ulna with anterior dislocation of the radial head. This is the most common fracture, occurring in 50 to 75 percent of instances. It is a common type of fracture in children (Fig. 11–71).

Type II. Fracture of the proximal ulna with a posterior or posterolateral dislocation of the radial head and a posterior angulation of the ulnar fracture (Fig. 11–71B). This is usually a more proximal fracture. It occurs most often in adults and represents about 10 to 15 percent of the Monteggia lesions.

Type III. Fracture of the ulna with a lateral or anterolateral dislocation of the radial head. This is a common type of fracture in children, representing 6 to 20 percent of Monteggia type lesions (Fig. 11–71C).

Type IV. Anterior dislocation of the radial head with fracture of the proximal third of the radius and ulna. This is the rarest of the Monteggia lesions and represents about 5 percent of cases (Fig. 11–71D).

In addition to these types, many variants of the fracture were described by Bado as well.[122] Variations of Type I fractures consist of (1) isolated anterior dislocation of the radial head in children; (2) fracture of the ulnar diaphysis with fracture of the neck and the radius; (3) isolated fractures of the neck of the radius; (4) fracture of the ulnar diaphysis and a more proximal fracture of the radial diaphysis;

(5) fracture of the ulnar diaphysis and olecranon with anterior dislocation of the radial head (Fig. 11–70A); and (6) fracture-dislocation of the elbow, including fracture of the ulnar diaphysis with or without variations of the fracture of the proximal radius. Variations of Type II fractures consist of epiphyseal fractures of the dislocated radial head or fractures of the neck of the radius. Usually these occur in children.

Mechanism of Injury. There have been three mechanisms proposed for this injury, and probably all three can give rise to one or the other of the types. These include

1. A direct blow to the posterior aspect of the ulna.

2. A fall on the outstretched hand with the elbow flexed by impact. This occurs with the forearm in pronation, causing a levering of the radius and fracture of the ulna.[130]

3. A hyperextension mechanism. This has been proposed by Tompkins,[145] as mentioned previously.

Probably all three mechanisms—direct blow, hyperpronation, and hyperextension—are implicated in this type of fracture.

Roentgenographic Findings. Adequate roentgenograms in two or more planes are particularly important in this injury since the dislocation of the radial head may be missed in a single view. Certainly in the severe cases the diagnosis is not difficult (Fig. 11–72). If the dislocation becomes inadvertently reduced at the time of positioning for the x-ray, the full severity of the injury may be missed. This occurred in 50 percent of the early cases.[144] In 1940, this incidence was reduced to 33 percent in a series reported in 1955 from the Mayo Clinic by Mobley and Janes.[135] It is currently approximately 16 percent, according to the most recent report by Reckling and Cordell.[141]

Treatment. In the child the fracture is usually able to be reduced and hence treated by nonoperative modalities. However, for the adult, surgical intervention is the treatment of choice. Since the early recommendations for this treatment in 1940, improved techniques of osteosynthesis have resulted in a more aggressive approach to the fracture with a concurrent decrease in the complication rate. In fact, a specific surgical approach to the region has been proposed by Boyd[124] for this specific injury. The most recent studies recommend such operative management (Fig. 11–72B and C).[122, 125, 139, 141]

Results. Boyd[124] reported 77 percent satisfactory results in the surgical management of these fractures. Reckling[140, 141] in 1968 and again in 1982 demonstrated that the results of treatment in the adult were best in those that underwent an anatomic reduction. However, only 9 of 40 of their patients obtained an excellent result. To some extent, the results depend on the type of fracture, which reflects the severity of the injury.

Complications. Radial palsy has been reported rather commonly as a sequela of this fracture.[125, 132, 135] It is most common with the Type III fracture. Median[132] and ulnar[125] palsies have also been reported. Malunion is uncommon today with the better fixation techniques available, but cross-union has been observed following this fracture (Fig. 11–73).

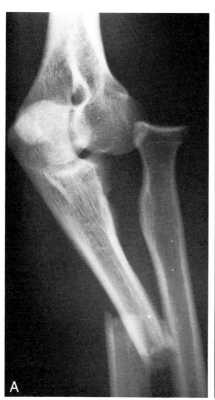
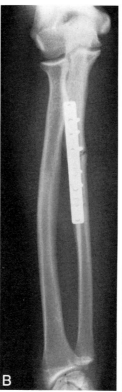
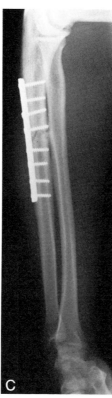

Figure 11–72. Classic Monteggia Type I fracture in an 18-year-old boy *(A)*. AP *(B)* and lateral *(C)* views showing fixation with plate. Notice the reduction of the radial head. (From Morrey, B. F. (ed.): The Elbow and Its Disorders. Philadelphia, W. B. Saunders Co., 1985.)

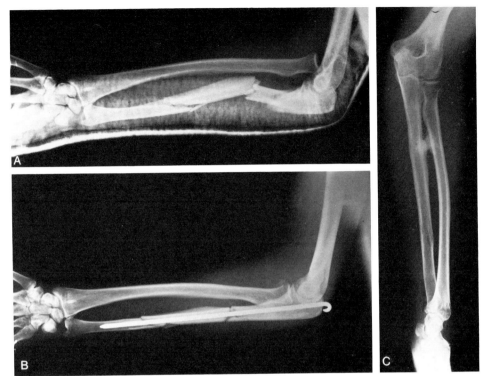

Figure 11–73. Segmental fracture of the ulna with anterior dislocation of the radial head *(A).* Treated with intramedullary fixation using a Rush rod *(B).* Synostosis occurred at the level of the proximal fragment *(C).* (From Morrey, B. F. (ed.): The Elbow and Its Disorders. Philadelphia, W. B. Saunders Co., 1985.)

RECONSTRUCTIVE SURGERY

Reconstructive surgery of the elbow is not a commonly indicated or frequently performed surgical procedure. In general, surgical intervention is offered in order to restore function that has been lost owing to pain, loss of motion, or instability resulting from rheumatoid or post-traumatic arthritis.[149, 150] Most reconstructive procedures are associated with a fairly high complication rate, and joint replacement is technically difficult. Thus, patients for reconstructive surgery must be carefully selected.

Patient Selection. Reconstructive surgery is performed only after the functional impairment and pain have been elicited by the history and after motion, strength, and stability have been evaluated both by physical examination and appropriate radiographic studies. In this regard, we should briefly discuss the preoperative evaluation and then turn to the postoperative assessment of elbow reconstructive surgery in more detail.

Preoperative Radiographic Assessment. Routine views are adequate to define the general condition of the joint, bone stock, and articular relationships. Tomography is useful for evaluating non-unions, loose bodies, and special conditions such as osteochondritis dissecans of the capitellum. Fluoroscopy may also be used to assess further the possibility of non-union. Arthrography is occasionally used to evaluate capsular and ligament integrity. The role of arthrography in demonstrating the presence of loose bodies has already been discussed.[9]

Postoperative Assessment. Only a limited number of reconstructive procedures are performed at the elbow. These are examined in the following sections.

Radial Head Resection and Synovectomy

Indications. Rheumatoid arthritis, infectious processes.

Radiographic Assessment. The radiograph demonstrates variable bone stock on the preoperative examination, but osteopenia is common. The joint is often reasonably well maintained; but because of prolonged or significant synovitis, the joint destruction may be moderate to marked.[157, 160] The operation is indicated, according to some, even with rather significant destruction of the joint. Hence, various grades of roentgenographic involvement have been identified and are observed before and after surgery (Fig. 11–74). A Silastic radial head implant is employed and recommended by some.[119] Progression of the disease regularly occurs after surgery but correlates poorly with symptoms (Fig. 11–74).

Interposition Arthroplasty (Functional or Anatomic Arthroplasty)

Indications. Post-traumatic arthritis, ankylosis.

Radiographic Appearance. The characteristic feature of the surgical procedure is to introduce a substance between the humerus and ulna after the joint has been surgically prepared, usually by release of soft tissue and distal humeral bone. The interposition substance may be fascia, fat, skin, Silastic, or other materials.[154, 159, 171] Since all these are radiolucent, it is not possible to distinguish the

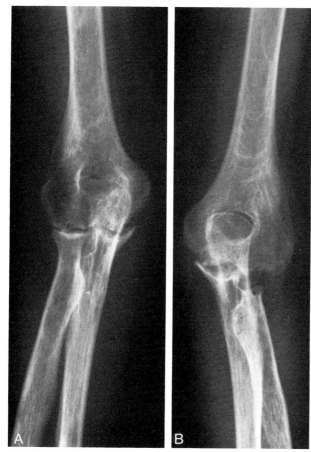

Figure 11–74. A 55-year-old female with rheumatoid arthritis and painful synovitis not responding to medical management (A). Seventeen months after a radial head resection and synovectomy the patient is without pain and has returned to work, although progression in the disease is evident on the radiograph (B).

interposed substance radiographically. The AP radiograph often demonstrates that a significant portion of the joint has been resected. The distal humerus is fashioned in such a manner as to provide a fulcrum against which the olecranon may articulate. These patients will frequently demonstrate some medial or lateral instability after the surgery (Fig. 11–75). The clinical and radiographic long-term follow-up studies reveal bony erosion or resorption and posterior subluxation in the severe cases.[159]

Arthrodesis

Indications. There are relatively few indications for elbow arthrodesis. The most frequent indication is probably a post-traumatic event in the young laborer or uncontrolled sepsis or tuberculosis.[51]

Technique. This joint in the past has been difficult to fuse, but with newer techniques the problem with non-union is less common. The bone ends may be fashioned to afford maximum contact, and bone bank or autogenous cancellous bone grafts

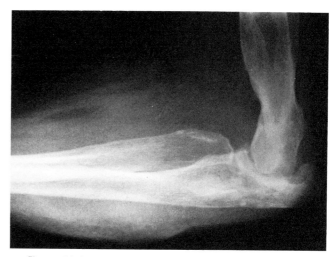

Figure 11–75. Interposition arthroplasty demonstrates distortion of the ulnohumeral joint. However, the patient had 90° of painless motion. Notice that the radial head is resected in this procedure.

may supplement the fusion. The bone ends are stabilized by some internal fixative device, for example, screws or plates (Fig. 11–76). An external fixator is employed for soft tissue problems or if the local bone stock is inadequate.

Results. The lateral x-ray is sufficient to demonstrate the position and integrity of fusion. Nonunion in the past approached 50 percent. If the lateral roentgenogram does not provide adequate information, tomograms or fluoroscopic techniques may be employed. The joint is usually fixed at about 90° flexion.[51]

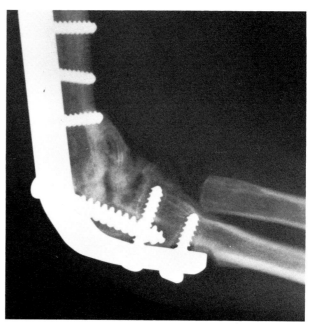

Figure 11–76. A plate used in arthrodesis of the elbow in approximately 75° of flexion. The plate can cause problems owing to a subcutaneous location, and sometimes it is removed later.

Total Elbow Arthroplasty

The precursors of total elbow anthroplasty consisted of custom-made devices designed to replace the distal humerus or proximal ulna. These devices were usually designed from x-rays of the uninvolved side and were used for patients with post-traumatic bone loss. These procedures were generally unsuccessful because of unpredictable relief of pain and predictable instability. In 1974, Stevens and Street reported on a humeral resurfacing device that seemed to provide a greater degree of stability and was applicable for the rheumatoid as well as the post-traumatic arthritic patient.[170] This device might be considered a precursor of the resurfacing total elbow arthroplasty as we know it today.

The semiconstrained prostheses include not only those that have an axis and therefore captive articulation but also some in which the articulation simply snaps together.[156] With this type of device, uncoupling of the snap-fit can occur. The exact incidence of this complication, however, has not been well worked out, though it does appear to be a related phenomenon. Insufficient time has elapsed since the introduction of these protheses to obtain an accurate analysis of this problem.

There are two basic types of artificial elbow joint. One is a resurfacing type of device, and the other is a coupled prosthesis. The selection of either of these depends upon the nature of the disease process and the preference of the surgeon.

Resurfacing Prosthesis

Indications. Rheumatoid arthritis, minimal bone loss after a traumatic injury in an individual over 60 years of age.[152, 160]

Biomechanics and Technique. There are currently three resurfacing devices present in the United States and several more around the world. The common feature of each is that the humeral and ulnar parts articulate to varying degrees, depending upon the degree of congruence of the ulnar component. This varies from 155° to over 200°, with obvious stability being imparted with the more constrained arc. Insertion of these prostheses requires removal of relatively little bone. They may or may not employ a humeral stem. The rationale is to avoid stress at the bone-cement interface and therefore to decrease the likelihood of loosening (Fig. 11–77).

Radiographic Assessment. The major evaluation of these joints is directed toward the stability of the joint itself. In the past, subluxation has been a problem with some of the designs, and the lateral radiograph is probably the most useful view to demonstrate this problem (Fig. 11–78). The AP radiograph is helpful in demonstrating the varus-

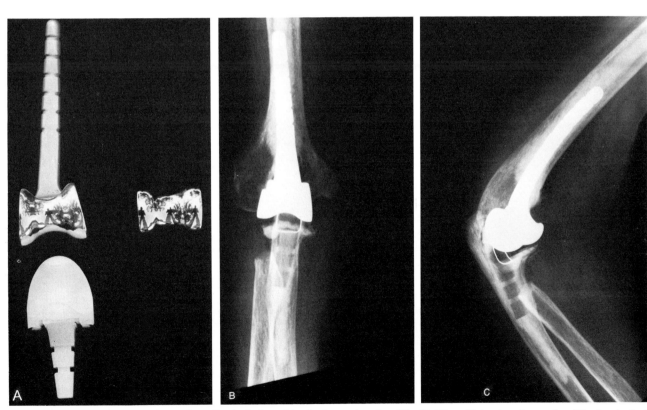

Figure 11–77. A resurfacing type of prosthesis designed by Dr. James London *(A),* with AP and lateral radiographs of the implanted device *(B* and *C).* (Courtesy of J. London.)

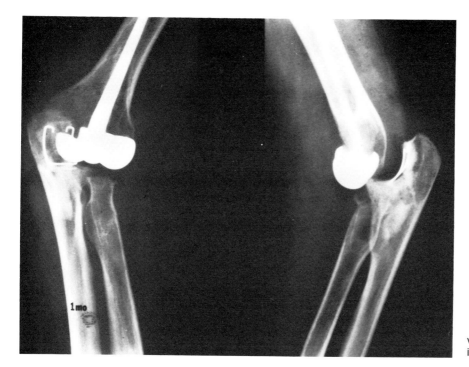

Figure 11–78. The resurfacing devices result in instability and dislocation in up to 5 to 10 percent of instances.

valgus angulation. It should be noted that if the patient has more than 15° flexion-contracture, the amount of varus-valgus angulation as measured from the x-ray or from clinical assessment will be spurious. Most components are cemented, and lucent lines are uncommon in the first 5 years.[153, 160] Flexion-contracture of greater than 30° may be seen with these devices.[169]

Coupled-Hinge Total Elbow Arthroplasty

Indications. Rheumatoid arthritis, post-traumatic arthritis, revision elbow surgery.

Biomechanics and Technique. The coupled type of total elbow arthroplasties are inherently stable, and all designs involve a humeral and ulnar medullary stem.[151] Some also provide a radial head implant. These prostheses are used when there is a greater amount of instability or greater joint deformity (Fig. 11–79). Because stability is provided by the prosthesis, stresses are transmitted to the bone-cement interface. Hence, the possibility of loosening is increased for these prostheses.[151, 155, 166] A proper cementing technique should demonstrate less than 1 mm of lucency in the AP and lateral projections, and the cement should extend past the

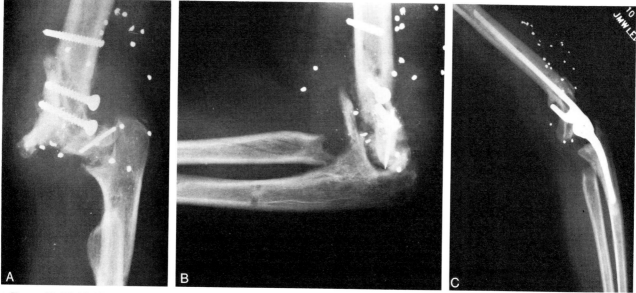

Figure 11–79. AP *(A)* and lateral *(B)* radiographs showing severe trauma. A stemmed prosthesis with an anterior phalanx combined with a bone graft *(C)* is the treatment of choice.

tip of the prosthesis.[166] A carefully placed lateral radiograph should show the prosthesis in true lateral profile. If this is not properly done, the so-called lateral radiograph will reveal an oblique projection of the prosthesis. If a revision device has been used, a longer stem of up to 8 inches may be employed.[163] It is thus imperative that the routine radiographs include the tip of the prosthesis in both the AP and the lateral view of all prosthetic replacement devices.

Results. The results of total elbow arthroplasty have been comparable to those reported for other joint replacements, provided that complications have not supervened. Relief of pain, therefore, is about 95 percent and the arc of motion that is obtained averages 30° to 130° of flexion and extension and 55° of pronation and supination.[165]

Complications. The elbow joint is a subcutaneous one, and many complications seem to relate to this anatomic feature.[163] Skin and wound healing was a problem in the early arthroplasties, but this has largely been resolved with improved technique.[156] Ulnar nerve injury occurs in 5 to 10 percent of instances, but loosening has been the major problem.[165] This complication has been reported in about 25 percent of tightly constrained joints[151, 155, 165] (Fig. 11–80), but it has been markedly reduced with the introduction of the semiconstrained joint. Loosening is uncommon in the resurfacing devices, but instability, as mentioned earlier, has been a problem.[152, 169] When a high-density polyethylene stem was used, fracture of the stem was regularly seen.[168] Material failure of the devices is not very common. However, if loosening has resulted in resorption of

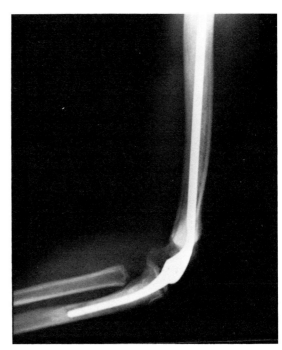

Figure 11–81. A long-stemmed device is now used for revision arthroplasty as well as in some initial implantations. Total elbow arthroplasty radiographs should include the tip of the prosthesis, thus necessitating the use of a larger cassette.

the bone, fractures have occurred about the tip of the prosthesis when this has become loose. These are not usually on the humeral side. The loosening results from forces that are directed posteriorly and superiorly. Thus, the tip of the prosthesis tends to migrate superiorly and anteriorly (Fig. 11–80). If a loose prosthesis requires revision, we employ a longer-stemmed device (Fig. 11–81). More recently, we have employed components that include an anterior hinge to provide rotatory and posterior displacement stability (see Fig. 11–79C).

A final but significant complication of total elbow arthroplasty is a high incidence of infection. This has been reported to occur in as many as 9 percent of cases in the Mayo Clinic experience.[164] The incidence is higher in patients with rheumatoid arthritis, though the evidence of radial lucency is not always present (Fig. 11–82). Because the deep infection is often associated with an intact component, and since removal of these components is necessary in order to clear the infection, fracture of the humerus or ulna is not uncommon in the treatment of these patients (Fig. 11–82B). Encouragingly, it has been reported that approximately 80 percent of patients with resection arthroplasties for infection gain reasonably functional extremities, with approximately 80 percent showing satisfactory results.[164] If a fracture has occurred at the time of removal, splinting the elbow results in fracture healing but also in some scarring of the resected joint (see Fig. 11–82B), which decreases the amount of stability that would ordinarily be expected.

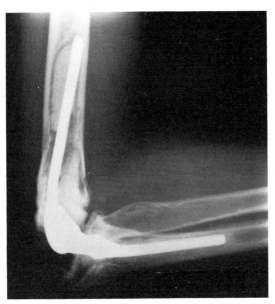

Figure 11–80. The most common complication with total elbow arthroplasty has been the loosening of the constrained devices. In this instance, generalized radiolucency is noted around the humeral component; however, the component appears to be stable.

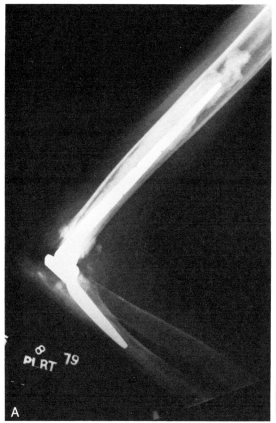
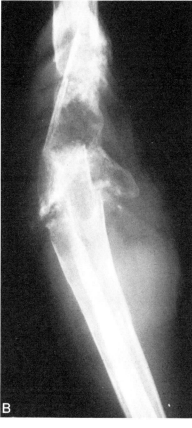

Figure 11–82. A total elbow arthroplasty that demonstrates a good cementing technique. However, this joint became infected *(A)*, resulting in a distal humeral fracture upon removal of the prosthesis *(B)*. Surprisingly and fortunately, the function of these joints even after resection and fracture is surprisingly good, with about 80 percent of function considered satisfactory.

REFERENCES

Anatomy

1. An, K. N., Hui, F. C., Morrey, B. F., et al.: Muscles across the elbow joint: A biomechanical analysis. J. Biomech. 14:659, 1981.
2. Atkinson, W. B., and Elftman, H.: The carrying angle of the human arm as a secondary sex characteristic. Anat. Rec. 91:49, 1945.
3. Beals, R. K.: The normal carrying angle of the elbow. Clin. Orthop. 119:194, 1976.
4. Ekholm, R., and Ingelmark, B. E.: Functional thickness variations of human articular cartilage. Acta Soc. Med. Upsal. 57:39, 1952.
5. Evans, E. M.: Rotational deformity in the treatment of fractures of both bones of the forearm. J. Bone Joint Surg. 27:373, 1945.
6. Gay, J. R., and Love, J. G.: Diagnosis and treatment of tardy paralysis of the ulnar nerve. J. Bone Joint Surg. 29:1087, 1947.
7. Guttierez, L. F.: A contribution to the study of the limiting factors of elbow fixation. Acta Anat. 56:146, 1964.
8. Hollinshead, W. H.: Anatomy for Surgeons. Vol. 3: The Back and Limbs. 3rd Ed. New York, Harper and Row, 1982.
9. Johansson, O.: Capsular and ligament injuries of the elbow joint. Acta Chir. Scand. (Suppl.) 287:1, 1962.
10. Loomis, L. K.: Reduction and after-treatment of posterior dislocation of the elbow: With special attention to the brachialis muscle and myositis ossificans. Am. J. Surg. 63:56, 1944.
11. Morrey, B. F., and Chao, E. Y.: Passive motion of the elbow joint. A biomechanical analysis. J. Bone Joint Surg. 58A:501, 1976.

12. Simon, W. H., Friedenberg, S., and Richardson, S.: Joint congruence. J. Bone Joint Surg. 55A:1614, 1973.
13. Thompson, H. C. III, and Garcia, A.: Myositis ossificans: Aftermath of elbow injuries. Clin. Orthop. 50:129, 1967.
14. Tillman, B.: A Contribution to the Functional Morphology of Articular Surfaces. In Bargmann, W., and Doerr, W., eds. Konorz, G., trans. Littleton, Mass., P.S.G. Pub. Co., 1978.

Routine and Special Radiographic Techniques

15. Arger, P. H. et al.: Lipohemarthrosis. A. J. R. 121:97, 1974.
16. Ballinger, P. W.: Merrill's Atlas of Roentgenographic Positions and Standard Radiologic Procedures. 5th Ed. St. Louis, C. V. Mosby, 1982.
17. Bassett, L. W., Mirra, J. M., Forrester, D. M., et al.: Post-traumatic osteochondral "loose body" of the olecranon fossa. Radiology 141:635, 1981.
18. Bernau, A., and Berquist, T. H.: Positioning Techniques in Orthopedic Radiology. Baltimore, Urban & Schwarzenberg, 1983.
19. Bledsoe, R. C., and Izenstark, J. L.: Displacement of fat pads in disease and injury of the elbow. A new radiographic sign. Radiology 73:717, 1959.
20. Bohrer, S. P.: The fat pad sign following elbow trauma. Clin. Radiol. 21:90, 1970.
21. Brown, R., Blazina, M. E., Kerlan, R. K., et al.: Osteochondritis of the capitellum. J. Sports Med. 2:27, 1974.
22. Eto, R. T., Anderson, P. W., and Harley, J. D.: Elbow arthrography with the application of tomography. Radiology 115:283, 1975.
23. Freiberger, R. H., and Kaye, J. J.: Arthrography. New York, Appleton-Century-Crofts, 1979.
24. Godefroy, D., Pallardy, G., Chevrot, A., et al.: Arthrography of the elbow: Anatomical and radiological consideration and technical considerations. J. Radiology, 62:441, 1981 (Fre.).
25. Greenspan, A., and Norman, A.: The radial head, capitellar

view. Useful technique in elbow trauma. A. J. R. *138*:1186, 1982.

26. Greenspan, A., and Norman, A.: The radial head, capitellar view. Another example of its usefulness. A. J. R. *139*:193, 1982.

27. Hudson, T. M.: Elbow arthrography. Radiol. Clin. North Am. *19*:227, 1981.

28. Kohn, A. M.: Soft tissue alterations in elbow trauma. A. J. R. *82*:867, 1959.

29. London, J. T.: Kinematics of the elbow. J. Bone Joint Surg. *63A*:329, 1981.

30. Mink, J. H., Eckhardt, J. J., and Grant, T. T.: Arthrography in recurrent dislocation of the elbow. A. J. R. *136*:1242, 1981.

31. Murry, W. A., and Siegel, M. J.: Elbow fat pads with new signs and extended differential diagnosis. Radiology *124*:659, 1977.

32. Norell, H. G.: Roentgenologic visualization of the extracapsular fat. Its importance in the diagnosis of traumatic injuries to the elbow. Acta Radiol. *42*:205, 1954.

33. Obermann, W. R., and Loose, H. W. C.: The os supratrochleare dorsale: A normal variant that may cause symptoms. A. J. R. *141*:123, 1983.

34. Pavlov, H., Ghelman, B., and Warren, R. F.: Double-contrast arthrography of the elbow. Radiology *130*:87, 1979.

35. Roback, D. L.: Elbow arthrography: Brief technical considerations. Clin. Radiol. *30*:311, 1979.

36. Rogers, L. F.: Radiology of Skeletal Trauma. New York, Churchill Livingstone, 1982.

37. Rogers, S. L., and MacEwan, D. W.: Changes due to trauma in the fat plane overlying the supinator muscle: A radiographic sign. Radiology *92*:954, 1969.

38. Smith, D. N., and Lee, J. R.: The radiological diagnosis of post-traumatic effusion of the elbow joint and its clinical significance: The displaced fat pad sign. Injury *10*:115, 1978.

39. Weisman, J., and Reimate, A.: Contrast arthrography in diagnosis of soft tissue injuries of the elbow joint. ROFO *136*:313, 1982.

40. Weston, W. J.: Arthrography. New York, Springer-Verlag, 1980.

41. Yousefzadeh, D. K., and Jackson, J. H.: Lipohemarthrosis of the elbow joint. Radiology *128*:643, 1978.

Trauma

42. Barnes, D. A., and Tullos, H. S.: An analysis of 100 symptomatic baseball players. Am. J. Sports Med. *6*:62, 1978.

43. Cirincione, R. J., and Baker, B. E.: Tendon ruptures with secondary hyperparathyroidism. A case report. J. Bone Joint Surg. *57A*:852, 1975.

44. Davis, W. M., and Jassine, Z.: An etiologic factor in the tear of the distal tendon of the biceps brachii. J. Bone Joint Surg. *38A*:1368, 1956.

45. Farrar, E. L. III, and Lippert, F. G. III: Avulsion of the triceps tendon. Clin. Orthop. *161*:242, 1981.

46. King, J. W., Brelsford, H. J., and Tullos, H. S.: Analysis of the pitching arm of the professional baseball player. Clin. Orthop. *67*:116, 1969.

47. Levy, M., Fischel, R. E., and Stern, G. M.: Triceps tendon avulsion with or without fracture of the radial head—a rare injury? J. Trauma *18*:677, 1978.

48. Linscheid, R. L., and Wheeler, D. K.: Elbow dislocations, JAMA *194*:1171, 1965.

49. Mains, D. B., and Freeark, R. J.: Report of compound dislocation of the elbow with entrapment of brachial artery. Clin. Orthop. *106*:180, 1975.

50. Match, R. M., and Corrylos, E. V.: Bilateral avulsion fracture of the triceps tendon insertion from skiing with osteogenesis imperfecta tarda. Am. J. Sports Med. *11*:99, 1983.

51. Morrey, B. F.: The Elbow and Its Disorders. Philadelphia, W. B. Saunders, 1985.

52. Morrey, B. F., Askew, L. J., An, K. N., et al.: Rupture of the distal biceps tendon: Biomechanical assessment of different treatment options. J. Bone Joint Surg. *67A*, 1985.

53. Norwood, L. A., Shook, J. A., and Andrews, J. R.: Acute medial elbow ruptures. Am. J. Sports Med. *9*:16, 1981.

54. Osborne, G., and Cotterill, P.: Recurrent dislocation of the elbow. J. Bone Joint Surg. *48B*:340, 1966.

55. Patrick, J.: Fracture of the medial epicondyle with displacement into the elbow joint. J. Bone Joint Surg. *28*:143, 1946.

56. Pritchard, D. J., Linscheid, R. L., and Svien, H. J.: Intra-articular medial nerve entrapment with dislocation of the elbow. Clin. Orthop. *90*:100, 1973.

57. Roberts, A. W.: Displacement of the elbow. Br. J. Surg. *56*:806, 1969.

58. Roberts, A. W.: Displacement of the internal epicondyle into the elbow joint. Lancet *2*:78, 1934.

59. Schwab, G. H., Bennett, J. B., Woods, G. W., et al.: Biomechanics of elbow instability: The role of the medial collateral ligament. Clin. Othop. *146*:42, 1980.

60. Thomas, T. T.: Fractures of the head of the radius. University of Pennsylvania. M. Bull. *18*:184 and 221, 1905.

61. Woods, G. W., and Tullos, H. S.: Elbow instability and medial epicondyle fractures. Am. J. Sports Med. *5*:23, 1977.

Humeral Fractures

62. Bryan, R. S.: Fractures about the elbow in adults. Instr. Course Lect. *30*:200, 1981.

63. Bryan, R. S., and Bickel, W. H.: T-condylar fractures of the distal humerus. J. Trauma *11*:830, 1971.

64. Bryan, R. S., and Morrey, B. F.: Extensive posterior exposure of the elbow. A triceps sparing approach. Clin. Orthop. *166*:188, 1982.

65. Cassebaum, W. H.: Open reduction of T- and Y-fractures of the lower end of the humerus. J. Trauma *9*:915, 1969.

66. Collert, S.: Surgical management of fractures of the capitellum humeri. Acta Orthop. Scand. *48*:603, 1977.

67. Corbett, R. H.: Displaced fat pads in trauma to the elbow. Injury *9*:297, 1978.

68. Edman, P., and Lohr, G.: Supracondylar fractures of the humerus treated with olecranon traction. Acta Chir. Scand. *126*:505, 1963.

69. Fowles, J. V., and Kassab, M. T.: Fracture of the capitellum humeri. Treatment by excision. J. Bone Joint Surg. *56A*:794, 1974.

70. Gejrot, W.: An intra-articular fracture of the capitellum and trochlea of the humerus with special reference to treatment. Acta Chir. Scand. *71*:253, 1932.

71. Grantham, S. A., Norris, T. R., and Bush, D. C.: Isolated fracture of the humeral capitellum. Clin. Orthop. *161*:262, 1981.

72. Horne, G.: Supracondylar fracture of the humerus in adults. J. Trauma *20*:71, 1980.

73. Hoyer, A.: Treatment of supracondylar fracture of the humerus by skeletal traction in an abduction splint. J Bone Joint Surg. *34A*:623, 1952.

74. Johansson, H., and Olerud, S.: Operative treatment of intercondylar fractures of the humerus. J. Trauma *11*:836, 1971.

75. Johansson, O.: Capsular and ligament injuries of the elbow joint. Acta Chir. Scand. (Suppl.) *287*:1, 1962.

76. Lansinger, O., and Mare, K.: Intercondylar T-fractures of the humerus in adults. Arch. Orthop. Trauma Surg. *100*:37, 1982.

77. Lipscomb, P. R., and Burleson, R. J.: Vascular and neural complications in supracondylar fractures of the humerus in children. J. Bone Joint Surg. *37A*:468, 1955.

78. McLaughlin, H. L.: Some fractures with a time limit. Surg. Clin. North Am. *35*:553, 1955.

79. Meyerding, H. W.: Volkmann's ischemic contracture associated with supracondylar fracture of the humerus. JAMA *106*:1138, 1936.

80. Milch, H.: Fracture of the external humeral condyle. JAMA *160*:641, 1956.

81. Milch, H.: Unusual fracture of the capitulum humeri and capitulum radii. J. Bone Joint Surg. *13*:882, 1931.

82. Mitsunaga, M. M., Bryan, R. S., and Linscheid, R. L.: Condylar non-unions of the elbow. J. Trauma *22*:787, 1982.

83. Mohan, K.: Myositis ossificans traumatica of the elbow. Int. Surg. *57*:475, 1972.
84. Reich, R. S.: Treatment of intracondylar fractures of the elbow by means of traction. J. Bone Joint Surg. *18*:997, 1936.
85. Rieth, P. L.: Fractures of the radial head—associated with chip fracture of the capitellum in adults: Surgical considerations. South. Surg. *14*:154, 1948.
86. Riseborough, E. J., and Radin, E. L.: Intracondylar T-fractures of the humerus in the adult. A comparison of operative and non-operative treatment in 29 cases. J. Bone Joint Surg. *51A*:130, 1969.
87. Smith, F. M.: Surgery of the elbow. Philadelphia, W. B. Saunders, 1972.
88. Smith, F. M.: Traction and suspension in the treatment of fractures. Surg. Clin. North Am. *31*:545, 1951.
89. Suman, R. K., and Miller, J. H.: Intercondylar fractures of the distal humerus. J. R. Coll. Surg. Edinb. *27*:276, 1982.
90. Van Gorder, G. W.: Surgical approach in supracondylar T-fracture of the humerus requiring open reduction. J. Bone Joint Surg. *22*:278, 1940.
91. Wilson, P. D.: Fracture and dislocations in the region of the elbow. Surg. Gynecol. Obstet. *56*:335, 1933.

Fractures of the Proximal Radius

92. Adler, J. B., and Shaftan, G. W.: Radial head fractures. Is excision necessary? J. Trauma *4*:115, 1964.
93. Arner, O., Ekengren, K., and VonSchreeb, T.: Fractures of the head and neck of the radius. A clinical and roentgenographic study of 310 cases. Acta Chir. Scand. *112*:115, 1957.
94. Arvidsson, H., and Johansson, O.: Arthrography of the elbow-joint. Acta Radiol. (Stockh.) *43*:445, 1955.
95. Bakalim, G.: Fractures of radial head and their treatment. Acta Orthop. Scand. *41*:320, 1970.
96. Bohl, W. R., and Brightman, E.: Fracture of a Silastic radial-head prosthesis: Diagnosis and localization of fragments by xerography. J. Bone Joint Surg. *63A*:1482, 1981.
97. Broberg, M., and Morrey, B. F.: Late excision of radial head fractures. In Press.
98. Broberg, M., and Morrey, B. F.: Treatment of radial head fracture and elbow dislocation. A long-term follow-up study. In Press, J. Bone Joint Surg. (Br).
99. Buxton, St., J. D.: Ossification in the ligaments of the elbow joint. J. Bone Joint Surg. *20*:709, 1938.
100. Carstam, N.: Operative treatment of fractures of the upper end of the radius. Acta Orthop. Scand. *19*:502, 1950.
101. Castberg, T., and Thing, E.: Treatment of fractures of the upper end of the radius. Acta Chir. Scand. *105*:62, 1953.
102. Conn, J., and Wade, P.: Injuries of the elbow: A ten-year review. J. Trauma *1*:248, 1961.
103. Edwards, G. E., and Rostrup, O.: Radial head prosthesis in the management of radial head fractures. Can. J. Surg. *3*:153, 1960.
104. Essex-Lopresti, P.: Fractures of the radial head with distal radio-ulnar dislocation. J. Bone Joint Surg. *33B*:244, 1951.
105. Harrington, I. J., and Tountas, A. A.: Replacement of the radial head in the treatment of unstable elbow fractures. Injury *12*:405, 1981.
106. Johnston, G.: A follow-up of one hundred cases of fracture of the head of the radius with a review of the literature. Ulster Med. J. *31*:51, 1962.
107. Keon-Cohen, B. T.: Fractures at the elbow. J. Bone Joint Surg. *48A*:1623, 1966.
108. Mackay, I., Fitzgerald, B., and Miller, J. H.: Silastic replacement of the head of the radius in trauma. J. Bone Joint Surg. *61B*:494, 1979.
109. Mason, J. A., and Shutkin, N. M.: Immediate active motion in the treatment of fractures of the head and neck of the radius. Surg. Gynecol. Obstet. *76*:731, 1943.
110. Mason, M. B.: Some observations on the fractures of the head of the radius with a review of one hundred cases. Brit. J. Surg. *42*:123, 1954.
111. Morrey, B. F., and An, K. N.: Articular and ligamentous contributions to the varus valgus stability of the elbow. J. Sports Med. *11*:315, 1983.

112. Neuwirth, A. A.: Nonsplinting treatment of fractures of elbow joint. JAMA *118*:971, 1942.
113. Odenheimer, K., and Harvey, J. P., Jr.: Internal fixation of fracture of the head of the radius. J. Bone Joint Surg. *61A*:785, 1979.
114. Poulsen, J. O., and Tophoj, K.: Fracture of the head and neck of the radius. Acta Orthop. Scand. *45*:66, 1974.
115. Radin, E. L., and Riseborough, E. J.: Fractures of the radial head. J. Bone Joint Surg. *48A*:1055, 1966.
116. Scharplatz, D., and Allgower, M.: Fracture-dislocations of the elbow. Injury *7*:143, 1976.
117. Stephen, I. B. M.: Excision of the radial head for closed fracture. Acta Orthop. Scand. *52*:409, 1981.
118. Sutro, C. J.: Regrowth of bone at the proximal end of the radius following resection in this region. J. Bone Joint Surg. *17*:867, 1935.
119. Swanson, A. B., Jaegar, S. H., and La Rochelle, D.: Comminuted fractures of the radial head. The role of silicone-implant replacement arthroplasty. J. Bone Joint Surg. *63A*:1039, 1981.
120. Taylor, T. K. F., and O'Connor, B. T.: The effect upon the inferior radio-ulnar joint of excision of the head of the radius in adults. J. Bone Joint Surg. *46B*:83, 1964.

Fractures of the Ulna

121. Aldredge, G. H., Jr., and Gregory, C. F.: Triceps advancement in olecranon fractures. J. Bone Joint Surg. *51A*:816, 1969.
122. Bado, J. L.: The Monteggia lesion. Clin. Orthop. *50*:71, 1967.
123. Beck, C., and Dabezies, E. J.: Monteggia fracture-dislocation. Orthopedics *7*:329, 1984.
124. Boyd, H. B.: Surgical exposure of the ulna and proximal third of the radius through one incision. Surg. Gynecol. Obstet. *71*:86, 1940.
125. Bryan, R. S.: Monteggia fracture of the forearm. J. Trauma *11*:992, 1971.
126. Colton, C. L.: Fractures of the olecranon in adults: Classification and management. Injury *5*:121, 1973.
127. Coughling, N. J., Slabaugh, P. B., and Smith, T. K.: Experience with the McAtee olecranon device in olecranon fractures. J. Bone Joint Surg. *61A*:385, 1979.
128. Daland, E. N.: Fractures of the olecranon. J. Bone Joint Surg. *16*:601, 1933.
129. Eriksson, E., Sahlen, O., and Sandohl, U.: Late results of conservative and surgical treatment of fractures of the olecranon. Acta Chir. Scand. *113*:153, 1957.
130. Evans, E. M.: Pronation injuries of the forearm with special reference to the anterior Monteggia fracture. J. Bone Joint Surg. *31B*:578, 1949.
131. Gartsman, G. M., Sculco, T. P., and Otis, J. C.: Operative treatment of olecranon fractures. J. Bone Joint Surg. *63A*:718, 1981.
132. Jessing, P.: Monteggia lesions and their complicating nerve damage. Acta Orthop. Scand. *46*:601, 1975.
133. Lou, I.: Olecranon fractures treated in the orthopedic hospital. Copenhagen, 1936–1947. A follow-up examination. Acta Orthop. Scand. *19*:166, 1949–1950.
134. MacAusland, W. R. Jr., and Wyman, E. T.: Fractures of the olecranon by longitudinal screw or nail fixation. Ann. Surg. *116*:293, 1942.
135. Mobley, J. E., and Janes, J. M.: Monteggia fractures. Proc. Staff Meet. Mayo Clin. *30*:497, 1955.
136. Monteggia, G. B.: Instituzioni Chirurgiche. Vol. 5. Milan, Maspero, 1814.
137. Muller, M. E., Allgower, M., Schneider, R., et al.: Manual of Internal Fixation. Techniques Recommended by the AO Group. 2nd Ed. New York, Springer-Verlag, 1979.
138. O'Donoghue, D. H., and Sell, L. S.: Persistent olecranon epiphysis in adults. J. Bone Joint Surg. *24*:677, 1942.
139. Penrose, J. H.: The Monteggia fracture with posterior dislocation of the radial head. J. Bone Joint Surg. *33B*:65, 1951.
140. Reckling, F. W.: Unstable fracture-dislocation of the forearm (Monteggia and Galeazzi lesions). J. Bone Joint Surg. *64A*:857, 1982.

141. Reckling, F. W., and Cordell, L. B.: Unstable fracture-dislocations of the forearm. The Monteggia and Galeazzi lesions. Arch. Surg. *96*:999, 1968.
142. Rettig, A. C., Waugh, T. R., and Evanski, P. M.: Fracture of the olecranon: A problem of management. J. Trauma *19*:23, 1979.
143. Rowe, C. R.: The management of fractures in elderly patients is different. J. Bone Joint Surg. *47A*:1043, 1965.
144. Speed, J. S., and Boyd, H. B.: Treatment of fractures of the ulna with dislocation of head of radius (Monteggia fracture). JAMA *115*:1699, 1940.
145. Tompkins, D. G.: The anterior Monteggia fracture. Observations on etiology and treatment. J. Bone Joint Surg. *53A*:1109, 1971.
146. Van der Kloot, J. F. V. R.: Results of treatment of fractures of the olecranon. Arch. Chir. Neerlandicum, *16*:237, 1964.
147. Wainwright, D.: Fractures of the olecranon process. Brit. J. Surg. *29*:403, 1942.
148. Weseley, M. S., Barenfeld, P. A., and Eisenstein, A. L.: The use of the Zuelzer hook plate in fixation of olecranon fractures. J. Bone Joint Surg. *58A*:859, 1976.

Reconstructive Surgery

149. Bryan, R. S.: Total replacement of the elbow joint. Arch. Surg. *112*:1092, 1977.
150. Coonrad, R. W.: History of total elbow arthroplasty. *In* Inglis, A. E. (ed.): Upper Extremity Joint Replacement. (Symposium on Total Joint Replacement of the Upper Extremity, 1979.) St. Louis, C. V. Mosby, 1982.
151. Dee, R.: Total replacement arthroplasty of the elbow for rheumatoid arthritis. J. Bone Joint Surg. *54B*:88, 1972.
152. Ewald, F. C.: Nonconstrained metal-to-plastic total elbow replacement. *In* Inglis, A. E. (ed.): Upper Extremity Joint Replacement. (Symposium on Total Joint Replacement of the Upper Extremity, 1979.) St. Louis, C. V. Mosby, 1982.
153. Ewald, F. C., Scheinberg, R. D., Poss, R., et al.: Capitello-condylar total elbow arthroplasty: Two to five year follow-up in rheumatoid arthritis. J. Bone Joint Surg. *62A*:1259, 1980.
154. Fromison, A. I., Silva, J. E., and Richey, D.: Cutis arthroplasty of the elbow. J. Bone Joint Surg. *58A*:863, 1976.
155. Garrett, J. C., Ewald, F. C., Thomas, W. H., et al.: Loosening associated with G.S.B. hinge total elbow replacement in patients with rheumatoid arthritis. Clin. Orthop. *127*:170, 1977.
156. Inglis, A. E., and Pellicci, P. M.: Total elbow replacement. J. Bone Joint Surg. *62A*:1252, 1980.
157. Inglis, A. E., Ranawat, C. S., and Straub, L. R.: Synovectomy and debridement of the elbow in rheumatoid arthritis. J. Bone Joint Surg. *53A*:652, 1971.
158. Kita, M.: Arthroplasty of the elbow using J-K membrane. An analysis of 31 cases. Acta Orthop. Scand. *48*:450, 1977.
159. Knight, R. A., and VanZandt, I. L.: Arthroplasty of the elbow: An end result study. J. Bone Joint Surg. *34A*:610, 1952.
160. Kudo, H., Iwano, K., and Watanabe, S.: Total replacement of the rheumatoid elbow with a hingeless prosthesis. J. Bone Joint Surg. *62A*:277, 1980.
161. Mackay, I., Fitzgerald, B., and Miller, J. H.: Silastic radial head prosthesis in rheumatoid arthritis. Acta Orthop. Scand. *53*:63, 1982.
162. Marmor, L.: Surgery of the rheumatoid elbow. Follow-up study of synovectomy combined with radial head excision. J. Bone Joint Surg. *54A*:573, 1972.
163. Morrey, B. F., and Bryan, R. S.: Complications of total elbow arthroplasty. Clin. Orthop. *170*:204, 1982.
164. Morrey, B. F., and Bryan, R. S.: Infection after total elbow arthroplasty. J. Bone Joint Surg. *65A*:330, 1983.
165. Morrey, B. F., and Bryan, R. S.: Prosthetic arthroplasty for the elbow. *In* McCollister, E. C. (ed.): Surgery of the Musculoskeletal System. New York, Churchill Livingstone, 1983.
166. Morrey, B. F., Bryan, R. S., Dobyns, J. H., et al.: Total elbow arthroplasty: A five-year experience at the Mayo Clinic. J. Bone Joint Surg. *63A*:1050, 1981.
167. Peterson, L. F. A., and Janes, J. M.: Surgery of the rheumatoid elbow. Orthop. Clin. North Am. *2*:667, 1971.
168. Rosenfeld, S. R., and Anzel, S. H.: Evaluation of the Pritchard total elbow arthroplasty. Orthopedics *5*:713, 1982.
169. Souter, W. A.: A new approach to elbow arthroplasty. Eng. Med. *10*:59, 1981.
170. Street, D. M., and Stevens, P. S.: A humeral replacement prosthesis for the elbow. J. Bone Joint Surg. *56*:1147, 1974.
171. Vainio, K.: Arthroplasty of the elbow and hand in rheumatoid arthritis: The study of 131 operations. *In* Chapchal, G. (ed.): Synovectomy and Arthroplasty in Rheumatoid Arthritis. Stuttgart, Georg Thieme Verlag, 1967.

FRACTURES OF THE SHAFTS OF THE RADIUS AND ULNA

12

CLAIRE E. BENDER • *DONALD C. CAMPBELL*

This chapter will discuss fractures of the shaft of both the radius and the ulna, fractures of the radius alone, and fractures of the ulna.

ANATOMY

The anatomy of the forearm is very complex (Fig. 12–1). Fractures of the forearm, therefore, create difficult treatment situations not seen in other diaphyseal long bones.

The ulna is a relatively straight bone. Its shaft or body has three borders, the interosseous (or lateral), anterior, and posterior, and three surfaces, the anterior, medial, and posterior. The radius is more complex, as it is composed of several angles and curves. There are three main curves in the normal radius. These can be quite variable. The largest curve is convex laterally in the middle three fifths of the bone. The second curve is convex dorsally in the distal fifth. The third is convex ventrally in the proximal fifth.[10] The body or shaft of the radius is somewhat triangular in shape, so that it presents three borders and three surfaces. Of the borders, the medial or interosseous is the best defined. The anterior border begins proximally at the tuberosity, runs obliquely across the front of the bone to its lateral side, and ends at the base of the styloid process. The posterior border is defined only in the middle third of the bone. The lateral, posterior, and anterior surfaces need no particular comment.[9]

The radius and ulna are relatively parallel but approximate at both ends. Proximally the elbow joint capsule envelops both bones, and the annular ligament, which surrounds the radial head, attaches on the ulna. Distally, the wrist joint capsule, the anterior and posterior radioulnar ligaments, and the fibrocartilaginous articular disk provide continuity. There are five complex joints associated with the forearm bones: (1) proximal radioulnar, (2) distal radioulnar, (3) ulnohumeral, (4) radiohumeral, and (5) radiocarpal.

The intraosseous ligament is located between the shafts of the radius and ulna. The strong oblique fibers of the fibrous tissue originate proximally on the radius and insert distally on the ulna. Proximal to the interosseous membrane there is a small band of fibrous tissue, the oblique cord. The interosseous membrane tends to resist independent upward movement on the radius.[9]

Complex muscle groups act across the forearm (Figs. 12–2 and 12–3). Fractures of the forearm thus result in complex deforming forces. The supinator, pronator teres, and pronator quadratus insert or originate solely on the radius or ulna. With fracture, these muscles tend to approximate the radius and ulna, with subsequent decrease in the interosseous space.

Other muscles cross the elbow or wrist joint, tending to produce pronation or supination. Pronators include the flexor carpi radialis, abductor polilicis longus and brevis, and extensor pollicis longus. Supinators include the biceps brachii.

Pronation and supination are the forearm motions. The movement of the radius around the ulna has been compared with the handle of a bucket. The radial head pivots in the annular ligament, while the distal end sweeps around the ulnar head (attached by the fibrocartilaginous articular disk).[3]

The radial, median, and ulnar nerves course through the soft tissues of the forearm.

The nutrient arteries of the radius and ulna are branches of the anterior interosseous artery (Fig. 12–4). The better defined chief nutrient canal of the radius is at the junction of the upper and middle thirds on the anterior surface and courses obliquely through the medial cortex.

ROENTGENOGRAPHIC EVALUATION

Although the clinical presentation of fracture of the forearm bones is usually quite obvious, thorough radiologic examination of the radius and ulna and adjacent wrist and elbow joints is mandatory. Standard views of the forearm of the patient include the AP and lateral projections (Fig. 12–5). The degree of shortening, angulation, rotation, and comminution should be noted.[1] The selected films must be long enough to include the adjacent elbow and wrist joints. The two views can be obtained either on one large film by alternately covering half the cassette with a lead mask or by using two separate 7 × 17 extremity cassettes.[4, 5] This is nec-

631

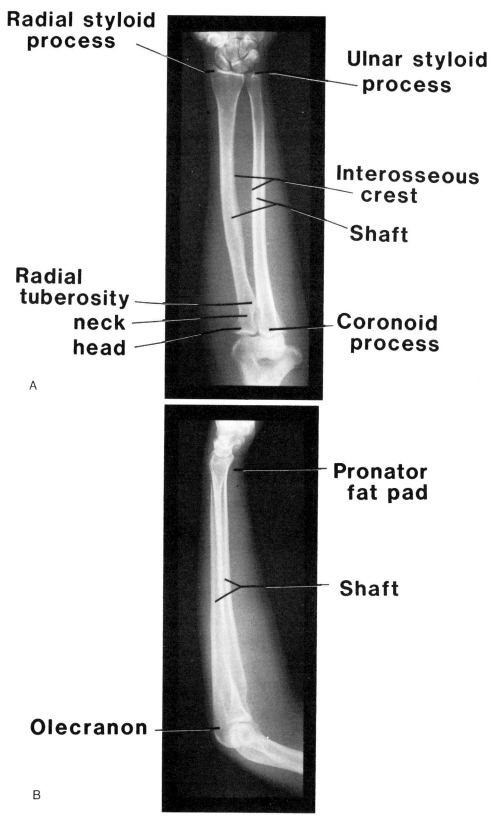

Figure 12–1. AP (*A*) and lateral (*B*) radiographs of radius and ulna.

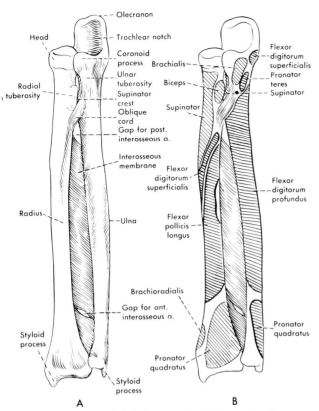

Figure 12–2. *A* and *B*, Anterior muscle attachments of forearm. (From Hollinshead, W. H.: Anatomy for Surgeons, Vol. 3: The Back and Limbs. 3rd Ed. Philadelphia, Harper and Row, 1982.)

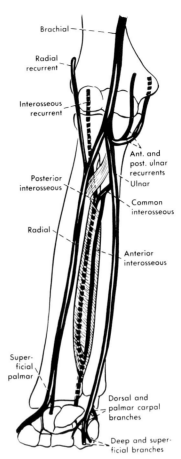

Figure 12–4. Arteries of forearm. (From Hollinshead, W. H.: Anatomy for Surgeons, Vol. 3: The Back and Limbs. 3rd Ed. Philadelphia, Harper and Row, 1982.)

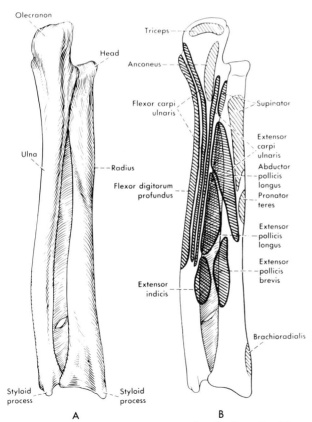

Figure 12–3. *A* and *B*, Posterior muscle attachments of forearm. (From Hollinshead, W. H.: Anatomy for Surgeons, Vol. 3: The Back and Limbs. 3rd Ed. Philadelphia, Harper and Row, 1982.)

essary to be certain of the position of the forearm and screen for detecting associated wrist and elbow pathology. If there is a clinical indication, separate views of the elbow and wrist, with proper centering, must be obtained.

The AP projection is made with the patient seated close to the extended elbow. The hand must be supinated to prevent superimposition of the distal radius and ulna. Immobilization may be necessary by placing a sandbag over the palm of the hand.

For the lateral projection, the patient is seated with the elbow and shoulder joints in the same plane and parallel to the table top. This permits the necessary superimposition of the proximal and distal radius and ulna. By flexing the elbow to 90°, the forearm is placed on the unmasked half of the cassette. In order to obtain a true lateral film, the thumb side of the hand must be up.

In immobilized patients with multiple severe injuries, films are made with the forearm at the patient's side. With severe forearm injuries or associated upper extremity injuries, accurate positioning of the forearm is impossible. In addition to the AP view, a cross-table lateral view can be taken.

The central beam is centered perpendicularly to the cassette. Lead aprons are used for gonadal shielding.

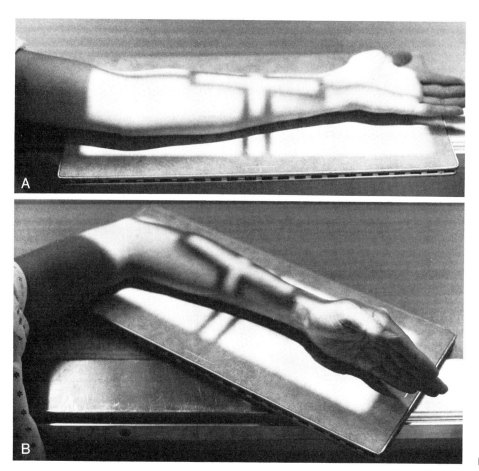

Figure 12–5. AP (*A*) and lateral (*B*) projections of forearm.

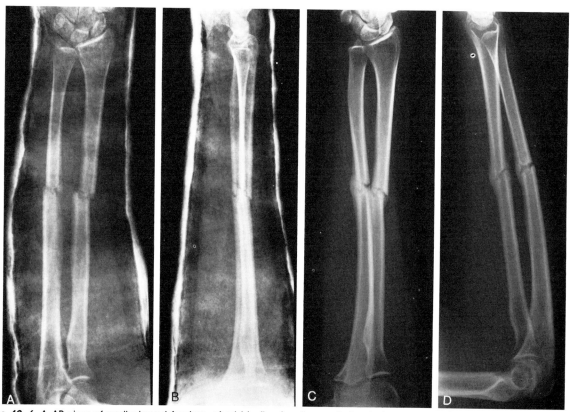

Figure 12–6. A, AP view of undisplaced fracture of midshafts of radius and ulna in long-arm cast. *B,* Lateral view. *C,* At 3-month follow-up, AP view shows healing fractures. *D,* Lateral view.

MECHANISM OF INJURY

A direct blow to the forearm, usually from some form of motor vehicle accident, is the most common mechanism of injury. A severe fall on the outstretched hand may also result in fractures to the shafts of the radius and ulna.

CLASSIFICATION

Fractures of either or both forearm bones are classified according to the level of fracture, degree of displacement and angulation, degree of comminution, and open versus closed wound. Each factor is of considerable importance in the treatment and prognosis.

In Smith and Sage's series of 555 forearm fractures in 338 adult patients, approximately 75 percent involved both bones, 15 percent involved the ulna alone, and 10 percent involved the radius alone.[17] About three fifths of the fractures involved the adjacent proximal and distal third of the shafts equally.

MANAGEMENT

Undisplaced fractures of the shafts of both the radius and ulna are rare.[1] Treatment usually consists of immobilization in a well molded long-arm cast, with the elbow flexed 90° and the hand in neutral position (Fig. 12–6).

The undisplaced fracture of the ulna alone, also called the nightstick fracture because the mechanism of injury is usually a direct blow, is fairly common. Treatment is by long-arm immobilization. Loss of position tends to be more common in the proximal half of the bone, where the forearm muscles attach.

Undisplaced fractures of the proximal radius alone are rare. The forearm muscles pad the area. Therefore, severe injuries to this area are likely to injure the ulna, too. Also, the anatomic position of the radius makes it less likely to receive a direct blow.

Because the fracture can become displaced even while immobilized, weekly AP and lateral roentgenograms must be obtained for the first several weeks. Each new set of films must be compared with the original films in order to exclude even the slightest displacement or rotation (Fig. 12–7).

Displaced fractures of the shafts of the radius and ulna are difficult and challenging to treat. The fractures are often rotated. If satisfactory results are obtained, longitudinal and rotational alignment must be maintained.

Good rotational alignment is necessary for a functional extremity. Generally fractures proximal to the pronator teres insertion on the radius result in supination of the proximal radial fragment of the supinators. In fractures distal to the insertion of the pronator teres, the major forces of the biceps and supinator muscles are neutralized, and therefore fragments are minimally displaced. Because the proximal ulnar fragment remains stable, the posi-

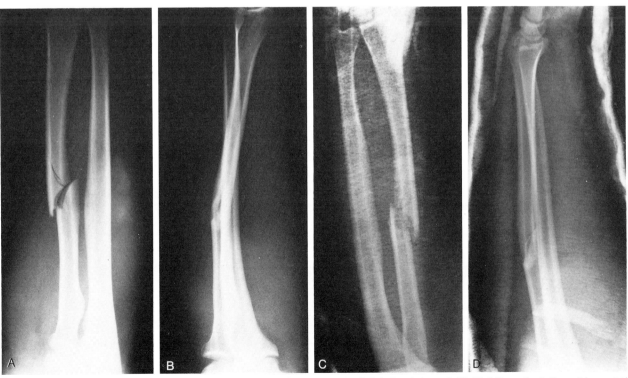

Figure 12–7. A, AP view shows minimally displaced fracture of radial shaft. B, Lateral view. C, Slight shift and rotation of fragments have occurred after cast application. AP view. D, Lateral view.

tion for immobilization must be governed by the position of this fragment. Thus, for satisfactory reduction the distal radial fragment must be rotated to align with the proximal fragment.[2]

Evans has described a method by which one can determine the correct rotational position in which to immobilize fractures of both the forearm bones.[7] He emphasizes standardized technique by obtaining AP views of both the involved elbow and the normal side. The elbow joint is flexed to 90°, and the tube is angled 20° toward the joint space. By locating the position of the radial tuberosity on the radiograph, the rotational position of the proximal radial fragment can be determined (Fig. 12–8), and thus the radial fragment can be appropriately reduced.

Closed treatment consists of a long-arm cast with the forearm in mild or full supination, depending upon whether the fracture is proximal or distal to the pronator teres, respectively. Closed reduction and treatment of displaced radial and ulnar shaft fractures has been disappointing, although Sarmiento has been a strong advocate of early functional bracing of forearm fractures and has reported satisfactory results in spite of imperfect reductions.[16]

Open reduction with some form of internal fixa-

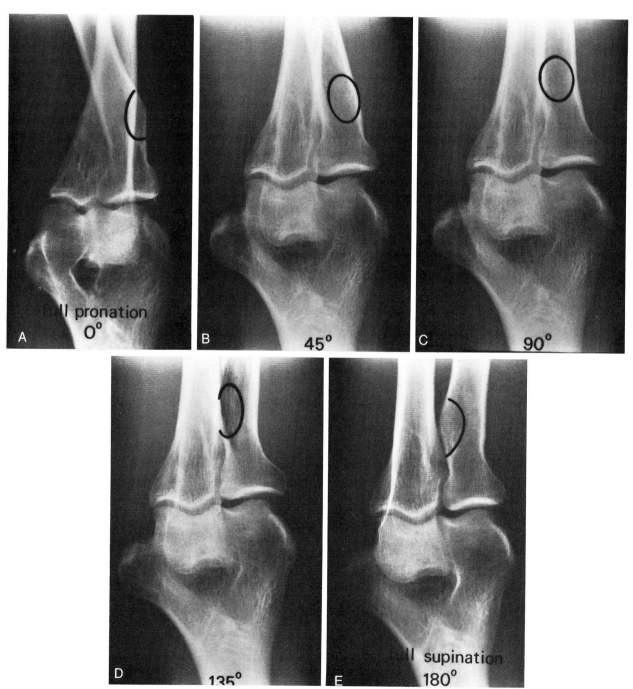

Figure 12–8. A–E, Location of radial tuberosity (outlined in black) determines the rotational position of the proximal radial fragment, which allows for proper reduction of distal radial fragment.

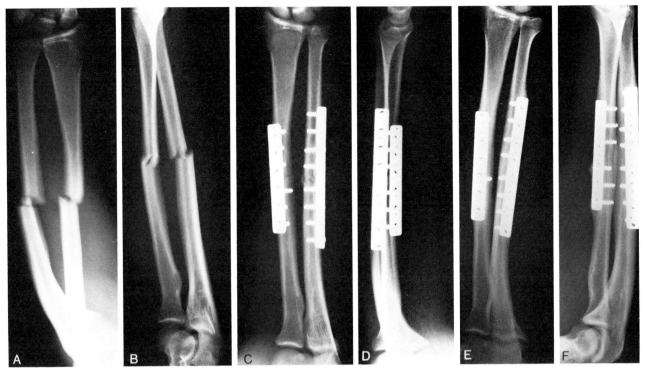

Figure 12–9. A and B, Moderately displaced fractures of midshafts of radius and ulna with pronation of distal fragments. C and D, 6-week films (AP and lateral views) of plate and screw fixation. E and F, 2-year follow-up (AP and lateral views). Fractures are healed.

tion offers the best chance for successful alignment and functional result. Various internal fixation devices include medullary nails (Rush pins, Kirschner wires, Steinmann pins, Lottes nails, Sage triangular nails), plate and screw fixation, and compression plating, with or without bone grafting (Fig. 12–9).

The most popular method of treatment of displaced fractures of the radius and ulna is compression plate fixation. Autogenous bone grafts are used if a significant degree of comminution is present. Anderson and colleagues reported satisfactory results with compression plate fixation in 240 patients with acute diaphyseal fractures of the radius and ulna.[2] Union occurred in 97.9 percent of radius fractures and 96.3 percent of ulna fractures. Satisfactory or excellent results were obtained in over 90 percent of the patients.

Follow-up roentgenographic evaluation for open reduction treatment is similar to that following closed reduction. With open reduction and internal fixation, however, early loss of reduction is unlikely; therefore, roentgenograms can be obtained at less frequent intervals. Because of the rigid fixation achieved, healing callus is reduced and radiographic evidence of healing is not as apparent. Long-arm cast immobilization may be used following open reduction and internal fixation if fixation is suboptimal or if the patient is unreliable. In those patients who are treated with casts, it has been observed that allowing a few days of gentle motion prior to casting will reduce stiffness following final cast removal.

Displaced fractures of the ulna alone rarely occur without fracture of the radius or radial head dislo-

cation. The likelihood of associated injury is greater as displacement increases.

The Monteggia fracture is a classic example of fracture of the ulna accompanied by other injury. This was originally described by Monteggia in 1814 as a "traumatic lesion distinguished by a fracture of the proximal third of the ulna and an anterior dislocation of the proximal epiphysis of the radius."[3] For this injury, Bado preferred the term Monteggia lesion, covering a group of four traumatic lesions having in common a dislocation of the radiohumeroulnar joint that is associated with a fracture of the ulna at various levels or lesions at the wrist.[3] Type I includes anterior dislocation of the radial head and fracture of the ulnar diaphysis at any level with anterior angulation (60 percent of the cases) (Fig. 12–10). Type II includes posterior or posterolateral dislocation of the radial head and fracture of the ulnar diaphysis with posterior angulation (15 percent of the cases). Type III (Fig. 12–11) includes lateral or anterolateral dislocation of the radial head and fracture of the ulnar metaphysis (20 percent of cases). Type IV includes anterior dislocation of the radial head, fracture of the proximal third of the radius, and fracture of the ulna at the same level. There are also several equivalent lesions that possess similar characteristics.

Detailed histories and careful examination of the lateral elbow roentgenogram are very important in the evaluation of these injuries. Unrecognized and untreated fractures may result in malunion with subsequent loss of function. Radiographically, the ulnar fractures are usually quite easy to detect. The dislocated radial head can easily be missed, how-

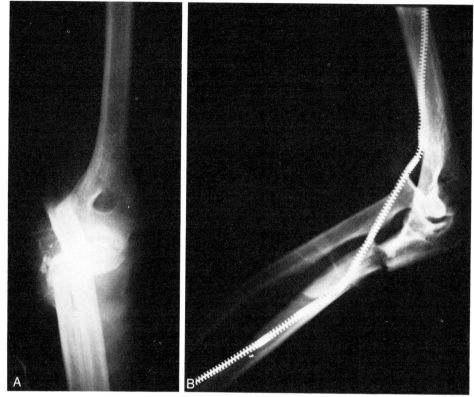

Figure 12–10. AP (*A*) and lateral (*B*) films of Type I Monteggia fracture with anterior dislocation of radial head.

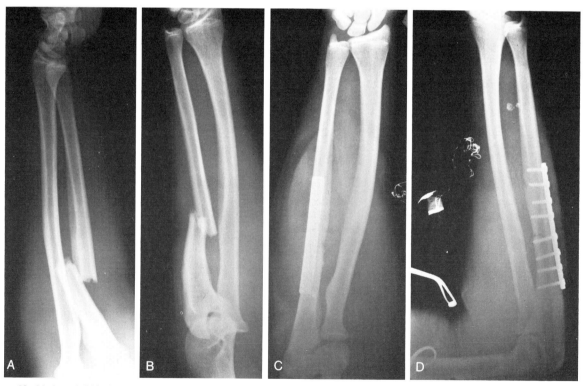

Figure 12–11. A and *B*, Variant of Type III Monteggia fracture with anterolateral dislocation of radial head and ulnar shaft fracture. *C* and *D*, Intraoperative AP and lateral films show excellent reduction.

ever. Reasons for this include (1) failure to include the elbow on the film, which occurs especially when the fracture involves the mid- or distal ulnar shaft; (2) failure to center the x-ray beam on the elbow joint, thereby producing image distortion; and (3) a low index of suspicion for this lesion.

Use of the radiocapitellar line is helpful in evaluation of the radial head. In any elbow film, a line bisecting the radial head must always pass through the capitellum.[8]

In 1929, Valdande described the solitary unstable fracture of the radius at the junction of the middle and distal thirds, known as the reverse Monteggia fracture.[18] In 1934, Galeazzi described the subluxation or dislocation of the distal radioulnar joint associated with this fracture. He further stressed that subluxation of the joint may be present initially or may occur during treatment.[13]

Other factors also contribute to the instability of this fracture. Shortening of the radius tends to occur because of the brachioradialis insertion on the radial styloid process. The pronator quadratus muscle action rotates the distal radial fragment toward the ulna. The weight of the hand pulls the distal fragment of the radius in a volar direction, and the action of the thumb abductors and extensors tends to deviate the wrist radially.[14] According to Galeazzi, this lesion is at least three times as common as the Monteggia fracture.

Radiologically the fracture usually has a transverse or short oblique configuration and is angulated (Fig. 12–12). Generally there is not significant comminution. If much fracture displacement has occurred, there will be dislocation of the distal radioulnar joint. The distal ends of the radius and ulna are normally parallel. On the AP film, there may be increased distance between the articulation of the distal radius and ulna, or there may be overlap owing to ligamentous injury. There may also be an avulsion fracture of the ulnar styloid.

On the lateral view the radius fracture is angulated dorsally, and the head of the ulna is prominent dorsally. Normally the projection of the distal ulna will overlie the posterior cortex of the distal radius. Although rare, damage to the ulnar nerve has been reported in this injury.[12]

Displaced fractures of the proximal two thirds of the radius are usually treated with compression plating or medullary nailing (Fig. 12–12D and E). Detection is important because untreated fractures may result in loss of pronation and supination.[6]

Closed treatment has led to poor results. Muscles acting across the distal forearm tend to displace the distal fragment. In order to maintain good pronation and supination, anatomic reduction must be obtained and held. The preferred method of treatment of these fractures, therefore, is open reduction and internal fixation with compression plating of the radial fracture. Temporary pin fixation of the radioulnar joint may be necessary. The pin must be removed before motion is instituted.

Open forearm fractures present special problems. When bone loss is minimal, treatment can proceed in the same way closed fractures are treated, once the soft tissue wounds are treated. For more serious injuries with soft tissue and bone loss, treatment is

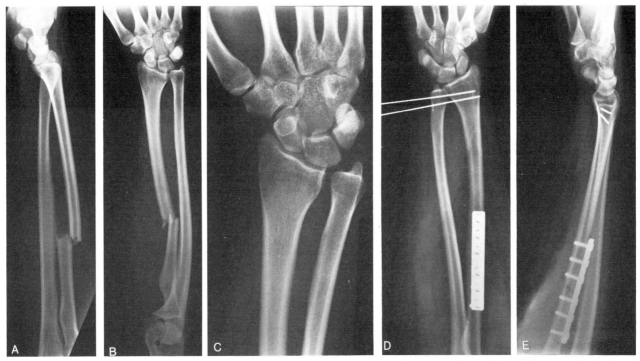

Figure 12–12. A and B, Galeazzi fracture (AP and lateral views) show radial shaft fracture with radial deviation of wrist. C, AP wrist view shows increased distance between ulna and radius, indicating ligamentous injury. D and E, Post-reduction films (AP and lateral).

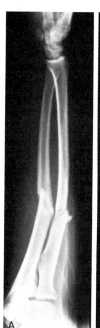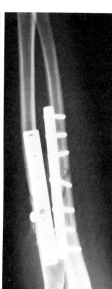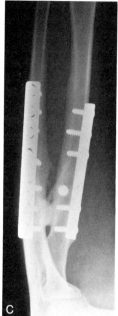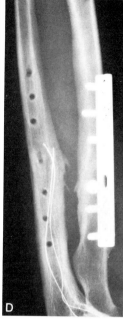

Figure 12–13. A, AP view of fractures of proximal shafts of radius and ulna. *B,* AP view of plate and screw fixation. Callus found on 2-month follow-up. *C,* Oblique film shows synostosis. Patient had no pronation or supination. *D,* Postoperative film shows removal of bony bridge and ulnar plate and screws. Good functional result.

much more involved. Following initial debridement of the wounds, stabilization of the fractures must be carried out. The use of external fixation devices, plates, or, occasionally, medullary devices may be useful. Treatment must then focus upon the soft tissue injuries. Muscle flaps, skin grafts, and free flap transfers of muscle—in some cases along with bone or skin—may be needed. When the soft tissue environment is satisfactory, definitive fixation of the fractures with bone grafting as necessary can be carried out.

Complications of fractures or treatment include non-union, malunion (including radioulnar synostosis) (Fig. 12–13), infection, nerve or vascular injury, or compartment injury. Nerve injuries have been reported in one sixth of forearm fractures.[17] The radial nerve is involved in three fifths of the injuries, with the remainder involving ulnar and medial nerves.

Thus, because of the complex anatomy and variety of forearm fractures, careful radiologic assessment of the radius and ulna is imperative. Attention must be directed not only to angulation and the degree of displacement but also to the correct rotational position of the forearm bones in the initial, early, and follow-up post-reduction films. Any degree of error will result in a corresponding loss of rotational movement.

REFERENCES

1. Anderson, L. D.: Fractures of the shafts of the radius and ulna. *In* Rockwood, C. A., and Green, D. P. (eds.): Fractures. Philadelphia, J. B. Lippincott Co., 1975.

2. Anderson, L. D., Sisk, F. D., Park, W., et al.: Compression plate fixation in acute diaphyseal fractures of the radius and ulna. J. Bone Joint Surg. *54A*:1332, 1979.
3. Bado, J. L.: The Monteggia lesion. Clin. Orthop. *50*:71, 1967.
4. Ballinger, P. W.: Merrill's Atlas of Roentgenographic Positioning and Standard Radiologic Procedures. 5th Ed. St. Louis, C. V. Mosby Co., 1982.
5. Bernau, A., and Berquist, T. H.: Orthopedic Positioning in Diagnostic Radiology. Baltimore, Urban and Schwarzenberg, 1983.
6. Crowe, J. E.: Acute bowing fracture of the forearm in children: A frequently missed injury. A. J. R. *128*:981, 1977.
7. Evans, E. M.: Rotational deformity in the treatment of fractures of both bones of the forearm. J. Bone Joint Surg. *27A*:L373, 1945.
8. Giustra, P. E.: The missed Monteggia fracture. Radiology *110*:45, 1974.
9. Hollinshead, W. H.: Anatomy for Surgeons. Vol. 3: The Back and the Limbs. 3rd Ed. New York, Harper and Row, 1982.
10. Jinkins, W. J. Lockhart, L. D., and Eggers, G. W. N.: Fractures of the forearm in adults. South. Med. J. *53*:669, 1960.
11. Patrick, J.: Study of supination and pronation, with especial reference to the treatment of forearm fractures. J. Bone Joint Surg. *28A*:737, 1946.
12. Poppi, M.: Fracture of the distal radius with ulnar nerve palsy. J. Trauma *18*:278, 1978.
13. Rang, M.: Anthology of Orthopaedics. Baltimore, Williams and Wilkins, 1966.
14. Reckling, F. W.: Unstable fracture-dislocation of the forearm (Monteggia and Galeazzi lesions). J. Bone Joint Surg. *64A*:999, 1982.
15. Rogers, L. F.: Radiology of Skeletal Trauma. New York, Churchill Livingstone, 1982.
16. Sarmiento, A., Cooper, J. S., and Sinclair, W. F.: Forearm fractures. Early functional bracing—a preliminary report. J. Bone Joint Surg. *57A*:297, 1975.
17. Smith, H., and Sage, F. P.: Medullary fixation of forearm fractures. J. Bone Joint Surg. *39A*:91, 1957.
18. Valdande, M.: Luxation en arriere du aibitus avec fracture de la diaphyse radiale. Bull. Mem. Soc. Nat. Chir. *55*:435, 1929.

THE HAND AND WRIST

13

MICHAEL B. WOOD ● *THOMAS H. BERQUIST*

This chapter, devoted to the hand and wrist, will attempt to summarize the pertinent normal and abnormal anatomic features of the distal upper extremity. Major emphasis will be placed on traumatic and post-traumatic conditions as well as on the more common congenital and arthritic conditions with radiographic significance. No attempt will be made to address those conditions of the hand and wrist that are of little radiographic significance in terms of diagnosis or assessment.

ANATOMY

Osteology

The wrist begins proximally at the distal metaphysis of the radius and ulna and extends distally to include the entire carpus. The term "wrist joint" is a misnomer, as the wrist includes a number of articulations. However, from the functional aspect these fall into three main articular groups: the distal radioulnar joint, the radiocarpal articulation, and the so-called midcarpal articulation.

The distal radial metaphysis and epiphysis is largely composed of cancellous bone with a relatively thin cortex. This structural arrangement, coupled with its liability to injury with falls on the outstretched hand, likely accounts for the frequency of fractures seen in this area. Its extreme radial aspect is elongated distally as a styloid process. The distal articular surface of the radius has two fossae for the scaphoid and lunate, respectively. These are separated by a variably defined vertical ridge. This surface of the radius is inclined 14° toward the ulna in the frontal plane and 12° toward the palmar

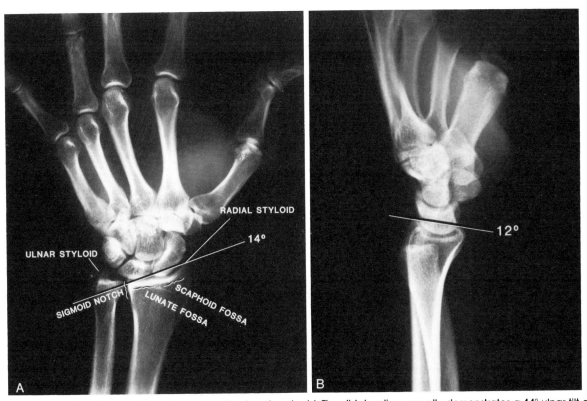

Figure 13–1. AP *(A)* and lateral *(B)* radiographs of the hand and wrist. The distal radius normally demonstrates a 14° ulnar tilt on the AP view *(A)* and 12° volar tilt on the lateral view *(B)*.

641

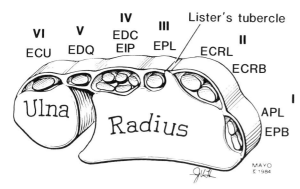

Figure 13–2. Ilustration of distal radius and ulnar en face demonstrating the first through sixth dorsal compartments. First compartment: abductor pollicis longus (APL) and extensor pollicus brevis (EPB). Second compartment: extensor carpi radialis longus (ECRL) and extensor carpi radiales brevis (ECRB). Third compartment: extensor pollicis longus (EPL). Fourth compartment: extensor indicis proprius (EIP) and extensor digitorum communis (EDC). Fifth compartment: extensor digiti quinti (EDQ). Sixth compartment: extensor carpi ulnaris (ECU).

surface in the lateral plane.[2] On the ulnar aspect of the distal radius is a separate concave joint surface called the sigmoid notch for articulation with the distal ulna (Fig. 13–1). The dorsal surface of the distal radius is characterized by a series of sulci and ridges that define the floor of the 1st through 4th dorsal tendinous compartments of the wrist. The most readily palpable protuberance of this surface is Lister's tubercle, which lies between the compartment of the radial wrist extensor tendons (2nd) and that of the extensor pollicis longus tendon (3rd). The 1st (most radial) dorsal compartment contains the tendons of the abductor pollicis longus and extensor pollicis brevis tendons, while the 4th compartment contains the extensor digitorum communis tendons to all fingers and the proprius tendons of the index digit (Fig. 13–2).

The distal ulna is also predominantly composed of cancellous bone but with a reasonably thick cortex. It has a spikelike well defined styloid process. Fracture of this process not infrequently accompanies a fracture of the distal radius. The ulnar head articulates with the distal radius, lunate, and triquetrum. It is usually separated from the latter two bones by an articular disk that represents a portion of the triangular fibrocartilage complex. The dorsal surface of the ulna has sulci for the 5th and 6th dorsal compartments of the wrist, which house the extensor digiti quinti and extensor carpi ulnaris tendons, respectively (Fig. 13–2). The position of

the distal articular surface of the ulna relative to that of the radius may have significance in certain clinical situations and is defined by the term "ulnar variance."[4, 5] In most patients it is either equal (neutral) or 1 mm shorter than the radius. Ulnar variance is positive if the ulnar articular surface is more distal than that of the radius. Conversely, it is negative if it lies more proximally (Fig. 13–3). The distal radioulnar joint in conjunction with the proximal radioulnar joint at the elbow permits rotation of the radius about the ulna in the process of forearm pronation and supination. Normally an arc of 160° to 180° of rotation is possible.[2]

The carpus functionally is composed of three anatomic groups (Fig. 13–4). The first, the proximal row, consists of the scaphoid, lunate, triquetrum, and overlapping pisiform. The scaphoid and triquetrum are firmly bound to the lunate by strong interosseous ligaments. The stability of these articulations is essential for normal wrist mechanics.[20] The proximal articular surfaces of these three bones should define a smooth unbroken arc in the frontal plane (Fig. 13–5). In this same projection the scaphoid tubercle will present a ringlike appearance in the distal half of the bone, and the lunate should appear "trapezoidal." The distance between the scaphoid and lunate or lunate and triquetrum

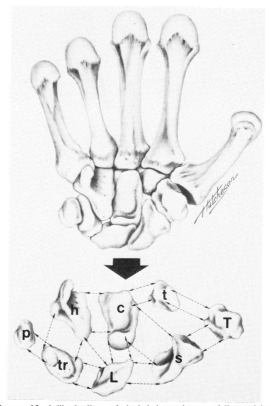

Figure 13–4. Illustration of skeletal anatomy of the wrist with bones detached below. The proximal carpal row: scaphoid (S), lunate (L), triquetrum (tr), and overlapping pisiform (p). The distal carpal row: trapezoid (t), capitate (c), and hamate (h). The trapezium (T) provides independent motion of the thumb. (From Dobyns, J. H., and Linscheid, R. L.: Fractures and dislocations of the wrist. *In* Rockwood, C. A., and Green, D. P.: Fractures. 2nd Ed. Philadelphia, J. B. Lippincott Co., 1984.)

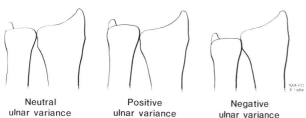

Neutral ulnar variance Positive ulnar variance Negative ulnar variance

Figure 13–3. Illustration of neutral, positive, and negative ulnar variance.

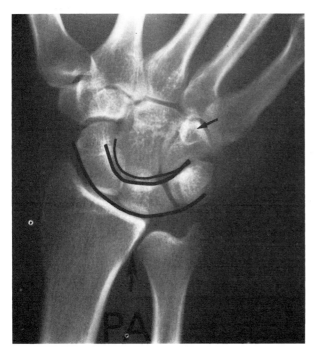

Figure 13–5. True PA view of the wrist. The proximal and distal carpal rows form concentric arcs. The normal distal radioulnar joint *(large arrow)* is 2 to 3 mm. The hook of the hamate is seen on end *(upper arrow)*.

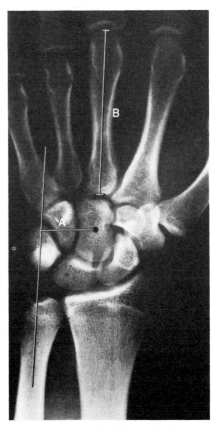

Figure 13–6. AP radiograph of the wrist demonstrating the carpoulnar distance. Normally the distance from a line parallel to the ulnar shaft to the midpoint of the capitate (A) divided by the length of the 3rd metacarpal (B) is 0.30 (± 0.03).

should be relatively constant in all positions of the wrist. Normally this distance should not exceed 2 mm.[3] The position of the scaphoid and lunate should be congruous with the scaphoid and lunate fossae of the distal radius. Ulnar translation of the carpus relative to the radius may be seen in conditions of chronic wrist synovitis and in disruption of the radiocarpal ligament complex, particularly if accompanied by dorsal subluxation of the distal ulna. This instability pattern is characterized by the presence of an apparent widened joint space between the lateral radial articular surface and the scaphoid as well as a decrease in the carpal ulnar distance.[21, 22] This latter term refers to the perpendicular distance between the midpoint of the head of the capitate and a line drawn through the midpoint of the ulna along its longitudinal axis on a PA radiograph. Normally the carpal ulnar distance should form a ratio of 0.30 (± 0.03) with the length of the 3rd metacarpal (Fig. 13–6). In the lateral plane with the wrist neutral, the lunate should generally be collinear with the radius and should appear symmetric within the lunate fossa. The scaphoid outline may be difficult to visualize owing to bony overlap. With the wrist in a neutral position, however, it should point obliquely in a palmar direction. A line drawn through its long axis should form an angle of 30° to 60° (mean 47°) with a line drawn through the axis of the lunate (Fig. 13–7).[2, 3] This angle is called the scapholunate angle and may be abnormal in certain collapse deformities of the wrist. The position of the scaphoid relative to the lunate, however, will vary with ulnar or radial

deviation of the wrist.[10, 18] This should be borne in mind when assessing the scapholunate angle. As the wrist moves from complete ulnar deviation to complete radial deviation, the scaphoid will subtend an arc of 40° (Fig. 13–8). The pisiform is a true sesamoid bone lying within the flexor carpi ulnaris tendon. It forms a synovial articulation with the

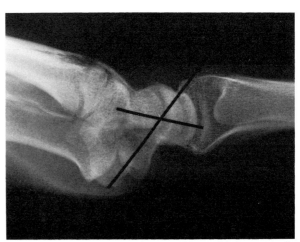

Figure 13–7. Normal lateral view of the wrist demonstrating the normal scapholunate axis (line through the long axis of the scaphoid and midlunate). This angle is normally 30° to 60°, with a mean of 47°.

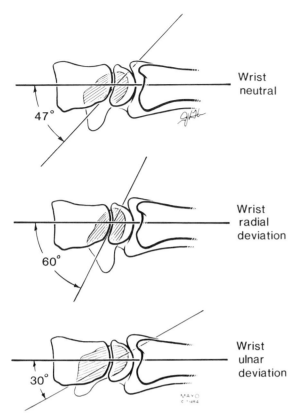

Figure 13–8. Illustration showing how the scapholunate angle changes with radial and ulnar deviation. The scaphoid subtends a 40° arc.

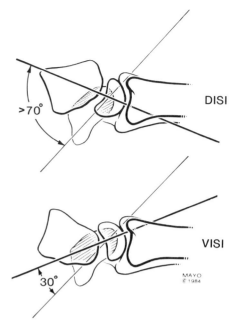

Figure 13–9. Illustration of collapse deformities: DISI (dorsal intercalated segment instability), VISI (volar intercalated segment instability).

triquetrum. Motion between the proximal carpal row and the forearm long bones is primarily associated with dorsiflexion (extension) and also contributes to radial and ulnar deviation.

The second anatomic group, the distal carpal row, consists of the trapezoid, capitate, and hamate. These too are tightly bound to each other by strong interosseous ligaments. The hook (hamulus) of the hamate will present an overlying ringlike appearance in the frontal projection (see Fig. 13–5). On the lateral view the capitate should articulate congruently with the lunate; with the wrist in a neutral position, these two bones along with the radius should be collinear[10] (see Fig. 13–7). This collinear relationship may be lost in certain collapse deformities of the wrist.

Two basic patterns of collapse deformity are recognized and are defined by the direction of the lunate relative to the capitate.[13] The first and most common is a DISI (dorsal intercalated segment instability) pattern. This is characterized on the lateral projection by the lunate appearing to be dorsiflexed on the radius and the capitate palmar flexed on the lunate (Figs. 13–9 and 13–10). DISI is most commonly associated with injuries that result in destabilization of the lunate to the scaphoid, for example, fractures of the scaphoid[6] and complete disruption of the scapholunate interosseous ligament. In such cases, therefore, an additional radiographic finding will be an exaggeration of the scapholunate angle.

The second major category of collapse deformity is in the opposite direction and is referred to as a VISI (volar intercalated segment instability) pattern. This type is characterized by the lunate assuming a palmar flexed position relative to the radius, with the capitate dorsiflexed relative to the lunate[12] (Figs. 13–9 and 13–11). It is most commonly associated with destabilization of the lunate and triquetrum (lunotriquetral interosseous ligament disruption), midcarpal sprains, rheumatoid arthritis, and exaggerated congenital ligamentous laxity in certain individuals. With this pattern a reduction of the scapholunate angle is frequently seen. It is important to emphasize that the diagnosis of either of these two collapse patterns can be made only on the basis of a true lateral x-ray with the wrist in a

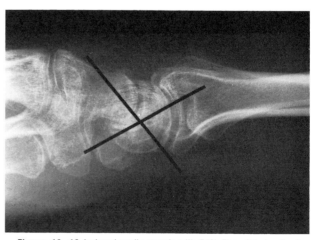

Figure 13–10. Lateral radiograph with DISI. The distal articular surface of the lunate is directed dorsally.

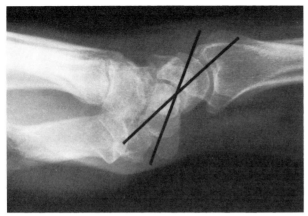

Figure 13–11. Lateral radiograph with VISI. The distal articular surface of the lunate is in a palmar direction, and the scapholunate angle is reduced.

neutral position. The diagnosis is further supported by the apparent persistence of the collapse pattern on true lateral radiographs obtained with the wrist in a fully extended and fully flexed position.

In the absence of a collapse pattern of the carpus, a fracture, or a loss of bone mass, the carpal height should be constant.[21, 22] This term refers to the distance between the base of the 3rd metacarpal and the distal articular surface of the radius along the axis of the 3rd metacarpal as determined on a PA x-ray. Normally the carpal height should be a ratio of 0.54 (± 0.03) when compared with the length of the 3rd metacarpal (Fig. 13–12). Motion between the proximal and distal carpal rows is primarily associated with palmar flexion and also contributes to radial and ulnar deviation.

The third anatomic component of the carpus is the thumb-axis, consisting of only one bone—the trapezium. This bone should appear generally cuboidal in both the frontal and lateral planes (see Fig. 13–1). Moreover, on the frontal projection the distal articular surface should appear as a shallow concavity that is congruous with the base of the 1st metacarpal.

Distal to the carpus are the five metacarpals. The 1st (thumb) metacarpal lies outside the plane of the others in an obliquely palmar direction. The structure of each is similar, with flared metaphyses proximally and distally composed chiefly of cancellous bone and a narrow diaphysis of cortical bone (see Fig. 13–4). This joint space of the 2nd and 3rd carpometacarpal articulations is usually poorly visualized on routine radiographs because of the amount of bony overlap. Moreover, these joints have essentially negligible motion.[8] The 4th and 5th carpometacarpal joints, however, usually do have a well defined joint space, which is best visualized on AP and oblique projections, and also have a range of motion between 15° and 40°.[7] Adjacent metacarpals are stabilized with respect to each other by strong proximal interosseous ligaments and by the transverse metacarpal ligaments distally. The metacarpal heads are roughly spherical. A lateral depression just proximal to the articular surface at the site of origin of the collateral ligaments may be seen on the Brewerton view (see section on Routine Radiographic Techniques and Fig. 13–26). This depression may be particularly obvious in rheumatoid arthritis and represents one of the x-ray diagnostic signs of this condition. The metacarpal head is eccentric in shape, with its palmar aspect broader than its dorsum. This configuration allows relaxation of the collateral ligaments with lateral motion for abduction of the fingers with the metacarpophalangeal joint in a position of extension. Conversely, flexion of the joint tightens the collateral ligaments and allows for little lateral motion. In all positions of the metacarpophalangeal joint, however, the respective articular surfaces should appear congruent.

The proximal and middle phalanges of the fingers are similar in structure, with flared proximal and distal ends composed chiefly of cancellous bone (see Fig. 13–1). The diaphysis consists predominantly of cortical bone and is cylindrical. The distal articular surface of the phalanges is bicondylar and is intimately congruent with its articular fellow on both frontal and lateral planes. The thumb lacks a middle phalanx and thus has only a single interphalangeal joint. The distal phalanx is foreshortened, with its distal end flared in the shape of a blunt arrowhead on the frontal projection.

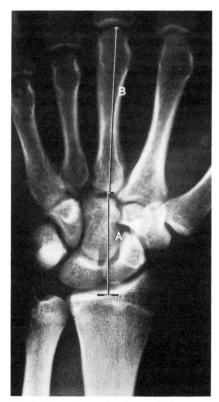

Figure 13–12. PA radiograph demonstrating carpal height measurement. The distance from the distal radial articular surface to the base of the 3rd metacarpal (A) divided by the length of the 3rd metacarpal (B) is 0.54 (± 0.03).

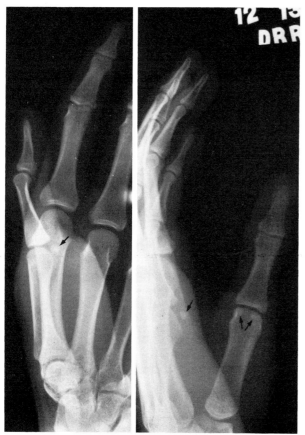

Figure 13–13. Two views of the thumb demonstrating paired sesamoid bones at the 1st metacarpophalangeal joint *(arrows)* and a single sesamoid at the 2nd metacarpophalangeal joint.

Small spherical sesamoid bones, although varying in position and number, are frequently seen in pairs volar to the metacarpophalangeal joints or the interphalangeal joint of the thumb (Fig. 13–13). Moreover, occasionally accessory ossicles can be visualized about the hand and wrist. At least sixteen accessory ossification centers have been reported.[16] The most significant of this group is probably the os centrali. If this ossification center fails to unite to the scaphoid, confusion with a so-called bipartite scaphoid may be possible. Another accessory ossicle described by some is the so-called "styloid bone" lying in the region of the 2nd and 3rd carpometacarpal joint. Whether this represents a true accessory ossicle or a reactive process is debatable, but it may present as a symptomatic carpe bosseau. Other well known accessory ossification centers are the lunula lying between the triquetrum and ulnar styloid and the os radiali externum at the distal end of the scaphoid. The order of ossification of the normal carpal bones is somewhat variable. However, in general the center of ossification appears for the capitate at 6 months, for the hamate at 6 to 18 months, for the triquetrum at 2 years, for the lunate at 4 years, for the trapezium at 5 years, for the trapezoid at 6 years, for the scaphoid at 5 to 6 years, and for the pisiform at 10 years.

Ligaments and Joint Capsules

A detailed description of all the various ligaments about the wrist and hand is beyond the scope of this chapter. However, a review of those ligaments most frequently associated with pathologic conditions or of particular radiographic significance will be emphasized. Because the wrist is composed of at least ten bones and allows a variety of degrees of motion, it naturally depends on a complex array of strong ligaments and soft tissue supports for its mechanical characteristics.

The stability of the distal radioulnar joint and a major component of the ulnocarpal articulation depends on the integrity of the triangular fibrocartilage complex.[10, 17] This so-called ligamentous complex consists of multiple components that blend imperceptibly into one another and include the triangular fibrocartilage proper, the ulnocarpal meniscus, the ulnar collateral ligament, and the volar and dorsal distal radioulnar ligaments (Fig. 13–14). The apex of the triangular fibrocartilage proper (or articular disk) originates from the base of the ulnar styloid process and fans out to insert broadly along the ulnar margin of the distal radius. Perforations may be seen in the central portion of the disk that may or may not be of clinical significance.[15, 17] The dorsal and volar margins of the fibrocartilage are thickened, blending with the respective radioulnar ligaments, capsular ligaments of the wrist, and lunotriquetral interosseous ligaments. The ulnocarpal meniscus component arises near the insertion of the articular disk on the radius and courses distally, inserting into the triquetrum and hamate. Its extreme ulnar aspect blends with the ulnar collateral ligament fibers. Other factors contributing to the stability of the distal radioulnar joint include the interosseous membrane of the radius and ulna, the extensor carpi ulnaris tendon and its retaining fibro-osseous sheath, and finally the degree of concavity of the sigmoid notch of the radius.

Both volar and dorsal extrinsic capsular ligaments contribute to the stability of the radiocarpal aspect of the wrist, but the former are of greatest clinical significance. Descriptions of the precise components and nomenclature of the capsular ligaments vary from author to author.[9, 14, 19] Hence, consider-

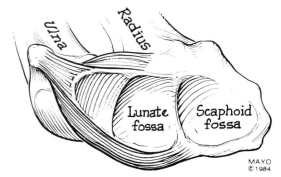

Figure 13–14. Illustration of triangular fibrocartilage complex.

able confusion exists in the literature regarding this topic. However, most agree on a general anatomic arrangement. The palmar capsular ligaments are most obvious when viewed intracapsularly. Basically they consist of two concentric arches originating from the volar radial lip of the radius and inserting into the triquetrum and triangular fibrocartilage complex (Fig. 13–15). The first arch is composed of the radiolunotriquetral ligament, which courses from the radius across the volar surface of the lunate, inserts into the volar surface of the lunate, and then inserts firmly on the triquetrum. The ulnotriquetral ligament then completes the arch. The second arch is made up of the radiocapitate ligament, which originates more laterally on the radius, passes across the waist of the scaphoid, and inserts into the capitate. This arch is completed by the capitotriquetral ligament and the ulnotriquetral ligament. Between these two arches is a rather thinned area of the volar wrist capsule known as the space of Poirier. In addition to the double ligamentous arch of the palmar capsule there is a short but stout radioscapholunate ligament (ligament of Testut). This structure arises from the volar lip of the radius and courses obliquely distally and dorsally to insert on the volar and middle aspect of the scapholunate interosseous ligaments. The dorsal capsular ligaments of the wrist are relatively thin and of lesser significance than their palmar counterparts. The most important components are the radiolunotriquetral and ulnotriquetral ligaments (Fig. 13–16). Both dorsal and volar complexes are reinforced by a radial and ulnar collateral ligament complex.

In addition to the extrinsic capsular ligaments, intrinsic intercarpal ligaments contribute to the sta-

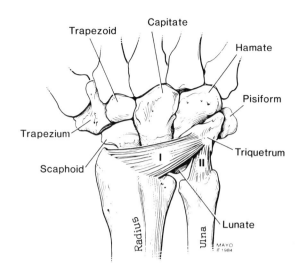

DORSAL

Figure 13–16. Dorsal ligaments of the wrist: I, radiolunotriquetral; II, ulnotriquetral.

bility of the radiocarpal and intercarpal articulations. These include the scapholunate and lunotriquetral interosseous ligaments in the proximal carpal row and both dorsal and volar interosseous ligaments connecting the hamate, capitate, trapezoid, and trapezium. The preserved integrity of the extrinsic capsular and intrinsic intercarpal ligaments is essential for normal wrist stability and mechanics.

Ligamentous support of the carpometacarpal articulations is provided by longitudinally oriented dorsal and volar carpometacarpal ligaments. These vary in location, number, and strength according to the joint involved.[8] The 1st carpometacarpal joint is relatively lax, allowing considerable motion in several degrees of freedom. Often its inherent instability is a source of clinical concern. The chief ligamentous support is provided by the palmar and dorsal oblique capsular ligaments. The former is strongest and most important. By contrast, the 2nd and 3rd carpometacarpal joints are extremely stable, with negligible motion. Strong short capsular ligaments pass from the trapezoid to both radial and ulnar condyles of the 2nd metacarpal on both the volar and dorsal aspects of the joint. The 3rd metacarpal base is stabilized by obliquely disposed dorsal ligaments passing from the trapezoid and capitate as well as by a volar ligament from the capitate and hamate. The 4th and 5th carpometacarpal joints have a moderate range of motion in the plane of flexion and extension and, therefore, are stabilized by less stout capsular ligaments. These arise on both dorsal and volar aspects from the capitate and hamate to the base of the 4th metacarpal and from the hamate alone to the base of the 5th metacarpal. The carpometacarpal articulations are further stabilized by strong transverse intermetacarpal ligaments between the bases of the 2nd through 5th metacarpals.[3] Moreover, these

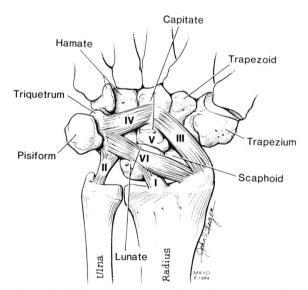

PALMAR

Figure 13–15. Palmar ligaments of the wrist: I, radiolunotriquetral ligament; II, ulnotriquetral ligament; III, radiocapitate ligament; IV, capitotriquetral ligament; V, space of Poirier; VI, ligament of Testut or radioscapholunate ligament.

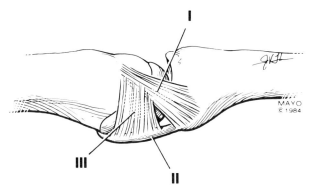

Figure 13–17. Metacarpophalangeal ligaments seen from the lateral view: I, collateral ligaments; II, volar plate; III, accessory collateral ligaments.

same metacarpals are weakly stabilized distally by distal transverse intermetacarpal ligaments.

Ligamentous support of the metacarpophalangeal joints is similar in all digits and depends primarily upon the collateral ligaments, the accessory collateral ligaments, and the fibrocartilaginous volar plate[9] (Fig. 13–17). The collateral ligaments are well defined capsular structures that arise from a dorsal position on either side of the metacarpal just proximal to its articular head. These structures then pass in a palmar and distal direction to insert onto the volar lateral aspect of the base of the proximal phalanx. The fibrocartilaginous volar plate arises from the base of the proximal phalanx and inserts into the volar aspect of the metacarpal just proximal to the articular surface. It is a thick unyielding structure distally but becomes thin and compliant more proximally. It is intimately associated with the distal intermetacarpal ligaments and proximal flexor-tendon-sheath pulley system. Between the collateral ligaments and the volar plate are the interconnecting fibers of the accessory collateral ligaments. Dorsal to the collateral ligaments the joint capsule is filmy and closely associated with the extensor apparatus. As such, the dorsal capsule contributes relatively little stability to the joint. The metacarpophalangeal articulation allows considerable lateral motion, particularly in a position of extension, owing to the eccentricity and relative spherical shape of the metacarpal head. Of particular clinical significance for collateral ligament injury is the metacarpophalangeal joint of the thumb. This joint is shrouded by a well defined extensor aponeurosis, or hood, which may become interposed with complete ruptures of the ulnar collateral ligament.

The ligamentous support of the interphalangeal joints is basically identical in all digits and is quite similar to the arrangement described earlier for the metacarpophalangeal joints.[11] The volar fibrocartilaginous plate of this joint, however, is thickened on its lateral extremes where it is most firmly attached to the base of the middle (or distal) phalanges.[1] Proximally the laterally thickened portions are inserted into the proximal phalanx in close association with the flexor-tendon-sheath pulley system and form the so-called checkrein ligaments. In contrast to the metacarpophalangeal joints, the interphalangeal joints are not eccentric and have little lateral motion. The collateral ligaments in the interphalangeal joint, therefore, are shorter and more rectangular in appearance. The dorsal capsule, although filmy, is reinforced at the base of the middle phalanx. In addition to the ligamentous structures discussed above and the inherent stability conferred by bony architecture, stability to all joints of the upper extremity is further augmented by musculotendinous structures crossing or inserting near the articulation. A detailed description of these structures, however, is of relatively little significance for radiographic evaluations. There are, however, certain specific clinical situations in which the musculotendinous anatomy is relevant, and these will be discussed later in this chapter.

ROUTINE RADIOGRAPHIC TECHNIQUES

There are numerous positioning techniques for evaluating the hand and wrist. Complex anatomy and subtle fractures often require multiple views for complete evaluation.

Hand

Routine evaluation of the hand requires PA, lateral, and oblique views.

PA Views. The PA view is obtained with the patient sitting and the hand positioned on one half of an 8 × 10 inch cassette. The remainder of the cassette is shielded, allowing a second view to be obtained. The fingers should be slightly spread and the palm laid flat against the cassette. The beam is perpendicular to the cassette and centered on the 3rd metacarpophalangeal joint (Fig. 13–18A).[23, 24] The hand, carpal bones, and distal radius and ulna are included on the film (Fig. 13–18B). Careful radiographic analysis will demonstrate uniform cortical margins along the diaphysis of the phalanges and metacarpals. The proximal metaphysis expands just distal to the cortex of the joint space. Asymmetry in the metaphysis is common with torus fractures. The carpometacarpal joints should be parallel and uniform in width.[31, 33] Fisher and colleagues describe an "M" configuration formed by the 2nd through 5th carpometacarpal joints.[31] Any disruption of this configuration suggests subluxation or dislocation (Figs. 13–19 and 13–20).

Oblique View. The hand is rotated superiorly about 45° (thumb up) with the fingers slightly spread. A sponge can be used to maintain the proper position (Fig. 13–21A). The central beam is perpendicular to the cassette and centered on the metacarpophalangeal joints. The oblique view more clearly demonstrates the metacarpal heads (Fig. 13–21B) and the 1st and 2nd carpometacarpal joints.

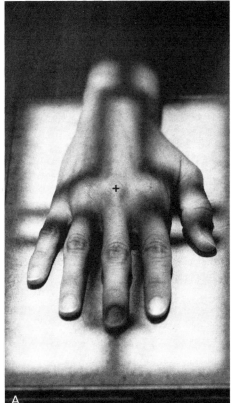

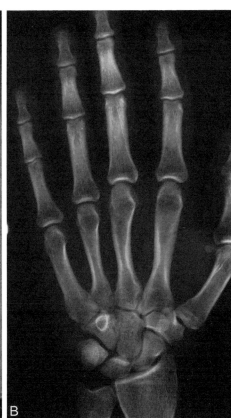

Figure 13–18. A, Patient positioned for PA view of the hand. The beam is centered perpendicular to the 3rd metacarpophalangeal joint (+). B, Normal radiograph of the hand. Note that the thumb is not entirely included on the film owing to "over-coning" from side to side.

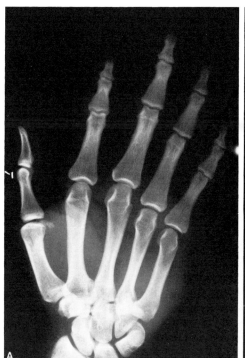

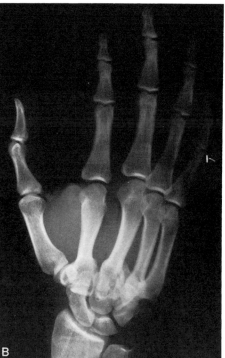

Figure 13–19. Radiographs of the right hand and wrist following trauma. The PA (A) and oblique views (B) demonstrate loss of the parallel configuration of the 2nd through 5th carpometacarpal joints due to dislocation. The lateral view (C) is essential in demonstrating the relationship of the articular surfaces (arrow).

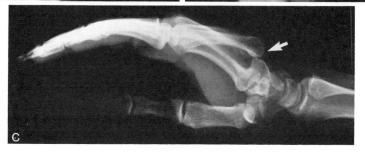

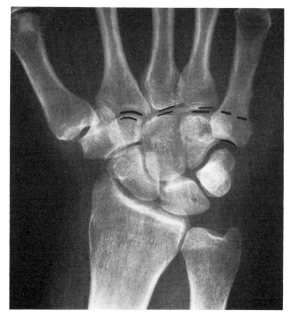

Figure 13–20. PA view of the hand. The carpometacarpal joints are parallel except in the case of the 5th. There is a dislocation of the 5th metacarpal.

Lateral View. The lateral view is obtained with the ulnar side of the hand adjacent to the cassette and the thumb and fingers extended (Fig. 13–22). The central beam is perpendicular to the cassette and centered on the metacarpophalangeal joints.

This view is useful in evaluating dislocations (Fig. 13–19B) and fracture-angulation.

Fingers

Overlapping of the metacarpals and phalanges is common on the lateral and oblique views. Obtaining views of the digit in question provides better detail. In this way subtle injuries are more easily detected.

Views of the individual fingers can be obtained with extremity cassettes or dental film (see Chapter 1, Routine Radiography). The finger being radiographed should be clearly marked on the film. The PA view is obtained with the finger flat on the cassette and the beam centered perpendicularly to the proximal interphalangeal joint (Fig. 13–23). The lateral view is essential in evaluating articular fractures (hyperextension volar plate fractures of the middle phalanx) and for determining the position and angulation of fractures.[24] This view is obtained with the ulnar side of the hand adjacent to the cassette and the finger separated by flexing the remaining digits (Figs. 13–23B and 13–24). This may require taping or props to assist in positioning. Centering is the same as in the PA view. The oblique view is obtained by rotating the hand as one would for the oblique view of the hand. The finger in question is isolated by flexing the remaining digits.

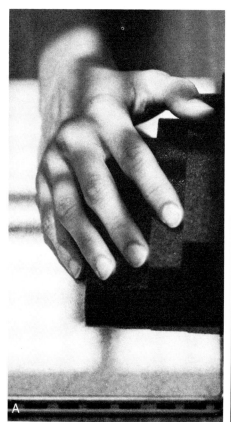
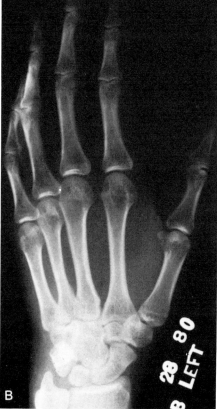
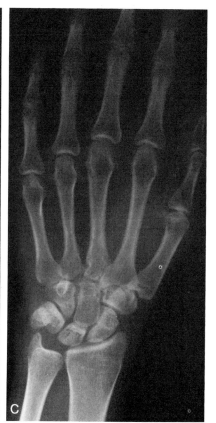

Figure 13–21. Hand positioned in the oblique view *(A).* Oblique radiograph *(B)* with PP view *(C)* for comparison. Note the overlap of the 3rd through 5th metacarpals and phalanges on the oblique view.

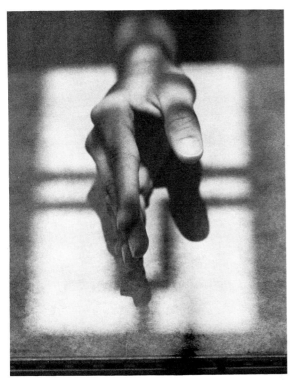

Figure 13–22. Hand positioned for the lateral view. The central beam is perpendicular to the cassette and centered on the metacarpophalangeal joints.

Thumb

The PA view of the thumb is obtained with the thumb elevated from the film and the ulnar side of the hand adjacent to the cassette (Fig. 13–25A). This results in some magnification. However, this position is much more easily maintained than the AP position, which requires that the hand be inverted with the dorsum of the thumb against the cassette.[23, 24] The central beam is perpendicular to the

Figure 13–23. A, Hand positioned for PA radiograph of the middle finger. The beam is centered on the proximal interphalangeal joint (+). The finger being examined is marked on the film with a lead number. B, Third finger positioned for lateral radiograph.

cassette and centered on the metacarpophalangeal joint.

The lateral view is obtained with the radial side of the thumb adjacent to the cassette and the fingers deviated to the ulnar side (Fig. 13–25B). The beam is centered on the metacarpophalangeal joint.

Figure 13–25C and D demonstrates the normal radiographic appearance of the thumb in the PA and lateral projections.

Special Views

Numerous additional views have been described.[23, 24] In our practice the Brewerton,[26, 37] Burman,[28] and stress views are commonly used.[13, 26, 33]

The Brewerton view is obtained by placing the dorsal aspect of the hand flat against the cassette (palm up) with the fingers flexed about 65° (Fig. 13–26A).[26] The beam is centered on the metacarpal heads, and the tube is angled 15° to the ulnar side of the wrist (Fig. 13–26B). The Brewerton view[26, 37] is useful in evaluating subtle arthritic abnormalities or fractures of the metacarpal heads.[26] The bases of the 4th and 5th metacarpals and hook of the hamate are also clearly demonstrated (Fig. 13–26C).

The Burman view improves visualization of the 1st carpometacarpal joint.[23, 28] The hand is hyperextended and rotated radially. The thumb is laid against the 8 × 10 inch cassette. The beam is angled 45° and centered on the base of the 1st metacarpal (Fig. 13–27A and B).

Stress views, especially of the 1st metacarpophalangeal joint, are frequently used to exclude ligament injury.[24, 25, 30] This study is more accurately performed fluoroscopically. Both thumbs should be in the PA position for comparison. Spot films are obtained in the neutral position and during radial and ulnar stress. Increase in the joint space on the stressed side (Fig. 13–28) or subluxation indicates ligament injury. Swelling and pain may reduce the

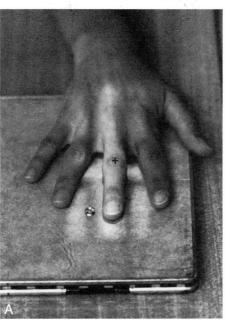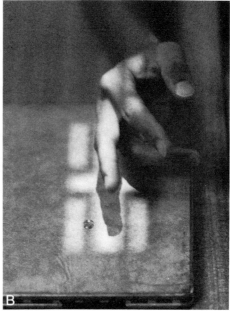

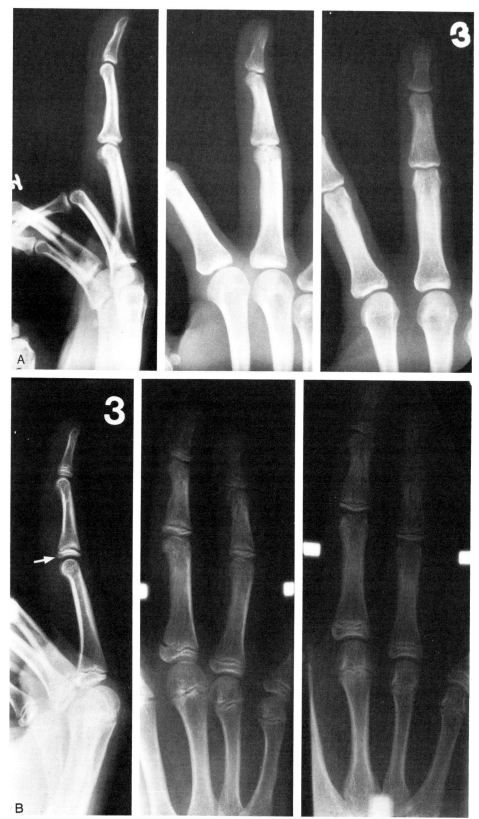

Figure 13–24. *A,* Normal PA, oblique, and lateral views of the middle finger. *B,* PA, lateral, and oblique views of the middle finger with a subtle volar plate fracture of the middle phalanx *(arrow).* The lateral view is most useful in evaluating hyperextension injuries.

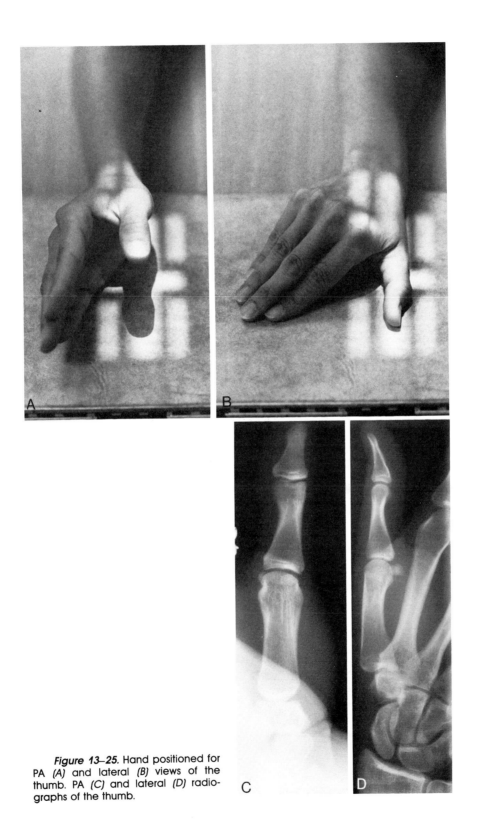

Figure 13–25. Hand positioned for PA *(A)* and lateral *(B)* views of the thumb. PA *(C)* and lateral *(D)* radiographs of the thumb.

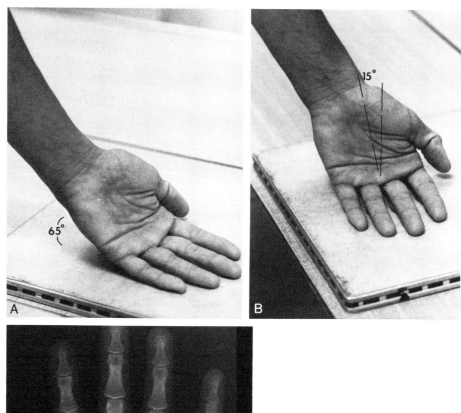

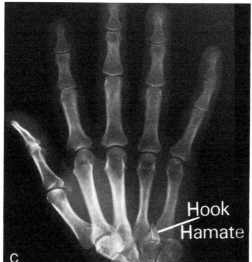

Figure 13–26. Brewerton view of the hand. *A*, The dorsum of the hand is against the cassette with the metacarpophalangeal joints flexed about 65°. *B*, The central beam is angled 15° to the ulnar side of the hand. *C*, Radiograph of the Brewerton view demonstrating the metacarpal heads, hook of the hamate, and 4th and 5th carpometacarpal joints.

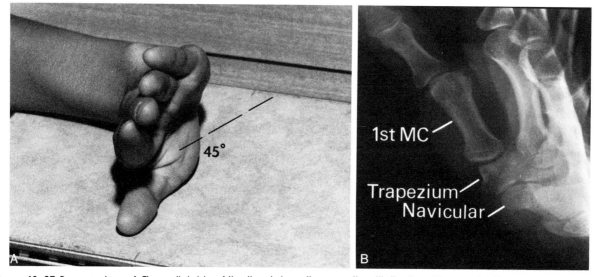

Figure 13–27. Burman views. *A*, The radial side of the thumb is on the cassette with the hand hyperextended. The beam is angled 45° and centered on the thenar eminence. *B*, The radiograph clearly demonstrates the articulations of the scaphoid (navicular), trapezium, and 1st metacarpal.

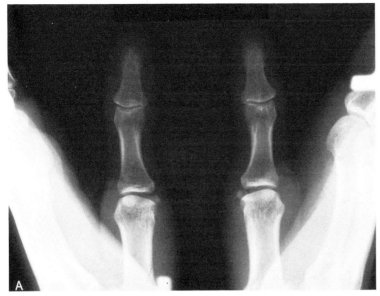

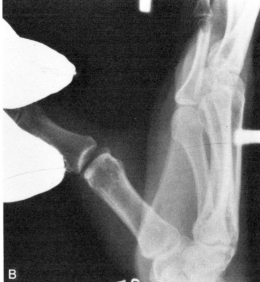

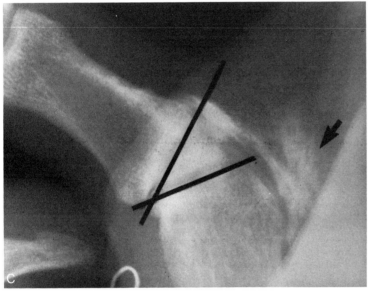

Figure 13–28. Stress views of the 1st metacarpophalangeal joint. *A,* PA views of both thumbs in neutral position. *B,* Radial stress demonstrates slight opening of the ulnar side of the joint. *C,* Arthrogram with anesthetic more clearly demonstrates the ulnar collateral ligament injury. Contrast material has extravasated through the ulnar ligament and into the capsular defect *(arrow).*

accuracy in the acute setting. Intra-articular injection of 1 percent lidocaine (Xylocaine) allows more accurate assessment. However, if this is needed, an arthrogram should be performed. The latter is more definitive (Fig. 13–28C). Use of local anesthetic results in an invasive procedure. Contrast material can be injected through the anesthetic needle. (See the following section, Arthrography of the Hand and Wrist.)

Wrist

PA, lateral, and oblique views are obtained following trauma.

PA View. Positioning for the PA view of the wrist is similar to that used for the PA view of the hand (Fig. 13–29; see Fig. 13–5) except that the beam is centered on the wrist instead of the metacarpophalangeal joints.

Careful examination of the PA view reveals sig-

nificant bony and soft tissue anatomy. If approached systematically, information regarding pathology and appropriate further views can easily be obtained.[24, 31, 32] Subtle fractures on the radial side of the wrist, especially the scaphoid, are easily overlooked. The navicular fat stripe is a useful structure in this regard. This fat plane lies between the radial collateral ligament and the tendon sheaths of the abductor pollicis longus and extensor pollicis brevis (Fig. 13–29). Though the fat plane is inconsistently seen in children, it is present in 96 percent of normal adults.[42] Terry and Ramin[42] noted absence or displacement of the fat stripe in 88 percent of fractures on the radial side of the wrist. These changes were noted in 87 percent of scaphoid fractures. Changes in the navicular fat stripe may be the only clue to a wrist fracture on the radial side (Fig. 13–29B).

The articular surfaces of the carpal bones should be parallel with 1 to 2 mm joint spaces.[2, 33, 34, 36] Any change in the joint space or shape of the carpal

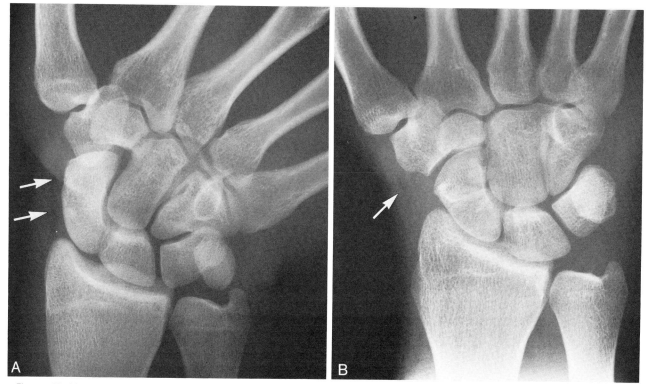

Figure 13–29. A, PA view of the wrist demonstrating the normal navicular fat stripe *(arrows)*. The hand is in slight ulnar deviation. Radial deviation may obliterate the fat stripe. B, Subtle scaphoid fracture with partial obliteration of the fat stripe *(arrow)*.

bones may indicate subluxation or dislocation. Three arcs can be drawn on the normal PA view (see Fig. 13–5). The first arc is formed by the proximal articular surfaces of the scaphoid, lunate, and triquetrum. The second arc is formed by the distal articular surfaces of these carpal bones. The third arc is formed by the proximal (convex) articular surfaces of the capitate and hamate. Any significant interruption of these arcs, other than where the trapezium, trapezoid, and pisiform are seen as overlapping structures on the PA view, suggests abnormality at the involved joint (Figs. 13–30 and 13–31). Flexion, extension, and radial and ulnar deviation result in significant changes in position and configuration (see treatment of motion views later in this chapter).

The distal radioulnar joint should also be clearly demonstrated on the PA view (see Fig. 13–5). This joint space normally measures about 2 mm.

Lateral View. Positioning for the lateral view is similar to that involved in the lateral view of the hand (see Fig. 13–22) except that the beam is centered on the wrist.

On the lateral view the normal pronator fat stripe (Fig. 13–32) can be seen passing proximally from the ventral surface of the radius. This normally lies within 1 cm of the cortical surface of the distal radius. Subtle radial fractures will cause displacement or obliteration of the fat plane (Fig. 13–33). This may be the only indication of fracture. Dorsal swelling is also best seen on the lateral view.

The relationship of the radius, lunate, capitate, and metacarpals is clearly demonstrated on the lateral view (see Figs. 13–7 and 13–32). The capitate

is firmly attached to the 3rd metacarpal. The convex proximal surface of the capitate articulates with the lunate, and the lunate articulates with the radius. A straight line can be drawn along the axis of the

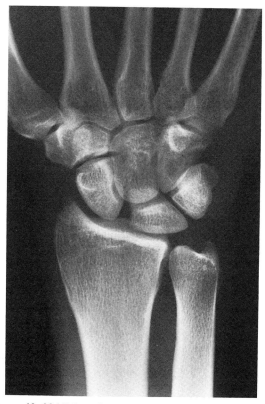

Figure 13–30. Widened scapholunate space due to ligament injury.

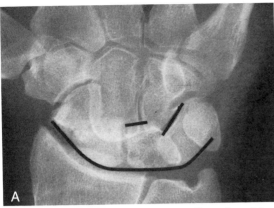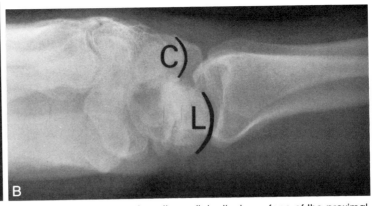

Figure 13–31. A, PA view of the wrist. Normally uninterrupted arcs can be drawn along the radial articular surface of the proximal carpal row and the articular surfaces of the midcarpal joints. On the true PA the radioulnar joint is well seen. Interruption of these arcs indicates abnormality at the level of the break in the arc. *B*, There is dorsal dislocation at the midcarpal joint, with the capitate (C) overriding the lunate (L).

radius, lunate, capitate, and 3rd metacarpal in the neutral position. However, slight flexion or extension will normally interrupt this line. The angle formed by the radius and scaphoid is normally about 136° (range 121° to 153°).[29] The scapholunate angle is normally about 45°.[2]

Oblique Views. For the external oblique view the position of the wrist should be similar to that used for the oblique view of the hand (see Fig. 13–21). The wrist is pronated approximately 45° from the PA position, and the beam is centered on the wrist. The radiograph (Fig. 13–34) demonstrates the scaphoid, trapezium, and 1st carpometacarpal articulation.[23, 24]

The internal oblique view is obtained by internally rotating the wrist 45°.[23, 24, 33] This view demonstrates the triquetropisiform articulation (Fig. 13–34). Normally this joint measures about 2 mm. If the wrist is flexed, the joint space may actually widen.

Subtle fractures of the radial and ulnar styloids are often only demonstrated on the oblique views.

Scaphoid View. The scaphoid is the most frequently fractured carpal bone. These fractures are often subtle. Therefore, a scaphoid view should be obtained initially if a fracture is suspected.

We routinely position the hand palm down on the cassette with the hand in ulnar deviation (Fig. 13–35). The thumb is extended and in line with the radius. The beam is centered on the scaphoid and is perpendicular to the cassette.[24] This clearly demonstrates the elongated scaphoid (Fig. 13–35*B* and *C*).

Variations of this technique have been described by Bridgman[27] and Stecher.[21]

Pisiform View. The pisiform view clearly demonstrates the pisiform and triquetropisiform articulation (Fig. 13–36). This technique is a variation of the external oblique view. The hand and wrist are rotated 30° externally from the lateral position.[24] The beam is centered on the ulnar side of the wrist and is perpendicular to the cassette.

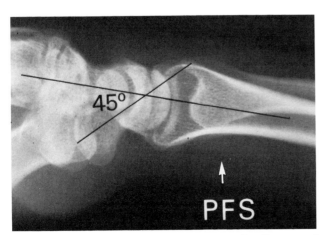

Figure 13–32. Lateral view of the wrist, showing the normal scapholunate angle (about 45°). The pronator fat stripe (PFS) is a useful indicator of distal radial fractures.

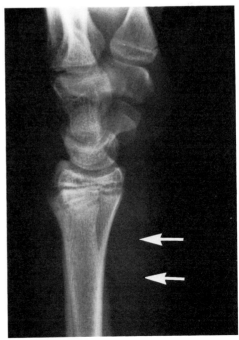

Figure 13–33. Subtle fracture of the distal radius. The displaced pronator fat stripe *(arrows)* was the only clue to the fracture.

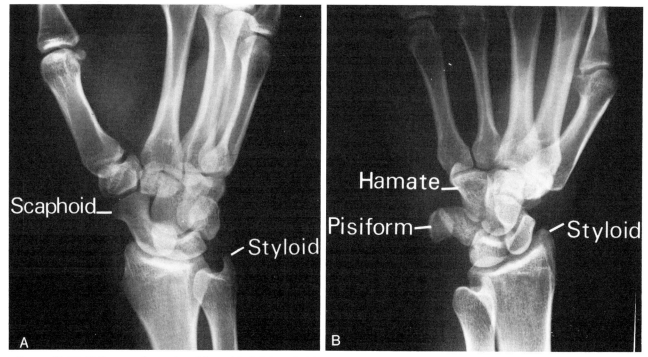

Figure 13–34. Oblique radiographs of the wrist. *A,* External oblique with the wrist externally rotated (pronated) 45°. The scaphoid, scaphotrapezial, and trapezoid–1st metacarpal articulations are well demonstrated. The 1st and 2nd carpometacarpal joints are also better demonstrated than on the PA view. *B,* The internal oblique (wrist rotated internally 45°) demonstrates the pisiform-triquetral articulation and the 4th and 5th carpometacarpal joints.

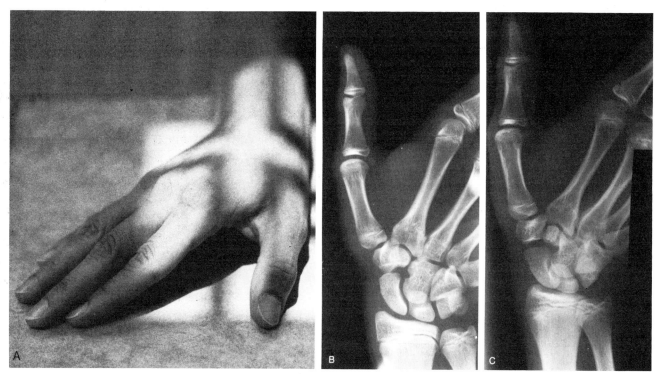

Figure 13–35. Scaphoid view. Hand positioned for scaphoid view of the wrist *(A).* Radiographs of the scaphoid in the PA *(B)* and slightly oblique *(C)* position. The scaphoid is clearly demonstrated and normal. There is a small chip fracture of the radial styloid with soft tissue swelling.

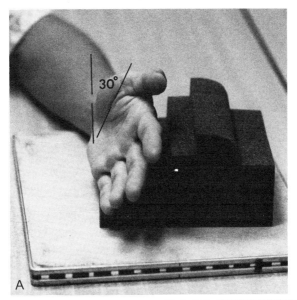

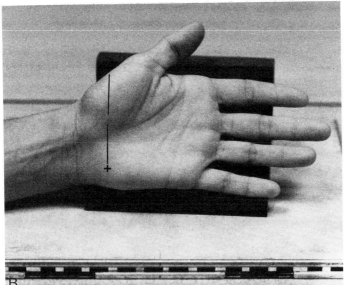

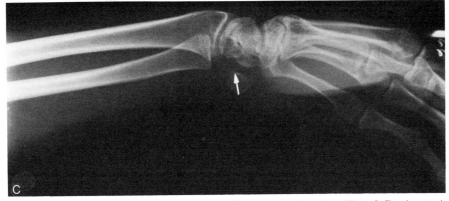

Figure 13–36. Pisiform view. *A,* The hand is externally rotated 30° from the lateral position. *B,* The beam is perpendicular and centered on the pisiform. *C,* Radiograph demonstrating an undisplaced fracture of the pisiform. The joint space is widened owing to hemorrhage and the slight flexion of the wrist.

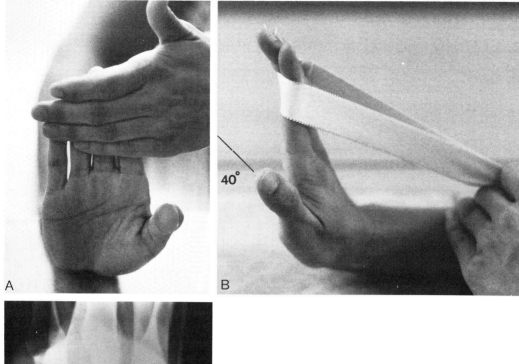

Figure 13–37. Carpal tunnel view. The hand is hyperextended and supported by the opposite hand *(A)* or a strap *(B)*. The tube is angled 40° off the horizontal table. The radiograph *(C)* demonstrates the carpal tunnel, hook of the hamate *(arrow)*, trapezium, pisiform, and 1st metacarpal base.

Carpal Tunnel View. Several methods have been described for obtaining this view. A simple technique involves hyperextending the hand with the base of the wrist against the cassette. The hand can be positioned using the opposite hand for support or by using a strap to maintain the hyperextended position. The tube is angled toward the wrist at 40° from the horizontal (tabletop) (Fig. 13–37*A* and *B*).[24, 35]

The radiograph (Fig. 13–37*C*) demonstrates the carpal tunnel and surrounding carpal structures. This is particularly useful in evaluating the hook of the hamate and soft tissue in the region of the carpal tunnel.[32]

Dorsal Tangential View. This projection was described by Lentino.[38] The dorsum of the hand is placed on the cassette, with the wrist maximally flexed (Fig. 13–38*A*). The central beam is angled 45° with the tabletop and centered 3 to 4 cm above the radiocarpal joint.

The radiograph (Fig. 13–38*B*) demonstrates the dorsal aspects of the proximal carpal row (scaphoid, lunate, and triquetrum). Definition of dorsal chip fractures, foreign bodies, and soft tissue calcifications is accomplished with this technique.[23]

Motion Studies. Bending views of the wrist are often obtained to evaluate subtle bony or ligamen-

tous injuries in patients with persistent pain. This series of radiographs includes the PA and lateral views. In addition, lateral views are obtained with maximal flexion and extension (Fig. 13–39), and PA views are obtained with radial and ulnar deviation (Fig. 13–40). Certain institutions also obtain lateral and AP clenched fist and oblique views.[34] In certain cases fluoroscopy with videotape or cineradiography may be helpful. These techniques allow review of the motion series for detection of more subtle abnormalities.[40]

The lateral dynamic views are obtained in the same manner as the views of the lateral wrist except that the wrist is flexed and extended. Dorsiflexion (hyperextension) and palmar flexion average 70° and 75°, respectively.[2]

With ulnar deviation (Fig. 13–40*B*) the scaphoid is elongated, and the lunate is more trapezoid in shape and articulates completely with the radius. During radial deviation (Fig. 13–40*D*) the lunate translates and only partially articulates with the radius. The scaphoid is foreshortened owing to palmar flexion. This provides a "ringlike" shadow distally that is similar to the ring sign seen with rotary subluxation. The scapholunate space (< 2 mm) does not change with radial and ulnar deviation unless ligament injury is present.

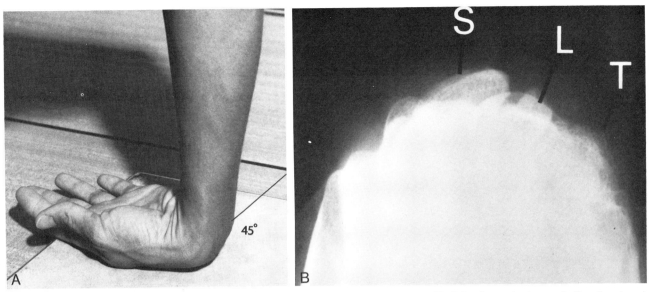

Figure 13–38. Dorsal tangential view. *A,* Hand positioned for dorsal tangential view (45°). *B,* Radiograph demonstrating the dorsal soft tissues and dorsal portions of the scaphoid (S), lunate (L), and triquetrum (T).

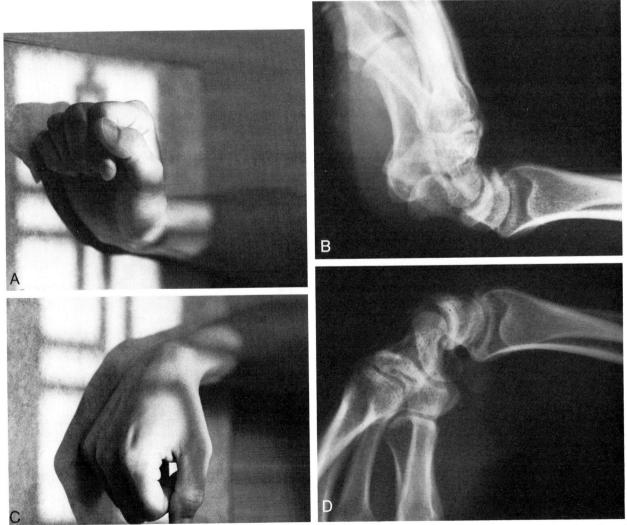

Figure 13–39. Lateral motion views of the wrist. *A,* Hand positioned for dorsiflexion lateral view with the beam centered on the wrist. *B,* Radiograph demonstrates the elongated scaphoid with slight dorsal rotation of the lunate. The degree of extension is normal (approximately 70°). *C,* Hand positioned for the palmar flexion lateral view. *D,* Radiograph on palmar flexion demonstrates normal flexion (approximately 75°). The scaphoid assumes a nearly vertical position.

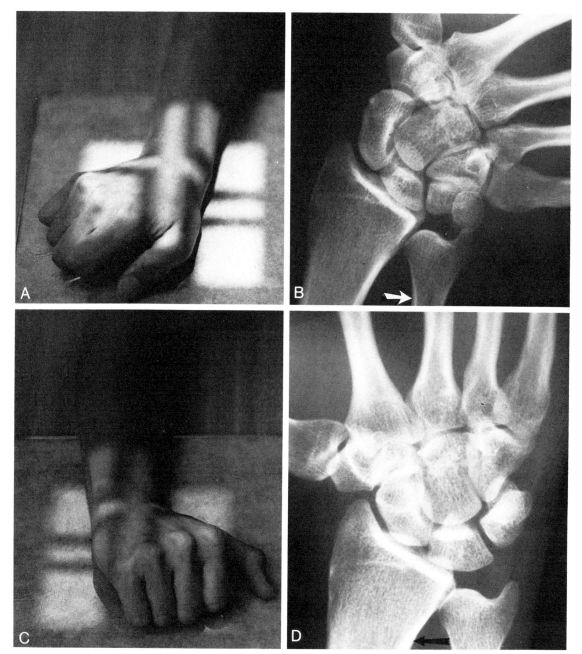

Figure 13–40. PA wrist view with radial and ulnar deviation. *A,* Hand with clenched fist and ulnar deviation. *B,* Radiograph showing ulnar deviation. The scaphoid is elongated. There is no increase in the joint space. *C,* Hand in radial deviation with clenched fist. *D,* Radiograph showing radial deviation. Normally the joint spaces do not increase. The lunate slides to the ulnar side of the radiocarpal joint and the scaphoid is rotated vertically, resulting in a foreshortened appearance.

The implications of this radiographic series will be discussed more fully in this chapter under carpal instability. The use of tomography and isotope studies in the hand and wrist will also be discussed later in this chapter.

ARTHROGRAPHY OF THE HAND AND WRIST

Wrist Arthrography

Wrist arthrography allows evaluation of the articular cartilage and synovium. The integrity of the ligaments, triangular cartilage, and joint compartments can also be assessed.

Arthrography is most commonly used to evaluate patients with post-traumatic wrist pain. Table 13–1 summarizes the indications for wrist arthrography.

Technique

The examination may be performed with the patient seated next to the fluoroscopic table or supine with the arm extended and the hand resting palm down. The latter method allows easier access

TABLE 13–1. Wrist Arthrography: Indications

Post-traumatic pain	Fracture union
Ligament injury	Periarticular masses
Triangular cartilage tears	Ganglia

to the patient and decreases the concern for syncopal attacks.

The dorsum of the wrist is prepared with a povidone-iodine (Betadine) preparation and sterile towels.

The radiocarpal joint is most frequently injected. The wrist is flexed over a cushion to open the dorsal radiocarpal joint (Fig. 13–41), and the injection site is checked by positioning the needle tip just distal to the radius and on the radial side of the scapholunate joint (Fig. 13–41). Care should also be taken not to inject the extensor tendon.[54] To assist in needle placement the dorsal joint space and distal radial tubercle are often easily palpated. A ½-inch 25-gauge needle is used to inject a small amount of 1 percent lidocaine (Xylocaine) in the skin. In most patients the same needle will easily reach the joint space and can be used to perform the procedure. If cultures are required or if the soft tissues are thicker, a 1½-inch 22-gauge needle may be required. Needle position and depth can be confirmed by gently rotating the wrist into the lateral position. The joint should be aspirated prior to the injection of contrast material. Cultures and synovial fluid analysis may be indicated. If infection is suspected and no fluid can be obtained, the joint should be flushed with nonbacteriostatic sterile saline and the aspirate sent for culture.[46] Injection of a small test dose of contrast material (meglumine diatrizoate) should demonstrate free flow away from the needle tip. When the proper position has been obtained, 1.5 to 3 ml of contrast material is injected. This should be performed slowly and observed fluoroscopically to confirm the site of any intercompartmental communication.[45]

Following the injection, the needle is removed, and the wrist is gently exercised under fluoroscopic guidance. Films are obtained in the PA, lateral, oblique, and bending (flexion, extension, radial and ulnar deviation) positions. In certain situations repeat films may be required after the initial films have been studied.

Double-contrast technique is rarely used in wrist arthrography. Occasionally trispiral tomography is used in conjunction with arthrography. In these cases epinephrine may be required (see Introduction to Arthrography in Chapter 1). Injection of the other compartments, particularly the distal radioulnar or intercarpal, may be necessary (Fig. 13–42). These compartments are easily entered fluoroscopically using a dorsal approach.

Normal Arthrographic Anatomy

The anatomy of the hand and wrist has been thoroughly discussed earlier in this chapter. The compartments of the wrist should be re-emphasized for proper arthrographic evaluation. These include

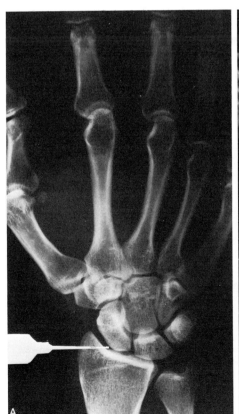 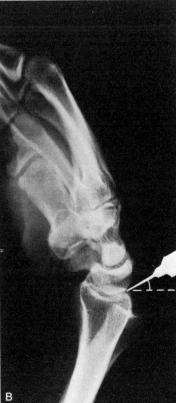

Figure 13–41. Radiograph simulating fluoroscopic appearance of needle positioning. *A*, The AP view demonstrates the proper needle position over the radiocarpal joint. The scapholunate space should be avoided. *B*, Lateral view with the wrist flexed. The needle tip should be angled proximally to ensure proper positioning in the radiocarpal joint.

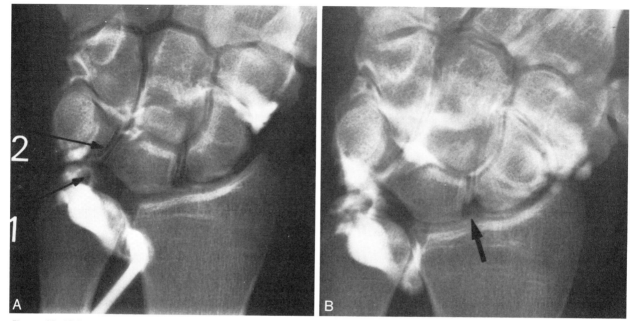

Figure 13–42. Patient with post-traumatic wrist pain and suspected abnormality of the radioulnar joint. *A,* With fluoroscopic guidance, the distal radioulnar joint was injected. Contrast left the radioulnar joint via a triangular cartilage tear (1) and entered the intercarpal joint via a defect in the lunotriquetral ligament (2). *B,* Scapholunate dissociation was also present (*arrow* marks widened joint). The complexity of the injury would not have been appreciated if the injection were not observed fluoroscopically.

the radiocarpal joint, distal radioulnar joint, intercarpal joint, carpometacarpal joints, 1st carpometacarpal joint, and pisotriquetral joint (Fig. 13–43).[46, 47, 50, 56]

Communications between the compartments of the wrist have been noted by numerous authors in normal patients (Table 13–2). The most common

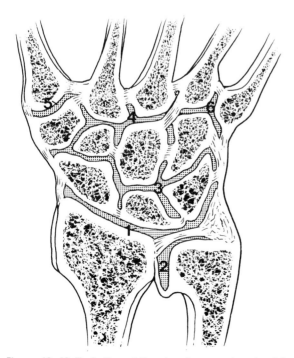

Figure 13–43. Illustration of the dorsal compartments of the wrist: 1, radiocarpal; 2, distal radioulnar; 3, intercarpal; 4, common carpometacarpal; 5, 1st carpometacarpal; and 6, outer carpometacarpal. The pisotriquetral articulation is located on the volar aspect of the wrist.

TABLE 13–2. Intercompartmental Communications of the Wrist

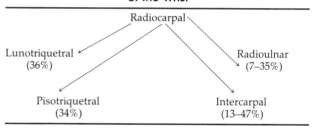

problem is differentiating communication between the radiocarpal and intercarpal compartments from a ligament tear in asymptomatic patients. Trentham and colleagues reported communication of the radiocarpal with the intercarpal and distal radioulnar joints in 20.5 percent of asymptomatic patients.[56]

Injection of the radiocarpal joint will normally demonstrate no communication with the intercarpal or distal radioulnar joint (see Figs. 13–42, 13–45, and 13–47). Communication with the pisotriquetral joint is commonly noted. Lewis[50] reported radiocarpal-pisotriquetral communication in 34 percent of the cadavers studied. Intracompartmental communications must be correlated with the clinical findings in each patient. Normal recesses are present in the prestyloid region and are volar to the distal radius (Fig. 13–44). The synovial lining is smooth. There is no communication with the tendon sheaths in the normal wrist. The triangular fibrocartilage is attached to the distal radius and ulnar styloid.[46, 50]

Abnormal Arthrogram

Trauma. As noted in Table 13–1, arthrography is most commonly performed to evaluate patients

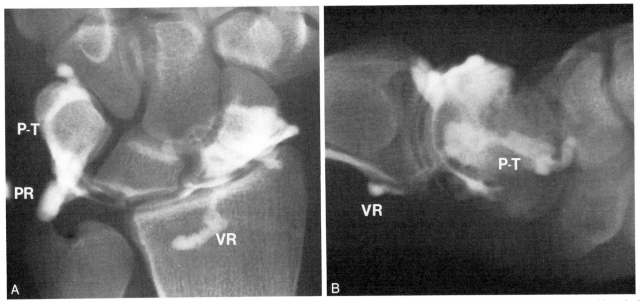

Figure 13–44. Normal wrist arthrogram. PA *(A)* and lateral *(B)* views demonstrate contrast in the radiocarpal joint. The pisotriquetral joint communication (P-T) is of no clinical significance. Normal recesses include the pre-styloid (PR) and volar radial recesses (VR).

with post-traumatic wrist pain or instability. In assessment of ligament injuries the arthrogram must be correlated with clinical findings, including the age of the patient. Patients with ligamentous disruption will demonstate communication between the compartments of the wrist. Most commonly the scapholunate ligament is involved. This results in communication between the radiocarpal and midcarpal joints. To be significant, point tenderness or other local symptoms should correlate with the area of abnormality on the arthrogram. The bones may also be malaligned. This may present with widening

or loss of the parallelism of the joint space (Fig. 13–45). In addition, a decrease in the radioscaphoid angle or the ring sign may be present (Fig. 13–46).[47] The latter is due to the vertical position of the scaphoid. In longstanding cases secondary degenerative changes are common, but these may require tomography for identification.

In patients with tears in the triangular cartilage, communication between the radiocarpal and distal radioulnar joints will be observed (Fig. 13–47). Tears

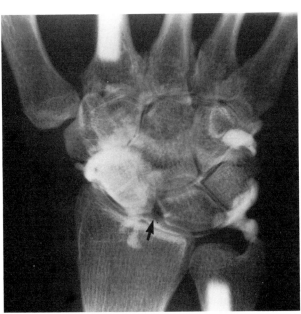

Figure 13–45. Scapholunate ligament disruption. There is communication between the radiocarpal and intercarpal compartments. Note the triangular configuration of the scapholunate space *(arrow).*

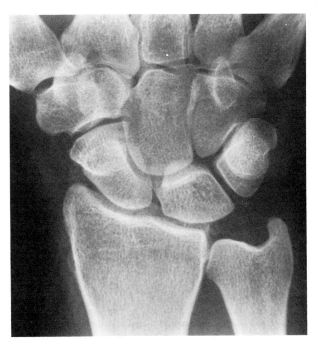

Figure 13–46. Chronic scapholunate ligament instability. PA view of the wrist demonstrates slight widening and a triangular configuration to the scapholunate joint. (The scaphoid is foreshortened with the ring sign.) Note that chondrocalcinosis is also present.

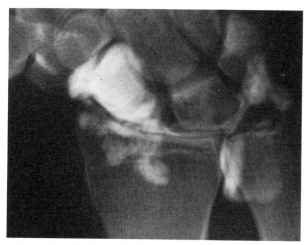

Figure 13–47. Wrist with chronic ulnar pain. Arthrogram (PA view) with injection of the radiocarpal joint demonstrates communication with the distal radioulnar joint, indicating a triangular cartilage tear.

in the triquetrolunate ligament may be associated with triangular cartilage tears (Fig. 13–42).

Occasionally local synovial irregularity or tendon communication may be evident.[54] Levinsohn and Palmer[49] noted triangular cartilage tears in 26 percent, radiocarpal-intercarpal communication in 30 percent, capsular lesions in 31 percent, lymphatic filling in 12 percent, and tendon sheath communication in 10 percent of patients with chronic post-traumatic pain.

Arthrography has also been used to differentiate fibrous union and true non-union of scaphoid fractures.[46]

Ganglia. Identification of periarticular ganglia may be difficult arthrographically. Frequently more contrast material (5 ml+) and repeat exercise are necessary. Communication is more frequent with the intercarpal than with the radiocarpal joint. Therefore, the intercarpal joint should be injected when a ganglion is suspected. If injection of the wrist fails to demonstrate the mass, a direct injection of the ganglion may be useful.

Andrén and Eiken[43] studied 59 patients and were successful in demonstrating 85 percent of volar and 44 per cent of dorsal ganglia arthrographically. The duct of the ganglion is often tortuous, causing a valvelike effect. This allows filling to occur more readily from the joint than by directly injecting the ganglion.

Arthritis. Arthrography may be useful in evaluation of early arthritic conditions, especially rheumatoid arthritis.[45, 46, 51, 52, 56] Arthritic changes are nonspecific. The most common finding is intercompartmental communication. Resnick[52] noted this finding in 92 percent of patients with a similar incidence of synovitis. Lymphatic filling may be evident in 32 to 42 percent of cases.[46, 52] Communication with tendon sheaths may occur in up to 25 percent of patients.[52]

Though the arthrographic findings may not be completely successful in differentiating the type of arthritis, synovial fluid analysis may be useful. This is especially true if infection is present.

Careful correlation of arthrographic findings with the clinical symptoms, proper injection technique, and fluoroscopic control of injection and exercise result in highly accurate, informative wrist arthrograms.

Arthrography of the Hand

Arthrograms of the hand are most commonly performed to evaluate ligament injury, instability, and cartilage abnormalities.[55] The technique is most often used to evaluate the 1st metacarpophalangeal joint of the thumb. Injury to the capsule and ulnar collateral ligament is common. This injury, formerly associated with gamekeepers, is commonly caused by skiing or other sporting injuries. The patient falls with the arm extended and the thumb forced into radial deviation. Subluxation or dislocation, resulting in weakness and decreased pinch strength, may occur.[25, 44] Bowers and Hurst[25] described associated chip fractures of the distal metacarpal in 55 of 109 cases.

Examination of the 2nd through 5th metacarpophalangeal joints and the proximal interphalangeal joints may also be required. Arthrography is equally effective, though less commonly requested, in evaluation of these articulations.

Technique

The examination is performed with the patient prone to avoid syncopal attack.[55] The joint is prepared using sterile technique. A ½-inch 25-gauge needle is used for the injection of local anesthetic and the contrast material. The injection site should be dorsal and contralateral to the side of suspected injury. Most commonly single-contrast technique is used. One to 1.5 ml of meglumine diatrizoate is injected. If ligament injury is not the primary concern, different techniques may be required. Study of the articular cartilage may be facilitated by double-contrast technique (0.1 to 0.3 ml of contrast material with 1 ml of air). Occasionally trispiral tomography or magnification technique may be useful.[55] Epinephrine is not used in the small joints because of the risk of vasospasm.[55]

The injection and post-injection filming should be fluoroscopically monitored. Films are taken in PA and lateral projections and with ulnar and radial stress. Hyperextended lateral views are obtained if hyperextension injury is suspected.

Normal Arthrographic Anatomy

The capsule of the metacarpophalangeal joint is straight to slightly concave laterally owing to the radial and ulnar collateral ligaments (Fig. 13–48). Proximally the capsule extends to a position near

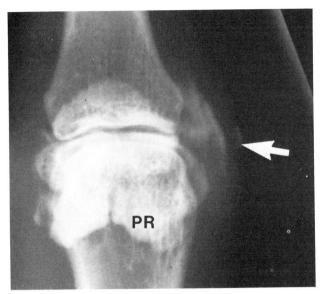

Figure 13–48. PA view of normal anatomy of the 1st meta-carpophalangeal joint. There is no extracapsular contrast on the ulnar side of the joint. The palmar recess (PR) extends more proximally. The distal aspect of the capsule is small. Slight extravasation at the injection site *(arrow)* should not be con-fused with a capsular tear.

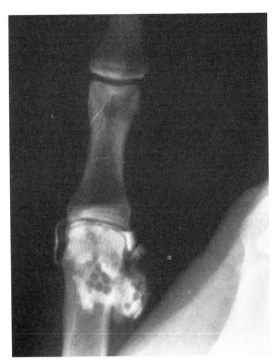

Figure 13–50. Ulnar capsular tear in right tumb. There is extravasation of contrast medium from the ulnar side of the capsule.

the metacarpal metaphysis, resulting in dorsal and palmar recesses (Fig. 13–49). A triangular plate extends into the palmar aspect of the joint (Fig. 13–50).[25, 44, 55]

Abnormal Arthrograms

Arthrograms are most accurate in the acute post-traumatic period. Extravasation of contrast material

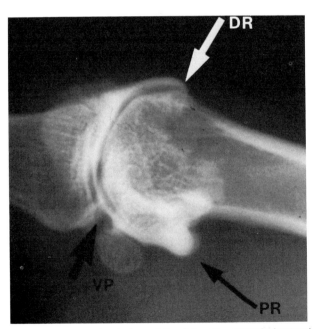

Figure 13–49. Lateral view of the 1st metacarpophalangeal joint. The palmar (PR) and dorsal (DR) recesses extend to the metaphysis. The volar plate (VP) projects into the margin of the palmar articular surface.

from the ulnar aspect of the capsule indicates cap-sular disruption with or without associated involve-ment of the ulnar collateral ligament (Fig. 13–50). If contrast material extends along the plane of the adductor pollicis muscle, a tear of the ulnar collat-eral ligament with involvement of the volar plate is more likely (Fig. 13–51).[25, 44]

In patients with chronic instability or old capsular tears, the arthrogram will demonstrate irregularity but extravasation may not occur. Chronic tears may fill in with fibrous tissue.

Examination of the interphalangeal joints is per-formed as easily and as accurately as in the case of the metacarpophalangeal joints. Ligament and cap-sule tears result in extravasation of contrast mate-rial. Associated periarticular fractures may occur.

Tenography of the hand and wrist is rarely indi-cated following trauma. Resnick[53, 54] has described this technique in evaluation of patients with rheu-matoid arthritis.

FRACTURES AND DISLOCATIONS

Distal Radius Fractures

Fractures of the distal radius likely account for the lion's share of significant trauma about the wrist. It is also the wrist bone that most frequently requires manipulative reduction and hence careful sequential radiographic monitoring. Most fractures of the distal radius fall into one of five eponymic categories.

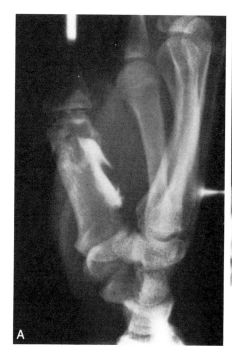

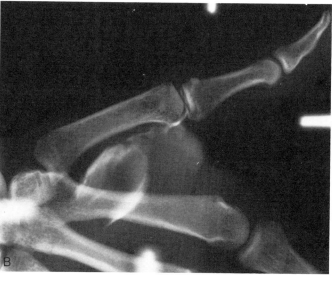

Figure 13–51. Ulnar collateral ligament tear involving the volar aspect of the capsule. PA *(A)* and lateral *(B)* views demonstrate extravasation with extension along the muscle planes of the thenar eminence.

Colles' Fracture Type

The Colles' fracture, first described by Abraham Colles in 1813 prior to the discovery of the x-ray, is undoubtedly the most common fracture of the distal radius.[2] This term is so well known that frequently, but incorrectly, it is applied to all bony injuries of the radius. The term Colles' fracture, however, should be restricted to those fractures of the distal radial metaphysis or epiphysis, with or without intra-articular involvement, that are either displaced and angulated or have the tendency to displace or angulate in the dorsal direction (Fig. 13–52).[2, 3] Most commonly, there is dorsal cortical comminution,

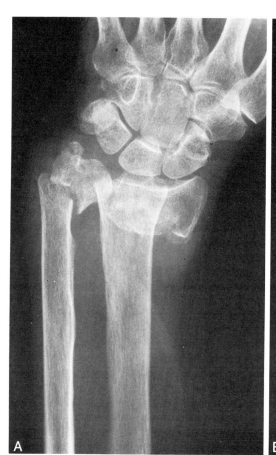

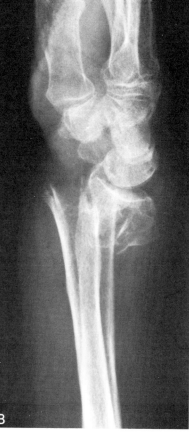

Figure 13–52. PA *(A)* and lateral *(B)* views of fractures of the distal radial and ulnar metaphysis with dorsal and radial displacement of the distal fragments.

THE HAND AND WRIST • 669

TABLE 13–3. Frykman Classification of Colles' Fracture[91]
(see Fig. 13–53)

Type	Fracture Location	Distal Ulnar Fracture
I	Extra-articular	Absent
II	Extra-articular	Present
III	Intra-articular involving radiocarpal joint	Absent
IV	Intra-articular involving radiocarpal joint	Present
V	Intra-articular involving distal radioulnar joint	Absent
VI	Intra-articular involving distal radioulnar joint	Present
VII	Intra-articular involving both radiocarpal and distal radioulnar joints	Absent
VIII	Intra-articular involving both radiocarpal and distal radioulnar joints	Present

but this is not a necessary feature of the fracture. There may or may not be an associated fracture of the ulnar styloid. There should be no demonstrable radiocarpal subluxation.

Radiographic evaluation can usually be adequately completed for this fracture with simple PA and lateral planar films. Interpretation, both pre- and post-reduction, should note the following characteristics of the fracture: (1) direction of displacement or angulation, if present (which, by definition, should be dorsal); (2) degree of comminution; (3) presence or absence of intra-articular involvement of the radiocarpal or distal radioulnar joint; (4) degree of apparent loss of radial length (or apparent positive ulnar variance); and (5) degree of loss of the ulnar inclination of the radial articular surface (normally 14°) on the PA projection and loss of the volar tilt of the articular surface (normally 12°)[2] on the lateral projection (see Fig. 13–1).

Classification. A classification of Colles' fractures may be quite adequately accomplished by a comprehensive description of its characteristics. This should include details, for example, regarding displacement, angulation, comminution, and presence or absence of intra-articular involvement. However, a numerical classification described by Frykman[91]

appears to be gaining widespread acceptance. This schema is based on the presence of intra-articular involvement of either the radiocarpal or distal radioulnar joint and the presence or absence of an associated ulnar fracture (Table 13–3) (Figs. 13–53 through 13–57). In addition to an anatomic classification as determined by radiographs, Colles' fractures may also be clinically classified as stable or unstable.[74] This grouping may be made by the surgeon at the time of reduction by the "feel" of the fracture or by demonstrated loss of position in the post-reduction period. Whether the fracture is stable or not will dictate the type of treatment and the degree of vigilance in monitoring the progress of healing. In general, those fractures with marked displacement, comminution, and intra-articular fracture lines will tend to be more unstable.

Mechanism of Injury. The mechanism of injury of the Colles' fracture is most usually a fall onto the outstretched hand. In an elderly patient with considerable osteoporosis, this may represent a relatively trivial trauma. However, in a younger patient a moderately violent force may be necessary to produce this fracture. In the latter instance, therefore, considerably more accompanying soft tissue injury can be anticipated, which may have implications in terms of the treatment options.

Treatment. The goal of treatment with the Colles'-type fracture is bony union in as close to an anatomic position as is possible and reasonable. Therefore, the minimally acceptable position will vary with the patient's age, other injuries, and other factors. In general, maintenance of radial length (neutral ulnar variance) (Fig. 13–57), 0° to 10° of palmar tilt of the articular surface (lateral projection) (Fig. 13–58), 14° of ulnar inclination of the articular surface (PA projection), and articular congruity are the criteria for evaluating adequacy of reduction. The stable fracture (nondisplaced, minimally displaced, or reduced with maintenance of position) is managed by cast immobilization. We generally prefer a position of forearm pronation and slight palmar flexion with ulnar deviation of the wrist for the

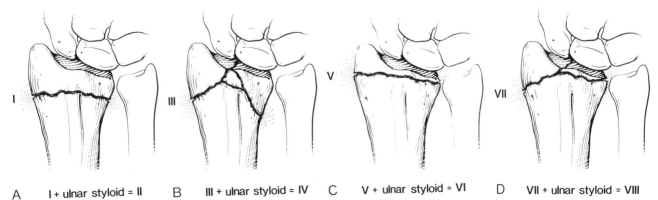

A   I + ulnar styloid = II   B   III + ulnar styloid = IV   C   V + ulnar styloid = VI   D   VII + ulnar styloid = VIII

Figure 13–53. Illustration of the Frykman classification. *A*, Type I: Fracture of the distal radius without articular involvement. If the ulnar styloid is also fractured, a Type II fracture results. *B*, Type III: Fracture involves the radiocarpal joint. If the ulnar styloid is also fractured, a Type IV fracture results. *C*, Type V: Fracture involves the distal radioulnar joint. If the ulnar styloid is also fractured, a Type VI fracture results. *D*, Type VIII: Fractures involving both the radiocarpal and distal radioulnar joint. If the ulnar styloid is also fractured, a Type VIII fracture results.

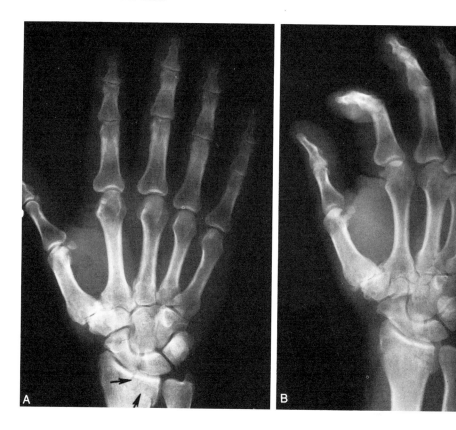

Figure 13–54. Frykman III fracture of the right wrist. AP *(A)* and oblique *(B)* views demonstrate a radial fracture *(A, arrows)* entering the radiocarpal joint. The ulnar styloid is not involved.

Figure 13–55. Frykman V fracture. Lateral *(A)* and PA *(B)* views of a distal radial fracture that enters the distal radioulnar joint. The ulnar styloid is not fractured.

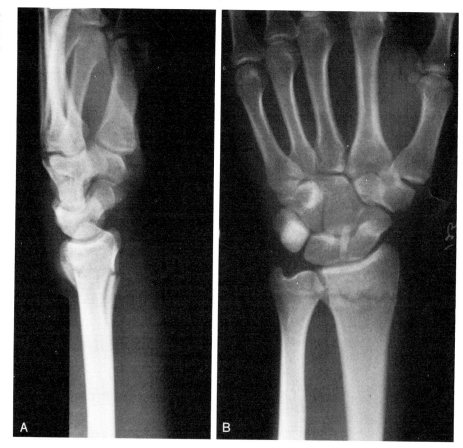

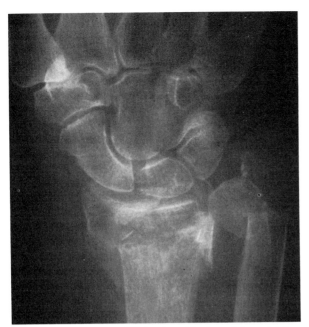

Figure 13–56. Frykman VIII fracture. PA view of the wrist shows a comminuted fracture of the distal radius involving the radio-carpal and distal radioulnar joints as well as an associated ulnar fracture.

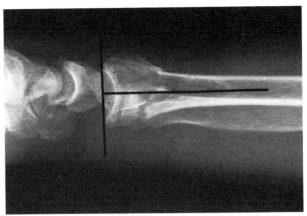

Figure 13–58. Lateral view of the wrist following reduction of a Colles' fracture. The distal radial articular surface is vertical (0°).

first 3 weeks. Thereafter a short-arm cast with the wrist in neutral position is used for an additional 3 weeks. Reduction, when necessary, is most easily achieved by longitudinal traction for approximately 10 minutes using finger traps and 8 to 10 lb of counterweight (Fig. 13–59). A gentle attempt at

manipulation involving a maneuver that extends the wrist, palmarly translates the distal fracture fragment, and palmarly flexes the wrist may be necessary. Close post-reduction monitoring by weekly serial PA and lateral x-rays for the first 3 weeks is advisable unless the fracture is initially nondisplaced and stable. The unstable fracture can be managed by reduction and cast immobilization but only with some uncertainty owing to the possibility of a loss of reduction in the first 2 weeks following the injury.

For this reason, we generally favor a more aggressive approach to management with this injury. Reduction is generally not difficult to achieve by

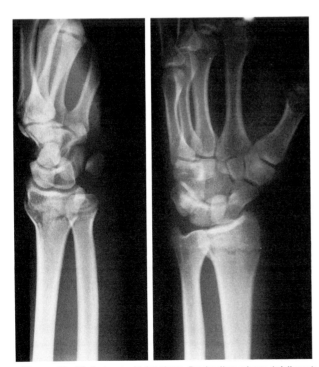

Figure 13–57. Frykman V fracture. Reduction views (oblique) show fracture of the distal radius with no loss of radial length and neutral ulnar variance.

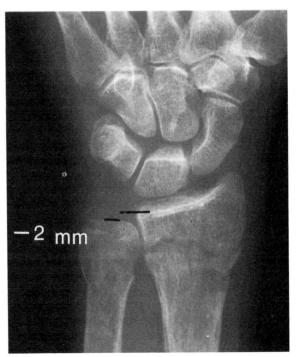

Figure 13–59. Reduced Colles' fracture in traction. Note 2-mm negative ulnar variance. The widened carpal joint spaces result from traction.

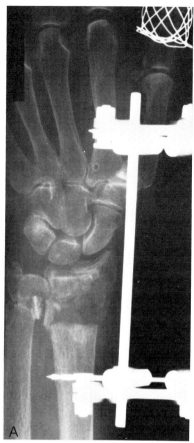

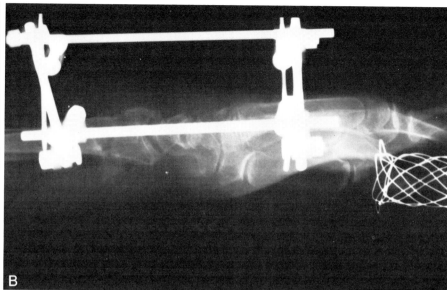

Figure 13–60. Post-reduction views of Frykman VIII fracture with finger traction and external fixation. (Same patient as in Fig. 13–55.) *A,* AP view shows no radial shortening with slight negative ulnar variance. *B,* Lateral view shows 0° distal radial angle.

the same method described above. Once reduced, the unstable Colles' variant may be secured by either percutaneous Kirschner wires across the fracture site or by exoskeletal fixation (Fig. 13–60). The latter may be carried out using a variety of available appliances. Four-pin fixation (two proximally in the radius and two distally in the base of the 2nd metacarpal, or one each in the base of the 2nd and 3rd metacarpals) is recommended.[71, 74] If exoskeletal means are used, the device should be maintained for at least 8 weeks before removal. Occasionally soft tissue interposition, volar cortical comminution,

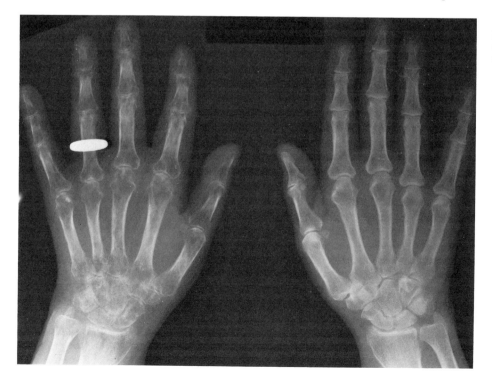

Figure 13–61. PA views of both hands and wrist. Classic Sudeck's atrophy on the left with marked osteoporosis.

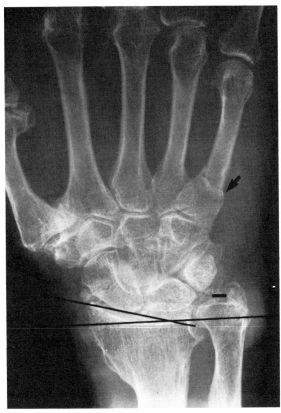

Figure 13–62. Old Colles' fracture of the right wrist with loss of radial length and reduced ulnar tilt. Note the fracture of the 5th metacarpal *(arrow)*.

or a depressed articular surface bone fragment may prevent closed reduction. In such cases, open reduction may be necessary. As the fracture heals, bone union or the presence of callus formation may be difficult to assess. Often the most reliable indicator of bony union will be maintenance of fracture position and absence of pain and tenderness.

Complications. Complications following a Colles' fracture are relatively frequent, with a reported rate of 35 percent.[72] The major problems relate to limited finger motion as a result of post-traumatic autonomic dysfunction syndrome (sympathetic dystrophy), median nerve compression, residual wrist pain and deformity, and wrist or forearm limitations in range of motion.[2] The first condition is often radiographically apparent by extreme bony rarefaction distal to the wrist (Fig. 13–61). The latter complications correlate fairly well with the adequacy of reduction (Figs. 13–62 and 13–63). Nonunion of the Colles' fracture is extremely rare.

Smith Fracture Type

The Smith fracture was described by Robert Smith, a Dublin contemporary of Colles, in 1847.[127] This injury was described without the aid of x-rays as "a fracture of the lower end of the radius with displacement of the lower fragment along with the carpus forewards and the head of the ulna backwards...." Most authors agree that this description

refers essentially to a "reverse Colles' fracture." Therefore, the term Smith fracture should be restricted to those fractures of the distal radial metaphysis or epiphysis, with or without articular involvement, that are displaced or angulated in the palmar direction (Fig. 13–64). There may or may not be an associated fracture of the ulnar styloid. There should be no radiocarpal subluxation. In the orthopedic literature there is, however, some confusion regarding the Smith fracture. Thomas has somewhat popularized a categorization of all palmarly displaced or angulated fractures of the distal radius, including the volar Barton-type fracture (to be discussed), as Smith-fracture variants.[145] We believe, however, that this classification groups together heterogeneous injuries. We recommend limiting usage of the term Smith fracture to the fracture described earlier. Adequate radiographic evaluation generally requires only PA and lateral planar films. Interpretation of the x-rays should note the same general characteristics as described for the Colles' fracture.

Classification. In general, the Smith fracture can be adequately classified as extra-, juxta-, or intra-articular, with or without displacement or comminution. The Thomas classification of the Smith fracture is perhaps too inclusive but is in moderately widespread use.[145] In this classification Type I is the classic Smith fracture through the distal radial metaphysis and is wholly extra-articular. Type II is a typical volar Barton-type fracture (to be discussed), and Type III is an oblique juxta-articular fracture with a greater degree of instability than that of Type I (Fig. 13–65).

Mechanism of Injury. The mechanism of injury as originally suggested by Smith was hyperflexion from a fall on the palmar flexed wrist. Others suggest that a blow to the dorsum of the wrist and hand or a hypersupination-type injury with a fall onto the extended wrist may reproduce this fracture type.[2]

Treatment. The goals of treatment and the criteria for an acceptable reduction are basically identical to those outlined for the Colles' fracture. Reduction is

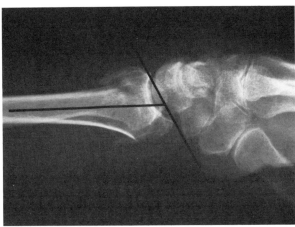

Figure 13–63. Lateral view of Colles' fracture deformity with dorsal tilt of the distal radius.

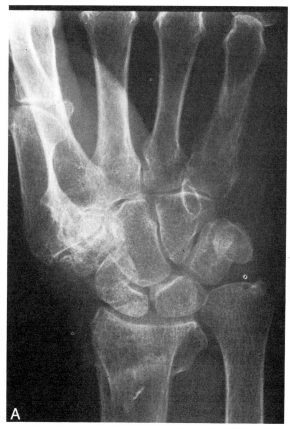

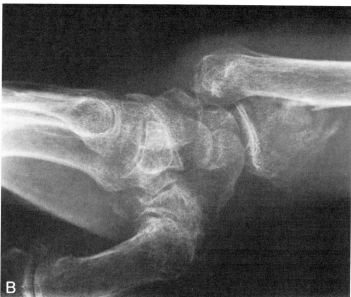

Figure 13–64. Juxta-articular fracture (Thomas Type III): Smith's fracture. PA *(A)* and lateral *(B)* radiographs demonstrate marked volar displacement of the distal radial fragment with considerable radial shortening and almost no ulnar tilt.

usually achieved by simple longitudinal traction, as discussed in the previous section. If a gentle manipulative reduction is also required, it is generally accomplished in a manner opposite to that of the Colles' fracture, i.e., hyperflexion followed by extension and dorsal translation of the wrist. Most often the typical extra-articular variety (Type I in

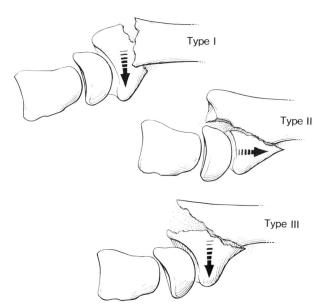

Figure 13–65. Thomas classification of Smith's fractures. Type I, extra-articular; Type II, volar intra-articular fracture; Type III, oblique juxta-articular fracture.

Thomas's classification) (Fig. 13–65) is stable following reduction and can be maintained in a long-arm cast that immobilizes the forearm in a position of supination with the wrist neutral. This position should be maintained for a period of 3 to 4 weeks followed by a short-arm cast with the wrist neutral for an additional 3 weeks. As with the Colles' fracture, serial x-rays to ensure maintenance of reduction in the cast for the first 3 weeks following injury are advised. Smith fractures with greater degrees of comminution or with obliquely directed juxta-articular fracture lines (Thomas Type III) may be unstable (Fig. 13–65). Such fractures may be candidates for percutaneous fixation or exoskeletal fixation, as previously described. Rarely is open reduction and internal fixation indicated.

Complications. The complications of the Smith fracture are virtually identical to those of the Colles' fracture. Residual subluxation of the distal radioulnar joint with pain or impaired grip strength is not uncommon.

Barton's Fracture Type

The Barton fracture is credited to John Rhea Barton, a Philadelphia surgeon who described this injury in 1838.[126] This term implies, in Barton's own words, "a subluxation of the wrist, consequent to a fracture through the articular surface of the carpal extremity of the radius." Therefore, by definition, this injury represents a marginal rim fracture of the radius that displaces along with the carpus, in this

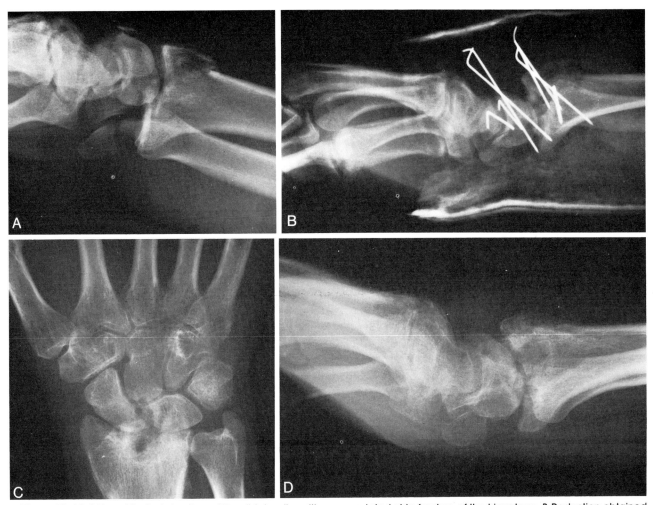

Figure 13–66. A, Dorsal Barton's fracture of the distal radius with an associated chip fracture of the triquetrum. B, Reduction obtained with K-wires. C, and D, PA and lateral views demonstrate advanced degenerative changes in the radiocarpal joint after healing.

way producing a fracture-subluxation (Fig. 13–66).[81] The latter feature, therefore, distinguishes this fracture from an intra-articular Colles' or Smith fracture. In his original description, Barton described the injury involving the dorsal or palmar lip of the radius. He believed the former to be more common. However, the palmar variety of this fracture is, in fact, more commonly seen. Furthermore, this variety is indeed the injury described by Thomas as a Type II Smith fracture (see Fig. 13–65). Considerable confusion is present in the literature regarding the terminology of Barton and reverse Barton fractures. The terms have been applied depending on whether the dorsal or palmar lip of the radius is fractured.[126, 146] We suggest that a distinction in terminology between palmar and dorsal Barton-type fractures will obviate any confusion in this regard.

Adequate radiographic evaluation generally requires only PA and lateral radiographs. It may be particularly important to obtain a high-quality true-lateral projection to appreciate the degree of carpal subluxation accompanying the fracture fragment. At times, particularly in assessing the adequacy of

reduction, lateral trispiral tomograms may be helpful to evaluate the articular congruity of the distal radius.

Classification. Adequate classification of the Barton fracture simply notes the location of the marginal fracture as palmar or dorsal, with or without comminution. By definition, the fracture is always intra-articular, exhibits some displacement, and is accompanied by a subluxation of the carpus.

Mechanism of Injury. The palmar Barton-type fracture (Fig. 13–67) probably occurs by a mechanism similar to that described for Smith-type injuries with perhaps an exaggerated degree of loading in compression across the wrist. The dorsal variety most often results from a fall that produces wrist extension and forearm pronation under compressive loading.

Treatment. Reduction by simple longitudinal traction as described earlier usually is readily achieved. Occasionally impaction of the fracture fragments may prevent adequate closed reduction. The major difficulty with this injury, however, is maintenance of a perfect reduction. Cast treatment may be suc-

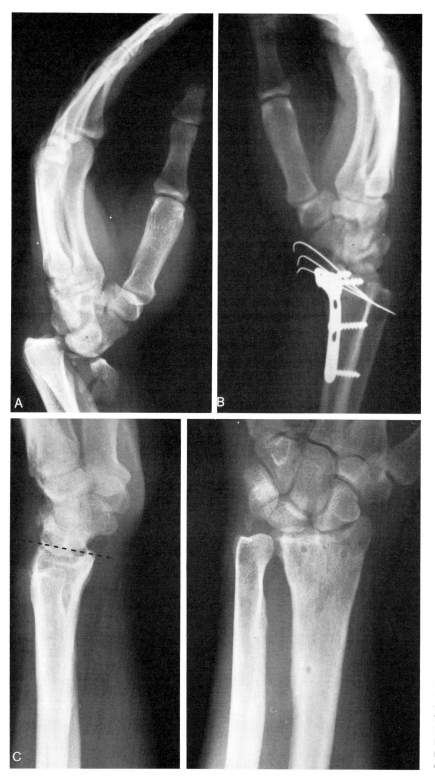

Figure 13–67. A, Lateral view of a comminuted volar Barton's fracture with considerable subluxation. *B,* The fragments are in good position following plate and K-wire fixation. *C,* Healed fracture following removal of the plate and screws. The distal radial angle is normal *(line).* There is slight negative ulnar variance with radiocarpal arthrosis.

cessful, particularly if the fracture is stable to a trial of gentle manipulation at the time of reduction. If so, the dorsal variety fracture should be immobilized in a long-arm cast in a position of forearm pronation and neutral position or slight wrist extension. Palmar flexion should be avoided, as this

appears to increase the tendency of the carpus to translate dorsally with recurrence of the subluxation. The palmar Barton fracture should be immobilized in the opposite position, that is, in a position of forearm supination and neutral or slight palmar flexion of the wrist.

If an anatomic closed reduction is not achieved, or if the fracture conveys the impression of marked instability at the time of reduction, some means of internal fixation is advised. For the dorsal variety, Kirschner wires placed percutaneously or under direct vision will often suffice for this purpose. The more common palmar variety is probably best managed by an open procedure with application of a volar buttress-type plate[85] and additional screw or pin fixation as needed (Fig. 13–67). Occasionally if the fracture is unstable but inappropriate for an open procedure, exoskeletal fixation as previously described may be indicated.

Complications. The same array of complications as outlined for the Colles' fracture may occur with this injury. The major late sequela of the Barton-type fracture, however, is residual radiocarpal subluxation and articular incongruity, leading to degenerative arthrosis of the wrist (Fig. 13–68).

Chauffeur's Fracture (Radial Styloid Fracture)

The chauffeur's fracture refers to an intra-articular fracture of the distal radius chiefly involving the radial styloid. The fracture line typically originates at the junction of the scaphoid and lunate fossae on the radial articular surface and courses laterally in a transverse or oblique direction. It may also be known by the eponym Hutchinson's fracture.[2, 3] It is best appreciated radiographically on a PA projection (Fig. 13–69A). The lateral projection may reveal few if any abnormalities (Fig. 13–69B).

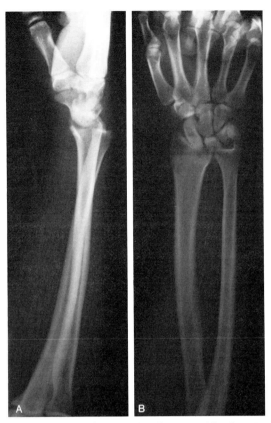

Figure 13–68. Lateral (A) and PA (B) views of the forearm in a patient with an old Barton's fracture. Note the radiocarpal subluxation. There is also dorsal subluxation of the distal radioulnar joint.

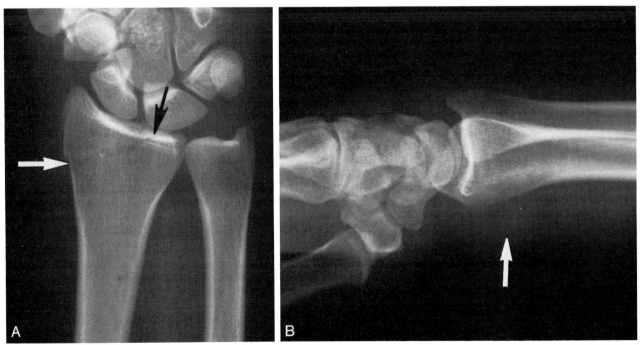

Figure 13–69. A, PA view of the wrist demonstrating a typical chauffeur's fracture (arrows). B, Lateral view of the wrist with chauffeur's fracture. Obliteration of the pronator fat stripe (arrow) is the only indication of injury.

Classification. This fracture may be simple or comminuted, displaced or undisplaced. By definition it is intra-articular. There should be no evidence of radiocarpal subluxation.

Mechanism of Injury. The likely mechanism of this fracture is direct axial compression transmitted through the scaphoid. Clinically this injury was associated decades ago with the backfire of the starting crank of an automobile engine.[84]

Treatment. If the fracture is nondisplaced or only slightly displaced (< 1 mm articular depression), simple cast immobilization is sufficient. Because the brachioradialis tendon inserts on the radial styloid, an above-elbow cast with the elbow in 90° of flexion is advisable at least for the first 3 weeks. Usually 6 weeks is sufficient for complete bony union. If the fracture is moderately displaced, manipulative reduction is required. If the fracture is stable, fixation may be possible with cast immobilization following reduction. However, in general, if reduction is required, percutaneous fixation with multiple Kirschner wires or open fixation with either Kirschner wires or screws is advised.

Complications. Complications are similar to those discussed for the other groups of distal radius fractures.

Galeazzi Fracture (Piedmont Fracture)

The Galeazzi fracture is included in this section, although it frequently falls outside of the topography of the wrist. This eponym refers to a fracture of the radius that usually, but not always, involves the diaphysis at the junction of the middle and distal thirds with an associated subluxation of the distal radioulnar joint.[2, 80, 117] The latter feature may not always be apparent at the time of initial injury and may not become apparent until treatment is under way (Fig. 13–70). Variants of the Galeazzi fracture include fractures involving the distal metaphysis (Fig. 13–71) or the more proximal diaphysis of the radius (Fig. 13–72) and cases involving fracture of the distal ulna in association with the radius injury. This injury is particularly important to recognize and differentiate from a Colles'-type fracture, since its treatment is quite different. Routine PA and lateral projections of the forearm are usually adequate to make the diagnosis. However, localized views of the wrist in the AP and true lateral positions may be necessary to evaluate the distal radioulnar joint (Fig. 13–70).

Classification. The fracture may be comminuted, but usually it is a simple oblique or transverse

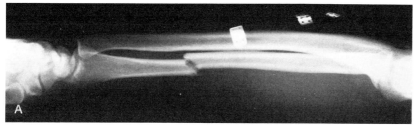

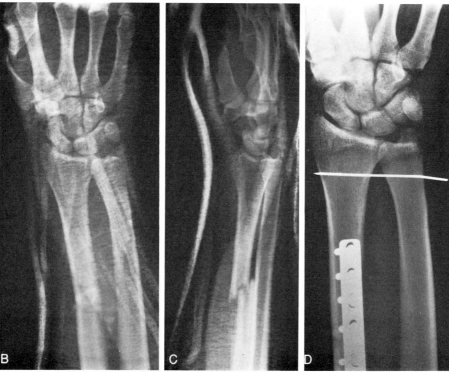

Figure 13–70. Galeazzi's fracture. Lateral view *(A)* of the forearm demonstrates a fracture of the radial diaphysis. PA *(B)* and lateral *(C)* views following casting show incomplete reduction of the radius. The distal radioulnar subluxation is subtle. *D,* The fracture was plated, and the distal radioulnar joint was internally fixed with a K-wire.

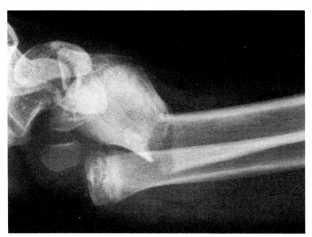

Figure 13–71. Galeazzi variant. There is a fracture of the distal radius metaphysis with dislocation of the distal radioulnar joint obvious on the lateral view.

fracture of the distal radial diaphysis. It may be initially nondisplaced. Displacement characteristically involves the distal radial fragment shortening and angulating in a radial direction by the pull of the brachioradialis.[2] Usually only the displaced va-

riety will exhibit significant radioulnar subluxation radiographically.

Mechanism of Injury. A fall onto the outstretched hand with hyperpronation of the forearm is the usual cause of this injury. Occasionally a direct blow on the dorsiradial aspect of the wrist may produce the fracture.

Treatment. Hughston has pointed out that closed treatment is unsatisfactory in 92 percent of cases.[103] Therefore, in nearly all cases this fracture should be managed by reduction and internal stabilization. In the usual instance involving the shaft of the radius, open reduction and internal fixation of the radius with a compression plate is recommended. The distal radioulnar joint can then be reduced with closed technique using forearm supination and fixed percutaneously with a Kirschner wire (see Figs. 13–70 and 13–72). The forearm should be maintained in a position of supination for 6 weeks following the operation. Then it should be further "protected" for 3 to 6 weeks by a short-arm cast or removable splint. Some authors advocate open repair of the distal radioulnar joint in such cases. If the injury is a variant of the typical Galeazzi fracture and involves the distal radial metaphysis, a

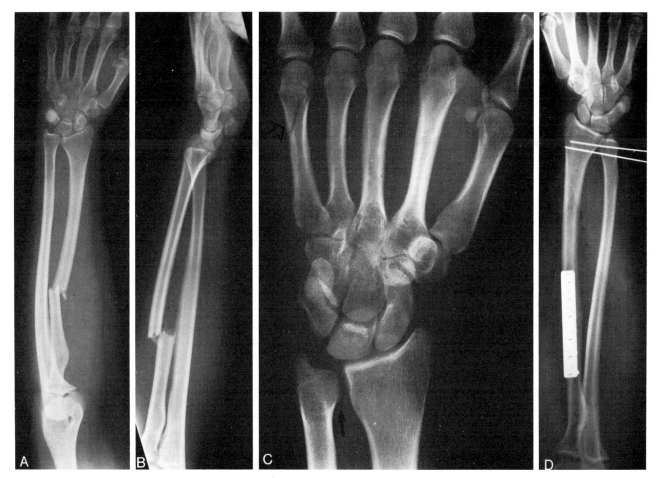

Figure 13–72. Galeazzi variant. AP *(A)* and lateral *(B)* views of the forearm demonstrate a proximal radial fracture. The AP view of the wrist *(C)* makes the distal radioulnar subluxation *(black arrow)* more obvious (i.e., it is widened). There is also an oblique fracture of the 5th metacarpal *(open arrow)*. *(D)* The fracture is internally fixed with plate and screws, and the distal radioulnar joint is fixed with K-wires.

compression plate may prove unsatisfactory for fixation. In such instances reduction followed by Kirschner-wire or exoskeletal fixation may be best. Again, distal radioulnar joint reduction by forearm supination and percutaneous fixation should not be overlooked.

Complications. The most frequent complication of the Galeazzi fracture is malunion of the radius and residual subluxation of the distal radioulnar joint. This results most often from inadequate treatment, usually because of failure to recognize the differences between this fracture and either the Colles' or Smith variety. In contrast to the injuries mentioned above, delayed union or non-union is not unusual.[103] If the fracture is seen late, chronic symptomatic subluxation of the distal radioulnar joint may require distal ulna excision.[82]

In addition to the fracture groups mentioned above, variations of any of these involving an accompanying fracture of the distal ulna can be seen. Strictly speaking, these are "distal both-bone forearm" fractures. Most often these represent an injury similar to the Galeazzi fracture, with bony rather than ligamentous damage to the distal ulna. Similar treatment principles as discussed earlier apply in this group as well.

Dislocations About the Distal Radius

Dislocations of the distal radioulnar joint, or rarely the radiocarpal joint, can be seen in the absence of an accompanying fracture of the distal radius.

Distal Radioulnar Joint—Dorsal Dislocation

This is the most common type of dislocation-subluxation of the distal ulna.[79, 98, 100] The usual cause is a hyperpronation injury to the wrist.[60] Clinically the patient maintains the forearm in a position of moderate pronation and resists supination. The distal ulna is usually dorsally prominent.[122] Radiographic evaluation may reveal only subtle abnormalities. On a true lateral view of the wrist, the distal ulna should appear dorsally displaced. Minor degrees of forearm rotation may obscure this finding, however. Perhaps of greater significance is the PA projection, which suggests overlap, widening, or incongruity of the distal radioulnar joint (Fig. 13–72C).[150] Images in the axial plane (CT or MRI) may be useful in diagnosing these injuries. If the dislocation is seen early, closed treatment by forearm supination and maintenance of this reduction through approximately 6 weeks of long-arm cast immobilization is usually satisfactory.[2, 60] Occasionally closed reduction is not successful, particularly if treatment is delayed. In such cases, open reduction, temporary Kirschner-wire fixation, and repair or reconstruction[104] of the damaged ligamentous structures may be indicated.

Distal Radioulnar Joint—Volar Dislocation

This injury results from a hypersupination stress to the forearm.[13, 154] Clinically, the patient presents with the forearm maintained in supination. The wrist appears narrowed in the lateral plane, and there may be a prominence or fullness over the palmar ulnar aspect of the wrist. Radiographic evaluation should suggest palmar displacement of the distal ulna on the lateral view and overlap of the distal radius and ulna in the frontal plane (Fig. 13–73). Reduction may be more difficult in this case than in the dorsal counterpart to this injury. It should be carried out by forearm supination with direct pressure in a dorsal direction over the displaced head of the ulna. Maintenance of reduction by long-arm cast immobilization with the forearm in a position of mild pronation should be continued for 6 weeks. If irreducible, open reduction and repair or reconstruction should be carried out.

Radiocarpal Dislocation

In the absence of significant bony injury to the distal radius or as a variant of a perilunate dislocation, radiocarpal dislocation is extremely rare.[87] Displacement of the carpus in both the palmar and dorsal direction has been more commonly reported with perilunate dislocation.[2, 3]

Carpal Fractures

Fractures of the carpus frequently involve multiple bones or a single bone in association with significant ligamentous injury. The possibility of such a combination of injured structures must be carefully kept in mind when evaluating these fractures.

Scaphoid

The scaphoid is the most frequently fractured carpal bone.[73, 83, 101, 149] Scaphoid fractures account for 70 percent and 55 percent of all carpal injuries in the Mayo and Böhler series, respectively.[2, 3] Whether justified or not, the prognosis for these injuries has a sinister reputation. Union rates ranging from 50 percent to 95 percent have been reported. Furthermore, one must be vigilant to rule out or recognize a "transcaphoid-perilunate dislocation" (to be discussed later) when evaluating the fractured scaphoid. Failure to recognize significant concomitant soft tissue injury may lead to serious errors in management.

If nondisplaced, fractures of the scaphoid may be difficult to detect on routine radiographs. The minimum requirements include PA, lateral, and scaphoid x-ray views. Air-gap magnification, particularly of the oblique projection, may enhance detail. Changes in the navicular fat stripe, as mentioned earlier in the section on Routine Radiographic Tech-

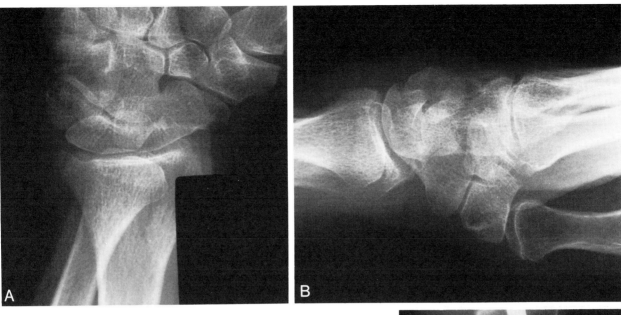

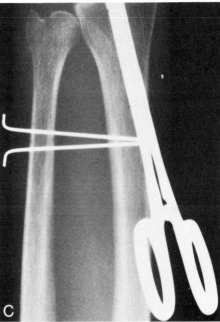

Figure 13–73. Volar dislocation of the distal radioulnar joint. *A,* The oblique view shows marked overlap of the joint space. *B,* The ulna is in a volar position on the lateral view. *C,* Reduction was accomplished using K-wire fixation. The towel clamp should have been adjusted prior to obtaining this operative film.

niques, may be noted. If a high index of clinical suspicion persists despite negative initial films, repeat x-ray evaluation at approximately 2 weeks following the injury may be indicated. Usually, but not always, a fracture line may be obvious at this stage. If there should still be some doubt as to the presence of a fracture following the second radiographic study, further evaluation using Tc-99m methyl diphosphonate bone scans and trispiral tomography may be indicated. Generally in such cases we recommend the use of a bone scan as a screening study and proceed with trispiral tomography only if there is an area of increased scintillation in the region of the scaphoid. Lack of an area of increased uptake in the carpus effectively rules out a fracture.

If the fracture is displaced, there is usually little difficulty in diagnosing the scaphoid fracture on routine radiographic views. However, trispiral tomography, particularly on the lateral plane, may be extremely helpful in assessing the degree of displacement or angulation of the fracture, the adequacy of an attempt at reduction, or the presence of any associated carpal instability patterns (Fig. 13–74). In general most displaced scaphoid fractures involving the waist (middle third) of the bone will tend to exhibit angulation of the distal fragment in a palmar direction, with resultant foreshortening of the carpal height, and dorsiflexion-instability pattern of the proximal scaphoid fragment and accompanying lunate.

Classification. The scaphoid fracture is most often classified by the location of the fracture line and its direction.[2, 3, 73, 133] Both of these factors have a bear-

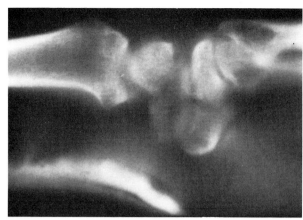

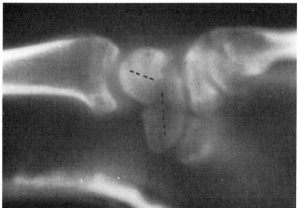

Figure 13–74. Lateral trispiral tomograms demonstrate a scaphoid fracture with volar flexion ("humpback deformity") of the distal fragment.

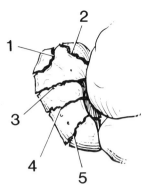

Figure 13–75. Illustration of typical zones of fracture in the scaphoid: 1, capsular attachment or tubercle; 2, distal articular surface; 3, fracture of the distal third; 4, waist fracture; and 5, proximal pole fracture.

ing on the prognosis as well as the approach to treatment. The fracture may be classified according to location as a proximal third, middle third, distal third, or tuberosity type (Fig. 13–75). The prognosis for union is worst, and the risk of ischemic necrosis of the proximal bony fragment is highest, in the proximal third type. Those fracture lines involving the distal third of the bone and tuberosity have the best prognosis and have the least risk of osteonecrosis (Fig. 13–76). The middle third fractures involving the waist of the scaphoid are intermediate in terms of prognosis.

The direction of the fracture line has been classified by Russe into three types (Fig. 13–77).[133] Type I is basically perpendicular to the long axis of the wrist and oblique to the long axis of the scaphoid (Fig. 13–77). Because it is perpendicular to the direction of the forces acting on it, most stresses acting on the fracture are compressive with little shear. This situation is most favorable for bony union. The Type II fracture line is perpendicular to the long axis of the scaphoid and oblique to that of the wrist (Figs. 13–77B and 13–78). A small shear vector acts on fractures of this sort, but most of the forces favor compression of the fracture. Type III is least favorable, with the fracture line tending to be

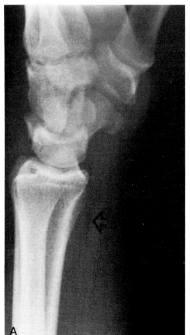

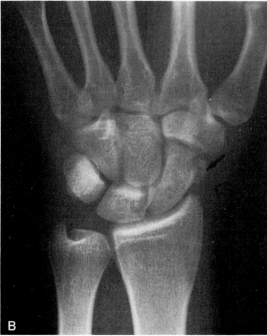

Figure 13–76. Lateral (A) and PA (B) views of a scaphoid tubercle fracture (black arrow). Note the minimal displacement of the navicular fat stripe on the PA view (open arrow). The pronator fat stripe on the lateral view (open arrow) is not displaced.

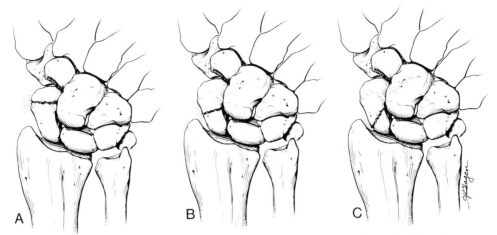

Figure 13–77. Russe classification of scaphoid fractures. *A,* Type I. *B,* Type II. *C,* Type III.

parallel to the long axis of the wrist (Fig. 13–77C). Stresses acting across the fracture tend to produce shearing vectors rather than compression. As a result, fracture displacement and non-union is highest with this type. Moreover, the Type III fracture is most common with proximal third fractures. This further exacerbates the unfavorable prognosis.

In addition to location and direction of the fracture line, the presence of comminution or displacement should be noted in classifying such injuries. Both have a negative effect in terms of prognosis.

Mechanism of Injury. A fall onto the outstretched hand is the most common mechanism leading to a fracture of the scaphoid. Wrist hyperextension injuries with other causes, for example vehicular accidents, may also be responsible. In the laboratory, fracture of the scaphoid is most consistently produced by wrist hyperextension in a position of

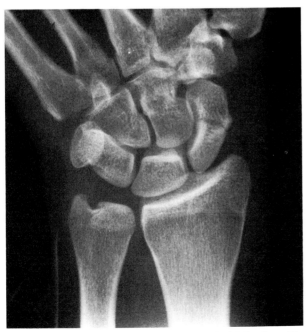

Figure 13–78. PA view of Russe II scaphoid fracture. The fracture is perpendicular to the axis of the scaphoid and oblique to the long axis of the wrist.

radial deviation.[151] Application of the deforming force more distally in the palm appears to produce a scaphoid fracture rather than a Colles'-type fracture.

Treatment. Treatment considerations will vary with the location of the fracture within the scaphoid bone, the degree of displacement, and the degree of associated soft tissue injury. The latter two factors are often related. In general, it is wise to consider all displaced fractures as inherently unstable, with a high percentage of these actually representing spontaneous partially reduced transscaphoid-perilunate dislocations.

Except under unusual circumstances, all nondisplaced scaphoid fractures should be treated by cast immobilization.[133, 149] In the distal third fracture or tuberosity fracture, a short-arm cast that immobilizes the wrist in a neutral position and utilizes a thumb-spica extension to the base of the thumb nail to place the thumb in moderate palmar abduction is satisfactory. In general, with this fracture type union will be complete in 4 to 8 weeks. Nondisplaced middle third and proximal third fractures present more of a challenge. Bony union requires more time, and avascularity of the proximal bone fragment must be considered. In the young individual with this fracture, an above-elbow cast with a similar thumb-spica extension is advised for the first 4 to 6 weeks. Thereafter, short-arm thumb-spica immobilization for 2 to 4 more months may be required. A small percentage of fractures will fail to unite even with this treatment. Such fractures may require further cast immobilization or bone grafting procedures to achieve union. In the older patient (i.e., over 50 years of age), an initial period of above-elbow cast immobilization is omitted because of concern for permanent limitation of the range of motion of the elbow.

The displaced fracture requires reduction. This is perhaps most easily achieved by longitudinal traction in finger traps followed by gentle manipulation. In all instances, once reduction is obtained a clinical test for the stability of the fracture is central for guiding further management. If reduction is ana-

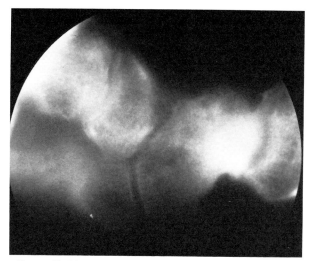

Figure 13–79. Lateral trispiral tomogram following reduction of the scaphoid fracture. The fracture is healing. The proximal dense appearance is due to the thickening of the tomographic slice, which includes the radial styloid.

tomic and post-reduction stability is achieved, then treatment as outlined earlier for the nondisplaced fracture is appropriate. Particular care in assessing post-reduction radiographs is important. Restoration of the scaphoid outline on PA and oblique projections with maintenance of the normal carpal height is essential. In the lateral projection palmar angulation of the distal fragment may be difficult to discern and is frequently overlooked. If this angulation remains, it may lead to healing in a "humpback" deformity (Fig. 13–74) and secondary distortion of the intercarpal relationships.[88] If routine lateral views leave room for doubt with regard to the adequacy of reduction in this case, trispiral tomographic evaluation may be indicated (Fig. 13–79).

If adequate reduction is possible but the reduction is unstable, a number of treatment options are possible. Above-elbow thumb-spica cast immobilization may be selected, but extreme vigilance is necessary for maintenance of reduction. This may require serial post-reduction radiographs. Alternatively, percutaneous Kirschner-wire fixation of the fracture or open reduction with screw or Kirschner-wire fixation may be appropriate (Fig. 13–80). Such unstable fractures may be frank or variants of forme fruste perilunate dislocations. As such, the extremely unstable variety may benefit from open repair of the injured ligaments (particularly the volar complex) in addition to fixation of the fracture. The unstable scaphoid fracture has a greater risk of non-union or delayed union. If there appears to be little progress toward union after 3 to 4 months of such treatment, bone grafting or the application of electrical stimulation methods may be appropriate.

If adequate reduction is not possible by closed means, open reduction is indicated. Internal fixation as outlined earlier and possibly repair of associated disrupted ligaments should be carried out.

Complications. The scaphoid fracture is generally associated with a litany of complications.[2, 3, 133, 149] However, if recognized early, reduced adequately, and treated appropriately over a sufficient period, uneventful healing can be expected in over 90 percent of cases.

Delayed union is perhaps the most common complication and is defined generally as failure of union within 3 months of the initiation of cast immobilization. It must be recognized, however, that a significant percentage of scaphoid fractures require 6 to 12 months of cast or splint immobilization to achieve union.[133, 149]

Non-union probably occurs in less than 10 percent of cases but is more prevalent in fractures of the middle or proximal thirds of the bone (Fig.

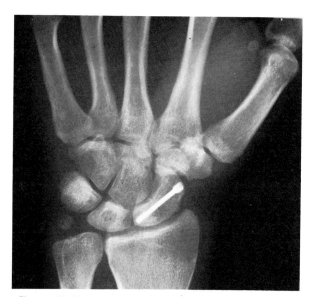

Figure 13–80. Internal fixation of scaphoid fracture with a Herbert screw.

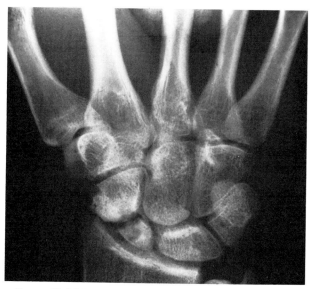

Figure 13–81. PA view demonstrating an old non-united fracture of the proximal scaphoid.

13–81), in Russe Type III fractures (vertical direction), in comminuted fractures, and in fractures with unstable reductions. The most common preventable factors associated with non-union include delay of diagnosis and inadequate treatment. Once non-union is established, its management usually takes the form of bone grafting or electrical stimulation modalities. The indications for one or the other of these approaches are not firmly established. If non-union persists despite either or both of these techniques, then further management, if indicated, may include radial styloidectomy, soft tissue arthroplasty of the pseudarthrosis site, scaphoid replacement arthroplasty, and limited wrist arthrodesis.[2]

Malunion most frequently results from failure to recognize an inadequate reduction. Usually this takes the form of palmar angulation of the distal fragment, producing the so-called "humpback" deformity. This situation may then lead to foreshortening of the carpal height, which in turn leads to an exaggerated scapholunate angle and a dorsal carpal instability pattern.[88]

Avascular necrosis of the proximal scaphoid fragment is most prevalent with fractures involving the proximal third of the scaphoid.[133] It may also be seen, but less frequently, in middle third fractures. It is distinctly unusual with fractures involving the distal third of the bone. Radiographically this condition is characterized by increased radiopacity of the avascular portion (Fig. 13–82). When such radiopacity is present, delayed union or non-union of the fracture is frequent. Revascularization occurs slowly over 1 to 2 years. Significant bony collapse of the avascular portion is unusual.

Radioscaphoid impingement or arthrosis may occur, particularly with malunited fractures or in those

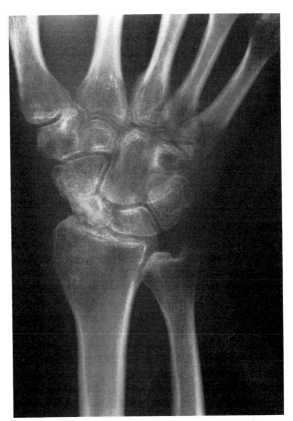

Figure 13–83. Old fracture of the scaphoid with degenerative arthritis at the junction of the radial styloid and scaphoid waist.

with a rather hypertrophic callus. It is most often between the tip of the radial styloid and the waist of the scaphoid (Fig. 13–83). If present, a limited radial styloidectomy or cheilectomy of the scaphoid may be indicated.

The other array of complications familiar to all wrist injuries, including limited wrist or digit range of motion, autonomic dysfunction syndrome (sympathetic dystrophy), and carpal tunnel syndrome, may also be seen.

Triquetrum

The triquetrum is the second most commonly injured carpal bone.[67] Most often these are dorsal avulsion injuries presumably at the site of the ulnotriquetral ligament insertion. More rarely fractures of the body of the triquetrum are seen.[62] Usually these are nondisplaced, and often they are comminuted. The diagnosis is usually made by routine PA, lateral, and oblique wrist radiographs (Fig. 13–84). Trispiral tomograms may be useful, particularly to assess displacement of fractures involving the body. Treatment of the dorsal avulsion fracture is symptomatic. A short-arm cast immobilizing the wrist in slight extension for 4 to 6 weeks is usually adequate. Fractures of the body that are nondisplaced are best treated by a long-arm cast for 4 to 6 weeks followed by a short-arm cast for 2 to 6 additional weeks or until evidence of union is pres-

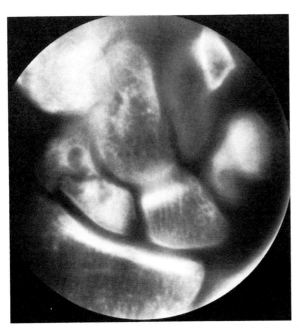

Figure 13–82. PA trispiral tomogram with a non-united scaphoid fracture and avascular necrosis of the proximal fragment.

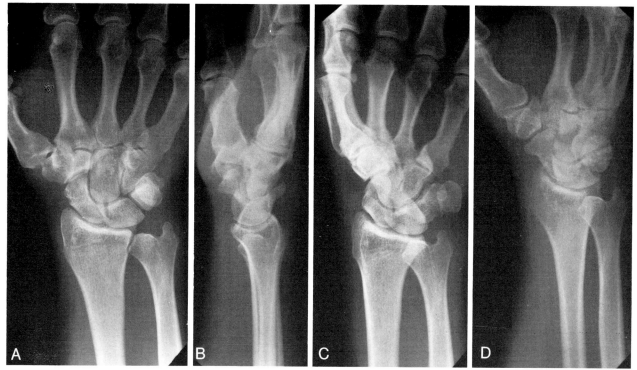

Figure 13–84. Fractured triquetrum demonstrated on PA *(A)*, lateral *(B)*, and oblique views *(C,* and *D)*. The fracture is most clearly seen on the lateral view. There is associated soft tissue swelling.

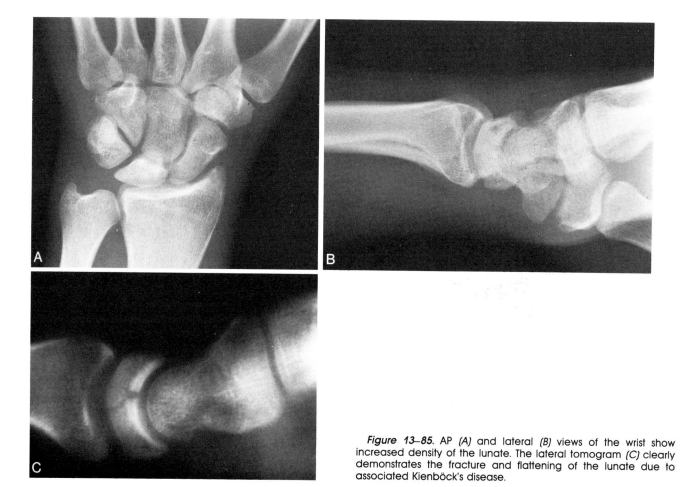

Figure 13–85. AP *(A)* and lateral *(B)* views of the wrist show increased density of the lunate. The lateral tomogram *(C)* clearly demonstrates the fracture and flattening of the lunate due to associated Kienböck's disease.

ent. Significantly displaced fractures may be candidates for open reduction and internal fixation.

Lunate

Considerable confusion and disagreement exist regarding fractures of the lunate and their relation to Kienböck's disease.[2, 3, 123] Some authors believe that the etiology of Kienböck's disease is a fracture of the lunate, whereas others believe that fracture and later fragmentation of the lunate is a consequence rather than a cause of Kienböck's disease. We believe that acute traumatic fracture of the lunate can occur and may or may not be followed by the typical radiographic findings of Kienböck's disease. We also believe that Kienböck's disease can be seen without a definite history of trauma and in the absence of radiographic evidence of lunate fracture. This condition will be discussed later in this chapter.

Fractures involving the body of the lunate may be extremely difficult to diagnose on routine radiographs. If a high index of clinical suspicion exists in spite of normal-appearing radiographs, further evaluation by trispiral tomography or bone scan may be warranted. The fracture line is usually disposed in the coronal plane (Fig. 13–85). The mechanism of injury of the lunate fracture is usually hyperextension. Direct axial compression has also been suggested. If the diagnosis is made in the absence of the typical radiographic changes suggesting Kienböck's disease, treatment is indicated. Nondisplaced fractures should be treated at least initially by long-arm cast immobilization. These fractures require careful vigilance to ensure that displacement does not occur from compressive loads within the cast. Because of the position of the lunate, compressive deforming forces as a result of finger motion are simply unavoidable. For this reason some authors suggest treatment by external fixation-distraction across the wrist similar to that described for the unstable Colles' fracture (Fig. 13–60). Displaced fractures of the lunate are likely best managed by open reduction and internal fixation with Kirschner wires or miniature screws. The chief complication following fractures of the lunate is the development of Kienböck's sequelae, as discussed later in this chapter.

Pisiform

Fractures of the pisiform usually result from a blunt blow. This occurs when the base of the hypothenar eminence is struck in a direct fall or when the hand is used as an ill-advised hammer. The fracture may be comminuted or simple. Displacement is usually not marked because this bone is enveloped in the tendon of the flexor carpi ulnaris. Although routine radiographs may reveal a fracture line, the fracture is best visualized on a lateral projection with the wrist in a position of 30° supination (pisiform view) (Fig. 13–86).[148] Closed symptomatic treatment in a short-arm cast is recommended.[67] The major late complication is arthrosis of the pisotriquetral joint, which may require excision of the pisiform.

Hamate

Fractures of the hamate may involve the body,[118] the distal articular surface as a component of a carpometacarpal fracture-dislocation,[99] or the hook (hamulus).[64] Fractures of the body are usually nondisplaced and can be diagnosed using routine AP, lateral, and oblique radiographs. These are stable injuries and can generally be managed adequately by short-arm cast immobilization for 4 to 8 weeks. Complications are unusual. Fractures involving the distal articular surface as a component of a carpometacarpal dislocation are suggested by routine wrist radiographs. Accurate delineation of the fracture may require trispiral tomography (Fig. 13–87). These are unstable injuries and hence usually require internal fixation after closed or open reduction. The major late complication is degenerative arthrosis of the carpometacarpal articulation, particularly if the fracture heals with residual articular incongruity or joint subluxation.

Fracture of the hook (hamulus) is the most common injury to the hamate.[67, 69, 70, 140] This is generally believed to be an avulsion fracture, presumably caused by the pull of the transverse carpal ligament that inserts on the hook of the hamate. It seems particularly prevalent in association with a dubbed golf swing.[147] The diagnosis is difficult to make on routine radiographs. A carpal tunnel view, however, may be helpful (Fig. 13–88A). Trispiral tomog-

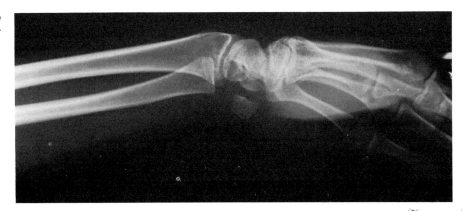

Figure 13–86. Pisiform view of the wrist demonstrating a minimally displaced pisiform fracture.

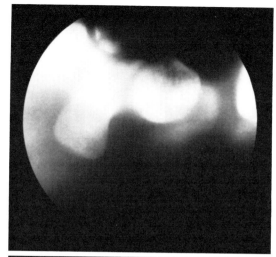

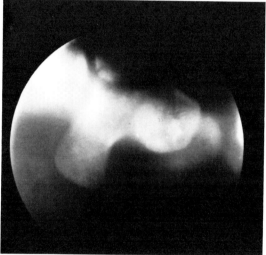

Figure 13–87. Lateral trispiral tomogram of the wrist with a combined fracture of the dorsal aspect of the hamate.

raphy is diagnostic in most instances; however, a localized bone scan may be useful in localizing the pathology prior to tomograms (Fig. 13–88B and C). Closed treatment by cast immobilization is unreliable for healing. Most authors recommend excision of the fractured fragment, although some suggest open reduction and internal fixation. Most complications of this injury result from failure to make the correct diagnosis. These include persistent pain, ulnar neuropathy, and attritional flexor tendon rupture.[78]

Capitate

Capitate fractures may involve the body, the distal articular surface as a component of a carpometacarpal fracture-dislocation, or the proximal pole.[2, 3, 57, 67] Fractures involving the body occur most commonly through the middle third and are transverse (Fig. 13–89). They are usually the result of a hyperextension injury. A direct blow over the dorsum of the capitate may also be responsible. Comminution may be present. Routine PA and lateral radiographs are usually sufficient to arrive at a

diagnosis. If the fracture is nondisplaced, short-arm cast immobilization for 6 to 8 weeks is usually adequate. If displaced, the fracture is likely to be unstable. In such cases, if reduction is adequate, vigilant cast immobilization may be successful. At least initially a long-arm cast is advised in such cases. Alternatively, the unstable capitate fracture may be treated by internal fixation, usually with Kirschner wires. Complications include non-union, delayed union, and avascular necrosis of the proximal fragment. Fractures involving the distal articular surface are similar to those described for the same location in the hamate as part of a carpometacarpal dislocation. However, in contrast to the hamate, where carpometacarpal motion is desired following healing, the capitate–3rd metacarpal articulation should be stable with essentially no motion.[8] Therefore, with extensive articular incongruity, treatment directed toward achieving an arthrodesis of the capitate–3rd metacarpal articulation may be justified.

Fractures of the proximal pole may be seen as isolated entities similar to middle third fractures as described earlier or as the so-called "naviculocapitate syndrome."[86, 116, 142] This injury, resulting from a hyperextension force to the wrist, is probably a variant of a perilunate dislocation. With it, fracture of the scaphoid and the proximal pole of the capitate occurs. On spontaneous reduction the latter rotates through 90° to 180°. Often this injury is overlooked, with the casual examiner directing his attention to the scaphoid fracture only, and with details of the proximal capitate fragment being obscured on routine radiographs. Trispiral tomography is diagnostic and should be carried out if there is any doubt regarding this syndrome (Fig. 13–90). Treatment requires open reduction and internal fixation of the capitate and scaphoid fractures. If the capitate fragment is extremely small, excision may be warranted. Avascular necrosis of the capitate fragment is not unusual. If seen late, excision of the fragment or capitolunoscaphoid arthrodesis may be indicated.

Trapezoid

Fractures of the trapezoid are uncommon.[2, 3, 67, 101] They may be seen as a component of a carpometacarpal fracture-dislocation.[99] In such instances, the comments directed to this same injury in the capitate apply. The major goal of treatment is stability of the trapezoid–2nd metacarpal articulation. This may require arthrodesis.

Trapezium

Fractures of the trapezium involve the body, the margin, or the ridge.[2, 3, 67, 76, 101] Those through the body are usually vertical and may result from direct axial compression on the thumb, hyperextension of the 1st metacarpal, or a blow to the adducted thumb (Fig. 13–91). Comminution and displacement may be present. In addition to routine PA, lateral, and oblique radiographs, x-ray evaluation should in-

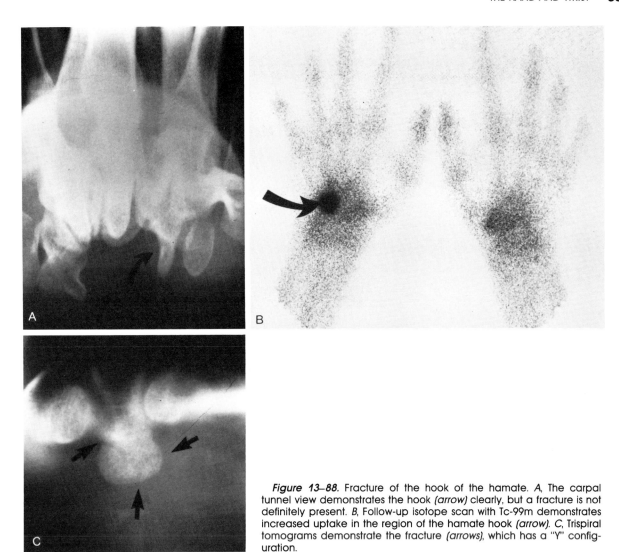

Figure 13-88. Fracture of the hook of the hamate. *A,* The carpal tunnel view demonstrates the hook *(arrow)* clearly, but a fracture is not definitely present. *B,* Follow-up isotope scan with Tc-99m demonstrates increased uptake in the region of the hamate hook *(arrow). C,* Trispiral tomograms demonstrate the fracture *(arrows),* which has a "Y" configuration.

Figure 13-89. Transverse fracture of the body of the capitate. The fracture is seen best on the PA view *(A, arrow)* and is difficult to detect on the lateral view *(B).*

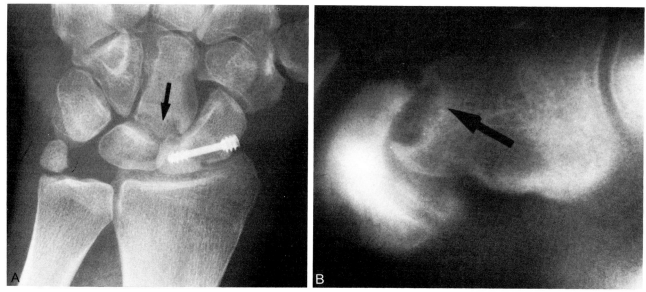

Figure 13–90. A, PA view of the wrist following fixation of the scaphoid fracture. *B,* The capitate fracture *(arrow)* was clearly seen only with tomography.

clude a true PA view of the 1st carpometacarpal joint and possibly trispiral tomograms. If the fracture is nondisplaced, short-arm thumb-spica cast immobilization with the thumb in moderate palmar abduction is usually adequate. If it is displaced, open reduction and internal fixation with the goal of anatomic articular reduction of both the scaphoid and the 1st metacarpal surfaces is recommended. The chief complication of this fracture is degenerative arthrosis of the basilar thumb joints.

Marginal fractures are not uncommon. Provided that they are not displaced, they are comparable in terms of treatment and prognosis to scaphoid tuberosity fractures (Fig. 13–92). If there is any displacement, careful radiographic scrutiny for evidence of subluxation of the joint should be carried out.

Fractures of the ridge of the trapezium are generally believed to be avulsion fractures at the site of

the transverse carpal ligament insertion. These may be difficult to visualize on routine radiographic views but can usually be seen on carpal tunnel views or trispiral tomograms. In terms of prognosis and treatment, they may be similar to fractures of the hook of the hamate. If the fracture is displaced or seen late, excision of the fracture fragment may be indicated.

Carpal Dislocations

Dislocations of the carpus are uncommon but most frequently are associated with a perilunate injury or a variant of this injury.[89, 96, 106, 114, 121, 134]

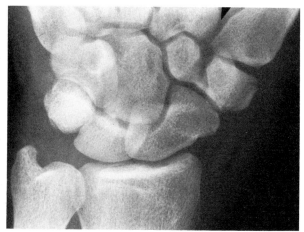

Figure 13–91. Oblique view of the wrist. There is a fracture of the trapezium with associated swelling. Note the associated widening of the bases of the metacarpals *(arrow)* and joint of the trapezium and trapezoid.

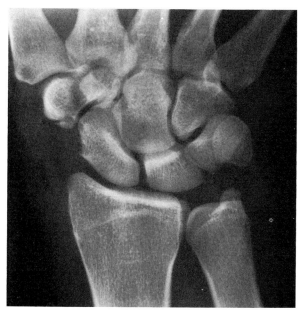

Figure 13–92. PA view of the wrist with a ridge fracture of the trapezium. Note the air in the soft tissues, indicating an open fracture.

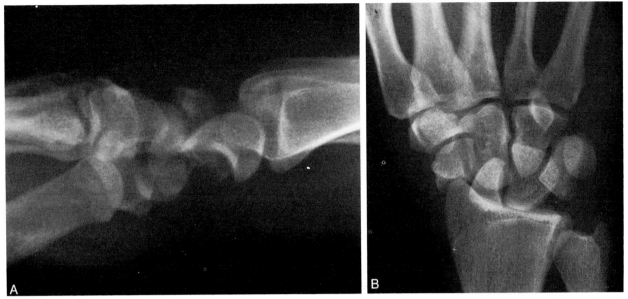

Figure 13–93. Trans-scaphoid perilunate dislocation of the wrist. *A,* The lateral view demonstrates volar flexion of the lunate, which no longer articulates with the capitate. *B,* PA view more clearly shows the scaphoid fracture with rotation of the proximal fragment. The capitate appears to articulate with the distal radius owing to its dorsal proximal position.

Dorsal Perilunate Dislocations and Variants

These injuries include a spectrum of findings varying with the degree of associated trauma and position of the force of impact on the wrist. Most are extreme hyperextension injuries resulting from a fall onto the dorsiflexed wrist.[96]

Trans-scaphoid Perilunate Dislocation. This is the most common type of perilunate dislocation. It is also known as de Quervain's fracture-dislocation. Typically the lunate and proximal scaphoid fragment remain in articulation with the distal radius, while the remainder of the carpus and the distal scaphoid fracture are displaced in a dorsal direction

(Fig. 13–93). Routine PA and lateral radiographs are usually adequate to suggest the injury. However, oblique views or tomograms may be necessary to clarify the diagnosis, particularly with regard to associated carpal fractures. Treatment requires reduction by closed or open means. Manipulative reduction is facilitated by strong longitudinal traction. The incidence of scaphoid malunion or nonunion following the injury is appreciable. For this reason, unless a perfect and stable closed reduction is achieved, many authors advocate stable internal fixation with or without open repair of the disrupted or attenuated volar radiocarpal ligament complex (Fig. 13–94).[2, 3]

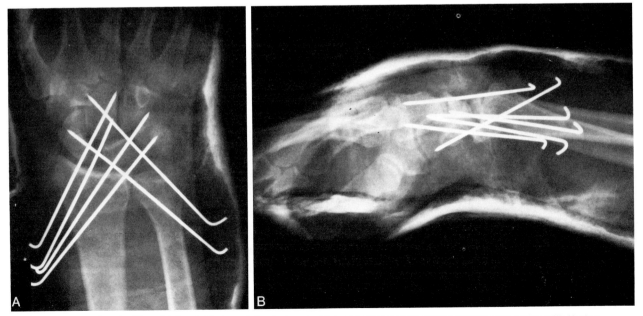

Figure 13–94. PA *(A)* and lateral *(B)* views following reduction of a trans-scaphoid perilunate dislocation with K-wires.

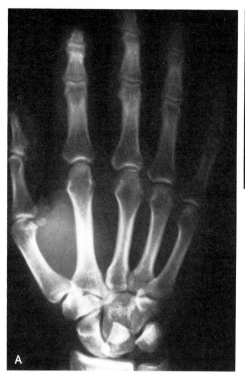
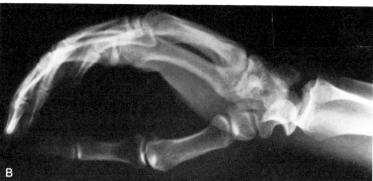

Figure 13–95. PA *(A)* and lateral *(B)* views of an anterior lunate dislocation. The scaphoid and triquetrum are in near normal position in the PA view. The lunate has lost its normal relationship with the radius, and the lunate appears triangular.

In addition to scaphoid non-union or malunion, late complications and sequelae include carpal instability deformities, limited range of motion of the wrist, median neuropathy, late degenerative arthritis, and occasionally avascular bony necrosis.

Dorsal Perilunate Dislocation. This dislocation is essentially the same injury as the trans-scaphoid–perilunate dislocation but without the scaphoid fracture. The volar radiocarpal ligament complex is completely disrupted. The mechanism of injury and treatment principles are the same. The most significant late sequela is residual carpal instability of the DISI variety (see Figs. 13–9 and 13–10).[2, 135]

Anterior (Volar) Lunate Dislocation. This injury is believed to represent a variant of the dorsal perilunate dislocation.[130] Presumably it results from a spontaneous reduction of the dorsally displaced carpus, which essentially settles on the lunate, displacing it in a palmar direction (Fig. 13–95). Closed reduction of this injury may be more difficult and requires direct pressure over the displaced lunate in a dorsal direction in addition to longitudinal traction. The mechanism of injury and treatment principles are as outlined earlier.

Perilunate Dislocation with Multiple Fractures. These are simply variants of the trans-scaphoid–perilunate injury. These may include any element or combination of elements, encompassing transradial styloid, trans-scaphoid, transcapitate, transtriquetral, and transulnar-styloid-perilunate dislocation.[153]

Volar Perilunate Dislocation and Variants

These injuries are extremely rare.[2, 3, 59] Most commonly they are associated with violent trauma that produces hyperflexion of the wrist. They can involve any combination of associated fractures or may lead to a posterior (dorsal) lunate dislocation by a mechanism similar to that described earlier. Treatment should aim for perfect reduction. If the dislocation is unstable following reduction, internal fixation with Kirschner wires, with or without open repair of the disrupted ligaments, is recommended. Complications following these injuries are frequent and include carpal instability, limited range of motion, avascular bony necrosis, and degenerative arthritis.

Dislocations of the Carpus Other Than Perilunate

Although rare, dislocation of virtually every carpal bone has been described.[105, 119, 125] These occur either as an isolated entity or in combination with other carpal dislocations or fractures (Fig. 13–96). The most common nonperilunar carpal dislocations involve the trapezoid[94, 109, 141] and the trapezium.[93, 136, 137] Trapezoid dislocations occur most commonly in the dorsal direction, presumably from a hyperflexion stress to the 2nd metacarpal. Palmar dislocations have also been described. Trapezial dislocations are most often associated with axial compression–adduction injuries. Associated marginal fracture is common.

Carpometacarpal Dislocation

Carpometacarpal dislocation or subluxation is most often associated with an accompanying fracture of the distal carpal row or metacarpal base (Fig. 13–97). These injuries may be difficult to define

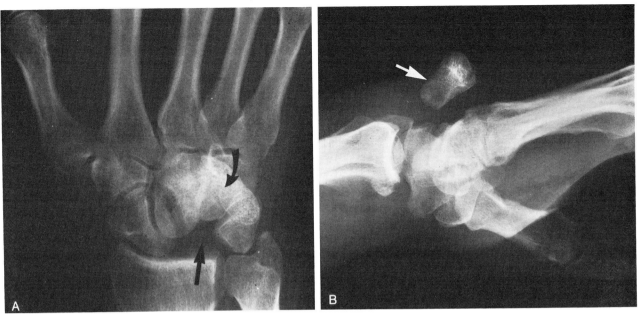

Figure 13–96. Isolated dorsal lunate dislocation. The PA view *(A)* shows absence of the lunate *(straight arrow)* with increased density *(curved arrow)* owing to bone overlap. The lateral *(B)* view demonstrates the dorsally located lunate *(arrow)*.

accurately on routine radiographs. Multiple oblique views or trispiral tomograms are often helpful. As an isolated injury without fracture, carpometacarpal dislocations are rare (see Fig. 13–20).[2, 120] Most commonly they involve multiple rays or the border rays.[102] The direction of displacement is usually dorsal, although volar dislocation has also been reported.[124] These dislocations, particularly when involving the 1st or 5th metacarpal, may be grossly unstable. If the dislocations are reducible but unstable, percutaneous fixation is recommended. If they

are irreducible, open reduction with internal fixation and possibly soft tissue repair is advisable, particularly with the thumb ray.

Metacarpal Fractures

Fractures of the metacarpals, particularly the 4th and 5th, are common.[3, 7, 132, 139] In spite of this, errors of either over- or undertreatment are not infrequent. Management considerations will de-

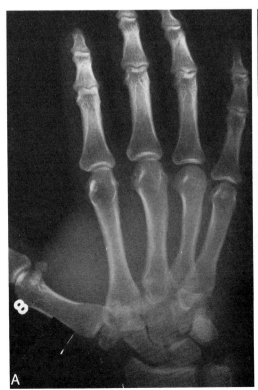

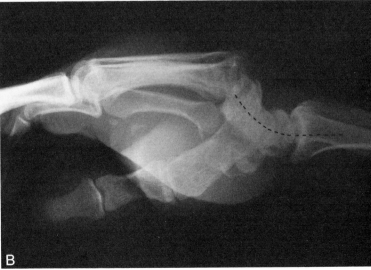

Figure 13–97. Dorsal carpometacarpal dislocation with an associated trapezial fracture. *A,* The PA view shows overlap of the carpometacarpal joints with comminution of the trapezium. *B,* The lateral view better demonstrates the position of the metacarpals *(dotted line).*

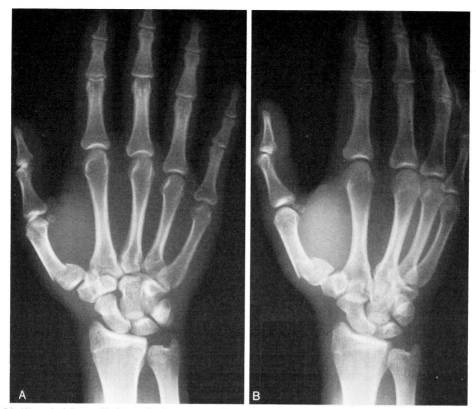

Figure 13–98. PA *(A)* and oblique *(B)* views of a transverse, slightly angulated fracture of the metaphysis of the 1st metacarpal.

pend upon a number of factors, which include the particular metacarpal involved, the type and location of the fracture line, the degree of displacement, the adequacy of rotatory alignment, and the presence of any associated soft tissue injury. In general, routine PA, lateral, and oblique radiographs are adequate for evaluation of these injuries. For both discussion and treatment purposes, metacarpal fractures should be considered in three subgroups—thumb, stable rays (2nd and 3rd metacarpals), and mobile rays (4th and 5th metacarpals). Within each of these groups, a similar fracture classification is applicable.

Thumb

The thumb metacarpal is highly mobile, with multiple degrees of freedom of motion at its basilar joint. Because of this freedom, considerable tolerance exists for fracture angulation and rotation. However, this same feature of high mobility of the basilar joint is offset by the requirement that the thumb transmit a high magnitude of compressive loads in pinch. This allows little tolerance for residual incongruity in the case of intra-articular fractures of the base.

Neck Fractures. These are uncommon. Displacement and instability are unusual. Symptomatic treatment by thumb-spica short-arm cast immobilization for 3 to 6 weeks is usually sufficient treatment.

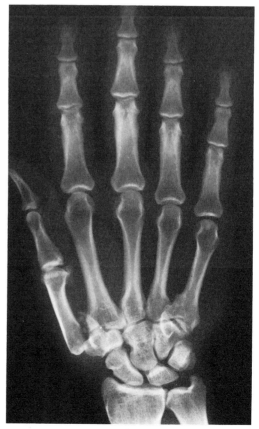

Figure 13–99. Bennett's fracture seen on a PA view of the hand.

Transverse Diaphyseal Fractures. These are also not common. Displacement may be present and require manipulative reduction. Angulation with the distal fragment flexed is usual. It should be corrected, although residual angulation of up to 20° may be acceptable. Rotatory alignment need not be anatomic provided there is not an excessive degree of clinical deformity. If the fracture is minimally displaced or stable following reduction, immobilization in a short-arm thumb-spica cast for 4 to 6 weeks is recommended. Unstable fractures may require percutaneous or open Kirschner-wire fixation. Continuous skeletal traction by a rubber band attached to a transverse Kirschner wire in the distal metacarpal fragment, which is anchored to an outrigger on a short-arm cast, may also be useful in certain cases. Irreducible fractures should be openly reduced and fixed with either Kirschner wires,[97] tension-band wires, or plate and screws.[63, 77, 111]

Spiral Diaphyseal Fractures. These are more fre-

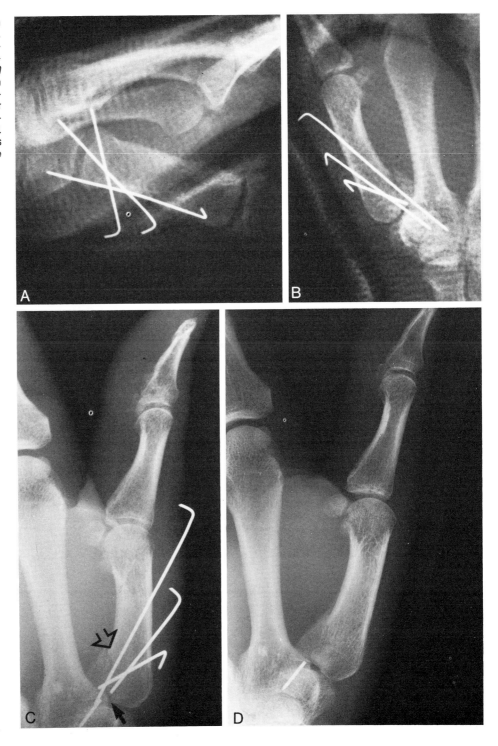

Figure 13–100. Internal fixation of Bennett's fracture with K-wires. PA *(A)* and lateral *(B)* views following reduction with three K-wires and splints. Lateral view *(C)* 5 weeks following reduction shows good position of the fracture *(open arrow)* and articular surface. There is fracture of a K-wire at the joint *(black arrow)*. Radiograph *(D)* taken 2 months after reduction shows that the fracture is healed.

quently unstable than transverse fractures. Internal fixation or skeletal traction is therefore often required. Otherwise these injuries do not differ from the transverse diaphyseal variety.

Extra-articular Proximal Metaphyseal Fractures. These fractures are relatively common (Fig. 13–98). They may be transverse or oblique and usually exhibit angulation in a dorsal direction. Displacement may be present. Angulation of up to 20° in the adult and 40° in the child is acceptable. Fractures of the transverse plane are usually readily reduced by longitudinal traction. Maintenance of reduction is usually possible through a well molded thumb-spica cast that secures the thumb metacarpal in moderate palmar abduction and extension. Cast immobilization is continued for 4 to 6 weeks. The oblique fracture variety is more unstable and commonly exhibits a tendency toward proximal migration of the distal fragment. This injury is readily reduced by longitudinal traction, but it is often difficult to maintain at length by cast immobilization alone. Such fractures, therefore, not infrequently require percutaneous Kirschner-wire fixation or continuous skeletal traction, as described above.

Intra-articular Basilar Fractures. These are the most common fractures seen in the thumb metacarpal.[3, 7, 132, 139] They also are the most demanding in terms of treatment, with little leeway for anything but anatomic reduction of the articular surface. Two basic fracture types, each with an attached eponym, are seen in this group.

The first, or Bennett's fracture, is actually a fracture-subluxation of the 1st carpometacarpal joint. Characteristically the fracture line is oblique and divides a smaller proximal fragment consisting of the volar (ulnar) lip of the 1st metacarpal base from the remainder of the metacarpal as the distal fragment (Fig. 13–99). The smaller proximal (volar or ulnar) fragment is anchored by the attached intermetacarpal and strong volar (ulnar) oblique ligament. It therefore remains undisplaced relative to the trapezium. But the larger distal fragment, consisting of essentially the entire 1st metacarpal, is characteristically unstable. It displaces proximally and falls into flexion. The proximal displacement is due primarily to the pull of the abductor pollicis longus and flexor pollicis longus tendons, while the fall into flexion is due to the action of the strong adductor pollicis muscle.

Reduction is usually possible by closed means and is accomplished by longitudinal traction on the thumb metacarpal accompanied by pronation. Maintenance of reduction by cast immobilization alone is very difficult and is unreliable. For this reason internal fixation with percutaneously placed Kirschner wires is recommended (Fig. 13–100). The wires do not necessarily need to cross the fracture line or directly fix the smaller proximal (volar) fragment to the remainder of the metacarpal. Fixation of the base of the metacarpal to the trapezium is usually adequate. If anatomic reduction is not possible by closed means, open reduction and fix-

ation by Kirschner wires is indicated. Following reduction and internal fixation, a short-arm thumb-spica cast should be worn for 4 to 6 weeks.

The second type of intra-articular basilar fracture of the 1st metacarpal is the Rolando fracture. This is by definition a comminuted injury, usually with a T or Y condylar component (Fig. 13–101). The principles of management for the Rolando fracture are the same as in the Bennett type described earlier. The degree of comminution, however, may preclude reasonable internal fixation by either percutaneous or open means. In such cases skeletal traction by a transverse Kirschner wire in the distal metacarpal may be indicated.

In all intra-articular fractures of the base of the 1st metacarpal, the major late complication is degenerative arthrosis of the 1st carpometacarpal joint. The risk of this complication is increased by residual articular incongruity or joint subluxation and in highly comminuted injuries.

Stable Metacarpal Rays—2nd and 3rd Metacarpals

The 2nd and 3rd metacarpals constitute the stable longitudinal axis of the hand. Because the position of these metacarpals is fixed with essentially no motion at the carpometacarpal joints, there is little compensatory potential to allow for fracture-rotation or angulation.

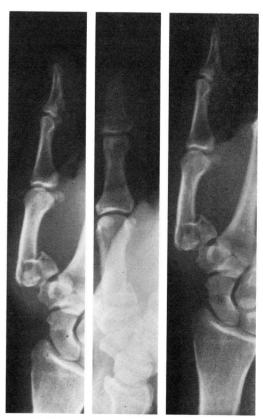

Figure 13–101. Complex displaced intra-articular fracture (Rolando type) of the 1st metacarpal base.

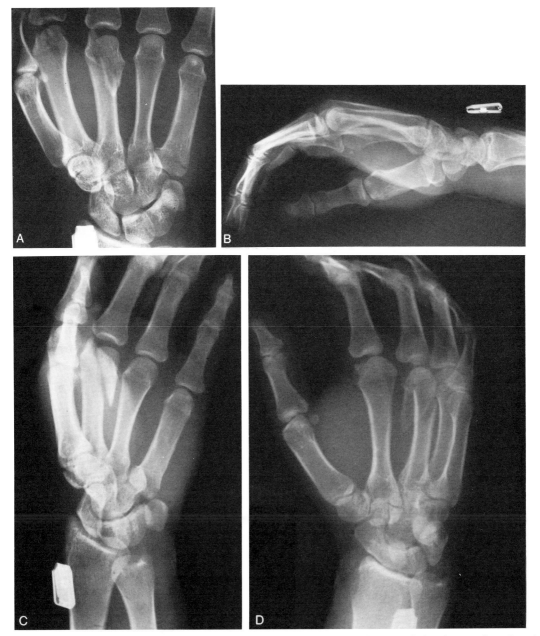

Figure 13–102. PA *(A)*, lateral *(B)*, and oblique *(C* and *D)* views of fractures of the 2nd and 3rd metacarpal necks extending into the articular surface. There is volar angulation of the 2nd metacarpal, shortening of the 3rd, and marked articular distortion. Note the subtle fracture of the base of the 5th metacarpal.

Neck Fractures. These are relatively common and usually result from axial compression or from a blow over the dorsum of the affected metacarpal. Displacement may be present. Characteristically the distal fragment falls into a position of palmar angulation as a result of the forces acting on the fracture from the intrinsic muscles and extrinsic flexor tendons (Fig. 13–102). Malrotation may be present. This is best assessed clinically rather than radiographically. Malrotation is characterized chiefly by overlap of the fingers on attempting to make a fist. In general, anatomic reduction of this fracture is required in the 2nd and 3rd metacarpals. This is usually readily achieved by longitudinal traction followed by a dorsally directed palmar pressure over the metacarpal head fragment and a palmarly directed dorsal pressure over the proximal fragment. If reasonably stable following reduction, the position can usually be maintained by application of a splint or cast. This secures the wrist in mild extension, the metacarpophalangeal joints in 60° to 70° of flexion, and the proximal interphalangeal joints in 10° to 15° of flexion. This position relaxes the deforming musculotendinous forces across the fracture site. If the position of reduction is moderately unstable, then percutaneous fixation with Kirschner wires may be indicated. Occasionally open reduction and internal fixation may be necessary if adequate reduction is otherwise not possible or if there is significant accompanying soft tissue injury requiring local wound care or skin coverage. Following reduction, splint or cast immobilization is continued for 3 to 6 weeks.

Transverse Diaphyseal Fractures. These fractures are less common than fractures of the neck region. They present, however, the same array of problems regarding angulation or rotation. The treatment principles are essentially the same as those described in the preceding section.

Spiral Diaphyseal Fractures. These fractures are similar to transverse diaphyseal fractures but have a greater tendency toward shortening, instability, and malrotation.

Extra-articular Proximal Metaphyseal Fractures. Such fractures may be oblique or transverse and are usually stable. If there is not marked displacement and if rotation is satisfactory, symptomatic treatment by simple cast or splint protection for 3 to 4 weeks is satisfactory. The latter may permit metacarpophalangeal joint motion. Occasionally open or closed reduction and internal fixation with multiple Kirschner wires may be necessary.

Intra-articular Basilar Fractures. These fractures are not common in the 2nd and 3rd metacarpals (Fig. 13–103). With such injuries, however, stability of the carpometacarpal joint is the goal of treatment. Therefore, if unstable and comminuted, internal fixation, possibly with an attempt at primary arthrodesis of the carpometacarpal joint, may be necessary.

Mobile Metacarpal Rays—4th and 5th Metacarpals

Owing to the mobility of the carpometacarpal joints of the 4th and especially the 5th rays, a moderate degree of latitude for fracture-angulation is permissible in these metacarpals.[3, 7, 139] For this reason anatomic reduction is less frequently necessary. However, malrotation or excessive displacement and shortening is not acceptable.

Neck Fractures. These are the most common metacarpal fractures and are particularly likely in the 5th ray. This injury is also known as the boxer's fracture, which implies that the common mechanism of injury is a direct axial compression force over the ulnar side of a clenched fist. Displacement usually is not excessive, but characteristically there is palmar angulation of the distal fragment (Fig. 13–104). The latter usually results from the deforming effects of the interosseus muscles and extrinsic digital flexors. Fracture-angulation in the lateral plane of up to 40° in the 5th metacarpal and up to 25° in the 4th is compatible with minimal functional limitation.[3] Greater degrees of angulation may be accepted in the child with significant growth potential, provided that no malrotation is present. The lateral view is essential in determining the degree of angulation (Fig. 13–104C and D).

Reduction, when required, is generally not a problem. In the usual situation with fracture-angulation but otherwise no displacement, a dorsally directed pressure over the distal fragment with

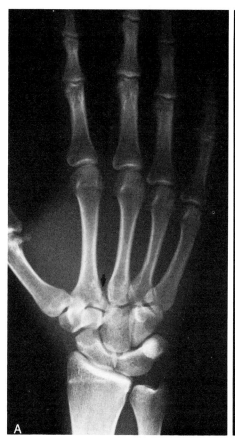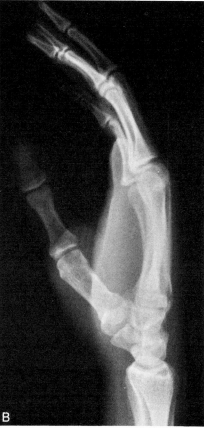

Figure 13–103. PA *(A)* and lateral *(B)* views of an intra-articular fracture *(A, arrow)* of the base of the 2nd metacarpal.

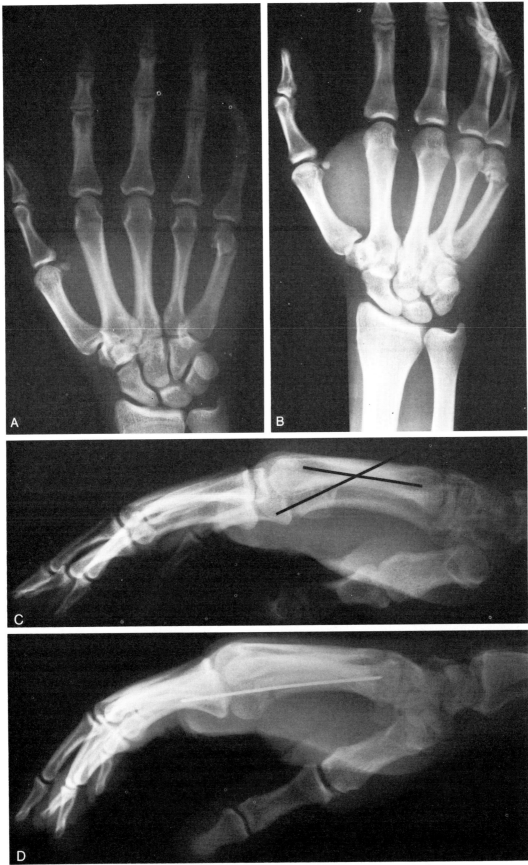

Figure 13–104. Boxer's fractures seen on the oblique *(A)* and AP *(B)* views. The degree of angulation is evaluated on the lateral view *(C)*. Following reduction with K-wire *(D)*, there is no angulation.

palmar counterpressure over the proximal fragment suffices. If complete displacement of the fracture is present, preliminary longitudinal traction may be necessary. Any malrotation must also be corrected with appropriate torsion on the distal bony fragment. Following reduction the ulnar two or three rays are immobilized in an ulnar gutter-type splint. This splint maintains the wrist in slight extension, the metacarpophalangeal joints in 60° to 70° of flexion, and the interphalangeal joints in 10° to 15° of flexion. Usually splinting is continued for about 3 weeks, followed by an additional 2 to 3 weeks of removable splint protection. Cautious active mobilization of the digits is permitted during this time. Grossly unstable fractures may require percutaneous internal fixation. This may be accomplished by the use of Kirschner wires passed transversely into the adjacent intact metacarpal or across the fracture site (Fig. 13–104D). This procedure is facilitated by the use of an image intensifier. If possible, the fixation hardware should avoid transfixing the metacarpophalangeal joint. Inability to achieve acceptable reduction by closed means, or extensive accompanying soft tissue injury, may be indications for open reduction and internal fixation with Kirschner wires or tension-band wires.

Transverse Diaphyseal Fractures. These fractures are less common but are associated with greater problems than injuries of the neck region (Fig. 13–105). Fracture union is less rapid, displacement and instability are more frequent, and angulation is less acceptable.[3, 7] The same principles of management as outlined for the neck fractures, however, are applicable to this injury.

Spiral Diaphyseal Injuries. These injuries are more prone to shortening, instability, and malrotation than transverse fractures of the mid-diaphysis (Fig. 13–106). It is not uncommon for multiple adjacent metacarpals to be affected. Internal fixation, either percutaneously or following open reduction, is frequently required.

Extra-articular Proximal Metaphyseal Fractures. These fractures are also not uncommon. They are usually impacted and stable and may be oblique or transverse. If there is no clinically apparent malrotation, reduction is rarely necessary. Because the interosseus muscles take their origin distal to the fracture, they do not represent a deforming force. Symptomatic treatment with a well molded splint or short-arm cast that permits metacarpophalangeal joint range of motion is usually adequate.

Intra-articular Basilar Fractures. Such fractures are particularly prevalent in the 5th metacarpal (see Figs. 13–102 and 13–103). In many respects this injury represents the 5th-ray counterpart of the Bennett fracture seen in the thumb.[3, 7] Instability, if

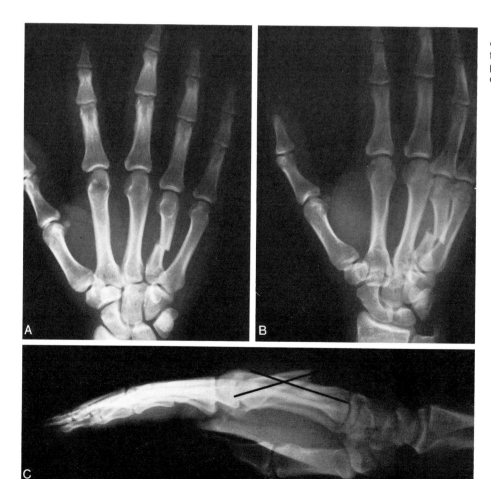

Figure 13–105. AP *(A)*, oblique *(B)*, and lateral *(C)* views of a displaced fracture of the 4th metacarpal diaphysis with shortening and dorsal angulation.

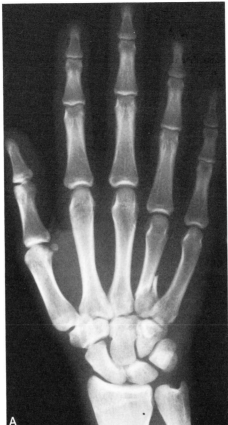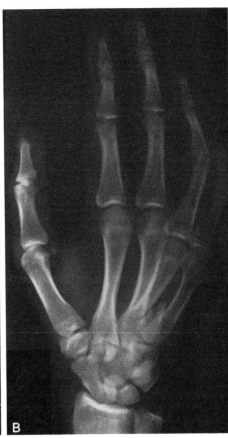

Figure 13–106. PA *(A)* and oblique *(B)* views of the hand with an overriding, shortened fracture of the proximal 4th metacarpal.

present, usually results from the pull of the extensor carpi ulnaris tendon, as it displaces the distal (metacarpal) fragment in a proximal direction. Treatment depends on the degree of articular incongruity and joint subluxation. In general, minor degrees of incongruity or subluxation are more tolerable in this case than with the same fracture type in the thumb metacarpal. However, greater amounts of articular incongruity and carpometacarpal joint subluxation are associated with greater risks of painful arthrosis. Therefore, an attempt at reduction is recommended for this injury when any obvious radiographic displacement is present. Except when impacted, this injury is frequently unstable. Therefore, percutaneous fixation with Kirschner wires should be used following reduction. In the nondisplaced or impacted fracture, immobilization for 3 to 4 weeks in an ulnar gutter-type splint, as previously described, or in a well molded short-arm cast is usually satisfactory. In such cases, however, vigilant radiographic monitoring of the fracture for the first 2 weeks is advisable to be certain that displacement within the splint or cast does not occur.

Complications of Metacarpal Fractures

The chief complications of metacarpal fractures are limited range of motion, malunion, arthrosis, and non-union. Limited joint range of motion is most commonly due to extension-contractures of the metacarpophalangeal joints and flexion-contrac-

tures of the proximal interphalangeal joints. These are often due to immobilization of the hand in an inappropriate position while awaiting fracture union. Occasionally these contractures can result from pericapsular fibrosis consequent to post-traumatic autonomic dysfunction (sympathetic dystrophy, Sudeck's atrophy). Furthermore, limited range of motion may be due to peritendinous adhesions of the extensor tendons. These may result from either associated soft tissue injury or adherence of the tendons to the fracture site.

With proper management malunion of the fracture is for the most part avoidable. Rotary malunion is the most frequent significant complication of this group. Arthrosis is mainly a complication of intraarticular fractures of the 1st or 5th metacarpal base. Non-union is unusual.

Metacarpophalangeal Joint Dislocations

Dislocations affecting the metacarpophalangeal joint are not frequent and usually are not accompanied by significant fracture. Occasionally small chip fractures at the site of collateral ligament or volar plate insertion or small shear fractures of the metacarpal head may be seen in association with this injury. Radiographically the lateral view of the involved joint is most useful. Most often the proximal phalanx is displaced dorsally relative to the metacarpal.[3, 61, 107, 112, 132] Displacement in the opposite direction has rarely been reported.[129, 156]

Dorsal Metacarpophalangeal Joint Dislocation

Dorsal metacarpophalangeal joint dislocation usually results from a hyperextension injury.[107, 112] It is most common in the thumb, where it may or may not be associated with an injury to the collateral ligaments (Fig. 13–107).[3, 66, 75, 138, 143] The dislocation may be simple or complex, with the latter term indicating an irreducible injury. Usually the volar fibrocartilaginous plate of the metacarpophalangeal joint is disrupted at its proximal attachment on the metacarpal and travels with the proximal fragment. It may be an impediment to reduction.

Most dorsal dislocations of the thumb metacarpophalangeal joint are reducible by closed means. This is most safely accomplished by initially extending the proximal phalanx and then, while maintaining this position, translating the proximal phalanx in a palmar direction. Straight longitudinal traction on the digit may impale the volar plate within the joint, thus converting a simple dislocation to a complex one.[3, 112] It should therefore be avoided. On post-reduction x-rays the joint space should be carefully evaluated. Incomplete reduction or widening of the joint space may indicate capsule or ligament interposition. Following satisfactory reduction the joint is clinically tested for stability. The period of subsequent immobilization will depend on the degree of post-reduction volar and collateral ligament stability. If the joint is markedly unstable in extension, or if a complete collateral ligament disruption is suspected, immobilization for as long as 6 weeks in a thumb-spica cast may be advisable. Failure to achieve a satisfactory closed reduction is an indication for open reduction. The most frequent complication of this injury is limitation of metacarpophalangeal joint range of motion. The most disabling complication, however, is residual ulnar or radial collateral ligament instability[138] or residual joint subluxation.

Dorsal metacarpophalangeal joint dislocation of the finger is most common in the index digit.[90, 107, 112] Unlike the thumb, a significant number of these injuries will not be amenable to closed reduction (Fig. 13–108). The same reduction maneuver and the same precautions regarding longitudinal traction as outlined above are applicable to finger metacarpophalangeal joint dislocation. If closed reduction fails, it is likely that the metacarpal head is "buttonholed" by the volar plate, the natatory ligament, and the flexor tendons and lumbrical muscle of the affected digit.[107] Open reduction of the complex dislocation is mandatory. Following reduction, the joint should be mobilized as early as the stability of the reduction permits. Preferably this should be within the first week. The most frequent late complication of dorsal metacarpophalangeal joint dislocation of the finger is limited range of motion. In contrast to the thumb, residual joint instability is infrequent and less of a functional impairment.

Volar Metacarpophalangeal Dislocation

Volar metacarpophalangeal dislocation is rare (Fig. 13–108). All reported cases have involved the fingers, and all have apparently been complex.[156] The pathologic feature blocking reduction has been variously reported as either an entrapped volar plate[129] or a dorsal capsular flap.[112, 156] The mechanism of injury has been reported as either a hyperextension injury or a hyperflexion injury with a palmar translation force. Open reduction, identification of the pathologic features, and repair of disrupted structures is advisable. Often this injury is seen late and requires either arthroplasty or arthrodesis.

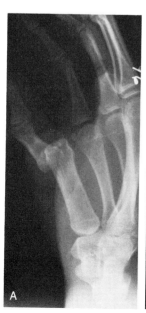
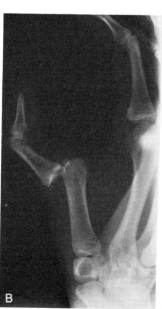
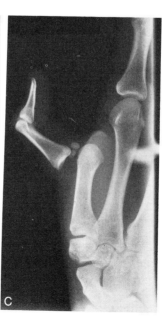

Figure 13–107. AP *(A),* oblique *(B),* and lateral *(C)* views of a dorsal dislocation of the 1st metacarpophalangeal joint.

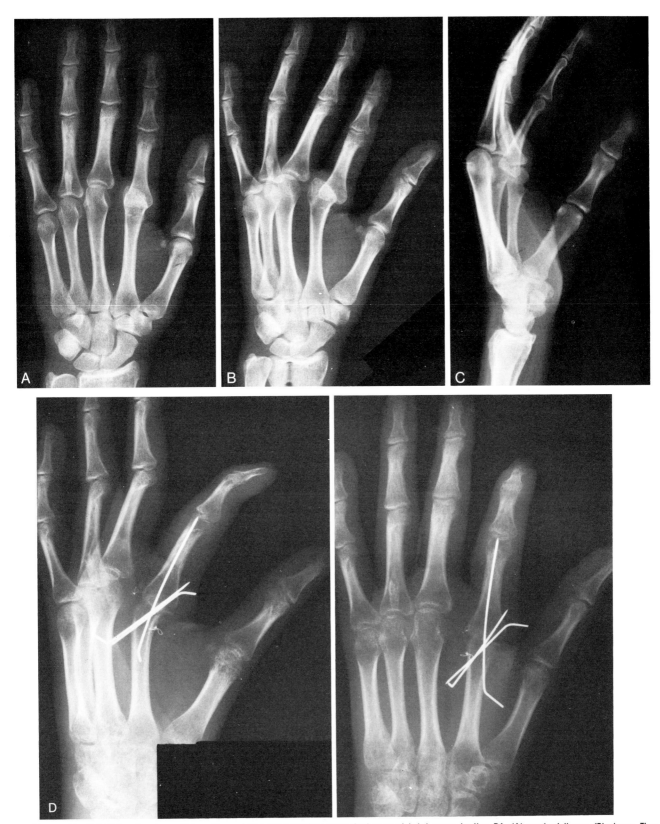

Figure 13–108. Volar fracture dislocation of the 2nd metacarpophalangeal joint seen in the PA *(A)* and oblique *(B)* views. The lateral view *(C)* is difficult to interpret owing to the bony overlap. *D,* Reduction required an arthrodesis with K-wire fixation.

Phalangeal Fractures

As a group, fractures of the phalanges are the most common fractures involving the hand.[3, 7, 68, 95, 132, 139, 144] As in the case of the metacarpals, management will depend upon a number of considerations. These include the particular phalanx fractured, the type and location of the fracture line, the degree of displacement or rotation, and the presence of associated soft tissue injury. Routine PA and lateral radiographs are usually adequate to evaluate these injuries. If possible, the involved finger should be separated from the other fingers to prevent overlap (see Figs. 13–110C and 13–116). Localized views of the injured phalanx using dental x-ray film may provide greater clarity.

Proximal Phalanx

Fractures of the proximal phalanx are more common than those of the middle or distal phalanges.[3] The adverse effects of malunion, shortening, and tendon adherence at the fracture site are more marked in the proximal phalanx than in the more distal fractures. The mechanism of injury in the proximal phalanx is widely varied and may include direct blows, sporting activities, falls, and vehicular injuries. Fractures of the proximal phalanx are best classified anatomically. Markedly comminuted fractures may have features of more than one type.

Distal Fractures. Unicondylar and bicondylar fractures of the distal portion of the proximal phalanx may be nondisplaced and appear innocuous (Fig. 13–109). However, they are frequently unstable as a result of traction on the fracture fragment from the attached collateral ligament. Furthermore, in the bicondylar type, compressive forces acting across the proximal interphalangeal joint can spread the two condyles apart. If nondisplaced, this fracture can often be adequately treated by splint protection. Complete immobilization of the digit for the first 3 weeks, however, is necessary. This usually requires a short-arm cast with attached aluminum splint. When the injury involves the ulnar two rays, an ulnar gutter-type cast or splint is required. Careful radiographic monitoring of the fracture position during this time is advised. If the fracture is displaced, there is little allowance for deviation from the normal without adversely affecting joint function. In such cases open reduction and fixation with Kirschner wires[95] or wire loop[92, 110] may be necessary (Fig. 13–109). Postoperative immobilization as outlined above should also be utilized. Protected motion of the digit may be initiated after 3 weeks. In most cases part-time splinting and avoidance of vigorous activities should be continued until 6 weeks after the injury.

Supracondylar fractures are extra-articular. If markedly displaced, they may clinically mimic a joint dislocation. If nondisplaced, the fracture is usually stable. It may be managed as outlined above for the condylar injury. If the fracture is displaced, reduction may be difficult to obtain owing to the small size of the distal fragment. However, if an anatomic reduction is accomplished, it is usually stable. If reduction is not possible by closed means, open reduction is indicated. In such cases or in cases of an unstable reduction, fixation by Kirschner wires[95] is indicated. Subsequent management is the same as outlined for the condylar fracture.

Diaphyseal Fractures. Transverse fractures of the diaphysis are quite common (Fig. 13–110). If the fractures are nondisplaced, they can almost always be managed by closed means. This usually requires a short-arm cast with an aluminum outrigger splint to maintain the wrist slightly extended, with the metacarpophalangeal joints flexed at 60° to 70° and the interphalangeal joints flexed at 10° to 15°. Angulation of the fracture, characteristically with the apex pointing in a palmar direction, is frequent (Fig. 13–111). This position results from the deforming forces of the intrinsic muscles, which act to flex the proximal fragment, and from the extrinsic extensor muscles, which act to extend the distal fragment. Angulation of more than 20° in the adult and 30° in the child should be corrected.[3, 7] If the fracture is otherwise not displaced, correction of the angulation and maintenance of reduction by an appropriate splint as outlined above are not difficult. If, however, the fracture is displaced as well as angulated, reduction may be difficult. It is most easily accomplished by applying longitudinal traction on the finger with the wrist extended, the metacarpophalangeal joints flexed, and the interphalangeal joints extended. Particular attention should be directed to proper rotatory alignment of the digit. Once the fracture is reduced, closed treatment as outlined above usually suffices. If closed reduction cannot be obtained, or if it is markedly unstable following reduction, open reduction and internal fixation with Kirschner wires or a tension-band wire loop may be indicated (Fig. 13–112). Internal fixation

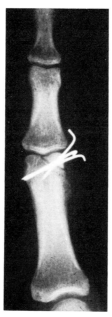

Figure 13–109. PA view of unicondylar fracture with K-wire fixation.

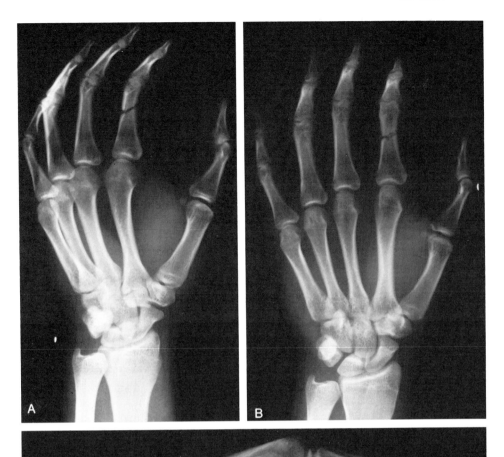

Figure 13–110. Oblique *(A)* and PA *(B)* radiographs of an undisplaced fracture of the proximal phalanx of the index finger. The lateral view *(C)* shows no angulation at the fracture site.

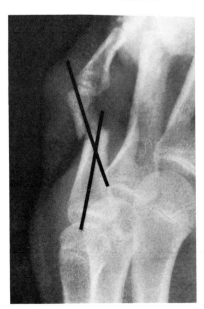

Figure 13–111. Angulated fracture of the 5th proximal phalanx. The lateral view demonstrates volar angulation.

may also be required in the unreliable patient or when significant associated soft tissue injury is present.

Spiral or oblique fractures of the diaphysis are more prone to shortening or malrotation than the transverse variety. A very long spiral fracture may extend into the epiphyseal region and impair joint motion by producing a bony block (see Fig. 13–135). Although reduction of this fracture type is not usually difficult, maintenance of reduction may be a problem. If this is the case, internal fixation by percutaneous Kirschner wires is recommended.[95] If open reduction is required, fixation by Kirschner wires, circlage wires, or small bone screws may be appropriate. The principles of management are otherwise similar to those described for the transverse diaphyseal fracture.

Proximal Fractures. Transverse fractures of the proximal metaphysis are common, particularly in the 5th digit in children. Displacement is usual, with angulation of the distal fragment dorsally and laterally and malrotation of the distal fragment in

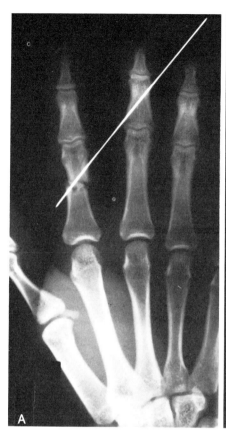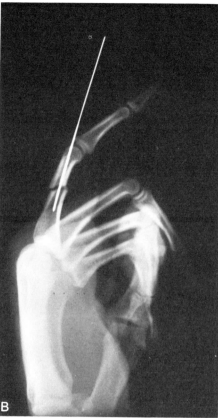

Figure 13–112. PA *(A)* and lateral *(B)* views of a fracture of the proximal phalanx with K-wire fixation. There is no angulation.

pronation. Closed reduction can usually be obtained. It is best carried out by maximally flexing the metacarpophalangeal joint to lock the small proximal fragment in position. The distal fragment may then be supinated and manipulated in a palmar and medial direction. Particular care should be taken to ensure proper rotatory reduction. Once reduced, this fracture is generally stable and should be immobilized for 3 weeks by a cast or splint in the position outlined in the preceding section. Continued part-time splint protection and limitation of activity are advisable until 6 weeks after the injury. Occasionally satisfactory closed reduction cannot be achieved. In such cases open reduction and internal fixation with Kirschner wires is recommended.

Proximal condylar fractures are more easily managed than their distal counterparts. They are usually insignificantly displaced and are often impacted and stable. If so, simple protection by taping the involved digit to its neighbor on the side of the injury may be adequate treatment. If the fragment is displaced (Fig. 13–113A), and particularly if it involves more than a third of the articular surface of the proximal phalanx, open reduction and internal fixation with Kirschner wires, a pullout suture, or a small bone screw may be necessary (Fig. 13–113B).

Proximal comminuted articular fractures are uncommon. This injury may or may not be stable. If the fracture is nondisplaced, motion of the involved metacarpophalangeal joint should be initiated as soon as the inherent stability of the fracture will permit. In such cases the clinical outcome is usually

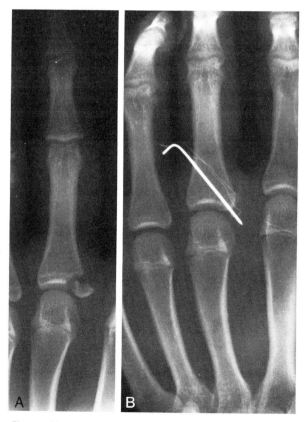

Figure 13–113. A, PA view demonstrates an intra-articular fracture of the base of the 3rd proximal phalanx. B, Radiograph demonstrating internal fixation with K-wire shows the fragment in excellent position.

favorable. If the fracture is displaced and it is feasible, an attempt to restore a congruous articular surface should be made. If the size of the major comminuted fragments is sufficient to permit purchase by a Kirschner wire, open reduction may be advisable. Otherwise longitudinal traction methods may be worthwhile, though some degree of residual arthrosis can be anticipated.

Middle Phalanx

For the most part the spectrum of fracture types seen in the middle phalanx is similar to that described for the proximal phalanx with the exception of those occurring about the base. The same general treatment principles as outlined in the preceding section apply to the middle phalanx. Moreover, in some respects management may be somewhat easier with middle phalangeal injuries. The more distal position of these fractures permits easier access for manipulative reduction and placement of percutaneous hardware. Furthermore, minor angulatory and rotatory deformity in the middle phalanx has less functional impact on the digit as a whole than a more proximally located deformity.

Volar Lip Proximal Base Fractures. In contrast to the proximal phalanx, the most common of the middle phalangeal fractures are those about the volar lip of the base. This fracture characteristically is associated with a direct axial "jamming" or hyperextension injury.[3, 7] It may be barely apparent radiographically (Fig. 13–114), or it may involve a sizeable portion of the proximal articular surface. If the latter is the case, when viewed laterally the fracture line characteristically courses obliquely in a dorsal and proximal direction. Treatment depends on the size of the bony fragment, the degree of displacement, and the presence or absence of volar proximal interphalangeal joint instability.

The small chip fracture without dorsal subluxation or volar instability (Fig. 13–114) may be treated symptomatically with a monarticular finger splint to rest the proximal interphalangeal joint in 20° to 30° of flexion. Range of motion exercises of the joint should be initiated early to prevent the develop-

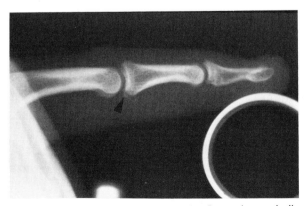

Figure 13–114. Lateral view of the index finger demonstrating a small volar plate fracture of the middle phalanx *(arrow)*.

ment of a flexion-contracture if there is no associated collateral ligament disruption. The recovery period with this injury may be surprisingly prolonged and depends upon the amount of associated traumatic joint synovitis.

The small chip fracture with either dorsal subluxation or significant volar instability of the proximal interphalangeal joint demands a considerably more vigilant management approach. In these cases the avoidance of subluxation of the joint takes precedence over the radiographic appearance of the volar chip fracture.[3, 7, 58, 65, 115] Indeed, the most significant pathologic lesion with this injury involves the volar fibrocartilaginous plate, which is not radiographically obvious.[65] This injury must be maintained in the minimum degree of flexion to prevent dorsal proximal interphalangeal joint subluxation. If the joint is statically splinted in this flexed position, there is a substantial risk of residual joint contracture. Therefore, management by extension block splinting is recommended.[3, 7, 115] This technique permits active proximal interphalangeal joint motion and full flexion but blocks extension just short of that which will allow dorsal joint subluxation. Over the 3- to 6-week period of treatment the degree of extension block is progressively diminished commensurate with healing and re-establishment of volar stability.

Management of the large volar lip fracture (Fig. 13–115) will depend upon the same joint instability considerations as well as factors related to articular surface incongruity. In general, displaced or undisplaced fractures involving less than one third of the articular surface may be managed in a manner similar to the small chip fracture. However, displaced fractures involving one third or more of the articular surface should be reduced with restoration of the articular congruity by either closed or open means.[155] Following reduction, management by extension block splinting, as outlined above, is recommended. The nondisplaced volar lip fracture involving more than a third of the articular surface is treated the same way.

The most significant complication of volar lip fractures of the middle phalanx is dorsal subluxation of the proximal interphalangeal joint (Fig. 13–115).[3, 7] This subluxation may result from inadequate treatment, failure to recognize joint subluxation in the course of treatment, or incorrect treatment by immobilization of the joint in full extension. The consequence of a dorsally subluxed joint is painful limitation of proximal interphalangeal joint motion.[58] An array of other complications may be seen with this fracture, the most common of which is limitation of joint motion as a result of capsular contracture. Late arthrosis as a result of a displaced articular fragment involving more than a third of the joint surface or traumatic chondrolysis is not infrequent. Finally, recurrent locking of the proximal interphalangeal joint in hyperextension may result from mild volar instability in the absence of dorsal joint subluxation.

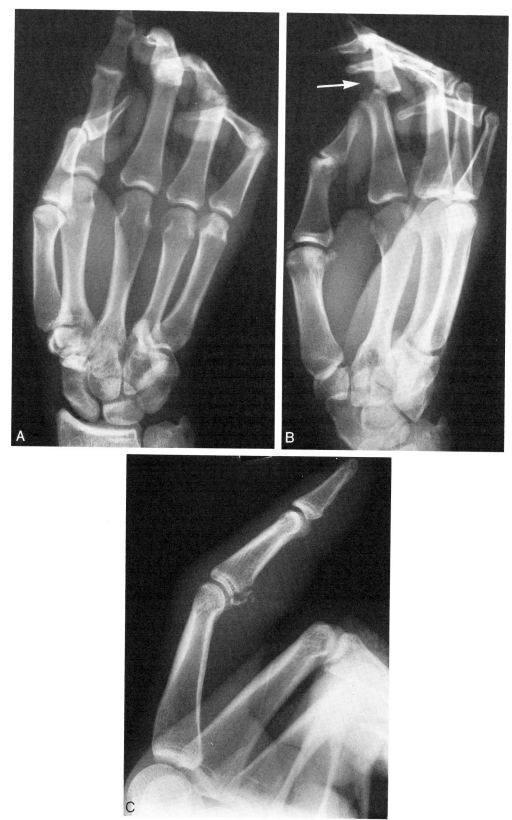

Figure 13–115. AP *(A)* and oblique *(B)* views of the right hand reveal a dorsal dislocation of the 2nd proximal interphalangeal joint *(B, arrow)*. There is also a chip fracture of the base of the 3rd proximal phalanx and a flexion deformity of the 5th proximal interphalangeal joint. Following reduction, the true lateral view *(C)* demonstrates the associated volar plate fracture.

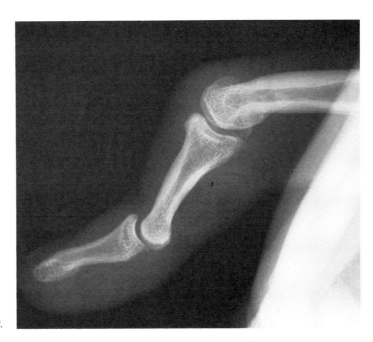

Figure 13–116. Boutonnière deformity.

Dorsal Lip Proximal Base Fractures. This fracture of the middle phalanx is much less common than the volar lip variety. However, it also demands a cautious approach. Usually this injury involves the insertion of the central extensor slip. If it is untreated or treated incorrectly, a boutonnière deformity of the proximal interphalangeal joint may result.[7, 132] This deformity is characterized by a flexion-contracture of the proximal interphalangeal joint and a hyperextension deformity of the distal interphalangeal joint due to an acquired imbalance of the extensor apparatus (Fig. 13–116). In addition to disruption of the extensor insertion into the middle phalanx, dorsal lip fractures may rarely be associated with volar subluxation of the proximal interphalangeal joint.

Appropriate management of the dorsal lip fracture will depend upon the size and degree of displacement of the fracture fragment, the integrity of the extensor mechanism, and the presence or absence of joint subluxation. The most frequent error of management is failure to distinguish this injury from the volar lip variety and to apply a splint that maintains the joint in a flexed position. This will result in further compromise of the extensor apparatus and will encourage fracture-displacement as well as volar joint subluxation. A small fracture fragment with or without displacement and with a complete, active proximal interphalangeal joint extension can be managed by monarticular splinting of the proximal interphalangeal joint in complete extension for 3 to 4 weeks. A patient with a similar fracture who is unable to actively extend the proximal interphalangeal joint completely most likely has disruption of the extensor mechanism. If maintenance of the joint in extension when it is passively straightened is possible, then management by splinting as described above is advised. In

this case, however, splinting should be continued for at least 6 to 8 weeks. In the case of a large fracture fragment (over a third of the articular surface), the fracture should be reduced closed, if possible, and splinted in extension until bony union is present. If closed reduction is not possible in patients unable to sustain the proximal interphalangeal joint in extension, or if volar proximal interphalangeal joint subluxation is present, then open reduction is recommended. Fixation of the dorsal lip fragment in such cases is usually possible with a pullout wire or with fine Kirschner wires. Complications of the dorsal lip fracture include joint contracture, boutonnière deformity, residual volar joint subluxation, and late joint arthrosis.

Comminuted Fractures of the Base. This injury may involve components of both dorsal and volar lip fractures as well as diffuse involvement of the proximal articular surface of the middle phalanx. Management considerations should be directed by restoration of a congruous articular surface without residual joint subluxation. Often this type of fracture may be so comminuted that little can be done to prevent late degenerative joint arthrosis. Treatment should be tailored to the patient and may include simple splinting, skeletal traction,[58] or open reduction and internal fixation.

Distal Phalanx

Fractures of the distal phalanx are extremely common, but with few exceptions these require little in the way of treatment and are not associated with a high incidence of disabling sequelae.

Tuft Fractures. These fractures are the most frequent injury to the distal phalanx (Fig. 13–117). The true incidence of the fracture is unknown because it may not be accompanied by pain sufficient to

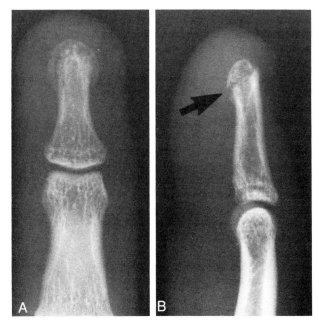

Figure 13–117. PA *(A)* and lateral *(B)* views of a minimally displaced tuft fracture of the distal phalanx.

warrant x-ray evaluation. Most often the mechanism of injury is a blunt crush to the fingertip. Frequently these fractures are accompanied by a nail-bed laceration, a nail-root avulsion, or a subungual hematoma that may obscure the underlying bony injury. Displacement may be present, particularly if there is a significant nail-bed laceration. However, most cases are minimally displaced and comminuted. They are often well stabilized by the overlying nail plate and the strong fibrous septa that characterize the fingertip tuft. Treatment is symptomatic, usually utilizing a thimble-type splint, and should be directed to any accompanying nail-bed injury. The latter may exceptionally require a manual "compressive" reduction of the bony injury. Tenderness in the fingertip may persist for some time and bear little relationship to the progress of fracture union. Non-union of the fracture may occur but is only rarely symptomatic. If it is, however, excision of the non-united fragment is usually curative.

Transverse Fractures. Transverse fractures of the distal phalanx are distinguished from tuft fractures by the absence of distal comminution. The mechanism of injury, however, is similar. These fractures are also often associated with nail-bed lacerations and nail-root avulsion. Reduction of the fracture usually facilitates management of the nail-bed injury. If the fracture is quite unstable, fixation with a fine smooth Kirschner wire may be helpful in the course of management of the nail-bed laceration. A variation of this injury, seen not infrequently in the child, is a displaced epiphyseal (Salter I or II) fracture of the distal phalanx (Fig. 13–118). An awareness of this fracture is quite important, since it is usually an open injury with displacement of the nail root. The unwary may mistakenly interpret

it as a mallet-finger deformity. In such cases, deep bony sepsis and a permanent nail deformity may result. Proper treatment requires thorough debridement, fracture reduction, relocation or excision of the nail root, and appropriate splinting.

Proximal Base Fractures. Like fractures of the middle phalanx, proximal base fractures of the distal phalanx are important. In contrast to the middle phalanx, however, the dorsal lip fracture of the distal phalanx is of the greatest clinical significance.

Dorsal Lip Fractures. Fractures of the dorsal lip of the distal phalanx constitute one of several members of the mallet-finger spectrum of injuries (Fig. 13–119). The terminal portion of the extensor apparatus of the finger is inserted into the dorsal lip region. Consequently a displaced fracture will result in the inability to extend the distal phalanx completely. The mechanism of injury is most commonly a hyperflexion stress applied to the distal phalanx.[3, 7, 132] Presumably in such a situation avulsion of the dorsal lip of the distal phalanx results from the pull of the extensor tendon, or else rupture of the extensor tendon itself occurs. Treatment of this injury depends primarily upon the size of the dorsal lip fragment and the presence or absence of volar joint subluxation.

A small dorsal lip fragment constituting less than 30 percent of the articular surface of the distal phalanx can usually be managed with closed techniques. Acceptable reduction is generally possible by simple distal interphalangeal joint hyperextension. Some authors feel that radiographic reduction of the bony fragment is irrelevant to the clinical result. An initial period of 3 to 4 weeks of biarticular splinting, with the proximal interphalangeal joint in 20° to 30° of flexion and the distal interphalangeal joint in maximum supple hyperextension, is our preference. This period is followed by monarticular splinting of the distal interphalangeal joint in com-

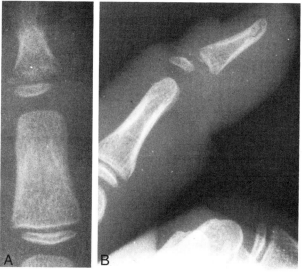

Figure 13–118. PA *(A)* and lateral *(B)* views of a displaced Salter II fracture of the distal phalanx.

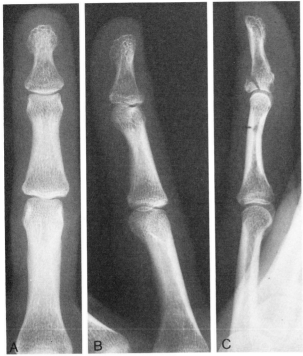

Figure 13–119. PA *(A)*, oblique *(B)*, and lateral *(C)* views of the 4th finger. The dorsal plate fracture is only clearly seen on the lateral view.

Dorsal lip fractures involving 30 percent or more of the articular surface should be reduced with restoration of articular congruity. If a satisfactory reduction is possible by simple hyperextension of the distal phalanx, further closed management as outlined above is acceptable. Failure to achieve congruous articular reduction, however, may be an indication for open reduction and fixation of the fracture, either by a pullout wire or by a Kirschner wire. Rarely volar subluxation of the distal phalanx may be associated with a large dorsal lip fracture. If this subluxation is present, the indications for open reduction and fixation are increased.

Volar Lip Fracture. Except in the thumb, volar lip fractures of the distal phalanx are unusual. They may or may not be associated with a large bony fragment and avulsion of the insertion of the flexor digitorum profundus tendon[108, 128, 152] (Fig. 13–120). If the latter occurs, dorsal subluxation of the distal interphalangeal joint may be present. Treatment usually depends on the presence or absence of associated flexor tendon injury. With an intact flexor tendon, simple monarticular symptomatic splinting of the distal interphalangeal joint in 20° to 30° of flexion is usually sufficient. The length of splint protection will depend upon any associated collateral ligament injury and the degree of traumatic synovitis. Late complications are unusual. If there is associated flexor tendon injury, tenorrhaphy or open reduction of an attached bony fragment is indicated. Late complications may occur and are usually related to dysfunction of the flexor apparatus.[108, 128, 152]

Comminuted Proximal Base Fractures. Comminuted fractures of the base of the distal phalanx may be seen. Treatment considerations are similar to those outlined for the same injury affecting the

plete extension or slight hyperextension for an additional 4 to 6 weeks. A further period of 3 to 4 weeks of monarticular night splinting is often helpful. The duration of splinting will vary but should be determined by the degree of tenderness at the fracture site, the integrity of distal interphalangeal joint extension, and the radiographic progress of fracture union.

Figure 13–120. PA *(A)* and lateral *(B)* views of dorsal dislocation of the 5th proximal interphalangeal joint with a volar plate fracture (50 per cent of articular surface).

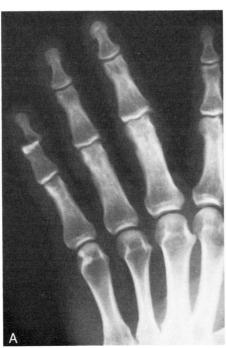
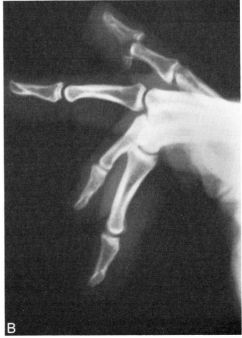

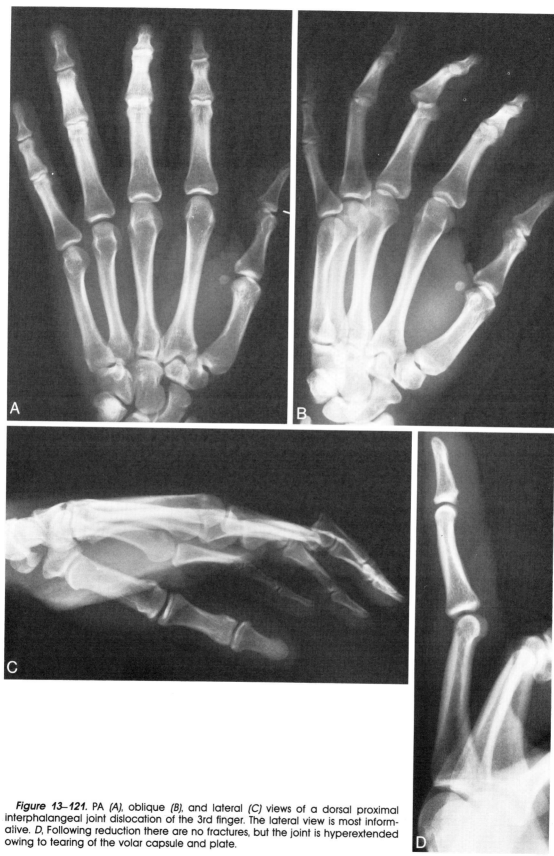

Figure 13–121. PA *(A)*, oblique *(B)*, and lateral *(C)* views of a dorsal proximal interphalangeal joint dislocation of the 3rd finger. The lateral view is most inform-ative. *D*, Following reduction there are no fractures, but the joint is hyperextended owing to tearing of the volar capsule and plate.

middle phalanx. However, in contrast to the middle phalanx, arthrodesis of the distal interphalangeal joint is often a viable and functionally satisfactory option in the highly comminuted fracture.

Complications of Phalangeal Fractures

General complications of phalangeal fractures are essentially the same as those involved in metacarpal fractures. These include limitation of range of motion, malunion, and non-union.[3] Complications peculiar to specific fracture types have been discussed in the preceding sections.

Dislocations of the Interphalangeal Joints

Dislocations affecting the proximal interphalangeal joint are extremely common.[3, 7, 115, 132] Less frequently this injury may occur in the distal interphalangeal joint. Often there may be accompanying bony injury, as in the dorsal or volar lip fractures of the middle phalanx discussed in the preceding sections. The dislocation almost always involves dorsal displacement of the middle on the proximal phalanx.

Dorsal Proximal Interphalangeal Dislocation

Dorsal proximal interphalangeal dislocation usually results from an axial compression or hyperextension injury to the fingertip (Fig. 13–121). In the absence of a displaced volar lip fracture there is disruption of the volar cartilaginous plate[65] and varying degrees of collateral ligament injury. Occasionally it is an open injury with a transverse palmar laceration. Reduction is usually possible by a maneuver identical to that described for dorsal dislocations of the metacarpophalangeal joints. Rarely the injury will be complex and require open reduction.

Following reduction, further management will be determined by the stability of the volar and collateral ligament structures. If the joint is stable in all planes, early mobilization is recommended, but the joint should be protected from repeat injury for at least 3 weeks. Collateral ligament instability may warrant splint immobilization of the proximal interphalangeal joint in 20° to 30° of flexion for 2 to 3 weeks followed by an additional 2 to 3 weeks of "buddy taping" to the neighboring finger. Volar instability may warrant the treatment approach outlined earlier for volar lip fractures of the middle phalanx, which is associated with dorsal proximal interphalangeal joint subluxation.

The most common complication of this injury is a residual flexion-contracture due to periarticular fibrosis. The most significant complication, however, is unrecognized dorsal joint subluxation and secondary arthrosis (Fig. 13–122). Occasionally recurrent volar instability may result with locking of

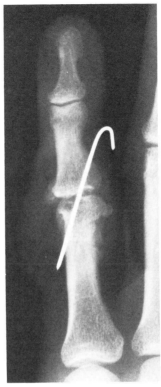

Figure 13–122. PA view of the left small finger following repair of instability. Note the severe degenerative change from improper treatment of the previous dislocation.

the digit in hyperextension, as described for the middle phalanx volar lip fracture.

Volar Proximal Interphalangeal Joint Dislocation

Volar proximal interphalangeal joint dislocation is rare and almost always associated with a displaced dorsal lip fracture of the middle phalanx. It usually results from a hyperflexion injury to the digit. Treatment should be operative with repair of the disrupted bony and soft tissue structures.

CHRONIC POST-TRAUMATIC CONDITIONS

The vast majority of traumatic afflictions of the hand and wrist have been discussed in the preceding section. There are in addition to this, however, a number of conditions of radiographic significance that are chronic and post-traumatic in origin. These are diagnosed or become symptomatic after one or more minor traumatic events.

Madelung's Deformity

Madelung's deformity is characterized by an exaggerated ulnar and volar inclination of the articular surface of the distal radius.[2] It is usually associated with a positive ulnar variance and a dorsal subluxation of the distal ulna (Fig. 13–123). This deformity

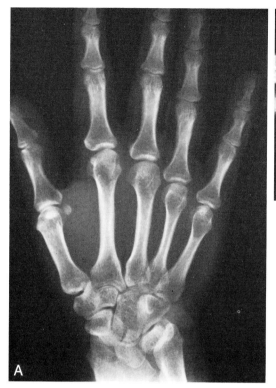

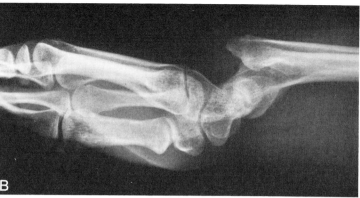

Figure 13–123. Madelung's deformity: PA *(A)* and lateral *(B)* views demonstrate marked ulnar and volar angulation of the distal radioarticular surface.

results from a deficiency of longitudinal growth of the most ulnar aspect of the distal radius. Most cases are probably congenital as a variant of epiphyseal dysplasia. However, in some cases direct trauma to the physis of the distal radius with a resultant asymmetric arrest of growth has been postulated.

Regardless of etiology, the diagnosis of Madelung's deformity is often made on the basis of a wrist x-ray obtained because of the complaint of wrist pain. Frequently the pain will be of an insidious onset, but it may also follow relatively minor repetitive trauma. Occasionally the presenting clinical complaint will be related to deformity or limitation of wrist motion. Surgical correction of the established deformity is only occasionally indicated[2, 3] and is limited to those cases with persistent wrist pain. This may involve excision of the subluxated distal ulna[82] or corrective osteotomy of the distal radius with or without distal ulna resection. If seen very early while the physis of the distal radius is still open, consideration can be given to radial dorsal epiphysiodesis or ulnar volar epiphysiolysis. Madelung's deformity may remain asymptomatic or only minimally symptomatic and be discovered as an incidental radiographic finding.

Tears and Disorders of the Triangular Fibrocartilage Complex

Tears of the triangular fibrocartilage complex may be diagnosed by wrist contrast arthrography (see Arthrography of the Wrist and Hand). These tears are characterized by communication of contrast material between the radiocarpal articulation and the distal radioulnar joint (see Figs. 13–42 and 13–47). The injury regularly occurs with certain more obvious conditions previously discussed (subluxation-dislocation of the distal radioulnar joint and most perilunate dislocations). However, triangular fibrocartilage complex tears are also common as an isolated entity.[15, 17] They may result from a single traumatic event or as an attritional tear from repetitive trauma. The true incidence of triangular fibrocartilage complex tears and the frequency of symptoms is unknown. The most common presenting complaint is pain over the ulnar aspect of the wrist with or without a "click," or crepitus. Treatment should be tailored to the patient and will range from symptomatic nonoperative management to surgical excision of a torn central fragment or repair of a peripheral rent.[17]

Ulnolunate Abutment Syndrome

The ulnolunate abutment syndrome may present with normal radiographs. However, a positive ulnar variance (see Fig. 13–3) and perhaps reactive changes over the ulnar articulation of the lunate may be present. The latter is characterized by either bony sclerosis or intraosseous cyst formation and, if present, is best visualized by trispiral tomograms (Fig. 13–124). Typically with this condition a bone scan may show increased scintillation activity about the ulnolunate region. In most cases a central perforation of the triangular fibrocartilage disk is present at the point of contact between the lunate and ulna.[17] Presumably this perforation is the result of

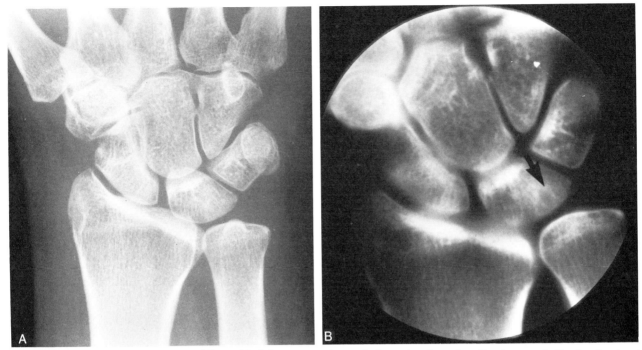

Figure 13–124. A, Normal PA view of the wrist. B, Tomogram demonstrates sclerosis and cystic changes in the lunate due to ulnolunate abutment syndrome.

attritional changes and should not be mistaken as the primary pathology. The most common clinical presentation with the ulnolunate abutment syndrome is pain over the ulnar aspect of the wrist. Although symptoms may be heralded by a single traumatic event, more often they occur insidiously or with a history of minor repetitive trauma. In most cases a trial period of nonoperative symptomatic treatment is warranted. However, if significant pain persists, surgical management by ulnar recession to a position of slight negative ulnar variance is warranted. In such cases the triangular fibrocartilage perforation may be ignored.

Avascular Necrosis of the Lunate (Lunatomalacia, Kienböck's Disease)[162, 163]

Kienböck's disease is not an uncommon cause of vague wrist pain, which may range from an annoying to a disabling degree. It may be associated with a single traumatic episode, and if so it is usually a result of a fall onto the outstretched wrist or a hyperextension injury. Conversely, the onset may be insidious or associated with repetitive minor trauma. In the early stages, routine radiographs may be normal. Later progressive x-ray changes occur. These are characterized initially by increased radiodensity of the lunate relative to the remaining carpal bones (Fig. 13–125).[160] Later, fragmentation and flattening may be seen. These ultimately progress to reconstitution and secondary osteoarthritic changes (Fig. 13–126). Lichtman has classified these radiographic changes for treatment purposes into four stages, as outlined in Table 13–4.[166]

The course of the progression of these changes

may be modified at any time, depending upon the speed of the revascularization process and the adequacy of bony reconstitution prior to marked collapse. Trispiral tomography is particularly useful for defining the radiographic changes (Fig. 13–126). Furthermore, in a few cases trispiral tomograms have revealed horizontal fracture lines following a traumatic episode prior to the development of the typical radiographic changes described above.[159] This finding has led some to postulate an acute fracture with consequent injury to the intraosseous

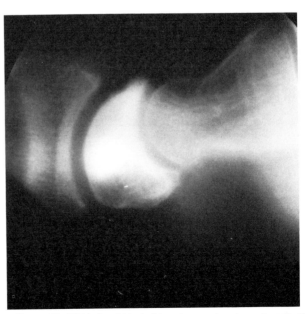

Figure 13–125. Lateral trispiral tomogram showing sclerosis of the lower lunate due to Keinböck's disease.

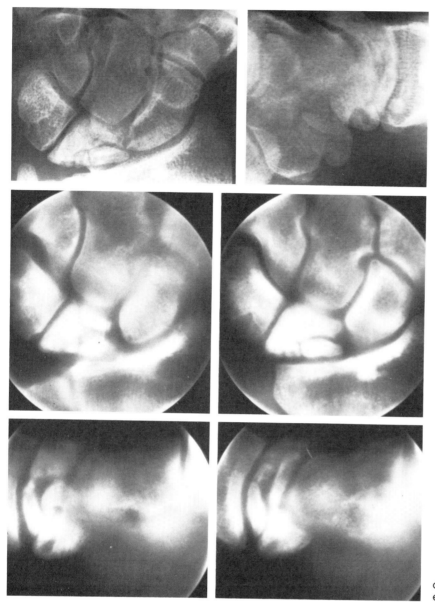

Figure 13–126. AP and lateral trispiral tomograms showing Stage III Keinböck's disease.

blood supply as the etiology of Kienböck's disease. An unusually high incidence of negative ulnar variance[5] has also been noted with this condition. This association has prompted others to postulate that the etiology of Kienböck's disease is a compression–stress concentration on the lunate by the distal

TABLE 13–4. Lichtman Classification of Stages of Kienböck's Disease

Stage I	Normal radiographic architecture and bone density. May be linear or compression fracture.
Stage II	Increased sclerosis of the lunate, but size, shape, and anatomic relationship of the bones not altered.
Stage III	Lunate collapse present with associated proximal migration of capitate and disruption of carpal architecture.
Stage IV	As in Stage III with generalized degenerative joint changes in the carpus.

radius without adequate ulnar support. Additionally, there are a number of cases without significant trauma, radiographic evidence of acute fracture, or negative ulnar variance. The etiology in these cases is unclear but appears in some way related to an intraosseous vascular insult.

Clinically most patients present with symptoms of wrist pain, but a relatively painless limitation of the wrist's range of motion or weakness of grip may also occur. With collapse of the lunate in later stages, symptoms of median neuropathy may predominate.[159] Occasionally the diagnosis is made as an incidental radiographic finding in a patient with an unrelated problem.

Treatment will vary with the stage of the disease and the severity of symptoms. Symptomatic nonoperative support is frequently adequate.[159, 162] However, if symptoms persist and limit function, surgical management should be considered. If bony collapse is not extreme and secondary degenerative changes are not present, procedures to decrease compressive loads or to alleviate stress concentrations on the lunate appear to be efficacious. These procedures may involve ulnar lengthening,[170, 175] radial shortening,[3] or scaphotrapezoidotrapezial arthrodesis.[3] If limited perilunate degenerative joint changes are present, Silastic or soft tissue lunate arthroplasty[159, 166, 173] appears worthwhile. With more advanced degenerative changes, total wrist arthroplasty, arthrodesis, or proximal row carpectomy[159, 161] may be required.

Avascular Necrosis of the Scaphoid (Preiser's Disease)

Avascular necrosis of the proximal portion of the scaphoid following fracture is relatively frequent and has been discussed earlier in this chapter. However, in the absence of a fracture or dislocation, avascular necrosis of the scaphoid is rare.[2, 3] Radiographically it is characterized by an increased radiopacity relative to the adjacent carpal bones.[160] Later fragmentation, bony collapse, and secondary degenerative arthritis may occur. In all suspected cases, trispiral tomography using 1- to 2-mm cuts through the scaphoid should be carried out to rule out an unrecognized scaphoid fracture (see Fig. 13–82). Treatment principles are similar to those outlined for the lunate.

Scapholunate Dissociation

Scapholunate dissociation (Fig. 13–127) is also not uncommon, but the diagnosis of this condition is frequently overlooked. For this reason it is often seen late, months or years after the original injury. Many authors regard scapholunate dissociation as the initial pathologic phase of the perilunate-dislocation spectrum of injuries.[96, 114] The mechanism of injury leading to scapholunate dissociation is usually one of wrist hyperextension resulting in at least a partial disruption of the volar radiocarpal ligament complex and scapholunate interosseous ligament.

Routine PA and lateral x-rays of the wrist may suggest the diagnosis but are often inadequate. For this reason we recommend a series of seven x-ray projections to define or rule out the diagnosis of scapholunate dissociation. This series[2, 3, 13, 167, 169] includes

"Palm-up" projections:	1. full ulnar deviation of wrist 2. neutral 3. full radial deviation of wrist 4. clenched-fist position
True lateral projections:	5. full-wrist palmar flexion 6. neutral 7. full-wrist dorsal flexion

The diagnosis of scapholunate dissociation is made by any of a number of characteristic x-ray findings. The most important finding is a diastasis exceeding 2 mm between the scaphoid and the

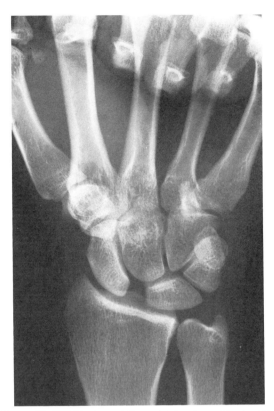

Figure 13–127. PA view of the wrist showing widening of the scapholunate space due to scapholunate dissociation.

lunate on any of the PA projections (Fig. 13–127).[13] This finding has been given the eponym of "Terry-Thomas sign" in recognition of the dental peculiarities of this British comedian.[2] The first-compression view is perhaps the most important in this regard. Supportive findings on the PA view should include a "ring sign" of the scaphoid as a result of the x-ray shadow of the scaphoid tubercle when viewed vertically (Fig. 13–128).[36, 89] The lunate may appear more triangular than quadrilateral. Furthermore, the opposing surfaces of the lunate and scaphoid may lose their parallel relationship and instead may appear to define a triangular space (Fig. 13–129). The carpal height is diminished. On the lateral projection of the wrist in neutral position there is usually a dorsiflexion-instability pattern (see Fig. 13–10), and in any of the lateral views the scapholunate angle may approach 90°. The supportive x-ray findings are particularly helpful when the scapholunate diastasis on the PA view is equivocal or falls within normal ranges.

The treatment of scapholunate dissociation is almost always surgical, particularly in the young patient prior to development of secondary degenerative changes. A detailed discussion of the array of surgical management options available for this condition is beyond the scope of this chapter. However, most involve the principle of scapholunate reduction and stabilization by tendon repair, reconstruction, or intercarpal arthrodesis (Fig. 13–130).[169, 174] If seen early and if a satisfactory closed

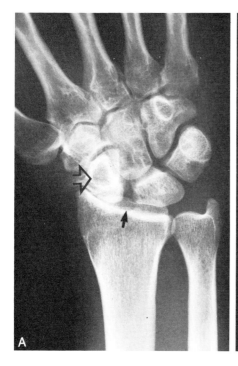
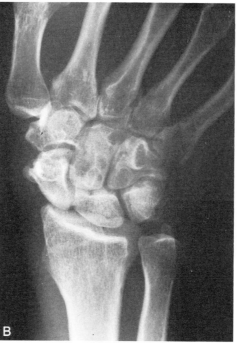

Figure 13-128. Old wrist injury with scapholunate dissociation. There is widening of the scapho-lunate space with radial deviation *(A).* The abnormality is less obvious with ulnar deviation of the wrist *(B).* Note the ring sign *(A, open arrow).*

manipulative reduction can be achieved, percutaneous fixation with multiple Kirschner wires and prolonged cast immobilization may be appropriate. If the condition is seen late and particularly if it is accompanied by degenerative joint changes, treatment will depend upon the level of symptoms. If pain is relatively minimal and not disabling, symptomatic nonoperative management is satisfactory. Those with more marked symptoms may require limited or total wrist arthrodesis, wrist arthroplasty, or proximal row carpectomy.

Lunotriquetral Instability

Lunotriquetral instability is less clearly defined than scapholunate instability but may be more common than previously appreciated. The diagnosis is usually made on the basis of the seven-projection

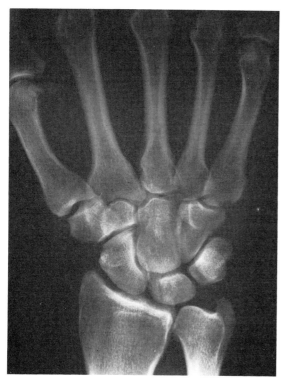

Figure 13-129. PA view of the wrist showing a triangular scapholunate joint.

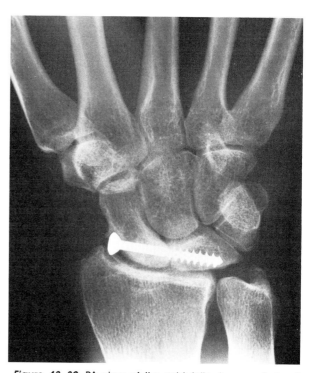

Figure 13-30. PA view of the wrist following scapholunate arthrodesis with screw fixation.

x-ray series previously described or by fluoroscopic examination of the wrist using cinematography or videotape. Unlike its scapholunate counterpart, a frank dissociation or diastasis between the lunate and triquetrum on the PA films is not often seen. However, on the lateral view a volar flexion-instability pattern in neutral position and a marked diminution of the scapholunate angle to less than 30° on at least one view is highly suggestive of this condition (see Fig. 13–11).[2] Arthrographic demonstration of contrast-material communication between the proximal and midcarpal joints through the lunotriquetral interval helps support the diagnosis (see Fig. 13–42). The principles of management are similar to those outlined for scapholunate instability.

Carpe Bosseau

Carpe bosseau is not a common deformity. It is clinically characterized by a firm mass or enlargement over the dorsum of the hand in the region of the 2nd or 3rd carpometacarpal joint.[157] The mass may or may not be painful or locally tender and is frequently mistaken for a ganglion cyst. Most authors agree that the "apparent" mass is actually a hypertrophic lipping of the 2nd or 3rd carpometacarpal joint (Fig. 13–131). It is usually associated with an acquired post-traumatic laxity of the respective carpometacarpal joints.[8] In some instances this condition has been attributed to a non-united chip fracture of the base of the 2nd or 3rd metacarpal, a congenital assessory ossicle,[158, 165] periostitis at the site of insertion of the radial wrist extensor tendons, or peritendinitis calcarea. If these latter etiologic factors occur, it is probably in the minority of cases. The carpe bosseau may be difficult to demonstrate on routine PA and lateral radiographs.

Oblique projection views, however, are often helpful. Lateral trispiral tomograms, although providing excellent visualization of the 2nd and 3rd carpometacarpal regions, are usually not necessary. Treatment will vary with the individual. The condition may be asymptomatic and represent a diagnostic problem only. Those cases with relatively mild pain and tenderness or of recent onset may require only local steroid injection. This is particularly true if periostitis or peritendinitis calcarea is thought to be an etiologic factor in the case. If pain is more marked and chronic, surgical treatment may be necessary. In such cases excision of a non-united chip fracture or accessory ossicle may be all that is required. However, in the more usual case in which the condition is due to carpometacarpal joint instability, arthrodesis of the involved carpometacarpal joint and dorsal cheilectomy of the hypertrophic marginal bone spur is the most reliable treatment.[2, 3, 8]

Turret Exostoses of the Phalanges

A phalangeal turret exostosis is a dorsal bony prominence of the middle or proximal phalanx that occasionally may be confused with a neoplasm.[3] It is post-traumatic in origin and is usually attributed to a blunt blow to the dorsum of the involved phalanx. It may result from ossification of a subperiosteal hematoma from any cause.

Boutonnière Deformity

The boutonnière deformity has been mentioned earlier in connection with fractures of the dorsal lip of the middle phalanx or volar dislocation of the proximal interphalangeal joint (Fig. 13–116). In most cases this deformity is not associated with either

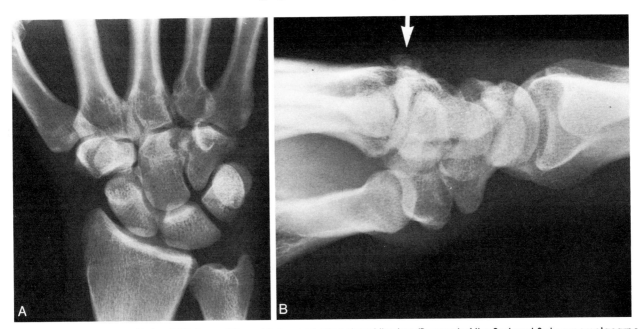

Figure 13–131. AP *(A)* and lateral *(B)* views of the wrist demonstrating dorsal lipping *(B, arrow)* of the 2nd and 3rd carpometacarpal joints (carpe bosseau).

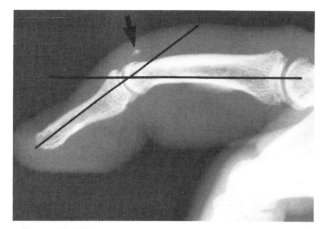

Figure 13–132. Lateral view of the finger demonstrates a small dorsal chip *(arrow)* with flexion of the distal interphalangeal joint (mallet deformity).

fracture or dislocation and results instead from a soft tissue injury at the insertion of the extensor central slip over the proximal interphalangeal joint.[65, 132, 139, 168, 171, 172] The mechanism of injury may be (1) a hyperflexion stress to the proximal interphalangeal joint, resulting in closed rupture of the extensor apparatus; (2) a gradual attenuation of the extensor apparatus from longstanding proximal interphalangeal joint synovitis; or (3) an open injury to the extensor apparatus over the proximal interphalangeal joint by penetrating trauma or a deep dorsal burn. The resultant deformity, when established, is characterized by a flexion-contracture of the proximal interphalangeal joint in association with a hyperextension-contracture of the distal interphalangeal joint. If the deformity is longstanding, secondary structural changes as a result of the joint contractures may be seen at either interphalangeal joint.[164] The same principles of treatment outlined for nondisplaced small dorsal lip fractures of the middle phalanx apply to this injury in the acute

or recent case. A discussion of treatment options for a chronic boutonnière deformity, however, is beyond the scope of this chapter.

Mallet Deformity (Baseball Finger)

Mallet-finger deformity has been previously mentioned in connection with fractures of the dorsal lip of the distal phalanx.[132, 139, 171] This same deformity is also frequently seen in the absence of fracture as a result of a rupture of the extensor tendon near its insertion into the distal phalanx. The mechanism of injury is usually a hyperflexion stress to the distal phalanx or a blow to the tip of the finger. This injury is especially common in sports. The mallet deformity is characterized by a flexion posture of the distal interphalangeal joint (Fig. 13–132). There may be varying degrees of hyperextension of the proximal interphalangeal joint, particularly in individuals with volar laxity of this joint. The same treatment principles outlined for small dorsal lip fractures of the distal phalanx apply to this injury in the acute or recent case. A discussion of late reconstructive procedures for a chronic deformity of this sort, however, is beyond the scope of this chapter.

Avascular Necrosis of Metacarpal Head

Rarely avascular necrosis of the metacarpal head following trauma can be seen in the absence of fracture. It is characterized radiographically by fragmentation and collapse of a portion of the metacarpal head (Fig. 13–133). Treatment will vary according to the digit involved, the age of the patient, and the extent of collapse and articular disruption.

Post-traumatic Degenerative Arthritis

Post-traumatic degenerative arthritis is common in the hand and wrist. It is particularly prevalent in

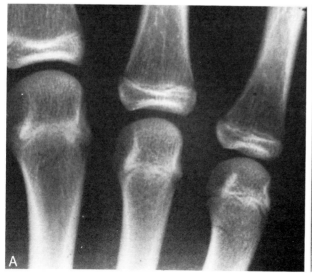 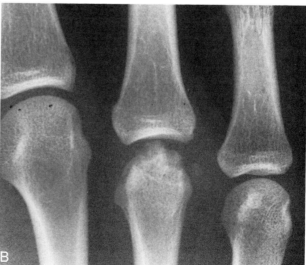

Figure 13–133. *A,* PA view of the 3rd and 4th metacarpal heads following a softball injury. There is no fracture. *B,* Eight months later there is avascular necrosis with collapse of the 4th metacarpal head.

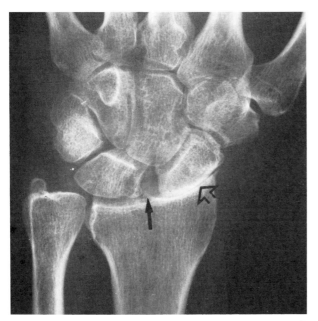

Figure 13–134. PA view of the wrist showing post-traumatic arthritis in the radiocarpal joint *(open arrow)* and an old scapholunate ligament tear with widening of the scapholunate joint *(black arrow).*

the distal interphalangeal joints, the 1st carpometacarpal joint, the scaphotrapezial joints, and the radiocarpal articulation (Fig. 13–134). It may be seen, however, at any joint following an intra-articular fracture or unreduced subluxation. A detailed discussion of the arthritides is beyond the scope of this text and will therefore be omitted.

POST-TRAUMATIC RECONSTRUCTION

Most of the traumatic conditions of the hand or wrist discussed in this chapter require some form of early treatment. However, the treatment rendered may not always lead to a satisfactory outcome, and in some instances the injury may go unrecognized or be inappropriately managed. Therefore, secondary surgical reconstruction may be necessary. A detailed description of reconstructive techniques and their indications for specific post-traumatic conditions is beyond the scope of this text. In general, however, reconstruction for post-traumatic conditions in the hand or wrist may be categorized into the following four groups: osteotomy, soft tissue stabilization, arthrodesis, or arthroplasty. An awareness of the basic principles involved with each of these groups may be pertinent to radiographic interpretation.

Osteotomy

Osteotomy is usually required to correct malunion of fractures (Fig. 13–135). It may additionally be useful for correction of congenital abnormalities (symptomatic ulnar variance, Madelung's deformity), to alter bone alignment for joint motion or stress concentration (radial shortening in Kienböck's disease), to position bones in certain fixed postures for functional considerations, and at times to facilitate surgical exposure of an underlying structure. The term osteotomy simply implies the sectioning of a bone by any means. Following bone

Figure 13–135. A, AP view of the left index finger with rotation and angular deformity as a result of an old fracture. B, The deformity was corrected with osteotomy using K-wire and band fixation.

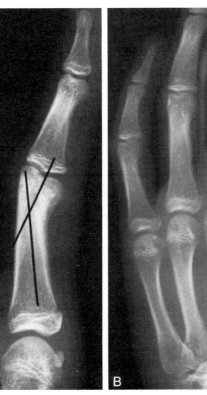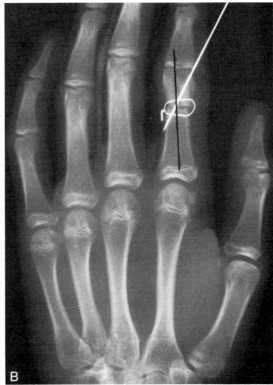

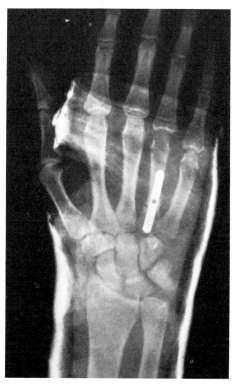

Figure 13–136. Fracture of the proximal 4th metacarpal with miniplate and screw fixation.

section, the position of the osteotomy is usually maintained by some means of internal fixation. In the small bones of the hand this is usually accomplished by smooth or threaded Kirschner wires. For longer bones, Steinmann pins of a similar configu-

ration but larger diameter than Kirschner wires may be used. Wire loops are applicable in certain situations and may be of the circlage type or the tension-band "Figure of 8" type. The former usually is placed along the central axis of the bone, while the latter is placed eccentrically over the "tension" side of the bone (the side opposite to where compressive bending moments are expected). Occasionally small bone screws, miniplates (Fig. 13–136), or external fixators may be preferred. For larger bones (radius or ulna), Kirschner wires, Steinmann pins, or wire loops may also be used, but compression plates and screws are more common (Fig. 13–72). These may be of any length or configuration. The chief complication of radiographic significance for osteotomy is delayed union or non-union. Routine views are usually insufficient to evaluate union. Tomography provides improved detail. However, differentiation of non-union from fibrous union is difficult.

Arthrodesis

The term arthrodesis implies bony fusion of a joint. It may also be applicable to a pseudarthrosis site. In general, arthrodesis is most often required for stabilization of a painful joint of any cause. It may also be a useful procedure for stabilization of an unstable joint (Fig. 13–137), particularly in certain paralytic disorders. Means of fixation for arthrodesis are similar to the hardware devices described in the preceding section. Bone-graft material may also be utilized at the arthrodesis site. The chief complication of radiographic significance for

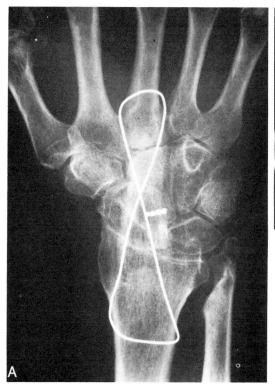
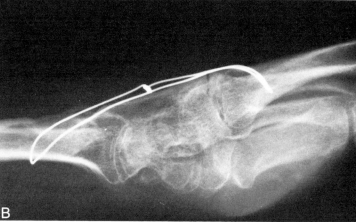

Figure 13–137. PA *(A)* and lateral *(B)* views following arthrodesis of the wrist. Bone graft dorsally with "Figure of 8" wire.

arthrodesis is delayed union or non-union. The evaluation of either of these complications may be aided by tomography and occasionally by arthrography.

Soft Tissue Stabilization

Soft tissue stabilization procedures are not infrequent. They are most often applied for reconstruction of symptomatic ligamentous disruptions (subluxation of the distal radioulnar joint,[104] scapholunate dissociation,[169, 174] proximal interphalangeal joint swan-neck deformity). The specific technique of soft tissue stabilization will vary widely. There are no particular radiographic features of such procedures.

Arthroplasty

Arthroplasty procedures utilized for salvage or reconstruction of the hand or wrist may be broadly categorized as resection or implant (prosthetic) arthroplasty. These are most frequently applicable for arthritic disorders, but they may also be required for reconstruction following post-traumatic articular incongruity or for correction of severe contractures. The more common resection arthroplasty procedures include excision of the distal ulna (Fig. 13–138),[82, 178] proximal row carpectomy,[161] excision of the trapezium (Fig. 13–139), or resection of metacarpal heads. Often some form of soft tissue interposition (e.g., a loop of tendon[177]) is used in conjunction with resection arthroplasty to prevent direct bone-to-bone contact or to minimize bony collapse into the resulting void.

A wide variety of implants are available for prosthetic arthroplasty. These fall into two broad categories—implants that act as spacers[173, 179] and implants that act as true articulating surfaces or hinges.[176] The spacer implants are more common and are more frequently used for metacarpophalangeal joint replacement (Fig. 13–140). The same

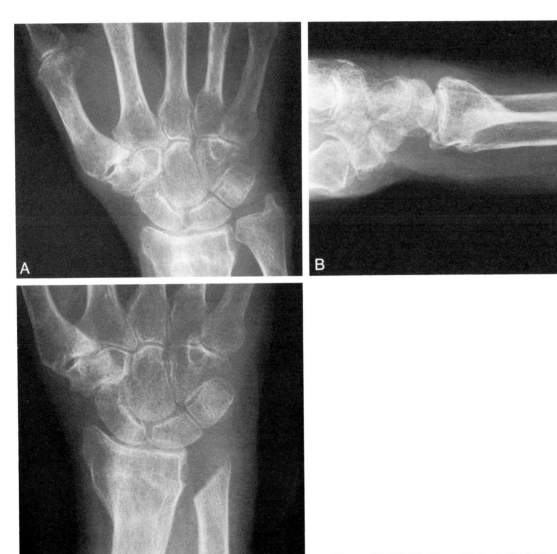

Figure 13–138. PA *(A)* and lateral *(B)* views of an old distal radial fracture with shortening of the radius and positive ulnar variance. PA radiograph *(C)* following resection of the distal ulna.

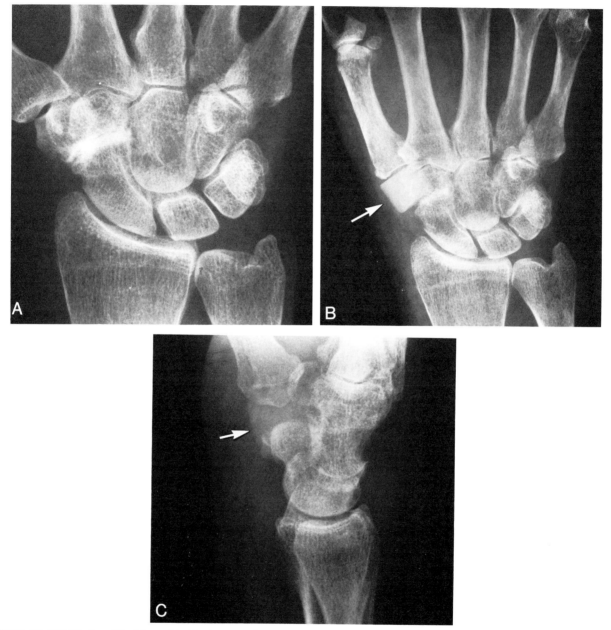

Figure 13–139. PA view *(A)* of the wrist with degenerative arthritis involving the scaphotrapezial articulation. PA *(B)* and lateral *(C)* views following prosthetic replacement *(arrows).*

type of implant is applicable for the purposes of proximal interphalangeal joint arthroplasty. Spacer implants are also available for total wrist replacement as well as lunate, scaphoid, trapezium, ulnar head, and 1st metacarpal base arthroplasty.

Articulating implants at this time appear to have a more limited application in the hand and wrist. In contrast to spacer implants, these generally require some means of stem-bone fixation. Usually this implies the use of methyl methacrylate cement or a porous surface–bone ingrowth stem design. Articulating implant arthroplasty is most commonly utilized for metacarpophalangeal joint or total wrist replacement (Figs. 13–141 and 13–142).

A variety of complications with radiographic significance may be noted with arthroplasty procedures. Excision arthroplasty may be associated with instability and subluxation of the pseudarthrosis. Prosthetic arthroplasty may be complicated by implant fracture, subluxation, or dislocation (Figs. 13–143 and 13–144). Erosion of the implant through bone may be seen late, particularly when firm bone-stem fixation is used. Deep sepsis involving the prosthesis may be characterized by a lucent zone of bone rarefaction about the implant stem, soft tissue swelling, and at times an exaggerated degree of periosteal ossification (Fig. 13–145).

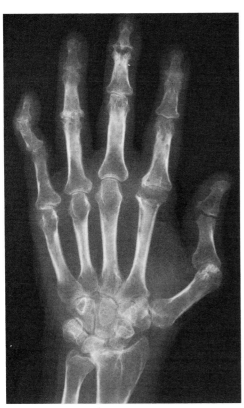

Figure 13–140. PA view of the hand and wrist with a 2nd metacarpophalangeal joint spacer (silicone) in place.

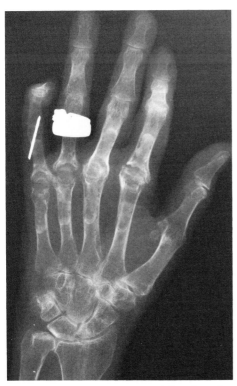

Figure 13–141. PA view of the right hand and wrist with implants (silicone) in the 2nd through 5th metacarpophalangeal joints. There are arthrodeses in the 1st metacarpophalangeal joint and the 5th interphalangeal joint.

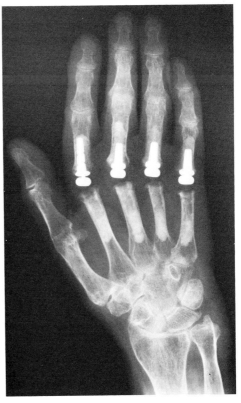

Figure 13–142. PA view of the hand and wrist with Steffee metacarpophalangeal joint replacements. There is a Mark III in the 2nd metacarpophalangeal joint and a Mark II in the 3rd through 5th metacarpophalangeal joints.

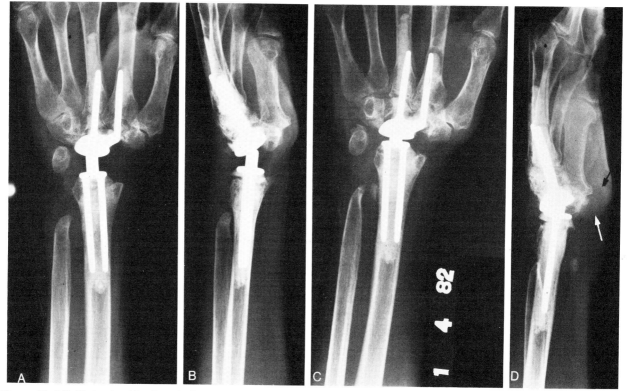

Figure 13–143. Bilateral wrist arthroplasties (Meuli total-wrist prosthesis). PA *(A)* and lateral *(B)* views following surgery are normal. Repeat radiographs were obtained 1½ years later owing to chronic pain. Note the compression of the components on the PA view *(C)* compared with the early radiograph *(A)*. On the lateral view *(D)* it is apparent that the plastic cup of the distal component *(arrows)* has become dislocated.

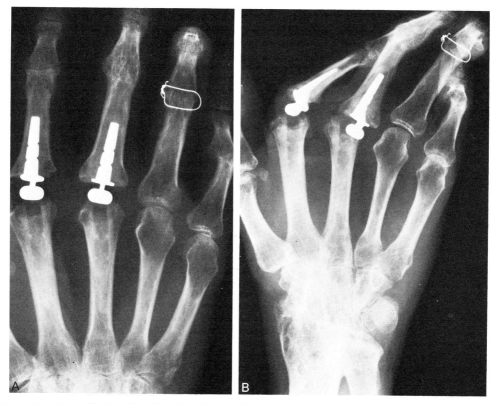

Figure 13–144. A, Arthroplasties (Steffee Mark III) of the 2nd and 3rd metacarpophalangeal joints. Follow-up radiograph *(B)* several years later demonstrates ulnar deviation with rotation of the 2nd and subluxation of the 3rd MCP joints.

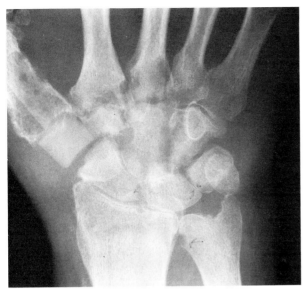

Figure 13–145. Infected prosthesis. AP view of the hand demonstrates bone destruction and periosteal new bone around the implant due to infection. There are numerous erosions in the carpal bones owing to infectious arthritis.

SUMMARY

Trauma is the most common etiologic factor leading to disability in the hand and wrist. Judicious radiographic evaluation is required for accurate assessment in practically all but the most minor of such injuries. Frequently serial radiographic evaluation is essential for directing the course of treatment and for following the healing process. A meaningful radiographic evaluation requires a comprehensive knowledge of the normal radiographic anatomy, an overview of the spectrum of pathology, and an awareness of the usual mechanisms of injury, appropriate treatment options, and relevant array of complications.

REFERENCES

Anatomy

1. Bowers, W. H., Wolf, J. W., and Nehil, J. L.: The proximal interphalangeal joint volar plate. I. An anatomical and biomechanical study. J. Hand Surg. 5:79, 1980.
2. Dobyns, J. H., and Linscheid, R. L.: Fractures and dislocations of the wrist. In Rockwood, C. A., Jr., and Green, D. P. (eds.): Fractures. Philadelphia, J. B. Lippincott Co., 1975.
3. Dobyns, J. H., Linscheid, R. L., Beckenbaugh, R. D., et al.: Fractures of the hand and wrist. In Flynn, J. E. (ed.): Hand Surgery. Baltimore, Williams & Wilkins Co., 1982.
4. Epner, R. A., Bowers, W. H., and Guilford, W. B.: Ulnar variance—the effect of wrist positioning and roentgen filming technique. J. Hand Surg. 7:298, 1982.
5. Gelberman, R. H., Solomon, P. B., Jurist, J. M., et al.: Ulnar variance in Kienböck's disease. J. Bone Joint Surg. 57:674, 1975.
6. Gilford, W. W., Bolton, R. H., and Lambrinudi, C.: The mechanism of the wrist joint with special reference to fractures of the scaphoid. Guy's Hosp. Rep. 92:52, 1943.
7. Green, D. P., and Rowland, S. A.: Fractures and dislocations in the hand. In Rockwood, C. A., Jr., and Green, D. P. (eds.): Fractures. Philadelphia, J. B. Lippincott Co., 1975.
8. Joseph, R. B., Linscheid, R. L., Dobyns, J. H., et al.: Chronic sprains of the carpometacarpal joints. J. Hand Surg. 6:172, 1981.
9. Kaplan, E. B.: Functional and Surgical Anatomy of the Hand. 2nd Ed. Philadelphia, J. B. Lippincott Co., 1965.
10. Kauer, J. M. G.: Functional anatomy of the wrist. Clin. Orthop. 149:9, 1980.
11. Landsmeer, J. M. F.: The proximal interphalangeal joint. Hand 7:30, 1975.
12. Lichtman, D. M., Schneider, J. R., Swafford, A. R., et al.: Ulnar midcarpal instability. Clinical and laboratory analysis. J. Hand Surg. 6:515, 1981.
13. Linscheid, R. L., Dobyns, J. H., Beabout, J. W., et al.: Traumatic instability of the wrist: Diagnosis, classification, and pathomechanics. J. Bone Joint Surg. 54A:1612, 1972.
14. Mayfield, J., Johnson, R., and Kilcoyne, R.: The ligaments of the human wrist and their functional significance. Anat. Rec. 185:417, 1976.
15. Mikic, Z. D.: Age changes in the triangular fibrocartilage of the wrist joint. J. Anat. 126:307, 1978.
16. O'Rahilly, R.: A survey of carpal and tarsal anomalies. J. Bone Joint Surg. 35A:626, 1953.
17. Palmer, A. K., and Werner, F. W.: The triangular fibrocartilage complex of the wrist—anatomy and function. J. Hand Surg. 6:153, 1981.
18. Seffafian, S., Melamed, J. L., and Goshgarian, G. M.: Study of wrist motion in flexion and extension. Clin. Orthop. 126:153, 1977.
19. Taleisnik, J.: The ligaments of the wrist. J. Hand Surg. 1:110, 1976.
20. Volz, R. G., Lieb, M., and Benjamin, J.: Biomechanics of the wrist. Clin. Orthop. 149:112, 1980.
21. Youm, Y., and Flatt, A. E.: Kinematics of the wrist. Clin. Orthop. 149:21, 1980.
22. Youm, Y., McMurthy, R. Y., Flatt, A. E., et al.: Kinematics of the wrist. I. An experimental study of radial-ulnar deviation and flexion-extension. J. Bone Joint Surg. 60A:423, 1978.

Routine Radiographic Techniques

23. Ballinger, P. W.: Merrill's Atlas of Roentgenographic Positions and Standard Radiologic Procedures. 5th Ed. St. Louis, C. V. Mosby, 1982.
24. Bernau, A., and Berquist, T. H.: Orthopedic Positioning in Diagnostic Radiology. Baltimore, Urban and Schwarzenberg, 1983.
25. Bowers, W. H., and Hurst, L. C.: Gamekeeper's thumb. Evaluation by arthrography and stress roentgenography. J. Bone Joint Surg. 59A:519, 1977.
26. Brewerton, D. A.: A tangential radiographic projection for demonstrating involvement of the metacarpal head in rheumatoid arthritis. Br. J. Radiol. 40:233, 1967.
27. Bridgman, C. F.: Radiography of the carpal navicular bone. Med. Radiogr. Photogr. 25:104, 1949.
28. Burman, M.: Anterioposterior projection of the carpometacarpal joint of the thumb by the radial shift of the carpal tunnel view. J. Bone Joint Surg. 40A: 1156, 1958.
29. Crittenden, J. J., Jones, D. M., and Santarelli, A. G.: Bilateral rotational dislocation of the carpal navicular. Radiology 94:629, 1970.
30. Curtis, D. J., and Downey, E. F., Jr.: A simple first metacarpophalangeal stress test. Radiology 148:855, 1983.
31. Fisher, M. R., Rogers, L. F., and Hendrix, R. W.: A systematic approach to identifying fourth and fifth carpometacarpal joint dislocations. A. J. R. 140:319, 1983.
32. Gandee, R. W., Harrison, R. B., and Dee, P. M.: Peritendinitis calcaria of the flexor carpi ulnaris. A. J. R. 133:1139, 1979.
33. Gilula, L. A.: Carpal injuries: Analytic approach and case exercises. A. J. R. 133:503, 1979.
34. Gilula, L. A., and Weeks, P. M.: Post-traumatic ligamentous instability of the wrist. Radiology 129:641, 1978.

35. Hart, V. L., and Gaynor, V.: Roentgenographic study of the carpal canal. J. Bone Joint Surg. 23:382, 1941.
36. Howard, F. M., Fahey, T., and Wojcik, E.: Rotary subluxation of the navicular. Clin. Orthop. 104:134, 1974.
37. Lane, C. G.: Detecting occult fracture of the metacarpal head: The Brewerton view. J. Hand Surg. 2:131, 1977.
38. Lentino, W., Lubetsky, H. W., Jacobson, H. G., et al.: The carpal bridge view. J. Bone Joint Surg. 39A:88, 1957.
39. Murry, W. T., Mueller, P. R., Rosenthal, D. I., et al.: Fracture of the hook of the hamate. A. J. R. 133:899, 1979.
40. Protos, J. M., and Jackson, W. T.: Evaluating carpal instability with fluoroscopy. A. J. R. 135:137, 1980.
41. Stecher, W. R.: Roentgenography of the carpal navicular bone. A. J. R. 37:704, 1937.
42. Terry, D. W., and Ramin, J. E.: The navicular fat stripe. A useful roentgen feature for evaluating wrist trauma. A. J. R. 124:25, 1975.

Arthrography of the Hand and Wrist

43. Andrén, L., and Eiken, O.: Arthrographic studies of wrist ganglions. J. Bone Joint Surg. 53A:299, 1971.
44. Engle, J., Ganel, A., Ditzian, R., et al.: Arthrograpy as a method of diagnosing tears of the ulnar collateral ligament of the metacarpophalangeal joint of the thumb ("gamekeeper's thumb"). J. Trauma 19:106, 1979.
45. Gilula, L. A., Totty, G. W., and Weeks, P. M.: Wrist arthrography: The value of fluoroscopic spot filming. Radiology 146:555, 1983.
46. Goldman, A. B.: The wrist. In Freiberger, R. H., and Kaye, J. J. (eds.): Arthrography. New York, Appleton-Century-Crofts, 1979.
47. Harrison, M. O., Freiberger, R. H., and Ranawat, C. S.: Arthrography of the rheumatoid wrist joint. A. J. R. 112:480, 1971.
48. Hudson, T. M., Caragal, W. J., and Kaye, J. J.: Isolated rotary subluxation of the carpal navicular. A. J. R. 126:601, 1976.
49. Levinsohn, E. M., and Palmer, A. K.: Arthrography of the traumatized wrist. Correlation of radiography and the carpal instability series. Radiology 146:647, 1983.
50. Lewis, O. J., Hamshire, R. J., and Buckneel, T. M.: The anatomy of the wrist. J. Anat. 106:539, 1970.
51. Ranawat, C. S., Harrison, M. O., and Jordan, L. R.: Arthrography of the wrist joint. Clin. Orthop. 83:6, 1972.
52. Resnick, D.: Arthrographic evaluation of arthritic disorders of the wrist. Radiology 113:331, 1974.
53. Resnick, D.: Roentgenographic anatomy of the tendon sheaths of the hand and wrist: Tenography. A. J. R. 124:44, 1975.
54. Resnick, D., and Dalinka, M. K.: Arthrography and tenography of the wrist. In Dalinka, M. K. (ed.): Arthrography. New York, Springer-Verlag, 1980.
55. Rosenthal, D. I., Murray, W. T., and Smith, R. J.: Finger arthrography. Radiology 137:647, 1980.
56. Trentham, D. E., Harrison, R. L., and Mosi, A. T.: Wrist arthrography: Review and comparison of normals, rheumatoid arthritis, and gout patients. Semin. Arthritis Rheum. 5:105, 1975.

Fractures and Dislocations

57. Adler, J. B., and Shaftan, G. W.: Fractures of the capitate. J. Bone Joint Surg. 44A:1537, 1962.
58. Agee, J. M.: Unstable fracture-dislocations of the proximal interphalangeal joint of the fingers: A preliminary report of a new treatment technique. J. Hand Surg. 3:386, 1978.
59. Aitkin, A. P., and Nalebuff, E. A.: Volar transnavicular perilunar dislocations of the carpus. J. Bone Joint Surg. 42A:1051, 1960.
60. Albert, S. M., Wohl, M. D., and Rechtman, A. M.: Treatment of the disrupted radio-ulnar joint. J. Bone Joint Surg. 45A:1373, 1963.
61. Baldwin, L. W., Miller, D. L., Lockhart, L. D., et al.: Metacarpophalangeal-joint dislocations of the fingers. J. Bone Joint Surg. 49A:1587, 1967.
62. Bartone, N. F., and Grieco, R. V.: Fractures of the triquetrum. J. Bone Joint Surg. 38A:353, 1956.
63. Belsole, R.: Physiologic fixation of displaced and unstable fractures of the hand. Orthop. Clin. North Am. 11:393, 1980.
64. Bowen, T. L.: Injuries of the hamate bone. Hand 5:235, 1973.
65. Bowers, W. H.: Management of small joint injuries in the hand. Clin. Orthop. 14:798, 1983.
66. Browne, E. Z., Dunn, H. K., and Snyder, C. C.: Ski pole thumb injury. Plast. Reconstr. Surg. 59:19, 1976.
67. Bryan, R. S., and Dobyns, J. H.: Fractures of the carpal bones other than lunate and navicular. Clin. Orthop. 149:107, 1980.
68. Burton, R. J.: Fractures of the proximal phalanx of the finger. Contemp. Surg. 11:32, 1977.
69. Cameron, H. U., Hastings, D. E., and Fournasier, V. L.: Fracture of the hook of the hamate. A case report. J. Bone Joint Surg. 57A:276, 1975.
70. Carter, P. R., Eaton, R. G., and Littler, J. W.: Ununited fracture of the hook of the hamate. J. Bone Joint Surg. 59A:583, 1977.
71. Cooney, W. P., Beckenbaugh, R. D., Bryan, R. S., et al.: External minifixators: Clinical applications and techniques. In Johnston, M. (ed.): Advances in External Fixation. Chicago, Year Book Medical Publishers, 1980.
72. Cooney, W. P., Dobyns, J. H., and Linscheid, R. L.: Complications of Colles' fractures. J. Bone Joint Surg. 62A:613, 1980.
73. Cooney, W. P., Dobyns, J. H., and Linscheid, R. L.: Fractures of the scaphoid: A rational approach to management. Clin. Orthop. 149:90, 1980.
74. Cooney, W. P., Linscheid, R. L., and Dobyns, J. H.: External pin fixation for unstable Colles' fractures. J. Bone Joint Surg. 61A:840, 1979.
75. Coonrad, R. W., and Goldner, J. L.: A study of the pathological findings and treatment in soft-tissue injury of the thumb metacarpophalangeal joint. J. Bone Joint Surg. 50A:439, 1968.
76. Cordrey, L. J., and Ferrer-Torells, M.: Management of fractures of the greater multangular. J. Bone Joint Surg. 42A:1111, 1960.
77. Crawford, G. P.: Screw fixation for certain fractures of the phalanges and metacarpals. J. Bone Joint Surg. 58A:487, 1976.
78. Crosby, E. B., and Linscheid, R. L.: Rupture of the flexor profundus tendon of the ring finger secondary to ancient fracture of the hook of the hamate: Review of the literature and report of two cases. J. Bone Joint Surg. 56A:1076, 1974.
79. Dameron, T. B.: Traumatic dislocation of the distal radioulnar joint. Clin. Orthop. 83:55, 1972.
80. Darrach, W.: Foreward dislocation at the inferior radioulnar joint with fractures of the lower third of the radius. Ann. Surg. 56:801, 1912.
81. De Oliveira, J. C.: Barton's fractures. J. Bone Joint Surg. 55A:586, 1973.
82. Dingman, P. V. C.: Resection of the distal end of the ulna (Darrach operation). End-result study of 24 cases. J. Bone Joint Surg. 34A:893, 1952.
83. Dunn, A. W.: Fractures and dislocations of the carpus. Surg. Clin. North Am. 52:1513, 1972.
84. Edwards, H. C.: Mechanism and treatment of backfire fracture. J. Bone Joint Surg. 8:701, 1926.
85. Ellis, J.: Smith's and Barton's fracture—a method of treatment. J. Bone Joint Surg. 47B:724, 1965.
86. Fenton, R. L.: The naviculo-capitate fracture syndrome. J. Bone Joint Surg. 38A:681, 1956.
87. Fernandez, D. L.: Irreducible radiocarpal fracture-dislocation and radioulnar dissociation with entrapment of the ulnar nerve, artery, and flexor profundus II-V—case report. J. Hand Surg. 6:456, 1981.
88. Fisk, G. R.: Carpal instability and the fractured scaphoid. Ann. Roy. Coll. Surg. 46:63, 1970.
89. Fisk, G. R.: An overview of injuries of the wrist. Clin. Orthop. 149:137, 1980.
90. Flatt, A. E.: Recurrent locking of an index finger. J. Bone Joint Surg. 40A:1128, 1958.
91. Frykman, G.: Fractures of the distal radius including se-

quelae—shoulder-hand-finger syndrome, disturbance in the distal radioulnar joint, and impairment of nerve function. Acta Orthop. Scand. (Suppl.) *108*:1, 1967.

92. Gingrass, R. P., Fehring, B., and Matloub, H.: Intraosseous wiring of complex hand fractures. Plast. Reconstr. Surg. *66*:383, 1980.

93. Goldberg, I., Amit, S., Bahar, A., et al.: Complete dislocation of the trapezium. J. Hand Surg. *6*:193, 1981.

94. Goodman, M. L., and Shankman, G. B.: Update: Palmar dislocation of the trapezoid—a case report. J. Hand Surg. *9*:127, 1984.

95. Green, D. P., and Anderson, J. R.: Closed reduction and percutaneous fixation of fractured phalanges. J. Bone Joint Surg. *55A*:1651, 1973.

96. Green, D. P., and O'Brien, E. T.: Classification and management of carpal dislocations. Clin. Orthop. *149*:55, 1980.

97. Grundberg, A. B.: Intramedullary fixation for fractures of the hand. J. Hand Surg. *6*:568, 1981.

98. Hamlin, C.: Traumatic disruption of the distal radioulnar joint. Am. J. Sports Med. *5*:93, 1977.

99. Hartwig, R. H., and Louis, D. S.: Multiple carpometacarpal dislocations: A review of four cases. J. Bone Joint Surg. *61A*:906, 1979.

100. Heiple, K. G., Freehafer, A. A., and Van't Hof, A.: Isolated traumatic dislocation of the distal end of the ulna or distal radioulnar joint. J. Bone Joint Surg. *44A*:1387, 1962.

101. Hill, N. A.: Fractures and dislocations of the carpus. Orthop. Clin. North Am. *1*:275, 1970.

102. Hsu, J. D., and Curtis, R. M.: Carpometacarpal dislocations of the ulnar side of the hand. J. Bone Joint Surg. *52B*:927, 1970.

103. Hughston, J. C.: Fracture of the distal radial shaft—mistakes in management. J. Bone Joint Surg. *39A*:249, 1957.

104. Hui, F. C., and Linscheid, R. L.: Ulnotriquetral augmentation tenodesis: A reconstructive procedure for dorsal subluxation of the distal radioulnar joint. J. Hand Surg. *7*:230, 1982.

105. Immermann, E. W.: Dislocation of the pisiform. J. Bone Joint Surg. *30A*:487, 1948.

106. Johnson, R. P.: The acutely injured wrist and its residuals. Clin. Orthop. *149*:33, 1980.

107. Kaplan, E. B.: Dorsal dislocation of the metacarpophalangeal joint of the index finger. J. Bone Joint Surg. *39A*:1081, 1957.

108. Lewis, H. H.: Dislocation of the lesser multangular: Report of a case. J. Bone Joint Surg. *44*:1412, 1962.

109. Liddy, J. P., and Packer, J. W.: Avulsion of the profundus tendon insertion in athletes. J. Hand Surg. *2*:66, 1977.

110. Lister, G. D.: Intraosseous wiring of the digital skeleton. J. Hand Surg. *3*:427, 1978.

111. Lucas, G. L.: Internal fixation in the hand: A review of indications and methods. Orthopedics *3*:1083, 1980.

112. MacLaughlin, H. L.: Complex "locked" dislocations of the metacarpophalangeal joints. J. Trauma *5*:683, 1965.

113. Maudsley, R. H., and Chen, S. C.: Screw fixation in the management of the fractured carpal scaphoid. J. Bone Joint Surg. *54B*:432, 1972.

114. Mayfield, J. K., Johnson, R. P., and Kilcoyne, R. K.: Carpal dislocations: Pathomechanics and progressive perilunar instability. J. Hand Surg. *5*:226, 1980.

115. McElfresh, E. C., Dobyns, J. H., and O'Brien, E. T.: Management of fracture-dislocation of the proximal interphalangeal joint by extension-block splinting. J. Bone Joint Surg. *54A*:1705, 1972.

116. Meyers, M. H., Wells, R., and Harvey, J. P., Jr.: Naviculo-capitate fracture syndrome. J. Bone Joint Surg. *53A*:1383, 1971.

117. Mikic, Z. D.: Galeazzi fracture-dislocations. J. Bone Joint Surg. *57A*:1071, 1975.

118. Milch, H.: Fracture of the hamate bone. J. Bone Joint Surg. *16*:459, 1934.

119. Minami, M., Hamazaki, J., and Ishii, S.: Isolated dislocation of the pisiform: A case report and review of the literature. J. Hand Surg. *9*:125, 1984.

120. Moore, J. R., Webb, C. A., and Thompson, R. C.: A complete dislocation of the thumb metacarpal. J. Hand Surg. *3*:547, 1978.

121. Morawa, L. G., Ross, P. M., and Schock, C. C.: Fracture and dislocations involving the navicular-lunate axis. Clin. Orthop. *118*:48, 1976.

122. Morrissy, R. T., and Nalebuff, E. A.: Dislocation of the distal radioulnar joint: Anatomy and clues to prompt diagnosis. Clin. Orthop. *144*:154, 1979.

123. Mouat, T. B., Wilkie, J., and Harding, H. E.: Isolated fracture of the carpal semilunar and Kienböck's disease. Br. J. Surg. *19*:577, 1932.

124. Nalebuff, E. A.: Isolated anterior carpometacarpal dislocation of the fifth finger: Classification and case report. J. Trauma *8*:1119, 1968.

125. Parks, J. C., and Stovell, P. B.: Dislocation of the carpal scaphoid: A report of two cases. J. Trauma *13*:384, 1973.

126. Peltier, L. F.: Eponymic fractures: John Rhea Barton and Barton's fractures. Surgery *34*:960, 1953.

127. Peltier, L. F.: Eponymic fractures: Robert William Smith and Smith's fractures. Surgery *45*:1035, 1959.

128. Reef, T. C.: Avulsion of the flexor digitorum profundus: An athletic injury. Am. J. Sports Med. *5*:281, 1977.

129. Renshaw, T. S., and Louis, D. S.: Complex volar dislocation of the metacarpophalangeal joint: A case report. J. Trauma *12*:1087, 1971.

130. Rosado, A.: A possible relationship of radio-carpal dislocation and dislocation of the lunate bone. J. Bone Joint Surg. *48B*:504, 1966.

131. Rose-Innes, A. P.: Anterior dislocation of the ulna at the inferior radioulnar joint. J. Bone Joint Surg. *42B*:515, 1960.

132. Ruby, L. K.: Common hand injuries in the athlete. Orthop. Clin. North Am. *11*:819, 1980.

133. Russe, O.: Fracture of the carpal navicular. J. Bone Joint Surg. *42A*:759, 1960.

134. Russell, T. B.: Intercarpal dislocations and fracture-dislocations. A review of 59 cases. J. Bone Joint Surg. *31B*:524, 1949.

135. Sebald, J. R., Dobyns, J. H., and Linscheid, R. L.: The natural history of collapse deformities of the wrist. Clin. Orthop. *104*:140, 1974.

136. Seimon, L. P.: Compound dislocation of the trapezium. J. Bone Joint Surg. *54A*:1297, 1972.

137. Siegel, M. W., and Hertzberg, H.: Complete dislocation of the greater multangulum (trapezium). J. Bone Joint Surg. *51A*:769, 1969.

138. Smith, R. J.: Post-traumatic instability of the metacarpophalangeal joint of the thumb. J. Bone Joint Surg. *59A*:14, 1977.

139. Stark, H. H.: Troublesome fractures and dislocations of the hand. Inst. Course Lect. *19*:130, 1970.

140. Stark, H. H., Jobe, F. W., Boyes, J. H., et al.: Fracture of the hook of the hamate in athletes. J. Bone Joint Surg. *59A*:575, 1977.

141. Stein, A. H.: Dorsal dislocation of the lesser multangular bone. J. Bone Joint Surg. *53A*:377, 1971.

142. Stein, R., and Siegel, M. W.: Naviculo-capitate fracture syndrome. J. Bone Joint Surg. *51A*:391, 1969.

143. Stener, B.: Displacement of the ruptured ulnar collateral ligament of the metacarpophalangeal joint of the thumb. J. Bone Joint Surg. *44B*:869, 1962.

144. Swanson, A. B.: Fractures involving the digits of the hand. Orthop. Clin. North Am. *1*:261, 1970.

145. Thomas, F. B.: Reduction of Smith's fractures. J. Bone Joint Surg. *39B*:463, 1957.

146. Thompson, G. H., and Grant, T. T.: Barton's fracture—reverse Barton's fracture: Confusing eponyms. Clin. Orthop. *122*:210, 1977.

147. Torisu, T.: Fracture of the hook of the hamate by a golf-swing. Clin. Orthop. *83*:91, 1972.

148. Vasilas, A., Grieco, R. V., and Bartone, N. F.: Roentgen aspects of injuries to the pisiform bone and pisotriquetral joint. J. Bone Joint Surg. *42A*:1317, 1960.

149. Verdan, C., and Narakas, A.: Fracture and pseudoarthrosis of the scaphoid. Surg. Clin. North Am. 48:1083, 1968.
150. Vesley, D. G.: The distal radioulnar joint. Clin. Orthop. 51:75, 1967.
151. Weber, E. R., and Chao, E. Y. S.: An experimental approach to the mechanisms of scaphoid waist fracture. J. Hand Surg. 3:142, 1978.
152. Wenger, D. R.: Avulsion of the profundus tendon insertion in football players. Arch. Surg. 106:145, 1973.
153. Weseley, M. S., and Barenfield, P. A.: Trans-scaphoid, transcapitate, transtriquetral, perilunate fracture-dislocation of the wrist. J. Bone Joint Surg. 54A:1073, 1972.
154. Weseley, M. S., Barenfield, P. A., and Bruno, J.: Volar dislocation of the distal radioulnar joint. J. Trauma 12:1083, 1972.
155. Wilson, J. N., and Rowland, S. A.: Fracture-dislocation of the proximal interphalangeal joint of the finger. Treatment by open reduction and internal fixation. J. Bone Joint Surg. 48A:493, 1966.
156. Wood, M. B., and Dobyns, J. H.: Chronic, complex volar dislocation of the metacarpophalangeal joint. J. Hand Surg. 6:73, 1981.

Chronic Post-Traumatic Conditions

157. Artz, T. D., and Posch, J. L.: The carpometacarpal boss. J. Bone Joint Surg. 55:747, 1973.
158. Bassoe, E., and Bassoe, H. H.: The styloid bone and carpe bosseau disease. Am. J. Roentgenol. 74:886, 1955.
159. Beckenbaugh, R. D., Shives, T. C., Dobyns, J. H., et al.: Kienböck's disease: The natural history of Kienböck's disease and consideration of lunate fractures. Clin. Orthop. 149:98, 1980.
160. Bobechko, W. P., and Harris, W. R.: The radiographic density of avascular bone. J. Bone Joint Surg. 52B:636, 1960.
161. Jorgensen, E. C.: Proximal-row carpectomy. An end-result study of 22 cases. J. Bone Joint Surg. 51A:1104, 1969.
162. Kienböck, R.: Uber traumatische Malazie des Mondbeins und ihre Folgezustande: Entartungsformen and Kompressionsfrakturen. Fortschr. Geb. Röntgen. 16:77, 1910.
163. Kienböck, R.: Concerning traumatic malacia of the lunate and its consequences: Degeneration and compression fracture. Clin. Orthop. 149:4, 1980.
164. Kleinert, H. E., and Kasdan, M. L.: Reconstruction of chronically subluxated proximal interphalangeal finger joint. J. Bone Joint Surg. 47A:958, 1964.
165. Koostra, G., Huffstadt, A. J. C., and Kauer, J. M. G.: The styloid bone. A clinical and embryological study. Hand 6:185, 1974.
166. Lichtman, D. M., Mack, G. R., MacDonald, R. I., et al.: Kienböck's disease: The role of silicone replacement arthroplasty. J. Bone Joint Surg. 59A:899, 1977.
167. Linscheid, R. L., Dobyns, J. H., Beckenbaugh, R. D., et al.: Instability patterns of the wrist. J. Hand Surg. 8:682, 1983.
168. Lovett, W. L., and McCalla, M. A.: Management and rehabilitation of extensor tendon injuries. Orthop. Clin. North Am. 14:811, 1983.
169. Palmer, A. K., Dobyns, J. H., and Linscheid, R. L.: Management of posttraumatic instability of the wrist secondary to ligament rupture. J. Hand Surg. 3:507, 1978.
170. Persson, M.: Casual treatment of lunatomalacia, further experience of operative ulna lengthening. Acta Chir. Scand. 100:531, 1950.
171. Posner, M. A.: Injuries to the hand and wrist in athletes. Orthop. Clin. North Am. 8:593, 1977.
172. Souter, W. A.: The problem of boutonnière deformities. Clin. Orthop. 104:116, 1974.
173. Swanson, A. B.: Silicone rubber implants for the replacement of the carpal scaphoid and lunate bones. Orthop. Clin. North Am. 1:299, 1970.
174. Taleisnik, J.: Posttraumatic carpal instability. Clin. Orthop. 149:73, 1980.
175. Tilberg, B.: Kienböck's disease treated with osteotomy to lengthen the ulna. Acta Orthop. Scand. 39:359, 1968.

Post-Traumatic Reconstruction

176. Beckenbaugh, R. D.: New concepts in arthroplasty of the hand and wrist. Arch. Surg. 112:1094, 1977.
177. Froimson, A.: Tendon arthroplasty of the trapeziometacarpal joint. Clin. Orthop. 70:191, 1970.
178. Lugnegard, H.: Resection of the head of the ulna in posttraumatic dysfunction of the distal radioulnar joint. Scand. J. Plast. Reconstr. Surg. 3:65, 1969.
179. Nalebuff, E. A., Millender, L. H., Goodman, M. J., et al.: Arthroplasty of the rheumatoid wrist with silicone rubber: An early evaluation. J. Hand Surg. 5:114, 1980.
180. Swanson, A. B.: Disabling arthritis at the base of the thumb. J. Bone Joint Surg. 54A:456, 1972.

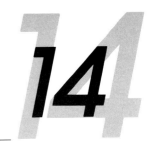

AN IMAGING APPROACH TO MUSCULOSKELETAL INFECTIONS

MANUEL L. BROWN • CURTIS B. KAMIDA
THOMAS H. BERQUIST • ROBERT H. FITZGERALD

Musculoskeletal infections may progress rapidly from their initial clinical presentation or may present with a slow, insidious course that complicates previous trauma or the placement of an orthopedic device. The forms of osteomyelitis covered in this chapter will include only the most common forms of infection. Hematogenous osteomyelitis, post-traumatic and postoperative infections, disk space infections, and septic arthritis will be considered.

OSTEOMYELITIS

Acute hematogenous osteomyelitis is primarily a disease of childhood, although neonates and adults are not spared.[79, 83, 161, 181] Hobo[71] described the vasculature of the metaphyses, where the narrowed capillaries take a very sharp turn back into themselves at the growth plate and end in a system of large sinusoidal veins. The presence of turbulent blood flow followed by slowing or stagnant blood flow, which occurs with these changes in vascular diameters, may allow bacteria an opportunity to reproduce, leading to infection. Attraction of the phagocytic activity of the tissue basal macrophages further enhances the opportunity for a nidus of sepsis in this location. This would account for the predilection of osteomyelitis for the metaphysis in children.

In addition to the depressed phagocytic function of reticuloendothelial cells on the venous side of the capillary loops, Hobo also identified a lack of phagocytic cells on the arterial side of the capillary loops.[71]

In the neonate the vascular supply tends to extend into the epiphysis, and this may explain the occurrence of osteomyelitis in the articular portion of long bones. However, with the appearance of the epiphyseal growth plate, infections are usually limited to the metaphysis of the long bones. In the adult, following closure of the epiphyseal growth plate the blood supply extends into the epiphysis and can allow infectious agents free access into the ends of long bones and the adjacent joint spaces.

Up to 30 percent of patients have acute infections in flat or irregular bones (ilium, vertebra, and calcaneus). Nixon[123] suggests that the vascular anatomy of these bones is similar to that encountered in the region of the growth plate of the tubular long bones and that it therefore serves as a metaphyseal equivalent.

In subacute and chronic forms of osteomyelitis the infecting organisms are present in the medulla and subperiosteal regions. The host's response to the infection process tends to isolate a portion of the bone from its vascular supply. This area of bone then becomes necrotic and may form a sequestrum. A reparative process may wall off this area, creating an involucrum about the necrotic sequestrum.

As mentioned, acute hematogenous osteomyelitis is distinctly uncommon in adult patients and usually occurs in patients with compromised defense mechanisms. However, acute hematogenous osteomyelitis in adults can follow urinary tract infections or genitourinary surgery by seeding of bacteria through Batson's venous plexus. The initial focus of this form of osteomyelitis is initially in the intravertebral disk space with later involvement of adjacent vertebrae.

Another form of adult hematogenous osteomyelitis occurs in the drug addict. These infections may well be due to a combination of self-inoculation and reduced resistance. In this group of patients the sites are often unusual. These include the sternoclavicular and sacroiliac joints and lumbar and cervical vertebrae. *Pseudomonas aeruginosa* is the commonest causal organism isolated from drug addicts who develop either septic arthritis or osteomyelitis.[148]

In post-traumatic patients there may be alteration of the host's defense mechanism from both the injury and the treatment that will allow bacterial colonization of the soft tissue and fracture site. In contrast to acute hematogenous osteomyelitis, the diaphysis is more frequently involved than the metaphysis.

Postoperative osteomyelitis is frequently associated with implantation of metal and other types of forearm bodies. In patients with total joint arthroplasty infections may be of a very low grade and proceed to chronic osteomyelitis. Although the exact mechanism is uncertain, Petty[134] has demonstrated that monomeric methyl methacrylate, which is released from the polymethyl methacrylate, has an adverse effect on the chemotactic and phagocytic functions of the host's white blood cells and that it is associated with abnormalities of serum complement activity and T-lymphocyte response. This may explain the prevalence of "nonpathogenic" organisms (*Staphylococcus epidermidis*) in such infections.

Routine Radiographic Evaluation

The earliest radiographic signs of an acute osteomyelitis are due to changes in the soft tissues. These radiographic signs are often subtle and comparison views of the clinically uninvolved contralateral limb can be of great help. Xeroradiography, magnification techniques, and tomography may detect early subtle changes more easily than routine techniques (see Chapter 1).

Capitano and Kirkpatrick[23] described the early changes in acute osteomyelitis. The first definitive change is small, local, deep soft tissue swelling adjacent to the site of the bone involvement (Fig. 14–1). This can occur as early as 2 to 3 days after the onset of infection.[78] This deep soft tissue swell-

ing is contiguous with the underlying bone and is identified on radiographs by a displacement of the deep muscle planes and fat lines that normally parallel the bony surface.[13, 29] Treatment with parenteral antibiotics at this stage usually results in complete resolution and no significant osseous destruction.[23, 29]

The second soft tissue change is obliteration of these same deep muscle planes and fat lines along with swelling of the deep musculature. This is due to edema of the soft tissues around the site of disease.[78] These changes occur initially in the deep layers and are followed by involvement of the more superficial muscles and lucent planes.[23] Recognition of this outward progression can help one distinguish between a primary bone infection and a cellulitis. In the latter, the subcutaneous tissues are involved earlier, with the deep muscle changes occurring at a later date.[78]

Since bone destruction cannot be detected on conventional radiographs until 35 to 50 percent of

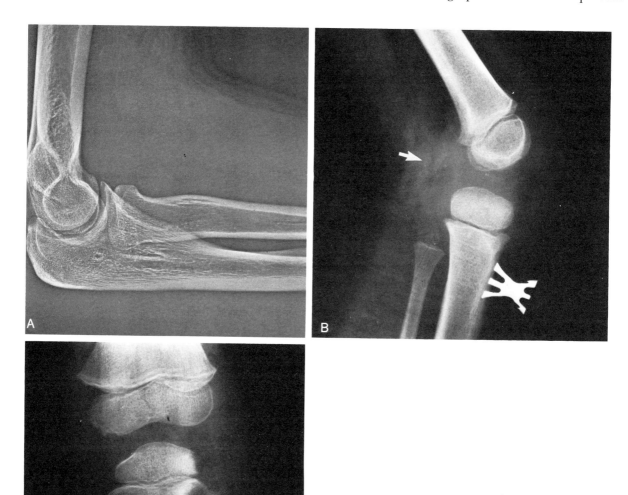

Figure 14–1. Soft tissue changes of osteomyelitis. *A*, Elbow xeroradiograph demonstrating diffuse soft tissue swelling with subcutaneous changes due to cellulitis. *B*, Lateral view of the knee demonstrating deep soft tissue changes (*arrow*) seen with early osteomyelitis. *C*, AP view of the knee demonstrating characteristic metaphyseal destruction with periosteal new bone formation due to osteomyelitis.

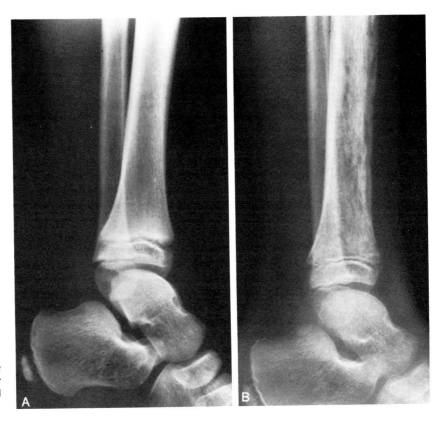

Figure 14–2. Radiographs taken at onset of clinical symptoms (*A*) and 14 days later (*B*) in a patient with osteomyelitis of the distal tibia.

the bone has been destroyed[13, 181] (Fig. 14–2), evidence of osseous involvement usually appears 10 to 14 days after the onset of the infection.[13, 23, 29, 41, 78] Therefore, the degree of true osseous involvement is considerably more than can be initially appreciated on conventional roentgenograms. The early bone changes are a mild rarefaction due to both hyperemia and actual destruction of trabecular bone.[23]

As mentioned previously, the initial sites of bacterial lodgement within bone can be explained on the basis of the varying vascular supply in the infant, child, and adult. In the infant, destruction of the unossified or poorly ossified epiphysis can be difficult to recognize on conventional radiographs.[19, 32, 48] Since the epiphysis in certain joints (e.g., the hips and proximal radius) is intrasynovial in location, extension of the infection can lead to a septic arthritis. Additional clues to the diagnosis of acute osteomyelitis in the infant include lucent defects in the metaphysis and periostitis.[145]

The destruction of trabecular bone in the child and adult extends in all directions. Horizontal extension through Howship's lacunae results in disruption of the cortex and elevation of the periosteum. A subperiosteal abscess is formed, and there is stimulation of periosteal new bone.[29] The periostitis can be seen as early as 3 weeks after the onset of infection.[38] The periosteum is tightly attached to the underlying bone in the adult, but the attachment in infants and children is relatively loose.[29] This results in a much more florid periosteal reaction in the infant and child when compared with the adult (Fig. 14–3). The periosteal reaction is not

necessarily in the same area as the bone destruction, since the inflammatory exudate can dissect below the periosteum for a considerable distance from the initial site of cortical rupture.[142, 169]

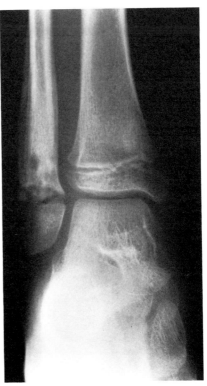

Figure 14–3. Acute osteomyelitis in a young child. The AP radiograph demonstrates metaphyseal lytic lesions with obvious periosteal reaction.

Improper treatment of acute osteomyelitis leads to subacute and chronic disease. This distinction is somewhat artificial,[158] and the roentgenographic findings vary depending on the type of organism, the patient's immunologic status, local trauma, and prior antibiotic therapy.[145] The periostitis seen in the early stages of disease may eventually lead to the formation of an involucrum that ultimately surrounds the shaft completely.[60] This shell of periosteal new bone will exhibit small holes or skip areas called "cloacae" (Fig. 14–4). Pathologic examination shows that these are areas of necrosis or small abscesses, which often extend into the adjacent soft tissues. These soft tissue abscesses from osteomyelitis will obliterate the adjacent fat planes, whereas neoplastic tumor masses will cause fat plane displacement.[120]

Sequestra are areas of necrotic bone deprived of their normal blood supply.[169] Radiographically such areas are seen as irregular osseous fragments that are often more dense than normal bone[13] and are commonly situated in the medullary aspect of a tubular bone (Fig. 14–5).[143] The increased density of such areas is primarily due to an absent blood supply and nonparticipation in the hyperemia, which results in osteoporosis in the adjacent vascularized bone.[143] The lucency surrounding such sequestra is due to granulation tissue[158] and pus.[21]

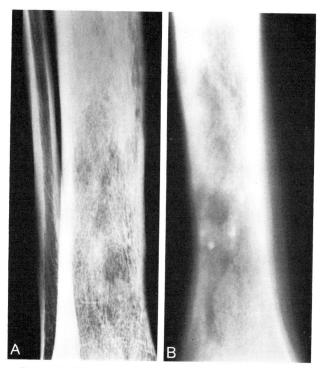

Figure 14–5. Radiograph (*A*) and tomogram (*B*) of the tibia. The small sclerotic sequestra are clearly defined on the tomogram.

The size of a sequestration is extremely variable. Sequestra can be very small or as large as the entire diaphysis.[120] Tomography is frequently required to demonstrate such sequestra (Fig. 14–5). It takes at least 3 weeks from the onset of infection until the appearance of the sequestra and involucrum.[13]

Occasionally, the infection will not produce areas

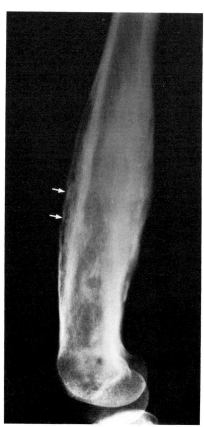

Figure 14–4. Lateral view of the femur in chronic osteomyelitis. Dense periosteal envelope with skip areas (*arrows*) anteriorly. (Courtesy of Dr. Gerald R. May, Mayo Clinic, Rochester, Minnesota.)

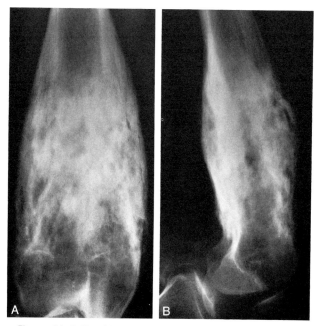

Figure 14–6. Garré's sclerosing osteomyelitis. AP (*A*) and lateral (*B*) views of the femur demonstrate dense cortical and medullary sclerosis.

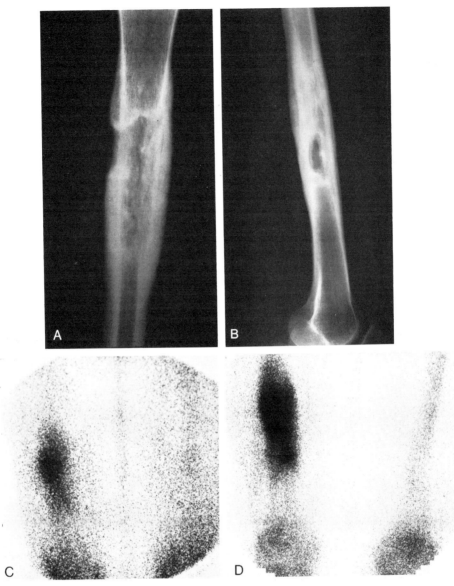

Figure 14–7. Chronic osteomyelitis. AP (*A*) and lateral (*B*) radiographs demonstrate cortical thickening with a lateral defect. Less sclerosis is evident in chronic osteomyelitis than in sclerosing osteomyelitis. Ga-67 (*C*) and Tc-99m (*D*) scans were positive.

of necrosis but will instead spread throughout an area of bone, resulting in a sclerotic, nonpurulent form of osteomyelitis[169] (Fig. 14–6). The eponym Garré's sclerosing osteomyelitis should more properly be reserved for this type of reaction,[181] but it is often carelessly applied to any form of chronic osteomyelitis exhibiting marked thickening of the periosteum and osseous eburnation[145] (Fig. 14–7). Garré's osteomyelitis is a rare condition and has a predilection for the mandible in patients under the age of 25.[26, 30, 74, 95] The considerable sclerosis may make radiographic diagnosis difficult. This condition can be confused with osteogenic sarcoma, osteoid osteoma, fibrous dysplasia, and Paget's disease, among others.[22, 26]

Clinically patients with Brodie's abscess, a related lesion, often have symptoms for weeks or months and are not systemically ill.[91, 117] *Staphylococcus aureus*

is the commonest cultured organism, but there is also a high proportion of sterile abscesses.[108] The classic description of a Brodie's abscess consists of a metaphyseal lesion with well defined margins, usually involving the tibia in young males prior to epiphyseal closure (Fig. 14–8*A*). Miller and colleagues reviewed 25 cases of Brodie's abscess and found only 5 (20 percent) in the classic location, although 60 percent were metaphyseal.[108] Involvement of the diaphysis, femoral neck, patella, and metatarsal head were all noted in their series. The degree of margin sharpness in their series was broad; some were well marginated and others barely perceptible.

The size of the abscess cavity will vary widely, in part owing to the success of the body's attempt at repair and the stage at which the initial diagnosis was made. Brodie's abscesses can range from 4 mm

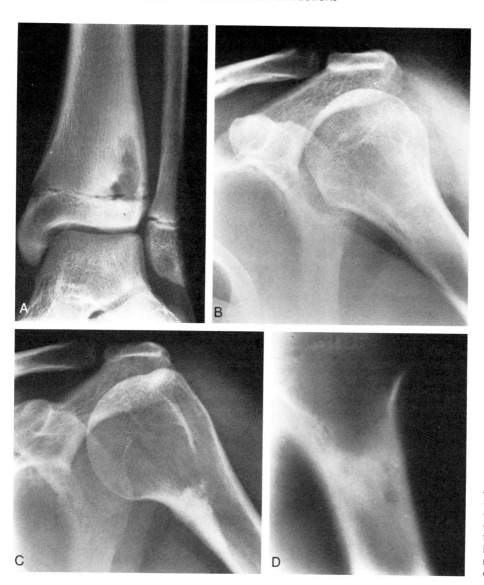

Figure 14–8. Brodie's abscess. AP view of the ankle (*A*) demonstrates classic tibial metaphyseal appearance. Tomography is frequently useful in better defining these lesions. AP views of humerus in internal (*B*) and external (*C*) rotation. Tomogram (*D*) more clearly defines the progress.

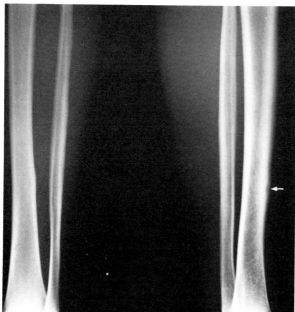

Figure 14–9. Brodie's abscess involving the distal tibial cortex (*arrow*).

to 4 or 5 cm[108, 145] (Figs. 14–8*B* to *D* and 14–9). Larger abscess cavities can disrupt the cortex, but a periosteal reaction in metaphyseal lesions is said to be uncommon.[13] Sequestration can be seen in up to 20 percent of cases.[108]

Involvement of the growth plate and extension from the metaphysis to the epiphysis can occur, although there is usually no resultant leg length discrepancy.[91, 108] Demonstration of a serpiginous channel connecting the metaphyseal lesion to the growth plate is said to be a relatively specific finding in Brodie's abscess[56] (Fig. 14–10).

Brodie's abscess can occur within the cortical bone of the diaphysis with an osteolytic area that is smaller than the lesions affecting the metaphysis[16] (Figs. 14–8*B* to *D* and 14–9). Cortical hyperostosis and more extensive periosteal new bone is seen with these variants.[54] Diaphyseal involvement may be more common in the older patient.[169]

In their discussion of Brodie's abscesses, Morrey and Peterson state that "this form referred to as subacute osteomyelitis by some authors is protean in presentation."[117] Its radiologic spectrum is also

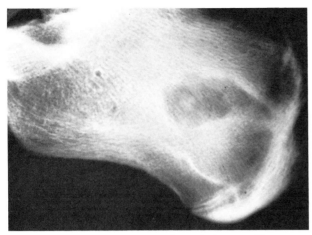

Figure 14–10. Calcaneal metaphyseal abscess with sequestration and serpiginous tract to the epiphysis.

extremely broad, with differences partly explained by variations in organism virulence, host resistance, and prior antibiotic therapy.

Sites of Infection

The majority of cases of osteomyelitis involve single areas in long bones of the lower extremity, particularly the lower femur and upper tibia.[83, 84, 117, 161, 190] Involvement of multiple sites is rare[32, 112, 117, 133, 190] except in neonates. Neonatal osteomyelitis usually exhibits multicentric involvement in patients who are not toxic.[19, 25, 48, 111, 126] This lack of clinical signs of infection places the burden of early

recognition on the radiologist, and a radiologic skeletal survey is indicated if a single site is initially identified.[19]

Osteomyelitis can involve flat bones, especially in areas bordering articular cartilage, fibrocartilage, or apophyseal growth plates. Nixon[123] terms these areas "metaphyseal equivalent locations." Unusual sites of osteomyelitis include the ribs, calcaneus, pelvis, and clavicle.[34, 114] Infection in these areas can be difficult to diagnose radiographically, and the sites are often confused with neoplasms[21, 34, 114] (Fig. 14–11).

Heroin addicts are predisposed to vertebral body osteomyelitis, which is the common site of involvement in the adult.[83, 85, 148] They also have frequent involvement of the sterno-articular region as well as the sacroiliac joints.[148] *Pseudomonas aeruginosa* is a common pathogen, while *Staphylococcus aureus* is the usual cause of most cases of acute hematogenous osteomyelitis.[41, 161]

Involvement of the hands and feet is usually from contiguous or soft tissue infections rather than from hematogenous spread.[107, 143, 176, 187] Osteomyelitis in the diabetic foot with vascular and neurologic disease can be especially difficult to diagnose. Injuries causing osteomyelitis of the hands and feet are often trivial and pass by unnoticed. The presence of periostitis is a valuable clue. There is usually no periosteal reaction with a neurotrophic change secondary to diabetes mellitus[102] (Fig. 14–12).

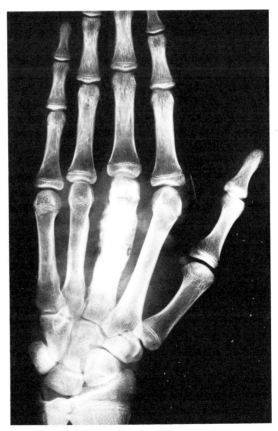

Figure 14–12. Tuberculous osteomyelitis. Note the dense periosteal reaction. (Courtesy of Dr. Gerald R. May, Mayo Clinic, Rochester, Minnesota.)

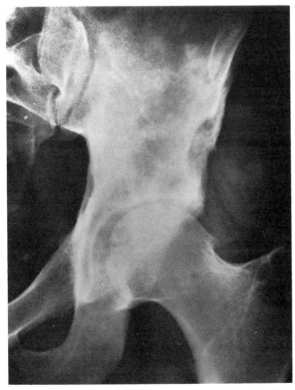

Figure 14–11. Post-traumatic osteomyelitis involving the ilium.

Complications and Sequelae

Chronic osteomyelitis follows acute osteomyelitis in 15 to 30 percent of patients.[12,79,112] Chronic osteomyelitis can also undergo carcinomatous degeneration in a very small percentage of cases. Roentgenographic examination usually shows more extensive destruction; however, it may be indistinguishable from chronic osteomyelitis alone[44] (Fig. 14–13). Malignant degeneration occurs in less than 2 percent of cases.[44, 182] Amyloidosis is no longer a major complication.[182]

Nuclear Imaging

It has only been in the last decade that nuclear medicine has been used in the workup of patients with known or suspected inflammatory disease of the musculoskeletal system. One of the major benefits of bone scanning is its high sensitivity for the early detection of osteomyelitis.[68, 118, 122, 127, 129, 153] This sensitivity has been demonstrated with a variety of radiopharmaceuticals. Strontium-87m scanning was performed in the early 1970's, and in a report by Staheli 18 out of 20 children with osteomyelitis, septic arthritis, or diskitis had a positive scan before any radiographic findings were shown.[167] Both flu-

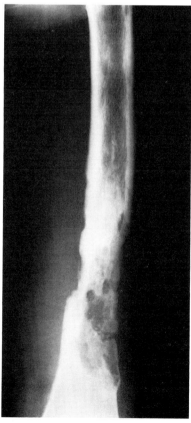

Figure 14–13. AP radiograph of the femur showing extensive destruction with a geographic distribution. Chronic osteomyelitis with squamous cell carcinoma.

orine-18 bone scanning[163] and technetium-99m pyrophosphate have been shown to be equally efficacious in the early identification of patients with osteomyelitis. Duszynski and colleagues, using Tc-99m pyrophosphate in 42 patients with suspected osteomyelitis, showed that early in the course of the disease there was only 1 true positive x-ray, whereas there were 18 false negative x-rays.[37] In their series the bone scan showed 18 true positives, 1 false positive, and only 1 false negative result. The use of bone scans for the early detection of osteomyelitis has been confirmed by many other reports.[39, 49, 66, 118, 122, 140]

In a recent large series, bone scintigraphy showed a sensitivity of 89 pecent with a specificity of 94 percent and an overall accuracy of 92 percent in a patient population with a prevalence of osteomyelitis of 44 percent[72] (Fig. 14–7). In another recent large series with a lower prevalence of disease (29 percent), the bone scan had a sensitivity of 76 percent, a specificity of 99 percent, and an overall accuracy of 93 percent, while the standard radiographic workup had a sensitivity of 24 percent, a specificity of 99 percent and an accuracy of 79 percent.[127] Similar findings have been reported for unusual sites of infection, such as pyogenic sacroiliitis,[12, 57] and unusual infections.[5, 55, 87]

One clinical problem that arises is the difficulty of distinguishing cellulitis from osteomyelitis. Gilday and colleagues[51] discussed the utility of comparing the early "blood pool" image, which is taken immediately after the tracer has been injected, with the standard delayed (2-hour) scan. The patient with typical osteomyelitis has a well defined area of increased uptake in the bone on both the early and delayed images. Cellulitis shows a diffuse increased uptake in both the "blood pool" and delayed scans, and septic arthritis shows a similar picture to cellulitis involving the joint alone. Maurer and colleagues[100] concluded that the addition of a radionuclide angiogram and immediate "blood pool" image to the standard delayed bone scan did not change the sensitivity in the detection of osteomyelitis but did lower the false positive rate from 25 percent to 6 percent. A similar result with a three-phase bone scan has been demonstrated in diabetic patients with suspected osteomyelitis.[128, 130]

Another clinical problem is the difficulty of distinguishing osteomyelitis from cellulitis and bone infarction in children.[39, 45, 49, 73, 153, 178, 179] Majd and Frankel[98] demonstrated that a normal "blood pool" scan with focal increased activity was a typical pattern for bone infarction in sickle cell crisis, whereas the previously mentioned patterns held true for osteomyelitis and cellulitis. Although the majority of cases of osteomyelitis can be detected with the standard delayed bone scan and the specificity of the scans can be improved in certain clinical situations with the addition of a radionuclide angiogram and early "blood pool" image, there have been a number of reports of normal bone scans or "cold" photopenic areas in early osteomyelitis[9, 45, 77, 98, 153, 170, 178] (Fig. 14–14). Murray, however, points

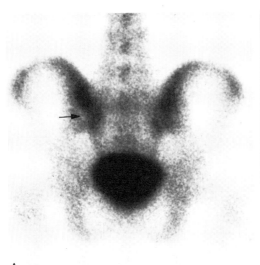

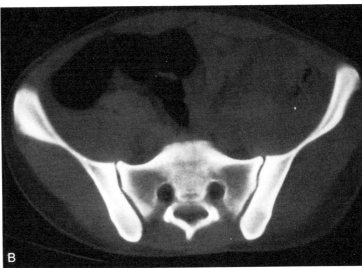

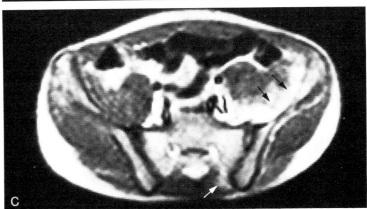

Figure 14–14. Young patient with suspected sacroiliac infection. *A,* Tc-99m scan demonstrates a "cold" spot in the inferior left sacroiliac joint (*arrow*). *B,* CT scan demonstrates a small irregularity of the sacrum that may be a small fracture. *C,* Magnetic resonance image clearly demonstrates soft tissue changes in the iliopsoas and posterior to the sacroiliac joint (*arrows*).

out that these photopenic areas may be just as diagnostically rewarding as the standard findings of increased uptake in osteomyelitis and septic arthritis.[119] Both Gilday[51] and Handmaker[65, 66] point out the need for high-quality studies and draw attention to the spectrum of findings characteristic of acute osteomyelitis. They both conclude that in a patient with a normal bone scan in whom there is a high clinical index of suspicion, a gallium scan should be performed; however, there is at least one case report of decreased gallium uptake in early acute osteomyelitis.[3]

While bone scanning is useful for childhood and adult osteomyelitis, there is some controversy as to its role in neonatal osteomyelitis.[19] Ash and Gilday[5] reported that only 6 out of 20 sites were positive on bone scanning in neonates with proven osteomyelitis. Mok and colleagues recommend that the bone scan be reserved for those cases of suspected neonatal osteomyelitis in which both the clinical and radiographic findings are equivocal.[111] However, a recent report by Bressler and Conway[18] showed that by using careful scintigraphic techniques they were able to identify all 25 sites of proven osteomyelitis. It would appear that in the child with normal x-rays and suspected osteomyelitis, even in the neonatal period, bone scintigraphy should be strongly considered.

Computed Tomography

Computed tomography has proved to be extremely useful in several clinical problem areas in evaluation of the musculoskeletal system (see Chapters 1, 3, and 4). Its role in infections of the musculoskeletal system is less well defined, however, especially for hematogenous osteomyelitis. The strength of the CT study is its ability to localize pathology in anatomically contiguous areas and its ability to detect small differences in attenuation. Kuhn and Berger's[92] preliminary experience suggests that CT may be helpful in the diagnosis of early osteomyelitis. In a study of 22 children they found that increased density of the medullary space was a good indicator of osteomyelitis (Fig. 14–15). They also noted that care must be taken in the positioning of the extremities, since a lack of symmetry (with more cancellous bone on one side and marrow on the other side) may be mistaken for osteomyelitis.

There are other limitations in using CT for the early detection of osteomyelitis. The marrow cavity is too small in the bones of the hands and feet to detect changes in attenuation. Also, increased attenuation of the marrow is not pathognomonic for osteomyelitis, as it may also occur in other disease processes, such as tumors, trauma, and marrow

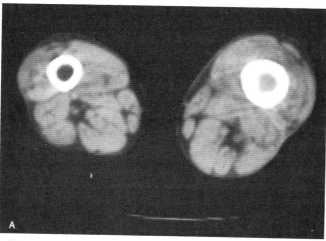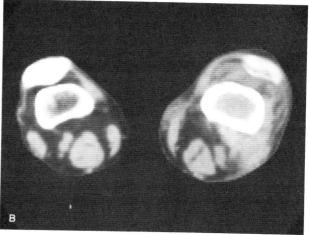

Figure 14–15. CT images in a patient with osteomyelitis. A, There is increased density in the medullary canal on the left with soft tissue swelling. B, The infection involves the joint space, resulting in an effusion. (Courtesy of Dr. R. A. McLeod, Mayo Clinic, Rochester, Minnesota.)

storage disease. However, CT does allow differentiation of soft tissue from bone involvement. Hermann and Rose[69] also noted that in infection there is an increase in the attenuation of the medullary marrow space in both acute and subacute phases of osteomyelitis. In chronic osteomyelitis the involucrum is well demonstrated, and they suggest that follow-up CT could be useful to differentiate healing from progression of osteomyelitis.

A CT scan can elucidate another sign of osteomyelitis described in three patients by Ram and colleagues,[138] namely gas within the medullary cavity. In all three patients the plain radiographs were not helpful, and the finding of gas in the marrow space on a CT image led to the diagnosis of osteomyelitis.

In an animal study Raptopoulos and colleagues[140] induced osteomyelitis in rabbits by direct inoculation of Staphylococcus aureus into the tibial metaphysis. Increased medullary attenuation was detected with a CT scan in 4 of 6 animals within the first week. This was approximately the same sensitivity as the indium-111 white blood cell scan (83 percent) in the first week in their series. Hald and Sudmann[63] have also shown that the change of CT numbers is an early indicator of osteomyelitis. Janson and associates[76] studied 20 patients with post-traumatic chronic osteomyelitis. CT found more sequestrations and demonstrated soft tissue disease better than plain films. Although CT was useful, they recommend that it be reserved for cases in which routine radiographic studies are inconclusive.

In general, CT imaging is not necessary for most cases of suspected osteomyelitis. Routine x-rays combined with radionuclide studies will be diagnostic in the majority of patients. In some patients with inconclusive studies and in patients with complex infectious processes,[41] CT may prove very useful.

Azouz[6] retrospectively reviewed patients in whom CT was performed when specific clinical problems were unsolved by standard radiographs, tomography, and nuclear bone scans. In this group the use of CT helped to visualize the entire articular surface on both sides of the involved joint as well as the periarticular soft tissue. Unexpected advanced septic sacroiliac joint involvement was demonstrated in two of three patients. CT can be very important in the workup. In this report[6] and in another report from Germany,[34] the authors reserve the use of CT for cases of osteomyelitis not clearly defined by plain films and nuclear studies, or for cases in which it is necessary to assess the periarticular soft tissues, especially if surgery is a consideration.

Magnetic Resonance Imaging

Early studies demonstrate that magnetic resonance imaging may be of particular value in the study of bone and soft tissue abnormalities.[10, 109, 110, 113] The medullary bone provides a high-intensity signal with little signal from normal cortical bone. Nerves, vessels, fat, and muscle are more easily differentiated with MRI than CT owing to improved contrast (see section on Magnetic Resonance Imaging in Chapter 1

A reduced signal (T1 weighted sequences) in the medullary bone is found in patients with osteomyelitis.[46] This may vary with different pulse sequences. In our experience the signal was decreased using partial saturation and inversion-recovery sequences but was increased with long T_R spin-echo sequences (SE, TE60, TR2000). Periosteal and soft tissue changes are easily detected. The findings are much more dramatic than with routine radiography or tomography (Fig. 14–16). Soft tissue and medullary changes are usually more clearly demonstrated with MRI than with CT images (Fig. 14–14). It is not yet certain if magnetic resonance imaging will detect changes more rapidly than nuclear imaging. Specificity is also in question. However, further work in T_1 and T_2 relaxation times may demonstrate improved tissue specificity compared with CT or isotope scans.

JOINT SPACE INFECTION

Routine Radiographic Evaluation

Although almost any organism has the potential to produce an infectious arthritis, the majority of joint space infections are due to *Staphylococcus aureus*.[82, 115, 136, 142, 144] Radiographs are usually not helpful in differentiating among the various causal organisms, and microbiologic isolation of the organism from aerobic and anaerobic incubation of clinical material is necessary for certain definitive diagnoses.[136, 142] Infectious arthritis usually affects a single joint; the most common sites of involvement include the knees and hips.[84] Polyarticular involvement can be seen in patients with rheumatoid arthritis on long-term corticosteroid therapy.[82] In

these patients an enlarging effusion and rapid bone destruction are useful clues in the diagnosis of a superimposed infection.[142]

The earliest roentgenographic sign seen in an infectious arthritis is soft tissue swelling in a periarticular location.[28, 186] This is accompanied by a joint effusion resulting from edema, swelling, and hypertrophy of the synovial membrane.[120, 142] Since infection of the synovial membrane precedes contamination of the synovial fluid (unless, of course, the cause of the infection is direct inoculation), an early joint aspiration may not reveal an organism.[145, 191] A sterile effusion can also occur on a sympathetic basis in a neighboring joint.[7]

In the hips, primarily in children, widening of the joint space is a good indicator of the presence of intra-articular fluid[67] (Fig. 14–17). However, a pyogenic arthritis can ultimately lead to loss of articular cartilage and joint space narrowing.[38, 132, 172] Therefore, it is important to understand the chronology of the infection (Fig. 14–18). Another sign of a septic arthritis involving the hip is obliteration of the para-articular fat planes, especially the obturator internus fat pad[67] (Fig. 14–17). In infants a large

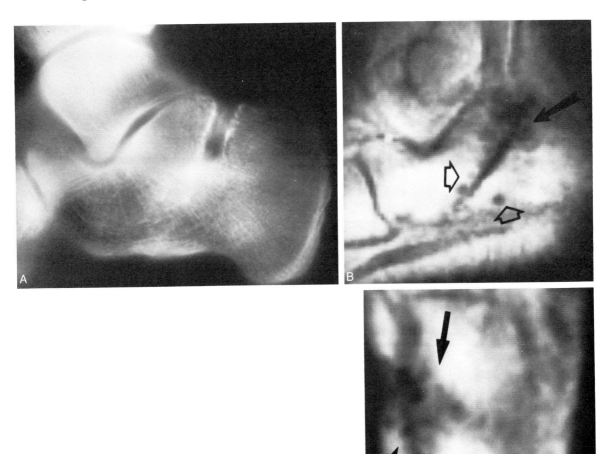

Figure 14–16. Osteomyelitis of the calcaneus. *A,* Lateral tomogram demonstrates a previous osteotomy defect. *B,* Sagittal magnetic resonance image in the same plane demonstrates considerable medullary (*open arrows*) and soft tissue (*black arrow*) changes due to osteomyelitis. *C,* Axial scan shows bone and soft tissue changes consistent with infection.

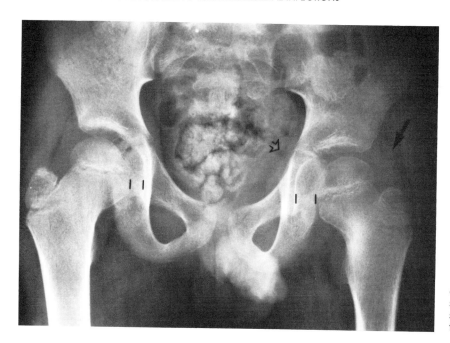

Figure 14–17. AP view of the pelvis in a child with septic arthritis. There is joint space widening, displacement of the fat stripes (*black arrow*), and obliteration of the obturator internus (*open arrow*).

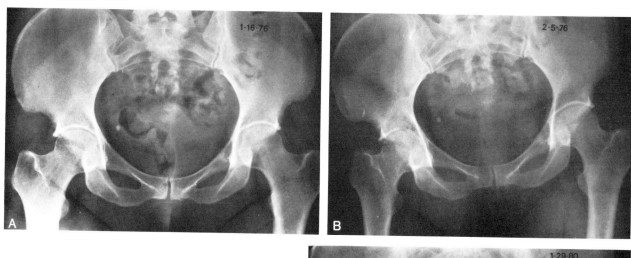

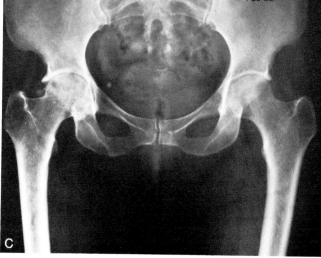

Figure 14–18. AP views of the pelvis in septic arthritis (right hip) due to *Staphylococcus aureus. A,* Film taken 1/16/76 shows minimal fat stripe displacement. *B,* Follow-up study 2/5/76 reveals marked joint space narrowing with early cortical destruction. *C,* Following successful treatment (1/29/80), degenerative arthritis developed in the involved hip.

effusion and marked capsular distention will cause lateral displacement of the femur and sometimes a pathologic dislocation along the physis.[15, 81, 97, 116] An arthrogram can help differentiate between a true dislocation and a pathologic epiphyseal separation.[53]

Knee effusions are best seen with a well positioned lateral view. Fluid accumulates initially in the suprapatellar bursa. When the fluid is pus, the boundary between the suprapatellar bursa and the quadriceps tendon becomes indistinct.[67] The posterior suprapatellar fat pad becomes compressed against the anterior femur and may be obliterated.[67] One of the most accurate signs is the "fat pad separation sign." This is the width of the base of the suprapatellar bursa, measured by taking the distance between the anterior suprapatellar fat pad and the posterior suprapatellar or prefemoral fat pad. In Hall's series,[64] 27 of 28 patients were correctly diagnosed as having an effusion when the width of the bursa was greater than 10 mm, and 64 of 65 were accurately diagnosed as having no effusion when the fat pad separation was less than 5 mm (see section on the lateral view of the knee in Chapter 6).

Increased intra-articular pressure from pus and proteolytic enzymes within the joint causes joint space narrowing owing to destruction of articular cartilage.[131, 154] This narrowing occurs within a few days after the start of the infection. It precedes any osseous changes,[38] which are not seen until 8 to 10 days from the onset of symptoms[120] (Fig. 14–18).

Early bone abnormalities include loss of the cortical outline of the subchondral bone and erosions at the margin of the joint where the synovium abuts bone without intervening protective cartilage.[38, 120, 145] Bone involvement is usually less severe than in primary osteomyelitis.[38, 120] Sequestrations are rare in patients with uncomplicated or primary infectious arthritis. It should be noted that septic arthritis can develop secondarily from osteomyelitis involving the epiphysis or intra-articular metaphysis.[142] In these instances, the findings of osteomyelitis will often be the predominant radiographic feature.

Osteoporosis in a periarticular or regional distribution is due to associated hyperemia and immobilization.[24, 120, 142] Periarticular calcification can also be seen and appears to be due to dystrophic calcification in necrotic tissue.[89, 162] The presence of gas within the joint should raise the possibility of a recent arthrocentesis as well as infection by *Escherichia coli* or *Clostridium welchii*.[11, 104, 177]

In summary, the radiographic findings of a joint effusion, rapid loss of articular cartilage, and loss of the subchondral cortical "white line" are characteristic for a pyogenic arthritis. Early treatment is necessary to prevent complications and sequelae, such as bony or fibrous ankylosis or growth disturbance. Unfortunately, once articular cartilage is destroyed, the joint space usually shows progressive narrowing owing to superimposed degenerative arthritis[115] (Fig. 14–18).

Nuclear Imaging

The radionuclide workup of a patient suspected of having a joint space infection should include an early "blood pool" image and a standard delayed scan.[52] Recently Kloiber and colleagues[88] studied the onset of acute hip pain in children. A photopenic area surrounding the joint space on the early "blood pool" scan was found to correlate with an effusion. Nine patients had diminished tracer on the affected side in the delayed scans. This resulted from compression of vessels due to a tense effusion (Fig. 14–14). Follow-up scans in 4 out of 5 patients reverted to normal after hip aspiration. One patient did not show normal activity after aspiration of the effusion. This proved to be due to infarction of the femoral head.

In transient synovitis 6 of 19 children had normal studies, whereas 10 of 19 patients had increased activity on delayed views.[88] In another series[70] children presenting with hip pain due to toxic synovitis had normal scans in 9 cases and increased activity over the affected joint in 3 cases. However, when there is a strong clinical suspicion of infectious (septic) arthritis, the addition of a gallium scan should be strongly considered. In an early report by Handmaker,[66] 4 patients with early acute septic arthritis had normal bone scans with positive gallium scans, while 2 patients with toxic synovitis had normal bone scans and normal gallium scans. Lisbona and Rosenthall[96] also reported on patients with septic arthritis. In 6 of 11 patients both gallium scans and bone scans were positive, but in 5 of the 11 patients the bone scan was negative whereas the gallium scan was positive. In their series they could differentiate between osteomyelitis, septic arthritis, and cellulitis in older children. In infants it was not possible to differentiate between these processes, but a diagnosis of a septic area was still possible. In their report they also noted that although the bone scan remains positive following adequate antibiotic therapy since it reflects the reparative process, gallium scans seem to revert to normal and parallel the clinical course during therapy. However, the same group[90] in a later series found that although the gallium scans did improve during the early period of therapy, over half of the patients showed low-grade persistent uptake after complete clinical resolution of infection. They hypothesized that this is due to a reparative process and that the gallium scan could not be used as an end point for antibiotic treatment of osteomyelitis.

In the patient with previous trauma or surgical intervention there is a major clinical problem in the diagnosis of superimposed infection. In trauma the radiographic anatomy is distorted, and the bone scan may stay positive for years.[151, 152] After total joint replacement the bone scan will remain positive for months[180] and will also be positive when the components become loosened or infected[50, 183, 189] (see the section on Total Hip Replacement in Chapter 4).

There have been reports of the utility of gallium scanning to diagnose or exclude sternal osteomyelitis after midline sternotomy.[40, 154, 156, 162, 164] In a small series Deysine and colleagues[31] demonstrated that gallium scans were useful in postoperative bone infections and detected early exacerbations of chronic osteomyelitis (Fig. 14–7). Rosenthall and colleagues[151] studied and described the pattern of uptake of both Tc-99m phosphate bone tracers and Ga-67 citrate following insertion of orthopedic devices. In their series spatially congruent uptake of Tc-99m MDP and mild to moderate gallium accumulation were seen in patients proven to be free of inflammatory disease. When there is spatially incongruent activity of Ga-67 and Tc-99m MDP, all patients proved to have osteomyelitis, cellulitis, nonspecific synovitis, or some combination thereof. They concluded that Tc-99m MDP–Ga-67 sequential imaging of orthopedic patients suspected of having infections will offer a more specific diagnosis than either of the tracers alone. A similar finding was made by Reing and colleagues,[141] who studied 79 patients with bone and gallium scanning and painful joint prostheses. Their results were 19 true positive scans, 59 true negative studies, and only 1 false negative study. Rushton and colleagues[152] also reported excellent results with sequential gallium and bone scintigraphy in patients with painful total hip replacement.

Using the criteria of moderate- to high-grade Ga-67 uptake or spatially incongruent gallium uptake when compared with sites of Tc-99m MDP uptake in a large series of patients suspected of having bone joint or soft tissue infections, Rosenthall and associates[150] reported a sensitivity of 72 percent, a specificity of 86 percent, and an accuracy of 80 percent. Using the same criteria, Merkel and colleagues[105] reported similar results in 101 patients with painful prosthetic joints. The sensitivity for detecting infection was 68 percent, the specificity 80 percent, and the accuracy 76 percent.

As noted above, gallium scanning alone or in combination with bone scanning still does not completely solve the complex problem of identifying infection in violated bone. Thakur and colleagues[174, 175] demonstrated that leukocytes could be labeled with In-111 oxine and retain their viability and function when reinjected. In a report on the use of In-111 oxine polymorphonuclear cells to localize infection, McDougall[101] reported that 4 of 4 patients with acute bone and joint infections were positive on scan. Sfakianakis[159,160] in a study on the diagnosis of occult sepsis with In-111 leukocytes and Ga-67 citrate had 2 true positive white blood cell scans and 32 true negative studies with no false positive or false negative studies for osteomyelitis. In their study, Propst-Proctor and colleagues[137] found a sensitivity of 98 percent, a specificity of 89 percent, and an overall accuracy of 93 percent in a series of 88 patients suspected of having osteomyelitis. Raptopoulos and colleagues[140] discussed the advantages of a white blood cell scan in the early detection of acute osteomyelitis in an animal model. Their study was interesting in that the white blood cell study was positive in 83 percent of the animals in a 1-week period of time, whereas only 22 percent of the Tc-99m MDP bone scans were positive within 1 week. Schauwecker and colleagues[156] suggest the use of In-111 white blood cell scans to increase the specificity of diagnosis of osteomyelitis in complicated cases in which the bone scan would be suspected to be positive owing to rapid bone turnover. Sfakianakis[159] studied 10 cases of chronic bone infection and reported that the bone scan had 100 percent sensitivity but only a 17 percent specificity, whereas the plain radiographs had a 75 percent specificity but only a 70 percent sensitivity. In his study both gallium and indium white blood cell scans had an 80 percent sensitivity but a poor specificity (42 percent for gallium and 58 percent for indium white blood cells).

Our experience is significantly different.[105, 106] In a prospective series of 50 patients presenting with symptoms suggestive of low-grade osteomyelitis, 44 had both Tc-99m MDP–Ga-67 citrate scans and In-111 white blood cell scans within 3 days. The In-111 white blood cell scan had a sensitivity of 82 percent, a specificity of 90 percent, and an accuracy of 85 percent; and all three observers in our study performed better on analysis of white blood cell scans than with the gallium scans. There are obviously mixed reports on the utility of In-111 white blood cell scanning for low-grade osteomyelitis, and a longer experience will be needed before its place in the workup of osteomyelitis is determined.

Computed Tomography and Magnetic Resonance Imaging

Computed tomography is rarely indicated for joint space infection. Routine radiography and isotope studies are usually sufficient. Following surgical procedures, such as joint replacement, the metal artifact with CT is significant. The result is loss of bone and adjacent soft tissue detail.

Magnetic resonance imaging provides information regarding effusion and synovitis. Following joint replacement there is less artifact, and therefore MRI may be useful (Fig. 14–19).

Aspiration and arthrography provide more information following arthroplasty (see Chapters 4 and 6).

SEPTIC SPONDYLITIS

Septic spondylitis is a general term broadly used to describe a spectrum of clinical findings that can be discussed as a single entity owing to similarities in roentgenographic appearance.[57, 60] At one end is the clinical syndrome of symptomatic narrowing of the disk space in a child with an elevated erythrocyte sedimentation rate.[17, 184] This syndrome has been called diskitis,[1, 43] intervertebral disk space

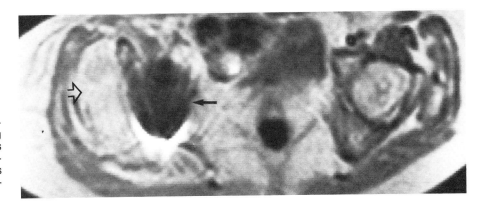

Figure 14–19. Magnetic resonance image of the hips following right total hip arthroplasty. There is some artifact (*black arrow*); however, the periarticular abscess (*open arrow*) is still well demonstrated.

infection,[135] infectious diskitis,[17] nonspecific spondylitis,[75] and intervertebral disk space inflammation.[165, 166] It most likely represents a low-grade infection of the intervertebral disk with secondary involvement of the adjacent vertebral bodies.[17, 149] Because of a difference in the nature of the blood supply to the disk,[27] the term pyogenic vertebral osteomyelitis is used to describe a similar radiographic appearance in the adult.[168] The adult form usually has a worse prognosis with a higher risk of paraplegia and death.[86]

In children and young adults until the age of 20 or 30, vascular channels actually perforate the vertebral end-plate.[27] Blood vessels passing through the hyaline cartilage of the disk permit perfusion of nutrients to disk cartilage.[36] These channels provide a pathway for blood-borne organisms to reach the intervertebral disk,[168] and diskitis in children is most likely due to actual hematogenous contamination of the intervertebral disk.[14, 166] *Staphylococcus aureus* is the commonest causal organism, but blood and biopsy cultures are not always positive, especially in the patient with long-standing symptoms.[166] Some authors have hypothesized a viral etiology.[43, 103] It should be noted that some consider childhood diskitis a post-traumatic phenomenon[1] or a noninfectious inflammation.

In the adult, the disk is relatively avascular and infection involving the disk is probably not the result of hematogenous spread. The primary infection occurs in the anterior subchondral area of the vertebral body and spreads rapidly to the disk.[14, 72, 145 168] In fact, Wenger[184] feels that even in children "diskitis" can represent a primary bone infection with secondary disk involvement. On the other hand, Kemp and associates[86] described 15 patients (ages 17 to 72 years) with what they felt represented isolated disk infection without previous trauma. They noted that other investigators have reported that the intervertebral disk did not become totally avascular even in the elderly, and they therefore concluded that a pyogenic infection of the intervertebral disk in adults differed from pyogenic osteomyelitis of the vertebral body in respective sites of origin. Because of the controversy, Resnick and Niwayama state, "Although the concept of hematogenous infection isolated to the interverte-

bral disk of the adult due to persistent normal or abnormal vascular channels is indeed intriguing, further documentation of this entity is required before its existence is truly established."[145] They feel that blood-borne organisms originally lodge in an anterior subchondral focus, probably through the venous plexus of Batson.[8] However, Wiley and Trueta showed that arterial spread through the nutrient branches of the posterior spinal arteries is more likely, since the vertebral venous plexus is a drainage system filling in a retrograde manner only with pressure.[188] Whatever the route, rapid spread to the adjacent intervertebral disk from the original subchondral focus causes early disk space involvement.[184] Naturally, direct penetrating trauma can violate the disk space itself and establish a "true" disk space infection. This infection is usually seen postoperatively.[57, 168]

Routine Radiographic Evaluation

The earliest radiographic finding in septic spondylitis in both children and adults is narrowing of the intervertebral disk space and adjacent soft tissue edema. This can be evident as early as 3 weeks after the onset of symptoms.[103] (Fig. 14–20). The degree of narrowing is variable and may not necessarily have prognostic value.[86] The lateral view is best for documenting changes in the height of the disk space[166] (Fig. 14–20). The majority of patients have involvement of a single disk space with the lumbar spine the commonest site of involvement.[33] In differentiating disk space infection from degenerative disk disease, the presence of a vacuum sign can be useful except in the rare cases involving gas-forming organisms.[128] The presence of the vacuum phenomenon should suggest a process other than infection[146] (Fig. 14–21). A narrowed disk space can also be seen after trauma in the battered child[171] and in Scheuermann's disease. In the latter condition, the erythrocyte sedimentation rate should be normal.[166]

The second radiographic sign is rarefaction of the adjacent vertebral bodies. This usually occurs approximately 6 weeks after the onset of symptoms[33] (see Fig. 14–20). This is closely followed by reactive

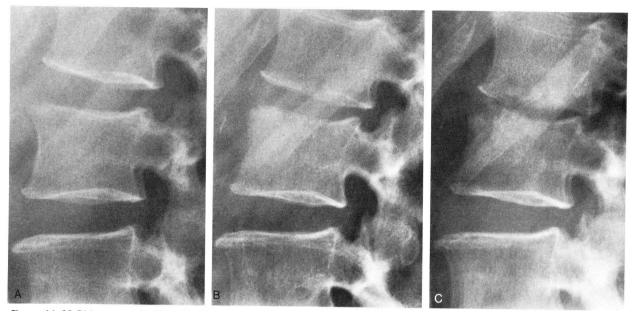

Figure 14–20. Disk space infection with *Staphylococcus aureus.* The initial spine films (*A*) were normal. Follow-up films several weeks later (*B*) demonstrate loss of detail in the end-plates and joint space narrowing. One month later (*C*) changes have progressed, and the disk space is obviously narrowed.

sclerosis of the subchondral bone adjacent to the involved disk space. This sclerosis is due to the deposition of new bone on existing trabeculae[86] (Fig. 14–22).

As more of the vertebral body is involved in the infection, lytic defects will appear within the vertebral body. These cavities are often best seen with tomography.[121, 166] Tomography will also demonstrate the characteristic relative sparing of the posterior elements.[61, 166] Most of the osseous destruction occurs in the anterior two thirds of the vertebral

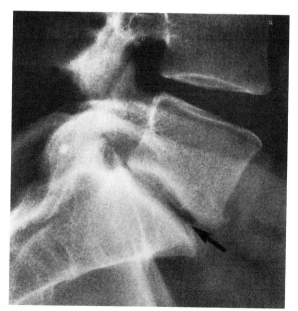

Figure 14–21. Lateral view of the lumbosacral interspace with vacuum sign due to degenerative disk disease. End-plates are intact.

body.[145] If the posterior elements are involved, tuberculosis should be considered.[120]

Soft tissue paraspinal masses are a variable finding, occurring in 18 to 23 percent of patients. The presence of a paraspinal mass may be helpful in differentiating pyogenic disease from tuberculosis,[33] although one large series found that this was not the case.[2] In fact, Allen's series of 12 nontuberculous and 33 tuberculous patients showed that no radiologic pattern was completely reliable in distinguishing tuberculous from nontuberculous infections.[2]

Some patients with septic spondylitis exhibit complete reconstruction,[47] while others progress to fusion of the vertebral bodies. Fusion occurs more commonly in children than in adults[86] except in the case of adult postoperative disk space infection, in which it may occur in almost all patients.[168] Scoliosis and kyphosis can occur as well as segmental or total vertebral body enlargement (vertebra magna).[166]

Nuclear Imaging

Disk space infections have been reported to occur in patients with a normal bone scan,[120, 121, 124, 125] and the false positive rate for bone scans in post-laminectomy patients with suspected disk space infection may be as high as 38 percent (Fig. 14–22). Gallium scanning of the suspected disk space infection has a sensitivity of 89 percent, a specificity of 85 percent, and an accuracy of 86 percent, as reported by Bruschwein and colleagues.[20] In an experimental animal model using rabbits and *Staphylococcus aureus*, Norris and colleagues found that although both Ga-67 and Tc-99m bone scans became

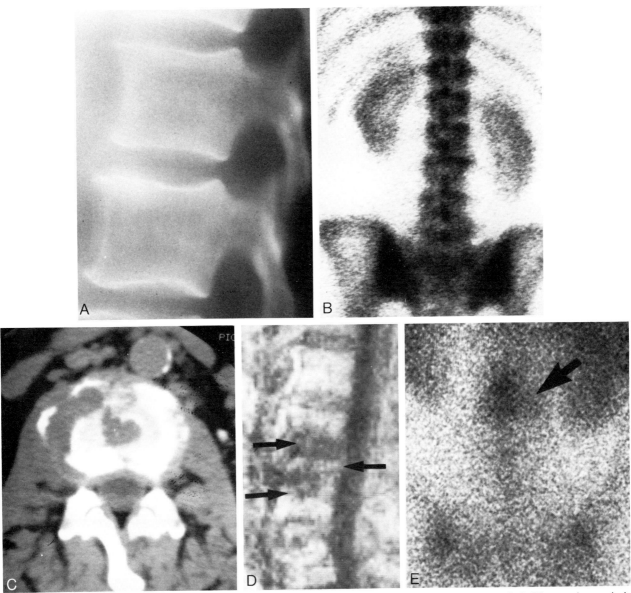

Figure 14–22. Disk space infection with *Candida. A,* Tomogram is normal. *B,* Tc-99m scan is also normal. *C,* CT scan demonstrates destruction of the vertebral body combined with soft tissue swelling. *D,* Sagittal magnetic resonance image demonstrates prolonged relaxation times in the vertebral end-plates (*double arrows*) and a narrowed disk space (*single arrow*). *E,* Indium-111 WBC scan was positive, indicating infection.

positive, the gallium scan became positive earlier in the course of the disease.[124]

Computed Tomography and Magnetic Resonance Imaging

On CT scans, lytic fragmentation of adjacent vertebral bodies is a characteristic appearance.[58, 135] Azouz[6] concludes that CT is useful "to assess the size, shape, and contents of the spinal canal, or to search for associated paravertebral soft tissue mass or abscesses."

As mentioned previously, in acute hematogenous osteomyelitis involving the long bones there is an increase in CT numbers (density). However, in pyogenic osteomyelitis of the spine the vertebral bodies show a drop in CT numbers,[80] as do the disk spaces themselves.[80, 92-94] In addition to the demonstration of vertebral osteomyelitis, CT can accurately localize epidural extensions[11, 58] and soft tissue abscesses. Following antibiotic therapy, bone density will increase, and soft tissue lesion sizes will decrease.[80]

The utility of CT in the workup of patients with tuberculous spondylitis is similar to that of CT in assessing the patient with the pyogenic lesion.[62, 92-94, 185]

Magnetic resonance imaging may be particularly suited to children, for there is no radiation with

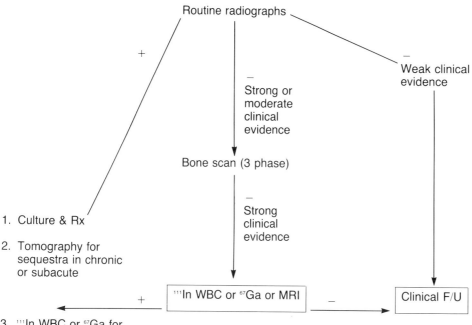

Figure 14–23. Diagnostic approach to osteomyelitis.

1. Culture & Rx

2. Tomography for sequestra in chronic or subacute

3. ^{111}In WBC or ^{67}Ga for activity in chronic or subacute

this imaging modality. Current techniques will demonstrate changes in the disk and vertebral bodies. However, changes are not specific, and resolution is less with MRI than with CT images.

The imaging workup of the patient with suspected septic spondylitis should start with conventional radiographs, including a lateral view of the area of concern. If the typical plain film findings are absent, a Ga-67 scan can be employed. This has a reported sensitivity of 85 percent[20] and will become positive earlier than the Tc-99m bone scan.[125]

Once the area of concern is localized, a CT scan of that region may then alleviate the necessity of myelography, or serial spine examinations.[42, 135] CT-guided aspiration of the disk space is also highly accurate.[58]

SUMMARY

In all infections except those associated with neonatal hematogenous osteomyelitis, the bone scan with TC-99m MDP is very sensitive. It misses only

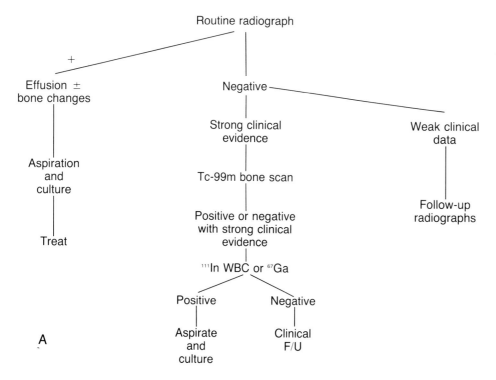

Figure 14–24. Diagnostic approach to joint space infection. *A,* No previous arthroplasty.
Illustration continued on opposite page

A

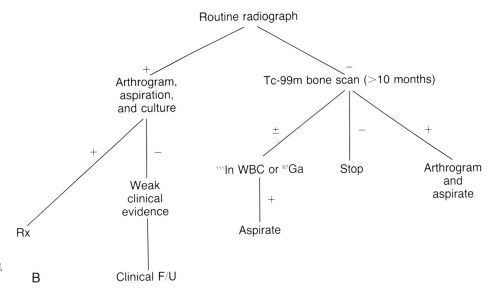

Figure 14–24 Continued. B, Previous arthroplasty.

a small percentage of early hematogenous osteomyelitis and early disk space infections. Its main drawback is a lack of specificity, and this can be improved by the three-phase bone scan that assesses vascularity. The addition of Ga-67 citrate scanning or In-11 white blood cell scanning appears to be very helpful in diagnosing infection that has been superimposed onto traumatized bone. These are also useful in cases in which surgical intervention would normally cause an increase in the uptake of the bone tracer.

The computed tomographic examination can supply valuable information unobtainable from other techniques in the patient with known or suspected musculoskeletal sepsis. In particular, early lesions may be detected when plain radiographs are negative and the radionuclide bone scans are nondiagnostic. The CT exam provides a detailed look at adjacent soft tissues and can help to determine if

surgical drainage should be a consideration in the septic patient.

Thus, imaging techniques can provide useful information and also guidance for diagnostic aspirations of joints and disk spaces. Figure 14–23 provides a suggested approach to the diagnosis of osteomyelitis. Isotope studies and magnetic resonance images will usually be positive before conventional radiographs. Tomography, In-111 white blood cell scans, and Ga-67 scans are useful in detecting activity in chronic or subacute cases. Since the diagnostic approach to evaluation of joint space disease depends upon the presence or absence of surgical appliances (joint replacements) (Fig. 14–24), isotope studies and arthrography are most accurate in this setting. Finally, computed tomography provides the most anatomic detail in study of disk space infection and also provides an excellent approach for aspiration (Fig. 14–25).

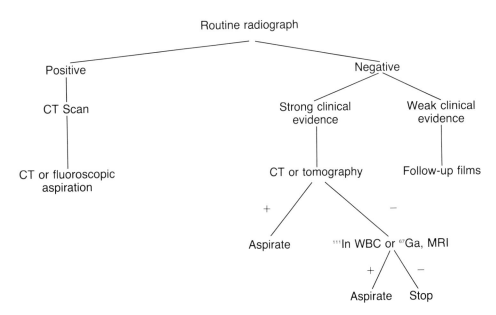

Figure 14–25. Diagnostic approach to disk space infection.

REFERENCES

1. Alexander, C. J.: The aetiology of juvenile spondylarthritis (discitis). Clin. Radiol. *21*:178, 1970.
2. Allen, E. H., Cosgrove, D., and Millard, F. J. C.: The radiological changes in infection of the spine and their diagnostic value. Clin. Radiol. *29*:31, 1978.
3. Ang, J. G. P., and Gelfand, M. J.: Decreased gallium uptake in acute hematogenous osteomyelitis. Clin. Nucl. Med. *8*:301, 1983.
4. Armbruster, T. G., Goergen, T. G., Resnick, D., et al.: Utility of bone scanning in disseminated coccidiodomycosis: Case report. J. Nucl. Med. *18*:450, 1977.
5. Ash, J. M., and Gilday, D. L.: The futility of bone scanning in neonatal osteomyelitis: Concise communication. J. Nucl. Med. *21*:417, 1980.
6. Azouz, E. M.: Computed tomography in bone and joint infections. Can. Assoc. Radiol. *32*:102, 1981.
7. Baker, S. B., and Robinson, D. R.: Sympathetic joint effusion in septic arthritis. JAMA *240*:1989, 1979.
8. Batson, O. V.: The function of the vertebral veins and their role in the spread of metastasis. Ann. Surg. *112*:138, 1940.
9. Berkowitz, I. D., and Wenzel, W.: "Normal" technetium bone scans in patients with acute osteomyelitis. Am. J. Dis. Child. *134*:828, 1980.
10. Berquist, T. H.: Magnetic resonance imaging: Preliminary experience in orthopedic radiology. Mag. Res. Imag. *2*:41, 1984.
11. Bliznak, J., and Ramsey, J.: Emphysematous septic arthritis due to E. coli. J. Bone Joint Surg. *58A*:138, 1976.
12. Blockey N. J., and Watson, J. T.: Acute osteomyelitis in children. J. Bone Joint Surg. *52B*:77, 1970.
13. Bonakdar-pour, A., Gaines, V. D.: The radiology of osteomyelitis. Orthop. Clin. North Am. *14*:21, 1983.
14. Bonfiglio, M., Lange, T. A., and Kim, Y. M.: Pyogenic vertebral osteomyelitis disk space infections. Clin. Orthop. *96*:234, 1973.
15. Borella, L., and Goobar, J. E., et al.: Septic arthritis in childhood. J. Pediatr. *62*:142, 1963.
16. Boriam, S.: Brodie's abscess. Ital. J. Orthop. Traumatal. *6*:373, 1980.
17. Boston, H. C. Jr., Bianco, A. J. Jr., Rhodes, K. H.: Disk space infections in children. Orthop. Clin. North Am. *6*:953, 1975.
18. Bressler, E. L., and Conway, J. J.: Bone scintigraphy in neonatal osteomyelitis. (abstract) Radiology *49*:35, 1983.
19. Brill, P. W., Winchester, P., Krauss, A. N., et al.: Osteomyelitis in a neonatal intensive care unit. Radiology *131*:83, 1979.
20. Bruschwein, D. A., Brown, M. L., and McLeod, R. A.: Gallium scintigraphy in the evaluation of disk-space infection: Concise communication. J. Nucl. Med. *21*:925, 1980.
21. Butt, W. P.: The radiology of infection. Clin. Orthop. *96*:20, 1973.
22. Cabanela, M., Sim, F. H., Beabout, J. W., et al.: Osteomyelitis appearing as neoplasms. Arch. Surg. *109*:68, 1974.
23. Capitano, M. A., and Kirkpatrick, J. A.: Early roentgen observations in acute osteomyelitis. A. J. R. *108*:488, 1970.
24. Clark, R. L., Cuttino, J. T. Jr., Anderle, S. K., et al.: Radiologic analysis of arthritis in rats after systemic injection of streptococcal cell walls. Arthritis Rheum. *22*:25, 1979.
25. Clarke, A. M.: Neonatal osteomyelitis: A disease different from osteomyelitis of older children. Med. J. Aust. *1*:237, 1958.
26. Collert, S., and Isacson, J. Chronic sclerosing osteomyelitis. Clin. Orthop. *164*:136, 1982.
27. Coventry, M. B., Ghormley, R. K., and Kernohan, J. W.: The intervertebral disc: Its microscopic anatomy and pathology. J. Bone Joint Surg. *27A*:105, 1945.
28. Curtis, P. H.: The pathophysiology of joint infections. Clin. Orthop. *96*:129, 1973.
29. Dalinka, M. K., Lally, J. F., Koniver, G., et al.: The radiology of osseous and articular infection. CRC Radiol. Nucl. Med. *7*:1, 1975.
30. Daramola, J. O., and Ajagbe, H. A.: Chronic osteomyelitis of the mandible in adults: A clinical study of 34 cases. Br. J. Oral Surg. *20*:58, 1982.
31. Deysine, M., Rafkin, H., and Teicher, I.: Diagnosis of chronic and postoperative osteomyelitis with gallium-67 citrate scans. Am. J. Surg. *129*:632, 1975.
32. Dich, V. Q., Nelson, J. D., and Hatalin K. C.: Osteomyelitis in infants and children. Am. J. Dis. Child. *129*:1273, 1975.
33. Digby, J. M., and Kersley, J. B.: Pyogenic non-tuberculous spinal infection. J. Bone Joint Surg. *61B*:47, 1979.
34. Dihlmann, V. W.: Koxale Computertomographie (KCT). ROFO *135*:333, 1981.
35. Donovan, R. M., and Shah, K. J.: Unusual sites of acute osteomyelitis in childhood. Clin. Radiol. *33*:222, 1982.
36. Doyle, J. R.: Narrowing of the intervertebral disc space in children. J. Bone Joint Surg. *42A*:1191, 1960.
37. Duszynski, D. O., Kuhn, J. F., and Afshani, E.: Early radionuclide diagnosis of acute osteomyelitis. Radiology *117*:337, 1975.
38. Edeiken, J.: Roentgen Diagnosis of Diseases of Bone. 3rd Ed. Baltimore, Williams and Wilkins, 1981.
39. Erasmie, U., and Hirsch, G.: Acute haematogenous osteomyelitis in children—the reliability of skeletal scintigraphy. Z. Kinderchir. *32*:360, 1981.
40. Feiglin, D. H., Detsky, A., and Simor, A. E.: The diagnostic value of gallium-67 in detection of postoperative sternal osteomyelitis (abstract). J. Nucl. Med. *24*:P64, 1983.
41. Ferguson, A. B.: Osteomyelitis in children. Clin. Orthop. *96*:51, 1973.
42. Firooznia, H., Rafii, M., Golimbu, C., et al.: Computed tomography of pressure sores, pelvic abscess, and osteomyelitis in patients with spinal cord injury. Arch. Phys. Med. Rehabil. *63*:545, 1982.
43. Fischer, G. W., Popich, G. A., Sullivan, D. E., et al.: Diskitis: A prospective diagnostic analysis. Pediatrics *62*:543, 1978.
44. Fitzgerald, R. H., Brewer, N. S., and Dahlin, D. C.: Squamous cell carcinoma complicating chronic osteomyelitis. J. Bone Joint Surg. *58A*:1146, 1976.
45. Fleisher, G. R., Paradise, J. E., and Plotkin, S. A.: Falsely normal radionuclide scans for osteomyelitis. Am. J. Dis. Child. *134*:499, 1980.
46. Fletcher, D. B., Scales, P. V., and Nelson, A. D.: Osteomyelitis in children: Detection by magnetic resonance. Radiology *150*:57, 1984.
47. Forsythe, M., and Rothman, R. H.: New concepts in the diagnosis and treatment of infections of the cervical spine. Orthop. Clin. North Am. *9*:1039, 1978.
48. Fox, L., and Sprunt, K.: Neonatal osteomyelitis. Pediatrics *62*:535, 1978.
49. Gelfand, M. J., and Silberstein, E. B.: Radionuclide imaging. Use in diagnosis of osteomyelitis in children. JAMA *237*:245, 1977.
50. Gelman, M. I., Coleman, R. E., and Stevens, P. M.: Radiography, radionuclide imaging, and arthrography in the evaluation of total hip and knee replacement. Radiology *128*:677, 1978.
51. Gilday, D. L.: Problems in the scintigraphic detection of osteomyelitis. Radiology *135*:791, 1980.
52. Gilday, D. L., Paul, D. J., and Paterson, J.: Diagnosis of osteomyelitis in children by combined blood pool and bone imaging. Radiology *117*:331, 1975.
53. Glassberg, G. B., and Ozonoff, M. B.: Arthrographic findings in septic arthritis of the hip in infants. Radiology *128*:151, 1978.
54. Gledhill, R. B.: Subacute osteomyelitis in children. Clin. Orthop. *96*:57, 1973.
55. Goergen, T. G., Resnick, D., and Lomonaco, A.: Radionuclide bone scan abnormalities in leprosy: Case reports. J. Nucl. Med. *17*:788, 1976.
56. Gohil, V. K., Dalinka, M. K., and Edeiken, J.: The serpiginous tract: A sign of subacute osteomyelitis. J. Can. Assoc. Radiol. *24*:337, 1973.
57. Goldman, A. B., and Freiberger, R. H.: Localized infections and neurotrophic diseases. Semin. Roentgenol. *14*:19, 1979.
58. Golimbu, C., Firooznia, H., and Rafii, M.: CT of osteomyelitis of the spine. A. J. R. *142*:159, 1984.

59. Gordon, G., and Kabins, S. A.: Pyogenic sarcoiliitis. Am. J. Med. 69:50, 1980.
60. Greenfield, G. B.: Radiology of Bone Diseases. 3rd Ed. Philadelphia, J. B. Lippincott, 1980.
61. Griffiths, H. E. D., and Jones, D. M.: Pyogenic infections of the spine. A review of 28 cases. J. Bone Joint Surg. 53:383, 1971.
62. Gropper, G. R., Acher, J. D., and Robertson, J. H.: Computed tomography in Pott's disease. Neurosurgery 10:506, 1982.
63. Hald, J. K., and Sudmann, E.: Acute hematogenous osteomyelitis. Early diagnosis with computed tomography. Acta Radiol. Diagn. 23:55, 1982.
64. Hall, F. M.: Radiographic diagnosis and accuracy in knee joint effusions. Radiology 115:49, 1975.
65. Handmaker, H.: Acute hematogenous osteomyelitis: Has the bone scan betrayed us? Radiology 135:787, 1980.
66. Handmaker, H., and Giammona, S. T.: The "hot joint"—increased diagnostic accuracy using combined ^{99m}Tc-phosphate and ^{67}Ga citrate imaging in pediatrics (abstract). J. Nucl. Med. 17:554, 1976.
67. Hayden, C. K., and Swischuk, L. E.: Para-articular soft tissue in infections and trauma of the lower extremity in children. A. J. R. 134:307, 1980.
68. Hemborg-Kempi, A., and van der Linden, W.: Scintigraphy with ^{99m}Tc-tripolyphosphate in the early diagnosis of osteomyelitis. Nuklearmedizin 15:53, 1976.
69. Hermann, G., and Rose, J. S.: Computed tomography in bone and soft tissue pathology of the extremities. J. Comput. Assist. Tomogr. 3:58, 1979.
70. Heyman, S., Goldstein, H. A., and Crowley, W.: The scintigraphic evaluation of hip pain in children. Clin. Nucl. Med. 5:109, 1980.
71. Hobo, T.: Zur Pathogenese der akuten haematogene Osteomyelitis mit berücksichtigen der Vitalfarbungslehre. Acta Sch. Med. Univ. Kioto 4:1, 1921.
72. Hooper, J., and Griffin, P.: Pyogenic osteomyelitis of the spine. Aust. NZ J. Surg. 46:367, 1976.
73. Howie, D. W., Savage, J. P., and Wilson, T. G.: The technetium phosphate bone scan in the diagnosis of osteomyelitis in childhood. J. Bone Joint Surg. 65A:431, 1983.
74. Jacobson, S., Hollender, J., and Lindberg, S., et al.: Chronic sclerosing osteomyelitis of the mandible. Oral Surg. 45:167, 1978.
75. Jamison, R. C., Heimlich, E. M., Miethke, J. C., et al.: Nonspecific spondylitis of infants and children. Radiology 77:355, 1961.
76. Janson, V. R., Kuhr, J., and Lackner, K.: CT-Diagnostik der chronischen Osteomyelitis. ROFO. 134:517, 1981.
77. Jones, D. C., and Cady, R. B.: "Cold" bone scans in acute osteomyelitis. J. Bone Joint Surg. 63B:376, 1981.
78. Jorup, S., and Kjellberg, S. R.: The early diagnosis of acute septic osteomyelitis, periostitis, and arthritis and its importance in the treatment. Acta Radiol. 30:316, 1948.
79. Kahn, D. S., and Pritzka, K. P.: The pathophysiology of bone infection. Clin. Orthop. 96:12, 1973.
80. Kattapuram, S. V., Phillips, W. C., and Boyd, R.: CT and pyogenic osteomyelitis of the spine. A. J. R. 140:1199, 1983.
81. Kaye, J. J., Winchester, P. H., and Frieberger, R. H.: Neonatal septic dislocation of the hip: True dislocation or pathological epiphyseal separation. Radiology 114:671, 1975.
82. Kelly, P. J.: Bacterial arthritis in the adult. Orthop. Clin. North Am. 6:973, 1975.
83. Kelly, P. J.: Osteomyelitis in the adult. Orthop. Clin. North Am. 6:983, 1975.
84. Kelly, P. J., Martin, W. J., and Coventry, M. B.: Bacterial (suppurative) arthritis in the adult. J. Bone Joint Surg. 52A:1595, 1970.
85. Kelly, P. J., Wilkowskie, C. J., and Washington, J. A. II.: Chronic osteomyelitis in the adult. Curr. Pract. Orthop. Surg. 6:120, 1975.
86. Kemp, H. B. S., Jackson, J. W., Jeremiah, J. D., et al.: Pyogenic infections occurring primarily in intervertebral discs. J. Bone Joint Surg. 55B:698, 1973.
87. Kimmel, D. J., and Klingensmith, W. C. III.: Unusual scintigraphic appearance of osteomyelitis secondary to atypical mycobacterium. Clin. Nucl. Med. 5:189, 1980.
88. Kloiber, R., Pavlosky, W., and Portner, O.: Bone scintigraphy of hip joint effusions in children. A. J. R. 140:995, 1983.
89. Kluge, R. M., Schmidt, M. C., and Barth, W. F.: Pneumococcal arthritis and joint calcification (abstract). Arthritis Rheum. 14:394, 1971.
90. Kolyvas, E., Rosenthall, L., and Ahronheim, G. A.: Serial ^{67}Ga-citrate imaging during treatment of acute osteomyelitis in childhood. Clin. Nucl. Med. 3:461, 1978.
91. Kozlowski, K.: Brodie's abscess in the first decade of life. Pediatr. Radiol. 10:33, 1980.
92. Kuhn, J. P., and Berger, P. E.: Computed tomographic diagnosis of osteomyelitis. Radiology 130:503, 1979.
93. Lardé, D., Mathieu, D., Frija, J., et al.: Spinal vacuum phenomenon: CT diagnosis and significance. J. Comput. Assist. Tomogr. 6:671, 1982.
94. Lardé, D., Mathieu, D., Frija, J., et al.: Vertebral osteomyelitis: Disk hypodensity on CT. A. J. R. 139:963, 1982.
95. Lichty, G., Langlais, R. P., and Aufdemorte, T.: Garré's osteomyelitis. Oral Surg. 50:309, 1980.
96. Lisbona, R., and Rosenthall, L.: Radionuclide imaging of septic joints and their differentiation from periarticular osteomyelitis and cellulitis in pediatrics. Clin. Nucl. Med. 2:337, 1977.
97. Lloyd-Roberts, G. C.: Suppurative arthritis of infancy. J. Bone Joint Surg. 42B:706, 1960.
98. Majd, M., and Frankel, R. S.: Radionuclide imaging in skeletal inflammatory and ischemic disease in children. A. J. R. 126:832, 1976.
99. Matin, P.: The appearance of bone scans following fractures including intermediate and long-term studies. J. Nucl. Med. 20:1227, 1979.
100. Maurer, A. H., Chen, D. C. P., and Camargo, E. E.: Utility of three-phase skeletal scintigraphy in suspected osteomyelitis: Concise communication. J. Nucl. Med. 22:941, 1981.
101. McDougall, I. R., Baumert, J. E., and Lantieri, R. L.: Evaluation of ^{111}In leukocyte whole-body scanning. A. J. R. 133:849, 1979.
102. Mendelson, E. B., Fisher, M. R., Deschler, T. W., et al.: Osteomyelitis in the diabetic foot: A difficult diagnostic challenge. Radiographics 3:248, 1983.
103. Menelaus, M. B.: Discitis. J. Bone Joint Surg. 46B:16, 1964.
104. Meredith, H. C.: Pneumoarthropathy: An unusual roentgen sign of Gram-negative septic arthritis. Radiology 129:642, 1978.
105. Merkel, K. D., Brown, M. L., and Fitzgerald, R. H.: Evaluating the painful prosthetic joint with sequential Tc-99m-MDP–Ga 67 (abstract). J. Nucl. Med. 24:P72, 1983.
106. Merkel, K. D., Brown, M. L., and Fitzgerald, R. H.: Prospective In-111 WBC scan vs. Tc-99m-MDP–Ga-67 scan for low-grade osteomyelitis. Final Report (abstract). J. Nucl. Med. 24:P72, 1983.
107. Michaeli, D.: Osteomyelitis with special reference to the hand. Prog. Surg. 16:38, 1978.
108. Miller, W. B. Jr., Murphy, W. A., and Gilula, L. A.: Brodie abscess: Reappraisal. Radiology 132:15, 1979.
109. Modic, M. T., Weinstein, M. A., Pavlicek, W., et al.: Nuclear magnetic resonance imaging of the spine. Radiology 148:757, 1983.
110. Modic, M. T., Weinstein, M. A., Pavlicek, W., et al.: Magnetic resonance imaging of the cervical spine: Technique and clinical observations. A. J. R. 141:1129, 1983.
111. Mok, P. M., Reilly, B. J., and Ash, J. M. Osteomyelitis in the neonate. Clinical aspects and the role of radiography and scintigraphy in diagnosis and management. Radiology 145:677, 1982.
112. Mollan, R. A., and Piggot, J.: Acute osteomyelitis in children. J. Bone Joint Surg. 59B:2, 1977.
113. Moon, K. L., Genant, H. K., Helnes, C. A., et al.: Musculoskeletal applications of nuclear magnetic resonance. Radiology 147:161, 1983.
114. Morrey, B. F., Bianco, A. J., and Rhodes, K. H.: Hematogenous osteomyelitis at uncommon sites in children. Mayo. Clin. Proc. 53:707, 1978.

115. Morrey, B. F., Bianco, A. J. Jr., and Rhodes, K. H.: Septic arthritis in children. Orthop. Clin. North Am. 6:923, 1975.

116. Morrey, B. F., Bianco, A. J., and Rhodes, K. H.: Suppurative arthritis of the hip in children. J. Bone Joint Surg. 58A:388, 1976.

117. Morrey, B. F., and Peterson, H. A.: Hematogenous pyogenic osteomyelitis in children. Orthop. Clin. North Am. 6:935, 1975.

118. Murphy, J., Anderson, N., and White, M.: Early diagnosis of acute osteomyelitis in childhood using radionuclide bone scanning. J. Irish Med. Assoc. 73:166, 1980.

119. Murray, I. P. C.: Photopenia in skeletal scintigraphy of suspected bone and joint infection. Clin. Nucl. Med. 7:13, 1982.

120. Murray, R. O., and Jacobson, H. G.: The Radiology of Skeletal Disorders. 2nd Ed. Edinburgh, Churchill Livingstone, 1977.

121. Musher, D. M., Thorsteinsson, S. B., Minuth, J. N., et al.: Vertebral osteomyelitis: Still a diagnostic pitfall. Arch. Intern. Med. 136:105, 1976.

122. Nelson, H. T., and Taylor, A.: Bone scanning in the diagnosis of acute osteomyelitis. Eur. J. Nucl. Med. 5:267, 1980.

123. Nixon, G. W.: Hematogenous osteomyelitis of metaphyseal equivalent locations. A. J. R. 130:123, 1978.

124. Norris, S., Ehrlich, M. G., and Keim, D. E.: Early diagnosis of disc-space infection using gallium-67. J. Nucl. Med. 19:384, 1978.

125. Norris, S., Ehrlich, M. G., and McKusick, K.: Early diagnosis of disk space infection with ⁶⁷Ga in an experimental model. Clin. Orthop. 144:293, 1979.

126. Ogden, J. A., and Lister, G.: The pathology of neonatal osteomyelitis. Pediatrics 55:474, 1975.

127. O'Mara, R. E., Wilson, G. A., and Burke, A. M.: Skeletal imaging in osteomyelitis (abstract). J. Nucl. Med. 24:P71, 1983.

128. Pare, D., and Katz, A.: Clostridia discitis: A case report. Arthritis Rheum. 22:1037, 1979.

129. Park, H. M., Wheat, J., and Siddiqui, A.: Scintigraphic evaluation of diabetic osteomyelitis: Concise communication. J. Nucl. Med. 23:569, 1982.

130. Park, H., Wheat, J., and Siddiqui, A. Three-phase bone scan in diabetic foot (abstract). J. Nucl. Med. 20:602, 1979.

131. Paterson, D.: Septic arthritis of the hip joint. Orthop. Clin. North Am. 9:135, 1978.

132. Paterson, D. C.: Acute suppurative arthritis in infancy and childhood. J. Bone Joint Surg. 52B:474, 1970.

133. Petersen, S., Knudsen, F. U., and Andersen, E. A., et al.: Acute hematogenous osteomyelitis and septic arthritis in childhood. Acta Orthop. Scand. 51:451, 1980.

134. Petty, W.: Influence of methylmethacrylate on bacterial phagocytosis and killing by human polymorphonuclear leukocytes. J. Bone Joint Surg. 60A:752, 1978.

135. Price, A. C., Allen, J. H., Eggers, F. M., et al.: Intervertebral disk-space infection: CT changes. Radiology 149:725, 1983.

136. Pritchard, D. J.: Granulomatous infections of bones and joints. Orthop. Clin. North Am. 6:1029, 1975.

137. Propst-Proctor, S. L., Dillingham, M. F., and McDougall, I. R.: The white blood cell scan in orthopaedics. Clin. Orthop. 168:157, 1982.

138. Ram, T. C., Martinez, S., and Korobkin, M.: CT detection of intraosseous gas: A new sign of osteomyelitis. A. J. R. 137:721, 1981.

139. Ranade, S. S., Shah, S., Advani, S. H., et al.: Pulsed nuclear magnetic resonance studies of human bone marrow. Physiol. Chem. Phys. 9:297, 1977.

140. Raptopoulos, V., Doherty, P. W., and Gross, T. P.: Acute osteomyelitis: Advantage of white cell scans in early detection. A. J. R. 139:1077, 1982.

141. Reing, C. M., Richin, R. F., and Kenmore, P. I.: Differential bone-scanning in the evaluation of a painful total joint replacement. J. Bone Joint Surg. 61A:933, 1979.

142. Resnick, D.: Infectious arthritis. Semin. Roentgenol. 17:49, 1982.

143. Resnick, D.: Osteomyelitis and septic arthritis complicating hand injuries and infections: Pathogenesis of roentgenographic abnormalities. J. Can. Assoc. Rad. 27:21, 1976.

144. Resnick, D.: Pyarthrosis complicating rheumatoid arthritis. Roentgenographic evaluation of 5 patients and a review of the literature. Radiology 114:581, 1975.

145. Resnick, D., and Niwayama, G.: Diagnosis of Bone and Joint Disorders. Vol 3. Philadelphia, W. B. Saunders, 1981.

146. Resnick, D., Niwayama, G., Guerra, J., et al.: Spinal vacuum phenomenon: Anatomical study and review. Radiology 139:341, 1981.

147. Robins, R. H. C.: Infections of the hand: A review based on 1000 consecutive cases. J. Bone Joint Surg. 34B:567, 1952.

148. Roca, R. P., and Yoshikawa, T. T.: Primary skeletal infections in heroin users: A clinical characterization, diagnosis and therapy. Clin. Orthop. 144:238, 1979.

149. Rocco, H. D., and Eyringe, S.: Infections of the intervertebral disk in children. Am. J. Dis. Child. 123:449, 1972.

150. Rosenthall, L., Kloiber, R., and Damtew, B.: Sequential use of radiophosphate and radiogallium imaging in the differential diagnosis of bone, joint, and soft tissue infection: Quantitative analysis. Diagn. Imaging 51:249, 1982.

151. Rosenthall, L., Lisbona, R., and Hernandez, M.: ⁹⁹ᵐTc-PP and ⁶⁷Ga imaging following insertion of orthopedic devices. Radiology 133:717, 1979.

152. Rushton, N., Coakley, A. J., and Tudor, J.: The value of technetium and gallium scanning in assessing pain after total hip replacement. J. Bone Joint Surg. 64B:313, 1982.

153. Russin, L. D., and Staab, E. V.: Unusual bone-scan findings in acute osteomyelitis: Case report. J. Nucl. Med. 17:617, 1976.

154. Salter, R. B., and Field, P.: Effects of continuous compression on living articular cartilage. J. Bone Joint Surg. 42A:31, 1960.

155. Sartoris, D. J., Moskowitz, P. S., Kaufman, R. A., et al.: Childhood diskitis: Computed tomographic findings. Radiology 149:701, 1983.

156. Schauwecker, D. S., Baker, M. K., and Burt, R. W.: Evaluation of postoperative sternum with Ga-67 and Tc-99M medronate (abstract). J. Nucl. Med. 24:P85, 1983.

157. Schauwecker, D. S., Mock, B. H., and Wellman, H. N.: Comparison of In-111 acetylacetone-labeled granulocytes, Ga-67 citrate, and 3-phase MDP skeletal imaging in complicated osteomyelitis (abstract). J. Nucl. Med. 24:P64, 1983.

158. Septimus, E. J., and Musher, D. M.: Osteomyelitis: Recent clinical and laboratory aspects. Orthop. Clin. North Am. 10:347, 1979.

159. Sfakianakis, G., Al-Sheikh, W., and Spoliansky, G.: Correlation of In-111-leukocyte (In-WBC) and Gallium-67 (Ga-67) scintigraphy with transmission computerized tomography (CT), ultrasonography (US), and plain radiography (R) in the diagnosis of focal infection (abstract). J. Nucl. Med. 24:P38, 1983.

160. Sfakianakis, G. N., Al-Sheikh, W., and Heal, A.: Comparison of scintigraphy with In-111 leukocytes and Ga-67 in the diagnosis of occult sepsis. J. Nucl. Med. 23:618, 1982.

161. Shandling, B.: Acute hematogenous osteomyelitis: A review of 300 cases treated during 1952–1959. S. Afr. Med. J. 34:520, 1960.

162. Shawker, T. H., and Dennis, J. M.: Periarticular calcification in pyogenic arthritis. A. J. R. 113:650, 1971.

163. Shirazi, P. H., Rayudu, G. V. S., and Fordham, E. W.: ¹⁸F bone scanning: Review of indications and results of 1,500 scans. Radiology 112:361, 1974.

164. Smith, P. W., Petersen, R. J., and Ferlic, R. M.: Gallium scan in sternal osteomyelitis. A. J. R. 132:840, 1979.

165. Smith, R. F., and Taylor, T. K.: Inflammatory lesions of intervertebral discs in children. J. Bone Joint Surg. 49A:1508, 1967.

166. Spiegel, P. G., Kengla, K. W., Isaacson, A. A., et al.: Intervertebral disk-space inflammation in children. J. Bone Joint Surg. 54A:284, 1972.

167. Staheli, L. T., Nelp, W. B., and Marty, R.: Strontium-87m scanning. Early diagnosis of bone and joint infections in children. JAMA 221:1159, 1972.

168. Stauffer, R. N. Pyogenic vertebral osteomyelitis. Orthop. Clin. North Am. 6:1015, 1975.

169. Steinback, H. L. Infections of bones. Semin Roentgenol. 1:337, 1966.

170. Sullivan, D. C., Rosenfield, N. S., and Ogden, J.: Problems

in the scintigraphic detection of osteomyelitis in children. Radiology 135:731, 1980.

171. Swischuk, L. E.: Spine and spinal cord trauma in the battered child syndrome. Radiology 92:733, 1969.

172. Tachdijian, M. O.: Pediatric Orthopedics. Philadelphia, W. B. Saunders, 1972.

173. Teates, C. D., and Williamson, B. R. J.: "Hot and cold" bone lesion in acute osteomyelitis. A. J. R. 129:517, 1977.

174. Thakur, M. L.: Indium-111: A new radioactive tracer for leukocytes. Exp. Hematol. 5:145, 1977.

175. Thakur, M. L., Coleman, R. E., and Mayhall, C. G.: Preparation and evaluation of 111-indium-labeled leukocytes as an abscess imaging agent in dogs. Radiology 119:721, 1976.

176. Tobias, R. H. C.: Infections of the hand: A review of 1000 consecutive cases. J. Bone Joint Surg. 34B:567, 1952.

177. Torg, J. S., and Lammot, T. R. III.: Septic arthritis of the knee due to *Clostridium welchii*. J. Bone Joint Surg. 50A:1233, 1968.

178. Trackler, R. T., Miller, K. E., and Sutherland, D. H.: Childhood pelvic osteomyelitis presenting as a "cold" lesion on bone scan: Case report. J. Nucl. Med. 17:620, 1976.

179. Treves, S., Khettry, J., and Broker, F. H.: Osteomyelitis: Early scintigraphic detection in children. Pediatrics 57:173, 1976.

180. Utz, J. A., Galvin, E. G., and Lull, R. J.: Natural history of technetium-99m MDP bone scan in asymptomatic total hip prosthesis (abstract). J. Nucl. Med. 21:P28, 1982.

181. Waldvogel, F. A., Medoff, G., and Swartz, M. N.: Osteomyelitis: A review of clinical features, therapeutic consid-erations and unusual aspects. N. Eng. J. Med. 282:198, 1970.

182. Waldvogel, F. A., and Papageorgion, P. S.: Osteomyelitis: The past decade. N. Eng. J. Med. 303:360, 1980.

183. Weiss, P. E., Mall, J. C., and Hoffer, P. B.: ^{99m}Tc-methylene diphosphonate bone imaging in the evaluation of total hip prostheses. Radiology 133:727, 1979.

184. Wenger, D. R., Bobechko, W. P., and Gilday, D. L.: The spectrum of intervertebral disc space infections in children. J. Bone Joint Surg. 60A:100, 1978.

185. Whelan, M. A., Naidich, D. P., and Post, J. D.: Computed tomography of spinal tuberculosis. J. Comput. Asst. Tomog. 7:25, 1983.

186. White, H.: Roentgen findings of acute infectious disease of the hip in infants and children. Clin. Orthop. 22:34, 1962.

187. Whitehouse, W. M., and Smith, W. S.: Osteomyelitis of the feet. Semin. Roentgenol. 5:367, 1970.

188. Wiley, A. M., and Trueta, J.: The vascular anatomy of the spine and its relationship to pyogenic vertebral osteomye-litis. J. Bone Joint Surg. 41B:796, 1959.

189. Williamson, B. R. J., McLaughlin, R. E., and Wang, G. J.: Radionuclide bone imaging as a means of differentiating loosening and infection in patients with a painful total hip prosthesis. Radiology 133:723, 1979.

190. Winters, J. L., and Canen, I.: Acute hematogenous osteo-myelitis: A review of 66 cases. J. Bone Joint Surg. 42A:691, 1960.

191. Wofsy, D.: Culture negative septic arthritis and bacterial endocarditis. Diagnosis by synovial biopsy. Arthritis Rheum. 23:605, 1980.

STRESS FRACTURES

THOMAS H. BERQUIST • KAY L. COOPER • DOUGLAS J. PRITCHARD

The term stress fracture has been applied to a variety of fractures that result from repetitive stress of a lesser magnitude than that required for an acute traumatic fracture. Daffner[8] states that a stress fracture results from muscular activity on bones rather than from direct trauma. Most stress fractures are fatigue fractures resulting from abnormal muscular tension on normal bone.[8, 11] These usually occur in the lower extremity in association with significant changes in physical activity. Fatigue fractures are commonly reported in military personnel.[20, 21, 39] Insufficiency fractures occur when normal stress or muscle tension acts on bone with abnormal elastic resistance.[8, 11, 46]

In the civilian population the patient frequently gives a history of starting a new activity, such as track or jogging. Usually several weeks after starting the activity the patient notes local pain. Symptoms are usually relieved by rest. If the activity is continued, the pain generally increases.[11] Table 15–1 lists the locations and related activity of common stress fractures.

TABLE 15–1. Common Stress Fractures*

Location	Etiology	References
Foot		
Metatarsals	Marching	18, 20, 21, 39
	Running	8, 20
	Ballet	11, 47
	Prior surgery	8, 17
Calcaneus	Jumping	25
	Marching	
	Running	20, 39, 52
	Recent immobilization	49
Tarsals	Long distance running	8, 11, 37
	Marching	8, 11, 37
Sesamoids	Standing, cycling, skiing	11, 21
Tibia		
Proximal	Running	14, 36
Mid-	Ballet	6, 9, 11, 13, 15, 47
Distal	Running	4, 20, 36, 47, 52
Fibula	Running	2, 4, 10, 20, 36
	Jumping (parachute)	21
Patella	Hurdling	8, 11, 13, 20
Femur		
Shaft	Running (long distance)	8, 22, 30, 36, 40
Neck	Running (long distance)	3, 8, 12, 36
	Ballet	11, 47
Pelvis (pubic arch)	Running	36
	Stooping	8, 21
	Bowling	4
	Gymnastics	11
Spine		
Vertebral arch (lumbar)	Lifting	8, 11
	Ballet	8
Spinous process (C,T)	Clay shoveling	21
Ribs		
1st	Back packing	4, 8, 21
Lower	Golf, cough	8, 42, 52
Clavicle	Radical neck surgery, tic	8, 21
Coracoid (scapula)	Trap shooting	45
Humerus	Baseball	4
Ulna	Baseball, pitchfork, wheelchair patients	8, 21
Hook of hamate	Golf, tennis, baseball	4, 8, 48
Metacarpals	Weight lifting, gymnastics	36

*After Daffner, R. H.: Stress fractures: Current Concepts. Skeletal Radiol. 2:221, 1978.

TABLE 15–2. Clinical Conditions Simulating Stress Fractures

Neoplasm
Infection
Tendinitis
Ligament injury
Gout
Pseudogout
Vascular occlusive disease (claudication)

Physical examination may reveal local tenderness or swelling over the fracture.[3, 11] Children may have slight temperature elevation.[11] Clinically most stress fractures arise distal to the knee. The importance of this finding lies mainly in the difficulty it presents for differentiating stress fractures from other entities. For example, stress fractures of the proximal tibia may result in periosteal new bone formation, leading the physician to suspect a primary bone tumor. Similarly, if the metatarsal is involved, there may be exuberant periosteal reaction that suggests either osteomyelitis or tumor. In either case the history of repetitive stress is helpful in suggesting the diagnosis. Table 15–2 lists clinical conditions that may simulate stress fractures.[11]

RADIOGRAPHIC EVALUATION

There are multiple imaging techniques available for evaluating musculoskeletal conditions. Unfortunately, detection of stress fractures may be difficult in the early stages except with isotope studies.[8, 20] Early diagnosis is especially important with stress fractures of the femoral neck; displacement of these fractures can occur, resulting in a significant increase in morbidity.[3]

Routine radiographs are almost always normal initially. Blickenstaff and Morris[3] described the phases of stress fractures. During the first 5 to 14 days osteoclastic resorption leads to local osteoporosis. This is followed by periosteal or endosteal callus. Swelling and increased vascularity accompany these changes. Continued activity results in fracture. The fracture defect may be primarily cor-

tical or trabecular. Greaney and colleagues[20] reported isotope findings in 250 military personnel. Twenty-three percent of the fractures were considered cortical and 77 percent cancellous. Routine radiographs were positive in only 40 percent of cortical and 26 percent of trabecular stress fractures. Cortical fractures may present with endosteal or periosteal callus, with or without a lucent cortical defect.[3, 6] Tomography is often necessary to define a fracture line. Stress fractures in cancellous bone may appear as a hazy area of increased density or a sclerotic line due to trabecular compression.[3]

Metabolic activity around stress fractures may allow isotope detection as early as 24 hours following the injury.[20] The bone changes must progress to cause a 30 to 50 percent change in the bone density before radiographs will be positive. This usually takes 10 to 21 days.[20, 38]

Classification of stress fractures may be useful in certain cases. Wilson and Katz[52] categorized fractures according to their radiographic appearance. Type I fractures present with a lucent line with no associated periosteal reaction; Type II fractures reveal cancellous sclerosis and endosteal callus; Type III fractures have external callus; and Type IV fractures present with a mixture of Types I through III.

Devas[11] divided stress fractures into compression and distraction categories. Compression fractures are equivalent to torus fractures. These most commonly occur in children and elderly patients and are most often located in the femoral neck and tibia. Distraction fractures are similar to greenstick fractures and may be transverse, oblique, or longitudinal. The transverse fractures are most significant in that complete fracture and displacement may occur.

Unfortunately stress fractures differ in their appearance depending upon location. Therefore, early diagnosis and appearance are important mainly in determining which fractures are likely to displace.[8, 40]

Attempts at earlier radiographic diagnosis of stress fractures with the use of magnification techniques, xeroradiography, and tomography have been useful in certain cases.[20, 37, 51] Magnetic resonance imaging may be useful in certain situations

TABLE 15–3. Distribution of Stress Fractures in Three Series (%)

Location	Orava et al.[36] (142 Patients)	Wilson and Katz[52] (250 Patients)	Greaney et al.[20] (250 Patients)
Foot			
Metatarsal	18.3	35.2	15
Calcaneus	—	28	23
Talus	—	—	7
Navicular	0.7	—	4
Tibia	53	24	39
Fibula	14.1	3.2	0
Femur	6.3	3.2	9
Pubic arch	1.4	.4	—
Spine	0.7	1	—
Ribs	—	5.6	—
Ulna	0.7		3 (Patella, cuboid, and cuneiform)
Humerus	1.4		
Metacarpals	1.4		

owing to the strong signal obtained from medullary bone. Detection of cortical changes is more difficult owing to the lack of signal.[2, 35]

Despite new imaging techniques isotope studies using Tc-99m remain most useful in early detection of stress fractures.[20] Greaney and colleagues[20] noted normal radiographs in 50 percent of their patients with stress fractures even during follow-up. Radiographic techniques are still extremely important in determining the nature of isotope abnormalities. Differential diagnostic challenges may occur with osteogenic sarcoma, chronic osteomyelitis, and osteoid osteoma.[8, 14, 28] Problems in diagnosis and treatment of stress fractures vary depending on the location and type of fracture.

DISTRIBUTION OF STRESS FRACTURES

Foot

Military recruits have provided a large controlled population for study of stress fractures. Wilson and Katz[52] studied 250 patients, and Greaney and colleagues[20] examined 250 Marine recruits. Orava and colleagues[36] reviewed stress fractures in 142 athletes and sportsmen. Though the statistics vary somewhat, most authors agree that stress fractures in the foot most commonly involve the metatarsals[43] (Table 15–3). "March" fractures are common in military recruits. Stress with marching is applied maximally to the 2nd and 3rd metatarsals (Fig. 15–1). Less commonly the 4th metatarsal is involved.[11, 43] Initial radiographs are usually normal. Follow-up films in 10 to 14 days often demonstrate a small lucent cortical defect or early periosteal change. Metatarsal stress fractures most commonly involve the mid- or distal shaft of the metatarsals (Fig. 15–2).

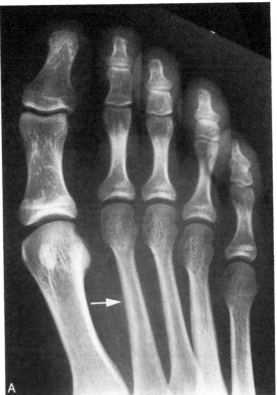

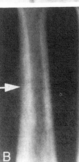

Figure 15–2. AP radiograph *(A)* and localized view *(B)* of the foot demonstrating a subtle midshaft stress fracture of the second metatarsal.

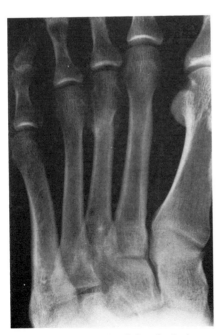

Figure 15–1. AP radiograph of the foot demonstrating a typical healing stress fracture of the third metatarsal neck.

Metatarsal stress fractures are not uncommon in civilians.[11, 36] These are usually the result of a change in the patient's footwear, walking, or running habits. For example, a patient who is relatively sedentary may assume a job that requires increased standing or walking. Pain with weight-bearing[17] may begin in the first few weeks after the change in activity. This pain is usually reproducible each time the activity is resumed. The pain is usually well localized. There is also an increased incidence of metatarsal stress fracture following bunionectomy.

Treatment of metatarsal stress fractures requires restriction of weight-bearing. These fractures essentially never displace and are of little consequence once the diagnosis is established.

Wilson and Katz[52] noted calcaneal stress fractures nearly as frequently as metatarsal fractures. Calcaneal stress fractures were most common in the Greaney series.[20] Associated stress fractures of the

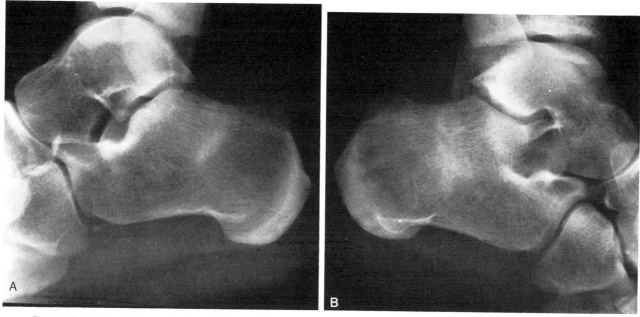

Figure 15–3. Lateral *(A)* and oblique *(B)* views of the calcaneus demonstrating bands of sclerosis due to stress fractures.

upper tibia medially were noted in 60 percent of military recruits.[20] This has been partially attributed to running and marching in combat boots.[18]

Calcaneal stress fractures occur less frequently in civilians, but again there seems to be an association between these fractures and footwear that increases heel stress. When asked to describe their pain, patients normally point to the medial and lateral sides of the heel rather than the plantar surface. Physical examination often reveals pain when the heel is squeezed.

Radiographically a hazy or speckled appearance may be noted first. This usually progresses to a sclerotic band if stress continues[20, 52] (Fig. 15–3). These findings may be more obvious using magnification technique or xeroradiography. Trabecular stress fractures rarely produce periosteal changes. Isotope scans will demonstrate a linear area of increased uptake. They may be positive within 24 hours and are almost invariably positive in 72 hours.[20, 32]

Treatment of calcaneal stress fractures is accomplished with a plastic heel cup and 4-inch foam rubber heel pad.

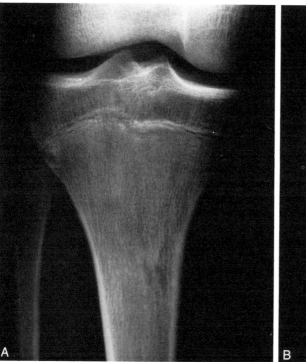
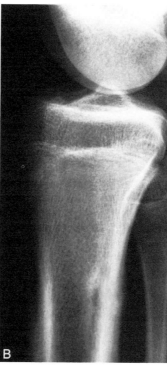

Figure 15–4. AP *(A)* and lateral *(B)* views of the proximal tibia demonstrating a typical stress fracture at the posteromedial junction of the metaphysis and diaphysis. There is early periosteal reaction.

Stress fractures involve the tarsal navicular, talus, phalanges, and sesamoids less frequently[36, 37, 51] (Tables 15–1 and 15–3). Tarsonavicular stress fractures, common in runners, are particularly difficult to diagnose.[19, 37] Pavlov and colleagues[37] accomplished diagnosis of tarsonavicular fractures with isotope scans and tomography. Isotope studies (Tc-99m), especially with the plantar view, were useful in localizing the abnormality, while tomograms were useful in defining the fracture. Tomograms were performed in the dorsiplantar projection with slight dorsiflexion. This allows a more tangential examination of the navicular.

Most navicular fractures are sagittal and involve the mid- and medial third of the navicular.[37, 51] In a series reported by Torg and colleagues,[51] treatment of navicular fractures was successful with non-weight-bearing. However, simple restriction of activity led to non-union in 7 of 9 patients.

Tibia

Tibial stress fractures are common in both military and civilian populations.[20, 36, 51] The incidence of tibial stress fractures in the series reported by Greaney was 73 percent.[20] Cortical involvement is much more common in the tibia.

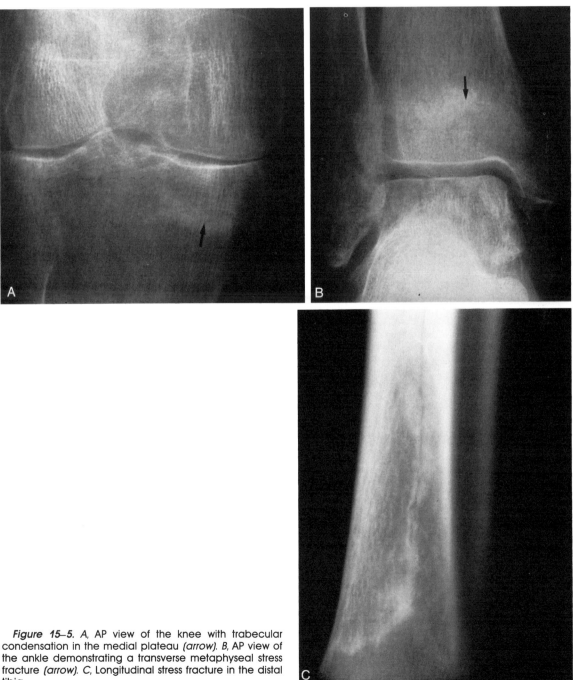

Figure 15–5. A, AP view of the knee with trabecular condensation in the medial plateau *(arrow). B,* AP view of the ankle demonstrating a transverse metaphyseal stress fracture *(arrow). C,* Longitudinal stress fracture in the distal tibia.

Stress fractures may arise anywhere along the length of the tibia. Classically they occur on the posteromedial aspect of the proximal tibia at the junction of the metaphysis and diaphysis (Fig. 15–4). However, variations are not uncommon (Fig. 15–5). Ballet dancers often develop stress fractures in the midtibia.[6, 14] Following total knee replacement, fractures occur in the medial tibial plateau. These fractures are most often associated with mal-

alignment and improper orientation of the component[41] (Fig. 15–6).

Almost any form of strenuous activity may precede stress fractures of the tibia; hence tennis, racquetball, and any form of running may be responsible. In the past, when the athlete first started training for a sport, leg pain was called "shin splints." It was recognized that this condition would not improve unless the activity was halted.

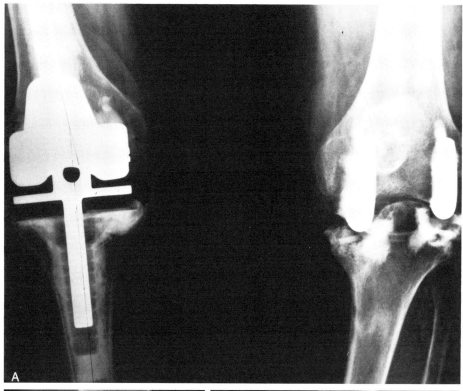

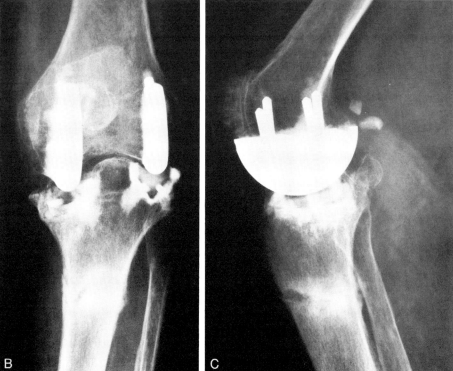

Figure 15–6. Bilateral total knee arthroplasty. Pain in left knee. Initial views *(A)* demonstrate sclerosis in the tibial plateau and periosteal changes in the left tibia medially. There is also trabecular sclerosis. Seven weeks later there is an obvious stress fracture in the upper tibia seen on the AP *(B)* and lateral *(C)* views.

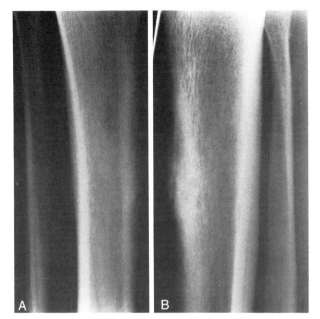

Figure 15–7. AP *(A)* and lateral *(B)* views of the midtibia. Osteosarcoma mimicking a stress fracture.

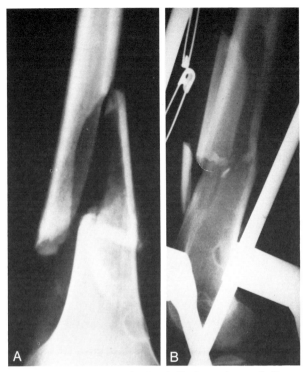

Figure 15–8. AP *(A)* and lateral *(B)* views demonstrating a displaced comminuted stress fracture.

Probably at least some of these cases were early stress fractures. Isotope studies will be positive soon after symptoms begin if a stress fracture is present.[20, 32, 38] Radiographs may remain negative for 2 to 3 weeks.[20] The earliest findings may be subtle periosteal reaction. Tomograms often demonstrate the fracture line and assist in differentiating a stress fracture from a primary bone tumor. The latter condition may be difficult to differentiate from a stress fracture if there is no clear-cut history of change in physical activity (Fig. 15–7).

Usually the pain present with stress fractures is sufficient to cause patients to restrict their activities voluntarily. This may be the only treatment neces-

sary. However, persistent pain with simple weight-bearing may indicate the need for more aggressive therapy, such as crutches or even a long-leg cylinder cast. Radiographic changes may be helpful in making this decision concerning therapy. Hallel and colleagues[22] described tibial fractures as Grade I if periosteal reaction involved one cortex, as Grade II if changes were circumferential, and as Grade III if the fracture was displaced. Tibial stress fractures rarely displace. However, Grade II fractures may

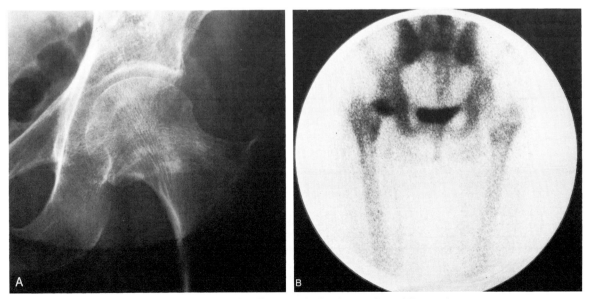

Figure 15–9. A, AP view of the hip demonstrates sclerotic zones in the trabeculae of the neck. B, Isotope scan demonstrates a femoral neck fracture.

require more aggressive therapy than the less extensive Grade I fracture.

Fibula

Stress fractures involve the fibula less frequently than the tibia. Orava[36] reported an incidence of 14.1 percent in 142 athletes with stress fractures. The fibula is a non-weight-bearing bone. Therefore, the fractures are due to muscle stress.[11, 52] This stress is most commonly applied with calf muscle contraction during running.[11] Fibular fractures can usually

be treated with reduction of the associated activity, since there are no weight-bearing stresses.

Femoral Shaft

Stress fractures of the femoral shaft are not common. Orava[36] reported an incidence of 2.8 percent in civilians. These fractures are more frequent in long-distance runners and occasionally in ballet dancers.[7, 29, 30, 47] Highly motivated well conditioned athletes tend to be at risk for this type of fracture.[22, 30] Luchini[30] reported femoral shaft fractures in long-distance runners who were totally asymptomatic

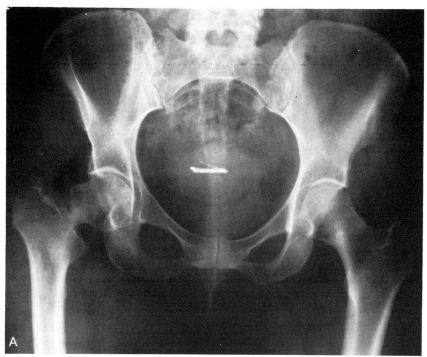

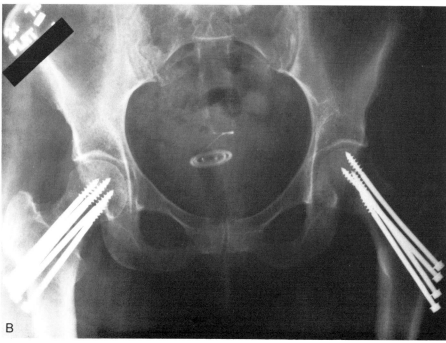

Figure 15–10. *A,* AP view of the pelvis with bilateral femoral neck stress fractures. The fracture on the right is complete with varus displacement. *B,* Pinning of both hips was necessary.

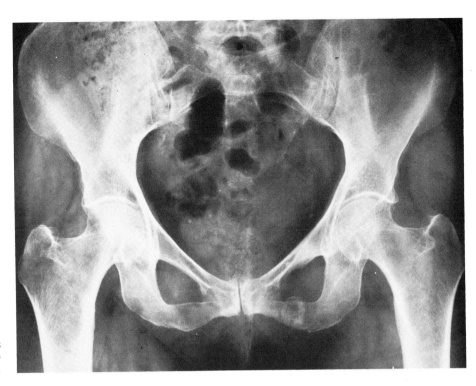

Figure 15–11. AP view of the pelvis demonstrating healing stress fractures of both pubic rami on the left.

prior to the fracture. This was attributed to muscle fatigue that resulted in transfer of stress to the femoral shaft. Early recognition of this fracture is important, as displacement tends to occur (Fig. 15–8). Treatment of femoral shaft fractures may require open reduction and internal fixation if such displacement occurs.

Femoral Neck

Stress fractures of the femoral neck are more common than diaphyseal stress fractures.[36] Detection may be difficult clinically (Fig. 15–9). The patient's pain will frequently be referred to the knee, and point tenderness may be difficult to elicit.[11, 40] Early diagnosis and treatment are essential, for progression of this type of fracture may lead to eventual displacement.[3, 11, 22] Classification of femoral neck fractures is useful in determining which fractures tend to displace.[3, 11, 34] Devas[11, 12] classified fractures as transverse or compressive. Compression fractures occur at the base of the femoral neck medially (calcar). They often present with localized osteoporosis that progresses to periosteal callus formation. This type usually occurs in younger patients.[34] Osteoid osteoma should be considered in this location as well. History and tomography are useful in differentiating these two conditions. Compression stress fractures usually do not displace and can be treated with non-weight-bearing.[34] Transverse fractures occur in older patients. Initially a defect in the superior cortex of the neck will be seen. This defect frequently progresses to a complete fracture and displacement. Devas noted displacement in 11 of 18 transverse fractures[11, 12] (Fig. 15–10).

Blickenstaff and Morris[3] classified femoral neck fractures according to radiographic appearance. A Type I fracture demonstrated callus only. Type II fractures demonstrated a fine calcar fracture with or without extension across the femoral neck. Type III fractures were displaced. Blickenstaff and Morris noted that once a fracture line was visible, internal fixation was indicated. Patients with Type I fractures were treated conservatively, requiring about 9½ weeks of hospitalization. Displaced fractures healed without complication only 20 percent of the time. The average hospital stay in Type III fractures was 59 weeks. Complications included malunion, non-union, and avascular necrosis.

Femoral neck stress fractures have also been noted following total knee replacement.[27] Most of these are probably insufficiency fractures that result from the application of normal stress to bone with abnormal elastic resistance.[46]

Pelvis

Stress fractures in the pelvis most frequently involve the pubic arch.[4, 8, 11] They may be related to running, gymnastics, and bowling[4, 8, 11] (Fig. 15–11).

Insufficiency fractures in this region are becoming more common as the incidence of joint replacement procedures increases. Owing to joint replacement, patients with severe rheumatoid arthritis are now able to walk and bear weight, but this in turn may lead to insufficiency fractures in the pubic arch and other locations.[31, 33, 46]

Pubic arch stress fractures tend to occur in older individuals. Patients frequently notice pain in the groin or hip with weight-bearing. Treatment consists of activity restriction or partial weight-bearing with crutches.

Other Locations

Stress fractures in the spine and upper extremities are uncommon compared with the lower extremity[24–26, 42, 45, 48] (Tables 15–1 and 15–3). Stress fractures may occur in the spinous processes of clay shovelers and in the lumbar pars in patients who repeatedly lift heavy weights.[8, 11, 20, 46, 52] Evaluation of the pars may be accomplished with isotope studies followed by localized (1 to 3 mm thick) tomograms. On occasion CT scanning may be used to evaluate the posterior elements (Fig. 15–12). This technique is especially helpful in excluding other bone and soft tissue abnormalities. Magnetic resonance imaging may provide even better sensitivity in soft tissue abnormalities.[2, 35]

Upper extremity stress fractures have been described in baseball players, golfers, and trap shooters (Table 15–1).[4, 8] Stress fractures of the ribs due to chronic cough and to golfing have also been described. Fractures of the first ribs can develop after prolonged use of heavy back packs.[4, 8]

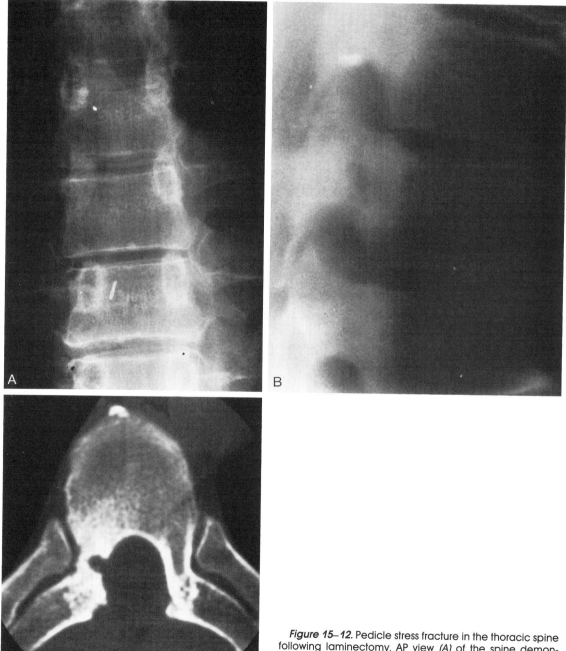

Figure 15–12. Pedicle stress fracture in the thoracic spine following laminectomy. AP view *(A)* of the spine demonstrates sclerosis of the pedicle. Lateral tomogram *(B)* and CT scan *(C)* demonstrate the changes to better advantage.

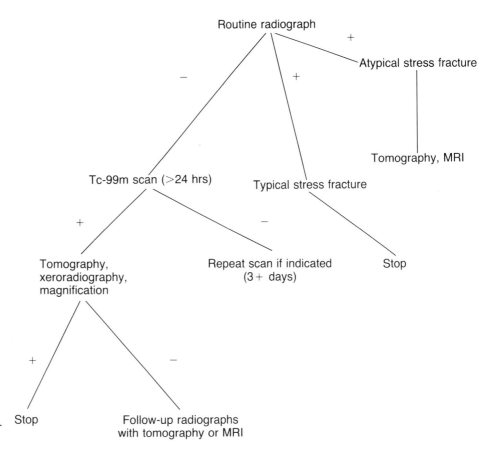

Routine radiograph

+

Atypical stress fracture

−

+

Tomography, MRI

Tc-99m scan (>24 hrs)   Typical stress fracture

+

−

Tomography,
xeroradiography,
magnification

Repeat scan if indicated   Stop
(3+ days)

+

−

Figure 15–13. An imaging ap-
proach to stress fractures.   Stop   Follow-up radiographs
with tomography or MRI

SUMMARY

The diagnosis of a stress fracture should be considered in patients presenting with pain after a change in activity, especially if the activity is strenuous and the pain is in the lower extremities. Since evidence of the stress fracture may not be apparent for weeks on routine radiographs, proper use of other imaging techniques will allow an earlier diagnosis (Fig. 15–13). Prompt diagnosis is especially important in the femur, where displacement may occur.

REFERENCES

1. Bargren, J. H., Tilson, D. H., Jr., and Bridgefort, O. E.: Prevention of displaced fatigue fractures of the femur. J. Bone Joint Surg. 53A:6, 1971.
2. Berquist, R. H.: Magnetic resonance imaging: Preliminary experience in orthopedic radiology. Mag. Res. Imag. 2:41, 1984.
3. Blickenstaff, L. D., and Morris, J. M.: Fatigue fracture of the femoral neck. J. Bone Joint Surg. 48A:6, 1966.
4. Bowerman, J. W.: Radiology and Injury in Sport. New York, Appleton-Century-Crofts, 1977.
5. Burrows, H. J.: Fatigue fractures of the fibula. J. Bone Joint Surg. 30B:266, 1948.
6. Burrows, H. J.: Fatigue infraction of the middle of the tibia in ballet dancers. J. Bone Joint Surg. 38B:83, 1956.
7. Butler, J. E., Brown, S. L., and McConnel, B. G.: Subtrochanteric stress fractures in runners. Am. J. Sports Med. 10:228, 1982.
8. Daffner, R. H.: Stress fractures. Skeletal Radiol. 2:221, 1978.
9. Darby, Capt. R. E.: Stress fractures of the os calcis. JAMA 200:1183, 1967.
10. Devas, M. B.: Longitudinal stress fractures. J. Bone Joint Surg. 42B:508, 1960.
11. Devas, M. B.: Stress Fractures. Edinburgh, Churchill Livingstone, 1975.
12. Devas, M. B.: Stress fractures of the femoral neck. J. Bone Joint Surg. 47B:728, 1965.
13. Devas, M. B.: Stress fractures of the patella. J. Bone Joint Surg. 42B:71, 1960.
14. Devas, M. B.: Stress fractures in children. J. Bone Joint Surg. 45B:528, 1963.
15. Devas, M. B., and Sweetnan, R.: Stress fractures of the fibula. J. Bone Joint Surg. 38B:818, 1956.
16. Farquharson-Roberts, M. A., and Fulford, P. C.: Stress fractures of the radius. J. Bone Joint Surg. 62B:194, 1980.
17. Ford, L. T., and Gilula, L. A.: Stress fractures of the middle metatarsals following the Keller operation. J. Bone Joint Surg. 59A:117, 1977.
18. Gilbert, R. S., and Johnson, H. A.: Stress fractures in military recruits—a review of twelve years' experience. Milit. Med. 131:716, 1966.
19. Goergen, T. G., Venn-Watson, E. A., Rossman, D. J., et al.: Tarsal navicular stress fractures in runners. A. J. R. 136:201, 1981.
20. Greaney, R. B., Gerber, F. H., Laughlan, R. L., et al.: Distribution and natural history of stress fractures in US Marine recruits. Radiology 146:339, 1983.
21. Grusd, R.: Pseudofractures and stress fractures. Semin. Roentgenol. 13:81, 1978.
22. Hallel, T., Amit, S., and Segal, D.: Fatigue fractures of the tibial and femoral shaft in soldiers. Clin. Orthop. 118:35, 1976.
23. Hartley, J. B.: "Stress" or "fatigue" fractures of bone. Br. J. Radiol. 16:255, 1943.
24. Kitchin, I. D.: Fatigue fracture of the ulna. J. Bone Joint Surg. 30B:622, 1948.

25. Kroening, P. M., and Shelton, M. L.: Stress fractures. A. J. R. *89*:1281, 1963.

26. Laferty, J. F., Winter, W. G., and Ganilaro, S. A.: Fatigue characteristics of posterior elements of vertebra. J. Bone Joint Surg. *59A*:154, 1977.

27. Lesniewski, P. J., and Testa, N. N.: Stress fractures of the hip as a complication of total knee replacement. J. Bone Joint Surg. *64A*:304, 1982.

28. Levin, D. C., Blazena, M. E., and Levina, E.: Fatigue fractures of the shaft of the femur: Simulation of malignant tumor. Radiology *89*:883, 1967.

29. Lombard, S. J., and Benson, D. W.: Stress fractures of the femur in runners. Am. J. Sports Med. *10*:219, 1982.

30. Luchini, M. A., Sarokhan, A. J., and Micheli, L. J.: Acute displaced femoral-shaft fractures in long distance runners. J. Bone Joint Surg. *65A*:689, 1983.

31. Marmor, L.: Stress fracture of the pubic ramus simulating a loose total hip replacement. Clin. Orthop. *121*:103, 1976.

32. Matin, P.: The appearance of bone scans following fractures, including immediate and long-term studies. J. Nucl. Med. *20*:1227, 1979.

33. McElwaine, J. P., and Sheehan, J. A.: Spontaneous fractures of the femoral neck after total replacement of the knee. J. Bone Joint Surg. *64B*:323, 1982.

34. Miller, F., and Wenger, D. R.: Femoral neck stress fracture in a hyperactive child. J. Bone Joint Surg. *61A*:435, 1979.

35. Moon, K. L., Genant, H. K., Helms, C. A., et al.: Musculoskeletal applications of nuclear magnetic resonance. Radiology *147*:161, 1983.

36. Orava, S., Puranen, J., and Ala-Ketola, L.: Stress fractures caused by physical exercise. Acta Orthop. Scand. *49*:19, 1978.

37. Pavlov, H., Tord, J. S., and Freiberger, R. H.: Tarsal navicular stress fractures: Radiographic evaluation. Radiology *148*:641, 1983.

38. Prather, J. L., Nusynowitz, M. L., Snowdy, H. A., et al.: Scintigraphic findings in stress fractures. J. Bone Joint Surg. *59A*:869, 1977.

39. Protzman, R. R., and Griffis, C. G.: Stress fractures in men and women undergoing military training. J. Bone Joint Surg. *59A*:825, 1977.

40. Provost, R. A., and Morris, J. M.: Fatigue fracture of the femoral shaft. J. Bone Joint Surg. *51A*:3, 1969.

41. Rand, J. A., and Coventry, M. B.: Stress fractures after total knee arthroplasty. J. Bone Joint Surg. *62A*:266, 1980.

42. Rasad, S.: Golfer's fracture of the ribs. Report of 3 cases. A. J. R. *120*:901, 1974.

43. Rogers, L. F., and Campbell, R. E.: Fractures and dislocations of the foot. Semin. Roentgenol. *13*:157, 1978.

44. Ross, D. J., Dieppe, P. A., Watt, I., et al.: Tibial stress fracture in pyrophosphate arthropathy. J. Bone Joint Surg. *65B*:474, 1983.

45. Sandrock, A. R.: Another sports fatigue fracture. Stress fracture of the coracoid process of the scapula. Radiology *117*:274, 1975.

46. Schneider, R., and Kaye, J. J.: Insufficiency fractures of the long bones occurring in patients with rheumatoid arthritis. Radiology *116*:595, 1975.

47. Schneider, H. J., King, A. Y., Brosnon, J. L., et al.: Stress injuries and developmental changes of lower extremities in ballet dancers. Radiology *113*:627, 1974.

48. Stark, H. H., Jobe, F. W., Boyes, J. H., et al.: Fracture of the hook of the hamate in athletes. J. Bone Joint Surg. *59A*:575, 1977.

49. Stein, R. E., and Stelly, F. H.: Stress fracture of the calcaneus in a child with cerebral palsy. J. Bone Joint Surg. *59A*:131, 1977.

50. Symeonides, P. P.: High stress fractures of the fibula. J. Bone Joint Surg. *62B*:192, 1980.

51. Torg, J. S., Pavlov, H., Cooley, L. H., et al.: Stress fractures of the tarsal navicular. J. Bone Joint Surg. *64A*:700, 1982.

52. Wilson, E. S., and Katz, F. N.: Stress fractures. An analysis of 250 consecutive cases. Radiology *92*:481, 1969.

53. Young, A., Kinsella, P., and Boland, P.: Stress fractures of the lower limb in patients with rheumatoid arthritis. J. Bone Joint Surg. *63B*:239, 1981.

16

INTERVENTIONAL ORTHOPEDIC RADIOLOGY

THOMAS H. BERQUIST • BRAD B. HALL

Fluoroscopy, computed tomography, ultrasound, and nuclear medicine provide the ideal tools to guide interventional procedures that can greatly assist the orthopedic surgeon and other clinicians. This section will discuss in-depth interventional radiographic procedures other than arthrography, thus providing the reader with the necessary information concerning techniques, indications, and complications related to these procedures. The discussion will include bone biopsy (including disk space aspirations), facet injections, sinograms, diskography, and nerve root sheath injections. These procedures assist in diagnosis, surgical planning, and most importantly, avoiding unnecessary surgery.

BONE BIOPSY

Advances in imaging techniques, including multidirectional tomography, nuclear medicine, CT scanning, and magnetic resonance imaging allow more accurate evaluation of bone lesions. However, because of sophisticated treatment protocols, tissue diagnosis is frequently required.[20] Open biopsy yields the large specimens required for histologic diagnosis; but the procedure is expensive, and morbidity and mortality are significant, especially in spinal lesions. Percutaneous needle biopsy allows cytologic and often histologic diagnosis with lower cost, morbidity, and mortality.[8, 9, 34, 35, 40] It is highly accurate; thus, open biopsy, especially of the spine, has become much less common.

Robertson and Ball reported a method of percutaneous needle biopsy in 1935.[38] Today, the literature contains data on more than 11,000 cases.[6, 11, 13-15, 17, 19, 20, 32, 34, 36, 39, 41] Experience since the 1930's has resulted in marked improvement in the types of needles available. These, along with the markedly improved imaging modalities available to the radiologist, make percutaneous biopsy more accurate. The incidence of complications is also lower.

Indications

The indications for percutaneous skeletal biopsies do, of course, vary with the institution and the type of practice (Table 16–1). Review of the literature

reveals that percutaneous biopsy is most commonly performed to obtain tissue confirmation in suspected metastasis. As a majority of metastatic lesions involve the spine,[1, 34] we are frequently called upon to biopsy patients with abnormal-looking vertebral bodies to exclude metastasis or to confirm metastasis in patients with unknown primary tumors.[34] Percutaneous biopsies are usually not indicated for patients in whom surgical exploration is contemplated. Biopsies are also helpful in detecting benign and malignant cystic lesions of bone or for differentiating between them.[16, 36] While DeSantos[16-18] and other authors[6, 32, 41] report increasing use of bone biopsy in primary bone tumors, especially for differentiating Ewing's or osteogenic sarcoma from infection, percutaneous biopsy of primary bone tumors is usually not performed in our practice. An exception may be made for reticulum cell sarcoma, for which chemotherapy and radiation are usually utilized rather than surgical removal.[1, 13, 17, 34, 37]

Material for histologic diagnosis in cases of metabolic bone disease can be obtained simply with a trephine biopsy needle. This allows one to obtain the necessary bone tissue (cortex-to-cortex) from the easily accessible iliac crest.[27] Simple aspiration is insufficient in the evaluation of metabolic bone disease, as the histologic specimens obtained are inadequate.[13, 37]

The third most common indication for needle biopsy is identification of organisms in various infectious processes. These infectious processes include osteomyelitis, disk space infection, and joint space infection. Depending upon the site of the infection and clinical setting, both tissue and material for culture can be obtained.[14, 34, 37]

Resnick[37] also describes the use of percutaneous closed biopsy in the identification of articular disorders, such as osteonecrosis and other arthritic conditions.

TABLE 16–1. Indications for Percutaneous Needle Biopsy

Metastasis (known primary, unknown primary)
Metabolic bone disease
Infection
Articular disease
Primary bone tumor (rare)
Open biopsy not possible

TABLE 16–2. Biopsy Locations: Percutaneous Skeletal Biopsy

Series	Location			
	Spine (including sacrum) (%)	Pelvis (%)	Ribs (%)	Other (%)
Debnam[14]	41	19	20	20
DeSantos[17]	19	29	9	43
Collins[10]	33	28	12	27
Murphy[34]	56	25	—	19
Mayo*	80	5	10	5

*Excluding metabolic bone disease as an indication.

Biopsy Locations

The frequency of various biopsy sites or locations varies significantly, depending upon the practice or institution. If biopsies are performed for metabolic bone disease, the iliac crest is the most common site. With the advent of interventional radiology and improved imaging modalities, the indications have now broadened to include metastatic disease, infection, and other orthopedic problems. At the present time, the most common indications for percutaneous biopsies in our practice are metastatic disease and infection, usually of the disk space. If one excludes metabolic bone disease, the majority of biopsies are performed on the vertebral body (80 percent), most commonly in the lumbar spine. Ten percent of biopsies involve the ribs, 5 percent involve the pelvis, and the remaining 5 percent involve the extremities. These figures are somewhat different from those presented by other authors in large series. The different series are presented in Table 16–2. Despite the higher percentage of spine biopsies performed at our institution, Table 16–2 shows that the majority of these biopsies are performed on the axial skeleton primarily because multiple metastases—the primary indication—occur most commonly in this region. There are several large series discussing percutaneous biopsy of the spine exclusively.[5, 13, 36, 38, 39, 43] In these series, a total of 2,905 vertebral biopsies were performed. The majority were in the lumbar region, although 106 biopsies were performed in the cervical region with no reported complications. We avoid using the technique on lesions in the cervical spine when possible, as the surrounding vascular and neural structures make it more difficult. In most instances, the diagnosis can be accomplished by combining laboratory data with findings from tomography, CT, and other imaging modalities.

Technique

The technical aspects of percutaneous bone biopsies vary significantly depending on the location of the lesion. Before a biopsy site is chosen, however, multiple factors must be taken into consideration (Table 16–3). The first and most important step in planning percutaneous needle biopsy of the skeletal system is to obtain adequate clinical data from the referring physician. This includes the background history and suspected clinical diagnosis (infection or metastasis, either with or without a known primary) as well as significant laboratory data, such as coagulation studies, that might indicate a bleeding disorder. If biopsy of a rib or a thoracic or upper lumbar vertebra is contemplated, the patient's pulmonary status should also be noted, as pneumothorax is a potential complication of biopsies in these locations. After the pertinent clinical data are obtained, radiographic features of the lesion to be examined by biopsy must be studied closely. Does the lesion look benign or malignant? Is it lytic or sclerotic? Does it involve the disk or joint space? The location of the lesion in question, be it spine, pelvis, or extremities, is also critical. With these data in hand, a rational approach to bone biopsy can then be planned to obtain optimal results with the least risk to the patient. The approach can perhaps best be discussed on the basis of whether the lesion is solitary or multiple.

With solitary lesions, the routine radiographs should be studied thoroughly to determine the nature of the lesion. If the lesion (Fig. 16–1A) involves an area of the spine and is not a suspected disk space infection, radioisotope scans are helpful in determining whether it is single or multiple (Fig. 16–1B). If, for example, the lesion is located in the upper thoracic region on the radiograph, the nuclear medicine scan may demonstrate a second lesion in a much more accessible location, such as the midlumbar region. If the isotope scan does demonstrate multiple lesions, radiographs (Fig.

TABLE 16–3. Skeletal Biopsy: A Planned Approach

Clinical data
    History
        Suspected diagnosis (infection, metastasis, known or unknown primary)
    Laboratory data
        Clotting studies
        Pulmonary function
Radiographic features
    Benign
    Malignant—solitary or multiple
    Lytic, sclerotic
    Location
        Spine (including sacrum)
        Pelvis
        Ribs
        Extremities

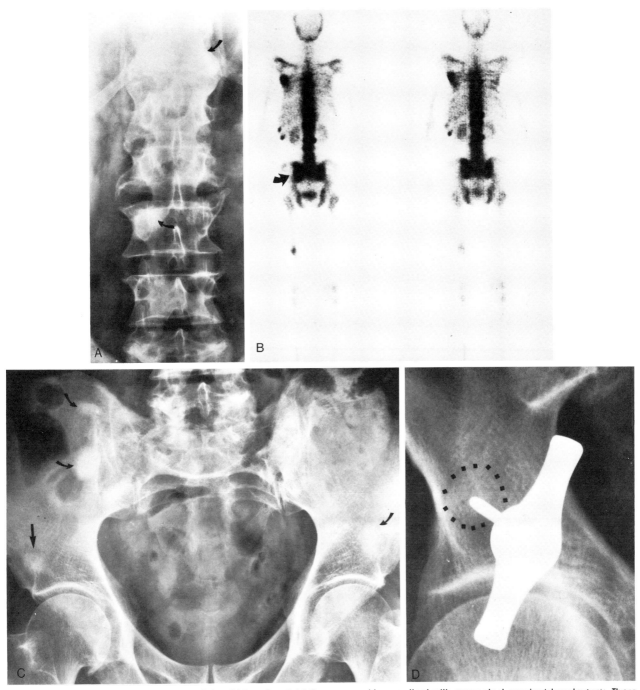

Figure 16–1. *A,* Blastic lesion in the pedicle of L3 on the right *(lower arrow)* in a patient with suspected carcinoid metastasis. There may be a second lesion in T12 *(upper arrow)*. *B,* Isotope bone scan (technetium) demonstrates multiple lesions. Rib, pelvic *(arrow)*, and right femoral lesions are more accessible. *C,* Pelvis film demonstrates multiple plastic metastases *(arrows)*, which are more easily biopsied than spinal lesions. *D,* Biopsy of the supra-acetabular lesion on the right confirmed the diagnosis of metastatic carcinoid.

16–1C and D) of other involved areas noted on the scan should be obtained to determine whether these lesions are accessible. In certain cases, tomography (Fig. 16–2) and CT scans may be helpful in determining the accessibility of the lesion and whether there is soft tissue involvement. If a soft tissue mass is present, biopsy may be accomplished more safely with a smaller needle (Fig. 16–3). Of course, a more accessible lesion, such as one in the pelvis, extremity, or rib, may also be identified with the isotope scan. Lesions seen on isotope scans, but not demonstrable with conventional radiographic techniques, are difficult to biopsy and yield fewer usable samples than lesions that can be identified on the radiograph.[13, 14]

If the solitary lesion noted in the spine is the only lesion present and the nuclear medicine studies are negative, CT can often be helpful in demonstrating the cortical and medullary characteristics of the lesion as well as any surrounding soft tissue mass.

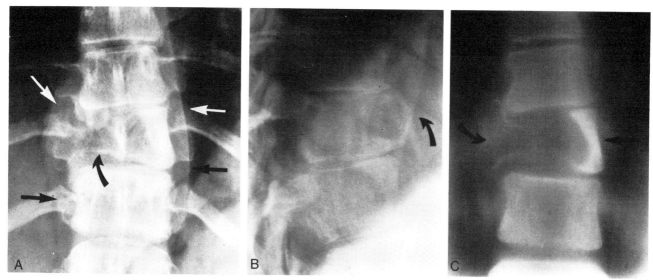

Figure 16–2. *A,* AP view demonstrates a destructive lesion *(curved arrow)* in T10 with an associated soft tissue mass *(straight arrows).* *B,* Lateral view demonstrates that the lesion predominantly involves the anterior body. *C,* Tomogram demonstrates a fine cortex on the right (allowing use of a smaller needle) compared with the more sclerotic left side. Tissue biopsy revealed malignant fibrous histiocytoma.

Recognition of these characteristics of the lesion helps not only in the choice of the proper needle (for example, a smaller needle may be used in soft tissue masses) but also in assessing whether the risks involved in performing the biopsy are so great that the procedure should not be performed. In certain situations, clinical history and radiographic appearance are such that empirical treatment with chemotherapy can be accomplished without biopsy if the risk to the patient is too great. This approach has been utilized by Hardy and colleagues.[25] They found that CT was of great value in planning percutaneous biopsies, and in 58 percent of the cases CT allowed cancellation of the biopsy either because it provided sufficient evidence for diagnosis or because it indicated that the biopsy would be more risky than anticipated therapy for the patient.

Biopsies of solitary lesions involving the pelvis, ribs, or extremities are usually less difficult and present fewer risks than a biopsy performed in the spine. Often the radiographic or tomographic fea-

tures alone are sufficient to suggest the diagnosis, and if the location of the lesion is accessible to biopsy, no further studies may be needed. If the lesion is sclerotic and medullary involvement or a soft tissue mass is in question, a CT scan may be helpful in determining the approach to the biopsy. Again, if a difficult approach is anticipated, a search by radioisotope scan for more accessible lesions should be considered.

In patients with multiple lesions metastasis is almost always the indication for biopsy, and in these situations one should utilize the available imaging modalities to choose the location that affords the safest approach. Again, radioisotope studies and CT scans offer alternative means to demonstrate the accessibility of the lesion and the needle of choice. The flow charts in Figure 16–4 and Table 16–3 should help in planning a rational approach to needle biopsy of the skeletal system that produces optimal results with the least morbidity and fewest possible complications.

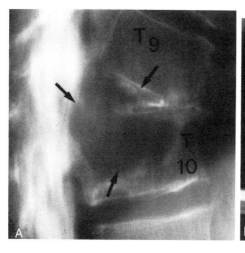

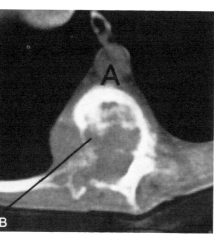

Figure 16–3. *A,* Tomogram demonstrates a destructive lesion in the lower thoracic spine *(arrows).* *B,* CT scan demonstrates a large soft tissue mass with interrupted cortex, allowing use of a smaller needle and more lateral approach (line indicates needle; A, aorta). Pleural space can be avoided more easily. Diagnosis was clear cell sarcoma.

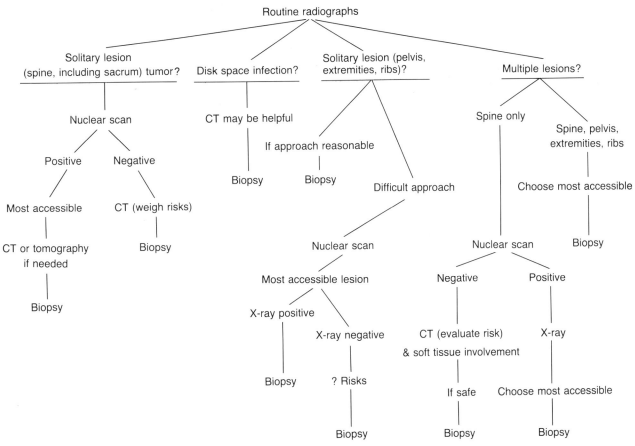

Figure 16–4. Imaging approach to a skeletal needle biopsy.

Needles and Positioning

There are many needles available for skeletal biopsy. As a rule of thumb, we prefer to perform the initial attempt with the smallest needle possible in order to minimize complications and patient discomfort. Small needles are effective in the case of lytic destructive lesions or lesions with associated soft tissue masses that can easily be detected and biopsied with CT if they are not visible on radio-graphs. Small needles are adequate in obtaining materials for cytologic analysis, and with proper technique histologic samples can also be obtained. We utilize 22-, 18-, and 16-gauge aspirating needles and 16-, 19-, and 21-gauge Surecut needles (Fig. 16–5). More difficult lesions may require a trephine type of biopsy needle that allows larger histologic specimens. If the cortex is relatively intact, the lesion sclerotic, or if a metabolic bone study is being requested (when a cortex-to-cortex specimen must

Figure 16–5. Aspirating needles for soft tissue and lytic musculoskel-etal lesions. Top to bottom: 18- and 16-gauge aspirating needle, 22-gauge Ciba needes, 16-gauge cut-ting needles.

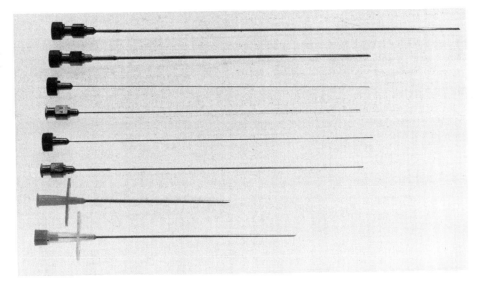

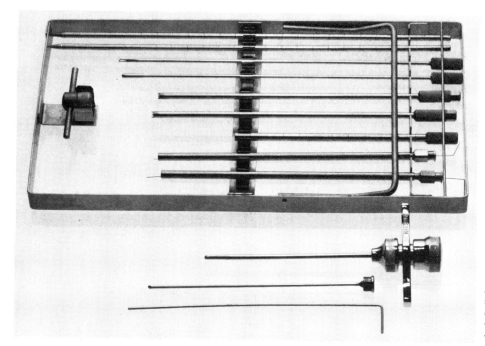

Figure 16–6. Craig (top) and Jamshidi (bottom) biopsy needle systems. The Craig needle includes a blunt trocar, guide, and wormer that are ideal for difficult vertebral lesions.

be obtained), we routinely use the Jamshidi needle or the Craig biopsy needle system (Fig. 16–6). Other available needles include Turkel, Ackerman, Vim-Silverman, and Westerman-Jensen needles, the latter of which have cutting blades to assist in obtaining tissue cores.[14, 15, 18, 21, 42]

When skeletal biopsies were first being performed, radiographs were utilized to check needle position. With the current imaging modalities of CT and conventional, C-arm, and biplane fluoroscopy, skeletal lesions can be identified, while the position of the needle is monitored continuously. These modalities increase accuracy, decrease morbidity, and reduce the time required to perform the procedure. We routinely use an overhead fluoroscopic table with a movable tabletop and image reverse to perform our skeletal biopsies. Biplane and C-arm fluoroscopic units are also available but are rarely needed. Following a thorough discussion of the patient's clinical problems and review of the radiographic and nuclear studies, the procedure and risks of the biopsy are discussed with the patient. Positioning of the patient on the fluoroscopic table depends upon the location of the lesion to be biopsied. The approach also differs depending upon the location of the lesion.

Skeletal Biopsy of Lesions of the Spine and Disks

Thoracic Spine from T3 to T9

The patient lies prone on the fluoroscopic table, and the skin over the biopsy site is prepared using sterile technique. The prone position is also used for CT-guided biopsies.

An entry point is chosen not more than 4 to 5 cm

from the spinous process in order to avoid entering the pleural space. The skin and soft tissues are anesthetized with lidocaine (Xylocaine). Anesthetic injection is carefully continued to the periosteum over the vertebral body to be biopsied. The anesthetic needle can be left in place to serve as a guide for the biopsy needle. This is particularly useful if the approach to the lesion is difficult. The biopsy is performed from the right side, if possible, to avoid striking the aorta with the needle. Because of the

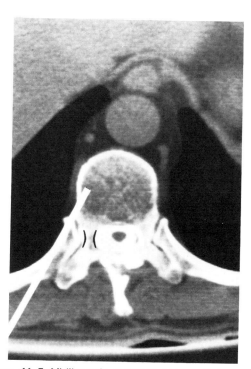

Figure 16–7. Midthoracic vertebral biopsy. Note angle of needle and position of lung and aorta. The pedicle, [ ] ( ) should be avoided.

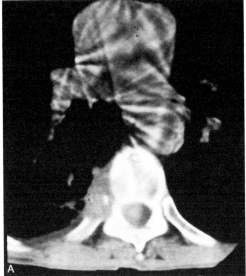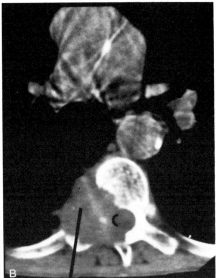

Figure 16–8. A, CT scan demonstrating a right paraspinal soft tissue mass. No neurologic deficit. B, Needle *(line)* must be positioned laterally to avoid hemorrhage near pedicle.

relatively steep angle with which the needle enters the vertebral body, care must be taken to avoid sliding along the vertebral body and entering the pleural space or posterior mediastinum (Fig. 16–7). This situation is most often encountered with sclerotic or blastic lesions, which are often difficult to penetrate. In these cases, a Craig needle or trephine needle of some type is almost always necessary. When possible, as in the case of lytic or destructive lesions, a smaller aspirating needle is used. One must also avoid penetrating too close to the pedicle (Fig. 16–7), especially in the destructive lesions, to avoid possible hematoma and cord injury (Fig. 16–8). In the past, metal markers were devised for measuring the proper angle of entrance,[37, 43] but in our practice fluoroscopy obviates the need for such devices. Another technique that is often helpful is utilization of a long exploring needle for administering the local anesthetic. The needle can be left in place to serve as a guide for either the trephine or aspirating needle that will actually be used for the biopsy. The patient can be rotated periodically to check exact needle position in different planes.

Lower Spine from T10 through the Sacrum

Biopsy is significantly less difficult in the lower thoracic and lumbar spine than in the upper thoracic or cervical region. Again, the patient is placed on the CT or fluoroscopic table in the prone position. The entrance point can be more lateral in these instances, approximately 6.5 to 7.5 cm from the midline. This results in less interference from the ribs and transverse processes and allows a more direct entry. Therefore, there is less chance of sliding along the cortical margin of the vertebral body (Fig. 16–9). Again, a long 20- or 22-gauge anesthetic needle is used to anesthetize the soft tissues and periosteum. The needle can then be left in place to

serve as a guide for the biopsy needle. Needle position is monitored carefully with the fluoroscope. The needle is most often placed into the vertebral body from the right side to avoid the aorta. The smallest needle possible is utilized. If an adequate specimen is not obtained in the initial aspiration, a second attempt can be made with a larger needle, such as the Jamshidi or Craig needle. With blastic lesions or lesions with an intact cortex and no soft tissue mass (in which CT may be definitive), a large needle is utilized initially.

The approach to disk biopsy or aspiration is similar to vertebral biopsy except that the disk is entered more easily. A 16-gauge needle is usually adequate (Fig. 16–10). The needle is fairly easily positioned except at the L5–S1 disk space. McCulloch has described a two-needle technique.[31]

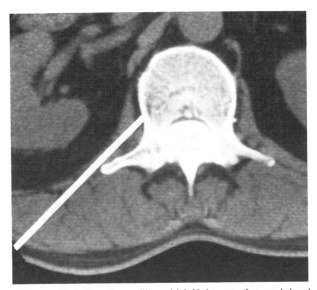

Figure 16–9. Needle position at L4. Note use of more lateral approach, which makes entering the vertebral body less difficult. Also, the pedicles and major vessels (aorta and vena cava) are well away from the needle tract.

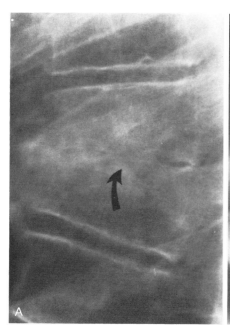 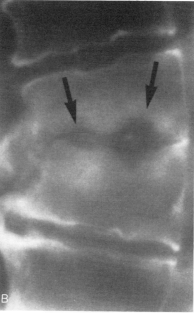

Figure 16–10. Lateral radiograph, *(A)* and lateral tomogram *(B)* of T8 disk space with marked end-plate irregularity *(arrows)* and a small sequestra.

This technique utilizes an 18-gauge needle that is placed adjacent to the disk space (L5–S1) posteriorly. A 22-gauge needle with the tip bent ½ to ¾ inch proximal from the tip is inserted into the first needle. This needle is used to enter the disk space.

Despite the relative ease with which lumbar vertebral bodies or disk spaces may be biopsied, care must be taken to avoid damage to the retroperitoneal structures, which may be injured by inadvertently initiating an overly lateral approach (Fig. 16–11). Again, fluoroscopic guidance usually allows visualization of the kidney. The L5 vertebral body may be difficult to approach owing to the iliac crest (Fig. 16–12). The needle must be directed caudally as well as vertically, requiring more care in positioning the patient and the needle. Also, in heavy patients the fluoroscopic images may not provide proper visualization. In these cases, CT may be required to monitor the biopsy. Sacral lesions are

often best studied with CT. If a soft tissue mass is present with an anterior lesion, it may be approached anteriorly with a fine (22-gauge) needle. This carries little risk to the patient. A large-bore needle should not be used from an anterior approach owing to the visceral structures lying in the path of the needle. If the lesion lies posteriorly, the choice of needles is less critical. If no soft tissue mass is present, a large-bore needle can be used.

Upper Spine from C1–T2

In our practice, we are rarely requested to biopsy cervical or upper thoracic lesions. Luckily, with today's imaging modalities, radiographic features, along with the clinical diagnosis, often obviate the need for skeletal biopsy. In the past, large series of biopsies in the cervical and upper thoracic region were accomplished with great accuracy. The dorsal lateral approach was used for the lower cervical spine, and a pharyngeal approach was used for the upper cervical spine.[39, 43]

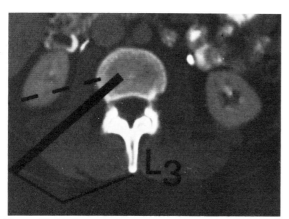

Figure 16–11. Biopsy in the upper lumbar region (L1–L3) may result in damage to retroperitoneal structures if the approach begins too far laterally *(dotted line)*. An approach of 6 to 7.5 cm lateral to the spinous process *(solid line)* will normally prevent this complication.

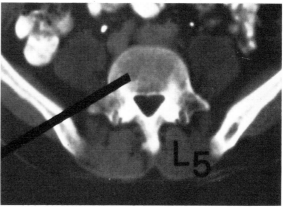

Figure 16–12. In most situations the needle for biopsy of L5 must be directed over the iliac crest.

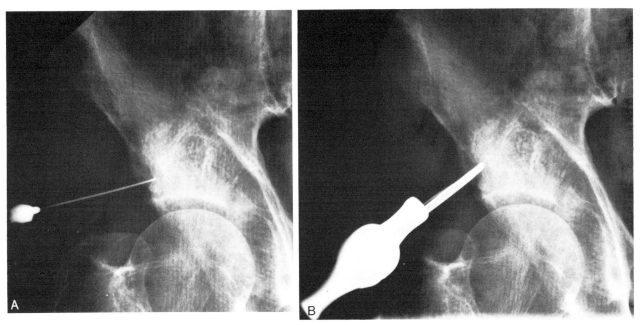

Figure 16–13. A, Anesthetic needle in place in the acetabular region of a suspected prostatic metastasis. B, Jamshidi needle positioned for biopsy (aligned with anesthetic needle). Histologic specimen proved to be metastatic prostatic carcinoma.

Other Sites for Skeletal Biopsy

Biopsies performed in other locations such as the rib, pelvis, and long bones are more easily accomplished than spinal biopsies because they are usually more accessible. One need only keep in mind the vascular and neural structures and choose the safest point of entry (Fig. 16–13).

Specimen Preparation and Evaluation

Regardless of the site of the biopsy, once the specimen has been obtained it must be properly handled. With fine needle techniques, smears are obtained and placed in 95 percent alcohol. The stylet is then passed through the needle, and any tissue fragments are placed in formalin for frozen section. These specimens and slides are taken immediately to the surgical pathologist to determine whether adequate tissue is present for diagnosis. If the diagnosis can be made from these specimens and the tissue is adequate, the procedure is terminated.

If the tissue specimen is inadequate, further attempts are made unless the patient's condition dictates otherwise. With disk space aspiration, a 16-gauge needle is usually adequate for obtaining aspirate and tissue samples. If a second attempt is required, a larger needle, such as the Craig or Jamshidi needle, is utilized. This, of course, is necessary with metabolic bone biopsies to obtain a cortex-to-cortex histologic core. If a large histologic core is obtained, it is placed in formalin to be decalcified and stained for further study. Any debris or liquid in the syringe can be cultured, if indicated. Again, smears are obtained for initial review. Aspirated blood and clot should also be studied. Hewes and colleagues[26] found osseous blood to be very useful microscopically. Electron microscopy may also be useful in cytologic studies.[7]

Diagnostic accuracy varies depending upon the patient's condition, the location of the lesion, the modality chosen to perform the biopsy, and the type of needle used. Accuracy rates vary from 73 to 94 percent (Table 16–4). Meyers[32] reports accuracy rates of 76 percent for benign tumors, 91 percent

TABLE 16–4. Percutaneous Skeletal Biopsy

Number of Procedures	Accuracy (%)	Imaging Modality	Series	Date
1078	73	Radiographs	O'Holeughi[36]	1969
100	93	Radiographs and fluoroscopy	Deeley[15]	1972
73	81	Fluoroscopy	Debnam[13]	1975
7165	74	Radiographs	Schajowicz[39]	1976
180	85	Nuclear scans and fluoroscopy	Collins[10]	1979
531	66–91	Fluoroscopy	Meyers[32]	1979
169	94	Fluoroscopy	Murphy[34]	1981
80	80	Fluoroscopy	El-Koury[20]	1983
120	72	Fluoroscopy	Tehranzadeh[41]	1983
222	78.6	Fluoroscopy	Ayala[6]	1983

for primary tumors, and 79 percent for metastatic lesions.

Pitfalls

In our experience, most biopsies have been performed on an outpatient basis. Patients have largely been able to tolerate the procedure without sedation or general anesthesia. Local anesthetic applied to skin, soft tissues, and periosteum is usually all that is required. Premedication with meperidine (Demerol) and diazepam (Valium) may be required occasionally.[2, 7, 8, 24] This is most commonly needed in patients with significant pain. If the patient is unable to maintain the necessary position for the biopsy, the test is not possible.

Biopsies can be obtained in most locations; however, the L5 level and upper thoracic region are more difficult than the pelvis or appendicular skeleton. In the thoracic region the needle tends to slide along the body owing to the steep angle employed to avoid the pleural space. Also, the adjacent ribs and mediastinal structures hinder the fluoroscopic image. CT guidance may provide the answer to this problem.[3] The iliac crest may cause difficulty in obtaining the ideal approach for biopsy of L5 (see Fig. 16–12).

Inaccuracy may result from an improper choice of needle for the type of lesion biopsied. Skeletal lesions with an associated soft tissue mass are most often successfully biopsied with Surecut or small aspirating needles. A 75 to 90 percent accuracy rate has been reported using small needles in soft tissue and destructive bone lesions.[4, 29] Choice of biopsy site in cystic or necrotic lesions may be assisted by injection of contrast material.[7] Use of blot preparations, smears, and a "wormer" with the Craig needle increase the chances for success.[6, 23] Blastic lesions may be very difficult to penetrate. Ayala[6] reported failure in 17 of 35 blastic biopsies. Jamshidi, Ackerman, and Craig needles provide better success. One may also biopsy bone immediately adjacent to the sclerotic area.

Complications

Major complications following bone biopsy are rare. Over 11,000 procedures have been performed, with significant complications occurring in only 0.2 to 1 percent.[30, 32, 34, 41] Serious neurologic complications such as paraplegia, paraspinal hematoma, meningitis, foot drop, and bladder dysfunction occurred in 0.08 percent of cases.[32, 34, 41] Other reported complications include pneumothorax (rib, thoracic, and L1 spine biopsies)[2, 5, 13, 34] and sinus tracts with tuberculous disk space infections.[5, 13, 34] Several deaths have been reported,[34] but in one case this was due to a myocardial infarct 48 hours after the procedure,[12] and the events may not have been related. Though spread of tumor cells along the needle tract theoretically could occur, this has not been a significant problem.[37, 44]

We have not experienced any major complications except pneumothorax. This occurred in 2 patients following thoracic vertebral biopsy. Most patients experience dull pain at the puncture site for 12 to 48 hours after the procedure. This rarely requires narcotic-strength analgesics.[27] Radiographically changes at iliac biopsy sites may be visible (exostoses or well circumscribed lucent zones).[22, 23] These changes have no clinical significance, but it is helpful to be aware of their etiology in order to avoid misinterpretation. Careful choice of patients with thorough knowledge of the history and careful utilization of the available modalities can help avoid complications. Of course, if the risks are weighed and determined to be too great, biopsy should be avoided.

SINOGRAPHY

Sinography is most often indicated for investigation of sinus tracts to determine the extent of soft tissue, bony, or articular involvement. Sinus tracts usually develop following chronic infections, often in postoperative patients. Complete evaluation of the extent of the tract and the degree of bony or articular involvement is paramount in planning the proper medical or operative therapy.[24]

Proper performance of the sinogram includes thorough investigation of the patient's cutaneous wound to determine the number and size of sinus tracts present. Multiple tracts may be present in postoperative patients, and all must be studied thoroughly. The patient is placed on the fluoroscopic table, and the area to be studied is thoroughly cleansed using sterile technique. After investigating the number and size of sinus tracts, the proper sized catheters can be chosen for the sinus tracts. When possible, we utilize small pediatric feeding tubes to catheterize the sinus tracts. Larger 5-French and 7-French angiographic catheters are occasionally required for investigation of larger sinus tracts (Fig. 16–14). When pediatric feeding tubes are utilized in shallow or superficial tracts, the end of the tube must be cut obliquely, as the normal feeding tube has several side holes but no end hole in its tip. Removing the tip also allows one to pass small guidewires into the sinus tract for better evaluation, if indicated.

Once the proper catheter has been chosen, it should be advanced into the sinus tract as far as can be comfortably tolerated by the patient. When some resistance is met, the position of the catheter or feeding tube is checked fluoroscopically, and a small amount of contrast material is injected. Many of the intravenously administered water-soluble contrast materials may be utilized for this study. We routinely use Hypaque (50 percent) or Conray. After initial injection, information can be obtained about the extent and complexity of the sinus tract. If the sinus tract is healing, nothing more than a superficial pocket may be identified. However, if

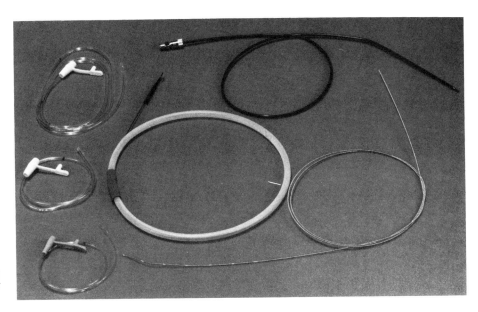

Figure 16–14. Pediatric feeding tubes and guidewires required for sinography.

the sinus tract is actually draining, there is usually a significant pocket, and several communications may be identified. If such is the case, catheters should be advanced in the direction of the tracts as far as possible with guidewires, if necessary, to determine the true extent of the sinus tract. Of course, care must be taken not to create any false channels with the catheter or guidewires. In determining the extent of sinus tracts, we have found it best to position the patient so that the catheter entry point is in the most superior position, thus utilizing gravity and also giving us the opportunity to compress the cutaneous entrance into the sinus tract. This helps prevent reflux of contrast material from the sinus tract onto the skin. This can be a problem, especially in small superficial sinus tracts that are partially closed.

In our practice, we are often presented with complex sinus tracts that have multiple branches and deep and superficial pocketing. These are extremely difficult for the surgeon to correct, and several further studies may be helpful in correcting the patient's clinical problem. If sinus tracts can be demonstrated to communicate with the joint, methylene blue can be injected into the joint, and the sinus tracts can then be better identified at the time of surgery. In complex extensive sinus tracts (Fig. 16–15), selective catheterization of the tracts is of value. This allows the surgeon to follow the catheters and thus both reduces the operating time and improves the chances for surgical success. If catheters are to be placed in a sinus tract, the catheterization should be accomplished as close as possible to the date of the planned surgical procedure, for following catheterization the patient occasionally develops a mild fever and some inflammatory response. It is to the patient's advantage not to have the catheters in place longer than is absolutely necessary.

Sinography, if carefully and meticulously performed, can be of great value to the surgeon in planning the proper mode of therapy. As mentioned earlier, most often these patients have a complex medical history, and any assistance that the radiologist can provide is valuable to the orthopedic surgeon.

DIAGNOSTIC AND THERAPEUTIC INJECTIONS

Radiologists are frequently called upon to inject or aspirate various joints, either for diagnostic or for therapeutic purposes. Injections of the shoulder, hip, ankle, and foot are commonly performed. These injections are easily accomplished with fluoroscopic guidance and can be efficiently performed on almost any joint that can be visualized fluoroscopically. Depending on the joint to be studied, an arthrogram may be obtained at the same time, aiding in the diagnostic portion of the procedure. The anatomic information provided by routine radiographs, tomography, and arthrography, along with the patient's response to injection of local anesthetic into the joint, can affect the orthopedic surgeon's plans for treatment. This might include the decision to manage the patient conservatively or to operate. Most injection techniques have been discussed in the arthrography sections of previous chapters.

Diagnostic and therapeutic injections are also commonly performed on patients with suspected facet syndrome. Low back pain is an extremely common clinical problem in orthopedic practice. Disk disease is most often considered in these patients, but diagnosis of the etiology of low back pain is a persistent problem, and disk disease does not explain the clinical setting in each case.[55] Facet arthropathy is an important cause of low back pain. Ghormley first coined the tern "facet syndrome" in 1933.[55] Many other authors have also confirmed the pathophysiologic basis of facet joint arthritis as a cause of low back pain.[45, 55, 73, 80]

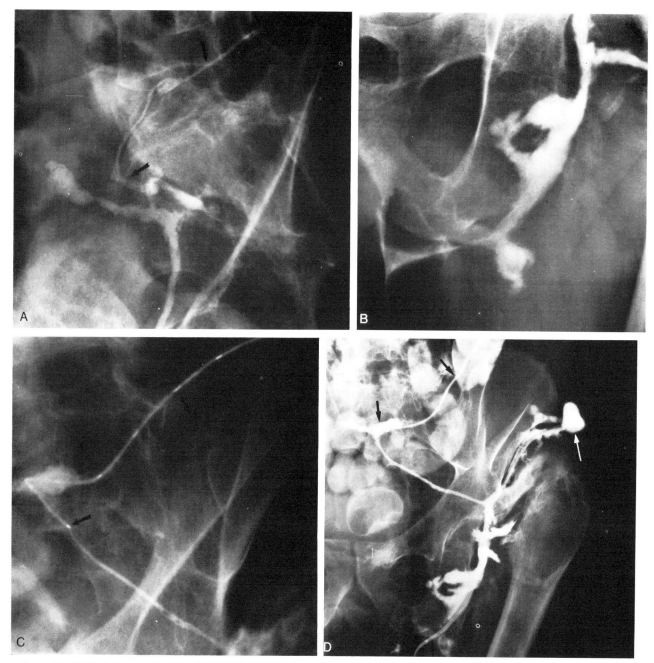

Figure 16–15. Girdlestone procedure in patient with chronic draining sinuses in the groin over the low back. *A,* Sinus tract extending from low back to presacral area *(arrows).* This communicated with a pocket that extended to the joint space. *B,* The sinus tract from the groin also communicated with the joint space. *C,* L-R torque guidewire in sacral sinus tract *(arrow)* prior to catheterization. *D,* Catheters in place from above *(upper arrows)* and below *(lower arrows)* allow the surgeon to follow the tracts more easily. Note contrast medium in the colon from previous CT scan.

Clinical diagnosis of facet syndrome can be imprecise, as the innervation of the facet joint is such that it is often difficult to predict exactly which facet joint may be involved. Radiographic findings often do not correlate with the patient's clinical symptoms. Many patients with extensive arthritic changes in the facet joints do not complain of low back pain, while patients with minor changes or no changes may have significant symptoms that may or may not be related to the facet joints. The facet joints are best demonstrated radiographically on the oblique views.[54] However, one must keep in mind that in progressing from L1 to L5, facet joints gradually become more oblique and laterally oriented. Thus, positioning may create the false impression of narrowed facet joints on the oblique view.

As one progresses caudally, it is not unusual for the lower lumbar facet joints to appear progressively more narrow. The normal facet joint, if viewed tangentially, is 2 to 3 mm wide with sharp margins and a well demarcated cortex (Fig. 16–16).

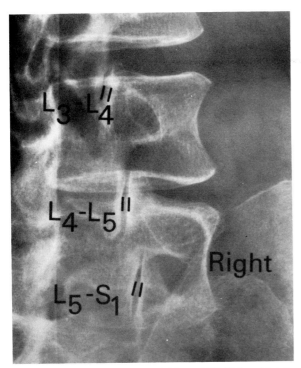

Figure 16–16. Normal L3–L4, L4–L5, and L5–S1 facet joints as seen on oblique radiograph. Note sharp joint margins and apparent progressive narrowing as one moves inferiorly from L3 to S1.

The earliest changes in arthritis appear to be sclerosis followed by progressive narrowing of the joint and bony eburnation at the margins of the joint (Fig. 16–17). With advanced stages, the joint may be totally obliterated and actually become ankylosed (Fig. 16–18).

CT studies may be of great value in studying patients with suspected facet syndrome.[48, 57] In Carrera's experience[48] and in ours as well, patients with normal CT scans do not usually respond to injection of the facet with local anesthetic. This would indicate that a normal CT scan suggests that the facet is not the site of pathology for the patient's symptom complex.[46–48]

Facet Joint Injections

Anatomy

To master the technical aspects of performing facet injections, it is imperative that one be familiar with the anatomy of the facet joint. The anatomic position and direction in which the facet joints of the cervical and thoracic region are aligned does not permit easy access for fluoroscopic imaging. The facet joints of the lumbar spine become more laterally and obliquely oriented as one moves caudally from L1 to L5 (Fig. 16–19). Facet joints are true synovial joints lined with synovial membrane and surrounded by a fibrous capsule. An important factor to keep in mind is the innervation of the facet joints. From the posterior rami a medial branch courses through a notch in the base of the transverse process at the inferior margin of the facet joint at the same level (Fig. 16–20). A medial branch then continues inferiorly and gives off several fibers to the superior aspect of the facet joint below. Therefore, each posterior ramus supplies two adjacent facet joints.[45, 76] This factor contributes to the somewhat difficult task of pinpointing the joint that is responsible for the patient's symptoms.

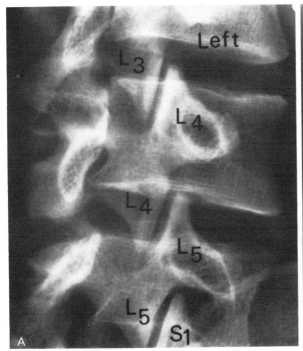
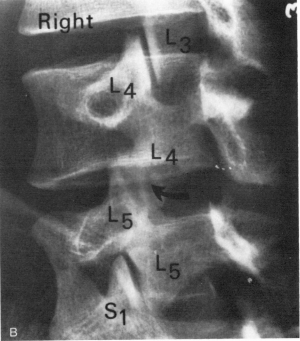

Figure 16–17. A, Early sclerosis and slight narrowing of L3–L4 facet joint on the right. *B,* There is marked narrowing of the L4–L5 facet joint on the right with bony eburnation. Symptoms were relieved with injection of the L3–L4 and L4–L5 facets.

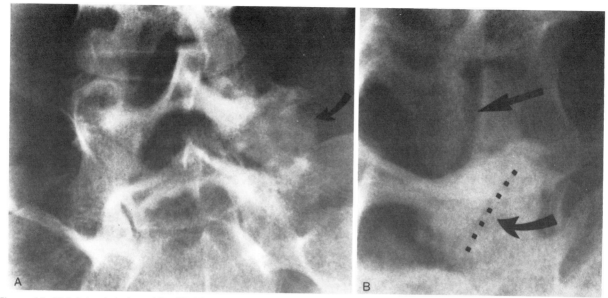

Figure 16–18. Total ankylosing of the L5–S1 facet joint on the left in an asymptomatic elderly male. *A,* AP view. *B,* Oblique view.

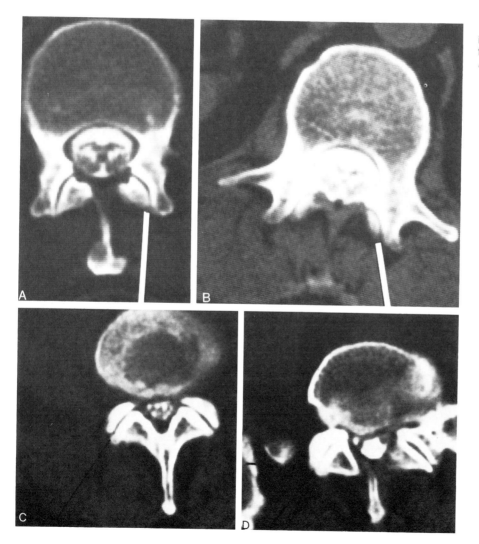

Figure 16–19. CT scans demonstrating progressive lateral oblique position of the lumbar facet joints. *A,* L2. *B,* L3. *C,* L4. *D,* L5.

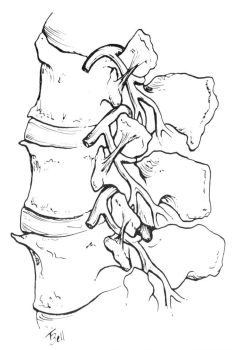

Figure 16–20. Innervation of the lumbar facets.

Indications

Review of the literature shows that patients referred for facet injection usually present with low back pain radiating to the buttock or down the leg. Symptoms suggesting disk protrusion are evaluated with electromyography and myelography. If these studies are normal and no neurologic deficit is present, facet syndrome is often considered. Differentiation between disk disease and facet syndrome can be difficult clinically.[46, 48, 51, 73] In a recent review of over 200 cases we also noted that facet syndrome was commonly encountered following laminectomy (25 percent of patients studied) and lumbar fusion, usually involving the facet joints immediately above the fusion site (Fig. 16–21). Response to injection is of great importance in planning conservative or surgical therapy.

Technique

Consultation with the clinician and review of available radiographs and CT scans are paramount in planning the site or sites to be injected. Depending upon the patient's clinical symptoms and the radiographic findings, multiple facet joints may be injected unilaterally or bilaterally. Occasionally clinical symptoms and radiographic findings indicate injection of only a single joint, whether unilaterally or bilaterally. Prior to the injection, it is important to discuss the patient's symptoms and to be certain whether they are intermittent or constant. If symptoms are intermittent, it is helpful to exercise the patient prior to the injection so that the pain is present at the time of injection.

The technique itself is quite simple. The patient is placed prone on the fluoroscopic table. Following sterile preparation of the injection sites, the patient is carefully rotated in order to position properly the facet to be injected (Fig. 16–19). It must be kept in mind that because of the orientation of the facets, only minimal rotation is usually needed in the upper lumbar spine. When injecting the L5–S1 facet joint, the patient is rotated with the side to be injected most superior. The skin overlying the facet joint is then injected with a small amount of local anesthetic, and a 22-gauge spinal needle is directed vertically into the joint. The position of the needle can be checked quickly and frequently with fluoroscopic guidance. With experience, the fibrous capsule of the facet joint can be palpated with a needle

Figure 16–21. A, AP radiograph of previous laminectomy of L4 on the left *(arrow)*. *B*, Unilateral facet arthrosis with narrowing and L4–L5 sclerosis on the left *(arrow)*.

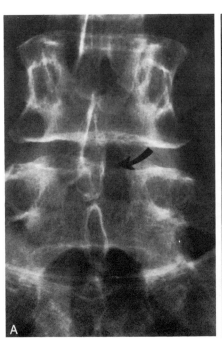

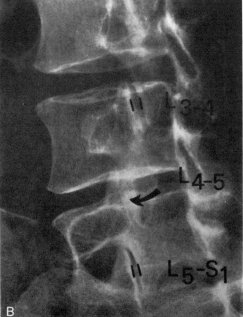

tip and easily punctured. Slight right-to-left rotation of the patient will allow one to detect either medial or lateral displacement of the needle tip on the bony margins of the facet joint.

Arthrography of facet joints has been advocated by other authors.[46, 51–53, 70] We have found that arthrography is not always necessary in checking for needle position if the above technique is utilized. Also, the arthrographic findings do not, in our experience, predict the response to facet injection. When the position of the needle tip is uncertain, 0.5 to 1 ml of Hypaque-M-60 can be injected to check the position of the needle tip. Once the needle is correctly positioned, the facet joint is injected with 1 to 2 ml of 0.25 percent bupivacaine (Marcaine) and betamethasone (Celestone). The suspension is mixed in a 2:1 ratio. While injecting the facet, the needle is moved up and down slightly. This facilitates the injection.

After the injection is completed, the patient is exercised or asked to perform certain range-of-motion exercises that have in the past tended to create the symptoms. In this way, one can detect if there has been any relief of the patient's symptoms. Marcaine is a long-acting anesthetic compared with the shorter acting Xylocaine, and it allows approximately 4 hours during which the radiologist and the referring clinician can evaluate the patient to determine the response to the injection. Complete relief of the patient's symptoms following the injection indicates that the patient's symptoms are related to the facet joint. This information assists the referring physician in selecting the appropriate conservative or operative therapy.

Results

In the last three years, over 200 patients with suspected facet syndrome have been studied in our department. The majority presented with low back pain radiating to the buttock or down the leg on the involved side. Most patients had also been studied with myelograms and electromyographs. Therefore, disk disease had been effectively excluded. Radiographic changes in these patients, when reviewed, revealed that 10 percent of the patients had normal routine radiographs, but in 90 percent, the radiographs were abnormal. In this latter group, the facets were sclerotic or narrowed, or there was associated degenerative disk disease, spondylolysis, or scoliosis. Slight instability with

TABLE 16–5. Facet Injection: Characteristics of 200 Patients at Mayo Clinic

Age range	17–68 yrs
Mean	44 yrs
Males	48%
Females	52%
Radiographs	
Abnormal	90%
Normal	10%

TABLE 16–6. Facet Injection: Results in 200 Patients at Mayo Clinic

Response to Injection	% of Patients
Mild (< 50% improved)	5
Moderate (> 50% improved)	11
Complete (essentially all symptoms resolved)	74
Pain (following injection)	4
No change	6

flexion and extension was also present in several cases. Table 16–5 summarizes the clinical and radiographic data.

Table 16–6 indicates the results achieved in this group of patients. Seventy-four percent received complete symptomatic relief following injection, implicating the facet joint as the cause for the patient's back pain. Best results were obtained if a single facet joint was involved (100 percent improved). Mild relief was noted in 5 percent and moderate relief in 11 percent of patients. There was no change in 6 percent, and in 4 percent of patients the pain actually increased. It should be kept in mind that distention of the facet joints can result in low back pain, as described by Mooney and Robertson.[73] Therefore, if the patient's symptoms are not derived from the facet joint, it is not surprising that distention of this joint may initially result in some increase in pain. We have also noted that following the anesthetic effect, the patient's symptoms usually recur prior to the steroid effect, and in several instances the patient's symptoms have actually been exacerbated by the introduction of steroids into the facet joints. In patients with complete relief following injection, the symptoms remained quiescent for days and up to 13 months. Symptoms in 2 patients recurred several months later, and repeat injections were again successful. In the majority of patients the procedure allows decisions to be made about subsequent surgical or conservative treatment. Carrera reported similar results in 20 patients; 13 obtained complete relief from facet injection (65 percent).[47] To date, there have been no complications from this procedure. Though it is theoretically possible to puncture the subarachnoid space, this has not occurred in our practice.[47] As we do not routinely perform arthrograms prior to facet injection, we avoid the hazard of overfilling the capsule prior to the injection of the anesthetic and Celestone. Nerve block, though possible, has also not occurred. Neurologic testing following injections reveals no evidence of nerve block.[47]

The significance of this diagnostic technique in diagnosis and treatment of patients with low back pain must not be minimized. In the series of patients we studied, 25 percent had previous laminectomy, and 10 percent had previous fusions. The use of facet injection as a diagnostic or therapeutic technique in these patients is helpful in determining the value of future operative intervention.

The sacroiliac joint may also present diagnostic problems to the clinician. This can be especially

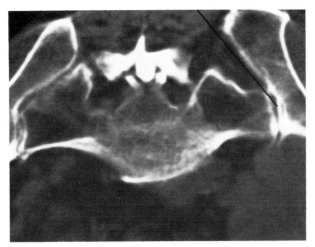

Figure 16–22. CT scan demonstrating angle *(line)* required to enter the sacroiliac joint.

puzzling after trauma to the lower back. Injection of the sacroiliac joint may aid the orthopedist in differentiating sacroiliac pain from low back pain. Instability of the sacroiliac joint with resulting pain should respond to injection and may require fusion. The injection of this joint, as with facet injections, can prove instrumental in planning operative or conservative therapy.

Injection of the sacroiliac joint can be accomplished simply. The patient is placed on the fluoroscopic table in the prone position with the involved joint rotated inferiorly. This allows a perpendicular needle approach below the posterior margin of the iliac crest (Fig. 16–22).[56] Marcaine or a combination of Marcaine and Celestone is injected (2 to 4 ml). If the needle position is in question, contrast material can be injected to confirm its location.

Diskography

Diskography of both the cervical and lumbar spine is a highly controversial diagnostic tool. The first reports of the clinical use of diskography appeared in the late 1940's.[58,67] In 1962, Collis and Gardner[50] claimed superiority in the detection of lumbar disk disease with diskography over lumbar myelography. Despite these claims, the technique never obtained general acceptance and usage in the United States.

The two studies published by Holt[59,60] in 1964 and 1968, in which he performed diskography on asymptomatic subjects and found abnormal roentgenographic appearances of the disks, discouraged widespread usage. His denouncement of the technique did not, however, discourage advocates outside of the United States. Since that time, a number of articles have been published supporting the use of both cervical[63,66,84] and lumbar diskography.[72,75,81] The true significance of diskography probably lies somewhere between these two schools of thought

and should be reserved for more difficult patients and selective preoperative situations.[78,83]

The use of lumbar diskography as a diagnostic tool will likely gain popularity in the United States soon. Now that chemonucleolysis has been given approval by the F.D.A., physicians will become familiar with the technique. An increase in the use of this diagnostic tool for purposes other than preparation for chymopapain injection is a likely sequel.

Indications

Although there is general agreement that the roentgenographic findings in diskography of the cervical spine are less reliable than the findings in diskography of the lumbar spine, the indications for use appear more clear cut in the case of cervical diskography. Simmons[81] and Kikuchi[63] feel that reproduction of symptoms during diskography is a reliable diagnostic tool for the localization of the level of symptomatic cervical disk degeneration in the patient who is nonresponsive to conservative treatment. The radiologic evidence of marked degeneration in a motion segment does not necessarily indicate that this level is the source of symptoms. Also, myelography and electromyography are of unreliable diagnostic value in the patient with symptomatic cervical disk degeneration. Difficulties in identifying the symptomatic level are probably responsible for doubts concerning the efficacy of anterior cervical fusion in patients with cervical disk degeneration but no evidence of impaired root conduction.[63] Kikuchi and colleagues[63] find that the combination of cervical diskography and selected nerve-root infiltration is helpful in the localization of the symptomatic level. The use of diskography in the diagnosis of disk herniation in the cervical spine has been advocated by Cloward,[49] Yamano,[84] Simmons,[81] and others. These authors feel that this technique is more accurate than clinical examination, routine radiography, and myelography.

The indications for lumbar diskography can be divided into four general areas: (1) localization of the symptomatic level in degenerative disk disease; (2) localization of a symptomatic pseudarthrosis; (3) determination of the necessary extent of a proposed spinal fusion; (4) before chemonucleolysis or diagnosis of a herniated nucleus pulposus producing sciatica.

Diskography may be useful in localizing the symptomatic level in a patient with mechanical low back pain secondary to either degenerative disk disease or scoliosis in the lumbar spine. Prior to performing fusion in either of these types of patients, it is essential to know that one is fusing the symptomatic motion segment(s). For example, in degenerative disk disease one may find that L5–S1 is markedly deteriorated on plain roentgenographs and that L4–L5 is relatively normal in appearance. Diskography may prove that the L4–L5 segment of the motion segment is producing the symptoms.

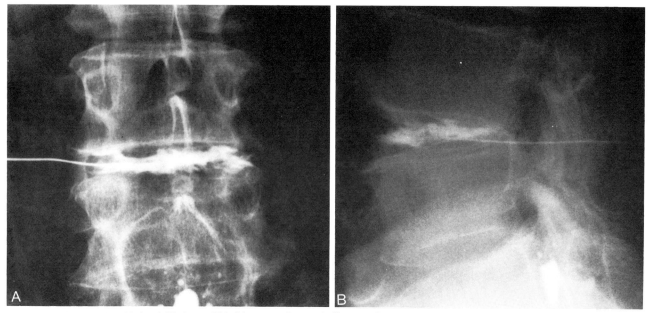

Figure 16–23. AP *(A)* and lateral *(B)* views of L4 diskogram demonstrating an abnormal disk. Symptoms were increased with injection.

Thus, a fusion of L5 to the sacrum alone will not benefit the patient (Fig. 16–23). In the patient with painful lumbar or thoracolumbar scoliosis, one must know prior to fusing the curvature whether or not the last two motion segments are contributing significantly to the production of pain. Kostuik[64,65] has found diskography to be extremely useful in adults with low back pain and scoliosis. Diskography in the preoperative assessment of these patients allowed a significant increase in the percentage of patients whose pain was relieved following surgical intervention.

The second indication for use of lumbar diskography is to localize a symptomatic pseudarthrosis in the lumbar spine.[78] Persistent pain following a lumbar fusion can be the result of a pseudarthrosis; however, not every pseudarthrosis is symptomatic. Pain reproduction on disk distention indicates the presence of a painful pseudarthrosis. The lack of pain reproduction indicates that the level is not responsible for the patient's complaints, and diskography at other levels may identify the origin of the pain.

The third indication is to determine the extent of a proposed spinal fusion. Fusing the lumbar spine places additional stress on the motion segment immediately above the level of fusion. Placing this added stress on a level with early disk degeneration will result in a rapid deterioration of that level and a return of symptoms within a few years of an otherwise successful operation. The roentgenographic appearance of the disk space is not totally reliable in the absence of unequivocal disk space narrowing.[77] Quinnell and Stockdale[77] found that not all claw-type osteophytes indicated disk degeneration, with 43 percent in their study showing normal disk characteristics. Traction spurs correlated much more highly with disk degeneration (89

percent association). Diskography at the level above a proposed fusion yields more reliable information concerning the status of the disk than plain radiographs (Fig. 16–24).

The role of lumbar diskography in the diagnosis of herniated nucleus pulposus, the fourth indication for its use, is a highly sensitive and controversial issue. In contrast to Holt[59] and others, who believe that it is of no value, Milette and Melanson[72] find lumbar diskography more sensitive than iophendylate (Pantopaque) myelography at the L5–S1 interspace. In their opinion diskography remains an ideal complementary examination to demonstrate normal or diseased disk morphology. They also feel that it is a valuable clinical test, since injection may reproduce the patient's symptoms. Their study indicated that diskography was at times critical in the surgeon's decision on whether to explore a disk.

With metrizamide myelography and the ever-increasing accuracy of computed tomography in the lumbar spine, it is doubtful that diskography will ever obtain a role more significant that that of a complementary examination following at least one and probably both of these tests in the difficult diagnostic case. It is our opinion that performing diskography on a patient who has not had myelography or computed tomography is inappropriate. This point cannot be overemphasized, particularly following the approval of chymopapain in the United States for the treatment of herniated nucleus pulposus that produces sciatica.

Diskography and/or disk distention can and should be used prior to chymopapain injection, but the patient should not be injected on the basis of diskographic findings alone. Diskography has no role in identifying neoplastic lesions of the spinal canal or the nerve roots. Failure to obtain the appropriate diagnostic study in the evaluation of patients with back and leg pain may result in the inappropriate injection of patients with lesions other than herniated nucleus pulposus as the source of their symptoms. Delay in obtaining an accurate diagnosis because of failure to obtain appropriate diagnostic studies can result in catastrophic problems for both patient and physician.

Technique and Interpretation

Needle insertion into the lumbar disk utilizing the posterolateral approach has already been described in this chapter.[71] The procedure may also be performed by the posterior or transdural approach. We prefer the posterolateral approach because it avoids puncture of the dura and the complication of postlumbar puncture headache. This is also the only accepted technique for administration of chymopapain intradiskally.

Diskography performed as a diagnostic tool should never be done with the patient under general anesthesia. The pain response during disk distention is probably the most important portion of the test. This would be eliminated if the patient were anesthetized.

The patient can be given intravenous sedation and the skin can be infiltrated locally with anesthetic to decrease the discomfort during needle insertion. Performing the test with the patient under local anesthesia has the advantage of a responsive patient who can notify the physician in the event of nerve root impalement by the needle. In the posterolateral approach the needle passes extremely close to the nerve roots as it exits from the neural foramen.

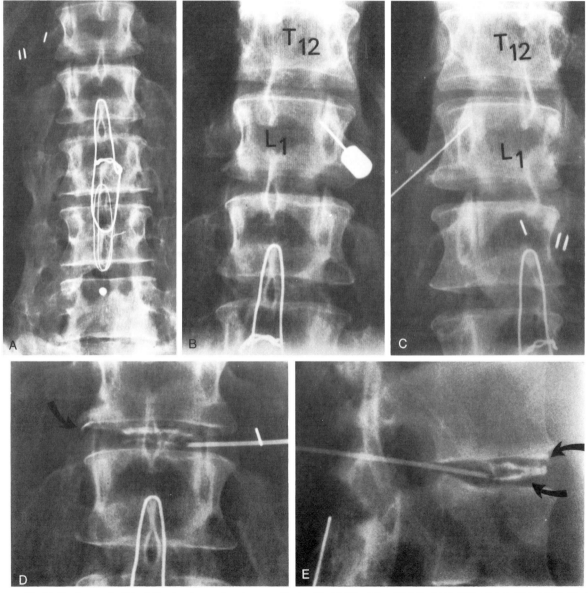

Figure 16–24. Radiograph *(A)* of the lumbar spine in a patient with continued midback pain following fusion of L2–S1. Facet injections *(B* and *C)* above the level of the fusion resulted in moderate improvement in symptoms. Diskogram *(D* and *E)* shows early degeneration *(arrows).* The symptoms were reproduced.

Cervical diskography, like lumbar diskography, must be performed under roentgenographic control. The use of the image intensifier or fluoroscope greatly facilitates the procedure. The use of mild sedation prior to performing the procedure, particularly in apprehensive patients, is advisable. The neck is prepared and draped in the usual sterile fashion. The skin is anesthetized just lateral to the trachea at the level of the disk to be punctured. The physician places his fingers in the groove between the carotid sheath and the trachea and gently presses down to the anterior surface of the cervical spine. The skin is punctured with a 2-inch 20-gauge needle, which is passed through the subcutaneous tissues until it makes contact with the spine. The periosteum and anterior longitudinal ligament as well as the prevertebral fascia are anesthetized. The position of the needle tip is adjusted and confirmed to be at the desired annulus under roentgenographic control. A 2 1/2-inch 25-gauge needle can then be inserted through the previous needle. This is passed through the annulus and into the nucleus pulposus. It is important that the anterior longitudinal ligament be infiltrated carefully with local anesthetic. It may be an irritable focus in degenerative disk disease. Injection into an asymptomatic disk may cause pressure on the inflamed anterior longitudinal ligament, giving rise to pain and a false postive test.[68]

Most people who utilize cervical diskography feel that at least the lower three motion segments of the cervical spine (C4–C5, C5–C6, and C6–C7) should be tested, since these are the disks most commonly affected. The order in which the disks are injected can be based upon percentages, going from the most commonly affected to the least commonly affected or in reverse order, depending on physician preference. We feel it is best to start with the disk least likely to be responsible for the patient's symptoms. If considerable pain results from testing one level, the chances that tests on the other levels will also produce pain is raised considerably. This finding has led Macnab[68] to utilize lidocaine as the distending agent; therefore, any pain produced is temporary. He advocates that the injection be stopped as soon as any discomfort is produced. The patient is then asked whether the pain is the same in character and location as his usual symptoms.

The normal cervical disk rarely accepts more than 0.2 mm of solution. Most people feel that the reproduction of symptoms by intradiskal injection or the "disk distention test" carries much greater significance that the diskogram itself. Therefore, many exclude the use of dye entirely.

There are many factors to be examined when interpreting lumbar diskography. The disk tests can be divided into three parts: (1) contrast, (2) disk distention, and (3) disk anesthesia. As already stated, the roentgenographic appearance of contrast diskography is probably the least reliable and useful portion of the test, except when one desires to confirm that a level is normal.

The disk distention test has three important elements. The first is the volume of fluid accepted. A normal lumbar disk will accept between 1 and 2 ml of fluid. When more fluid is easily accepted, the annulus is incompetent. The resistance to injection is also important. The first 1 to 2 ml of fluid should be received or accepted easily. If one encounters considerable resistance, the position of the needle should be checked again. More than likely the needle is in the annulus or endplate of the vertebra. The needle tip position should be readjusted. A normal disk will have a marked firm endpoint after injection of 1 to 2 ml of fluid.

The reproduction of pain or lack of pain produced with disk distention is the most important element of the disk distention test and also probably of lumbar diskography as a whole. Injection of the normal disk usually causes some local discomfort. Injection of an abnormal disk causes more pain. During injection of the symptomatic disk, the patient feels discomfort that is typical of the patient's usual back pain both in character and location.

After the disk distention portion of lumbar diskography, it is often helpful to wait for a few minutes and then slowly inject the symptomatic disk with an anesthetic solution. Relief of a patient's symptoms for an appropriate length of time can add significantly to the physician's knowledge in regard to the source of the patient's pain and the reliability of both the patient and the test. When interspace anesthetization dramatically relieves the patient of his previous pain and produces a temporary marked improvement in back motion, it is reasonable to assume that the injected disk (whether previously resected or not) is a major source of the patient's disability.[83]

Complications

The insertion of a needle into a disk may potentially introduce bacteria and lead to resultant diskitis. In his extensive experience with the procedure, Wilkinson reported 2 cases of diskitis out of 1,000 patients who had undergone multilevel lumbar diskography.[83] Patrick[75] reported 1 case in which he felt diskography might have led to the extrusion of additional disks and endplates into the spinal canal. He reasoned that "injection of Hypaque may have brought about disruption of the cartilaginous endplates above and below, leading to the intervertebral protrusion of nuclear material."[75] The use of the posterolateral or extradural approach eliminates the possibility of postlumbar puncture headaches. This is, however, a significant potential complication of the straight posterior transdural approach.

Nerve Root Infiltration

In his classic article, "Negative Disk Exploration," Macnab in 1971 stated that "in those instances in which the myelogram fails to reveal any abnormality and there are no neurologic defects to localize the root involved, a selective nerve root infiltration with local anesthetic, differential epidural injections, and the like may demonstrate the level of the lesion and indicate the type of lesion to be expected."[69] Since that time, a number of authors have described the use of selective nerve root sheath injections in the evaluation of patients with radicular symptoms for whom more conventional techniques are not diagnostic of the etiology.[61,62,79,82] Patients who have poor postoperative results, recurrent radiculopathy, and lumbar canal or lateral foraminal recess stenosis are the usual candidates for this technique. In pseudoclaudication, selective nerve root sheath infiltration is helpful in determining which nerve roots are responsible for the symptoms and which should be decompressed.

Kikuchi, Macnab, and Moreau used infiltration of cervical nerve roots with local anesthetic to localize the level of symptomatic cervical disk degeneration in patients presenting with cervicobrachial pain but without evidence of impaired conduction in the nerve root.[63] The authors found that a combination of this technique with cervical diskography made cervical fusion a rational treatment for segmental instability in the absence of evidence for compression of the root.

The technique for insertion of the needle into the lumbar, first sacral, and cervical nerve root sheaths is well described in the literature.[61,62,79,82] When the needle touches the nerve root, the patient experiences a sudden sharp radiating pain. At this point the patient is asked whether this pain is similar to his or her usual symptoms. Contrast medium is then injected and should be seen to flow proximally and distally, confirming that the needle tip is inside the nerve root sheath. Macnab and others do not feel that the radiculographic findings are usually helpful in localizing the lesion, but Tajima and colleagues feel that it frequently is helpful.[82] Local anesthetic is then injected. If the symptomatic root is blocked, the patient will experience relief of symptoms. The patient is examined and an effort is made by the physician and patient to reproduce earlier positive findings (for example, pain with walking in the case of pseudoclaudication). Some patients will experience a temporary neurologic deficit consisting of numbness or even motor deficit. The pain-free state wears off over a period of time, depending on the volume, concentration, and type of anesthetic used. This temporal relationship can be helpful in assessing the reliability of some of the more difficult patients' subjective responses.

The only complication of selective nerve root sheath injections reported is aggravation of symptoms for 1 to 2 days.[82]

REFERENCES

Bone Biopsy and Sinography

1. Ackerman, W.: Application of the trephine for bone biopsy. JAMA 184:11, 1965.
2. Ackerman, W.: Vertebral trephine biopsy. Am. J. Surg. 143:573, 1956.
3. Adapon, B. D., Logada, B. D., Lim, E. V. A., et al.: CT-guided biopsy of the spine. J. Comput. Assist. Tomogr. 5:73, 1981.
4. Adler, O., and Rosenberger, A.: Fine needle aspiration of osteolytic metastatic lesions. A. J. R. 133:15, 1979.
5. Armstrong, P., Chalmers, A. H., Green, G., et al.: Needle biopsy of the spine in suspected disk space syndrome. Br. J. Radiol. 51:333, 1978.
6. Ayala, A. G., and Zornesa, J.: Primary bone tumors: Percutaneous needle biopsy. Radiology 149:675, 1983.
7. Berkman, W. A., Chowdhury, L., Brown, N. L., et al.: Value of electron microscopy in cytologic diagnosis of fine needle biopsy. A. J. R. 140:1253, 1983.
8. Cohen, M. A., Cornoya, J., and Finkelstein, J. B.: Percutaneous needle biopsy of long-bone lesions facilitated by use of a hand drill. Radiology 139:750, 1981.
9. Coley, B. L., Sharp, G. S., and Ellis, E. B.: Diagnosis of bone tumors by aspiration. Am. J. Surg. 13:215, 1931.
10. Collins, J. D., Bassett, L., Main, G. D., et al.: Percutaneous biopsy following positive bone scan. Radiology 132:439, 1979.
11. Craig, F. S.: Vertebral body biopsy. J. Bone Joint Surg. 38A:93, 1956.
12. Cramer, L. E., Kahn, C., and Stan, A. H.: Needle biopsy of bone. Surg. Gynecol. Obstet. 118:1253, 1964.
13. Debnam, J. W., and Staple, T. W.: Needle biopsy of bone. Radiol. Clin. North Am. 13:157, 1975.
14. Debnam, J. W., and Staple, T. W.: Trephine bone biopsy by radiologists. Radiology 116:607, 1975.
15. Deeley, T. J.: The drill biopsy of bone lesions. Clin. Radiol. 23:536, 1972.
16. DeSantos, L. A., and Edeiken, B. S.: Intralesional injection of contrast media for percutaneous needle biopsy of bone. Radiology 143:789, 1982.
17. DeSantos, L. A., Lukeman, J. M., Wallace, S., et al.: Percutaneous needle biopsy of bone in the cancer patient. A. J. R. 130:641, 1978.
18. DeSantos, L. A., Murry, J. A., and Ayala, A. G.: The value of percutaneous needle biopsy in management of primary bone tumors. Cancer 43:735, 1979.
19. Edieken, B., and DeSantos, L. A.: Percutaneous needle biopsy of the irradiated skeleton. Radiology 146:653, 1983.
20. El-Koury, G. Y., Terepka, R. H., Mickelson, M. R., et al.: Fine-needle aspiration biopsy of bone. J. Bone Joint Surg. 65A:522, 1983.
21. Ellis, L. D., Jensen, W. N., and Westerman, M. P.: Needle biopsy of bone and marrow. Arch. Intern. Med. 114:213, 1964.
22. Gilsany, V., and Grunebaum, M.: Radiographic appearance of iliac marrow biopsy sites. A. J. R. 128:597, 1977.
23. Gilula, L. A., Destouset, J. M., and Murphy, W. A.: Valuable use for the "worm" of the Craig skeletal biopsy set. Radiology 142:787, 1982.
24. Griffiths, H. J.: Interventional radiology: The musculoskeletal system. Radiol. Clin. North Am. 17:475, 1979.
25. Hardy, D. C., Murphy, W. A., and Kula, G.: CT in planning percutaneous bone biopsies. Radiology 134:447, 1980.
26. Hewes, R. C., Vigorita, V. J., and Freiberger, R. H.: Percutaneous bone biopsy: The importance of aspirated osseous blood. Radiology 148:69, 1983.
27. Johnson, K. A., Kelly, P. J., and Jowsey, J.: Percutaneous biopsy of the iliac crest. Clin. Orthop. 123:34, 1977.
28. Lallie, A. F.: Roentgen-guided aspiration of skeletal lesions. J. Can. Assoc. Radiol. 21:71, 1970.
29. Legge, D., Ennes, J. T., and Dempsey, J.: Percutaneous biopsy of solitary lesions of bone. Clin. Radiol. 29:497, 1975.
30. Mankin, H. J., Lange, T. A., and Spancer, S. S.: Hazards of biopsy on patients with malignant primary bone and soft tissue tumors. J. Bone Joint Surg. 64A:1221, 1982.
31. McCulloch, J. A., and Waddell, G.: Lateral lumbar discography. Br. J. Radiol. 51:498, 1978.
32. Meyers, M. H., Patzakis, M. J., Terry, R., et al.: Closed biopsy of musculoskeletal lesions. J. Bone Joint Surg. 61A:375, 1979.
33. Murphy, W. A.: Exostosis after iliac bone marrow biopsy. A. J. R. 129:1114, 1977.
34. Murphy, W. A., Destouset, J. M., and Gilula, L. A.: Percu-

taneous skeletal biopsy 1981: A procedure for radiologists—results, reviews and recommendations. Radiology *139*:545, 1981.

35. Nordenstrom, B.: Percutaneous biopsy of vertebrae and ribs. Acta Radiol. Scand. *11*:113, 1971.

36. O'Holeughi, C. E.: Aspiration biopsy of the spine. J. Bone Joint Surg. *51A*:1531, 1969.

37. Resnick, D., and Niwayama, G.: Diagnosis of Bone and Joint Disorders. Philadelphia, W. B. Saunders, 1981.

38. Robertson, R. C., and Ball, R. K.: Destructive spine lesions: Diagnosis by needle biopsy. J. Bone Joint Surg. *17*:749, 1935.

39. Schajowicz, F., and Hokama, J.: Aspiration biopsy in bone lesions. Cancer *54*:139, 1976.

40. Simon, M. A.: Biopsy of musculoskeletal tumors. J. Bone Joint Surg. *64A*:1253, 1982.

41. Tehranzadeh, J., Freiberger, R. H., and Ghelman, B.: Closed skeletal needle biopsy: A review of 120 cases. A. J. R. *140*:113, 1983.

42. Tenopus, J., and Silverman, I.: Importance of biopsy in tumor diagnosis. Radiology *36*:56, 1931.

43. Valls, J. D., Holenghirce, and Schajowicz, F.: Aspiration biopsy in diagnosis of lesions of vertebral bodies. JAMA *136*:376, 1948.

44. Van Schreeb, T., Arner, A., Skodsted, G., et al.: Renal adenocarcinoma: Is there risk of spreading tumor cells on diagnostic puncture? Scand. J. Urol. Nephrol. *1*:270, 1967.

Diagnostic and Therapeutic Injections

45. Bradgley, C. E.: The articular facets in relation to low back pain and sciatic radiation. J. Bone Joint Surg. *23*:481, 1941.

46. Carrera, G. F.: Lumbar facet arthrography and injection in low back pain. Wis. Med. J. *78*:35, 1979.

47. Carrera, G. F.: Lumbar facet joint injection in low back pain and sciatica. Radiology *137*:665, 1980.

48. Carrera, G. F., Williams, A. L., and Haughton, V. M.: Computed tomography in sciatica. Radiology *137*:433, 1980.

49. Cloward, R. B.: Cervical diskography. A. J. R. *79*:563, 1958.

50. Collis, J. S. Jr., and Gardner, W. J.: Lumbar discography. An analysis of 1000 cases. J. Neurosurg. *19*:452, 1962.

51. Destouset, J. M., Gilula, L. A., Murphy, W. A., et al.: Lumbar facet injection: Indication, technique, clinical correlation, and preliminary results. Radiology *145*:321, 1982.

52. Dory, M. A.: Arthrography of the cervical facet joints. Radiology *148*:379, 1983.

53. Dory, M. A.: Arthrography of the lumbar facet joints. Radiology *140*:23, 1981.

54. Gehweeler, J. A., and Daffner, R. H.: Low back pain: The controversy of radiologic examination. A. J. R. *140*:109, 1983.

55. Ghormley, R. K.: Low back pain with special reference to the articular facets with presentation of an operative procedure. JAMA *101*:1773, 1933.

56. Hendrix, R. W., Lin, P. P., and Kane, W.: Simplified operation and injection technique for the sacroiliac joint. J. Bone Joint Surg. *64A*:1249, 1982.

57. Hermanus, N., de Becher, D., Baleriaux, D., et al.: The use of CT scanning for the study of the posterior lumbar intervertebral articulations. Neuroradiology *24*:159, 1983.

58. Hirsch, C.: An attempt to diagnose the level of the disk lesion clinically by disc puncture. Acta Orthop. Scand. *18*:132, 1948.

59. Holt, E. F. Jr.: Fallacy of cervical discography. JAMA *188*:799, 1964.

60. Holt, E. F. Jr.: The question of lumbar discography. J. Bone Joint Surg. *50A*:720, 1968.

61. Hoppenstein, R.: A new approach to the failed back syndrome. Spine *5*:371, 1980.

62. Kemper, J. F., and Smith, B. S.: Nerve-root injection. J. Bone Joint Surg. *56A*:1435, 1974.

63. Kikuchi, S., Macnab, I., and Moreau, P.: Localization of the level of symptomatic cervical disc degeneration. J. Bone Joint Surg. *63B*:272, 1981.

64. Kostuik, J. P.: Decision-making in adult scoliosis. Spine *4*:521, 1979.

65. Kostuik, J. P.: Recent advances in treatment of painful adult scoliosis. Clin. Orthop. *147*:238, 1980.

66. Laun, A., Lorenz, R., and Angoli, A. L.: Complications of cervical discography. J. Neurosurg. Sci. *25*:17, 1981.

67. Lundbloom, K.: Diagnostic puncture of intervertebral disks in sciatica. Acta Orthop. Scand. *17*:231, 1948.

68. Macnab, I.: Cervical spondylosis. Clin. Orthop. *109*:69, 1975.

69. Macnab, I.: Negative disk exploration. J. Bone Joint Surg. *53A*:891, 1971.

70. Maldaque, D. A., Mathuren, P., and Malghems, J.: Facet joint arthrography in lumbar spondylolysis. Radiology *140*:29, 1981.

71. McCulloch, J. A., and Waddell, G.: Lateral lumbar discography. Br. J. Radiol. *51*:498, 1978.

72. Milette, P. C., and Melanson, D.: A reappraisal of lumbar discography. J. Can. Assoc. Radiol. *33*:176, 1982.

73. Mooney, J., and Robertson, J.: The facet syndrome. Clin. Orthop. *115*:149, 1976.

74. Oppenheimer, A.: Disease of the apophyseal articulators. J. Bone Joint Surg. *20*:285, 1938.

75. Patrick, B. S.: Lumbar discography: A 5-year study. Surg. Neurol. *1*:267, 1973.

76. Pedersen, H. E., Blunck, C. F. J., and Gardner, E.: The anatomy of the lumbosacral posterior rami and meningeal branches of the spinal nerves. J. Bone Joint Surg. *38A*:377, 1956.

77. Quinnell, R. C., and Stockdale, H. R.: The significance of osteophytes on lumbar vertebral bodies in relation to discographic findings. Clin. Radiol. *33*:197, 1982.

78. Rothman, R. H., and Simeone, F. A.: Lumbar disk disease. *In* Rothman, R. H., and Simeone, F. A. (eds.): The Spine. Philadelphia, W. B. Saunders, 1982.

79. Schultz, H., Lougheed, W. M., Wortzman, G., et al.: Intervertebral nerve-root in the investigation of chronic lumbar disc disease. Can. J. Surg. *16*:217, 1973.

80. Shealy, C. N.: Facet denervation in the management of back and sciatic pain. Clin. Orthop. *115*:159, 1976.

81. Simmons, E. H., and Segil, C. M.: An evaluation of discography in the localization of symptomatic levels in discogenic disease of the spine. Clin. Orthop. *108*:57, 1975.

82. Tajima, T., Furukawa, K., and Kuromochi, E.: Selective lumbosacral radiculopathy and block. Spine *5*:68, 1980.

83. Wilkinson, H. A.: The failed back syndrome: Etiology and Therapy. New York, Harper and Row, 1983.

84. Yamano, Y.: Disk herniation of cervical spine. Arch. Orthop. Trauma Surg. *96*:271, 1980.

Index

Page numbers in *italics* refer to illustrations. Page numbers followed by (t) refer to tables.

Abdomen, radiographic technique chart on, *4–5*
Absorptiometry, dual photon, *23–24, 23–25*
  single photon, 22, *22–23*
Acetabular fracture, 210–214, *210–215*, 210t
  classification of, 210–211, 210t
  complex, 212–214, *214–215*
    CT in, 214, *215*
    vertical cleft fracture in, 214, *215*
  elementary, *210–214*, 211–212
    anterior column fracture in, 212, *214*
    CT in, *210*, 211
    femur position in, 211, *211*
    posterior column fracture in, 211–212, *212*
    transverse fracture in, 212, *213*
Acetabular labral tears, hip arthrography in, 257, *260*
Acetabulum, anatomy of, 184
  fracture of. See *Acetabular fracture.*
Acromegaly, bone mineral quantitation in, 27, *27*
Acromioclavicular joint, anatomy of, 503
  arthrography for, 541–542
  dislocation of, 549, *549–550*, 549t
  routine radiography of, 510–513, *511–512*
Adhesive capsulitis, shoulder arthrography in, 532–533, *532–533*, 532t
Alar ligament, 100–102, *101–102*
ALRI test, in ligamentous injuries of knee, 338t
Angiography, 34–36
  equipment in, 34–35
  indications for, 35–36
  technique in, 35, *36*
Ankle, 407–452
  arthrography of, 418–425, 418t, *419–424*. See also *Ankle arthrography.*
  arthroplasty of, *491–493*, 491–494. See also *Ankle arthroplasty.*
  fracture of, 427–443. See also *Ankle fracture.*
  gross anatomy of, 407–408, *407–409*
  ligamentous injury of, *443–451*, 443–452. See also *Ankle ligamentous injury.*
  routine radiography for, 408–415, *409–413*
    AP view in, 408, *409*
    lateral view in, 408–410, *410–411*
    mortise view in, 410–411, *411*
    oblique views in, 411, *412*
    stress views in, 411–415, *412–413*
Ankle arthrography, 418–425, 418t, *419–424*
  abnormal, *420–424*, 420–425
  anterior talofibular ligament tear in, 420, *420–421*
  in calcaneofibular ligament injury, *421*, 421–422
  in medial ligament injury, 422, *422–423*
  in persistent pain, 423, *424*
  indications for, 418t
  ligaments in, 420

Ankle arthrography (*Continued*)
  normal anatomy in, 419–420, *419–420*
  technique in, 418–419, 418t, *419*
  tomography with, *423*, 424
Ankle arthroplasty, *491–493*, 491–494
  complications of, *491–493*, 492
  indications for, 494
  results of, 491–492
  types of, 491, *491*
Ankle fracture, 427–443
  bimalleolar, *436–437*, 438–439
  classification systems for, *428*, 429–435, 429t, *430–435*
  comminuted, *440*, 442
  complications of, 442–443, *442–443*
  fibular fracture in, 428, *428*
  Lauge-Hansen classification for, 429, 429t, *430–432*
  medial malleolar, 428, *428*
  pathologic anatomy in, *427–428*, 427–429
  preferred classification for, 434–435
  prognosis in, 435–437
  single malleolar, displaced, *435*, 438
    undisplaced, *434–435*, 437–438
  sites of disruption in, *427, 428*
  syndesmosis measurement in, 428, *428*
  tibial plafond, *440–441*, 441–442
  treatment in, 434–443, 437–443
  trimalleolar, *438–439*, 440–441
  Weber classification for, 433–435, *434*
Ankle ligamentous injury, 443–451, *443–452*
  anatomy in, *443–444*, 444–445
  classification and pathologic anatomy in, 446–448, *446–449*
  complications in, *451*, 451–452
  function and, 445
  mechanism of injury in, *445*, 445–446
  routine radiography in, 448–450, *449–450*
  treatment in, 450–451
Annulus fibrosus, 98–99
Anterior drawer sign, ligamentous injuries of knee and, 332, *333*
Apical ligament, 100, *101–102*
Arachnoid, 104
Artery of Adamkiewicz, *102*, 103
Arthritis, hip arthrography in, *256*, 256–257
Arthrography, 40–45. See also individual joints.
  complications in, 43
  contrast material in, 43
  equipment in, 41–43, *42*
  joints commonly studied in, 41t
  subtraction technique in, 43–45, *44*, 44t–45t
Articular evaluation, imaging techniques in, 45t
Atlanto-occipital dislocation, *127*, 127–128

Atlantoaxial dislocation, 129–131, *129–132*
Atlantoaxial region, ligamentous anatomy of, 100–102, *101*
Atlas, anatomy of, 94, *95*
    fracture of, 128–129, *128–129*, 128t
        management of, 148
Avulsion fracture, 54, *54*
Axis fracture, 132–137
    associated injuries in, 137, *137*
    classification of, 133, *133*
    management of, 149–150, *149–150*
    os odontoideum in, 136, *136*
    retropharyngeal soft tissue swelling in, 133, *133*
    type I, 133, 133t, *134*
    type II, 133, *135*
    type III, 136

Barton's fracture, 674–677, *675–677*
Baseball finger, 720, *720*
Bennett's fracture, 694–695, *696*
Biceps tendon abnormalities, shoulder arthrography in, 533–534, *533–534*
Biopsy, bone, 767–776. See also *Bone biopsy.*
Bladder, 187, *188*
    in pelvic fracture, 225, *225*, 226t
Bone, biomechanics of, 64–65, 64t
    compression vs tension in, 64
    fracture and, 64–65
    nonisotopic nature in, 64
    viscoelasticity in, 64
    blood flow in, 60–61, 61t
    compression-plate fixation and, 70
    intramedullary nail fixation and, 72–74
    vascular supply of, *58–60*, 59–60
        afferent or arterial, *58–59*, 59
        anastomoses in, 60
        centrifugal flow in, 59–60, *60*
        efferent or venous, 59
        nutrient artery in, 60
Bone biopsy, 767–776
    complications in, 776
    indications for, 767, 767t
    locations for, 768, 768t
    needles and position in, *771*, 771–772
    of lower spine, 773–774, *773–774*
    of thoracic spine, 772–773, *772–773*
    of upper spine, 774
    percutaneous, 775t
    specimen preparation and evaluation in, 775–776
    technique in, 768–772, 768t, *769–771*
Bone graft, bone induction in, 68
Bone mass, normal, *25*, 25–26
Bone mineral quantitation, 20–28
    clinical relevance of, 20–21
    different methods in, 21t
    dual photon absorptiometry in, *23–24*, 23–25
    dynamics of mineral changes and, 21–22, 21t
    fracture threshold and, 26
    in hip fracture, 27
    in metabolic bone disease, 27, *27*
    in osteoporosis, 26, *26–27*
    normal bone mass and, *25*, 25–26
    single photon absorptiometry in, 22, *22–23*
Bone morphogenic protein, 68
Bone scan, 16–20, *17–20*
    in bone vascularity assessment, 19, *20*
    in infection, 19
    in trauma, 18–19, *18–20*
    in tumors, 17–18, *17–18*
    instrumentation in, 17
    radiopharmaceuticals in, 16–17
Boutonnière deformity, 719–720
Bowing fracture, 51–53, *52*

Brachial artery, 569, *569*
Brachialis, *582*, 582–583
Brodie's abscess, 735–737, *736–737*

Calcaneal fracture, 470–481
    articular, 475–481
        classification of, 475–476, *475–476*
        complications of, *480*, 480–481
        results of, 476t, 480
        treatment of, 476–480, 476t, *477–479*
    beak, 474–475, *475*
    classification of, 470–472, 471t, *472*
    mechanism of injury in, 472
    of anterior process, 473–474, *473–474*
    of sustentaculum tali, 472–473
    of tuberosity, 472
    radiographic evaluation in, 472
    stress fracture of, 757–758, *758*
    treatment of, 472–481
Calcaneofibular ligament injury, ankle arthrography in, *421*, 421–422
Calcaneus, anatomy of, 470, *470–471*
    fracture of, 470–481. See also *Calcaneal fracture.*
Capitate fracture, 688, *689–690*
Capitellar fracture, 604–606, *605*
Capitotriquetral ligament, 647, *647*
Carpal height, 645, *645*
Carpal ulnar distance, 643, *643*
Carpe bosseau, 719, *719*
Carpometacarpal joint, anatomy of, 645
    dislocation of, 692–693, *693*
Carpus, anatomy of, 642–645, *642–645*
    dislocation of, 690–693, *691–693*
    dorsal intercalated segment instability pattern of, 644, *644*
    first anatomic group in, 642–644, *642–644*
    fractures of, 680–690, *682–690*. See also individual bones.
    ossification of, 646
    second anatomic component of, 644–645, *644–645*
    third anatomic component of, 645
    volar intercalated segment instability pattern of, 644, *644–645*
Cervical pillar fracture, 140, 140t, *141–142*
Cervical spine, articular facets in, 94
    radiographic technique chart on, *4*
    radiography in trauma to, 104–115
        AP view in, 108–109, *111*
        C7 vs T1 in, *104*, 105
        disk space evaluation in, 107, *108*
        flexion and extension views in, *114*, 114–115
        interspinous distance widening in, 108, *108*
        lateral view in, *104–110*, 105–108, 105t
        normal anatomic relationships in, *105*, 106
        normal cervical lines in, 106–108, *107*
        normal lordotic curve in, 106–108, *107*
        oblique view in, 109, *112*
        odontoid view in, 109, *110–111*
        pillar view in, 109, *113*, 114
        prevertebral fat stripe in, 106, *107*
        soft tissues in, 106, *106*
        swimmer's views in, 108, *110*
    spinous processes of, 92
    transverse processes of, 92
    trauma to, 121–155. See also *Cervical spine trauma.*
    upper, ligamentous anatomy of, 100–102, *101*
Cervical spine trauma, 121–155
    associated injuries in, 147–148, 147t
    fractures and dislocations in, 127–148
        atlantoaxial region, 129–131, *129–132*
        atlanto-occipital region, 127, *127–128*
        atlas, 128–129, *128–129*
        axis, 132–137, *133–137*

Cervical spine trauma (*Continued*)
  fractures and dislocations in, management of, *152–153*, 152–154
    vertebral arch, 138–140, *138–142*
    vertebral body, 140–144, *143–144*
  management of, 148–155
    atlas and axis injury in, 148–150, *148–150*
    dislocation and fracture-dislocation in, *152–153*, 152–154
    extension injury in, 154–155
    lower cervical spine injury, 150–155, *151–154*
    sprains in, 150–152, *151*
    vertebral body fractures in, *154*, 155
  mechanism of injury in, 121–127
    classification of, 121, 121t
    compressive hyperflexion as, 123, *123–124*
    compressive shearing force as, 123
    disruptive hyperflexion as, 122, *122*
    flexion teardrop injury as, 123, *124*
    flexion-rotation as, 122, *122–123*
    hyperextension as, 124–125, *125–126*
    hyperflexion as, 121–124, *122–124*
    lateral radiography for, 123–124, *124*
    ventral compression as, 125, *126*
  subluxation and fracture dislocation in, 144–147, *145–147*
    anterior ligament injury in, 147
    bilateral locking of facets in, 144–147, *147*
    flexion teardrop type, 147
    posterior ligament injury in, 144, *145–146*
    unilateral locking or perching of facets in, 144, *146*
Cervical vertebra, anatomy of, 91–92, *93*
  C2, 94, *96*
  C3 through C6, 94, *97*
  C7, 94, *97*
Cervical vertebral arch fracture, 138–140, *138–142*, 138t
Cervical vertebral body fractures, 140–144, *143–144*, 143t. See also *Vertebral body fractures, cervical.*
Chauffeur's fracture, *677*, 677–678
Chest, radiographic technique chart on, *5*
Chondromalacia, knee arthrography in, 355–356
  shoulder arthrography in, *536*, 537
Chondromalacia patellae, 315
Chopart's joint dislocation, *468–469*, 469–470
Clavicle, anatomy of, *499*, 499–500
  fracture of, 551–552, *551–554*
  routine radiography of, *512–513*, 513
Coccyx, anatomy of, 183
  fracture and fracture-dislocation of, 206
Collateral ligaments, arthrography for, *344*, 345, *346*, 354
Colles' fracture, 668–673, *668–673*
  classification of, 669t
  complications of, *672–673*, 673
  mechanism of injury in, 669
  treatment of, 669–673, *671–672*
Compartment syndrome, in tibial fracture, 404
Compression-plate fixation, 68–72
  adverse effects of, 71–72, *71–72*
  biomechanics of, 70–71
  bone blood flow and, 70
  bone porosity in, 71, *71*
  bone refracture after, 72
  Eggers plate in, 68–69
  external fixation vs, 78–80
  historical, 68–69
  intramedullary nail fixation vs, 75–78, *77–78*
  mechanism of action in, 69
  morphologic findings of primary bone healing in, 69–70
  plate types in, *68*
  stiff vs flexible, 71

Computed tomography, 28–31
  equipment in, 28–29, *28–29*
  in spinal trauma, 118, *120*
  indications for, *30*, 31
  techniques in, *29*, 29–30
Conus medullaris, 104
Cruciate ligament, *297–298*, 297–299
  arthrographic anatomy of, 345, *348*
  injury to, anterior, 331–332
    arthrography for, 353, *354*
    posterior, 339–340
Cuboid fracture, 484, *484*
Cuneiform fracture, 484, *484*

Diagnostic and therapeutic injections, 777–787
  diskography in, 783–786
  facet joint injections in, 779–783
  nerve root infiltration in, 786–787
Diagnostic techniques, 1–50. See also individual techniques.
  angiography, 34–36
  arthrography, 40–45
  bone mineral quantitation, 20–28
  magnetic resonance imaging, 31–34
  myelography, 36–40
  radiography, magnification, 10–11
    routine, 1–6
  skeletal scintigraphy, 16–20
  tomography, 6–9
    computed, 28–31
  ultrasound, 14–16
  xeroradiography, 11–14
Disk space infection, imaging in, *749*
Diskography, 783–786
  complications in, 786
  indications in, 783–785, *784–785*
  technique and interpretation in, 785–786
Dislocation, radiographic description of, 56–57, *57.* See also individual types.
Dual photon absorptiometry, 23–24, *23–25*
Dura, spinal, 103

Elbow, 579–629
  anatomy of, *579–582*, 579–583
    muscle groups in, 581–582, *582*
    neurovascular structures in, *582*, 582–583
  arthrography for, 587–594, *588–594*
    abnormal, *591–594*, 593–594
    indications for, 588, 588t
    normal, *590*, 593
    technique in, *588–589*, 588–593, 588t
  arthroplasty for, 623–625, *623–626*
    complications in, 625, *625–626*
    coupled hinge total, 624–625, *624–626*
    results of, 625
    resurfacing prosthesis for, 623–624, *623–624*
  carrying angle of, 579, *580*
  humeral fracture of, 599–611. See also *Humeral fracture.*
  ligament injury in, 595, *595–598*, 598
  reconstructive surgery for, 621–625, *622–626*
    arthrodesis in, 622, *622*
    interpositional arthroplasty in, 621–622, *622*
    radial head resection and synovectomy in, 621, *622*
  routine radiography in, 583–587, *583–587*
    AP view, *583*, 583
    assessment of, *586–587*, 587
    axial view, *586*, 587
    lateral view, 583, *584*
    oblique view, 583–584, *585*
    radial head view, 584, *585*, 587

Elbow (*Continued*)
soft tissue injury in, 594–595
tendon injury in, *598, 598–599*
trauma to, 594–599, *595–598*
External fixation, 78–80, *79*
compression-plate fixation vs, 78–80
imaging techniques in, 45t
phases of fracture healing in, 78
External rotation recurvatum test, 339
Extremity, radiographic technique chart on, *5*

Facet joint injection, 779–783, *780–783*
anatomy in, 779, *780–781*
indications for, 781, *781*
results in, 782–783, 782t, *783*
technique in, *780*, 781–782
Facet syndrome, 778
Femoral artery, common, 185, *187*
superficial and deep, 185, *187*
Femoral condyle, osteochondral fracture of, *319*, 319–320
supracondylar fracture of, 322–325, *323–324*
classification of, 323, *323*
internal fixation in, 325
treatment of, 323–325, *324*
Femoral neck fracture, 234–247
classification of, 235, *235*, 235t
complications of, 244–247, *245–246*, 245t
avascular necrosis as, 244–247, *245–246*, 245t
non-union of, 247
radiographic evaluation of, 235–236, *236–238*
treatment of, 236–244
endoprosthesis in, 244, *244–245*
impacted fracture of, 237–239, *239–240*
internal pin fixation in, 241–243, *243–244*
total hip arthroplasty in, 243
unstable fracture of, 239, *243*
Femoral shaft fracture, 281–291
classification and mechanism of injury in, 282–283
ipsilateral hip injury in, 291, *291*
radiographic technique in, 283, *284*
treatment in, 283–291
bone grafts as, 290, *290*
cast brace as, 285, *286*
complications of, 290–291, *291*
Ender nail in, 287, *287*
internal fixation as, 285–290, *286–290*
Küntscher intramedullary nail in, *286–287*, 287
plate fixation in, *289*, 290
traction and casting as, 284–285, *285–286*
wire fixation in, *288*, 289
Femur, anatomy of, 281–282, *281–282*
ipsilateral fracture of tibia and, 330–331
radiographic technique chart on, *5*
stress fracture in, *761–762, 762–763*
Fibula, anatomy of, 393–395, *393–395*
arterial supply of, 394–395, *395*
muscles of, 394, *394*
nerve supply of, 395
stress fracture in, 762
Fibular fracture, 395–405. See also *Tibial fracture.*
Filum terminale, 104
Finger. See *Phalanx.*
Flexion-rotation drawer sign, 338t
Floating knee, 330
Foot, routine radiography for, *413–418*, 415–418
AP view in, *413–414*, 415
axial calcaneal view in, *416*, 416–417
lateral view in, 415–416, *416*
oblique view in, 415, *415*
sesamoid view in, 417–418, *418*
subtalar view in, 417, *417*
stress fracture in, *757–758, 757–759*

Foramen transversarium, 92, *93*
Forearm, anatomy of, 631, *632–633*
Forefoot injury, *481–490*, 481–491. See also individual types.
Fracture, avulsion, 54, *54*
biomechanics of, 64–65
complete, 53–54, *54–55*
compression, 54, *54*
depressed, 54, *54*
greenstick, 51, *52*
growth plate or physeal, 53, *53*
incomplete, 51–53, *52–53*
insufficiency, 54
intracapsular, 51, *52*
microfracture or bowing, 51–53, *52*
pathologic, 54, *55*
radiographic description of, 54–57, 55t
division of shaft into thirds, 54–55, 55f
fragment distraction and angulation in, 55–56, *56*
fragment rotation in, 56, *56*
impaction in, 55, *56*
stress, 54, *55*
subtle, 51, *51*
torus, 51, *52*
types of, 51–54, *51–55*
Fracture fixation, 68–80. See also individual types.
compression plate fixation, 68–72
external fixation, 78–80
intramedullary nail, 72–75
Fracture healing, 51–90
biologic signal for, 66–68, *67*
bone-inductive, 67–68
electrical, 66–67, *67*
biomechanics of, 64–68
breaking strength in, 65, *65*
callus area in, 66
compression-plate fixation and, 68–72
external fixation and, 78–80
intramedullary nail fixation and, 72–78
phases of, 57–59, *58*
physiology of, *61*, 61–64
blood flow in, 61, *61*
cellular response in, 63–64, 63t
efferent sources of blood supply in, 61–62
endosteal vs periosteal callus in, 63
medullary vs periosteal blood supply in, 62
oxidative metabolism in, 63
oxygen tension in, 62–63
periosteal vs endosteal blood supply in, 62
vascular dilatation in, 62
vascular response in, *61*, 61–63
union and non-union in, 80–86
White's biomechanical stages of, 66, *66*
Fracture non-union, 80–86
avascular, 83, *84*
definition of, 80–81
diagnosis and classification of, 82–83, *82–84*
electrical stimulation in, 86, *86*
etiologic factors in pathogenesis of, 81–82, 81t
hypervascular, 83, *83*
radiographic findings in, 82, *82*
scintigraphy in, 82, *83*
tomographic findings in, 82, *82*
treatment modalities in, 83–86, *83–86*
Fracture threshold, 26
Fracture union, 80–81, *81*

Galeazzi fracture, *638*, 639, *639*, *678–679*, 678–680
Gallium-67 citrate, 16
Gastrointestinal anatomy, 187–189, *188*
Genitourinary anatomy, 187–189, *188*
Genitourinary system, in pelvic fracture, 223–226, *224–225*, 226t

Glenohumeral dislocation, *544–548, 544–549*
  anterior, *544–546, 545–546*
  complications of, 548–549
  posterior, 546–547, *547*
  superior and inferior, 547–548, *548*
Glenohumeral joint, anatomy of, *502, 502–503*
Gluteal artery, superior, 186, *187*
Greenstick fracture, 51, *52*
Growth plate fracture, 53, *53*

Hamate, fracture of, 687–688, *688–689*
Hamulus, fracture of, 687–688, *688–689*
Hand, 641–730
  anatomy of, 641–648, *641–648*. See also individual
    parts.
  arthrography of, 666–667, *667–668*
  chronic post-traumatic conditions of, 713–721
  degenerative arthritis in, 720–721, *721*
  post-traumatic reconstruction of, 721–725, *721–727*
    arthrodesis in, 722, *722–723*
    arthroplasty in, 723–725, *723–727*
    osteotomy in, 721–722, *721–722*
    soft tissue stabilization in, 723
  routine radiographic techniques for, 648–655, *649–
    655*
    Brewerton view in, 651, *654*
    Burman view in, 651, *654*
    lateral view in, 650, *651*
    oblique view in, 648, *650*
    PA view in, 648, *649–650*
    stress view in, 651, 655, *655*
Hangman's fracture, 128, 128t, *136, 136–137*
  management of, 149–150, *149–150*
Hip, anatomy of, *185*
  arthrography of, 253–260. See also *Hip arthrography.*
  dislocation and fracture-dislocation of, 226–234. See
    also *Hip dislocation and fracture-dislocation.*
  fat planes of, 184, *186*
  genitourinary and gastrointestinal anatomy in, 187–
    189, *188*
  ligaments and articulations of, 183–184, 183t, *184–
    186*
  muscle insertions of, 184, *186*
  neuroanatomy of, 187, *187*
  periarticular anatomy of, 184, *186*
  routine radiography in, 196–197
    AP view in, *196*, 196–197, 197t
    Judet views in, 197, *198–200*
    lateral view in, 197, *201*
    oblique view in, 197, *202*
  vascular anatomy of, 185–187, *186*
Hip arthrography, 253–260
  for removal of loose bodies, 257, *257–259*
  in acetabular labral tears, 257, *260*
  in arthritis, 256, *256–257*
  in enlarged iliopsoas bursa, 260, *260*
  indications for, 253, 254t
  technique in, 253–255, *255*
  with normal anatomy, 255–256, *256*
Hip dislocation and fracture-dislocation, 226–234
  classification of, 227–230, 227t, *228–230*, 229t
    anterior, 230, *230–231*
    Pipkin, 229–230, 229t, *230*
    posterior, 227–230, 227t, *228–230*, 229t
  complications of, 234, 234t
  radiographic evaluation of, 230–233, *231–232*, 232t
    AP view in, *227–232, 231–232*
    oblique view in, 232, 232t
  treatment of, *233*, 233–234
Hip fracture, bone mineral quantitation in, 27
Hip joint replacement, 260–274
  accuracy of radiographic techniques in, 274, 274t
  anteversion or retroversion of femoral components
    in, *262–263*, 263, 263t

Hip joint replacement (*Continued*)
  cement evaluation in, *262*, 262–263
  complications of, 261, 261t
  painful, diagnostic approach to, 274, 274t
  plain film evaluation in, 263–266, *264–267*, 264t
    component loosening and, 264–265, *264–266*, 264t
    infection and joint-related symptoms and, 265–
      266, *266–267*
  radionuclide scan in, 270–274, *272–273*
    component loosening and, 271, *272*
    infection and, 271, *273*
  routine radiography in, 261–263, *262–263*, 263t
  subtraction arthrography in, 267–270, *268–272*
    component loosening and, 268–271, *269–270*
    infection and joint related symptoms and, 270,
      272
    resurfacing arthroplasty and, 270, *270–271*
    technique in, 267–268, *268*
Humeral fracture, 599–611
  capitellar, 604–606, *605*
  condylar, 606–607, *606–607*, 611
  epicondylar, *600–601*, 601–602
  proximal, *541–543*, 542–544, 542t
  supracondylar and transcondylar, *599–600, 599–601*
  T and Y condylar, 602–603, *602–605*
Humeral shaft fracture, 567–577
  anatomy in, 567–569, *567–569*
  management of, 573–576, *573–577*
    delayed, 575–576, *575–577*
    initial, 573–574, *573–575*
    internal fixation in, 574, *575*
  mechanism of injury and classification in, 569–571
  radiographic evaluation in, 570–572, *571–573*
Humerus, distal, anatomy of, 579, *579*
  proximal, *501*, 501–502
Hypercortisolism, bone mineral quantitation in, 27,
  27
Hyperparathyroidism, bone mineral quantitation in,
  27, *27*
Hyperthyroidism, bone mineral quantitation in,, 27,
  27
Hypoparathyroidism, bone mineral quantitation in,
  27, *27*

Ileofemoral ligament, 184, *185*
Iliac artery, common, 185, *187*
  internal and external, 185, *187*
Iliac spine, avulsion fracture of, 203, *204*
Iliofemoral ligaments, 184, *186*
Iliolumbar artery, 186, *187*
Iliolumbar ligaments, 183, *184*
Iliopsoas bursa, enlarged, hip arthrography in, 260,
  260
Iliopsoas fat plane, 184, *186*
Ilium, anatomy of, 181, *183*
Indium-111–labeled autologous white blood cells, 16–
  17
Innominate bone, 181, *183*
Insufficiency fracture, 54
Internal fixation device, imaging techniques for, 45t
Interphalangeal joint, ligaments of, 648
  dislocation of, *712–713, 713*
    dorsal proximal, *712–713, 713*
    volar proximal, 713
Intertransverse ligament, spinal, 99, *100*
Interventional orthopedic radiography, 767–788. See
  also individual techniques.
Intramedullary nail fixation, 72–75
  biomechanics of, 74–75
  bone blood flow and, 72–74
  compression-plate fixation vs, 75–78, *77–78*
  delayed union in, 73
  fluted nail in, 75
  historical data, 72

Intramedullary nail fixation (*Continued*)
 intramedullary reaming in, 73–74
 loose-fitting vs tight-fitting, 73
 morphologic findings in, 74
 nail types for, 72, *73*
 unfixed fractures vs, 75
Intraspinous ligament, 99, *100*
Iophendylate, 36
Ischiofemoral ligaments, 184, *186*
Ischium, anatomy of, 181–182, *183*

Jefferson fracture, 128–129, *128–129*
Jerk test, in ligamentous injuries of knee, 338t
Joint space infection, 741–744
 computed tomography and magnetic resonance imaging in, 744, *745*
 diagnostic approach in, *748–749*
 nuclear imaging in, 743–744
 routine radiography in, 741–743, *742*
Jones fracture, 485–486

Kienböck's disease, *715–716*, 715–717, 716t
Knee, 293–391
 anatomy of, 293–301
 arthrography of, 341–361. See also *Knee arthrography.*
 arthroplasty of, 367–383. See also *Knee arthroplasty.*
 arthroscopy of, 361–367. See also *Knee arthroscopy.*
 biomechanics of, 301–303, 367–370
 bone in, 293
 floating, 330
 fractures about, 319–331. See also individual fractures.
 ligamentous injuries of, 331–341
  anterior drawer sign in, 332, *333*
  arthrography in, 333
  avulsion fracture in, 333, *334*
  bracing in, 340, *341*
  classification of, 336
  combined instability in, 339–340
  diagnosis of, 332–333, 332t, *333–336*
  frequency of, 332t
  history and physical exam in, 332
  instability types in, 334–337
  lateral capsular avulsion sign in, 333, *335*
  natural history of, 331–332
  notch or impression defect in, 333, *335*
  primary repair in, 340–341
  rotatory instability in, 337–339, 338t
  straight or single-plane instability in, 337
  stress radiographs in, 333, *336*
  treatment of, 340–341, *341*
 ligamentous restraints of, 301t
 ligaments of, 295–299
  anterior, 299
  cruciate, *297–298*, 297–299
  lateral, 296–297, *296–297*
  medial, 295–296, *295–296*
 meniscus of, 293–294, *294*
 muscle of, 299–300, *300*
 osteochondral fracture of, *319*, 319–320
 patella of. See *Patella.*
 radiographic technique chart on, *5*
 radiography in, 303–309
  AP view in, 303, *303*
  lateral view in, 303–305, *304–305*
  notch view in, *306*, 306–307
  oblique view in, 305–306, *305–306*
  patellar view in, 307, *307*
  stress views in, 307–309, *308*
 restraints of, 293, 293t
 vascular supply of, 300–301

Knee arthrography, 341–361
 after knee arthroplasty, 359–361, *360*
 articular cartilage in, 345, *347*
 collateral ligaments in, *344*, 345, *346*
 cruciate ligament in, 345, *348*
 for articular abnormalities, *355*, 355–356
 for chondromalacia of patella, 355–356
 for degenerative meniscal lesions, 352–353, *353*
 for discoid menisci, 350–352, *351–352*
 for intra-articular loose bodies, 355–356
 for ligament abnormalities, 353–355, *354*
 for meniscal tears, 348–350, *349–350*
 for osteochondritis dissecans, 355
 for popliteal cysts, 356, *357*
 for synovial abnormalities, 356–357, *356–358*
 for synovial plicae, 357, *357*
 indications for, 341t
 joint capsule in, 345, *348*
 meniscal abnormalities in, 348–353, *349–353*
 meniscal anatomy in, 343–345, *344–346*
 meniscal tear in, 358, *359*
 normal anatomy in, 343–348, *344*
 patient position for meniscus in, 343, *343*
 pitfalls in, 357–359, *358–359*
 positioning errors in, 358, *358–359*
 stress lateral view in, 343, *344*
 technique in, 341t, 342–343, *342–344*
Knee arthroplasty, 367–383
 biomechanics in, 367–370
 cruciate ligament retention in, 368–369
 gait analysis in, 368
 knee arthrography after, 359–361, *360*
 lucent lines after, 379
 preoperative evaluation in, 379, *379–380*
 prosthetic choices in, *368–377*, 370–377
  biologic fixation in, 376–377, *376–377*
  constrained, 370, *371*
  moderately constrained, 370, *370–371*
  revision, 371, *372–374*
  rigid hinge, 376
  total condylar, 374, 376
  unconstrained, *368–369*, 370, 376
  unicompartmental, *375*, 376
  variable axis, *375*, 376
 prosthetic design in, 367–368
 prosthetic loosening in, 379
 radiographic studies in, 379–383, *380–383*
 technique in, 378–379, *378–380*
 tibial component loosening in, 369–370
Knee arthroscopy, 361–367
 accuracy of, 361, 361t
 for degenerative joint disease, 366–367, *367*
 for removal of loose bodies, 364–365, *364–365*
 for osteochondritis dissecans, 365–366, *365–366*
 for partial meniscectomy, 363
 for patellar disorders, 366–367, *367*
 for peripheral meniscal tears, 363–364, *364*
 for synovial disorders, 366, *366*
 improved visualization in, 361, *361–362*
 in acute knee injuries, 362, *362*
 in medial fibrous plica, 362, *363*
 in synovial plicae, 362–363
 indications for, 361
 routine preparation and equipment for, 361, *361*

Ligament of Wrisberg, 293
Ligamentum flavum, 99, *100*
Ligamentum nuchae, 99, *100*
Lisfranc fracture, *481–483*, 481–484
Lister's tubercle, 642, *642*
Longitudinal ligament, anterior spinal, 99, *100*
 posterior spinal, 99, *100*
Loose bodies, hip arthrography for removal of, 257, *257–259*

Losee test, in ligamentous injuries of knee, 338t
Lumbar spine, articular facets in, 94
  radiographic technique chart on, *4–5*
  radiography in trauma to, *115–117,* 116–118
  Scotty dog view of, *117,* 118
  spinous processes of, 92
  transverse process of, 92, *94*
  trauma to, 155–172. See also *Thoracolumbar trauma.*
  unfused ossification center of, 91, *92*
Lumbar vertebra, anatomy of, 91–92, *93,* 98, *98*
Lumbosacral plexus, 187, *187*
Lunate, avascular necrosis of, *715–716,* 715–717, 716t
  dislocation, anterior, 692, *692*
    dorsal, 692, *693*
  fracture of, *686,* 687
Lunatomalacia, *715–716,* 715–717, 716t
Lunotriquetral instability, 718–719

Madelung's deformity, 713–714, *714*
Magnetic resonance imaging, 31–34
  advantages and disadvantages of, 32t
  clinical applications of, *32–34,* 33–34, 33t
  equipment in, 33
  principles of, *31,* 31–33
Magnification radiography, 10–11, *10–11*
Malgaigne fracture, *208,* 209
Mallet deformity, 720, *720*
March fracture, 757, *757*
Median nerve, *568,* 569
Meniscal arthrography, 348–353, *349–353*
  anatomy in, 343–345, *344–346*
  for degenerative lesions, 352–353, *353*
  for discoid menisci, 350–352, *351–352*
  for meniscal tears, 348–350, *349–350*
Meniscus, 293–294, *294*
  in tibial condyle fracture, 326
Metabolic bone disease, bone mineral in, 27, *27*
Metacarpal anatomy, 645
Metacarpal fracture, 693–701
  complications of, 701
  of mobile rays (4th and 5th), 698–701, *699–701*
  of stable rays (2nd and 3rd), 696–698, *697–698*
  of thumb, 694–696, *694–696*
Metacarpal head, avascular necrosis of, 720, *720*
Metacarpophalangeal joint, ligaments of, 648, *648*
Metacarpophalangeal joint dislocation, 701–703, *702–703*
  dorsal, 702, *702–703*
  volar, 702, *703*
Metatarsal fracture, 485–486, *485–488,* 486t
  stress and, 757, *757*
Metatarsophalangeal arthrography, *424,* 425
Metrizamide, 36
Mineral, bone. See *Bone mineral.*
Monteggia fracture, 619–620, *619–621,* 637–639, *638*
  reverse, *638,* 639, *639*
Musculoskeletal infection, imaging in, 731–753. See also individual types.
Myelography, 36–40
  contrast agents in, 36–37
  indications for, 39–40, 39t, *40–41*
  normal anatomy in, *38–39,* 39
  positioning effects in, 37
  technique in, *37–38,* 37–39

Navicular fat stripe, 655, *656*
Navicular fracture, *466–469,* 466–470
  acute, *466–467,* 467
  Chopart's joint dislocation in, *468–469,* 469–470
  stress and, 468
Navicular stress fracture, 759

Nerve root infiltration, 786–787
Nucleus pulposus, 98–99

Obturator internus fat plane, 184, *186*
Obturator ring, double fracture of, *205*
Occipital condylar fracture, 127
Occipitocervical dislocation, 148
Odontoid fracture, 132–136, *133–136*
  management of, *148,* 148–149
Olecranon, articular cartilage of, 579, *581*
Olecranon fracture, 613–618
  classification of, *613,* 613–614
  complications of, 616–618, *617–618*
  compression screw in, 615, *615*
  displaced, 614–618, *615–618*
  fragment excision in, 616, *617*
  mechanism in, 613
  plate fixation in, 615–616, *616*
  radiographic evaluation of, 614, *614*
  tension band wiring in, 614, *615*
  treatment of, 614
Os odontoideum, 136, *136*
Osteochondritis dissecans, knee arthrography in, 355
  knee arthroscopy in, 365–366, *365–366*
Osteomyelitis, 731–741
  complications and sequelae in, 738, *738*
  computed tomography in, 739–740, *740*
  diagnostic approach in, 748
  etiology of, 731
  infection sites in, 737, *737*
  magnetic resonance imaging in, 740–741, *741*
  nuclear imaging in, 738–739, *739*
  routine radiography in, 732–737
    Brodie's abscess in, 735–737, *736–737*
    Garre's osteomyelitis in, *734,* 734–735
    in chronic disease, 735, *735*
    involucrum in, 734, *734*
    osseous involvement in, 732–733, *733*
    periosteal reaction in, 733, *733*
    sequestra in, 734, *734*
    soft tissue changes in, 732, *732*
Osteoporosis, bone mineral quantitation in, *26,* 26–27

Palmar capsular ligaments, 647, *647*
Patella, 293, 309–319
  anatomy of, 309–310, *309–310*
  apprehension test of, 311–312
  biomechanics of, *310,* 310–311
  chondromalacia of, 355–356
  disorders of, knee arthroscopy for, 366–367, *367*
  examination of, 311–315
  fracture of, 320–322, *320–323*
    classification of, 320, *320*
    internal fixation in, 321, *322*
    patellectomy in, 321–322, *322–323*
    treatment of, 320–322, *322–323*
  fragmentation of, 310, *310*
  instability of, 317–318
  osteochondral fracture of, *319,* 319–320
  Q-angle of, 311, *311*
  radiography of, *312–315,* 313–315
    axial, *312–314,* 313–314
    congruence angle in, 314, *314*
    Ficat view in, *312,* 313
    Jaroschy or Hughston view in, *312,* 313
    lateral patellar displacement and, 314, *315*
    lateral patellofemoral angle in, 314, *314*
    lateral view, 313
    Laurin view in, *312,* 313
    Merchant view in, *312,* 313
    patellofemoral index in, 314, *314*

Patella (*Continued*)
  radiography of, previous dislocation and, 315, *315*
    Settegast skyline view in, *312*, 313
    sulcus angle in, 313–314, *314*
  shapes of, 309–310, *309–310*
  stabilizers of, 309
  subluxation of, 317–318
  vascular supply of, 309
Patella alta, *312*, 313
Patellar-tendon-bearing cast, 398
Patellofemoral angle, lateral, 314, *314*
Patellofemoral index, 314, *314*
Patellofemoral ligament, 299
Patellofemoral pain syndrome, 315–317, *316*
  basal degeneration in, 316
  classification of, 316, *316*
  etiology of, 316, *316*
  radiologic evaluation in, 316–317
  treatment of, 317
Pathologic fracture, 54, *55*
Pelvic fracture, 202–226
  classification of, 203–214, 203t
    avulsion, 203, *204*
    class I, 203–206, *204–206*
    class II, 206–208, *207*
    class III, 208–209, *209–210*
    class IV, 210–214, *210–215*
    Connally-Hedberg, 203, 203t
    Key-Conwell, 203, 203t
    Tile-Pennal, 203, 203t
    Watson-Jones, 203, 203t
  complex, 202, 202t
  complications of, 220–226
    adjacent or distant fracture, 222–223, 223t
    delayed, 226, 226t
    genitourinary, 223–226, *224–225*, 226t
    head, chest, abdomen injury, 226
    in complex fractures, 221t
    neurologic, 223, *223*, 223t
    pelvic hemorrhage, 221–222, *222*
  computed tomography in, 30, *31*
  treatment of, 214–220
    class I, 214–216, *216*
    class II, 217–218
    class III, *216*, 218
    class IV, 217–221, *218–220*
  stress fracture, 216, *216*
Pelvic region, radiographic technique chart on, *5*
Pelvis, 181–279
  anatomy of, 181–189
  fracture of, 202–226. See also *Pelvic fracture.*
  ligaments and articulations of, 183–184, 183t, *184–186*
  neuroanatomy of, 187, *187*
  routine radiography in, 189–195
    anatomic landmarks in, 189, *189*
    AP angled view in, 192, *192–193*
    AP view in, *189–191*, 189–192
    lateral view in, 193, *193–195*
  skeletal anatomy of, 181–183, *183*
  stress fracture in, *763*, 763–764
  vascular anatomy of, 185–187, *187*
  weight–bearing forces of, 181, *182*
Pericapsular fat plane, of hip, 184, *186*
Perilunate dislocation, dorsal, 691–692, *691–692*
  volar, 692
Peritoneum, 187, *188*
Peroneal tenography, *425–426*, 425–427
  abnormal, *425–426*, 427
  normal anatomy in, *425*, 427
  technique in, 425–427
Phalangeal fracture, 486, *488–489*, 489, 704–713
  complications of, 713
  distal, 709–713

Phalangeal fracture (*Continued*)
  distal, proximal base, 710–713, *711*
    comminuted, 711–712
    dorsal lip, 710–711, *711*
    volar lip, 711, *711*
  transverse, 710, *710*
  tuft fracture, 709–710, *710*
  middle, 707–709, *707–709*
    comminuted, 709
    dorsal lip proximal base, 709, *709*
    volar lip proximal base, 707, *707–708*
  proximal, 704–707
    diaphyseal, 704–705, *705–706*
    distal, 704, *704*
    proximal, 705–707, *706*
Phalanx, anatomy of, 645–646, *646*
  fracture of, 704–713. See also *Phalangeal fracture.*
  routine radiographic techniques for, 650, *651–652*
  turret exostosis of, 719
Physeal fracture, 53, *53*
Pia mater, 103–104
Piedmont fracture, 678–679, *678–680*
Pillar fracture, cervical, 140, 140t, *141–142*
Pisiform, fracture of, 687, *687*
Pivot shift test, in ligamentous injuries of knee, 338t
Poirier's space, 647
Popliteal cysts, knee arthrography in, *356*, 357
  ultrasound in, 15–16, *16*
Posterior oblique ligament, 295, *296*
Post-reduction radiographs, imaging techniques in, 45t
  interpretation of, 57, 57t
Preiser's disease, 717
Pseudarthrosis, 80
Pubic bone, anatomy of, 181, *183*
Pubic ligaments, 183
Pubic ramus, inferior, fracture of, *205*
Pubic symphysis, diastasis of, 207, *208*

Q-angle, 311, *311*
Quadriceps tendon injury, arthrography for, 355

Radial and ulnar shaft fracture, 631–640. See also *Ulnar and radial shaft fracture.*
Radial fracture, distal, 667–680
  Barton type, 674–677, *676*
  chauffeur (radial styloid), 677, *677–678*
  Colles' type, 668–673, *668–673*
  Galeazzi type (piedmont), *678–679*, 678–680
  Smith type, *664*, 673–674
  head, posterior fat stripe in, 51, *51*
  proximal, *608–612*, 611–613
  shaft, pronator fat stripe in, 51, *51*
  styloid, *677*, 677–678
Radial nerve, *568*, 568–569, 582, *582*
Radiation protection, in routine radiography, 6
Radiocapitate ligament, 647, *647*
Radiocarpal joint, dislocation of, 680
Radiographic technique chart, 4–5, *4–5*
Radiography, magnification, 10–11, *10–11*
  routine, 1–6
    equipment for, 1, *2*
    kilovoltage vs centimeter body thickness in, 3, *4*
    object position within x-ray beam in, 6, *6*
    radiation protection in, 6
    radiographic technique chart in, 4–5, *4–5*
    screen-film combinations in, 2, *2–6*, *2–6*
Radiolunotriquetral ligament, 647, *647*
Radiopharmaceuticals, in bone scanning, 16–17
Radioscapholunate ligament, 647, *647*

Radioulnar joint, distal, dislocation of, *679*, 680
Radius, anatomy of, 631, *632–633*
    distal, anatomy of, 641–642, *641–642*
    fracture of. See *Radial fracture.*
    proximal, 579, *580*
Rectum, pelvic, 189
Ribs, radiographic technique chart on, *5*
Rolando fracture, 696, *696*
Rotator cuff tear, arthritis in, 557, *557*
    plain film findings in, 522t, 524
    reconstructive surgery of, 554–557
    shoulder arthrography in, 529–531, *530–531*

Sacroiliac ligaments, 183
Sacrolumbar ligaments, 183, *184*
Sacrospinous ligaments, 183
Sacrotuberous ligaments, 183
Sacrum, anatomy of, 98, *99*, 182–183
    isolated transverse fracture of, 204–206, *206*
    radiography in trauma to, 118, *118*
Salter-Harris fracture, 53, *53*
Scaphoid, avascular necrosis of, 717
Scaphoid fracture, 680–685, *682–685*
    classification of, 681–683, *682–683*
    complications of, 684–685, *684–685*
    diagnosis of, 680–681, *682*
    mechanism of injury in, 683
    treatment of, 683–684, *684*
Scapholunate axis, 643, *643*
Scapholunate dissociation, 717–718, *717–718*
Scapula, anatomy of, *500*, 500–501
    fracture of, 552–554, *554–556*
    routine radiography of, 509–510, *510*
Sciatic nerve, 187, *187*
    anatomy of, 184, *186*
Scintigraphy, skeletal, 16–20, *17–20*. See also *Bone scan.*
Scotty dog view, *117*, 118
Screen-film combinations, phosphor materials used in, 2, *2*
    relative speed index for, 2, *2*
Seatbelt injury, 159–161, *160–161*
Semimembranous muscle, 300, *300*
Sesamoid bones, 646, *646*
Sesamoid fracture, 489, *490*
Shin splints, 760
Shoulder, 499–566. See also individual parts.
    anatomy of, *499–504*, 499–506
    arthrography for, 523–539. See also *Shoulder arthrography.*
    arthroscopy for, 539–540, *539–540*
    articular anatomy of, *502*, 502–503, 503t
    biomechanics of, 504–506
    bursae of, 503t
    bursography for, *540*, 540–541
    computed tomography for, 521, *522*
    fracture of, computed tomography in, *30*, 31
    neurovascular anatomy of, 503–504, *504*
    osteology of, *499–501*, 499–502
    radiographic technique chart on, *4*
    radionuclide scanning for, 520–521, *521*
    reconstructive surgery of, 554–562, *557–563*
        in cuff tear arthritis, 557, *557*
        in radiation necrosis, 560, *560*
        in rheumatoid arthritis, 557–559, *557–559*
        in rotator cuff tear, 554–557
        in traumatic arthritis, 559–560, *560*
        postoperative analysis of, 560–562, *561–563*
    routine radiography of, 506–509
        AP view in, *505*, 507
        axillary view in, 508–509, *509*
        bicipital groove view, *515*, 516

Shoulder (*Continued*)
    routine radiography of, for recurrent dislocation, 516, *516*
        posterior oblique view in, *506–507*, 507–508
        scapular Y-view in, 508, *508*
        soft tissue, 518
        Stryker notch view in, 517, *518*
        West Point view in, 516–517, *517*
    tomography for, 518–520, *519*
    trauma to, *541–556*, 542–554. See also individual types.
    ultrasonography for, 520
Shoulder arthrography, 523–539
    abnormal, 529–536, *530–537*
    complications in, 538–539
    cystic changes in, *524*, 525
    double tuberosity sign in, 525, *525*
    for adhesive capsulitis, 532–533, *532–533*, 532t
    for articular cartilage abnormalities, 534–536, *535–537*
    for biceps tendon abnormalities, 533–534, *533–534*
    for chondromalacia, 536, *537*
    for rotator cuff tear, 529–531, *530–531*
    for synovitis, 535, *536–537*
    humeroacromial distance in, 523, *524*
    indications for, 522t, 523
    inferior acromial surface spurring in, *525*, 526
    normal, 528–529, *528–529*
    pitfalls in, 537–538
    soft tissue calcification in, *526*, 526
    subtraction, 536–537, *538*
    technique in, 522t, 526–528, *527–528*
Sigmoid colon, pelvic, 189
Single photon absorptiometry, 22, *22–23*
Sinography, 776–777, *777–778*
Skeletal evaluation, imaging techniques in, 45t
Skeletal scintigraphy, 16–20, *17–20*. See also *Bone scan.*
Skull, radiographic technique chart on, *4*
Smith fracture, 673–674, *674*
Soft tissue evaluation, radiographic techniques in, 44t
Spinal accessory ligament, *101–102*, 102
Spinal cord, anatomy of, 103–104
Spine, 91–180
    anatomy of, 91–104. See also individual anatomic parts.
        AP and lateral views in, 91, *91*
        ligamentous, 98–102
        neurovascular, 102–104
        osteology in, 91–98
    blood supply of, 102–103, *102–103*
    bone biopsy of, 772–774, *772–774*
    cervical. See *Cervical spine.*
    lumbar. See *Lumbar spine.*
    nerves of, 104
    stress fracture in, 764, *764*
    thoracic. See *Thoracic spine.*
    trauma to, radiographic evaluation in, 104–121. See also individual spinal segments.
Spondylitis, septic, 744–748
    computed tomography in, 747–748
    magnetic resonance imaging in, 747–748
    nuclear imaging in, 746–747, *747*
    routine radiography in, 745–746, *746–747*
Spondylolisthesis, 172–177
    etiology of, 173, 173t
    foreshortening of spine in, 174–175, 174t–175t
    grading in, 175, *175*
    treatment of, 176–177
Spondylolysis, 172–177
    etiology of, 173, 173t
    treatment of, 176–177
Sternoclavicular joint, anatomy of, 503
    dislocation of, 549–551
    routine radiography of, 513–516, *514–515*

Straddle fracture, *208*, 209
Stress fracture, 54, *55*, 755–766
    clinical conditions simulating, 756t
    common types of, 755t
    distribution of, 756t, *757–764*
    imaging approach to, *765*
    in femur, *761–762*, *762–763*
    in fibula, 762
    in foot, *757–758*, *757–759*
    in pelvis, *763*, *763–764*
    in spine, 764, *764*
    in tibia, *758–761*, *759–762*
    radiographic evaluation of, 756–757
Styloid bone, 646, *646*
Subtalar dislocation, *465*, 466
Superficial medial ligament, 295
Supracondylar process, 568, *568*
Suprapatellar intracapsular fracture, lipohemarthrosis
    in, 51, *52*
Supraspinous ligament, 99, *100*
Synovial disorders, knee arthroscopy in, 366, *366*
Synovial plicae, knee arthrography in, 357, *357*
    knee arthroscopy in, 362–363

Talar dislocation, *465*, 466
Talar fracture, 453–466
    body, *462–464*, 462–466
        classification of, 462, *462*
        diagnosis of, 462–463, *463*
        treatment of, 463–466, *464*
    neck, 459–462
        classification of, *458–460*, 459–460
        diagnosis of, 460–461, *461*
        mechanism of injury in, 459
        results in, 461–462, *461–462*
    transchondral, 453–458
        classification of, 454–455, *455*
        diagnosis of, 455
        mechanism of injury in, *454*, 454
        radiographic diagnosis of, *455–456*, 456
        results of, 458
        treatment of, *456–457*, 456–458
Talofibular ligament, anterior, anatomy of, *444*, 445
    injury to, ankle arthrography in, *420*, 420–421
    posterior, *444*, 445
Talus, 452–466
    anatomy of, 452, *452–453*
    fracture of, 453–466. See also *Talar fracture.*
    function of, 453
    gross anatomy of, 407–408, *408–409*
Tarsometatarsal fracture, *481–483*, 481–484
    anatomy of, 481, *481–482*
    classification of, *482*
    mechanism of injury in, 482, *482*
    treatment of, 483–484, *484*
Tarsonavicular stress fracture, 759
Technetium pertechnetate (Tc-99m), 16
Testut's ligament, 647, *647*
Thoracic spine, articular facets in, 94
    radiographic technique chart on, *4*
    radiography in trauma to, *114*, 115–116
    spinous processes of, 92
    transverse processes of, 92
    trauma to, 155–172. See also *Thoracolumbar trauma.*
Thoracic vertebra, 94–95, *97*, *98*
    anatomy of, 91–92, *93*
Thoracolumbar trauma, 155–172
    management of, 165–172
        bursting fracture in, 168, *170–171*, 172
        compression fracture in, *167*, 168
        decompression in, 166
        flexion injuries in, *167–169*, 168
        flexion-distraction injury in, 168, *168–169*

Thoracolumbar trauma (*Continued*)
    management of, flexion-rotation injury in, 168, *169*
        shear injury in, 172, *172–173*
        spinal instability in, 166
    mechanism of injury in, 155–165
        anterior wedge fracture as, 156–158, *156–158*,
            156f, 158f
        burst fracture as, 161, *164*
        flexion-distraction as, 158–159, *159*
        flexion-rotation as, 161, *162–163*
        hyperextension as, 161–164
        hyperflexion as, 156–161, *156–161*
        lateral wedge fracture as, 158, *158*
        minor fracture as, 165, *165–166*
        seatbelt injury as, 159–161, *160–161*
        shearing as, 164–165, *165*
        three-column approach to, 156, *156*
        vertical compression as, 161, *164*
Thumb, routine radiography for, 651, *653*
Thumb metacarpal fracture, 694–696, *694–696*
    extra-articular proximal metaphyseal, 696
    intra-articular basilar, *694–696*, 696
    neck, 694
    spiral diaphyseal, 695–696
    transverse diaphyseal, 695
Tibia, anatomy of, 393–395, *393–395*
    arterial supply of, 394–395, *395*
    ipsilateral fracture of femur and, 330–331, 330f
    muscles of, 394, *394*
    stress fracture in, *758–761*, *759–762*
Tibial condyle fracture, 325–330
    associated injuries in, 325–326
    classification of, 326–327, *327*
    diagnosis of, 325
    mechanism of injury in, 327, *327*
    meniscus tears in, 326
    nonoperative treatment in, *327*, 327–328
    operative treatment in, 328–330, *329*
    tomography in, 325, *326*
    treatment in, *327*, 327–330, *329*
Tibial fracture, 395–405
    alignment in, 397
    angulation in, 397, *398*
    anterior compartment syndrome in, 404
    AO plate fixation in, 400–401, *401*
    cast wedging in, *398*, 398–399
    closed reduction in, 398–399, *398–399*
    complications in, 404
    electrical stimulation in, 404
    Fischer fixation in, 400, *401*
    Hoffman fixation in, 400, *400*
    intramedullary nailing in, 401, *402*
    management of, 397–404, *398–404*
    mechanism of injury and classification of, 395–396
    multiple screw fixation in, *403*, 404
    patellar-tendon-bearing cast in, 398
    prognosis for healing in, 404, *404*
    radiographic evaluation in, 396–397, *396–397*
    shortening and fragment distraction in, 397
    Steinman pins in, 399
Tomography, 6–9
    blurring and section thickness in, 7, *7*
    computed, 28–31. See also *Computed tomography.*
    equipment in, 6
    fixation devices and, 8, *9*
    in spinal trauma, 118, *119*
    linear motion in, 7, *9*
    technique in, 6–7, *7*
    trispiral motion in, 7, *9*
    tube motion in, *7–10*, 7–9
Torus fracture, 51, *52*
Trans-scaphoid perilunate dislocation, *691*, 691–692
Trapezium, fracture of, 688–690, *690*
Trapezoid, fracture of, 688
Trauma, bone scan in, 18–19, *18–20*
    computed tomography in, *30*, 31

Triangular fibrocartilage complex, 646, *646*
  tears and disorders of, 714
Triceps, 582
Triquetral fracture, 685–687, *686*
Trochanteric fracture, 247–253
  avulsion, 251
  classification of, *247–250*, 247–251
  intertrochanteric, 247–249, *247–249*, 248t
  subtrochanteric, 249–250, *250*, 250t
  treatment of, 251–253, *251–254*
Tumor, bone scan in, 17–18, *17–18*

Ulna, anatomy of, 631, *632–633*
  distal, anatomy of, 642, *642*
Ulnar and radial shaft fracture, 631–640
  anatomy in, 631, *632–633*
  classification in, 635
  closed treatment of, 636
  complications of, 640, *640*
  compression plate fixation in, 637
  management in, *634–640*, 635–640
  mechanism of injury in, 635
  open, *638*, 639–640, *640*
  open reduction in, 636–637, *637*
  roentgenographic evaluation in, 631–633, *634*
  rotational alignment in, 635–636, *636*
  undisplaced, *634–635*, 635
Ulnar collateral ligament, 581, *581*
Ulnar fracture, proximal, 613–614, *613–614*
  classification of, *613*, 613–614
  displaced, 614–618, *615–618*
  mechanism of, 613
  Monteggia, 619–620, *619–621*
  radiographic evaluation in, 614, *614*
  treatment of, 614
Ulnar nerve, 582, *582*
Ulnar variance, 642, *642*
Ulnolunate abutment syndrome, 714–715, *715*
Ulnotriquetral ligament, 647, *647*
Ultrasound, 14–16, *15–16*
  in popliteal cyst, 15–16, *16*
  orthopedics applications for, 14–15, *15*
  static and real-time scanners in, 14
Urethra, female, *188*, 189
  in pelvic fracture, 223–225, *224–225*, 226t
  male, *188*, 188–189

Vertebra, cervical, 94, *95–97*. See also *Cervical vertebra.*
  lumbar, 98, *98.* See also *Lumbar vertebra.*
  ossification centers of, 91, *92*
  thoracic, 94–95, *97, 98.* See also *Thoracic vertebra.*
Vertebral arch fracture, cervical, 138–140, *138–142*, 138t

Vertebral body, 91, *93*
Vertebral body fractures, cervical, 140–144, *143–144*, 143t
  burst type, 143, *144*
  chip type, 142, *143*
  compression, 142, *143*
  management of, *154*, 155
  sagittal, 143–144
  triangular, 142, *143*

Wrisberg's ligament, 293
Wrist, 641–730
  anatomy of, 641–648, *641–648.* See also individual parts.
  arthrography of, 662–666, *663–666.* See also *Wrist arthrography.*
  chronic post-traumatic conditions of, 713–721
  degenerative arthritis in, 720–721, *721*
  intercompartmental communications in, 664, 664t
  ligaments of, 646–647, *646–647*
  post-traumatic reconstruction of, 721–725, *721–727.* See also *Hand, post-traumatic reconstruction of.*
  routine radiographic techniques for, 655–662, *656–662*
    carpal tunnel view in, 660, *660*
    dorsal tangential view of, 660, *661*
    lateral view in, 656–657, *657*
    motion studies of, 660, *661–662*
    oblique views in, 657, *658*
    PA view, 655–656, *656–657*
    pisiform view in, 657, *659*
    scaphoid view in, 657, *658*
Wrist arthrography, 662–666, *663–666*
  abnormal, 664–666, *665–666*
  for arthritis, 666
  for ganglia, 666
  for trauma, 664–666, *665–666*
  indications in, 663t
  normal anatomy in, 663–664, *664–665*
  technique in, 662–663, *663–664*

Xeroradiography, 11–14, *12–13*
  advantages and limitations of, 12–14
  equipment and principles of, 12
  for nonopaque foreign bodies, 13, *13*
  indications for, 12t
  process in, *12*
  tomographic sections with, *13*, 13–14

Zona orbicularis, 184